The Textbook of Pharmaceutical Medicine

Fifth edition

Edited by

John P Griffin BSc, PhD, MBBS, FRCP, FRCPath, FFPM

Director, Asklepieion Consultancy Ltd.,
Visiting Professor, University of Surrey Postgraduate Medical School
Former Director, Association of the British Pharmaceutical Industry, London
Formerly Professional Head of the Medicines Division, DHSS, London

and

John O'Grady MD, FRCP, FFPM, FBIRA, MRCPath

Visiting Professor of Clinical Pharmacology, University of London

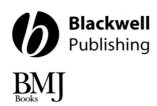

Blackwell Publishing

BMJ Books

Blackwell Publishing, Inc., 350 Main Street, Malden, Massachusetts 02148-5020, USA
Blackwell Publishing Ltd, 9600 Garsington Road, Oxford OX4 2DQ, UK
Blackwell Publishing Asia Pty Ltd, 550 Swanston Street, Carlton, Victoria 3053, Australia

First three editions were published by The Queen's University of Belfast
First edition published in 1993
Second edition published in 1994
Third edition published in 1998
Fourth edition published in 2002
Second impression of Fourth edition published in 2002
Fifth edition published in 2006
2   2007

Library of Congress Cataloging-in-Publication Data

The textbook of pharmaceutical medicine / edited by John P. Griffin and John
O'Grady.—5th ed.
p. ; cm.
Includes index.
ISBN 978-0-7279-1840-6 (hardback)
1. Pharmacology, Experimental.
[DNLM: 1. Drug Approval. 2. Clinical Trials. 3. Pharmacology. QV 771 T3445 2005]
1. Griffin, J. P. (John Parry) II. O'Grady, John, Professor.

RM301.25.T49 2005
615'.1—dc22   2005015284

ISBN 978-0-7279-1840-6

A catalogue record for this title is available from the British Library

Set Chennai, India by Newgen Imaging Systems (P) Ltd
Printed and bound by Replika Press Pvt. Ltd, India

Commissioning Editor: Mary Banks
Development Editor: Veronica Pock
Production Controller: Debbie Wyer

For further information on Blackwell Publishing, visit our website:
http://www.blackwellpublishing.com

Contents

Contributors

Christine H Bendall, Solicitor, Arnold & Porter, London, UK

Carole Bradley BSc(Hons) MSc, Manager, Health Economics and Reimbursement, Boehringer Ingelheim (Canada) Ltd, Burlington, Ontario, Canada

Alan G Davies MBBS MRCP(UK) MD (London), Therapeutic Director, Kendle International Inc, Crowthorne, Berkshire, UK

Anand S Dutta PhD, Department of Academic Affairs, Hope Hospital, Salford, UK

A Peter Fletcher MBBS PhD MFPM, Independent Consultant Little Maplestead, Essex formerly Senior Prinicipal Medical Officer, DOH

Andrew P Grieve, Statistical and Consulting Centre, Pfizer Global Research and Development, Sandwich, UK

Jane R Griffin BA(Hons) MSc, Head, Health Economics and Outcomes Research, Boehringer Ingelheim UK Ltd, Bracknell, UK

John P Griffin BSc PhD MBBS FRCP FRCPath FFPM, Asklepieion Consultancy Ltd, Welwyn, Hertfordshire, UK. Formarly Head of UK Regulatory Authority

Gavin Halbert BSc PhD CChem MRSC MRPharmS, Director, Cancer Research UK Formulation Unit, Department of Pharmaceutical Sciences, University of Strathclyde, Glasgow, Scotland, UK

Dean WG Harron BSc PhD FRPharmS MPSNI, Professor, School of Pharmacy, The Queen's University of Belfast, Northern Ireland, UK

Darrall L Higson MB ChB FFPM, formerly Medical Director, Global Switch & Innovations, GlaxoSmithKline Consumer Healthcare, Uxbridge, Middlesex, UK

Janice Hirshorn BSc (Hons) PhD FAICD, Consultant, Rose Bay, NSW, Australia

Christopher JS Hodges MA (Oxon) PhD FSALS, Consultant, CMS Cameron McKenna, London, UK; Associate Fellow, University of Oxford, Oxford, UK

D Michael Humphreys MB ChB FFPM, Consulting Pharmaceutical Physician, formerly Corporate Medical Advisor, Corporate Department Medical Affairs, Boehringer Ingelheim, Ingelheim-am-Rhein, Germany

Peter Barton Hutt, Senior Counsel Covington and Burling, Washington DC USA; Lecturer in Food and Drug Law, Harvard Law School, Cambridge MASS Former Chief Counsel to the US Food and Drug Administration (FDA)

Judith K Jones MD PhD, President, The Degge Group; President, The Pharmaceutical Education and Research Institute; Adjunct Professor of Pharmacology, Georgetown University, Washington DC, USA

Yuichi Kubo, Daiichi Pharmaceutical Co Ltd, Tokyo, Japan

Valeria Molnar Clinical Pharmacology Consulting, Torquay, UK

Deborah Monk B Pharm Dip Hosp BA, Director of Scientific and Technical Affairs, Medicines Australia, Deakin, ACT, Australia

John O'Grady MD FRCP FFPM FBIRA MRCPath, Visiting Professor of Clinical Pharmacology, University of London, UK

John Posner BSc PhD MBBS FRCP FFPM, Independent Consultant in Pharmaceutical Medicine, John Posner Consulting, Beckenham, UK

Paul Rolan MBBS MD FRACP FFPM DCPSA, Professor of Clinical and Experimental Pharmacology, Medical School, University of Adelaide Adelaide SA 5005 Australia

Rashmi R Shah BSc MBBS MD FRCP FFPM, Pharmaceutical Consultant, formerly Senior Clinical Assessor, Medicines and Healthcare products Regulatory Agency (MHRA), London, UK

Susan Shaw MBBS BSc MRCPsych, Consultant Psychiatrist, Chelsea and Westminster Hospital, London, UK

Richard N Spivey Pharm D PhD, Senior Vice President, Corporate Technology Policy, Pharmacia, Peapack, New Jersey, USA

Peter D Stonier BA MB ChB Bsc PhD MRCPsych FRCP FRCPE FFPM, Medical Director, Amdipharm plc, Basildon, UK

David J Tweats C. Biol BSc PhD FRCPath FIBiol, Professor, Centre for Molecular Genetics and Toxicology, School of Biological Sciences, University of Wales, Swansea, UK

William Vodra Senior Partner, Arnold & Porter, Washington DC, USA

William Wardell MA(Oxon), President, Wardell Associates International, Princeton, New Jersey, USA

Amanda Wearing MA (Oxon), Solicitor, Arnold and Porter, London, UK

Roger A Yates MA MB BChir MRCP(UK) FFPM DCPSA Independent Consultant in Pharmaceutical Medicinal, Ray Cander Ltd, Wilmslow, Cheshire, UK

John H Young MBBS FRCP FRCPath FFPM, Medical Director, Merck Sharp and Dohme Ltd, Hoddesdon, UK

Preface

This book has grown considerably since the first edition in 1993. The fifth edition is the most comprehensive of all editions to date and reflects the increasing complexity of the speciality. The enthusiastic uptake of this book is a tribute to The Faculty of Pharmaceutical Medicine of The Royal Colleges of Physicians of the United Kingdom who have done so much to sponsor the discipline leading to the discipline achieving the status of specialist recognition.

However, we have been aware that the book has appealed to a much wider audience than those for whom it was initially written, namely those studying for the Diploma of Pharmaceutical Medicine. It is now the standard text used by courses in pharmaceutical medicine in both Europe and the Unites States.

Widening the scope of the textbook to cover all aspects of the speciality's Higher Medical Training (HMT) programme has also increased the usefulness of the book to those working in National Drug Regulatory Authorities, as well as those involved in the economics of healthcare, pharmaceutical marketing and NHS purchasing of medical products.

Acknowledgements

We would like to thank all those who have contributed in any way to this book, either to the current fifth edition or previous editions. We owe the success of this book to every one of its contributors, who have produced work of the highest quality promptly from edition to edition.

We would particularly like to pay tribute to those contributors who are no longer with us: Dr John Domenet, Professor Ken McRea, Professor PF D'Arcy and Professor Lou Lasagna – whose expertise will be greatly missed.

We would also like to record our great appreciation to Mary Banks who steered this book through its fourth and fifth editions, and to her colleague at Blackwell Publishing, Veronica Pock.

Finally, we would like to thank the World Medical Association, The European Medicines Evaluation Agency and the Association of the British Pharmaceutical Industry for permission to reproduce their various documents as appendices to this book. All others who allowed us to quote or use their material are acknowledged in the text, however, a general thanks is appropriate at this point.

John P Griffin
John O'Grady

The Editors

Professor John P Griffin BSc PhD MBBS FRCP MRCS FRCPath FFPM graduated in medicine at the Royal London Hospital, where he was also in clinical practice. He was a lecturer in Physiology at King's College, London and held the post of Head of Clinical Research at Riker Laboratories from 1967 to 1971. Professor Griffin joined the then Medicines Division of the Department of Health, now Medicines Healthcare Agency (MHRA) London, as a Senior Medical Officer, in 1971, and was subsequently appointed Medical Assessor to the Committee on Safety of Medicines. From 1977 to 1984, Professor Griffin was Senior Principal Medical Officer and Professional Head of Medicines Division in addition to being Medical Assessor to the Medicines Commission. As the Professional Head of Medicines Division he also attended the Scientific Sub-Committee of the Veterinary Products Committee of the Ministry of Agriculture, Food and Fisheries. During this time he was a member of the EC committee on Proprietary Medicinal Products and Chairman of the CPMP's Working Party on Safety Requirements.

From 1976 to 1984 John Griffin served on the Joint Formulary Committee of the British National Formulary, during which period the first eight issues of the current format were produced.

John Griffin was the director of the Association of the British Pharmaceutical Industry from 1984 to 1994. During this time he was a member of the Executive Board of the European Federation of the Pharmaceutical Industries' Associations and IFPMA. He chaired the ICH Safety Working Group from 1988 to 1994 and presented papers at ICH1 and ICH2 in the plenary sessions.

Since June 1994, John Griffin has run his own independent consultancy company, which has provided independent and impartial advice to governments on the development of a pharmaceutical policy, and to national trade associations and individual companies. John Griffin is Visiting Professor in Pharmaceutical Medicine at the University of Surrey, and is also Honorary Consultant Clinical Pharmacologist at the Lister Hospital in Hertfordshire, UK.

Professor Griffin is on the Board of the Faculty of Pharmaceutical Medicine, was Chairman of the Board of Examiners of the Faculty of Pharmaceutical Medicine of the Royal College of Physicians for 7 years, and is currently Academic Registrar and serves on the Task Force on Specialist Medical Training in Pharmaceutical Medicine. He has served on a number of Royal College of Physicians, London Working Parties including that on the 'Development of Clinical Pharmacology and Therapeutics in a Changing World'.

Professor Griffin is the author and co-author of over 250 publications on adverse drug reactions and iatrogenic disease, aspects of neurophysiology and clinical pharmacology and toxicology and drug regulation. Notable among his publications are the following four standard texts:

- *Iatrogenic Diseases* Oxford University Press, 1st edn 1972, 3rd edn 1986; jointly with Prof PF D'Arcy.
- *A Manual of Adverse Drug Interactions* John Wright Bristol, 1st edn 1975; Elsevier Press Amsterdam, 5th edn 1997; jointly with Prof PF D'Arcy.
- *The Textbook of Pharmaceutical Medicine* The Queen's University of Belfast Press, 1st edn 1993, 2nd edn 1994, 3rd edn 1998, 4th edn 2002 published by the *BMJ* Publishing Group in 2002.

• *Medicines, Research, Regulation and Risk* The Queen's University of Belfast Press, 1st edn 1989, 2nd edn 1992.

From 1991 to 2003 he served as Editor in Chief of *Adverse Drug Reactions and Toxicological Reviews*, a peer-reviewed journal produced quarterly by Oxford University Press.

Professor John O'Grady MD FRCP FFPM FBIRA
MRCPath, after graduating in medicine, trained in general medicine and also in clinical pharmacology and therapeutics to achieve specialist registrations. He held medical appointments at the Radcliffe Infirmary in Oxford, Royal Postgraduate Medical School, Hammersmith Hospital, Hospital for Nervous Diseases Queen's Square, London and St Bartholomew's Hospital, London.

Formerly Head of Clinical Pharmacology at Wellcome Research Laboratories, then Medical Director Rhone-Poulenc and Visiting Professor at the University of Cape Town, South Africa. He was later a Director of Imperial Cancer Research Technology Ltd, Visiting Professor of Clinical Pharmacology and Therapeutics at the University of Vienna, Austria, the University of Cape Town, South Africa and a member of the British Pharmacopoeia Commission.

Professor O'Grady is Examiner of the Royal College of Physicians, Faculty of Pharmaceutical Medicine. He is a Fellow of the Royal Statistical Society and Visiting Professor of Clinical Pharmacology, University of London.

He has published widely in the field of medicine, in clinical pharmacology and therapeutics and in pharmaceutical medicine. He is editor of several books dealing with drug effects in man and with medicines and the law.

PART I

Research and development

CHAPTER 1

1

Discovery of new medicines

Anand S Dutta

1.1 Introduction

Ancient civilisations, like modern society, had a keen interest in the health of man and other animals. Continuation of this interest over a period of time led to the discovery of a large number of therapeutic agents primarily from the natural sources; many of the natural sources are still being used as lead structures for the discovery of new drugs.[1] In more recent times (~50 years), with the involvement of a large number of pharmaceutical companies and many academic institutions, progress in the understanding of disease processes and mechanisms to control or eliminate the disease has accelerated. Similarly, despite the advances and achievements of the last 50 years, the need to discover treatments for existing and evolving diseases has also increased. This is primarily due to the inadequacies of the current medicines. In many cases the treatment only leads to symptom relief, and in various other cases, the cure is associated with undesirable side effects. In some cases (e.g. infectious diseases such as tuberculosis, malaria and HIV), resistance/tolerance to the existing treatments may develop, thus making them ineffective against the infecting bacteria, parasite or the virus.[2] New infectious agents such as SARS, hepatitis C, human herpes virus-6, -7 and -8 are also appearing.[3] In addition, with the changing environmental factors, lifestyle and increasing life span, more and more pathological abnormalities that require new treatments are being identified. For example, obesity and a number of cardiovascular diseases may have their origins in altered (more prosperous?) lifestyle habits including environmental and psychosocial factors and diet.[4–6] Changing social attitudes are also creating markets for the so-called lifestyle drugs. Although the term 'lifestyle drug' is applied currently to drugs such as sildenafil for erectile dysfunction and minoxidil or finasteride for baldness, the precise definition of lifestyle drugs is a subject of debate.[7] Increasing knowledge about the underlying causes of diseases is enabling the discovery of more selective and less toxic drugs. Progress in molecular biology (e.g. sequencing of human genome, proteomics, pharmacogenomics and protein engineering) is creating new avenues for the understanding of precise disease mechanisms (biochemical pathways) and discovery of new targets based on new disease pathways. Advances in this field are expected to lead to highly selective and efficacious medicines. Recombinant technologies are enabling the synthesis of larger biologically active proteins in sufficient quantities. Proteins and monoclonal antibodies are therefore becoming more important and common as therapeutic agents. Equally important is the progress being made in the fields of combinatorial chemistry, enabling the synthesis of millions of compounds, high-throughput screening technologies and other automation techniques facilitating more rapid drug discovery. In the longer run, a combination of all the new developments is likely to generate safer and more effective medicines not only for the existing diseases but also for the diseases of the future which may become more important as a consequence of changes in lifestyle, and increasing age.

Malaria (caused in humans by single-celled *Plasmodium* protozoa parasites), tuberculosis (caused by *Mycobacterium tuberculosis*) and leprosy (caused by *Mycobacterium leprae*) can be considered examples of 'older' diseases still in need of more effective and cheaper treatments.[8-14] Each year, 300–500 million people contract malaria and about 2–3 million die. A number of medicines, including chloroquine, 4-aminoquinolines, atovaquone, malarone, halofantrine, mefloquine, proguanil and artemisinin derivatives are available. Three main types of vaccines, based on the three major phases of the parasite's life cycle, are being developed: anti-sporozoite vaccines designed to prevent infection (pre-erythrocytic vaccines), anti-asexual blood stage vaccines (anti-invasion and anti-complication) designed to reduce severe and complicated manifestations of the disease and transmission-blocking vaccines aimed at arresting the development of the parasite in the mosquito itself. A number of vaccines are in phase I and phase II clinical trials. Monoclonal antibodies against specific malarial antigens are being explored for diagnostic and potential therapeutic purposes. In addition, efforts are also being made to shed light on the origin of the development of resistance in specific cases. Discovery of complete genome sequences of the human malarial parasite *Plasmodium falciparum* and the malaria-transmitting mosquito *Anopheles gambiae* is likely to enhance the discovery of antimalarial drug candidates. Like malaria, tuberculosis and leprosy are more common in less-developed countries. Tuberculosis is the second leading cause of death worldwide, killing nearly 2 million people each year. Multidrug-resistant tuberculosis continues to be a serious problem, particularly among some countries of Eastern Europe, China and Iran.[15] Currently available drugs for tuberculosis include isoniazid, rifampicin, pyrazinamide and ethambutol. The first-line drugs against leprosy are rifampicin, clofazimine and dapsone. Other drugs like minocycline, the macrolide clarithromycin and the fluoroquinolones pefloxacin and ofloxacin are all highly active against *M. leprae* but are rarely used in field programmes because of their cost.

1 Celecoxib

2 Rofecoxib

3 Valdecoxib

Bone disorders like arthritis and osteoporosis are examples of diseases that are becoming increasingly important with the ageing population.[16-18] Anti-inflammatory glucocorticoids like prednisolone and methylprednisolone and immunosuppressants such as cyclosporin-A and dexamethasone are used for the treatment. Although the treatment options have increased recently, most of these therapies focus on addressing the symptoms rather than the underlying causes of the disease. For example, cyclooxygenase-2 (COX-2) inhibitors such as celecoxib (**1**), rofecoxib (**2**, recently withdrawn from the market), etoricoxib,[19] valdecoxib[20] (**3**) and parecoxib (prodrug of valdecoxib) are being marketed as safer non-steroidal anti-inflammatory drugs (NSAIDs).[21-23] Although the older NSAIDs are highly effective as analgesic, antipyretic and anti-inflammatory agents, long-term ingestion causes gastric lesions. The discovery that the COX enzyme, which catalyses the conversion of arachidonic acid to prostaglandin H_2 (common biosynthetic precursor to prostaglandins and thromboxane – mediators of physiological and pathological processes, including pain, fever, inflammation),[24] exists in two isoforms, with COX-2 being the primary isoform at sites of inflammation, led to a suggestion that inhibition of this isoform accounts for the therapeutic benefit of NSAIDs whereas inhibition of COX-1 results in adverse effects. The newer COX-2 selective agents appear to have a superior gastrointestinal (GI) safety profile. COX-2 inhibitors are also being investigated for the prevention and treatment of colorectal cancer.[25] In addition to COX-2 inhibitors, inhibitors of matrix metalloproteinases (MMPs) are emerging for the treatment of many diseases including arthritis. Enzymes that degrade the extracellular matrix are normally controlled by a set of tissue inhibitors that, if disrupted, will allow the enzymes to work unchecked, degrading the matrix and promoting not only arthritis but also tumour growth and metastasis. Another treatment option is the inhibition of tumour necrosis factor-α (TNF-α), an inflammation-promoting cytokine associated with multiple inflammatory events, including arthritis. Anti-TNF-α therapies are already in the market. Finally, a variety of genes that code for antiarthritic proteins are under investigation.

Recently, the process of drug discovery has been expanded to cover a range of molecular biology, biotechnology and medicinal chemistry (including combinatorial chemistry) techniques. The newer disciplines like genome analysis, proteomics and bioinformatics are likely to lead to many new targets (receptors, enzymes, etc.) and therapeutically important proteins. Techniques like combinatorial chemistry and high-throughput screening are expected to identify hits/leads against various therapeutically important receptors and enzymes. Depending upon the knowledge available on the receptor or the enzyme of interest, the hits/leads can then be modified in a random, semi-rational or rational manner to generate the drug candidates.

Like the chapter in the fourth edition of this book,[26] this chapter includes a short account of the historical aspects[27] and a short introduction to some of the newer disciplines. The main theme/objective of this chapter is to give an idea about the changing disease patterns, which may be reflected in the discovery process,

4 Fexofenadine

5 Ranitidine

6 Esomeprazole

examples of receptor agonists and antagonists, enzyme inhibitors, including signal transduction inhibitors and inhibitors of protein–protein interaction that have been discovered by random and 'semi-rational/rational' approaches, antibody and protein therapeutics and currently available drugs for more widespread diseases. This enables one to understand actual drug discovery procedures and the science that has led to many drugs currently in the market. Examples include

- COX inhibitors (1–3)
- angiotensin-converting enzyme (ACE) inhibitors (antihypertensives such as captopril and lisinopril)
- histamine H_1 receptor antagonists (anti-allergic compounds such as fexofenadine (4))
- histamine H_2 receptor antagonists (acid secretion inhibitors such as cimetidine and ranitidine (5))
- proton pump inhibitors (acid secretion inhibitors such as omeprazole and esomeprazole (6))[28,29]
- nuclear peroxisome proliferator activated receptor-γ activators such as pioglitazone (7)[30] and troglitazone (type 2 diabetes mellitus treatments)

7 Pioglitazone

8 Atorvastatin

9 Ezetimibe

10 Zanamivir

11 Donepezil

12 Montelukast

13 Sildenafil

14 Orlistat

15 Quetiapine

16 Olanzapine

- lipid lowering agents such as atorvastatin (**8**) and rosuvastatin and cholesterol absorption inhibitor ezetimibe (**9**)[31]
- anti-influenza treatments like zanamivir (**10**)[32]
- acetylcholinesterase inhibitors such as donepezil (**11**) for the treatment of Alzheimer's disease
- selective and competitive inhibitor of the cysteinyl leukotrienes (LTC$_4$, LTD$_4$ and LTE$_4$) such as zafirlukast and montelukast (**12**) for the treatment of asthma
- sildenafil (**13**; an inhibitor of phosphodiesterase type 5 used for erectile dysfunction)[33]
- antiobesity compound orlistat (**14**)
- atypical antipsychotic agents such as quetiapine (**15**) and olanzapine (**16**).

Table 1.1 Leading causes of death and disability worldwide (1990–2020)

Rank	1990	2020
1	Ischaemic heart disease	Ischaemic heart disease
2	Cerebrovascular disease	Unipolar major depression
3	Lower respiratory infections	Road traffic accidents
4	Diarrhoeal diseases	Cerebrovascular disease
5	Perinatal disorders	Chronic obstructive pulmonary disease
6	Chronic obstructive pulmonary disease	Lower respiratory infections
7	Tuberculosis (HIV excluded)	Tuberculosis
8	Measles	War injuries
9	Road traffic accidents	Diarrhoeal diseases
10	Lung, tracheal and bronchial cancer	HIV

In 1990, just over 50 million died worldwide (53% males); 10.912 million in the developed world and 39.554 million in the developing regions.

It may be useful to mention at this stage that many of the highly successful drugs launched in the last 25 years were discovered in the pre-genomic era, and the real contribution of all the new technologies mentioned above remains to be proven. In some cases, the drug was initially investigated for different indications. For example, sildenafil was being investigated in the clinic as an antianginal drug when its beneficial effects in improving erectile function were observed.

1.2 Market Needs and Changing Disease Patterns

From the point of view of the discovery of new medicines, it is important to project changing disease patterns and markets so that the new drugs may become available early. Currently, the developed world accounts for 11–12% of the global burden from all causes of death and disability but >90% of health expenditure; most of the remainder is spent in the form of public-health aid. The Global Burden of Disease Study initiated in 1992 by the World Bank in collaboration with the World Health Organisation (WHO) has sought to quantify mortality, life expectancy and risk factors for different regions of the world and to project trends in mortality and disability in 2020. Of the 10 leading causes of death and disability in 1990 (Table 1.1), those due

to ischaemic heart disease, cerebrovascular disease, cancer and lower respiratory infections are in the established market economies, whereas most deaths due to diarrhoea, communicable diseases, maternal and perinatal conditions and nutritional deficiencies are in the developing world. Overall, in the developed regions, only 6.1% deaths were due to communicable (infectious and parasitic diseases), maternal, perinatal and nutritional conditions, and deaths due to non-communicable diseases (e.g. cardiovascular, cancer) and injuries accounted for 86.2% and 7.6%, respectively. Considering disability alone in the developed regions, the leading causes in 1990 were unipolar major depression, iron-deficiency anaemia, falls, alcohol abuse, chronic obstructive pulmonary disease, bipolar disorder, congenital anomalies, osteoarthritis, schizophrenia and obsessive-compulsive disorder. Absence of cancer from the top 10 killers of 2020 reflects use of a disability-adjusted measure used in the study rather than discovery of a magical cure, although, new medicines and regimes have increased survival rates in cancer patients. Indeed, the fact that the analysis of GI cancer is organ based while cancers affecting the respiratory system are lumped together also distorts the above analysis. Thus, deaths due to all cancers affecting the respiratory system (lung, trachea and bronchi) have been aggregated to make this the 10th leading cause of mortality. Aggregating all the data for the bowel (oesophageal, stomach and colorectal tumours) would elevate GI cancer to the eighth place. Similarly liver disease (cirrhosis plus cancer) at 1.38 million would rank as the ninth leading cause of death.

Health trends over the next 20 years will be largely determined by ageing of the world's (female) population, a 40% fall in third-world deaths from communicable, perinatal and nutritional causes, and a 77% increase in non-communicable diseases, including a 180% increase in tobacco-attributable mortality. The potential for so-called lifestyle drugs, for example, anti-smoking treatments, is also apparent. While the drug industry may not be quite so aware of opportunities in relation to trauma, it has recognised the threats posed both by psychotic illness and AIDS. The prediction that depression will rank second in terms of disability-adjusted life years creates opportunity for drugs directed at peripheral as well as central sites such as those targeting the brain–gut axis.

1.3   Historical Aspects

1.3.1   Early discoveries

A number of early medicines, including morphine, atropine, salicylic acid and quinine were isolated from plants. Over the years the search for therapeutic agents was widened to isolate products from living agents such as bacteria, fungi, sea animals and even human beings. The important discoveries from this research not only include anti-infective agents like penicillin and tetracyclin but also many other hormones and transmitters. Ivermectin (a drug used to treat tropical filariasis), amphotericin B, lovastatin (HMGA-CoA reductase inhibitor), insulin, heparin (anticoagulant), paclitaxel (anticancer), artemisinin (antimalarial) and cyclosporin-A and FK506 (immunosuppressants) are other examples originating from natural sources.[34] Many of the biologically active peptides like oxytocin, vasopressin, adrenocorticotropic hormone (ACTH), insulin, calcitonin,

luteinising hormone releasing hormone (LHRH), growth hormone and erythropoietin are important examples of compounds isolated from humans and other animals that have led to medicines currently used in clinical practice. In addition, discoveries of many other agents like adrenaline, histamine, tyramine, tryptamine and γ-aminobutyric acid (GABA) and their receptors have led to extremely important medicines.

Many other early discoveries were primarily based on low-throughput random screening approaches. The mechanism of action was later rationalised when additional biochemical and pharmacological information became available. Examples of early drugs include sulpha drugs which led to the discoveries of several other classes of drugs.[27] For example, the active metabolite of the sulphonamide prontosil (**17**) inhibits the enzyme carbonic anhydrase, leading to an increase in natriuresis and the excretion of water. Sulphanilamide (**18**) gave rise to better carbonic anhydrase inhibitors such as acetazolamide and later led to more effective diuretics such as hydrochlorothiazide and furosemide (**19**). Further chemistry in the field led to the development of sulphonylureas like tolbutamide (**20**), which is used in the treatment of type 2 diabetes.

$$H_2N-SO_2 \text{—} \bigcirc \text{—} N=N \text{—} \bigcirc \text{—} NH_2$$
$$H_2N$$

17 Prontosil

$$H_2N-SO_2 \text{—} \bigcirc \text{—} NH_2$$

18 Sulphanilamide

19 Furosemide

$$Me \text{—} \bigcirc \text{—} SO_2\text{-}NH\text{-}CO\text{-}NH\text{-}(CH_2)_3Me$$

20 Tolbutamide

1.4 Impact of New Technology on Drug Discovery

1.4.1 Receptor subtypes

Since the idea of a receptor as a selective binding site for chemotherapeutic agents was developed, huge progress has been made in the identification, characterisation and classification of receptors and receptor subtypes. In addition, knowledge has been gained about the downstream signalling pathways, most often involving transcription factors that ultimately act on DNA and result in altered gene expression. Mapping the key signalling molecules in biochemical pathways and attempting to modulate their effects is resulting in new areas of drug discovery. The early assumptions that a ligand acts at one receptor are no longer tenable and it is now well established that many endogenous ligands act at different receptor subtypes. The availability of more selective synthetic ligands and cloning and amino acid sequencing technologies have shown that different receptor subtypes exist for most of the receptors. The situation is further complicated by the existence of different receptor subtypes in different tissues in the same species, and by structural differences in receptor subtypes in different species of animals. Many recent studies have indicated that G-protein-coupled receptors (GPCRs) form homo-oligomeric and hetero-oligomeric complexes and these complexes ('new receptors') have functional characteristics that differ from homogeneous populations of their constituent receptors.[35] Thus, the accumulated knowledge has not only provided many challenges for the drug discovery process but has also opened a way to many new drug discovery targets and much more selective treatments.

From the point of view of drug discovery, ligands acting at the G-protein-coupled receptors have resulted in most successful drug candidates.[36–38] Some of the examples illustrating how receptor research has led to more selective drugs and enhanced our understanding of the roles played by various receptor subtypes in disease processes are mentioned below. Early examples of different receptor subtypes that led to clinically useful drugs include α and β adrenoreceptors and histamine H_1 and H_2 receptor subtypes. One of the more complicated and extensively studied area of receptor subtypes is the field of 5-hydroxytryptamine (5-HT; serotonin) receptors.[39–42] The seven receptor subtypes, 5-HT_1 to 5-HT_7, have been characterised using selective ligands (agonists and antagonists); cloning and amino acid sequencing techniques have been used to define molecular structures and intracellular transduction mechanisms. Several of the more selective compounds have reached the market for the treatment of various disorders of the nervous system. For example, several selective 5-HT_3 antagonists (e.g. ondansetron (**21**), granisetron, tropisetron, nazasetron (**22**) and ramosetron) are marketed for the management of nausea and vomiting induced by cancer chemotherapy and radiotherapy. Tryptamine 5-$HT_{1B/1D}$ receptor agonists such as sumatriptan (**23**), almotriptan, frovatriptan, zomitriptan (**24**), rizatriptan (**25**), naratriptan and eletriptan are marketed for the treatment of migraine. 5-HT_3 receptor antagonist alosetron (diarrhoea-predominant irritable bowel syndrome) (**26**) and 5-HT_4 receptor partial agonists mosapride (**27**) (relief of GI symptoms in patients with gastritis, gastro-oesophageal reflux, dyspepsia) and tegaserod

21 Ondansetron

22 Nazasetron

$MeNHSO_2CH_2$ $CH_2CH_2NMe_2$

23 Sumatriptan

24 Zomitriptan

25 Rizatriptan

26 Alosetron

27 Mosapride

28 Tegaserod

29 Ziprasidone

30 Sertindole

31 Risperidone

32 Aripiprazole

33 H_3 agonist

(constipation-predominant irritable bowel syndrome) (**28**) are marketed for various GI conditions. Many other 5-HT receptor ligands with dopamine receptor activity have been marketed as antipsychotic agents. Examples of this class of compounds include quetiapine (**15**), olanzapine (**16**), ziprasidone (**29**), sertindole (**30**), risperidone (**31**) and aripiprazole (**32**).[43]

In case of the histamine receptor ligands, H_1 and H_2 receptor antagonists such as fexofenadine

(**4**, anti-allergic) and ranitidine (**5**, acid secretion inhibitor) are highly successful drugs. However, other two receptor subtypes (H_3 and H_4) have only been identified relatively recently and ligands (e.g. **33–35**) to these receptor subtypes are currently being identified in order to explore the role of these subtypes in pathological processes.[44–46]

Other more recent examples of new receptor subtypes include neurokinin, melanocortin and somatostatin receptor subtypes. Neurokinins (substance P, neurokinin A and neurokinin B) act at three receptor subtypes: NK_1, NK_2 and NK_3. Selective ligands are being

34 H$_3$ antagonist

35 H$_4$ antagonist

36 MC-1 receptor agonist

37 MC-4 receptor agonist

38

39

explored for the treatment of pain, asthma, depression and the like. The natural melanocortic peptides are derived from the precursor peptide pro-opiomelanocortin (expressed in the pituitary) by proteolytic cleavage in three regions of the protein generating ACTH, and α-, β- and γ-melanocyte stimulating hormone (MSH) peptides. Pro-opiomelanocortin also generates a number of other peptides including enkephalin and β-endorphin. Five melanocortin receptor subtypes (MC$_1$–MC$_5$) belonging to the G-protein-coupled receptor family have been cloned (40–60% sequence identities) and selective ligands for the receptor subtypes have been synthesised.[47–49] Early pharmacological studies have indicated that drugs selective for MC$_1$ receptor may be useful for the treatment of inflammatory conditions, whereas compounds selective for the MC$_4$ receptor may be useful for controlling eating behaviour and body weight. Compounds **36** and **37** were identified as receptor subtype 1 and 4 agonists, respectively, by traditional screening and medicinal chemistry approaches. The melanocortin

receptor subtype 1 agonist showed a dose-dependent decrease in TNF-α production in a murine lipopolysaccharide-induced cytokine accumulation model. These biological effects are very different from the involvement of MSH and ACTH in skin pigmentation and secretion of corticosteroids, respectively.

Cloning studies have also identified five receptor subtypes of somatostatin [Ala-Gly-Cys-Lys-Asn-Phe-Phe-Trp-Lys-Thr-Phe-Thr-Ser-Cys, a cyclic peptide with a disulphide bridge], a peptide discovered in 1971–2 and shown to be an inhibitor of growth hormone, insulin, glucagon and gastric acid secretion. Screening of heterocyclic β-turn mimetic libraries (based upon the Trp-Lys motif found in the turn region of somatostatin) against a panel of the five cloned human somatostatin receptors (hSST$_1$–hSST$_5$) led to the development of somatostatin receptor ligands such as those shown in structures **38–40** that bind to the five receptor subtypes.[50] Compound **38** is relatively more selective for the hSST$_2$ receptor subtype and **39** shows higher affinity against hSST$_3$ and hSST$_5$ subtypes. The turn

40

41 hSSTR$_1$ selective

42 hSSTR$_2$ selective

43 hSSTR$_3$ selective

44 hSSTR$_4$ selective

45 hSSTR$_5$ selective

receptors regulated release of growth hormone from the rat anterior pituitary gland. Some of the recent information has shown that the five receptor subtypes may fall into two classes or groups. One class (SRIF$_1$) appears to comprise SST$_2$, SST$_3$ and SST$_5$ while the other class (SRIF$_2$) consists of the other two recombinant receptor subtypes (SST$_1$ and SST$_4$).

More recently, attention has also been focused on orphan G-protein-coupled receptors, a family of plasma membrane proteins involved in a broad array of signalling pathways.[53,54] Novel members of the orphan G-protein-coupled receptors have continued to emerge through cloning activities as well as through bioinformatic analysis of sequence databases. Their ligands are unidentified and their physiological relevance remains to be defined. Methods are being developed to identify ligands acting at these receptors. One of these approaches identifies ligands by purification from biological fluids, cell supernatants or tissue extracts. The discoveries of endothelin (a vasoconstrictor peptide) and nociceptin (an orphan opioid-like receptor ligand) are examples of this type. Ligands can also be identified by screening the orphan receptor against a number of diverse chemical libraries. Once identified, the ligand is used to clarify the physiological and pathological roles of the receptor, followed by the discovery of other agonist and antagonist analogues by medicinal chemistry approaches.

Currently the drug discovery process has progressed beyond the receptor stage and

mimetic **40** is more potent at the hSST$_5$ receptor subtype. In another series of compounds, library screening followed by studies of structure–activity relationships led to the development of compounds selective for the hSST receptor subtypes (**41–45**).[51,52] *In vitro* experiments using these selective compounds demonstrated the role of the hSST$_2$ receptor in inhibition of glucagon release from mouse pancreatic α-cells and the hSST$_5$ receptor as a mediator of insulin secretion from pancreatic β-cells. Both subtypes of various steps that result from the interaction of the receptor with a specific ligand have been characterised. One of the more important processes, signal transduction, converts the external signals induced by hormones, growth factors, neurotransmitters and cytokines into specific internal cellular responses (e.g. gene expression, cell division or even cell suicide). The process involves a cascade of enzyme-mediated reactions inside the cell that typically include phosphorylation and dephosphorylation of proteins (kinases and phosphatases) as mediators of downstream processes. Signal transduction inhibitors are currently being developed for the treatment of a number of diseases, including cancer and inflammation.

1.4.2 Genomics

Genetic factors influence virtually every human disorder (e.g. Alzheimer's and Parkinson's diseases, diabetes, asthma and rheumatoid arthritis) by determining disease susceptibility or resistance and interactions with environmental factors. Gene transfer research ('gene therapy') holds promise for treating disorders through the transfer and expression of DNA in the cells of patients. Initial concept of gene therapy was focused on the treatment of genetic diseases (e.g. cystic fibrosis, Duchenne's muscular dystrophy and Gaucher's disease) but the field has now been expanded and many more options like cancer, cardiovascular diseases, arthritis, type 1 diabetes (e.g. non-insulin glucose lowering genes, gene(s) capable of restoring glucose-regulated production of insulin and neogenesis and regeneration of pancreatic islets), neurodegenerative disorders, X-linked severe combined immunodeficiency[55] and infectious diseases, including acquired immunodeficiency syndrome (AIDS), are being considered.[56–60] Cancer treatment options are most advanced and include suicide gene therapy, tumour suppressor gene therapy, cytokine gene therapy and expression of 'prodrug activating enzymes' with the ability to convert a nontoxic 'prodrug' administered to the patient into a cytotoxic agent at the tumour site. Although many gene therapy clinical trials

have started, several important issues, including efficient delivery of the genetic material to the required sites, along with other chemical, biological, safety, toxicity and ethical issues have not yet been fully resolved. From the point of view of drug discovery, mapping of the human genome is only the first step. It is likely that even when the human genomic sequencing has been fully completed and all genes have been identified, a substantial fraction of these, possibly up to 50%, will have complex biochemical or physiological functions. Therefore, only a proportion (about 20% of the genome) will be amenable to pharmacological exploitation.[61] Another major problem is the involvement of many genes and environmental factors in various diseases. For example, with the exception of some diseases or traits resulting principally from specific and relatively rare mutations (e.g. cystic fibrosis), most of the genetic disorders (e.g. cardiovascular diseases, diabetes, rheumatoid arthritis and schizophrenia) develop as a result of a network of genes failing to perform correctly, some of which might have a major disease effect but many a relatively minor effect. Complex diseases and traits result principally from genetic variation that is relatively common in the general population. Along with the role of multiple genes and environmental factors in various diseases, problems exist with gene 'redundancy' at the functional level.[62] Thus, completion of the human genome will not provide an immediate solution to the genetics of complex diseases. This can only be achieved by documenting the genetic variation of human genomes at the population level within and across ethnic groups and by characterising mutant genes. For further progress it is therefore essential to identify the function of each gene in the normal and disease situation and establish a link with the expressed protein (before and after post-translational modification) and its role in a disease pathway. This process and further phenotypic analysis through detailed biology will then lead to new validated targets for drug discovery by traditional methods or treatment options using gene therapy or protein products.

Since the complete genome of *Haemophilus influenzae* was published, sequencing of genomes from a wide range of organisms, from bacteria to man, has continued apace. Initial sequencing and analysis of the human genome has been published.[63,64] Another more recent example includes the genome sequence of *Escherichia coli* O157:H7, implicated in many outbreaks of haemorrhagic colitis.[65] The functional characterisation of microbial genomics will have a significant impact on genomic medicine (new antimicrobial targets and vaccine candidates) and on environmental (waste management, recycling), food and industrial biotechnology.[66,67] In addition to the work on human and microbial genomes, progress is also being made on the sequencing of the mouse and rat genomes.[68] Data from rodent species should speed the discovery of genes and regulatory regions in the human genome and make it easier to determine their functions. In addition, these sequences may have significant impact on the disease models since these animals are most often used in the early discovery and pre-clinical testing of new drugs.[69] Comparative genomics and proteomics studies between various genomes may also lead to additional information useful for various stages of the drug discovery process.[70]

There are three main approaches to mapping the genetic variants involved in a disease: functional cloning, the candidate-gene strategy and positional cloning. In functional cloning, identification of the underlying protein defect leads to localisation of the responsible gene (disease–function–gene–map). An example of functional cloning is the finding that individuals with sickle cell anaemia carried an amino acid substitution in the β chain of haemoglobin. Isolation of the mutant molecule led to the cloning of the gene encoding β globin.

In the candidate-gene approach – the most frequently used approach adopted to identify the predisposing or causal genes in the complex and multigenic and multifactorial diseases – genes with a known or proposed function, with the potential to influence the disease phenotype, are investigated for a direct role in disease. In a small number of cases of type 2 diabetes, candidate-gene studies have identified mutations in,

for example, the genes encoding insulin and the insulin receptor.

Marker genes not related to disease physiology and genome-wide screens are the starting points for mapping the genetic components of the disease. The aim is first to identify the genetic region within which a disease-predisposing gene lies and, once this is found, to localise the gene and determine its functional and biological role in the disease (disease–map–gene–function).

The introduction of functional genes for the restoration of normal function or the transfer of therapeutic genes to treat particular diseases such as cancer or viral infections is of growing interest. The hurdles to overcome inefficient gene therapy include successful transfer of the therapeutic genes, appropriate expression levels associated with sufficient duration of gene expression and the specificity of gene transfer to achieve therapeutic effects in the patient. Viral vectors are still among the most efficient gene transfer vehicles.[71–73] Because of the comparatively long history of characterisation of particular viruses and their genomes, their valuable characteristics for target cell infectivity, transgene capacity and accessibility of established helper cell lines for the production of recombinant virus stocks to infect target cells, the most commonly used vectors are developed from retroviruses, lentiviruses, adenovirus, herpes simplex virus and adeno-associated virus. The advantages of retroviral vectors (stable integration into the host genome, generation of viral titres sufficient for efficient gene transfer, infectivity of the recombinant viral particles for a broad variety of target cell types and ability to carry foreign genes of reasonable size) are accompanied by several disadvantages (e.g. instability of some retroviral vectors, possible insertional mutagenesis by random viral integration into host DNA, the requirement of cell division for integration of Moloney murine leukaemia virus-derived retroviral vectors and targeting of retroviral infection and/or therapeutic gene expression). In addition to the viral transfection procedures, non-viral transfection procedures (e.g. liposomes, gene gun and DNA conjugates) are also being developed.[74,75] In a recent example, human monocyte-derived dendritic cells were transfected with genes encoding tumour-associated antigens.[71] The transfection was achieved by dimerisation of a 35 amino acid cationic peptide (Lys-Lys-Lys-Lys-Lys-Lys-Gly-Gly-Phe-Leu-Gly-Phe-Trp-Arg-Gly-Glu-Asn-Gly-Arg-Lys-Thr-Arg-Ser-Ala-Tyr-Glu-Arg-Met-Cys-Asn-Ile-Leu-Lys-Gly-Lys), and then using a complex of this dimeric peptide with plasmid DNA expression constructs. Injection of transfected dendritic cells expressing a tumour-associated antigen protected mice from lethal challenge with tumour cells in a model of melanoma.

Identification of the genes which provide structural and regulatory functions in an organism are likely to be useful in obtaining genetically modified (transgenic) animals using gene knock-out or knock-in strategies.[76] The transgenic animals are useful in determining the physiological functions of genes, identification and validation of new molecular drug targets, generation of animal models of disease for the testing of novel therapeutic strategies and early recognition of toxicological effects.[77] In a number of cases, a direct correlation between the gene knock-out phenotype and the efficacy of drugs which modulate that specific target has been demonstrated.[78] Using gene knock-out methodology and phenotypic studies, a number of new targets have been suggested in cancer and neurological, metabolic, cardiovascular, immunological and bone disorders.

1.4.3 Pharmacogenomics and toxicogenomics

Because different patients with the same disease symptoms respond differently to the same drug, both in terms of therapeutic benefits and side effects, understanding of the relationships between gene variations and the effect of such variations on drug responses within individuals is likely to lead to tailor-made therapies for specific population of patients. For example, a variety of antihypertensive and congestive heart failure drugs are now available, including calcium antagonists, ACE inhibitors, β-blockers, diuretics, α-blockers, centrally

acting antihypertensives and, more recently, AT_1 receptor antagonists. Although all of these agents are effective in lowering blood pressure in most cases, there are significant differences between their therapeutic and side-effect profiles. A better knowledge of the mechanisms that influence the efficiency of the drugs in different individuals, and understanding why some patients can tolerate the drug better than others may lead to more efficacious drugs with a better side-effect profile. The variation of the individual's response to such drugs may be caused by either the heterogeneity of the mechanisms underlying hypertension, inter-individual variations in the pharmacokinetics of drugs (genetic polymorphisms in drug metabolising enzymes) or a combination of both.

The likely benefit of more efficacious tailor-made drugs with fewer side effects has led to the development of the science of pharmacogenomics, a name given to any drug discovery platform that attempts to address the issues of efficacy and toxicity in individuals based on the influence of inheritance on variable drug response.[79] The concept of individual variation at the molecular level is not new. Proteins obtained from different individuals have been known to have different amino acid sequences. These protein isoforms originate either by genomic variation at the level of the actual gene sequence or by variation in expression which results from changes in the promoter and control elements that regulate expression. Alleles differ from each other in structural features, such as single base pair changes, or as a result of rearrangements or deletions of entire gene portions. Depending on the structure of regulatory sequences, some alleles may be expressed at very high levels, while others may be repressed. Similarly, depending on variation at the critical points in the assembly of genes, splicing variants may result from alternative arrangement of building blocks. Technologies that enable the monitoring of gene expression under different circumstances (based on high-throughput sequencing and screening approaches) are currently being developed and will enable systematic investigations of the patterns of gene expression between normal and disease states in a statistically meaningful way along with the expression of the relevant proteins in different individuals. In addition, the potential of using single-nucleotide polymorphisms to correlate drug regimens and responses is also being investigated.[80] The availability of precisely located single-nucleotide polymorphic sites spanning the genome holds promise for the association of particular genetic loci with disease states. This information, together with high-throughput gene-chip technologies, will offer new opportunities for molecular diagnostics and monitoring of disease predisposition in large sections of the population. It will also allow much earlier preventive treatment in many slowly evolving diseases.

Toxicogenomics uses global gene expression analysis studies to detect expression changes that influence, predict or help define drug toxicity.[81] The principle behind the technique relies on the identification of toxicity-related gene expression signatures (fingerprints) of known compounds and comparing these to gene-expression profiles of new, similar compounds. Similarities between the two sets of compounds may predict the toxic potential of unknown compounds. It is expected that toxicogenomics will reduce failure rates of drugs by helping select the right compounds for development early on and by accelerating toxicology testing and identifying suitable biomarkers amenable to screening using the generated data.

Several toxicogenomic databases are currently being built. A substantial amount of data has already been generated in animal models with known toxicants, mainly hepatotoxins, proving that gene expression analysis can provide information to allow classification of compounds according to their mechanism of toxicity as well as identifying cellular pathways related to the toxic event. More recently, this global gene expression analysis has been applied to the evaluation of nephrotoxicity, genotoxicity and testicular toxicity. In addition to the classification of compounds based on gene expression fingerprints obtained from tissue samples after exposure to toxicants, information has also been obtained about the underlying mechanisms of toxicity. Identification of genes and/or pathways

that are modulated by certain toxicants provides insight into possible mechanisms of toxicity. Much further work, such as quality of databases and relationship between gene expression and dose-dependent induction of toxicity, still needs to be done before the techniques become fully acceptable.

1.4.4 Proteomics

The control mechanisms in health and disease are found at the protein level and, as mentioned above, genome sequencing does not provide sufficient information at the protein level. The tertiary structure and the type and extent of post-translational modifications (e.g. glycosylation and phosphorylation) of a protein are critical to its function and cellular localisation but this information is not encoded in the protein's corresponding DNA. An additional complication between genes and proteins is the existence of alternative splice variants of mRNA which give rise to isomeric proteins that might contribute to regulatory processes in the cell. The processing of proteins may also be different in various tissues under different conditions. Some proteins may give rise to biologically active fragments and some may exert diverse functions in collaboration with other proteins. Therefore, the complete structure and function of an individual protein cannot be determined by reference to its gene sequence alone. Thus, beyond genomics it is essential to compare the protein content of cells/tissues/organs in the normal and disease situation and to generate functional information on proteins required for various drug discovery processes. Proteomics is any protein-based approach that provides new information about proteins on a genome-wide scale and addresses these difficulties by enabling the protein levels of cellular organisation to be screened and characterised.[82,83] In a high-throughput manner, a large number of proteins from normal and disease samples (cells and tissue extracts) are separated on the basis of their charge and molecular weight by two-dimensional electrophoresis, and the amino acid sequences of proteins and their post-translational modifications are identified by mass spectrometry. The separated proteins are then stained and the maps of protein expression are digitally scanned into databases. The protein expression maps can be used to study cellular pathways and the perturbation of these pathways by disease and drug action. Thus, an understanding of cellular pathways and protein changes resulting from the disease and drug actions not only lead to new drug targets but can also provide early markers for diseases and early indications of drug toxicity.[84] It should be emphasised, however, that characterisation of a different protein in a disease state does not necessarily mean that it plays a causal role or represents a potential therapeutic target. In many cases, the new protein may be a consequence of the disease rather than the cause. Further studies are required to check whether the activity of a candidate target eliminated by molecular/cellular techniques could reverse the disease phenotype. Moreover, even when a potential therapeutic target has been identified and a molecule capable of disrupting it has been obtained, we cannot assume that it will constitute an effective treatment for the disease under investigation. Alternative metabolic routes may provide cells with ways of circumventing blocked pathways.

The potential benefit of proteomics in predicting toxicity at an early stage may lead to accelerated drug discovery programmes. A comparison of the protein profiles of normal tissue with those of tissue treated with a known toxic agent might give an indication of the drug's toxic activity. Similarly, identification of a known toxic protein in drug-treated tissues may give an idea about the toxicity of the drug. As a first approach, an examination of liver and kidney, which are the major sites for metabolism and excretion of most drugs, before and after the drug administration may provide early indications about events that might result in toxicity. Proteomic analysis of the serum, where the majority of toxicity markers released from susceptible organs and tissues throughout the entire body collect, can be utilised to identify serum markers (and clusters thereof) as indicators of toxicity. These serum markers could subsequently be used to predict the response of each individual and allow

tailoring of therapy whereby optimal efficacy is achieved while minimising adverse side effects. Surrogate markers for drug efficacy could also be detected by this procedure and could be used for identifying patient classes who will respond favourably to a drug.

There is currently some debate about the ability of the techniques being used to detect all the proteins present in a given sample. It is possible that global proteome displays based on two-dimensional gel electrophoresis are largely limited to the more abundantly expressed and stable proteins. Thus, important classes of regulatory proteins involved in signal transduction and gene expression, for example, and other proteins of lower abundance remain undetected by current methodologies. Proteins of lower abundance are more likely to be detected by separating these from high-abundance proteins. The disadvantage of this strategy, however, is that it requires much larger amounts of protein, and many additional separations, and therefore may be impractical for studies of small cell populations or tissue samples. Efforts are underway to develop advanced proteomic technologies that do not rely upon two-dimensional gel electrophoresis.

After the discovery of protein maps and characterisation of individual proteins, the most important aspect of proteomics is to define protein function. Although new proteins are likely to include receptors, ligands, enzymes, enzyme inhibitors, signalling molecules and pathways that may be therapeutic targets, precise functions of the individual proteins have to be identified. To discover and monitor the relevance of a protein to a disease-related process, it is also important to find where, when and to what extent a protein is expressed. Many approaches are being used to discover protein function.[85,86] Structural homology methods may be used to ascribe function to some proteins, since it is known that proteins of similar function often share structural homology (tertiary structure). Another approach to defining protein function is chemical proteomics (or chemical genomics),[87] which is the identification of small molecules that interact with the proteins by screening new proteins against diverse chemical libraries using methods such as nuclear magnetic resonance (NMR) spectroscopy, microcalorimetry or microarrays. Another method for identifying ligand-binding sites involves scanning the surface of a protein molecule for clefts. In many cases, the largest cleft is the known primary binding site for small ligands. Further information about the ligand structures that can be accommodated in the binding site can be obtained by various computational methods like DOCK or HOOK. Some of the proteins likely to have known enzyme activity or enzyme inhibition properties can be identified by using screens for generic enzyme activities. Chemical proteomics techniques, which involve the use of chemical probes (synthetic small molecules) designed to covalently attach to proteins of interest and allow purification and/or identification, have also been used to identify new protease drug targets.[88] Along with the structural and chemical library methods, several 'non-homology' methods are being developed to identify protein functions.[89] These are computational methods that take advantage of the many properties shared among functionally related proteins, such as patterns of domain fusion, evolutionary co-inheritance, conservation of relative gene position and correlated expression patterns. Protein function is defined by these methods in terms of context, that is, which cellular pathways or complexes the protein participates in, rather than by suggesting a specific biochemical activity. Large-scale functional analysis of new proteins can be accomplished by using peptide or protein arrays, ranging from synthetic peptide arrays to whole proteins expressed in living cells.[90] Comprehensive sets of purified peptides and proteins permit high-throughput screening for discrete biochemical properties, whereas formats involving living cells facilitate large-scale genetic screening for novel biological activities. Protein arrays can be engineered to suit the aims of a particular experiment. Thus, an array might contain all the combinatorial variants of a bioactive peptide or specific variants of a single protein species (splice variants, domains or mutants), a family of protein orthologues

from different species, a protein pathway or even the entire protein complement of an organism.

Access to structural information on a proteome-wide scale is not only important for ascribing protein function but may also be useful in target validation and medicinal chemistry on hits/leads requiring structural information for rational design processes. The most straightforward strategy for predicting structure is to search for sequence similarity to a protein with a known three-dimensional structure.[91–94] Additional information can be obtained by identifying known and novel folds in a protein. There are databases of structural motifs in proteins which contain data relevant to helices, β-turns, γ-turns, β-hairpins, ψ-loops, β-α-β motifs, β-sheets, β-strands and disulphide bridges extracted from proteins, which can be used for comparison. Novel folds can be identified by employing *ab initio* approaches used for prediction of protein structure. With the aim of extracting further information from protein sequences, sequence motif libraries have been developed. Advances in X-ray crystallography, particularly the use of synchrotron radiation sources, and NMR spectroscopy also allow more rapid determination of protein structures. Using protein crystals in which methionine residue is replaced by selenomethionine and multi-wavelength synchrotron experiments, electron-density maps for proteins can be generated in less than an hour instead of the weeks of experimental time required for a conventional crystallography structure determination.[95] Despite great improvements in X-ray crystallography techniques, the rate-limiting step in structure determination remains the expression, purification and crystallisation of the target protein.

Many problems still remain to be solved before protein function can be confidently assigned by using the above techniques. For example, the idea of 'one gene–one protein–one function' is not valid in many cases and increasing numbers of proteins are found to have two or more different functions.[96] The multiple functions of such moonlighting proteins can vary as a consequence of changes in cellular localisation, cell type, oligomeric state or the cellular concentration of a ligand, substrate, cofactor or product. Multidrug transporter *P*-glycoprotein (a large 170 kDa cell-surface molecule encoded by the human *MDR1* gene) is an example of a protein with multiple functions. It is well established that *P*-glycoprotein can efflux xenobiotics from cells and is one mechanism that tumour cells use to escape death induced by chemotherapeutic drugs. Recent observations have raised the possibility that *P*-glycoprotein and related transporter molecules might play a fundamental role in regulating cell differentiation, proliferation and survival. *P*-glycoprotein encoded by *MDR1* in humans and *Mdr1a* in mice can regulate an endogenous chloride channel. This activity of *P*-glycoprotein can be inhibited by phosphorylation by protein kinase C. *MDR1 P*-glycoprotein has also been proposed to play a role in phospholipid translocation and cholesterol esterification. Functional *P*-glycoprotein has also been suggested to play a role in regulating programmed cell death (apoptosis).[97]

1.4.5 Bioinformatics and data-mining technologies

The availability of genomic data and the corresponding protein sequences from humans and other organisms together with structure/function annotations, disease correlations and population variations require sophisticated data management systems (databases) for analytical purposes. Proteomics-oriented databases include data on the two-dimensional gel electrophoresis maps of proteins from a variety of healthy and disease tissues. Bioinformatic systems (computer-assisted data management and analysis) are used to gather and analyse this information in order to attach biological knowledge to genes, assign genes to biological pathways, compare the gene sets of different species, understand processes in healthy and disease states and find new or better drugs.[98] The currently available techniques have the capability to translate a given gene sequence into a protein structure, complete with prediction of secondary structure and database comparisons.

Progress is being made in devising systems that provide information on biological function derived from sequencing and functional analysis. In addition to the gene/function analysis studies, the need for data-mining techniques (defined as 'the nontrivial extraction of implicit, previously unknown and potentially useful information from data') is becoming necessary in order to deal with the enormous amount of information that the industry collects in individual databases (ranging from, e.g. databases of disease profiles and molecular pathways to sequences, chemical and biological screening data, including structure–activity relationships (SARs), chemical structures of combinatorial libraries of compounds, individual and population clinical trial results). A large number of companies are developing data-mining applications (software), which can identify cause-and-effect relationships between data sets and group together data points or sets based on different criterion. A time-delay data-mining approach is used when complete data set is not available immediately and in complete form, but is collected over time. The systems designed to handle such data look for patterns, which are confirmed or rejected as the data set increases and becomes more robust. This approach is geared towards analysis of long-term clinical trials and studies of multicomponent modes of action. It is also possible to overlay large and complex data sets that are similar to each other and compare them. This is particularly useful in all forms of clinical trial meta-analyses, where data collected at different sites over different time periods, and perhaps under similar but not always identical conditions, need to be compared. Here, the emphasis is on finding dissimilarities, not similarities. Predictive data-mining programmes are available for making simulations, predictions and forecasts based on the data sets analysed.

1.4.6 Combinatorial chemistry and high-throughput screening

One of the earliest approaches to drug discovery was the random screening process. More recently, significant efforts were directed towards rational/semi-rational approaches. However, recent advances in high-throughput screening and synthesis techniques, coupled with large-scale data analysis and data management methods, have shifted the balance towards testing libraries of 'diverse' chemical compounds in multiple screens (>20 000 compounds in a week) in the shortest possible time. This approach is expected to provide leads much more quickly for optimisation using combinatorial synthesis methods (targeted libraries) to generate drug candidates. Starting from the solid-phase peptide synthesis in the early 1960s, which opened the way to chemical synthesis on solid supports, automated synthesis of diverse organic compounds has now become routine in many laboratories. Assays have been developed that make use of fluorescently labelled reagents (e.g. receptors, ligands and enzyme substrates) allowing the rapid optical screening of large collections of compounds. Assays using microtitre plates (96–384 wells in each plate) have been designed to enable small quantities of compounds to be tested at a much-reduced cost in terms of the reagent use.

In the early phase of the work, combinatorial libraries and screening procedures had many problems, primarily because the main focus of the work was on the number of compounds produced in a mixture, with little regard for their quality. Over the years, many improvements have been made in the library design process.[99] The attention has now shifted to smaller high-quality libraries of discrete compounds, using various data-mining technologies,[100] new parallel and combinatorial approaches,[101] and filters for lead-like or drug-like properties,[102,103] as well as avoiding non-selective or promiscuous inhibitors. Due to the importance of natural products to early drug discovery process, many natural product-like libraries containing natural product scaffolds, including carbohydrates, steroids, fatty acid derivatives, polyketides, peptides, terpenoids, flavonoids and alkaloids, have been prepared and investigated in various screens. Advances in analytical chemistry have enabled the routine high-throughput purification of

compounds by mass-triggered preparative liquid chromatography.[104,105] Although the quality of leads discovered directly from combinatorial libraries is steadily increasing, it is clear that parallel synthesis is even more powerful at the lead optimisation phase, when a series of related compounds needs to be made and tested rapidly.

1.4.6.1   Combinatorial synthesis

Combinatorial chemistry is having a major impact in generating libraries containing large numbers of compounds in a relatively short period of time using solid-phase synthesis technologies. In addition, it is possible to buy ready-made libraries built around specific molecular themes and consisting of many thousands of compounds, and to test these libraries in high-throughput screening systems using automated, off-the-shelf instrumentation and reagents. The technique of combinatorial biocatalysis is also used to obtain diverse libraries.[106] This approach takes advantage of natural catalysts (enzymes and whole cells), as well as the rapidly growing supply of recombinant and engineered enzymes, for the direct derivatisation of many different synthetic compounds and natural products. The types of reactions catalysed by enzymes and micro-organisms include reactions which can introduce functional groups (e.g. carbon–carbon bond formation, hydroxylation, halogenation, cyclo additions, addition of amines), modify the existing functionalities (oxidation of alcohols to aldehydes and ketones, reduction of aldehydes or ketones to alcohols, oxidation of sulphides to sulphoxides, oxidation of amino groups to nitro groups, hydrolysis of nitriles to amides and carboxylic acids, replacements of amino groups by hydroxyl groups, lactonisation, isomerisation, epimerisation, dealkylation and methyl transfer) or addition onto functional groups (esterification, carbonate formation, carbamate formation, glycosylation, amidation and phosphorylation). Currently available technologies allow these biocatalysis reactions to be carried out in aqueous and non-aqueous solvents.

Techniques to screen individual compounds or mixtures in solution or still attached to the solid support are available. The main advantage of screening single compounds in solution (most commonly used technique in the past) is that activity can be directly correlated with chemical structure. Screening mixtures of compounds has the advantage that fewer assays need to be performed and at the same time fewer synthetic steps are required to generate mixtures. However, it is not possible to synthesise mixtures which contain entirely different structures without compromising synthetic efficiency. Screening of mixtures can lead to false positives due to additive or co-operative effects of weakly active compounds. Thus, the most active mixture may not contain the most potent compound. An additional disadvantage of testing mixtures is that once an active mixture has been identified, the exact structure of the active compound, in most cases, can only be obtained by extensive deconvolution studies. There are some procedures like the positional scanning approach which enable the active compound to be identified directly from screening. This method depends on the synthesis of a series of subset mixtures which contain a single building block (substituent) at one position and all the building blocks at the other positions. The structure of the most active compound is then assigned by selecting the building block from the most active subset at each position. The structure is confirmed by synthesis.

The most widely used solid-phase method for the synthesis of libraries (originally used for peptides) has been termed the 'split-mix', 'divide, couple and recombine' and 'one bead–one compound' method. The resin beads display a linker to which the building blocks are sequentially attached, to effectively grow molecules. As a first step, different batches of resin are reacted individually with a unique set of reagents (first set of building blocks); the resins are then combined and deprotected to liberate another reactive group. The resin is then divided into several components and each component is reacted individually by the second building block. This 'divide, couple and recombine' strategy is continued until all the building blocks have been added. The resin batches are not combined after the final building blocks have been added. This strategy results in a resin library in which a single

compound is attached to an individual bead. When a synthesis is complete, cleavage at the linker releases the molecule(s) from the bead(s). The screening of single beads, or the compounds derived from single beads, corresponds to screening of single compounds. Screening of these libraries can quickly identify the preferred last building block in the most active set. The subset library is then re-synthesised by keeping this preferred final building block constant and screened to identify the penultimate preferred building block in each set. This deconvolution process, or iterative re-synthesis and screening, is repeated in order to define all of the positions. The deconvolution process has to be repeated each time the library is tested in a new screen. Several different approaches have been investigated to avoid this inconvenient and time-consuming deconvolution method. One of these, using tagging/encoding strategies, involves introduction of chemical tags at each stage of the 'split-mix' synthesis either before the addition of each building block during the synthesis or before the subsequent mixing step. At the end of the synthesis, any individual bead will possess a compound made up from a single combination of building blocks and an associated tag sequence with a specific tag corresponding to each building block. The identity of the compound on a single bead can be determined simply by analysing the tagging sequence. The original tagging methods, oligonucleotides [read by polymerase chain reaction (PCR) amplification and DNA sequencing] and peptides (read by Edman microsequencing), have now been replaced by using binary coding with chemical tags. This tagging strategy increases the number of steps in the synthesis of each library but allows more rapid identification of the active hits.

1.4.6.2 Library design
The design strategy may vary according to the information available on the target and the purpose of the library.[107] For example, when the class of target is known (e.g. an enzyme with a known mechanism of action and/or structural information or a known or similar receptor type/subtype), library design may

be started from a known pharmacophore. For example, aspartyl proteinases like renin, HIV and cathepsin D proteases are inhibited by compounds containing a statine residue, a known transition-state analogue. Several libraries based on statine or a hydroxyethylamine core have been prepared and investigated against other aspartyl proteinases. The use of synthetic positional-scanning combinatorial libraries offers the ability to rapidly test and evaluate the extended substrate specificities of proteases.[108] For example, a fluorogenic tetrapeptide positional-scanning library (containing a 7-amino-4-methylcoumarin-derivatised lysine) in which the P_1 amino acid was held constant as a lysine and the P_4–P_3–P_2 positions were positionally randomised was used to investigate extended substrate specificities of plasmin and thrombin, two of the enzymes involved in the blood coagulation cascade. The optimal P_4 to P_2 substrate specificity for plasmin was P_4-Lys/Nle/Val/Ile/Phe, P_3-Xaa and P_2-Tyr/Phe/Trp. The optimal P_4 to P_2 extended substrate sequence determined for thrombin was P_4-Nle/Leu/Ile/Phe/Val, P_3-Xaa and P_2-Pro. By three-dimensional structural modelling of the substrates into the active sites of plasmin and thrombin, it was possible to identify potential determinants of the defined substrate specificity. This method is amenable to the incorporation of diverse substituents at the P_1 position (all 20 proteinogenic and other non-proteinogenic amino acids) for exploring molecular recognition elements in various new uncharacterised proteolytic enzymes.

A similar approach can be adopted when a lead ligand has been identified by random screening. The structural template in the lead is modified to generate a targeted library. Many libraries have been synthesised around the so-called 'privileged structures' which have shown activity against various targets. For example, compounds based on a benzodiazepine core have shown activity against a number of G-protein-coupled receptors. However, when there is little information, or when entirely different structural leads are required, a larger diverse library is likely to be more suitable to increase the chance of success. The chemical diversity between the different members of the library is also very important to cover a wide chemical area and increase chances of success. In addition to some simple rules like incorporating acidic, basic, hydrophilic and hydrophobic groups of different sizes, a large number of computer-based methods are available for diversity analysis. Information is also available on the so-called drug-like molecules that tend to have certain properties. For example, $\log P$, molecular weight and the number of hydrogen bonding groups have been correlated with oral bioavailability.[109] Analysis of a large number of compounds from the World Drug Index establishment resulted in the 'rule of five' based on the assumption that compounds meeting these criteria have entered human clinical trials, and therefore must possess many of the desirable characteristics of drugs. A high percentage of compounds contained ≤ 5 hydrogen bond donors (expressed as the sum of OHs and NHs), ≤ 10 hydrogen bond acceptors, ≤ 500 relative molecular weight and $\log P$ of ≤ 5.[110] Along with these measures, it is also desirable to exclude functional groups that tend to be undesirable because of chemical reactivity, for example, alkylating and acylating groups, and other unstable groups leading to metabolism (solvolysis or hydrolysis).[111]

The availability of complex, large and diverse chemical libraries and ultrahigh-throughput screening technologies also provides an option whereby the biological pathways and proteins do not have to be fully characterised before starting the screening process. A number of pre-selected, incompletely characterised, disease-associated protein targets can be screened against many different libraries. Using the whole cell systems and libraries containing membrane-permeable compounds, it is possible to identify compounds which perturb a cellular process or system, followed by identification of proteins required in cell function. From the perspective of drug discovery, this approach offers the means for the simultaneous identification of proteins that can serve as targets for therapeutic intervention ('therapeutic target validation') and small molecules that can modulate the functions of

46 5-HT$_6$ receptor ligand

47 Fibrinogen receptor antagonist

48 PPARα agonist

49 PPARδ agonist

50 VLA4 antagonist

these therapeutic targets ('chemical target validation'). The overall process differs from the traditional methods of drug discovery in which the biological methods are first used to select and characterise protein targets for therapeutic intervention, followed by chemical efforts to determine whether the protein target can be modulated by small molecules.

1.4.6.3 Examples of compounds discovered by library approaches

Over the years, with improving design and screening processes, the success rate for the discovery of 'hits' and 'leads' from various high-throughput, project-directed and thematic libraries has increased significantly. A large number of examples are mentioned in two recent reviews.[112,113] Other examples include ligands for the five somatostatin receptor ligands (see Section 1.3.1), fibrinogen receptor antagonist, PPARα, PPARδ and very late antigen (VLA-4) antagonists shown in **46–50**.

1.4.7 Structure-based drug design

The entire process of structure-based drug design requires identification and characterisation of

a suitable protein target, determination of the structure of the target protein, the availability of an easy and reliable high-throughput screening assay, identification of a lead compound, development of computer-assisted methods for estimating the affinity of new compounds, and access to a synthetic route to produce the designed compounds.[114] Progress has been made on many of these aspects. For example, expression systems are now available that allow the production of large amounts of naturally occurring proteins and modified proteins like isotope-labelled proteins required for NMR studies and proteins containing residues like selenomethionine (in place of methionine) that simplify the determination of the X-ray structure. Advances in automation technologies have resulted in increasing the synthesis and screening capabilities. From the point of view of design, more important aspects of 'rational design' strategy involve methods of using the information contained in the three-dimensional structure of a macromolecular target and of related ligand–target complexes, and predicting novel lead compounds. A variety of 'docking' programmes now exist that can select from a large database of compounds a subset of molecules that usually includes some compounds that bind to the selected target protein.[115,116] One such programme, DOCK, systematically attempts to fit each compound from a database into the binding site of the target structure, such that three or more of the atoms in the database molecule overlap with a set of predefined site points in the target-binding site. The newer computational methods are aimed at using the information contained in the three-dimensional structure of the unligated target to design entirely new lead compounds *de novo*, as well as to construct large virtual combinatorial libraries of compounds that can be screened computationally (virtual screening) before going to the effort and expense of actually synthesising and testing them.

The *de novo* design of structure-based ligands involves fragment positioning methods, molecule growth methods and fragment methods, coupled to database searches.[117] The fragment positioning methods determine energetically favourable binding site positions for various functional group types or chemical fragments. In the molecule growth methods, a seed atom (or fragment) is first placed in the binding site of the target structure. A ligand molecule is successively built by bonding another atom (or fragment) to it. Fragment positioning methods can also be coupled to database searching techniques either to extract from a database existing molecules that can be docked into the binding site with the desired fragments in their optimal positions or for *de novo* design.

Once a lead compound has been found by some means, an iterative process begins, which involves solving the three-dimensional structure of the lead compound bound to the target, examining that structure and characterising the types of interactions the bound ligand makes, and using the computational methods to design improvements to the compound. A large number of examples that demonstrate the utility of this approach exist in the literature. Many inhibitors of enzymes, for example, renin, HIV protease and thrombin, have been optimised using this approach.

1.4.8   Virtual screening

The virtual screening strategy involves construction or 'synthesis' of molecules on the computer.[118] The number of 'synthesised' compounds is limited by synthesising focused libraries (e.g. a hydroxamate library of matrix MMP inhibitors) and concentrating on reactions that will work in high yield with reagents that are easily accessible and incorporating 'drug-like' properties. Synthetic accessibility can be checked using programmes such as computer-aided organic synthesis or computer-aided estimation of synthetic accessibility. As molecules are constructed, a variety of filters are applied to 'weed out' compounds that do not meet certain criteria (e.g. similarity and diversity analysis, presence of undesirable functional groups, molecular weight and lipophilicity). Once a virtual library has been created and the undesirable compounds removed, the next step is to generate three-dimensional conformations for each molecule. Since most molecules are quite flexible, a multi-conformer docking approach is adopted. In this strategy, a set of conformations (typically 10–50) is generated and then each conformer is docked as a rigid molecule into the target enzyme or receptor, which is held fixed throughout. None of the docking approaches can take into account the important conformational changes that take place during the binding process of the ligand to its receptor. Before the three-dimensional conformational analysis, it is also useful to get two-dimensional 'shape' and 'distance' information to remove molecules that cannot possibly match the active site.

The factors taken into account for searching the virtual library include:

1. Knowledge about compounds that interact with the target, for example, substrates, known classes of inhibitors, antagonists and agonists, SAR within various series, pharmacophores deduced from compound classes.
2. Knowledge about receptor structure and receptor–ligand interactions, for example, homology models, X-ray and/or NMR structures, thermodynamics of ligand binding, effect of point mutations and dynamic motions of receptor and ligands.
3. Knowledge about drugs in general, for example, chemical structures and properties of known drugs, rules of conformational analysis and thermodynamics of receptor–ligand interactions.

In the early stages of the project when leads do not exist, computational methods can be used to select a diverse set of compounds from a large virtual library. If a compound shows activity, then other similar compounds from the library are synthesised and tested. If a lead already exists at the start of the programme, the size of the virtual library can be reduced by selecting a subset of compounds that are similar to the lead.

1.4.9 NMR, X-ray and mass spectroscopic techniques

As a first step in structure-based design, the three-dimensional structure of the target macromolecule (protein or nucleic acid) is determined by X-ray crystallography, NMR spectroscopy or homology modelling. Many examples of this type of research are well known in the literature.[119,120] However, it should be emphasised that even after many cycles of the structure-based design process, when a compound that binds to the target with high affinity has been developed, it is still a long way from being a drug on the market. The compound may still fail in animal and clinical trials due to factors such as toxicity, bioavailability, poor pharmacokinetics (absorption, metabolism and half-life) and lack of efficacy.

In the lead generation phase, NMR methods are first used to detect weak binding of small molecule scaffolds to a target. The binding information is subsequently used to design much tighter binding inhibitors, or drug leads.[121] SAR by NMR was the first NMR screening method disclosed in the literature.[122] This is a fragment-based approach wherein a large library of small molecules is screened using two-dimensional ^{1}H or ^{15}N spectra of the target protein as a readout. From spectral changes one can identify the compounds binding to the target. After deconvolution and identification of the active compound(s), a second screen of close analogues of the first 'hit' is performed to optimise binding affinity to the first subsite. In order to identify small molecules that bind to another site on the target molecule, the screen is then repeated with the first site saturated.

If small molecule fragments are identified that occupy several neighbouring subsites, one can then, based on the known structure, synthesise compounds that incorporate the small molecule fragments with various linking groups. If linked effectively, resulting compounds may have affinities for the target that are even stronger than the products of the binding constants of the individual unlinked fragments. As an example of the approach, several small fragments (**51**, **52**) were discovered as ligands for the FK506-binding protein (K_i values 2–9500 μM). Linking these fragments led to more potent compounds like **53** (K_i 49 nM).

The SHAPES strategy technique, like the above methods, relies on monitoring ligand signals to determine which compounds in a mixture bind a drug target.[123] The method uses standard one-dimensional line broadening and two-dimensional transferred nuclear Overhauser effect measurements to detect binding of a limited (<200) but diverse library of soluble low molecular weight scaffolds to a potential drug target. The scaffolds are derived largely from shapes or frameworks, most commonly found in known therapeutic agents, and as such represent approximations to 'successful' regions of diversity space. This approach was used to identify p38 inhibitors. In the initial screen, the

51 K_i 2 μM

52 K_i 100 μM

53 K_i 49 nM

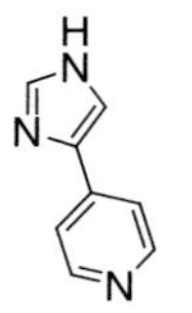

54

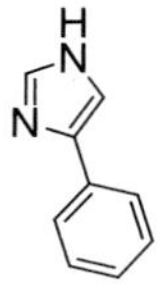

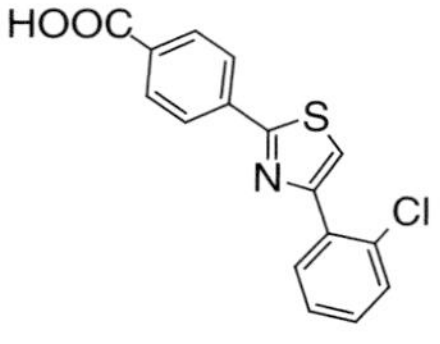

HOOC

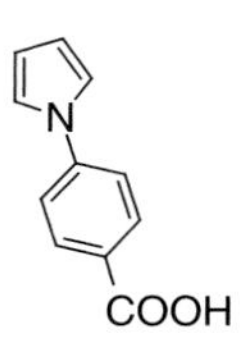

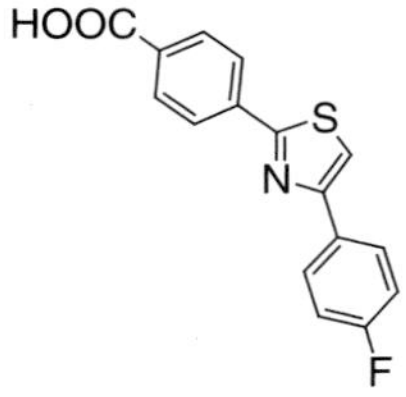

58 200 μM

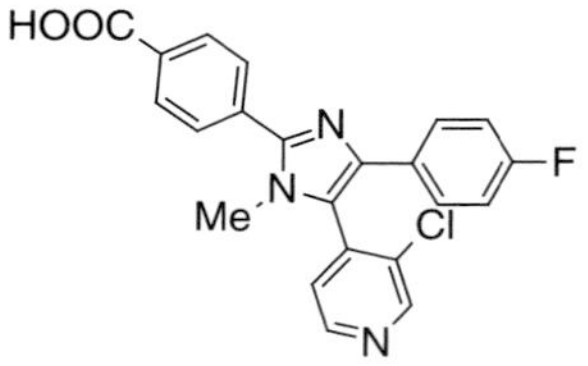

55

HOOC

Me

59 200 nM

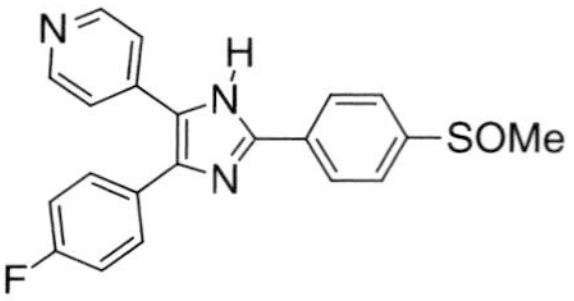

COOH

56

SOMe

F

60

HOOC

Cl

57

simple imidazole core did not appear to bind to p38. However, several tethered bicyclic compounds containing an imidazole (or close derivative) and an aryl moiety (pyridyl, phenyl or benzoic acid) (54–57) exhibited weak binding (200 μM to 2 mM). Since imidazole by itself did not bind, it was used as a core to fuse two of the tethered bicyclics or their derivatives, creating tricyclic molecules with aryl derivatives as side chains and the imidazole as the binding core. Two such compounds (58, 59) showed improved binding. Further modifications resulted in more potent trisubstituted imidazoles like 60 (K_i approximately 200 nM in a p38 enzyme assay).

Unlike in the past when X-ray crystallography was used to study the structures of proteins and ligands, the technique is now being incorporated in all aspects of drug discovery, including lead identification, structural assessment and optimisation. Crystallographic screening methods are being developed enabling experimental 'high-throughput' sampling of up to thousands of compounds per day. One such technique, CrystaLEAD, has been used to sample large ($\geq 10\,000$) compound libraries and to detect ligands by monitoring changes in the electron-density map relative to the unbound form.[124] By careful design of the library, the technique leads to identification of the bound molecule from the primary data (electron-density map) and eliminates the need for the deconvolution process. The electron-density map yields a high-resolution picture of the ligand–protein complex and the resulting information on the ligand–target interactions can be used for structure-directed optimisation. As an example, the method was used for the discovery and optimisation of an orally active series of urokinase inhibitors for the treatment of cancer. The initially identified weaker 5-aminoindole and 2-aminoquinoline leads

61

62

63

64

(**61**, **62**, K_i values 50–200 μM) were optimised. One of the 2-aminoquinoline inhibitor (**63**, K_i 0.37 μM) demonstrated oral bioavailability (38%). The 2-naphthamidine derivative (**64**) did not show oral bioavailability.

In addition to its application in drug discovery, crystallographic screening may also be applied in the structural genomics field, where crystal structures will become available even in the absence of functional characterisation of the protein. In such cases, the ligands discovered could facilitate target validation, assay development and the assignment of function.

1.4.10 Pharmacokinetics

The issues related to pharmacokinetics – drug absorption, distribution, metabolism, excretion – have always been important to the success of the drug discovery process. In many cases, not enough attention was paid to these factors in the early stages of the discovery

process, leading to failures in the late stages of development. To avoid expensive late-stage failures and to cope with the high-throughput synthesis and screening technologies that result in many hits/leads, efforts are being directed to identify absorption, distribution, metabolism and excretion (ADME) problems at an early stage of the discovery process.[125] High-throughput ADME assays are being developed to differentiate between the large number of hits that are now routinely identified from screening compound collections and compound libraries.[126] The techniques making this possible include liquid chromatography/mass spectrometry and liquid chromatography/tandem mass spectrometry due principally to enhanced sensitivity, selectivity and ease of automation relative to traditional analytical methods. Many *in vitro* ADME screens (e.g. metabolic stability assays, plasma protein binding, solubility and log P screens) may be performed in microtitre plate format and it is at the time of biological screening that several daughter plates may also be generated for high-throughput ADME. It has become common practice to determine cytochrome P450 inhibition, blood levels after intravenous and oral administration and identification of metabolites at an early stage. Some of this information may be useful in the lead optimisation process so that chemistry can be directed to overcome the problems. Bioavailability studies may be particularly important for evaluating the significance of the *in vivo* biological results, especially, if the results are negative or less convincing. Although the ADME studies may be valuable in highlighting the shortcomings of the early hits/leads, these may sometimes result in inappropriate rejection of a lead. In many cases, the physicochemical and toxicological properties of the early hits/leads may be very different from that of the optimised drug candidates.

1.4.11 Imaging

Major advances have been made in imaging techniques such as magnetic resonance imaging (MRI) nuclear tomographic imaging, X-ray computed tomography, positron emission tomography and single-photon-emission computed tomography.[127–136] The entire body can now be imaged in exquisite anatomical detail leading to greatly improved capacity to detect pathologic processes. Main advantages of imaging techniques include direct visualisation of disease processes, the ability to quantitate changes over time and the non-invasive nature of the techniques. For example, MRI allows the precise localisation of the site of vascular occlusion, quantification of ensuing perfusion and the oxygenation deficit in stroke patients. Similarly, MRI can provide anatomical detail of brain tumours and can also reveal the biology, cellular structure and vascular dynamics of a tumour.[137] Functional MRI has been used increasingly to map the modulatory effects of psychopharmacological agents on cognitive activation of large-scale networks in the human brain.[138] Such pharmacological MRI studies can be informative about pharmacodynamics, specific neurotransmitter mechanisms that underlie the adaptivity of neurocognitive systems to variation in task difficulty and familiarity, and changes in neurophysiological drug effects associated with genetic variation, neuropsychiatric disorders and normal ageing. These imaging techniques have become essential tools for the diagnosis of central nervous system disorders and are used increasingly for the evaluation of a variety of diseases (e.g. cancer, vascular diseases, musculoskeletal diseases and developmental abnormalities). New tissue and antigen-specific contrast agents and radioligand tracer molecules are being continuously developed. Discovery of improved therapies for neurological disorders and/or drugs acting on the brain is particularly likely to depend on access to imaging modalities to aid early clinical studies.

1.5 Examples of Drug Discovery

This section covers the discovery of many successful drugs in the market, together with some others, which did not make it to the market for various reasons. Although medicinal chemistry along with structural (e.g. X-ray and NMR spectroscopy) and modelling studies have

played a major part in all the cases, the starting leads and the final drugs were not always obtained by totally rational design processes. The structure–activity studies in the most relevant *in vitro* and *in vivo* models have played a significant role in converting the initial lead into the final drug that reached the market. Even today, because of the complexities of the drug discovery process, a totally rational approach leading to a marketed drug is not possible. In each of the examples discussed below, chosen to include different design strategies, an attempt has been made to highlight the origins of the starting leads and the various rational/semi-rational discovery steps used in the optimisation process. Several interesting points emerge from the examples mentioned below. One of the more interesting and recent developments has been the discovery of non-peptide antagonists and agonists acting at the peptide receptors. Although non-peptide antagonists have been obtained in many cases [e.g. ACTH, angiotensin, bradykinin, cholecystokinin (CCK), gastrin and LHRH], agonists have only been obtained in a few cases (e.g. angiotensin and bradykinin). These agonist/antagonist discoveries show how small chemical changes can convert an antagonist to an agonist and thus highlight the importance of the screening process. In a chapter of this size, it is not possible to cover the topics in detail and to include all the SAR and modelling data and original references. Recent references to reviews have been included. These can be used to trace original publications. Details of some of the peptide-based topics have been published previously.[139,140]

1.5.1 Receptor ligands (agonists and antagonists)

1.5.1.1 Early examples
In the past, a number of discoveries have been made in the absence of any knowledge about the receptors or ligands. One of the earliest examples of this kind is morphine (**65**) which was used for many years as an analgesic agent (as a constituent of opium, extracted from the poppy plant, *Papaver somniferum*) without

65 Morphine

66 Diazepam

67 Dopamine, adrenaline and noradrenaline

68 Salbutamol

any knowledge about its mechanism of action. Only in the last 30 years have various opiate receptor subtypes (e.g. μ-, δ-, κ- and σ-receptors) been identified. In addition, endogenous opiate-like peptides, for example, enkephalins (Tyr-Gly-Gly-Phe-Met and Tyr-Gly-Gly-Phe-Leu) and endorphins have been isolated and character-ised. Many other opiate peptides have been isolated from different species, and enormous numbers of receptor-selective analogues (agon-ist and antagonist) have been synthesised in the hope of finding analgesic agents without the side effects associated with morphine. How-ever, no such compound has yet reached the market. Although there are some reports about peptides acting at the benzodiazepine receptor, the story of morphine and enkephalins is the only example so far where a non-peptide (morphine) acting at a peptide receptor was known before the peptide ligand (enkephalin) was isolated. In all the other examples (described below), the endogenous peptide ligand was isolated first from natural sources and the non-peptide lig-ands were obtained later by random screening or semi-rational approaches.

Another example of drug discovery without much knowledge of the receptor or the lig-and is the discovery of benzodiazepines initially obtained by random (*in vivo*) screening of com-pounds for anxiolytic activity. The compounds were later found to act as modulators of GABA at its receptor. Many years later, the discovery and characterisation of benzodiazepine recep-tors from brain tissue led to the development of *in vitro* receptor-binding assays and drugs like Diazepam (**66**). In a similar manner, histam-ine had been recognised as a chemical mes-senger and shown to stimulate acid secretion many years before the discovery of its receptors. Discovery of antihistamine compounds resulted

in the classification of four receptor subtypes (H_1, H_2, H_3 and H_4). Histamine acting via H_1 receptors causes contraction in some smooth muscles (e.g. in the gut, the uterus and the bronchi) and relaxation in other smooth muscles (e.g. in some blood vessels) causing hypotension. Physiologically, histamine plays a role in regu-lating the secretion of gastric acid by stimulating the parietal cells to produce the acid. This effect is mediated by H_2 receptors. The role of H_3 and H_4 receptor is much less defined. Extensive work on antihistamine compounds has resulted in many successful drugs like fexofenadine (Allegra) (**4**), cimetidine and ranitidine (**5**).

In many cases, including the adrenergic recep-tors, the nature of the ligand/transmitter (**67**, dopamine R1 = R = H; epinephrine (adren-aline) R1 = OH, R2 = Me; norepinephrine (noradrenaline) R1 = OH, R2 = H) was known before starting the drug discovery pro-grammes. The availability of many synthetic analogues led to receptor classification (α- and β-adrenergic receptors and other subtypes) and selective ligands. Many of these, like salbutamol (**68**, a β_2-selective agonist) used as a bron-chodilator for the treatment of asthma, proprano-lol (**69**, a non-selective β-antagonist) and atenolol (**70**, a selective β_1-antagonist) both used for the

69 Propranolol

70 Atenolol

71 Tamoxifen

72 Toremifene

73 Droloxifene

treatment of angina and hypertension, have been successful drugs.

1.5.1.2 Selective oestrogen receptor modulators (oestrogen antagonists and aromatase inhibitors)

Another example of drug discovery in the absence of any significant knowledge about the receptors has been the discovery of selective oestrogen receptor modulators.[141,142] Like the examples above, the structures of the ligands were known and utilised, in some cases, for the discovery of drugs on the market. The discovery of selective oestrogen receptor modulators (agonists and antagonists) highlights the impact of developing science in any area of drug discovery as new information emerges and new indications become obvious. In the case of oestrogen, over the years it has become clear that it is important not only in the growth, differentiation and function of tissues of the reproductive system but also importantly in its role in maintaining bone density and protecting against osteoporosis. It also has beneficial effects in the cardiovascular (cardioprotective) and central nervous system (protecting against Alzheimer's disease). In addition, the two isoforms of oestrogen receptor (ERα and ERβ) belonging to a family of nuclear hormone receptors that function as transcription factors on binding to their respective ligands have been identified. Thus, tissue-selective oestrogen receptor modulators ranging from full agonist activity to pure antioestrogenic activity may be useful in the treatment and prevention of osteoporosis, treatment of breast cancer

and may reduce the risk of cardiac disease and Alzheimer's disease.

Tamoxifen (**71**), a non-steroidal, antioestrogen demonstrates antiproliferative effects in the breast and is widely used for the treatment of breast cancer.[143] However, it does not show antioestrogenic properties in all the tissues. For example, tamoxifen acts as an agonist on bone, liver and the endometrium. This mixed antagonist/agonist profile leads to many advantages in cancer patients. As an antagonist, tamoxifen prevents oestrogen-induced proliferation of breast ductal epithelium and breast cancer, and as an agonist in bone and liver, it prevents bone loss in post-menopausal women and reduces cholesterol levels. However, the oestrogenic effects in the endometrium in post-menopausal women can result in an increased risk of endometrial cancer. Many other tamoxifen analogues like toremifene (**72**) and droloxifene (**73**) show similar selectivity profile. The activity of raloxifene (**74**) is also similar to that of tamoxifen, except on the endometrium where it possesses less agonist activity. In comparison with the above, mixed

74 Raloxifene

75 Fulvestrant

76 OS-689 (+)-enantiomer

77 Formestane

78 Exemestane

79 Anastrozole

80 Letrozole

agonist/antagonist compounds, the steroidal, antioestrogen fulvestrant (**75**) demonstrates a pure antioestrogenic profile in all tissues. One of the more recent compounds, OS-689 (+)-enantiomer (**76**), has been reported to have good affinity for the oestrogen receptor. It decreased serum cholesterol in rats and prevented the loss of total bone mineral density of the distal femur but had only marginal effects on the uterus and breasts.[144]

As an alternative to blocking the actions of oestrogen by compounds like tamoxifen, similar biological/clinical effects can be obtained by inhibiting aromatase, the enzyme that catalyses the final and rate-limiting step in oestrogen synthesis (conversion of androgens into oestrogens).[145] Steroidal compounds such as formestane (**77**) and exemestane (**78**) that are structurally related to the natural substrate of aromatase, and non-steroidal compounds such as anastrozole (**79**), letrozole (**80**), fadrozole and vorozole have been developed as aromatase

inhibitors. Many of these are currently in use for the treatment of breast cancer.

1.5.1.3 LHRH agonists and antagonists

In more recent times, efforts have been directed towards finding receptor agonists and antagonists acting at the peptidergic receptors. In most of these cases (including LHRH), naturally occurring ligands were first isolated from various animal species, including humans, and crude receptor preparations were then used to screen for other agonist and antagonist ligands. Extensive structure–activity studies are carried out to identify the regions responsible for binding to the receptor and intrinsic activity. In general, SAR studies involve the synthesis of a large

Table 1.2 LHRH antagonists in various stages of clinical trials

Name	Chemical structure
Abarelix	Ac-D-Nal-D-Phe(*p*-Cl)-D-Pal-Ser-MeTyr-D-Asp-Leu-Lys(iPr)-Pro-D-Ala-NH$_2$
Acyline	Ac-D-Nal-D-Phe(*p*-Cl)-D-Pal-Ser-Aph(Ac)-D-Aph(Ac)-Leu-Lys(iPr)-Pro-D-Ala-NH$_2$
Antarelix	Ac-D-Nal-D-Phe(*p*-Cl)-D-Pal-Ser-Tyr-D-hCit-Leu-Lys(iPr)-Pro-D-Ala-NH$_2$
Cetrorelix	Ac-D-Nal-D-Phe(*p*-Cl)-D-Pal-Ser-Tyr-D-Cit-Leu-Arg-Pro-D-Ala-NH$_2$
Degarelix	Ac-D-Nal-D-Phe(*p*-Cl)-D-Pal-Ser-Aph(Hor)-D-Aph(Cbm)-Leu-Lys(iPr)-Pro-D-Ala-NH$_2$
Ganirelix	Ac-D-Nal-D-Phe(*p*-Cl)-D-Pal-Ser-Tyr-D-hArg(Et$_2$)-Leu-hArg(Et$_2$)-Pro-D-Ala-NH$_2$
Iturelix/Antide	Ac-D-Nal-D-Phe(*p*-Cl)-D-Pal-Ser-Lys(Nic)-D-Lys(Nic)-Leu-Lys(iPr)-Pro-D-Ala-NH$_2$
Ornirelix	Ac-D-Nal-D-Phe(*p*-Cl)-D-Pal-Ser-Lys(Pic)-D-Orn(6-Anic)-Leu-Lys(iPr)-Pro-D-Ala-NH$_2$

number of analogues by carrying out deletion studies (eliminating one or more amino acids from the chain), amino acid replacements by natural and unnatural amino acids, peptide bond replacements and synthesis of conformationally restricting cyclic peptides. These studies are often followed by conformational studies using various spectroscopic and modelling techniques. Based on the results, further modifications are carried out in a semi-rational manner to obtain compounds with desired properties.

LHRH [Pyr-His-Trp-Ser-Tyr-Gly-Leu-Arg-Pro-Gly-NH$_2$] is secreted from the hypothalamus and its action on the pituitary gland leads to the release of luteinising hormone and follicle stimulating hormone. Both of these hormones then act on the ovaries and testes and are responsible for the release of steroidal hormones. Early studies indicated that chronic administration of potent agonist analogues leads to tachyphylaxis or desensitisation of the pituitary receptors, leading finally to a suppression (not stimulation) of oestrogen and testosterone. This finding has led to the use of potent LHRH agonists in the treatment of hormone-dependent tumours. The LHRH antagonists are also expected to be useful for the treatment of these tumours

but progress in the antagonist field has been relatively slow. Potent antagonists have been obtained by multiple amino acid substitutions in various positions of the LHRH molecule and a number of the best antagonists have between five and seven amino acid residues replaced by unnatural amino acids. These combinations of multiple substitutions were arrived at in a stepwise manner starting from the first antagonist, [des-His^2]-LHRH. Most of the peptide GnRH antagonists in various stages of clinical trials are shown in Table 1.2. Based on some of the recent animal data, degarelix (**81**) appears to have the best profile. In castrated male rats injected subcutaneously (sc) with degarelix (FE200486) (2 mg/kg), plasma concentrations of degarelix remained above 5 ng/mL until day 41. At a dose of 2 mg/kg, it maintained testosterone at castrate levels for 49 days. Rats sacrificed on day 45 had considerably reduced prostate, seminal vesicles and testes weights. Degarelix was less potent than other antagonists in histamine-releasing assays.

For the discovery of potent LHRH agonist and antagonist analogues, a large number of analogues were synthesised by incorporating amino acid changes in single and

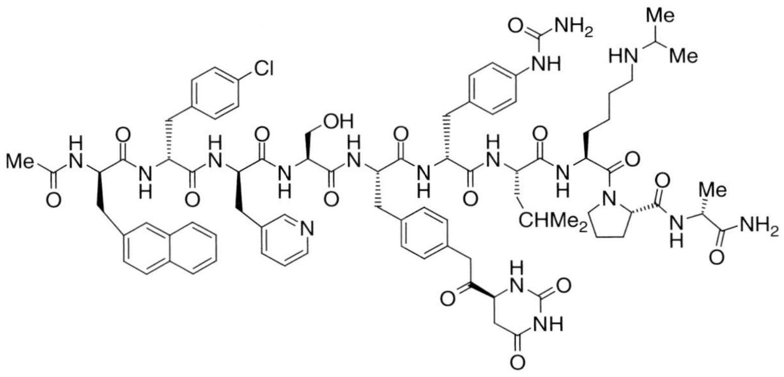

81 Degarelix

multiple positions.[146,147] The most important structure–activity findings that led to these compounds were

1. Replacement of the C-terminal glycinamide residue (-NHCH$_2$CONH$_2$) by a number of alkyl amide (-NH-R) or aza amino acid amide residues [-NH-N(R)-CONH$_2$] (two- to three-fold improvement in potency);
2. Substitution of the glycine residue in position 6 by D amino acid residues [e.g. D-Ala, D-Leu, D-Arg, D-Phe, D-Trp, D-Ser(Bu^t)] (two- to 100-fold improvement in potency);
3. A combination of D amino acids in position 6 and an ethylamide or azaglycine amide in position 10.

The effects of multiple changes were not always additive. A combination of many of these changes has led to the discovery of potent agonists, which are currently on the market, for the treatment of prostate and breast cancer and some non-malignant conditions such as endometriosis and uterine fibroids. The marketed drugs include Zoladex {[D-Ser(Bu^t)^6, Azgly^{10}]-LHRH},[148,149] Leuprolide {[D-Leu^6, des-Gly-NH$_2^{10}$]-LHRH(1–9)NHEt}, Nafarelin {D-Nal(2)^6]-LHRH}, Buserelin {[D-Ser(Bu^t)^6, des-Gly-NH$_2^{10}$]-LHRH(1–9)NHEt} and Triptorelin {[D-Trp^6]-LHRH}.

The potential of LHRH agonists in human medicine has been greatly enhanced by the development of convenient formulations for the

82

delivery of these peptides. The most successful of these have been the biodegradable poly(d,l-lactide-co-glycolide) depot formulations which release the drug over a period of 1–3 months. A biodegradable poly(d,l-lactide-co-glycolide) sustained release formulation of 'Zoladex' can deliver 3.6–10.5 mg of the peptide over a period of 1–3 months. The formulation consists of a homogeneous dispersion of the drug (20% w/w) in a rod of the polymer and is administered by subcutaneous injection.

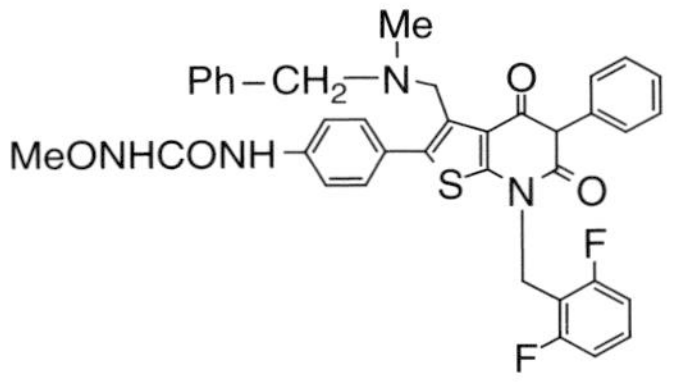

Non-peptide antagonists of GnRH, discovered by random screening approaches, are further behind the peptide antagonists in terms of clinical development. Takeda compound TK-013 (**82**) is most advanced. Other major companies have recently published data on their non-peptide antagonists (**83**). However, due to the availability of longer acting (1–4 months) depot formulations of GnRH agonists already in the market and the possibility of depot formulations of peptide antagonists and longer acting compounds like degarelix, the need for orally active compounds is debatable.

83

1.5.1.4 Somatostatin agonists and antagonists

The cyclic peptide somatostatin [Ala-Gly-Cys-Lys-Asn-Phe-Phe-Trp-Lys-Thr-Phe-Thr-Ser-Cys, disulphide bridge between Cys^3 and Cys^{14}] and the 28 amino acid precursor containing 14 additional amino acid residues [Ser-Ala-Asn-Ser-Asn-Pro-Ala-Met-Ala-Pro-Arg-Glu-Arg-Lys] at the N-terminus were isolated from the extracts of bovine and porcine hypothalamus, respectively. Both peptides are associated with a large number of biological activities, including the inhibition of growth hormone, insulin, glucagon and gastric acid secretion. Thus, somatostatin may play an important role in many physiological and pharmacological systems.[150] Five human receptor subtypes ($hSSTR_1$–$hSSTR_5$) of somatostatin have been characterised. There is now emerging evidence for additional somatostatin receptor subtypes. The realisation that somatostatin acts through multiple receptors suggested the possibility that somatostatin may also achieve functional selectivity by acting through a specific receptor subtype to control a specific action. Large number of analogues have, therefore, been synthesised in the hope of finding drugs for various diseases. These analogues are being used to define specific functions of various receptor subtypes. However, the process of linking specific functions to receptor subtypes has proved to be much more difficult.[151,152] The task has been made even more difficult by the finding that somatostatin and its receptor subtypes are widely distributed in the body.

Examples of compounds which have reached the market include octreotide [sandostatin, D-Phe-cyclo(Cys-Phe-D-Trp-Lys-Thr-Cys)-Thr-ol],

lanreotide [D-Nal-cyclo(Cys-Tyr-D-Trp-Lys-Val-Cys)-Thr-NH$_2$] and vapreotide (RC-160) [D-Phe-cyclo(Cys-Tyr-D-Trp-Lys-Val-Cys)-Trp-NH$_2$]. Daily and slow release depot formulation of octreotide have been used for the treatment of growth-hormone secreting pituitary tumours, thyrotropin secreting pituitary adenomas, pancreatic islet cell tumours and carcinoid tumours that express somatostatin receptors.[153] A long-acting formulation of octreotide administered to acromegalic patients for 18 months (once every 4 weeks) suppressed growth hormone and insulin-like growth factor levels in all the patients, and signs and symptoms of acromegaly improved during treatment. Reduction of the pituitary tumour was seen in all previously untreated patients.

Progress towards small cyclic peptides that are equipotent or more potent than somatostatin was made in several steps. Early SAR established that the Ala^1-Gly^2 residues and the disulphide bridge were not essential for biological activity. Amino acid substitution studies indicated that replacements of Lys^4 by Arg, Phe, Phe(F$_5$) or Phe(p-NH$_2$) residues; Asn^5 by Ala or D-Tyr; Phe^7 by Tyr; Trp^8 by D-Trp, D-Trp(5-F), D-Trp(6-F), D-Trp(5-Br); Phe^{11} by Phe(p-I) or NaI(2) and Cys^{14} by D-Cys gave compounds that were either equipotent or more potent than the parent peptide. Amino acid substitutions in other positions gave less potent analogues. For example, most of the analogues obtained by substituting the Phe^6 and Phe^7 residues, except by other aromatic amino acids like Phe(p-Cl), Phe(p-I) and Tyr, were less potent (<10%) than somatostatin. Deletion of the C-terminal carboxyl group or its replacement by an ethylamide group also resulted in compounds equipotent to somatostatin. An equally important finding, useful in designing smaller peptides, emerged by deleting various amino acid residues. Compounds lacking Lys^4 and Asn^5 were found to retain significant biological activity whereas compounds lacking Phe^6, Trp^8, Lys^9, Thr^{10}, Phe^{11}, Thr^{12} were relatively poor agonists. The deletion and substitution studies led to much smaller peptides like cyclo(Aha-Phe-Phe-D-Trp-Lys-Thr-Phe), cyclo(Pro-Phe-D-Trp-Lys-Thr-Phe) and cyclo(Pro-Phe-D-Trp-Lys-Val-Phe). The most

(CH₂)₂——NHCO——(CH₂)₃

HN Tyr-D-Trp-Lys-Val—N Thr-NH₂

84

H₂C——S——CH₂

D-Phe Phe-D-Trp-Lys-Thr—N Thr-ol

85

potent analogue cyclo(MeAla-Tyr-D-Trp-Lys-Val-Phe) was 20–50-fold more potent than somatostatin in inhibiting growth hormone, 70 times more potent in inhibiting insulin and >80 times more potent in inhibiting glucagon. Other more potent cyclic peptides containing a disulphide bridge, D-Phe-Cys-Phe-D-Trp-Lys-Thr-Cys-Thr(ol), D-Phe-Cys-Tyr-D-Trp-Lys-Val-Cys-Thr-NH₂, D-Phe-Cys-Tyr-D-Trp-Lys-Val-Cys-Trp-NH₂ and D-Phe-Cys-Tyr-D-Trp-Lys-Val-Cys-Thr-NH₂, were 80–200 times more potent than somatostatin. Since the discovery and availability of cloned multiple receptors, additional SAR studies have led to more receptor-selective agonist and antagonist analogues. For example, the cyclic peptide [Cys-Lys-Phe-Phe-D-Trp-Phe(*p*-CH₂NH-CH(CH₃)₂-Thr-Phe-Thr-Ser-Cys, disulphide bridge] was a potent agonist at human SSTR₁ receptors and the N(α-Me)benzylglycine containing analogue cyclo[(R)-βMeNphe-Phe-D-Trp-Lys-Thr-Phe] is a hSSTR2 selective agonist. The hSSTR2 agonist selectively inhibited the release of growth hormone in rats (equipotent to sandostatin) but had no effect on the inhibition of insulin at the same dose. Cyclo-Phe(N-aminoethyl)-Tyr-D-Trp-Lys-Val-Phe(N-carboxypropyl)-Thr-NH₂ (PTR 3046; **84**), a backbone-cyclic somatostatin analogue, and the lanthionine octapeptide (**85**) displayed high selectivity for the SSTR5 receptor.

In comparison with the agonist analogues, very few antagonists of somatostatin have been obtained by amino acid substitution. Two

octapeptide derivatives, 4-NO₂-Phe-c(D-Cys-Tyr-D-Trp-Lys-Thr-Cys)-Tyr-NH₂ and Ac-4-NO₂-Phe-c(D-Cys-Tyr-D-Trp-Lys-Thr-Cys)-D-Tyr-NH₂ (inactive at the SST₁ and SST₄ receptor subtypes; high affinity at the SSTR₂ and SSTR₅ receptor subtypes), inhibited somatostatin-mediated inhibition of cAMP accumulation in a dose-dependent manner. The more potent antagonist, [Ac-4-NO₂-Phe-c(D-Cys-Tyr-D-Trp-Lys-Thr-Cys)-D-Tyr-NH₂], displays a binding affinity to SSTR₂ comparable with that observed for the native hormone. H-Nal-c[D-Cys-Pal-D-Trp-Lys-Val-Cys]-Nal-NH₂ was also a more selective hSST₂ receptor antagonist.

1.5.1.5 Angiotensin agonists and antagonists (peptides and non-peptides)

The renin–angiotensin system has been one of the most active fields of research for antihypertensive drugs.[154,155] Angiotensin II and other members of the angiotensin family are produced by the processing of a protein called α₂-globulin or angiotensinogen which is synthesised in the liver and found in the blood. The protein is first cleaved by the enzyme renin to generate a decapeptide angiotensin I [Asp-Arg-Val-Tyr-Ile-His-Pro-Phe-His-Leu], which is further cleaved by the ACE to produce octapeptide angiotensin II [Asp¹-Arg-Val-Tyr-Ile-His-Pro-Phe⁸], which is a potent vasoconstrictor.

Angiotensin II acts at two receptor subtypes (AT₁ and AT₂). In the case of the agonist analogues, one of the most significant change has been the replacement of the N-terminal Asp by Sar (N-methylglycine) to give [Sar¹]-angiotensin II, which in a number of *in vitro* tissue preparations was 1.5–2.5 times more potent than the natural ligand. AT₂ receptor selective analogues were obtained by modifications at the N- and C-terminal ends of the peptide. The N-terminally modified compounds [Me₂Gly¹]-, [Me₃Gly¹]- and [Me₃Ser¹]-angiotensin II were >1000-fold more potent at the AT₂ receptor subtypes. The analogue modified at positions 1 and 8, [Sar¹,Phe⁸]-angiotensin II was 345-fold more potent than angiotensin II at the AT₂ receptor. Modifications of the

C-terminal dipeptide (Pro[7]-Phe[8]) of [Sar[1],Val[5]]-angiotensin II with constrained aromatic (Tic) and hydrophobic (Oic) amino acids led to analogues with negligible affinity for the AT_1 receptor, but nanomolar affinity for the AT_2 receptor. The most potent and AT_2-selective analogue of the series was Sar-Arg-Val-Tyr-Val-His-Phe-Oic (IC_{50}s 240 and 0.51 nM at the AT_1 and AT_2 receptors, respectively). A conformationally restricted analogue of angiotensin II, [hCys[3], hCys[5]]-angiotensin II, was equipotent to angiotensin II in displacing [^{125}I]-angiotensin II from rat uterus membranes and in inducing contractions in the rabbit aortic rings (pD_2 8.48). Conformational analysis studies indicated that the cyclic peptides like analogues (e.g. c[hCys[3,5]]-angiotensin II) may assume an inverse γ-turn conformation; thus, amino acid residues 3–5 in angiotensin II were substituted with different turn mimetic residues. Most of the analogues were either inactive or much less potent than angiotensin II.

Antagonists of angiotensin II were initially obtained by eliminating the side chain from the C-terminal phenylalanine residue. Antagonist like [Gly[8]]-angiotensin II which competitively blocks the myotropic action of both angiotensin I and angiotensin II in *in vitro* test systems but did not antagonise the pressor response to angiotensin II in anaesthetised cats were further modified in position 8 to give more potent antagonists, for example, [Ile[8]]-angiotensin II. A combination of positions 5 and 8 changes along with the N-terminal changes (Sar[1]) discovered in the case of agonist series of compounds gave more potent antagonists like [Sar[1],Ala[8]]-angiotensin II, [Sar[1],Ile[8]]-angiotensin II (pA_2 9.48) and [Sar[1], Pen(SMe)[5],Ile[8]]-angiotensin II. [Sar[1],Thr(Me)[5],Ile[8]]-, [Sar[1],β-MePhe[5],Ile[8]]- and [Sar[1],His[5],Ile[8]]-angiotensin II were more potent than [Sar[1],Ile[8]]-angiotensin II in the *in vivo* rat blood pressure test. In the cyclic series of antagonists, except [Sar[1],hCys[3],hCys[5],Ile[8]]-angiotensin II, many other cyclic compounds, for example, [Cys[1,5],Ile[8]]-, [D-Cys[1],Cys[5],Ile[8]]-, [Sar[1],Cys[5,8]]-, [Sar[1],Cys[5],D-Cys[8]]- and [Sar[1], hCys[5],D-Cys[8]]-angiotensin II, were much less potent.

86 Losartan

87

Non-peptide antagonists of angiotensin II were obtained by random screening approaches. Despite all the progress achieved in discovering potent agonist and antagonist analogues and the ligand receptor information derived from the above compounds, it was not possible to design non-peptidic molecules by this rational design procedure. The discovery from a random screening lead of DuP753 (Losartan, **86**), which is selective for AT_1, opened the way to non-peptide antagonists. The SAR studies indicated that a considerable variation was allowed in the chemical structures of the antagonists. The synthetic medicinal chemistry approaches identified various replacements for the imidazole and the biphenyl tetrazole groups and highlighted chemical changes which led to AT_1- or AT_2-selective or mixed (AT_1 and AT_2) receptor antagonists. Compound **87** (L-162,389) is an example of a mixed antagonist (AT_1 and AT_2 binding affinities 2–4 nM). In a macrocyclic series of analogues, **88** bound primarily to the AT_1 receptor (AT_1 and AT_2 receptor IC_{50} values 23 and 4000 nM, respectively) whereas a very similar analogue **89** bound to both the receptors with similar affinity (IC_{50}s 20–30 nM).

Another interesting aspect of the non-peptide agonist/antagonist structure–activity studies has been the identification of both agonists and antagonists in the same series of compounds by minor structural modifications. For example,

88

89

90 Agonist

91 Agonist

92 Valsartan

93 Candesartan

94 Ibresartan

95 Eprosartan

compound **90** was an agonist and a similar analogue that differs chemically by only a single methyl group (**87**) was an antagonist. Another close analogue (**91**) also displayed agonist activity. At present, it is not possible to predict changes that lead to agonist/antagonist analogues by any rational design approaches. Only by screening the compounds in appropriate tests can selective compounds with the desired biological profile be identified. A large amount of chemical effort in the angiotensin antagonist field has led to the discovery of many successful drugs like losartan (**86**), valsartan (**92**), candesartan (**93**) ibresartan (**94**), eprosartan (**95**), telmisartan and olmesartan for the treatment of high blood pressure and other cardiovascular complications.

1.5.1.6 Bombesin/neuromedin agonists and antagonists

Semi-rational approaches Four subtypes of the bombesin receptor have been identified (gastrin-releasing peptide [GRP] receptor, neuromedin B receptor, the orphan receptor bombesin receptor subtype 3 and bombesin receptor subtype 4). The roles of individual receptor

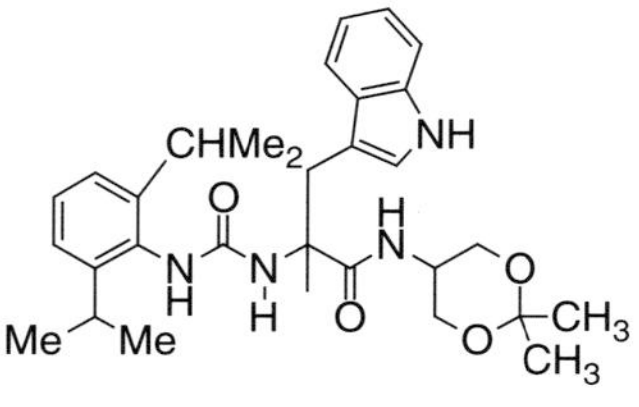

96

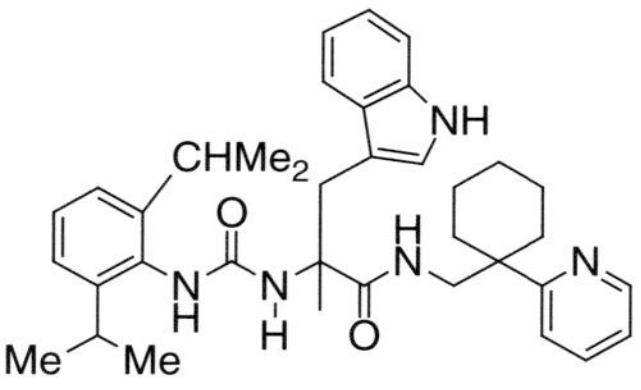

97

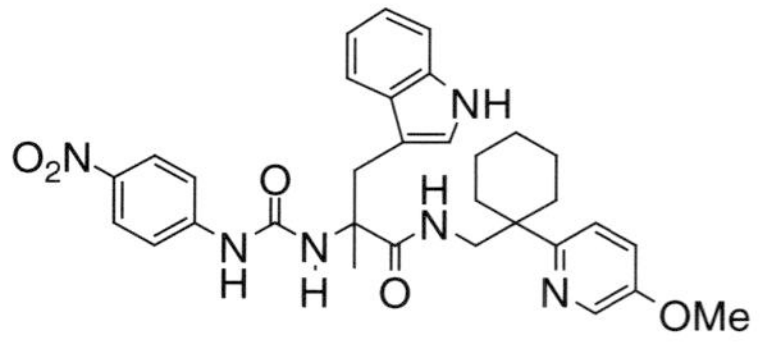

98

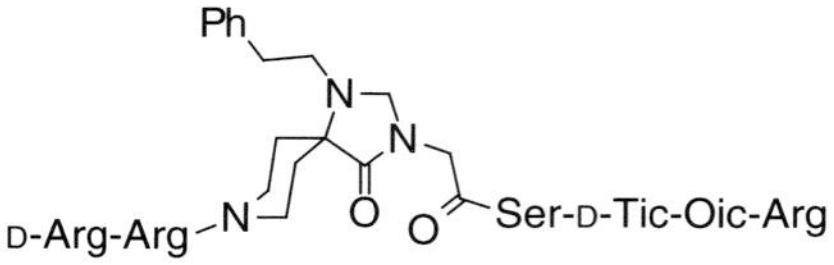

99

subtypes are under investigation and selective ligands for these receptor subtypes are being synthesised. Systematic SAR studies have provided many receptor antagonists.[156] A semi-rational approach was used for the discovery of non-peptide antagonists of neuromedin B. The role of each amino acid side chain was defined by alanine scanning in bombesin(7–14)-octapeptide, Ac-Gln-Trp-Ala-Val-Gly-His-Leu-Met-NH$_2$ (minimum active fragment), and indicated that Trp^8, Val^{10} and Leu^{13} were most important for the binding affinity to the receptors. A search, within the company compound collection, was then initiated for various templates containing Trp, Val/Leu types of side chains. This led to a moderately active lead (96). Changes at the C-terminal end led to more potent (S) α-methyl-Trp derivative (97). Additional chemical modifications on 97 resulted in a series of 'balanced' neuromedin-B preferring (BB$_1$)/GRP preferring (BB$_2$) receptor ligands, as exemplified by PD 176252 (98). Compound 98 displaying a BB$_2$ receptor affinity of 1 nM while retaining sub-nanomolar (0.17 nM) BB$_1$ receptor affinity and is a competitive antagonist at both the receptor subtypes.

1.5.1.7 Bradykinin agonists and antagonists

Bradykinin (Arg-Pro-Pro-Gly-Phe-Ser-Pro-Phe-Arg) is a vasoactive peptide, which mediates vasodilation, increases vascular permeability, smooth-muscle contraction, recruitment of inflammatory cells, induction of pain and hyperalgesia. The effects of bradykinin are mediated by the B$_2$ receptor. Because of its role in mediating pain and inflammation, a number of potent and selective non-peptide antagonists for the B$_2$ receptor have been identified in recent years.[157] Peptide SAR studies resulted in potent bradykinin B$_2$ receptor antagonists like HOE 140 [D-Arg-Arg-Pro-Hyp-Gly-Thi-Ser-D-Tic-Oic-Arg]. Replacement of some of the amino acids by substituted 1,3,8-triazaspiro[4,5]decan-4-one-3-acetic acids in the B$_2$ receptor antagonist D-Arg-Arg-Pro-Pro-Gly-Phe-Ser-D-Tic-Oic-Arg gave potent B$_2$ receptor antagonists like 99 (NPC18521, K_i 0.15 nM), which contains a phenethyl group at position 1 of the spirocyclic mimetic. Another example of a pseudopeptide analogue is compound NPC18884 (100), which contains three arginine residues. Given intraperitoneally or orally, compound 100 inhibited bradykinin-induced leucocytes influx and exudation. The effects lasted for up to 4 h and were selective for the bradykinin B$_2$ receptors. At similar doses, compound 100 had no significant effect against the inflammatory responses induced by des-Arg^9-bradykinin, histamine or substance P.

Like angiotensin II, non-peptide B$_2$ receptor antagonists and agonists of bradykinin were obtained by random screening approaches. Chemical modifications on random screening leads like 101 led to non-peptide antagonists

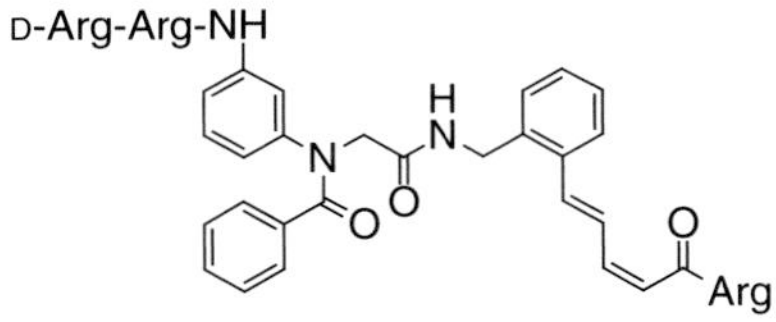

100

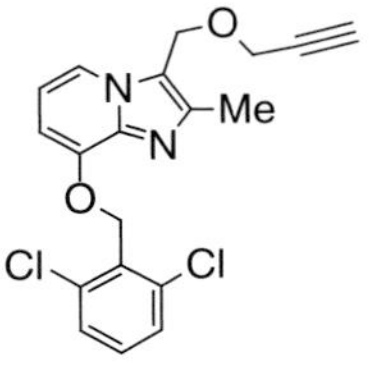

101

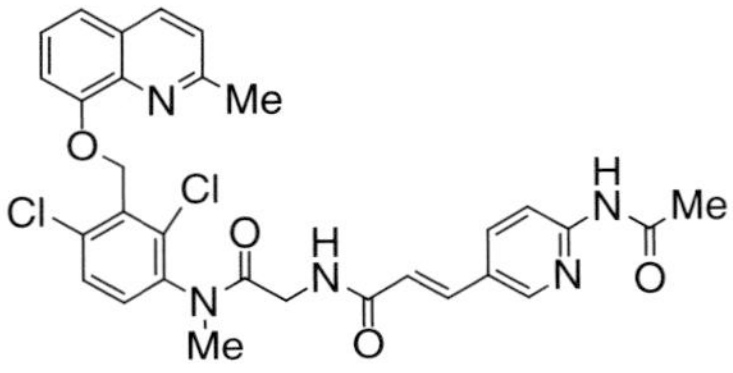

102 Antagonist

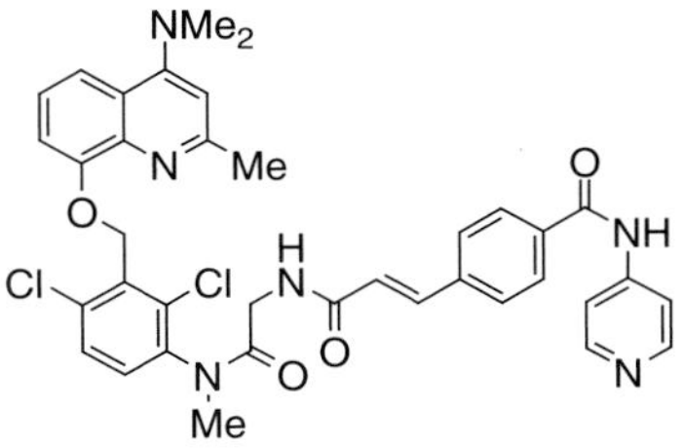

103

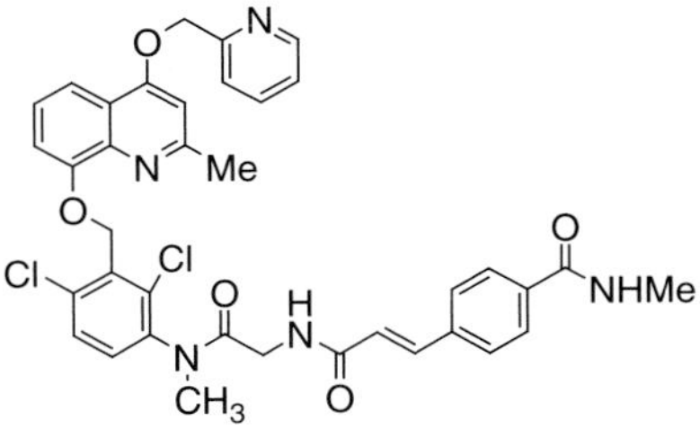

104 Agonist

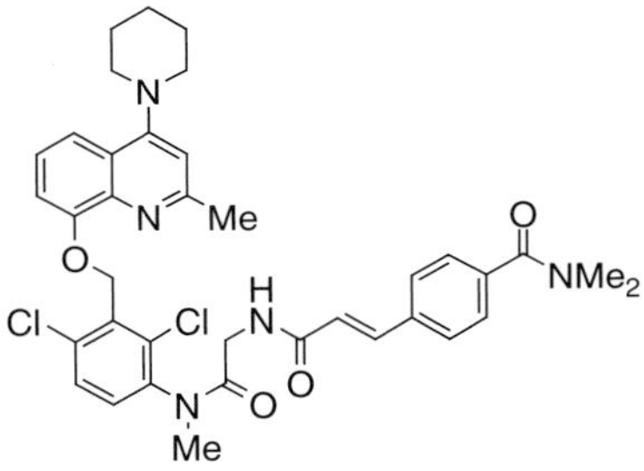

105 Partial agonist

like **102–105** that were active in a number of *in vitro* and *in vivo* (e.g. bradykinin-induced bronchoconstriction and carrageenin-induced paw oedema) test systems.[158] The non-peptide agonist **104** bound with high affinity to the B_2 receptor (IC_{50} 5.3 nM) had no binding affinity for the B_1 receptor, and at concentrations between 1 nM and 1 μM, it stimulated phosphatidylinositol hydrolysis in Chinese hamster ovary cells permanently expressing the human bradykinin B_2 receptor. The response was antagonised by the B_2 receptor selective antagonist Hoe 140. Intravenous administration of bradykinin or the agonist (**104**) (both at 10 μg/kg) caused a fall in blood pressure. However, the duration of the hypotensive response to **104** was significantly longer than the response to bradykinin. Another non-peptide compound **105** was a partial agonist.

1.5.1.8 CCK agonists and antagonists

CCK, a 33 amino acid regulatory peptide hormone, regulates motility, pancreatic enzyme secretion, gastric emptying, and gastric acid secretion in the GI tract and is involved in anxiogenesis, satiety, nociception and memory and learning processes in the nervous system.[159] Antagonists of CCK are being sought as therapeutic agents for various GI disorders, anxiety and obesity. A number of peptide and non-peptide ligands acting at CCK_A and/or CCK_B receptors have been described. Peptidomimetic agonist and antagonist analogues of CCK were obtained from the C-terminal tetrapeptide of CCK/gastrin (Boc-Trp-Met-Asp-Phe-NH_2) and analogues like Boc-Trp-MeNle-Asp-Phe-NH_2 and by synthesising conformationally constrained analogues by replacing the Trp-Met/Trp-MeNle dipeptides. The diketopiperazine derivative **106** and the constrained cyclic pseudopeptide CCK_B agonist **107** [(*S*) at the α-carbon of the aminononane moiety

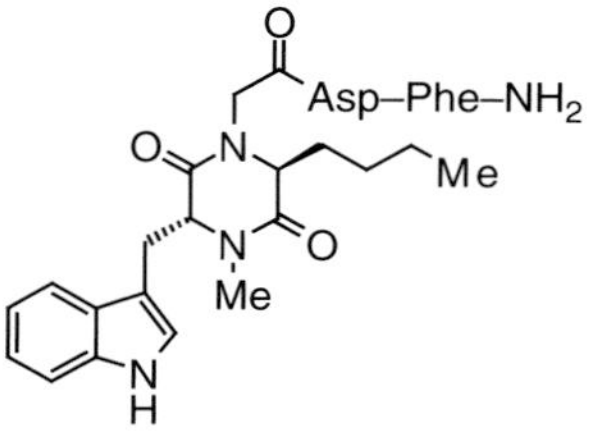

106

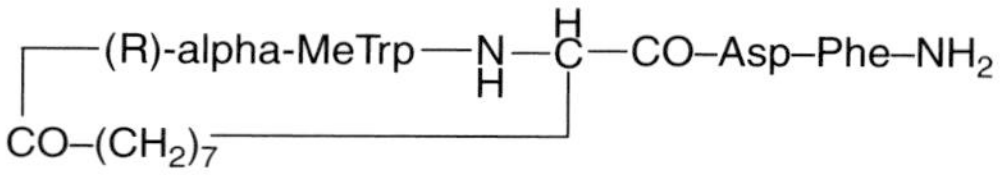

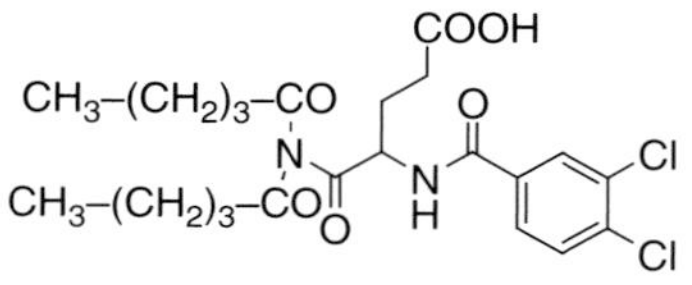

108 Lorglumide

107

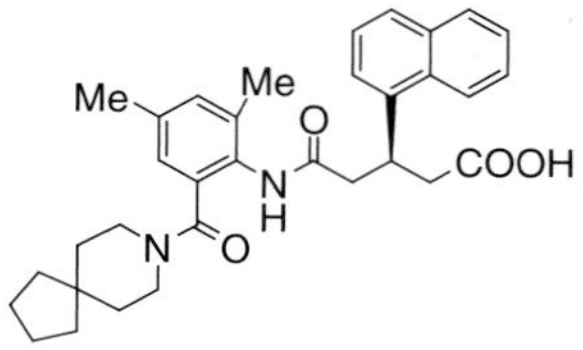

109 Itriglumide

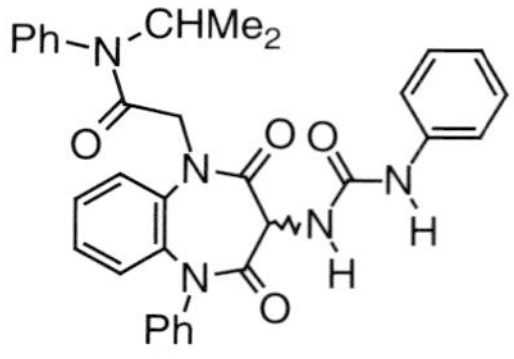

110

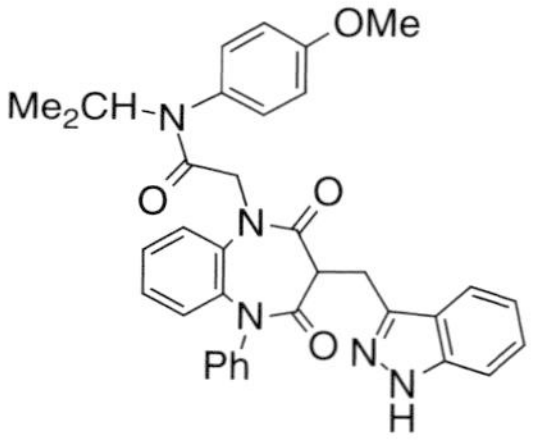

111

(CCK$_A$/CCK$_B$ = 147)] exhibited full CCK$_B$ receptor agonist properties and increased gastric acid secretion in anaesthetised rats.

Some of the early non-peptide antagonists of CCK$_A$ and CCK$_B$ receptors were glutamic acid derivatives. Benzoyl-glutamic acid dipropylamide (proglumide), a weak gastrin antagonist, was marketed for the treatment of ulcers. Further work on this series of compounds led to CCK$_A$ antagonists like lorglumide (**108**) and CCK$_B$ receptor antagonists like itriglumide (**109**). Non-peptide CCK agonists and antagonists based on a benzodiazepine skeleton were obtained by random screening and lead optimisation approaches. 1,5-Benzodiazepine derivatives like **110** were shown to be agonists and antagonists of CCK$_A$ and CCK$_B$. The substitution pattern at the anilinoacetamide nitrogen played an important role for the activity. While compounds with a hydrogen or methyl substituent were weak antagonists of CCK-8, the ethyl, propyl (**110**), n-butyl and cyanoethyl derivatives were agonists. Compound **110** displayed 86% CCK-8 functional activity in the guinea pig gallbladder assay at 30 μM (CCK-8 = 100% at 1 μM) and showed similar affinity for CCK$_A$ and CCK$_B$ receptors. When given orally to rats, the CCK$_A$ agonist (**111**) (GW5823) reduced food intake to 40% of that in vehicle-control treated animals. When administered orally, the CCK$_B$/gastrin antagonist YF476 (**112**) inhibited gastric acid secretion in a pentagastrin-induced

acid secretion model and displayed a long duration of action (>6 h at a dose of 100 nmol/kg). In addition to the benzodiazepine derivatives, a number of other chemically distinct CCK antagonists have been prepared starting from the random screening leads. The nine-membered ring analogue (**113**) was a potent CCK$_B$/gastrin antagonist (rat stomach pK_B 9.08, mouse cortex pIC$_{50}$ 8.3). In comparison, analogues containing six-, seven- and eight-membered rings were poor CCK$_B$/gastrin receptor antagonists. Although, many of the compounds have reached various stages of clinical trials, none of the compounds has yet reached the market.

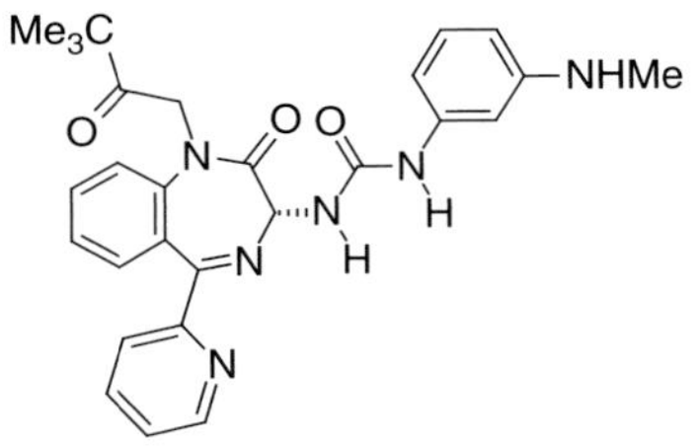

112

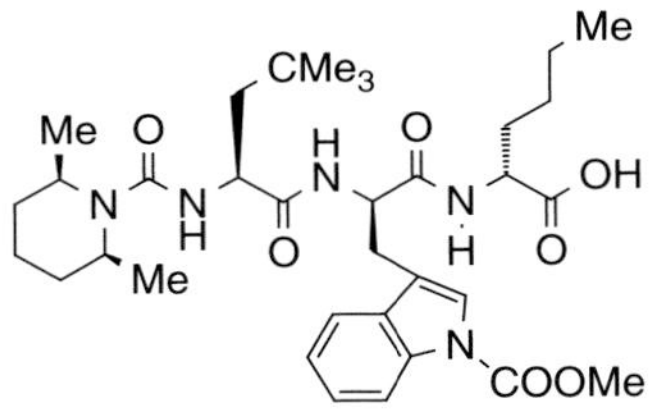

115

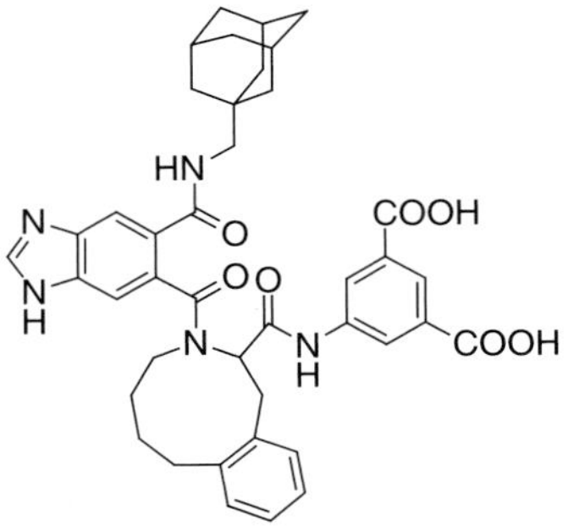

113

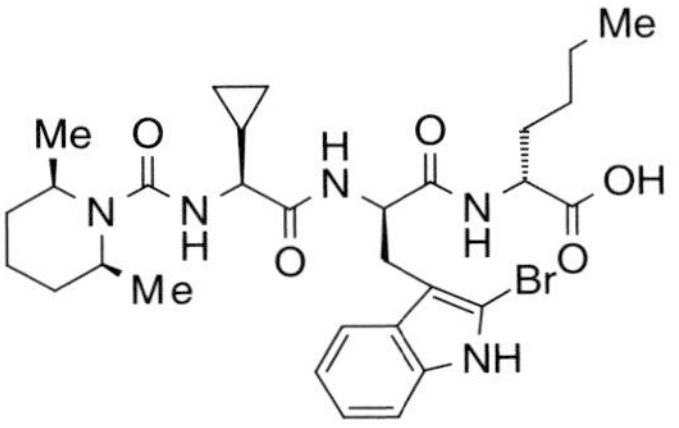

116

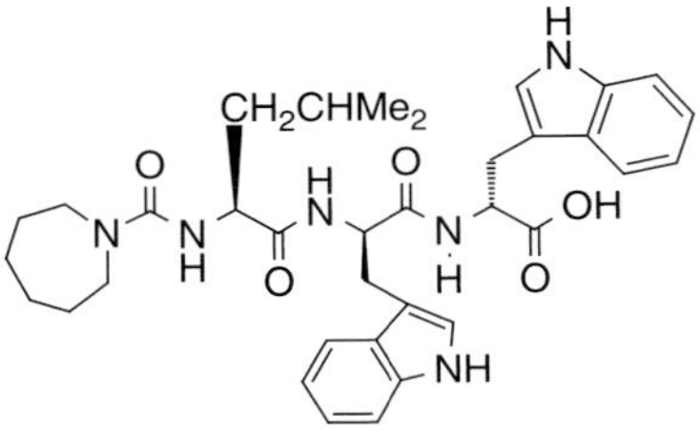

114

1.5.1.9 Endothelin antagonists

Endothelin, a 21 amino acid peptide, is one of the most potent vasoconstrictor peptides that was isolated initially from the conditioned medium of cultured endothelial cells.[160] The peptide has been associated with many physiological and pathological functions, including chronic heart failure, ischaemic heart diseases, hypertension, atherosclerosis, pulmonary hypertension, chronic renal failure and cerebrovascular spasm after subarachnoid haemorrhage.[161,162] Antagonists of endothelin-1 are, therefore, being sought for various cardiovascular disorders.[163] Two receptor subtypes (ET_A and ET_B) have been identified for this family of peptides. The ET_A receptor binds ET-1 and ET-2 with greater affinity than it does ET-3, whereas the ET_B receptor binds all three isoforms with equal affinity. Leads for antagonist design have originated from natural sources, from rational design approaches and by random screening. ET_A and ET_B receptor selective antagonists were obtained from cyclic pentapeptides of microbial origin like the ET_A-selective peptide BQ123 [c(D-Val-Leu-D-Trp-D-Asp-Pro)]. Linear tripeptide derivatives were subsequently developed as ET_A [BQ485 (114)] or ET_B [BQ788 (115)] receptor selective or non-selective (116, BQ928) antagonists. In the BQ123 series, amino acid replacements converted the ET_A selective antagonist BQ123 to ET_B selective and non-selective antagonists. For example, c(D-t-Leu-Leu-2-chloro-D-Trp-D-Asp-Pro) and c(D-Pen(Me)-Leu-2-bromo-D-Trp-D-Asp-Pro) were nearly equipotent at both the receptors, and c(D-Pen(Me)-Leu-2-cyano-D-Trp-D-Asp-Pro) was much more potent at the ET_B receptor. In the cis-(2,6-dimethylpiperidino) carbonyl-Leu-D-Trp-D-Nle series of analogues, the 2-bromo-D-Trp, 2-chloro-D-Trp and 2-methyl-D-Trp analogues were potent antagonists at both receptors while the 2-cyano-D-Trp and 2-ethyl-D-Trp analogues were more potent at the ET_B receptor.

Antagonists similar to compounds 114–116 were also discovered by using a rational

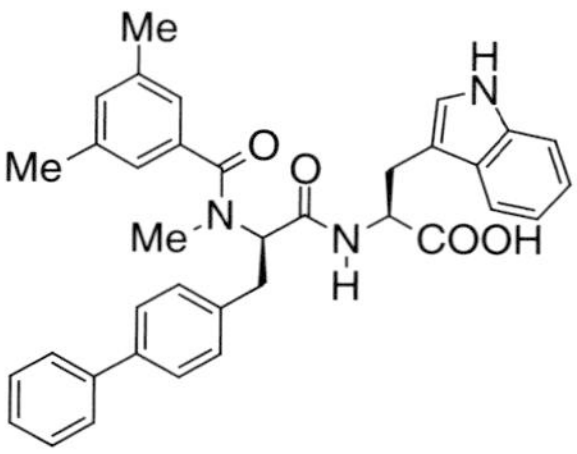

117

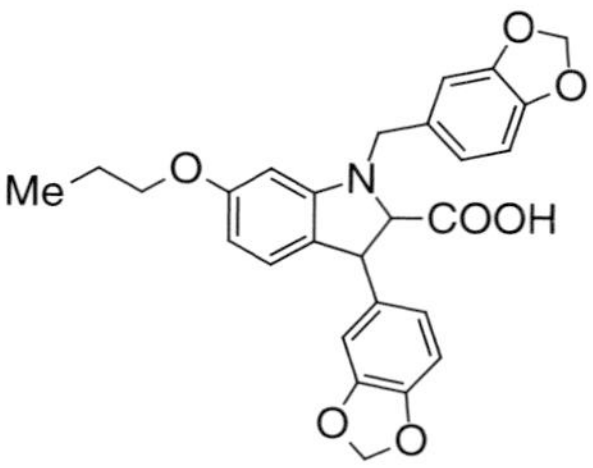

119

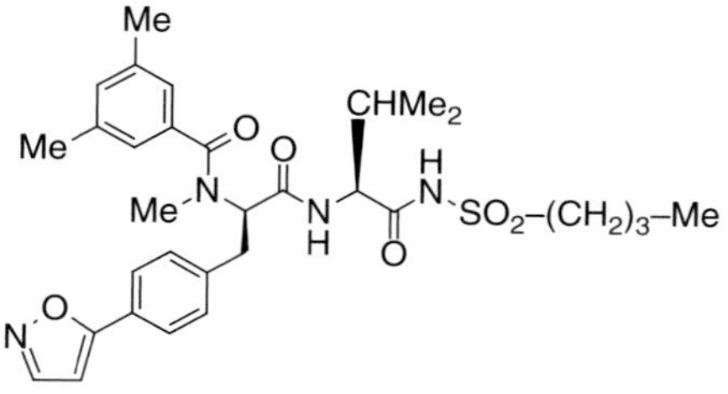

118

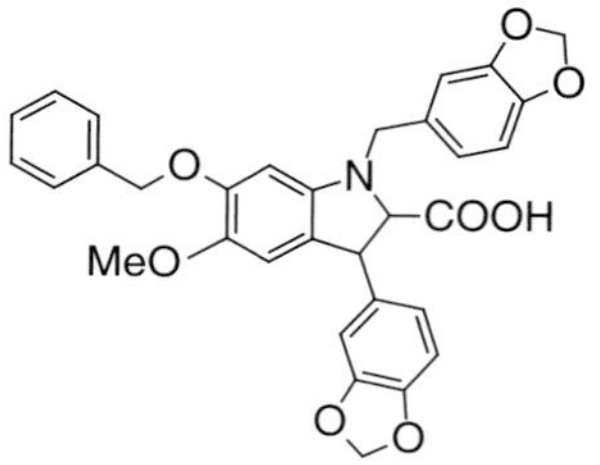

120

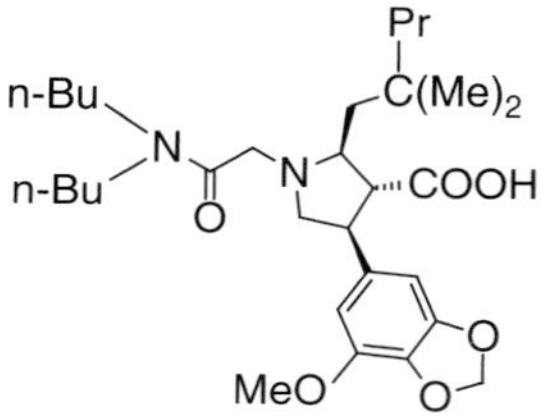

121

approach starting from the endothelin C-terminal dodecapeptide derivative, succinyl-Glu-Ala-Val-Tyr-Phe-Ala-His-Leu-Asp-Ile-Ile-Trp. Replacing each of the amino acid in turn with glycine indicated that Phe[14], Ile[19,20] and Trp[21] were the most important residues. Based on this evidence, a series of compounds having an aromatic moiety attached through a spacer to the amino group of the Trp residue were synthesised. Further work, around the initial weak antagonist lead, N-*trans*-2-phenylcyclopropanoyl-Trp, resulted in a 400-fold selective ET_B antagonist (**117**). Replacement of the biphenylalanine residue by 2-naphthylalanine, Met, Leu, Ile, Cha, Thr or ethylglycine gave antagonists that were two to four-fold more potent at the ET_B receptor. The D-Phe-Val derivative (**118**) displayed similar affinity for ET_A and ET_B receptors (K_i 1–2 nM).

Non-peptide antagonists of endothelin were discovered by random screening approaches. A comparison of compounds **119** and **120** demonstrates that it is possible to obtain selective and non-selective compounds in the same series by chemical modifications. Carboxyindoline derivative **119** was about 100-fold more selective ET_A receptor antagonist and compound **120** was a non-selective antagonist. Another series of

ET_A-selective antagonists included a more selective (>25 000-fold) pyrrolidine carboxylic acid derivatives A-216546 (**121**). A-216546 was orally available in rat, dog and monkey and blocked endothelin-1-induced presser response in conscious rats. Replacement of the dialkylacetamide side chain in **121** resulted in a complete reversal of receptor selectivity, preferring ET_B over ET_A. Compound **122** (A-308165) demonstrated over 27 000-fold selectivity favouring the ET_B receptor. So far one of the endothelin ET_A-receptor antagonists bosentan (**123**) has reached the market for the treatment of pulmonary hypertension. Several other compounds have either failed in the clinic or are in various stages of development (e.g. sitaxsentan (**124**) and **125**).[164]

122

123 Bosentan

124 Sitaxsentan

125

1.6 Enzymes and Enzyme Inhibitors

Although most of the enzyme-based drugs are inhibitors of enzymes, a number of enzyme preparations have also been developed as drugs for the treatment of a number of diseases.[165] The development of enzymes as therapeutics has been made easier due to the advances in biotechnology. Most successful example of enzyme therapy includes various preparations of plasminogen activators (thrombolytic or fibrinolytic agents) such as a bacterial protein streptokinase and two plasminogen activators that occur naturally in blood, the tissue-type (tPA) and the urokinase-type (uPA) plasminogen activators. These plasminogen activators do not have a direct fibrinolytic activity and their therapeutic action is via limited proteolytic cleavage of the inactive plasminogen to fibrinolytic plasmin. In contrast, streptokinase possesses no enzymatic activity of its own but acquires its plasminogen activating property by complexing with circulatory plasminogen or plasmin. The resulting high-affinity 1:1 stoichiometric complex (i.e. the streptokinase–plasminogen activator complex) is a high-specificity protease that proteolytically activates other plasminogen molecules to plasmin. Examples of marketed fibrinolytic enzyme drugs that are used as antithrombolytic agents for the treatment of stroke and myocardial infarction[166–170] include anisoylated human plasminogen-streptokinase (eminase), single-chain tissue plasminogen activators (recombinant human tissue plasminogen activator alteplase and reteplase) and double-chain recombinant tPA (duteplase).

Other successful examples of enzyme therapeutics include recombinant form of human α-galactosidase A (Agalsidase-β and Agalsidase-α) for the treatment of Fabrey disease, a recombinant form of urate oxidase (rasburicase, a highly potent uricolytic agent that catalyses the oxidation of uric acid to allantoin, a water-soluble product that is readily excreted via the kidney) for the treatment and prophylaxis of acute hyperuricaemia (to prevent acute renal failure), modified version of glucocerebrosidase (Alglucerase and Imiglucerase) for the treatment of type I Gaucher's disease, recombinant human deoxyribonuclease I (Dornase-α) for the treatment of cystic fibrosis, a polyethylene glycol conjugate of L-asparaginase (pegaspargase, Oncaspar) for combination therapy in acute lymphoblastic leukaemia, human α_1-proteinase inhibitor (Aralast) for the treatment of emphysema and pegadamase bovine (Adagen; bovine adenosine deaminase) for the treatment of patients afflicted with a type of severe combined immunodeficiency disease.

Antibody-directed enzyme prodrug therapy (ADEPT) illustrates a further application of enzymes as therapeutic agents in cancer. A monoclonal antibody carries an enzyme specifically to cancer cells where the enzyme activates a prodrug, destroying cancer cells but not normal cells.

1.6.1 Converting enzyme inhibitors

Many biologically active peptides are obtained from their precursors by the actions of converting enzymes (zinc metallopeptidases). For example, ACE cleaves a dipeptide from the C-terminus of angiotensin I to generate the pressor peptide angiotensin II. In addition, some of the biologically active peptides (e.g. bradykinin, atrial natriuretic peptide (ANP) and enkephalins) are degraded by the converting enzymes into inactive fragments. These enzymes are important in controlling many physiological and pathological processes. In the case of the peptides that, in some pathological conditions, produce undesirable effects (e.g. vasoconstriction in the case of angiotensin II and endothelin and inflammatory responses in case of TNF-α), it is beneficial to prevent the formation of such peptides from their precursors by inhibiting the enzymes involved in the process (e.g. ACE, endothelin and TNF-α converting enzyme). On the other hand, in the case of peptides producing therapeutically beneficial effects (e.g. enkephalins and atrial natriuretic factor, ANF), inhibiting the enzymes, which inactivate these peptides (e.g. enkephalinase and atriopeptidase), is likely to lead to an increased biological half-life of the peptide and thus extend the duration of action. From the point of view of drug discovery, ACE inhibitors, which prevent the formation of a pressor peptide angiotensin II, have been the most successful examples. From the point of view of medicinal chemistry, the lessons learned from the ACE story have been very useful in the design of inhibitors of many other metalloproteinases like enkephalinase, atriopeptidase and MMPs.

ACE (peptidyl dipeptidase, EC 3.4.15.1), known to catalyse the hydrolysis of dipeptides from the C-terminus of polypeptides, belongs to a family of zinc metalloproteinases, which require a zinc atom in the active site. In these enzymes, a combination of three His, Glu, Asp or Cys residues creates a zinc-binding site. The first major step in the discovery of ACE inhibitors was the isolation of bradykinin potentiating peptides like BPP5$_a$ (Pyr-Lys-Trp-Ala-Pro) and SQ20881 (Pyr-Trp-Pro-Arg-Pro-Gln-Ile-Pro-Pro) from the venoms of the Brazilian snake, *Bothrops jaraca* and the Japanese snake, *Agkistrodon halys blomhoffii*. SAR studies on these peptides indicated that a number of pentapeptide analogues of BPP5$_a$, for example, Pyr-Lys-Phe-Ala-Pro, were equipotent to the parent peptide in inhibiting ACE. However, smaller di- or tri-peptides, for example, Gly-Trp, Val-Trp, Ile-Trp, Phe-Ala-Pro and Lys-Trp-Ala-Pro were less potent. Although SQ20881 was studied extensively in the clinic, it could not be used as a drug due to lack of oral activity. Progress towards the orally active ACE inhibitors was made after the discovery of D-benzylsuccinic acid as an inhibitor of another zinc metalloprotease, carboxypeptidase A. This led to the synthesis of proline derivatives by combining the features present in venom peptides and benzylsuccinic acid. One of the early compounds, succinylproline, was only a weak inhibitor of ACE (~150-fold less potent than SQ20881). Further modifications in this series led to 2-D-methylsuccinyl-proline and 2-D-methylglutaryl-proline (five- and 10-fold less potent, respectively, than SQ20881). Replacement of the carboxyl group by a thiol group (a better zinc-ion ligand) resulted in potent ACE inhibitors like captopril (2-D-methyl-3-mercaptopropanoyl-proline, **126**) which produced dose-related inhibition of the pressor response to angiotensin I in normotensive male rats and produced marked antihypertensive effects in unanaesthetised Goldblatt two-kidney renal hypertensive rats. Captopril was the first ACE inhibitor to reach the market for the treatment of high blood pressure.

126 Captopril

127 Enalapril

128 Lisinopril

129 Fosinopril

Since the discovery of captopril, a number of other analogues either containing a different chelating group or a proline replacement have been found to be potent inhibitors of ACE. Some of this work was based on a hypothetical model of the substrate (angiotensin I) binding at the active site of the enzyme. In the case of the ACE inhibitors containing a thiol function (e.g. captopril), the thiol group interacts with the zinc ion and the methyl group binds at the S_1' subsite. The proline residue binds at the S_2' subsite and the C-terminal carboxyl group of the proline residue interacts with a positively charged group present in the enzyme. Over the years, medicinal chemistry approaches involving modifications of the chelating group and different groups binding in the S_1' and S_2' subsites have resulted in many potent inhibitors of ACE, including captopril (126), enalapril (127) and lisinopril (128), which have become highly successful drugs for the treatment of hypertension and some other cardiovascular disorders. The design of phosphorus-containing ACE inhibitors, for example, fosinopril (129), was based on the structure of phosphoramidon, [N-(α-L-rhamnopyranosyloxy-hydroxyphosphinyl)-Leu-Trp], an inhibitor of another zinc metalloproteinase (thermolysin) isolated from a culture filtrate of *Streptomyces tanashiensis*. In addition to the ACE inhibitors mentioned above, many others like alacepril, perindopril, delapril, quinapril, ramipril, benazepril, cilazapril, imidapril,

trandopril, temocapril, moexipril, spirapril and zofenopril are in the market for the treatment of hypertension, heart failure, heart attack and kidney failure.

Since the discovery of early ACE inhibitors, additional information has become available indicating that ACE is a complex two-domain enzyme, comprising of an N- and a C-terminal domain, each containing an active site with similar but distinct substrate specificities and chloride-activation requirements. Currently available ACE inhibitors show some degree of selectivity for the C-terminal domain inhibition. High-resolution crystal structure of human testis ACE (tACE; containing only the C-terminal domain with one catalytic site) has become available providing an opportunity for the discovery of N- and C-terminal domain-selective inhibitors.[171] The selective inhibitors may have much improved clinical profile. In addition to tACE, a human homologue of ACE (ACE2; cloned from a human heart failure cDNA library) has recently been identified with a more restricted distribution than ACE, and is found mainly in heart and kidney. In contrast to ACE, ACE2 has only one active enzymatic site and functions as a carboxypeptidase rather than a dipeptidyl carboxypeptidase. Instead of cleaving dipeptide residues from the C-terminal end of the peptide, ACE2 cleaves a single residue from angiotensin I to generate angiotensin(1–9), and degrades angiotensin II to the vasodilator angiotensin(1–7). ACE2 is insensitive to classic ACE inhibitors. The importance of ACE2 in normal physiology and pathophysiological states is currently under investigation.[172,173] It has been hypothesised that ACE2 might protect against increases in blood pressure and that ACE2 deficiency leads to hypertension.

In comparison with the effort required for the discovery of ACE inhibitors, the progress in identifying potent inhibitors of the enkephalin degrading dipeptidyl-carboxypeptidase (enkephalinase) (used as analgesics) and ANF degrading enzyme (used as antihypertensive agents) was more rapid due to similarities between the enzymes. However, the similarities resulted in problems in achieving selectivity. The differences in the S_1' and S_2' subsites of metalloproteinases were exploited to achieve selectivity. The first potent inhibitor of enkephalinase (thiorphan, 130), was about 30-fold more potent against enkephalinase ($K_i \sim$ 4 nM) than against ACE. Another inhibitor, kelatorphan (131), was a potent inhibitor of enkephalinase and dipeptidylaminopeptidase and a weak inhibitor of aminopeptidase. Inhibitors like glycoprilat (132) and their orally active prodrugs were potent inhibitors of ACE and enkephalinase; they prevented angiotensin I-induced pressor responses in rats and also increased urinary water and sodium excretion. Dual inhibitors of ACE and neutral endopeptidase were anticipated to provide additional benefits in cardiovascular diseases in comparison with ACE inhibitors alone due to the importance of the natriuretic peptide system in the pathogenesis of heart failure.[174–176]

Recombinant B-type natriuretic peptide [nesiritide, Ser-Pro-Lys-Met-Val-Gln-Gly-Ser-Gly-Cys-Phe-Gly-Arg-Lys-Met-Asp-Arg-Ile-Ser-Ser-Ser-Ser-Gly-Leu-Gly-Cys-Lys-Val-Leu-Arg-Arg-His (disulphide bridge containing cyclic peptide)] is already approved for the treatment of acutely decompensated congestive heart failure in patients who have dyspnoea at rest or with minimal activity. The agent causes arteries and veins to dilate, alleviating symptoms by improving blood movement around the heart without a change in heart rate. Many dual inhibitors (vasopeptidase inhibitors) have been synthesised and investigated in cardiovascular disorders.[177,178] Until recently, omapatrilat (BMS 186716) was the most advanced ACE and NEP inhibitor in clinical trials. Although pre-clinical studies in experimental models of hypertension and heart failure and a few clinical trials demonstrated some pharmacological advantages, none of the vasopeptidase inhibitors, including omapatrilat has reached the market.

It has been much more difficult to achieve complete selectivity in the case of inhibitors of MMPs (e.g. collagenases, stromelysins and gelatinases), a family of zinc-containing proteinases involved in extracellular matrix remodelling and degradation. At least 20 members of this enzyme family, subdivided into collagenases (MMP-1, -8, -13 and -18), gelatinases (MMP-2 and -9), stromelysins (MMP-3, -10 and -11) and membrane-type (MMP-14, -15, -16 and -17) families, have been reported. These enzymes have been implicated in diseases like rheumatoid arthritis, osteoarthritis, cancer and multiple sclerosis.[179–181] Work is also ongoing to discover novel antibacterial agents by designing inhibitors of bacterial metalloenzymes. This approach has been successfully applied to the discovery of in vivo active antibacterial agents that are inhibitors of bacterial peptide deformylase and UDP-3-O-(R-3-hydroxymyristoyl)-N-acetylglucosamine deacetylase.[182] Many inhibitors of MMPs were identified with different levels of selectivity against various MMPs. One of these inhibitors (marimastat, 133) was extensively studied in the clinic for the treatment of

130 Thiorphan

131 Kelatorphan

132 Glycoprilat

133 Marimastat

pancreatic, lung, brain and stomach cancers but failed to demonstrate efficacy in humans. Despite the failure of marimastat in the clinic, new compounds continue to be designed and developed.[183–185]

1.6.2 Aspartyl protease (renin and HIV protease) inhibitors

Aspartyl proteases are a family of enzymes which, in general, cleave peptide bonds between bulky hydrophobic amino acid residues. The cleavage of the peptide bond is mediated by a general acid–general base catalysis mechanism using the carboxyl groups of the aspartic acid residues at the active site. Enormous progress has been made in the discovery and optimisation of the pharmacokinetic properties of the inhibitors. Since the antihypertensive market is well served by a number of orally active agents like β-blockers, ACE inhibitors and angiotensin II antagonists, and the condition is chronic, requiring long-term treatment, it is essential to have orally active inhibitors for this indication. Many of the potent and selective renin inhibitors are now approaching the appropriate level of oral bioavailability after more than 25 years of research. In contrast, by using all the chemical information available in the case of renin inhibitors, it has been possible to discover potent, orally bioavailable HIV protease inhibitors in a relatively short period of time, and many of these are already highly successful drugs.

1.6.2.1 Renin inhibitors

A number of chemical approaches have been used in the design of renin inhibitors. In the absence of the purified enzyme, most of the early search for inhibitors was carried out using crude renin preparations. The amino acid sequences

of mouse, rat and human renin were obtained later on either by using the traditional isolation and sequencing techniques or by using cDNA methodology. Various three-dimensional models of renin were constructed in the early stages based on the X-ray structures of other similar aspartyl proteases, for example, endothiapepsin and penicillopepsin. Later on the X-ray crystal structure of recombinant human renin was reported. The inhibitor design process has been based on some of these models.

Initial design of the inhibitors was based on a rational design strategy using the renin substrate as a starting point. Some of the early studies indicated that the octapeptide of horse angiotensinogen (His-Pro-Phe-His-Leu-Leu-Val-Tyr), cleaved slowly by renin between the Leu-Leu residues, was a weak competitive inhibitor of renin. This led to the modifications in the P_1 and P'_1 positions (Leu-Leu) of this peptide. The early work indicated that the two leucine residues could be replaced by other natural and unnatural amino acids (e.g. Phe, D-Leu). Many of the resulting analogues like His-Pro-Phe-His-Leu-D-Leu-Val-Tyr, His-Pro-Phe-His-Phe-Phe-Val-Tyr and Pro-His-Pro-Phe-His-Phe-Phe-Val-Tyr-Lys though more potent than the original substrate-based compounds were still weak inhibitors of renin. More potent inhibitors were obtained by replacing the peptide bond between the two leucine residues. Many of these peptides, for example, Pro-His-Pro-Phe-His-Pheψ(CH₂NH)Phe-Val-Tyr-Lys, His-Pro-Phe-His-Leuψ(CH₂NH)Val-Ile-His and Pro-His-Pro-Phe-His-Leuψ(CH₂NH)Val-Ile-His-Lys (H-142), were potent and selective inhibitors of human renin. The two peptides containing a reduced Leu-Val peptide bond were 800–1000 times more potent inhibitors of human renin (IC_{50} 10–190 nM) than of dog renin (IC_{50} 10–150 mM) and H-142 did not inhibit cathepsin D up to a concentration of ~700 mM. One of the smaller peptides, Boc-Phe-His-Chaψ(CH₂NH)Val-NHCH₂CH(Me)-Et, approached the potency of H-142 in inhibiting human renin and was effective in lowering blood pressure in salt-depleted cynomolgus monkeys at a dose of 0.1–0.5 mg/kg. Unlike the reduced peptide bond

[-ψ(CH$_2$NH)-] analogues, replacement of the scissile peptide bond by -CH$_2$O-, -COCH$_2$-, -CH$_2$S- and -CH$_2$SO- did not lead to enhanced potency. The reduced peptide bond analogue, H-142, has been studied extensively in various animal and human models. At a dose of 1 and 2.5 mg/kg/h, H-142 produced a dose-related reduction in plasma renin activity and reduced the circulating levels of angiotensin I and II.

Another important step in the discovery of potent inhibitors of renin was the isolation of a naturally occurring aspartyl protease inhibitor pepstatin (Iva-Val-Val-Sta-Ala-Sta [Sta = (3S,4S)-4-amino-3-hydroxy-6-methylheptanoic acid]), which was a relatively poor inhibitor of human renin but a potent inhibitor of pepsin. Incorporation of the statine residue in the angiotensinogen octapeptide resulted in potent inhibitors of renin. His-Pro-Phe-His-Sta-Val-Ile-His and Iva-His-Pro-Phe-His-Sta-Leu-Phe-NH$_2$ were equipotent to H-142 as inhibitors of human plasma and kidney renin. Another similar compound, Iva-His-Pro-Phe-His-Sta-Ile-Phe-NH$_2$, was a five-fold more potent inhibitor of human plasma and kidney renin than was H-142. However, the statine analogue was much less selective. In comparison with H-142, the statine analogue was about a 300-fold more potent inhibitor of dog renin. The statine residue [-NH-CH(CH$_2$CHMe$_2$)-CH(OH)-CH$_2$CO-] in the above transition-state analogues was modified in various ways to assess the importance of the side-chain isobutyl group, the hydroxyl group and the methylene group. In general, replacement of the isobutyl side chain (occupying the P$_1$ position) by cyclohexylmethyl or benzyl groups resulted in more potent compounds. The hydroxyl and the methylene groups of statine were not essential for the renin inhibitory activity. Several analogues containing difluorostatine, difluorostatone, norstatine [(2R,3S)-3-amino-2-hydroxy-5-methylhexanoic acid], cyclohexylnorstatine [(2R,3S)-3-amino-4-cyclohexyl-2-hydroxybutyric acid], aminostatine (3,4-diamino-6-methylheptanoic acid) and α, α-difluoro-β-aminodeoxystatine were potent inhibitors of human renin.

134

135

136

Incorporation of the hydroxyethylene, dihydroxyethylene and other statine-like residues in place of the scissile peptide bond in substrate-based analogues, along with other amino acid or non-peptide changes at the N- and C-termini, led to more potent, selective and relatively small molecular weight inhibitors of renin. Examples of such compounds include compounds 134–137. Ro 42-5892 was effective in lowering blood pressure in sodium-depleted marmosets and squirrel monkeys after oral administration (0.1–10 mg/kg). The indole-2-carbonyl derivative (135, JTP-3072) caused significant reduction in blood pressure in marmosets at an oral dose of 10 mg/kg for up to 3 h. Compounds like 136 showed some oral absorption. Compound 137 (IC$_{50}$ 1.4 nM) displayed oral activity in a sodium-depleted normotensive cynomolgus monkey at a dose of 3 mg/kg.

Conformational analysis of the binding mode of one of the inhibitors has indicated that the S$_1$ and S$_3$ pockets constitute a large contiguous,

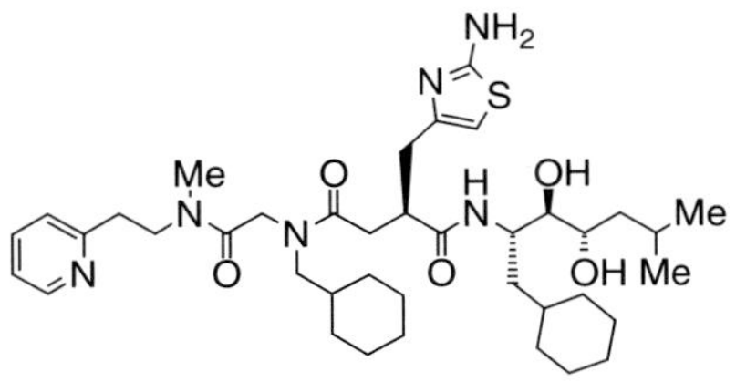

137

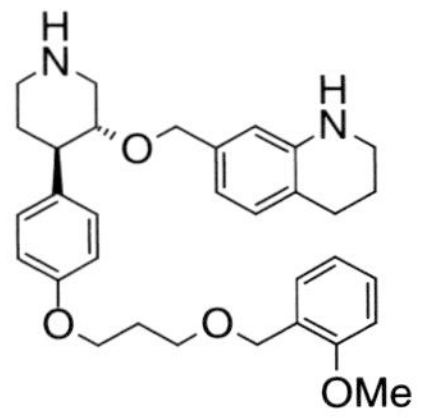

140

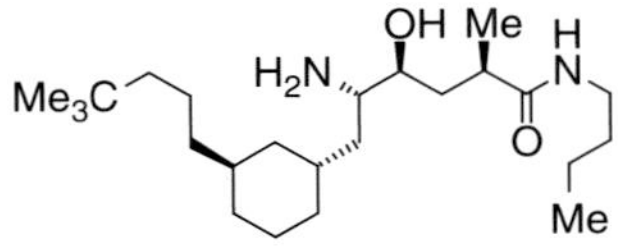

138

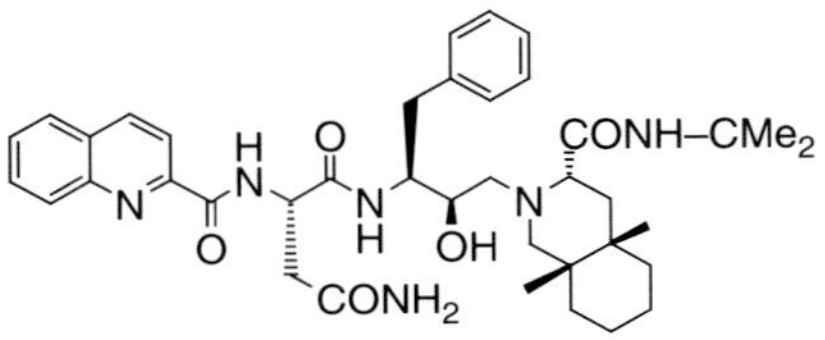

141 Saquinavir

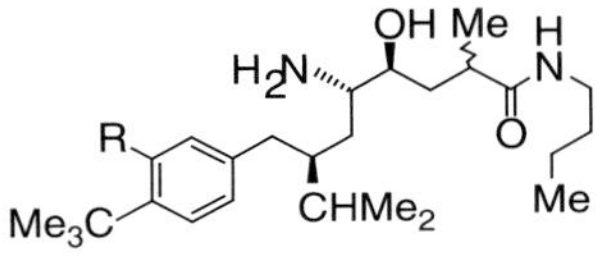

139

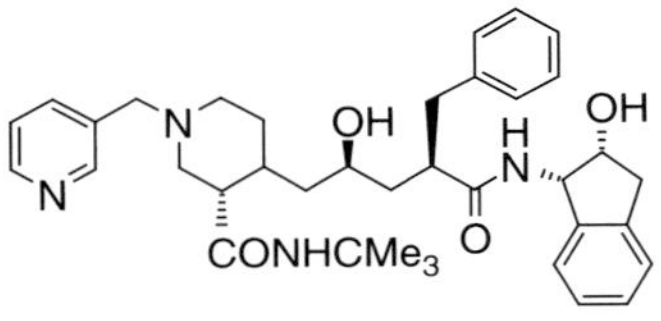

142 Indinavir

hydrophobic binding site accommodating the P_1 cyclohexyl and the P_3 phenyl groups in close proximity to each other. This led to the synthesis of δ-amino hydroxyethylene dipeptide isosteres lacking the P_4–P_2 peptide backbone. Compound **138** was a moderately potent inhibitor of human renin (IC_{50} 300 nM). Non-peptide inhibitors like compound **139**(R = -OCH$_2$COOCH$_3$, -OCH$_2$CONH$_2$ or -OCH$_2$SO$_2$CH$_3$) were 15–50-fold more potent inhibitors than **138**. Random screening approaches led to non-peptide inhibitors like the tetrahydroquinoline derivative **140** [IC_{50} 0.7 nM (recombinant human renin) and 37 nM (human plasma renin)], which displayed long-lasting (20 h) blood pressure lowering effects after oral administration (1 and 3 mg/kg) to sodium-depleted conscious marmosets. The piperidine derivative also inhibited plasmepsin I and II from *P. falciparum*.

1.6.2.2 HIV protease inhibitors

In comparison with the discovery of renin inhibitors, the task of discovering inhibitors of HIV protease has been relatively easy. This is primarily because many of the approaches used

successfully in the design of renin inhibitors were also applicable in the design of HIV protease inhibitors.[186] In addition, samples of both HIV-1 and HIV-2 proteases (99 residue peptides), obtained by chemical synthesis and recombinant technology, were available in the early stages of the programme, along with the three-dimensional structure of the HIV-1 protease. Like renin, HIV protease was found to prefer a hydrophobic amino acid (Leu, Ile, Tyr, Phe) in the P_1 position of the substrate and was inhibited by pepstatin. However, unlike renin, incorporation of the statine residue in the P_1 position of the substrate, or the replacement of the scissile peptide bond in the substrate-like peptides by a -CH$_2$NH- group, did not lead to potent inhibitors. Potent inhibitors of the enzyme were obtained by replacing the scissile peptide bond by a hydroxymethylcarbonyl, hydroxyethylamine, hydroxyethylurea or a hydroxyethylene group. Many such compounds like amprenavir, lopinavir, saquinavir (**141**), indinavir (**142**), ritonavir (**143**), nelfinavir (**144**) palinavir (**145**)

143 Ritonavir

146 Atazanavir

144 Nelfinavir

147

145 Palinavir

148

and atazanavir (**146**)[187] have either reached the market or are in the late stages of clinical trials. In order to overcome the problem of viral resistance, computational studies using HIV-1 protease mutants (Met[46]Ile, Leu[63]Pro, Val[82]Thr, Ile[84]Val, Met[46]Ile/Leu[63]Pro, Val[82]Thr/Ile[84]Val and Met[46]Ile/Leu[63]Pro/Val[82]Thr/Ile[84]Val) and known inhibitors of the enzyme were used to design inhibitors with better binding affinity towards both mutant and wild-type proteases. Several such compounds inhibited wild-type and mutant HIV protease, blocked the replication of laboratory and clinical strains of HIV type 1 and maintained high potency against mutant HIV selected by ritonavir *in vivo*.

Many other non-peptide inhibitors of HIV protease (dihydropyrone, cyclic urea and sulphamide series of compounds) were obtained by modifications of random screening leads. Examples of these include a cyclic sulphone derivative **147** and **148** (PNU-140690) that showed activity against a variety of HIV type 1

laboratory strains, clinical isolates and other variants resistant to other protease inhibitors.

1.6.3 Thrombin inhibitors (serine protease)

Thrombin, a serine protease, cleaves fibrinogen into fibrin to create a fibrous plug and also amplifies its own production through the activation of factor XI and cofactors V and VIII. Thrombin also plays a crucial role in the activation of platelets through the cleavage of the protease-activated receptors on the platelet surface. Antagonists of G-protein-coupled protease-activated receptor PAR$_1$ have been synthesised to study the role of thrombin PAR$_1$ receptor in thrombosis and vascular injury.[188] Thrombosis is the most common cause of death in the industrialised world and, whether through venous thromboembolism, myocardial infarction or stroke, ultimately involves the inappropriate activity of thrombin.[189] Although anticoagulants like warfarin, heparin, low-molecular weight heparin and hirudin are available for treating diseases like deep vein thrombosis, these agents suffer significant disadvantages and their use has to be carefully monitored.[190–192] Orally available thrombin inhibitors may provide several advantages, and for this reason, such agents have been sought for a long time for the treatment of venous thromboembolism and for prophylactic prevention of venous thromboembolism after large-joint orthopaedic surgery in high-risk patients.

Thrombin inhibitors like D-Phe-Pro-Arg-chloromethylketone and D-Phe-Pro-Arg aldehyde have been known for a long time. However, the compounds lacked oral bioavailability. A semi-rational approach was adopted to modify P_1–P_3 positions to improve potency, selectivity and pharmacokinetic properties. Changes in individual positions were followed by multiple changes and synthesis of conformationally restricted analogues. Substitution of the C-terminal arginine aldehyde moiety (P_1 position) in D-Phe-Pro-Arg aldehyde by p-amidinobenzylamine resulted in thrombin inhibitors comparable in potency to the transition-state aldehyde analogue and much less potent (130–400 000-fold) against trypsin, plasmin, tissue plasminogen activator and urokinase. Incorporation of a conformationally restricted analogue of arginine in the P_1 position, along with a six- or seven-membered lactam sulphonamide moiety at P_3–P_4 positions, also resulted in inhibitors that showed much more selectivity against serine proteases like factor Xa and trypsin. Inhibitor **149** containing conformationally restricting moieties in the P_3–P_2 region showed improved pharmacokinetics in the rat (61% oral bioavailability, elimination half-life 1 h). A chemically similar inhibitor (**150**) inhibited thrombus formation when administered orally (30 mg/kg; bioavailability 55%, 4 h duration) 1 h before induction of stasis.

A number of P_3 position modified thrombin inhibitors exhibited oral bioavailability in rats and dogs, and were efficacious in a rat FeCl$_3$-induced model of arterial thrombosis. Compounds like **151** and the corresponding

149

150

151

analogues with an unprotected amino group at the N-terminus, showed selectivity (300–1500-fold selectivity for thrombin compared with trypsin) and oral bioavailability (40–76%) in rats or dogs. The arylsulphonylpropargylglycinamide derivative **152** (K_i values 5, 19 000, >30 000, >200 000 and >200 000 nM against thrombin, factor Xa, trypsin, plasmin and tissue plasminogen activator, respectively) also demonstrated oral activity at a dose of 30 mg/kg in rats. Compound **153** containing a Phe(p-CH$_2$NH$_2$) residue in the P_1 position was one of the more potent and selective inhibitor of thrombin (K_i values 6.6 and 14 200 nM against thrombin and trypsin, respectively), and showed good oral bioavailability in rats (~70%) but low oral bioavailability in dogs (10–15%). Some of the modified D-Phe-Pro-Arg aldehyde analogues like melagatran (**154**) are undergoing clinical evaluation. An orally available prodrug form of melagatran (ximelagatran)

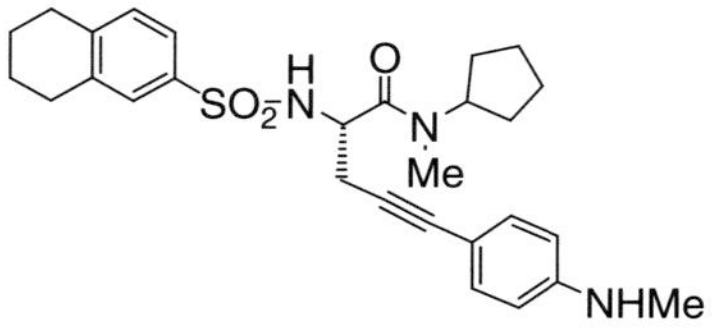

152

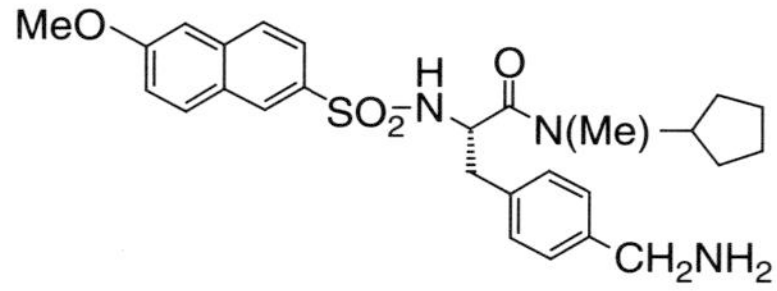

153

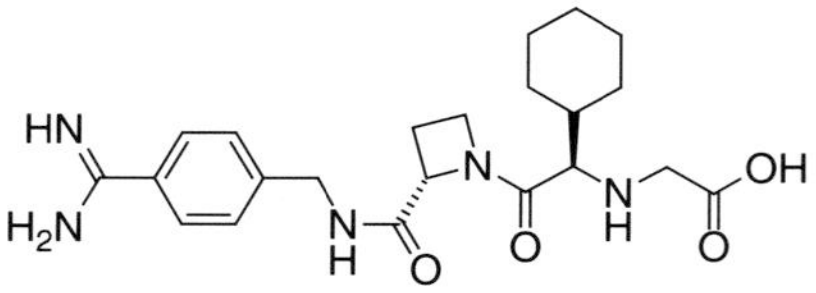

154 Melagatran

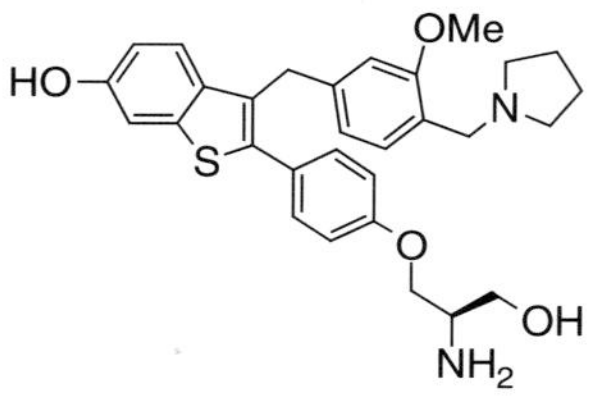

155

156

has been approved for marketing in some countries.

Non-peptide inhibitors of thrombin (obtained by random screening procedures) include compounds based around benzothiophene (e.g. 155) and other ring systems and cyclic and linear oligocarbamate derivatives (e.g. 156). The benzothiophene derivative 155 showed antithrombotic efficacy in a rat model of thrombosis after infusion (ED_{50} 2.3 mg/kg/h). The cyclic oligocarbamate tetramer 156 inhibited thrombin with an apparent K_i of 31 nM.

1.6.4 Ras protein farnesyltransferase inhibitors

Cysteine farnesylation of the ras oncogene product Ras is required for its transforming activity and is catalysed by the enzyme protein farnesyltransferase. The enzyme catalyses the transfer of a farnesyl group from farnesyl diphosphate to a cysteine residue of the protein substrate such as Ras. The enzyme recognises a tetrapeptide sequence [Cys-A-A-X (A is an aliphatic amino acid and X is Met, Ser, Ala, Cys or Gln)] at the C-terminus of the protein. A closely related enzyme, geranylgeranyltransferase, recognises the Cys-A-A-X motif when X is either Leu or Phe, but transfers a geranylgeranyl group from geranylgeranyl diphosphate. Inhibition of farnesyltransferase represents a possible method for preventing association of Ras p21 to the cell membrane, thereby blocking its cell-transforming capabilities. Such inhibitors may have therapeutic potential as anticancer agents.[193,194]

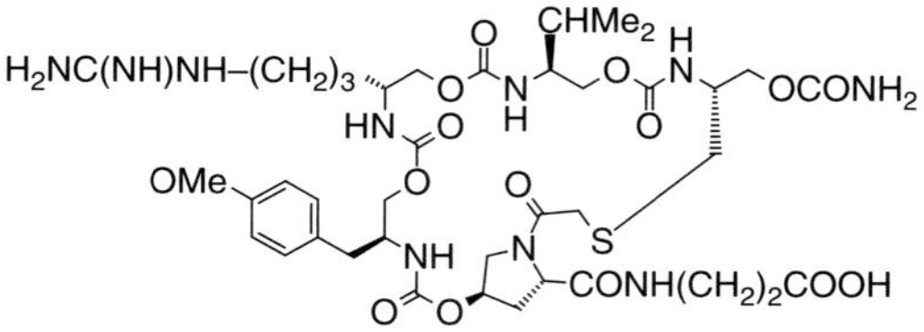

'Semi-rational' design approaches for the discovery of farnesyltransferase inhibitors were based on the tetrapeptide Cys-Val-Phe-Met. SAR studies, followed by the synthesis of conformationally restricted analogues, led to inhibitors like 157, which was effective in prolonging the survival time in athymic mice implanted intraperitoneally with H-ras-transformed RAT-1 tumour cells. A non-thiol inhibitor incorporating an N-alkyl amino acid residue (158, methyl ester prodrug) showed activity in several in vivo tumour models. Further medicinal chemistry approaches on these modified peptides, including the synthesis of a library of secondary benzylic amines led to orally active methionine derivatives like 159, which attenuated tumour growth in a nude mouse xenograft model of human pancreatic cancer. The methyl ester prodrug (160) suppressed the growth of human lung adenocarcinoma A-549 cells in nude mice by 30–90% in a dose-dependent manner.

157

161

158

162

159

163

160

164

Random screening approaches also provided inhibitors of the enzyme. SAR studies on the random screening lead Z-His-Tyr(OBn)-Ser(OBn)-Trp-D-Ala-NH$_2$ (PD083176) (IC$_{50}$ 20 nM), including the replacement of the N-terminal Z group and the histidine and Trp residues, led to less potent peptides. However, substitution of the Tyr(OBn) and Ser(OBn) residues did not have much effect on the enzyme inhibitory activity. Based on the SAR and truncation studies, potent inhibitors of farnesyltransferase like 161 were obtained. The Z-His derivative 161 inhibited isolated farnesyltransferase but was about 4000-fold less potent against geranylgeranyltransferase-1. Compound 161 was also active in athymic mice implanted with H-ras-F cells. When administered intraperitoneally (150 mg/kg/day once daily) for 14 consecutive days after tumour implantation, the tumour growth was inhibited by ~90%. Random screening approaches followed by medicinal chemistry also resulted in chemically distinct farnesyltransferase inhibitors. Examples include compounds like 162–165. Compound 162 was orally active in several human tumour xenograft models in the nude mouse, including tumours of colon, lung, pancreas, prostate and urinary bladder. Although many compounds like 162–165 are in various stages of clinical trials, none of the farnesyltransferase inhibitors has yet reached the market.

165

1.6.5 Protein kinase inhibitors

The protein kinases are a family of proteins (serine/threonine and tyrosine kinases) involved in signalling pathways regulating a number of cellular functions, such as cell growth, metabolism, differentiation and death. Examples of protein tyrosine kinases include intracellular domains of transmembrane growth factor receptors, such as epidermal growth factor (EGF) receptor,[195,196] platelet-derived growth factor receptor,[197] vascular endothelial growth factor (VEGF) receptor[198,199] and fibroblast growth factor receptor,[200] and cytosolic kinases, such as src, abl and lck. Examples of serine/threonine kinases include mitogen-activated protein kinase,[201–204] Jun kinase and cyclin-dependent kinases[205–210] and glycogen synthase kinase.[211–213] Signal transduction via these proteins occurs through selective and reversible phosphorylation of the substrates by the transfer of γ-phosphate of ATP (or GTP) to the hydroxyl group of serine, threonine and tyrosine residues. A large number of protein kinases (>150) have been identified from mammalian sources, and the human genome is expected to provide many more in the future. Selective inhibitors of these enzymes are expected to be useful in a number of diseases like cancer, inflammatory disorders, diabetes and neurodegenerative disorders and, for this reason, this is one of the most active areas of pharmaceutical research at the present time.[211–221] With approaches based on monoclonal antibodies and synthetic small molecules, inhibitors of kinases are being developed.

A recent example of the antibody-based approach is the discovery of a monoclonal antibody against human EGF receptor (HER2), a family of EGF-receptor tyrosine kinases, including the EGF receptor. Many epithelial tumours, including breast cancer, express excess amounts of these proteins, particularly HER2. HER2 is a tyrosine kinase receptor with extracellular, transmembrane and intracellular domains. Initially, several monoclonal antibodies against the extracellular domain of the HER2 protein were found to inhibit the proliferation of human cancer cells that over-expressed HER2. The antigen-binding region of one of the more effective antibodies was fused to the framework region of human IgG to generate a 'humanised' monoclonal antibody. The antibody (trastuzumab, Herceptin) was investigated alone and in combination with chemotherapy in women with metastatic breast cancer that over-expressed HER2. Compared with chemotherapy alone, treatment with chemotherapy plus trastuzumab was associated with significantly higher rate of overall response and a longer time to treatment failure.[222] Treatment with trastuzumab was associated with some side effects (chills, fever, infection and cardiac dysfunction). A humanised monoclonal antibody cetuximab (C225) has not yet reached the market.

Two of the small molecule inhibitors, gefitinib (**166**, EGF receptor kinase inhibitor) and imatinib (**167**, Bcr-Abl receptor kinase inhibitor), have reached the market. Although many of the starting leads for kinase inhibitors were obtained by random screening approaches, further medicinal chemistry was aided by the availability of a number of crystal structures and other modelling approaches.[223,224] The design of irreversible inhibitors like **168** was also based on modifications of the same basic skeleton.[225] Irreversible EGFR tyrosine kinase inhibitor **168** inhibited human tumour xenografts when dosed as infrequently as once per week, and a single dose eliminated the level of EGFR phosphorylation in tumours for longer than 72 h. Examples of VEGF receptor kinase (anti-angiogenic agents), fibroblast growth factor receptor kinase, p56[Lck] kinase and Aurora kinase included ZD4190 (**169**), PD173074 (**170**), BMS-279700 (**171**) and VX-680 (**172**), respectively. Direct measurement of tumour vascular endothelial permeability,

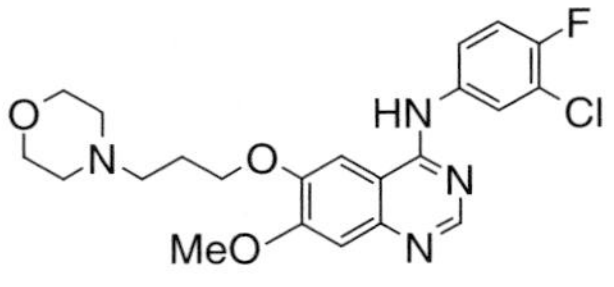

166 Gefitinib

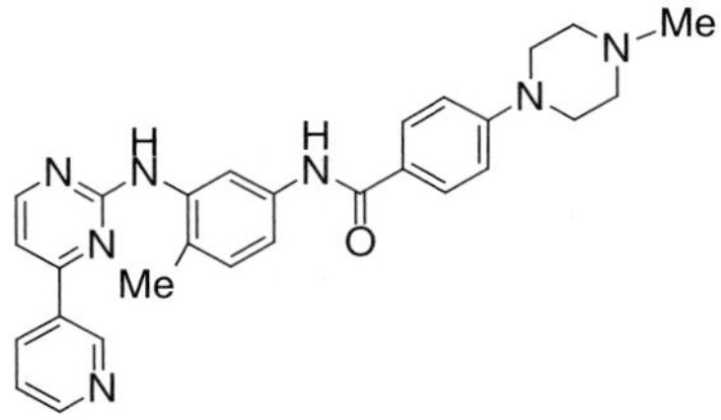

167 Imatinib

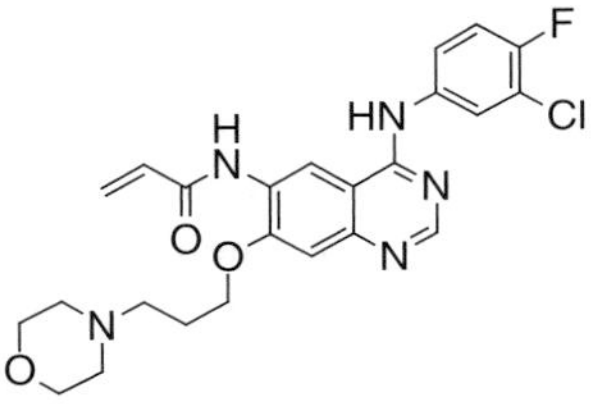

168

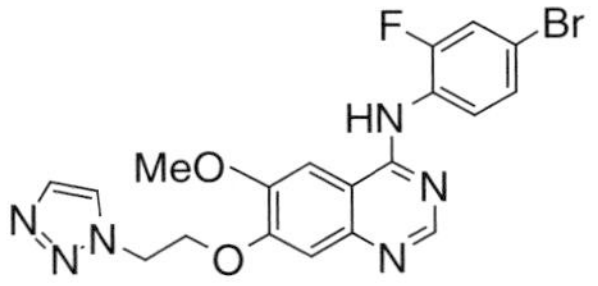

169

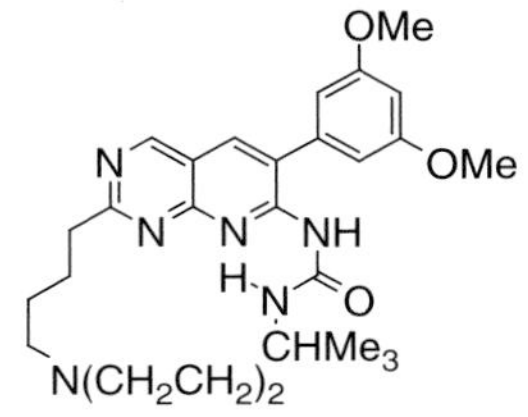

170

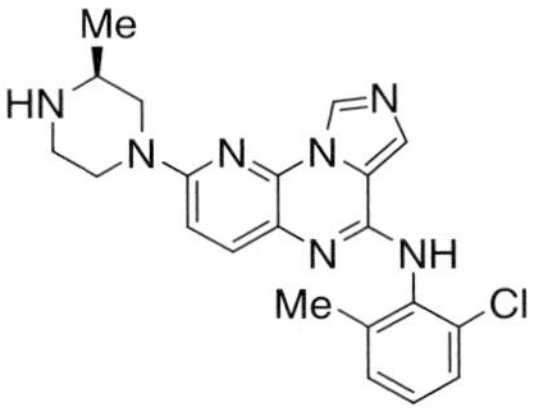

171

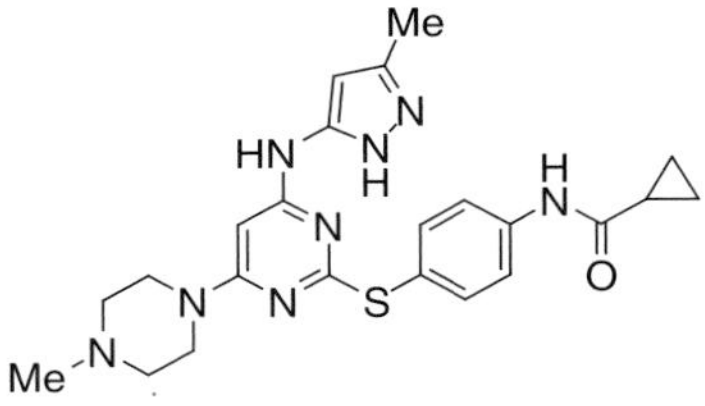

172

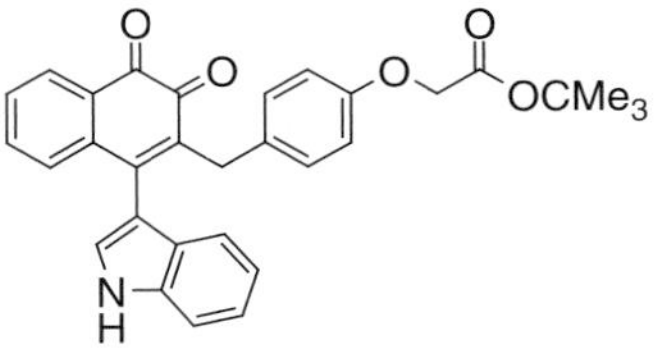

173

using contrast medium-enhanced MRI indic-ated that acute ZD4190 treatment produced measurable changes in vascular permeability at doses which yielded antitumour activity dur-ing chronic administration. BMS-279700 blocked the inflammatory cytokines (interleukin, IL-2 and TNF-α) *in vivo*.[226] The Aurora kinase inhib-itor VX-680 inhibited tumour growth in a vari-ety of *in vivo* xenograft models, leading to regression of leukaemia, colon and pancreatic tumours.[227]

In addition to receptor tyrosine kinases, which catalyse the formation of phosphate ester bond, protein phosphatases also play an important role in regulating signalling pathways. They hydrolyse the phosphate ester bond on tyr-osine and serine/threonine residues, thus creat-ing a balance between the phosphorylated and non-phosphorylated states. Inhibitors of pro-tein phosphatases are also being designed as treatment for various diseases mentioned above for protein receptor kinases.[228–233] Chemically, many leads were identified initially from nat-ural products as protein phosphatase inhibitors. Subsequently, combinatorial and other chemical approaches led to many compounds like **173** and **174** that act as inhibitors, but so far, none of these agents has reached the clinic.

174

1.7 Protein–Protein Interaction Inhibitors

Many physiological and pathological processes are mediated by protein–protein interactions. The proteins involved in cell adhesion have been most widely studied. The interactions between integrin (a family of at least 24 transmembrane glycoprotein heterodimers formed by the non-covalent associations between 18 α and 8 β subunits) family of heterodimeric cell-surface receptors and their protein ligands are fundamental for maintaining cell function, for example, by tethering cells at a particular location, facilitating cell migration or providing survival signals to cells from their environment. Ligands recognised by integrins include extracellular matrix proteins (e.g. collagen and fibronectin), plasma proteins like fibrinogen and cell-surface molecules like transmembrane proteins of the immunoglobulin family and cell-bound complement. A number of integrins and their ligands have been associated with many disease processes involved in cardiovascular (e.g. thrombosis involving platelet aggregation), inflammation, cancer (e.g. metastasis) and bone disorders.[234–238] The discovery of platelet aggregation inhibitors by blocking the interaction of platelet glycoprotein IIb/IIIa with its natural ligands fibrinogen and von Willebrand factor is described as an example of protein–protein interaction inhibitors.

Novel inhibitors of glycoprotein IIb/IIIa and fibrinogen/van Willebrand interaction include injectable peptides (e.g. integrilin, 175) and orally active peptidomimetics that act as competitive inhibitors and a monoclonal antibody c7E3 (abciximab) that irreversibly binds to GP IIb/IIIa.

Clinically, the antibody c7E3 has been shown to be effective in reducing 30-day and 6-month clinical events after high-risk coronary intervention. Administered intravenously, circulating abciximab has a plasma half-life of less than 10 min. However, the antibody binds tightly to platelets and provides receptor blockade up to a period of 15 days.

The design of peptide and non-peptide inhibitors of platelet aggregation was based on the early observations that the integrins recognise peptide sequences like Arg-Gly-Asp present in the larger protein ligands like fibronectin and vitronectin. This led to the synthesis of a large number of analogues containing the Arg-Gly-Asp tripeptide or the chemical features of the tripeptide side chains (e.g. the guanidino function and the carboxyl group).[239] SAR studies indicated that a basic functional group that mimics the side chain of the arginine and a carboxylic acid group mimicking the Asp side chain are critical to the receptor-binding and platelet aggregation activities of these compounds. In addition, a lipophilic group near the carboxylic acid function was found to enhance the potency of the antagonists. These findings led to the synthesis of more stable cyclic peptides like integrelin and many other compounds containing different non-peptide templates to hold the important functional groups in the proper spatial arrangements. All these approaches have resulted in potent, injectable or orally active platelet aggregation inhibitors. Examples of compounds that have reached the market include the antibody abciximab, the injectable peptides integrelin (175) and tirofiban (176). Many of the orally active compounds like lamifiban[240] (177), sibrafiban[241] (178), xemilofiban, orbofiban and tirofiban have been studied extensively in the clinic. However, most of these have failed in the late stages of development.

In addition to the well-known examples of IIb/IIIa, antagonists of other integrins like $\alpha_v\beta_3$ (vitronectin receptor), $\alpha_v\beta_5$, $\alpha_v\beta_6$, $\alpha_4\beta_1$ and $\alpha_4\beta_7$ have been synthesised. The design of $\alpha_v\beta_3$ receptor antagonists was based on IIb/IIIa antagonists. Therefore, some of the early compounds were antagonists of both $\alpha_v\beta_3$ and IIb/IIIa.

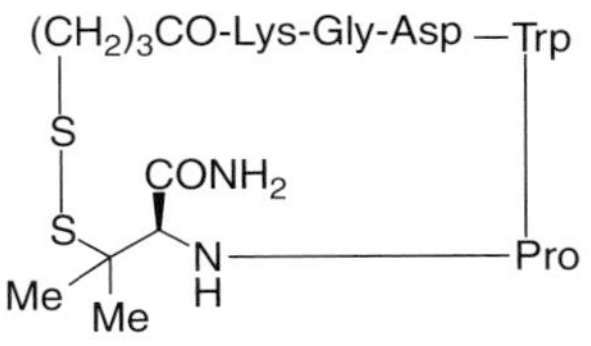

175 Integrilin

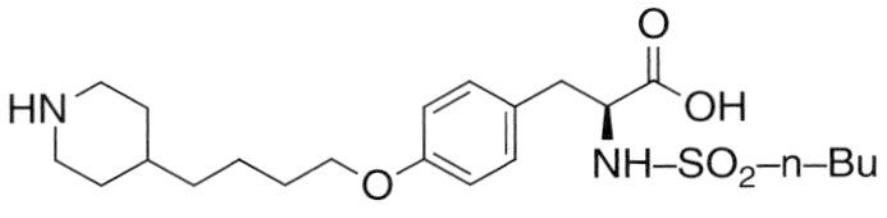

176 Tirofiban

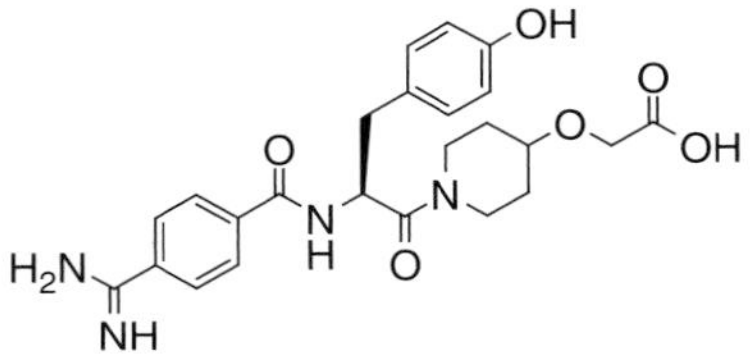

177 Lamifiban

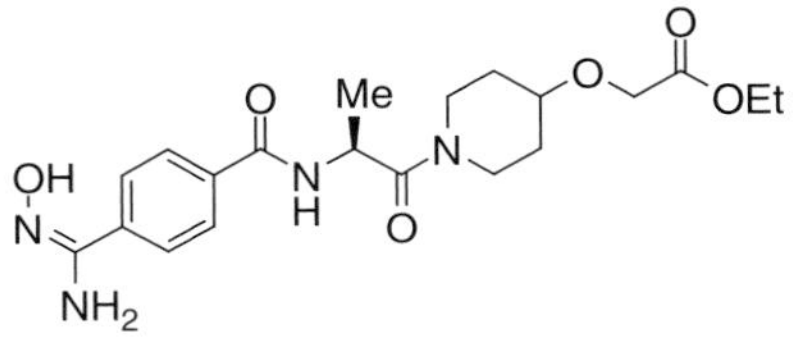

178 Sibrafiban

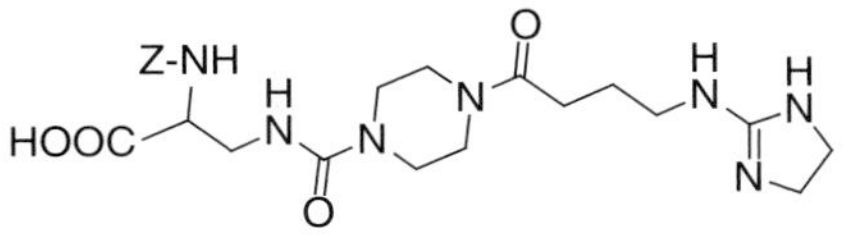

179

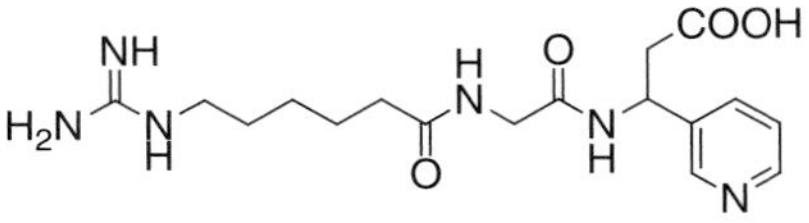

180

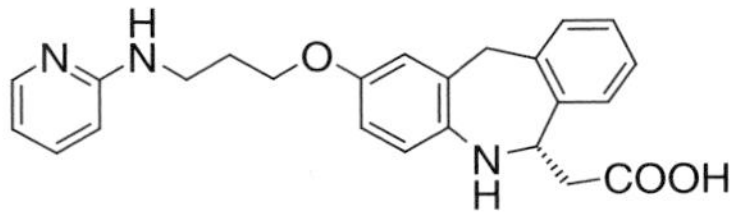

181

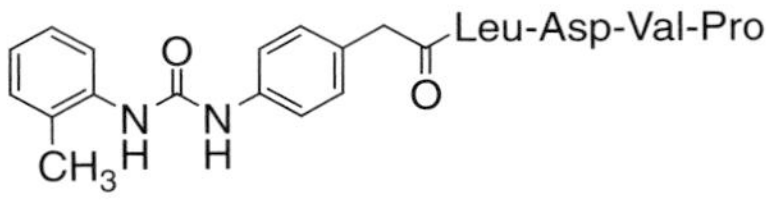

182

Analogues like **179** and **180** were more selective against $\alpha_v\beta_3$ receptor. For example, the diaminopropionic acid derivative **179** was >500-fold more potent against $\alpha_v\beta_3$ integrin than against $\alpha_v\beta_5$, $\alpha_5\beta_1$ and GPIIb/IIIa integrins. Compound **180** (SC56631) blocked osteoclast-mediated bone particle degradation. Further, medicinal chemistry led to non-peptide vitronectin receptor antagonists with oral activity. For example, compound (**181**) SB265123 (K_i 4.1 nM for $\alpha_v\beta_3$, 1.3 nM for $\alpha_v\beta_5$, 18 000 nM for $\alpha_5\beta_1$, and 9000 nM for $\alpha_{IIb}\beta_3$) displayed 100% oral bioavailability in rats, and was active *in vivo* in the ovariectomised rat model of osteoporosis.

1.7.1 $\alpha_4\beta_1$ and $\alpha_5\beta_1$ antagonists

Cyclic peptide inhibitors of VLA-4 and fibronectin/vascular cell adhesion molecule (VCAM-1) interaction, for example, c(Ile-Leu-Asp-Val-NH(CH$_2$)$_5$CO) were reported. Several of these inhibitors like c(Ile-Leu-Asp-Val-NH(CH$_2$)$_5$CO), c(Ile-Leu-Asp-Val-NH(CH$_2$)$_4$CO) and c(MePhe-Leu-Asp-Val-D-Arg-D-Arg) blocked VLA-4/VCAM-1 and VLA-4/fibronectin interaction in *in vitro* assays and inhibited oxazolone and ovalbumin-induced contact hypersensitivity responses in mice.[242–244] The compounds did not affect cell adhesion mediated by two other integrins, VLA-5 ($\alpha_5\beta_1$) and leucocyte function-associated antigen (LFA-1; $\alpha_L\beta_2$). *p*-Aminophenylacetyl-Leu-Asp-Val derivatives containing various non-peptide residues at the N-terminal end are reported as inhibitors of integrin $\alpha_4\beta_1$. In various integrin adhesion assay, compound **182** showed activity against $\alpha_4\beta_7$, $\alpha_1\beta_1$, $\alpha_5\beta_1$, $\alpha_6\beta_1$, $\alpha_L\beta_2$ and $\alpha_{IIb}\beta_3$ integrins at much higher concentrations. Other inhibitors of LFA-1 and its ligand integrin-type cell adhesion molecule (ICAM-1) and VLA-4 and endothelial vascular cell adhesion molecule (VCAM-1) were described in recent reviews.[245,246]

In addition to the inhibitors of integrins and their ligands, research is also ongoing to find

183 SP-4206

185

184

small molecule compounds that are able to interfere interactions of other proteins and their receptors. Some success has been achieved in this field.[247] An example of this is the discovery of an inhibitor of cytokine IL-2 and its receptor. Extensive use of site-directed mutagenesis studies to identify IL-2 residues important for interaction with the receptor followed by modelling, X-ray crystallography and fragment-based discovery approach led to the conversion of a weak inhibitor Ro26-4550 ($IC_{50} = 3$–$6\,\mu M$) to a potent inhibitor SP-4206 (**183**, $IC_{50} = 30\,nM$) that binds to IL-2 and prevents its interaction with the IL-2 receptor. Random screening approaches have resulted in the discovery of reversible inhibitors (e.g. **184**) of cell-surface proteins B7-1 and B7-2 (found on antigen-presenting cells) and CD28, found on the T-cell, reducing T-cell activation. Several inhibitors of B-cell lymphoma (BCL2) and $BCL\text{-}X_L$ (anti-apoptotic proteins) to the pro-apoptotic protein BAK have been discovered by various approaches like virtual screening, high-throughput screening and ligand-based design techniques. Information about the binding of $BCL\text{-}X_L$ to the 16 amino acid BH3 domain of BAK was obtained using NMR. Compound (**185**) represents one example of a $BCL\text{-}X_L$ and BAK inhibitor.

1.8 Protein and Antibody Therapeutics

Many successful protein products, including antibodies, have been marketed over the years for the treatment of a number of diseases. One of the oldest examples of a protein product is insulin, still one of the most successful drugs after 70–80 years of its discovery. Early insulin preparations, derived from natural sources, are being replaced by recombinant human insulin preparations and new formulations are being marketed that provide a more gradual and continuous release profile and maximise glucose control in diabetic patients.[248]

The new genomic/proteomic discoveries will result in many more therapeutic protein products (including monoclonal antibodies and therapeutic vaccines) for the treatment of many diseases, including autoimmune, inflammatory and infectious diseases and cancer.[249–251] These protein/antibody products pose different sets of problems compared with the traditional small molecular weight products. Many of these are highly glycosylated proteins, and precise molecular structures, including secondary and tertiary protein structures, of these agents cannot be defined. The choice of expression systems and growth conditions for the production of these agents has a big impact on the quality of the final product. Although many highly sophisticated analytical techniques are used for the characterisation of these protein products, it is still not possible to achieve the level of characterisation achieved with the small molecule products.[252] Safety and clinical testing in animals present additional problems. Several biopharmaceuticals are species-specific in terms of their biological effects, and may induce immune reactions in animals. These agents, except orally active vaccines, are administered parenterally (subcutaneous injections or infusion) and it is often difficult to define precise pharmacokinetic-pharmacodynamic properties. Many problems associated with the development of protein products (e.g. production, characterisation, administration/formulation) are being overcome gradually. Various techniques like pegylation[253] and N-glycosylation are used to increase biological half-life of protein products. Successful protein products marketed in the last 15–20 years include interferones, granulocyte-macrophage colony-stimulating factor (GCSF), thrombopoietin,[254] erythropoietin,[255] parathyroid hormone,[256] recombinant human parathyroid hormone N-terminal fragment (1–34) (teriparatide),[257] tinzaparin (a low molecular weight heparin formed by the enzymatic degradation of porcine unfractionated heparin),[258] etanercept and several others listed in Table 1.3. Etanercept is a soluble, dimeric, fusion protein consisting of the two copies of the extracellular ligand-binding portion of the human TNF p75 receptor linked to the constant portion of human immunoglobulin G_1. It binds to TNF, thereby blocking its interaction with cell-surface receptors and attenuating its pro-inflammatory effects in rheumatoid arthritis and psoriasis.[259,260] Etanercept appears to have greater affinity for TNF than infximab (a monoclonal antibody against TNF). Etanercept is administered subcutaneously twice a week to rheumatoid arthritis patients. A 36 amino acid peptide (enfuvirtide) has recently been marketed for the treatment of HIV aids. The peptide binds to a region of the envelope glycoprotein 41 of HIV-1 that is involved in the fusion of the virus with host cell membrane and specifically prevents the fusion of the virus gp41 glycoprotein with the CD4 receptor of the host cell.[261,262]

Along with the protein products mentioned above, significant progress has also been made in the discovery and marketing of antibodies.[263,264] Development of the hybridoma technology allowed the production of rodent monoclonal antibodies that are the product of single clone of antibody-producing cells and have only one

antigen-binding specificity. However, the therapeutic use of rodent monoclonal antibodies in humans is limited by their immunogenicity. Using genetic engineering and expression systems, it is now possible to produce chimeric, humanised and totally human antibodies as well as antibodies with novel structures and functional properties.[265] Like the protein products mentioned above, production, formulation and characterisation of antibodies also presents significant challenges.[266] Currently available antibodies are used for the treatment of many diseases like cancer,[267,268] rheumatoid arthritis,[269] Crohn's disease, spondyloarthropathies, psoriasis, allograft rejection[270] and respiratory diseases.[271] Compared with small molecule drugs, antibodies are very specific and are less likely to cause toxicity based on factors other than the mechanism of action. Bound to a target, therapeutic antibodies can deliver a toxic payload, act as agonists or antagonists of receptors or as neutralisers of ligands.[272,273] All of the antibodies that are currently on the market are produced in mammalian cell cultures. Chimeric, humanised and phage-display-derived monoclonal antibodies need to be produced from recombinant genes reintroduced into mammalian cells to enable proper folding and glycosylation. These time-consuming steps are not required for human antibodies from genetically engineered mice, as these can be produced directly from the original hybridomas. Development of transgenic animals such as goats or cows, which are engineered to produce monoclonal antibodies in their milk, may offer an economical alternative.[274–276]

Examples of antibodies in the market include trastuzumab (anti-HER2 monoclonal antibody), rituximab, natalizumab (α_4-integrin antibody),[277] abciximab, infximab (targets TNF-α in Crohn's disease and rheumatoid arthritis), alemtuzumab, adalimumab (TNF-α antibody for the treatment of rheumatoid arthritis) and efalizumab (anti-CD11a monoclonal antibody for the treatment of psoriasis).[278] Rituximab is a mouse/human chimeric anti-CD20 monoclonal antibody used for the treatment of various lymphoid malignancies. As CD20 antigen is found on the surface of

Table 1.3 Protein products in the market since 1987

Protein product	Treatment indication
Nesiritide – recombinant B-type natriuretic peptide (32 amino acid peptide with one disulphide bridge)	Heart failure
Carperitide – recombinant α-hANP	Congestive heart failure
Anact C – Human plasma-derived activated protein C concentrate	Deep vein thrombosis, pulmonary thromboembolism due to congenital protein C deficiency
Drotrecogin α (activated) – recombinant human activated protein C	Reducing mortality in patients with severe sepsis (sepsis associated with acute organ failure)
Protein C concentrate (Human)	Purpura fulminans and coumarin-induced skin necrosis in patients with severe congenital protein C deficiency
Anakinra – recombinant version of human IL-1 receptor antagonist	Rheumatoid arthritis patients failing to respond to disease-modifying antirheumatic drugs
Darbepoietin α – long-acting erythropoietin preparation	Anaemia in patients with chronic renal failure
Peginterferon α-2a – pegylated interferone derivative	Chronic hepatitis C
Interferon Alfacon-1 – 30% identity with IFN-β and 60% identity with IFN-ω	Chronic hepatitis C
Interferon β-1a	Relapsing form of multiple sclerosis
Interferon β-1b – recombinant, stable analogue of human interferon-β	Relapsing remitting multiple sclerosis
Interferone γ-1α – recombinant	Cutaneous T-cell lymphoma
Interferon γ-1b – recombinant	Chronic granulomatous disease
γ- Interferon – recombinant	Rheumatoid arthritis
NovoMix 30 – combination of 30% soluble insulin aspart/70% insulin aspart protamine crystals	Diabetes
Insulin lispro – fast-acting, recombinant human insulin analogue	Diabetes
Recombinant glucagon	Insulin-induced hypoglycaemia; emergency treatment for severe hypogycaemic reactions
OCT-43 (Octin) – recombinant variant of IL-1β (Cys^{71} replaced by Ser)	Mycosis fungoides and antitumour in malignant skin tumours and in the treatment of aplastic anaemia and myelodysplastic syndrome
IL-2 – stable rDNA IL-2	Antineoplastic – renal cell carcinoma
Tasonermin – recombinant TNF	Soft tissue sarcoma of the limbs
Lepirudin – recombinant, modified hirudin	Myocardial infarcts, unstable angina and cardiovascular events
Parnaparin – low MW heparin	Anticoagulant
Reviparin – low MW heparin	Prevention of deep vein thrombosis and pulmonary embolism following surgery
Enoxaparin – low MW heparin	Antithrombotic

continued

Table 1.3 Continued

Nartograstim – recombinant GCSF derivative	Chemotherapy-induced leukopaenia
Filgrastim – recombinant human GCSF	Adjunct to cancer chemotherapy for patients with non-myeloid malignancies
Pegfilgrastim – conjugate of recombinant methionyl-GCSF and monomethoxypolyethylene glycol	Decreasing the incidence of infections, as manifested by febrile neutropaenia, in patients with non-myeloid malignancies receiving myelosuppressive anticancer drugs
Sargramostin – recombinant GCSF	Immunostimulant – cancer patients after autologous bone marrow transplant
Somatomedin-1 – insulin-like growth factor-1	Growth disorders in children; hereditary Laron-type dwarfism
Somatotropin – recombinant, modified human growth hormone	Growth failure in children due to a lack of endogenous growth hormone secretion
Somatropin – recombinant growth hormone	Hypopituitary dwarfism and other disorders resulting from growth hormone deficiencies
Epoetin delta, gene-activated human erythropoietin	Anaemia related to renal disease in patients receiving dialysis and in patients who have not yet undergone dialysis to elevate and maintain red blood cell production
Erythropoietin – recombinant erythropoietin	Anaemia associated with renal transplant or end-stage renal disease
EGF – recombinant	Healing of the corneal epithelium following various corneal diseases

malignant and normal B lymphocytes, treatment with rituximab induces lymphopaenia in most patients, but the effects are reversible (6–9 months after therapy).[279] Administered once a week by intravenous infusion, rituximab is approved for the treatment of aggressive non-Hodgkin's lymphoma in combination with cyclophosphamide, doxorubicin, vincristine and prednisone chemotherapy. Recent studies have demonstrated the efficacy of rituximab in several refractory autoimmune disorders including rheumatoid arthritis, systemic lupus erythematosus, immune thrombocytopenic purpura, chronic cold agglutinin disease, IgM-mediated neuropathies and mixed cryoglobulinaemia.[280]

Cetuximab is a chimeric monoclonal antibody highly selective for the EGF receptor that induces a broad range of cellular responses (e.g. inhibits cell cycle progression, apoptosis, reduction in growth factors like EGF, TGF-α and VEGF) that enhance tumour sensitivity to radiotherapy and chemotherapeutic agents. The antibody has

a longer half-life (79–129 h) and is administered once a week by intravenous infusion. It is indicated for the treatment of colorectal cancer in combination with irinotecan.[281,282] Alemtuzumab is an unconjugated, humanised, monoclonal antibody directed against the cell-surface antigen CD52 on lymphocytes and monocytes. It is administered by intravenous infusion (three times a week) for 12 weeks for the treatment of B-cell chronic lymphocytic leukaemia in patients previously treated with alkylating agents and refractory to fludarabine.[283]

Basiliximab is a mouse/human chimeric monoclonal antibody with specificity and high affinity for the α-subunit of the IL-2 receptor. The antibody acts as an IL-2Rα antagonist and inhibits IL-2-mediated activation and proliferation of T lymphocytes. It is indicated for the prevention of acute organ rejection in adult and paediatric renal transplant recipients in combination with other immunosuppressive agents like ciclosporin, azathioprine, mycophenolate mofetil

Table 1.4 Examples of antibodies currently on the market

Antibody (generic name)	Indication (target)
Rituximab	Non-Hodgkin's lymphoma, rheumatoid arthritis (CD20)
Ibritumomab	Non-Hodgkin's lymphoma (CD20)
Tositumomab	Non-Hodgkin's lymphoma (CD20)
Trastuzumab	Metastatic breast cancer, non-small-cell lung cancer, pancreatic cancer [HER-2/neu (p183^{neu})]
Gemtuzumab Ozogamicin	Acute myelogenous leukaemia (CD33)
Alemtuzumab	Chronic lymphocytic leukaemia, multiple sclerosis (CDw52)
Cetuximab	Colorectal cancer
Bevacizumab	Colorectal cancer
Endrecolomab	Colorectal cancer (17-A1)
Adrecolomab	Colorectal cancer (EpCAM)
Infiximab	Crohn's disease, rheumatoid arthritis (TNF-α)
Adalimumab	Rheumatoid arthritis (TNF-α)
CDP-870	Crohn's disease, rheumatoid arthritis (TNF-α)
Natalizumab	Crohn's disease, multiple sclerosis (VLA4β_1)
Omalizumab	Allergic asthma (IgE)
Muromonab	Organ transplant rejection (CD3)
Daclizumab	Kidney transplant rejection (CD25), leukaemia
Basiliximab	Kidney transplant rejection (CD25)
Epratuzumab	Autoimmune diseases (CD22)

and corticosteroids.[284] Abciximab is an antibody fragment that inhibits platelet aggregation and leucocyte adhesion by binding to the glycoprotein IIb/IIIa, vitronectin and Mac-1 receptors. It reduces the short- and long-term risk of ischaemic complications in patients with ischaemic heart disease undergoing percutaneous coronary intervention; it is administered by intravenous infusion for 12 h.[285]

An example of targeted delivery of cytotoxic agents to tumours is gemtuzumab. In this case, calicheamicin, a potent cytotoxic agent that causes double-strand DNA breaks, resulting in cell death, is conjugated to monoclonal antibodies specific for tumour-associated antigens. The tumour-specific antibody directs the cytotoxic agent to the tumour cells, thereby reducing damage to other cells in the body.[286] Examples of many other therapeutic antibodies are listed in Table 1.4 along with their clinical indications.

1.9 Examples of Currently Available Drugs for Major Diseases

1.9.1 Infectious (bacterial, fungal and viral) diseases

A large majority of drugs used today to treat infections caused by various Gram-negative and Gram-positive strains of bacteria are derivatives of penicillin and cephalosporin like cefdinir,[287] carbapenems like fropenem, meropenem, ertapenem and panipenem, erythromycin and its semi-synthetic derivatives like telithromycin,[288,289] aminoglycosides, glycopeptide antibiotics like vancomycin and teicoplanin,[290] lipopeptide antibacterials like daptomycin[291] and rifamycin. Only quinolones like ciprofloxacin, levofloxacin[292] and gatifloxacin (**186**) and linezolid (**187**) have originated from recent synthetic efforts. All major antifungal agents (triazole and imidazole

186 Gatifloxacin

187 Linezolid

188 Torasemid

derivatives like fluconazole and itraconazole) inhibit the fungal ergosterol biosynthetic pathway that is necessary for the fungal cell viability. Inhibitors of *N*-myristoyltransferase are currently being designed as a new class of antifungal agents.[293] Echinocandin derivatives like micafungin (β-(1,3)-D-glucan synthase inhibitors interfering with fungal cell wall synthesis), derived from a naturally occurring compound isolated from the culture broth of the fungus *Coleophoma empetri*, have been introduced recently into the market for the treatment of invasive aspergillosis, *Candida albicans* and non-albicans *Candida* spp. These agents are administered by infusion and are claimed to be superior to fluconazole.[294] The current antiviral drugs are either reverse transcriptase (required for the replication of the HIV genome) inhibitors like retrovir, abacavir, emtricitabine[295] and tenofovir[296] or inhibitors of HIV protease (e.g. saquinavir, amprenavir, lopinavir, nelfinavir, indinavir and ritonavir) blocking the processing of *gag* and *gag-pol* polyproteins that are required for viral maturation. Recently, inhibitors of both influenza A and B virus neuraminidase (sialidase) isoenzymes, zanamivir (**11**) and oseltamivir, have been developed for the treatment of influenza.[297]

1.9.2 Cardiovascular disorders

In addition to the thiazide diuretics like hydrochlorothiazide (**19**) and chlorthalidone used in the treatment of hypertension for a long time,[298] a few newer diuretics such as azosemide and torasemid (**188**) have been introduced for

the treatment of hypertension. Understanding of the adrenergic amines and their receptors (α and β), the renin–angiotensin system and calcium channels (e.g. dihydropyridine-sensitive, voltage-dependent calcium channels, L-type voltage-gated Ca channels) has been responsible for the discovery of the most important drugs in the fields of hypertension, angina and congestive heart failure. Examples of β-blockers with varying degree of selectivity include propranolol (**69**), atenolol (**70**), arotinolol, bisoprolol, bevantolol, tertatolol, nipradilol, amosulalol, dilevalol, carvedilol, tilisolol and nebivolol. Combinations of β-blockers and diuretics have also been marketed. Following the discovery of the first ACE inhibitor captopril (**126**), which demonstrated that the renin–angiotensin system was important in the control of hypertension in a large majority of patients, many other ACE inhibitors like enalapril (**127**), lisinopril (**128**), alacepril, perindopril, delapril, quinapril, ramipril, benazepril, cilazapril, fosinopril, imidapril, trandopril, temocapril, moexipril, spirapril, and zofenopril were marketed for the treatment of hypertension, heart failure, etc. Following the success of ACE inhibitors, antagonists of angiotensin II (e.g. losartan (**86**), valsartan (**92**), candesartan (**93**), telmisartan, irbesartan (**94**), eprosartan (**95**), olmesartan) were marketed for the treatment of hypertension and heart failure either alone or in combination with diuretics. Calcium antagonists like amlodipine (**189**), felodipine, nitrendipine, nisoldipine, isradipine, nilvadipine, manidipine, efonidipine, benidipine, lacidipine, barnidipine, aranidipine, lercanidipine,[299] cilnidipine and azelnidipine[300] have also been successful drugs for controlling blood pressure. Platelet aggregation inhibitors (e.g. adenosine diphosphate P2y, receptor antagonists like clopidogrel (**190**) and fibrinogen/GPIIb/IIIa interaction inhibitors like eptifibatide and tirofiban (**176**)) are being used in various

189 Amlodipine

190 Clopidogrel

191 Simvastatin

thrombotic disorders. A few new antithrombotic agents like factor Xa inhibitor fondaparinux (a synthetic pentasaccharide)[301] and a thrombin inhibitor ximelagatran (a prodrug of melagatran, **154**)[302] have been marketed recently. Anticoagulants like warfarin, heparin, low-molecular weight heparin and hirudin are also available for treating diseases like deep vein thrombosis.

Inhibition of the enzyme HMG-CoA reductase has provided the most successful drugs for lowering low-density lipoproteins and elevating high-density lipoproteins. After the success of the first inhibitors like lovastatin and simvastatin (**191**),[303] many other HMG-CoA reductase inhibitors [e.g. pravastatin, fluvastatin, atorvastatin (**8**, currently the best selling drug in the world) and rosuvastatin] were marketed. These cholesterol lowering agents have been shown to have a significant beneficial effect on adverse outcomes of death, heart attack and stroke.[304] Although HMG-CoA reductase inhibitors mentioned above have established a huge market (>$15 billion), current statins are associated with toxicity concerns (cerivastatin was recently withdrawn). Other agents like ezetimibe (**9**, inhibitor

of dietary cholesterol absorption) are just entering the market. Work is ongoing to discover clinically useful inhibitors of the cholesteryl ester transfer protein as cholesterol lowering agents.[305,306] This protein plays a critical role not only in the reverse cholesterol transport pathway but also in the intravascular remodelling and recycling of high- lipoprotein particles.

1.9.3   Diabetes and obesity

Diabetes is rapidly becoming one of the more common diseases. There are 120 million diabetics worldwide and this number is estimated to increase to greater than 200 million by 2010 and 300 million by 2025. Complications associated with diabetes (retinopathy, nephropathy, neuropathy and macro- and microangiopathy) lead to blindness, kidney failure, limb amputation and cardiovascular disease. The need for antidiabetic drugs is, therefore, likely to increase significantly.[307] From a mechanistic viewpoint, most therapies for the treatment of diabetes can be grouped into one of four categories: insulin or insulin secretagogues; enhancers of insulin action (decrease insulin resistance); inhibitors of hepatic glucose production or inhibitors of glucose absorption. Insulin (from natural and recombinant sources) is currently the most successful drug for treating diabetes. Insulin secretagogues that act by stimulating pancreatic β-cells to secrete insulin, for example, glibenclamide (**192**), glipizide, gliclazide and glimepiride (**193**) (sulphonylurea derivatives, blockers of ATP-sensitive K$^+$ channel in the pancreatic β-cells) and non-sulphonylurea derivatives like repaglinide (**194**) are used for the treatment of type 2 diabetes.[308] The newer agents have a rapid onset and short duration of action, and may improve glycaemic control without inducing prolonged hyperinsulinaemia that has been associated with weight gain and hypoglycaemic episodes.

Thiazolidinediones are the newer agents that favourably influence insulin sensitivity and possibly also pancreatic β-cell function.[309] The biological response of thiazolidinediones is mediated by binding to the nuclear peroxisome proliferator-activated receptor-γ (PPAR)

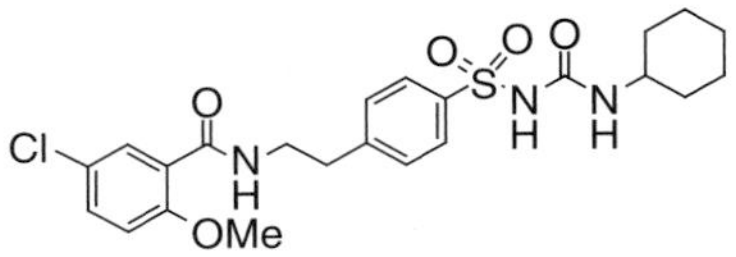

192 Glibenclamide

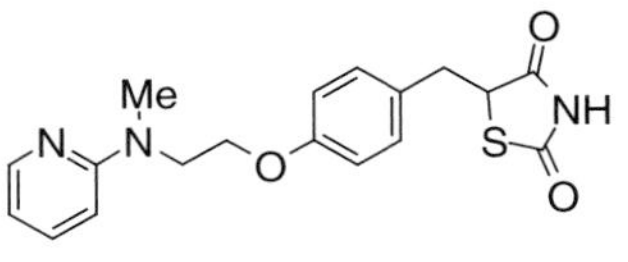

195 Rosiglitazone

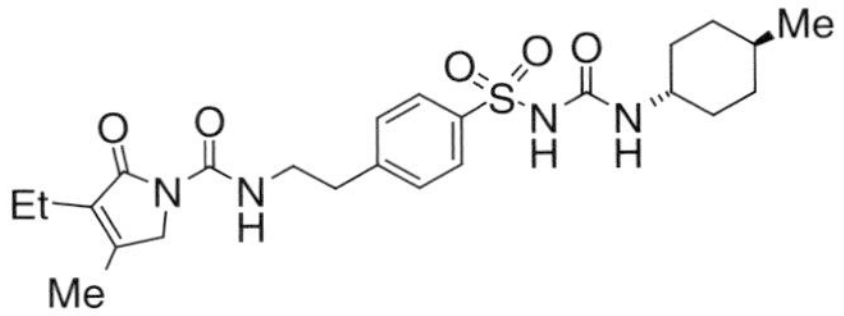

193 Glimepiride

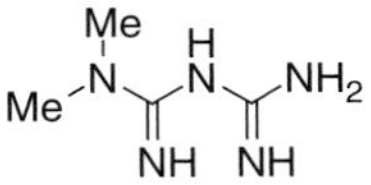

196 Metformin

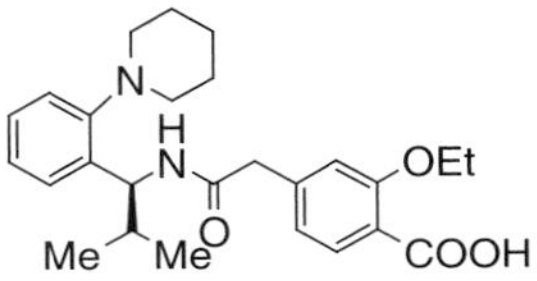

194 Repaglinide

and activating transcription of genes that, among others, regulate adipocyte differentiation and adipogenesis as well as glucose and lipid metabolism. The peroxisome-proliferator-activated receptors are a subfamily of the 48-member nuclear-receptor superfamily and regulate gene expression in response to ligand binding. Various fatty acids serve as endogenous ligands for PPARs, whereas some members of the superfamily (farnesoid X receptors) bind bile acids and others (liver X receptors) bind oxysterols. Three PPARs, designated PPAR-α, PPAR-δ (also known as PPAR-β), and PPAR-γ, have been identified to date.[310] Involvement of PPAR receptors in various cardiovascular diseases has been discussed in many recent reviews.[311–314] Although a number of thiazolidinediones like pioglitazone (**7**), troglitazone, rosiglitazone (**195**) and ciglitazone have reached the market for the treatment of type 2 diabetes, some toxicity problems still exist with this class of compounds, and one of the compounds (troglitazone, Rezulin) was voluntarily withdrawn from the market in the United Kingdom (possible adverse effects on the liver) but remains on the market in the United States and Japan with increased monitoring of liver function in patients.

Metformin (**196**) is the currently prescribed drug for the inhibition of hepatic glucose production. While the molecular target for this drug has not been identified, its primary mode of action seems to be the inhibition of hepatic gluconeogenesis. More recent discoveries in the treatment of diabetes include intestinal α-D-glucosidase inhibitors and aldose reductase inhibitors. Islet transplantation and pancreatic regeneration strategies are also being investigated for the treatment of diabetes.[315,316]

Only one new anti-obesity agent (orlistat, **14**), inhibitor of GI lipases required for the lipolysis and digestion of dietary fat, has been marketed recently. Earlier compounds had many safety concerns and some, for example, dexfenfluramine (inhibitor of presynaptic release of serotonin, reuptake inhibitor, 5-HT$_{1B}$ receptor agonist and a postsynaptic 5-HT$_{2c}$ receptor agonist) were later withdrawn due to the side effects of primary pulmonary hypertension, brain serotonin neurotoxicity and valvular heart disease. Many gut and brain hormones have been implicated in obesity. Examples include CCK, ghrelin, leptin, orexins, neuropeptide Y and peptide YY. Ghrelin stimulates, and glucagon like peptide-1, oxyntomodulin, peptide YY, CCK and pancreatic polypeptide inhibit, appetite.[317,318] Many receptor selective agonist and antagonist analogues of the above gut and brain hormones have been investigated as anti-obesity agents but none has come to the market yet.

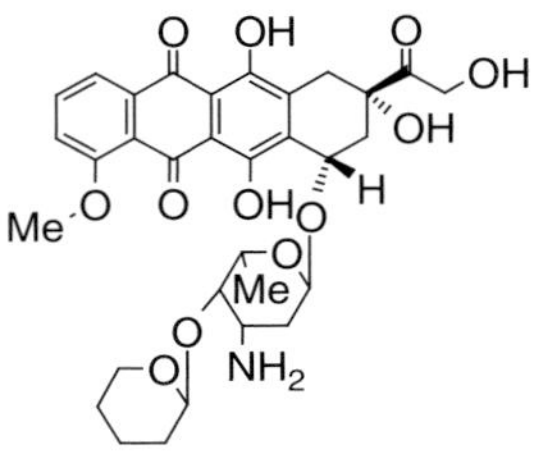

197 Pirarubicin

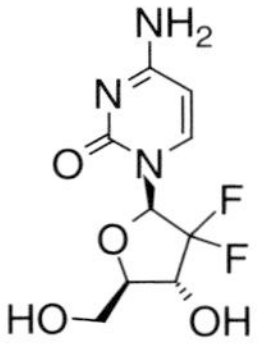

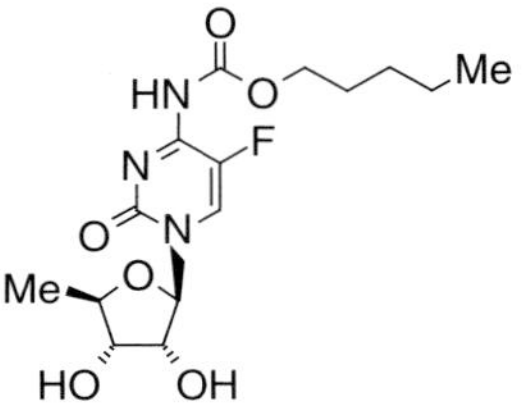

199 Capecitabine

198 Gemcitabine

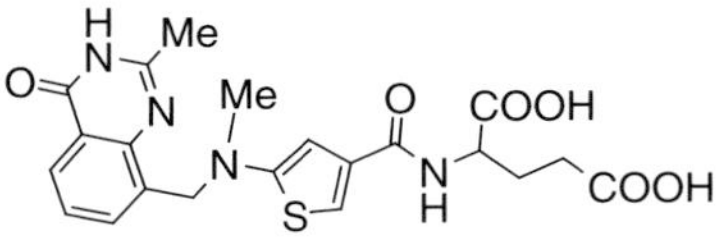

200 Raltitrexed

1.9.4   Cancer

Many of the earlier cytostatic or cytotoxic drugs (inhibitors of DNA or RNA synthesis) used for the treatments of various cancers were derived either from naturally occurring cytotoxic compounds like doxorubicin or were nucleoside derivatives. Doxorubicin and its liposomal formulations have been in the market for a long time. Examples of other antineoplastic anthracene derivatives based on doxorubicin, which act as DNA synthesis inhibitors, include epirubicin, pirarubicin (**197**), idarubicin and mitoxantrone. These agents are indicated for various cancers including lung,[319] breast, ovarian, prostate,[320] gastric, pancreatic,[321] colorectal, head and neck and brain tumours and Hodgkin's disease. Examples of nucleoside antineoplastic agents and their prodrugs with similar clinical indications include compounds like 5-fluorouracil (5-FU; thymidylate synthase inhibitor), gemcitabine (**198**) and capecitabine (**199**). Capecitabine is an orally active prodrug, which is converted to 5-FU by a three-step enzymic process. It passes intact through the intestinal mucosa, is converted first by carboxyesterase to 5′-deoxy-5-fluorocytidine in the liver, then by cytidine deaminase to 5′-deoxy-5-fluorouridine in the liver and tumour tissues and finally by thymidine phosphorylase to 5-FU

in tumours. Although some of these agents are safer than others, toxicity still remains a problem with these agents. Other thymidylate synthase inhibitors like raltitrexed (**200**) have also been developed and are indicated for the treatment of advanced colorectal cancer.[322] In addition to the above cytotoxic/cytostatic agents, several platinum-containing antineoplastic agents, for example, cisplatin, carboplatin, oxaliplatin[323] and nedaplatin, reacting with nucleophilic sites on DNA and causing cytotoxicity, are also being used for treating a variety of cancers, including head and neck, small-cell and non-small-cell lung, oesophageal, prostatic, testicular, ovarian, cervical, bladder and uterine cancers.[324,325]

More recent developments in cancer therapy have been based on the understanding of the growth factors/hormones involved in tumour growth and more detailed understanding of the cell cycle. The hormonal approach has led to many antioestrogens, acting as receptor antagonists [e.g. tamoxifen (**71**), toremifene (**72**), droloxifene (**73**), raloxifene (**74**) and fulvestrant (**75**)] or aromatase inhibitors [e.g. formestane (**77**), exemestane (**78**), anastrazole (**79**) and letrazole (**80**)], for the treatment of breast cancer, and many antiandrogens [e.g. flutamide, nilutamide and bicalutamide (**201**)] for the treatment of prostate cancer. Agents that can simultaneously block oestrogen in females and testosterone in males, for example, goserelin [Pyr-His-Trp-Ser-Tyr-D-Ser(But)-Leu-Arg-Pro-AzGly-NH2],[148,149] buserelin and leuprolide have been developed

201 Bicalutamide

202 Irinotecan

203 Topotecan

both for the treatment of breast and prostate cancer. Availability of taxol from natural sources has led to the discovery of antitumour agents like paclitaxel[326] and docetaxel possessing anti-microtubule actions (promote microtubule assembly and induce formation of stable, non-functioning microtubules) leading to cell death. Examples of other marketed antitumour agents include drugs that inhibit topoisomerase I [e.g. irinotecan (**202**) and topotecan (**203**)] and II (e.g. sobuzoxane)[327] or deliver a cytotoxic antibiotic like calicheamicin by using an antibody-targeted approach. Gemtuzumab ozogamicin is an example of antibody-targeted antineoplastic agent for the treatment of patients with acute myeloid leukaemia. This immunoconjugate consists of an anti-CD33 humanised mouse monoclonal antibody (IgG4) linked via a bifunctional linker to the cytotoxic antibiotic calicheamicin. Once the anti-CD33 binds to its antigen expressed on acute myeloid leukaemia blast cells, a complex is formed that is internalised, eventually releasing the calicheamcin derivative inside the cell. More recently, antibody- or small-molecule-based inhibitors of receptor tyrosine kinases [e.g. gefitinib (**166**), imatinib (**167**) and trastuzumab] have become available as antitumour agents. Work is ongoing to obtain clinically useful farnesyltransferase inhibitors for the treatment of various forms of cancer.[194] Evidence is also accumulating that selective inhibitors of COX-2 may be effective in the prevention and treatment of cancer.[328–330]

1.9.5 Neurological disorders

This has been one of the more difficult and complex area of medicinal research. Many diseases of the brain like personality disorders[331,332] and repair processes after brain injury[333,334] are poorly understood and for many others the treatments are not satisfactory. Most of the treatments are based on transmitters like GABA, dopamine, 5-hydroxy-tryptamine, central adrenergic and cholinergic systems and glutamate receptors. Work based on these transmitters has led to treatments for Parkinson's disease,[335] depression,[336,337] schizophrenia,[338] bipolar disorder[339] and migraine.[340] The emergence of multiple receptors (e.g. 5-HT$_{1-7}$ and their subtypes and dopamine D$_{1-5}$) for various transmitters and a deeper understanding of the role played by these transmitters and their receptors in controlling various neurological processes is resulting in more selective and efficacious drugs. For example, although the newer drugs against Parkinson's disease are still primarily based on dopamine, newer dopamine agonists like pergolide, ropinirole (**204**), pramipexole (**205**) and talipexole display varying levels of selectivity for D$_2$ receptor subtypes with weak or no significant activity at α_2 adrenergic, 5-HT$_1$, 5-HT$_2$ benzodiazepine, GABA, α_1 and β adrenoreceptors. Based on the differences in selectivity, the side-effect profiles of these agents are different to each other. Orally active catechol-O-methyltransferase inhibitors like tolcapone and entacapone (**206**) are used as adjuncts to levodopa therapy. Selective serotonin uptake inhibitors [e.g. fluoxetine (**207**), paroxetine (**208**), sertraline (**209**), citalopram (**210**), escitalopram (S isomer of citalopram)], noradrenaline uptake inhibitors like reboxetine (**211**), dual serotonin/noradrenaline uptake inhibitors

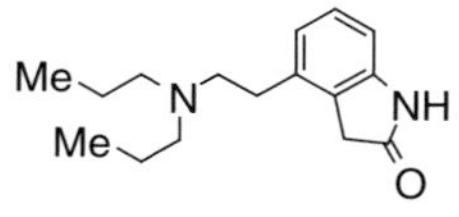

204 Ropinirole

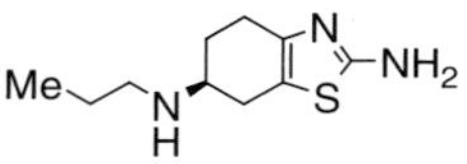

205 Pramipexole

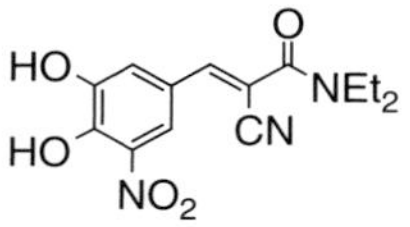

206 Entacapone

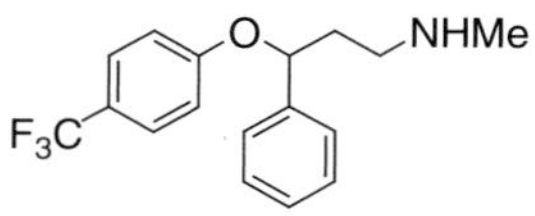

207 Fluoxetine

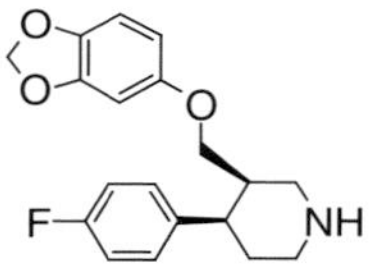

208 Paroxetine

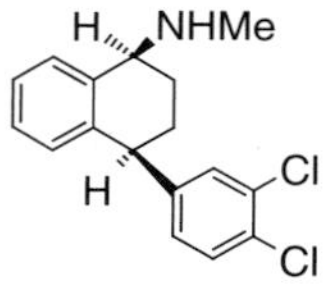

209 Sertraline

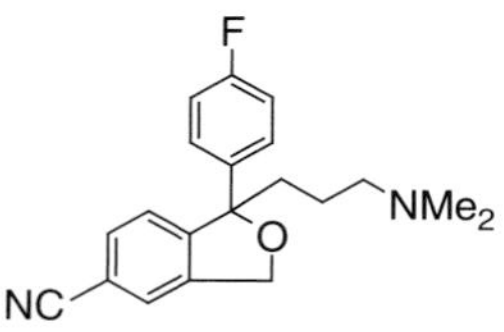

210 Citalopram

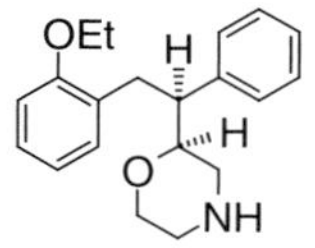

211 Reboxetine

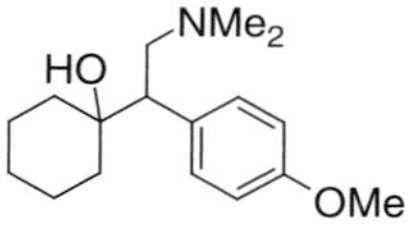

212 Venlafaxine

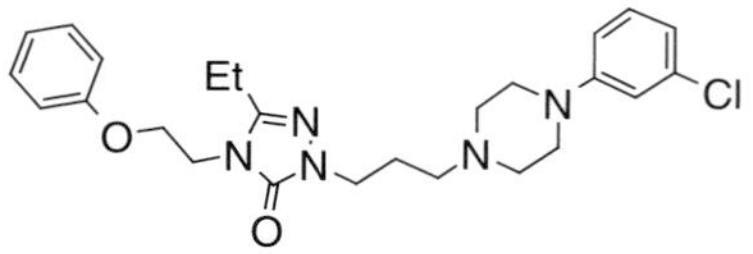

213 Nefazodone

In comparison with traditional antipsychotic agents (e.g. haloperidol, fluphenazine and chlorpromazine), which were thought to exhibit their beneficial effects almost exclusively through a blockade of central dopaminergic (D_2) receptors in the mesolimbic region of brain, newer 'atypical' antipsychotic agents have been developed to inhibit more selectively dopamine and 5-HT receptor subtypes. For example, clozapine is a more selective antagonist of 5-HT_{2A}, 5-HT_{2D} and 5-HT_6 receptors, in addition to greater D_4 and D_2 receptor blockade. Improvements in the side-effect profile (less extrapyramidal symptoms) has led to the acceptance of newer agents like quetiapine (**15**), olanzapine (**16**), ziprasidone (**29**), sertindole (**30**), risperidone (**31**) and perospirone (**214**) as atypical antipsychotic agents. In addition to 5-HT and dopamine receptor activities, quetiapine is a strong antagonist of histamine H_1 receptors. Newer agents like aripiprazole (**32**) are just entering the market. Selective 5-HT_3 antagonists [e.g. ondansetron (**21**), granisetron, tropisetron, nazasetron (**22**), ramosetron and dolasetron] are marketed as antiemetics and selective 5-$HT_{1B/1D}$ receptor antagonists [e.g. sumatriptan (**23**), zomitriptan (**24**), naratriptan, almotriptan, rizatriptan (**25**) and eletriptan] and dopamine D_2 antagonist like

[(e.g. milnacipran and venlafaxine (**212**)] and compounds acting as both a potent 5-HT_2 receptor antagonist and as a serotonin reuptake inhibitor [(e.g. nefazodone (**213**)] are currently marketed as antidepressant drugs.

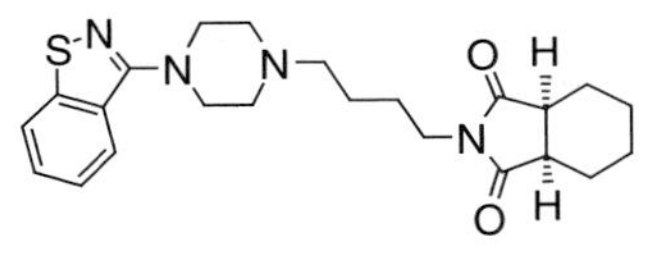

214 Perospirone

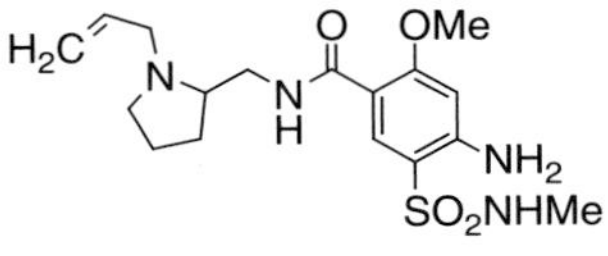

215 Alpiropride

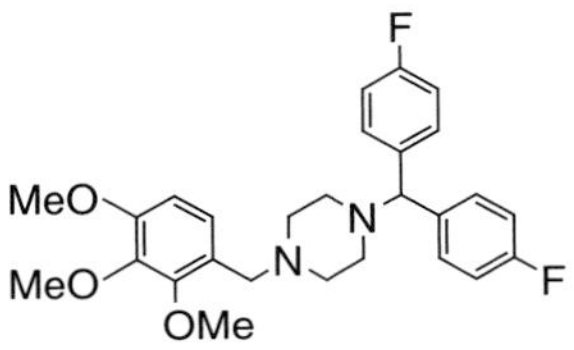

216 Lomerizine

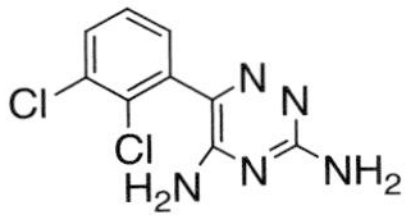

217 Lamotrigine

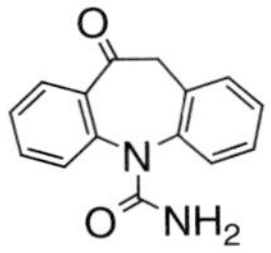

218 Oxcarbazepine

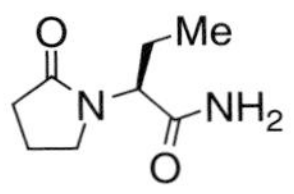

219 Levetiracetam

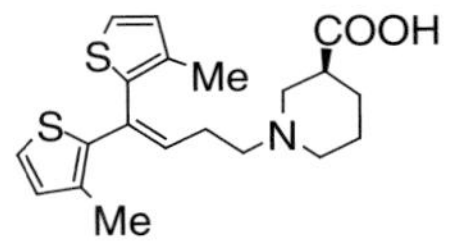

220 Tiagabine

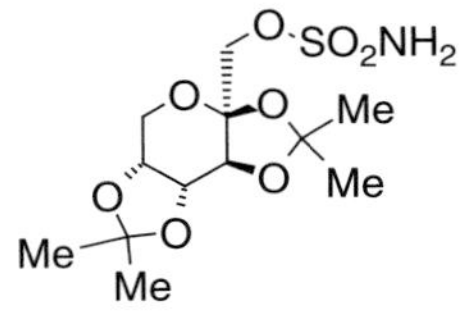

221 Topiramate

topiramate (**221**), felbamate and gabapentin are antiepileptic drugs on the market acting by somewhat different mechanisms.[341,342] Due to lack of effects on other uptake or receptor systems, tiagabine (inhibitor of GABA synaptosomal uptake) is expected to have a reduced potential for neurological side effects. In particular, it does not have benzodiazepine-like sedative effects. Topiramate appears to act by blocking voltage-sensitive sodium channels to raise the action potential threshold and block the spread of seizure, enhancing GABA activity at post-synaptic GABA receptors and reducing glutamate activity at post-synaptic AMPA-type receptors, and is also a carbonic anhydrase inhibitor. Anti-anxiety drugs are primarily based on benzodiazepine drugs like diazepam (**66**). Newer analogues include etizolam (thienodiazepine anxiolytic) and flutazolam (**222**), mexazolam, flutoprazepam and metaclazepam (all benzodiazepine anxiolytics). Several benzodiazepine and non-benzodiazepine hypnotic drugs [e.g. zopiclone, xolpidem (**223**), rilmazafone (**224**), cinolazepam, zeleplon (**225**)] are available for the treatment of sleep disorders. Alzheimer drugs on the market include reversible or irreversible inhibitors of acetylcholinesterase like donepezil (**11**), rivastigmin (**226**) and tacrine (**227**).[343–345] Although these drugs improve the symptoms of Alzheimer's disease, the underlying cause of the dementing process is not altered. The role of interferon-β as a disease-modifying drug for the treatment of relapsing–remitting multiple sclerosis is now

alpiropride (**215**) and a dual sodium and calcium channel blocker (especially a functional blocker of L-type voltage-sensitive calcium channels) lomerizine (**216**) are used for the treatment of migraine.

Vigabatrin (irreversible GABA aminotransferase inhibitor), zonisamide, lamotrigine (**217**) (glutamate inhibitor), oxcarbazepine (**218**), levetiracetam (**219**), piracetam, tiagabine (**220**),

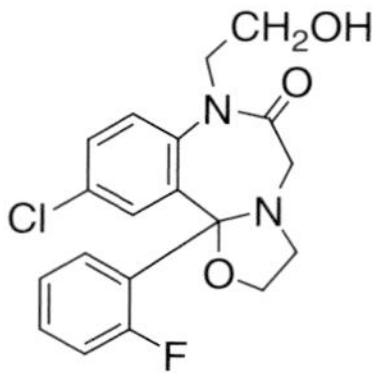

222 Flutazolam

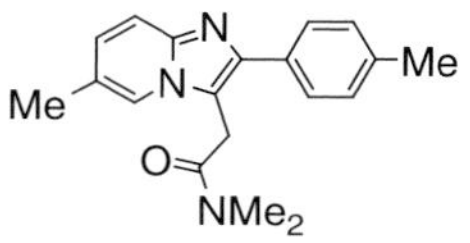

223 Xolpidem

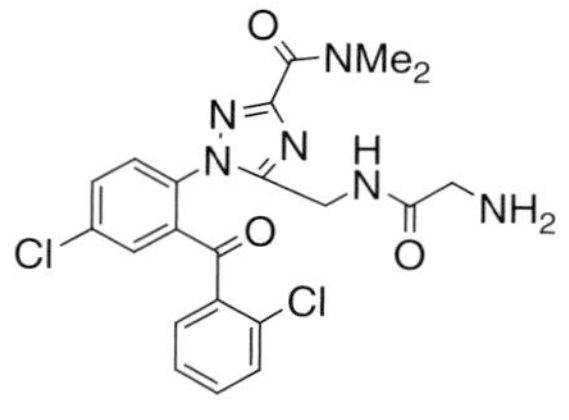

224 Rilmazafone

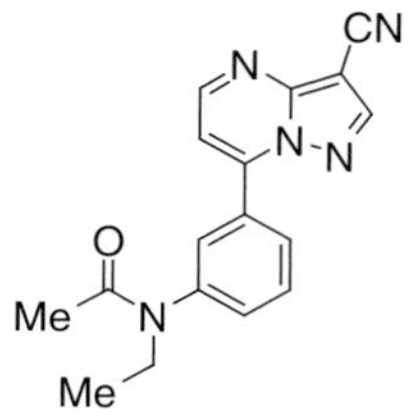

225 Zeleplon

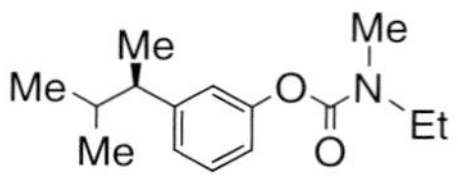

226 Rivastigmin

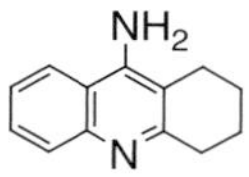

227 Tacrine

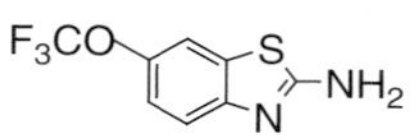

228 Riluzole

well established, and its efficacy has been demonstrated in large-scale clinical trials.[346] However, the drug is effective in a small population of patients. Other treatments of multiple sclerosis include glatiramer acetate (Copaxone).[347] The drug is a synthetic copolymer with an amino acid composition based on the structure of myelin basic protein, one of the autoantigens implicated in the pathogenesis of MS and experimental autoimmune encephalomyelitis. Some benefits in multiple sclerosis patients were observed with cannabis extract.[348] Riluzole (**228**), an antagonist of excitatory amino acids that blocks pre-synaptic release of glutamate and an antagonist of NMDA-induced acetylcholine release, is one of the drugs currently used for the treatment of motor neurone disease.[349]

In addition to the medicines mentioned above, a number of opiate- and non-opiate-based analgesics, including COX-2 inhibitors,[350–353] anaesthetics (e.g. propofol, desflurane, sevoflurane, ropivacaine, levobupivacaine and remifentanil), neuromuscular blockers (e.g. rocuronium bromid, zemuron, cisatracurium, doxacurium,

mivacurium chloride), attention deficit/hyperactivity disorder treatments (methylphenidate and dexmethylphenidate) are available and affective treatments for preventing and treating addiction are being developed.[354–356]

1.9.6 Inflammatory disorders (including arthritis, asthma and other allergic diseases)

Many steroidal and NSAIDs are in the market for use in various forms of rheumatoid and osteoarthritis and relief of pain associated with these conditions. Examples of non-steroidal anti-inflammatory agents include ibuprofen, dexibuprofen [(S)-isomer of ibuprofen], ketoprofen, laxoprofen, piketoprofen, pimaprofen, flunoxaprofen, indomethicin, tenoxicam, piroxicam (**229**), droxicam and ampiroxicam (both prodrugs of piroxicam) and aceclofenac (**230**). These agents have been associated with GI toxicity. The problem has been overcome to some extent with

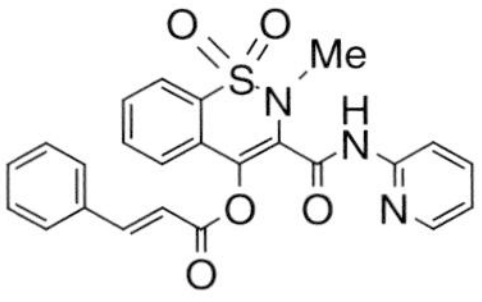

229 Piroxicam

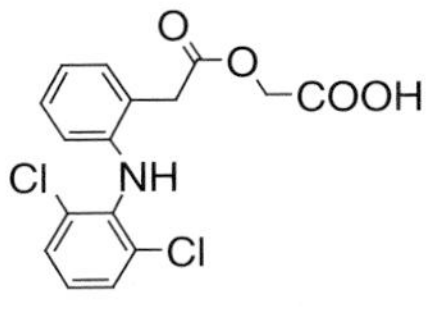

230 Aceclofenac

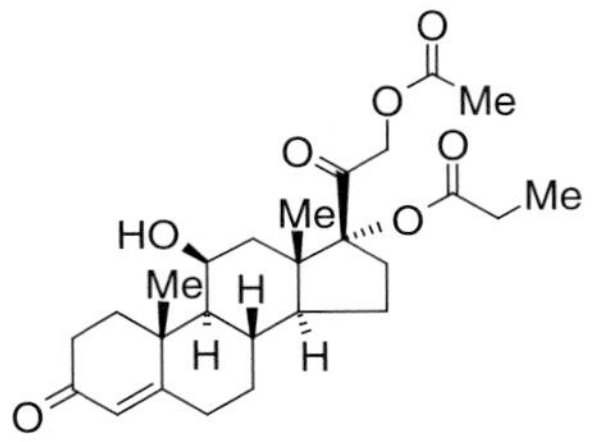

231 Hydrocortisone

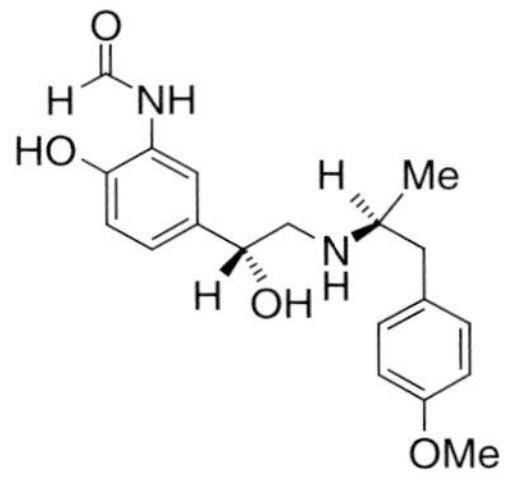

232 Formoterol

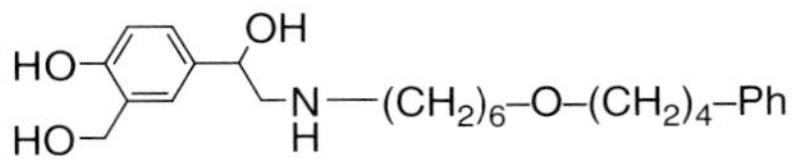

233 Salmeterol

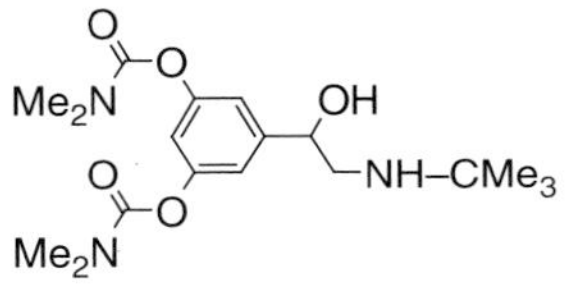

234 Bambuterol

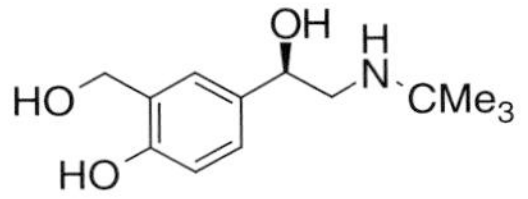

235 Levalbuterol

the discovery of selective COX-2 inhibitors like celecoxib (**1**), rofecoxib (**2**, recently withdrawn), parecoxib, valdecoxib (**3**) and etoricoxib, starting with the discovery of meloxicam.[357] Many topical steroidal anti-inflammatory agents like prednicarbamate, mometasone, hydrocortisone (**231**), halobetasol, deprodone, betamethasone are used for the treatment of cutaneous inflammatory disorders such as eczema and psoriasis, corticosteroid-responsive dermatoses and arthritis; inhaled steroids have been used for various allergic conditions including asthma and seasonal rhinitis. In addition to inhaled steroids, the most successful drugs for the treatment of asthma and chronic bronchitis include inhaled β_2-selective adrenergic agonists [e.g. formoterol (**232**), mabuterol, salmeterol (**233**), terbutaline and its prodrug bambuterol (**234**), salbutamol (**68**), levalbuterol (**235**) – acting as bronchodilators] and the newer, orally active leukotriene antagonists like montelukast (**12**) zafirlukast and pranlukast. Combinations of corticosteroids like budesonide and β_2-selective adrenergic agonists like formoterol are used

as bronchodilators for the treatment of asthma and chronic obstructive pulmonary disease in the form of various inhaler devices.[358] Antihistamines (inhibitors of histamine release or selective H_1-receptor antagonists) have been the most successful drugs for the treatment of various allergic conditions and many of the nonsedating H_1-receptor antagonists [e.g. cetrizine, levocetirizine (**236**), fexofenadine (**4**), loratadine (**237**), desloratadine, ebastine, levocabastine, olopatadine and betotastine] have become blockbuster drugs. Thromboxane receptor antagonists (e.g. seratrodast and ramatroban) and 5-lipoxygenase inhibitors (e.g. zileutron) have only made a limited impact.

In addition to the small molecular weight drugs, various antibodies (adalimumab, rituximab, omalizumab), a recombinant form of human IL-1-receptor antagonist (anakinra) and a recombinant fusion protein comprising the

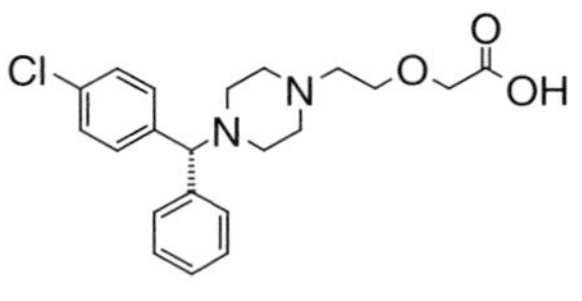

236 Levocetirizine

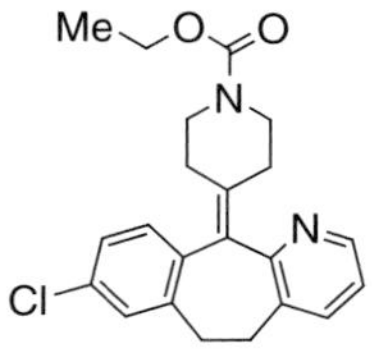

237 Loratadine

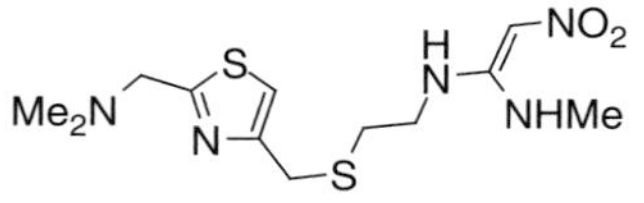

238 Nizatidine

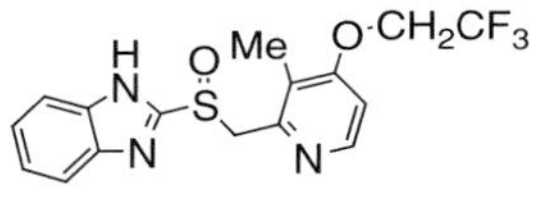

239 Lansoprazole

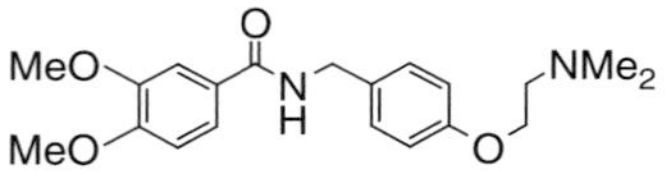

240 Itopride

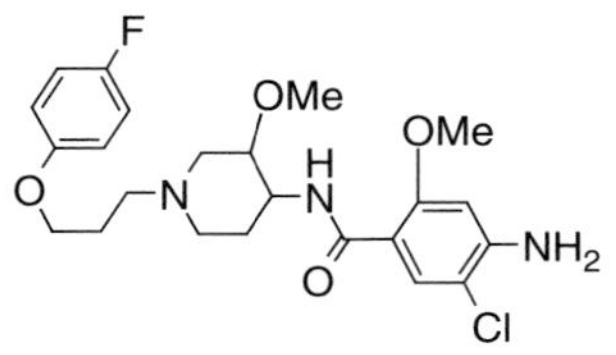

241 Cisapride

1.9.7 GI diseases

Major anti-ulcer drugs are either histamine (H_2) receptor antagonists [e.g. cimetidine, ranitidine (**5**), famotidine, roxatidine, lafutidine, ebrotidine and nizatidine (**238**)] or proton pump inhibitors [omeprazole, lansoprazole (**239**), pantoprazole, rabeprazole and esomeprazole (**6**)], which demonstrate selective inhibitory effect on the H^+, K^+-ATPase – an enzyme system involved at the secretory surface of the stomach's parietal cells responsible for the secretion of gastric acid. Currently, proton pump inhibitors are the main treatment for gastrooesophageal reflux disease.[367] Other marketed drugs for GI diseases include prostaglandin-based compounds, 5-HT$_4$ partial agonists like mosapride (**27**) for relief of GI symptoms in patients with gastritis, gastrooesophageal reflux, dyspepsia and tegaserod (**28**) for constipation-predominant irritable bowel syndrome[368] and dopamine D$_2$-receptor antagonists like itopride (**240**) and cinitapride (anti-ulcer agents), enkephalinase inhibitor (acetorphan, antidiarrhoeal – acting at the µ opiate receptor) and 5-HT$_3$ receptor antagonists like alosetron (**26**) (diarrhoea-predominant irritable bowel syndrome in women). Drugs like cisapride (**241**), used in the treatment of reflux oesophagitis, constipation and a variety of GI motility disorders, are thought to act by enhancing acetylcholine release in the mysenteric plexus of the gut. Mechanism of action of drugs like balsalazide (**242**), used for the treatment of mild to moderate attacks of ulcerative colitis, is not clearly understood but the drug is cytoprotective and has anti-inflammatory properties. An anti-TNF-α antibody infliximab has been introduced recently for the treatment of Crohn's disease.[369,370] Other drugs

soluble human p75 TNF receptor linked to the Fc portion of human IgG1 (enbrel) have become available recently (see Section 1.7 for protein and antibody products) for the treatment of rheumatoid arthritis.[280,359–362] These agents are usually compared with methotrexate in clinical trials. Signal transduction pathways involved in inflammation, including mitogen-activated protein kinases, nuclear factor-kappa B (NF-κB), Janus kinases, are currently being studied to identify new targets for rheumatoid and osteoarthritis.[363–365] Orally bioavailable inhibitors of the mitogen-activated protein kinase and NF-κB pathways have been designed and are currently being evaluated.[366]

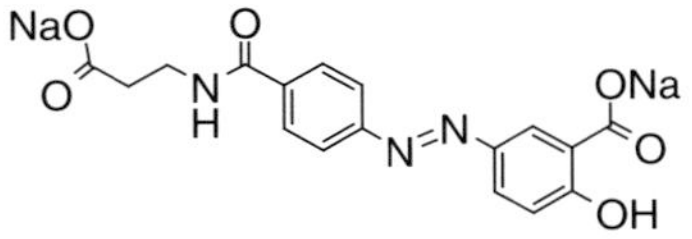

242 Balsalazide

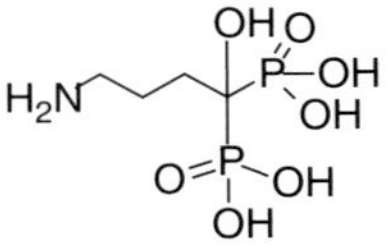

243 Alendonate

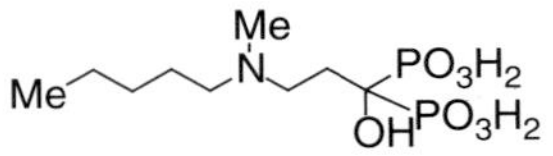

244 Ibandronic acid

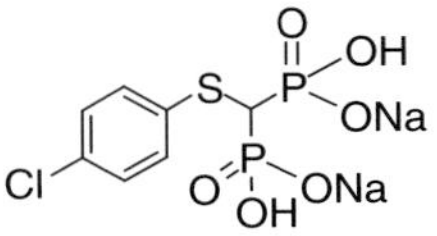

245 Tiludronate

indicated for the treatment of Crohn's disease include budesonide, sulphasalazine, methotrexate, 6-mercaptopruine, azathioprine, mycophenolate mofetil (inhibitor of type 2 inosine monophosphate dehydrogenase), tacrolimus (calcineurin inhibitor), leflunomide. Antibodies like CDP-571 (recombinant humanised monoclonal antibody directed against TNF-α), CDP-870 (completely humanised anti-TNF-α Fab fragment that is linked to a polyethylene glycol molecule), onercept (human, genetically engineered, recombinant TNF p55 receptor monomer), adalimumab (recombinant fully human IgG1 monoclonal antibody directed against TNF-α) and natalizumab (recombinant IgG4 humanised monoclonal antibody) are in the late stages of clinical trials.[370]

1.9.8 Bone disorders

Except for some of the earlier drugs like calcitonin, most of the newer agents are bisphosphonates (bone resorption inhibitors – presumably reducing the bone resorption of calcium by inhibiting the formation and attachment of osteoclasts) that are used for the treatment of Paget's disease, hypercalcaemia of malignancy and osteoporosis. Examples of some of the recently launched bisphosphonates include alendonate (**243**), ibandronic acid (**244**), incadronic acid, risedronate, zoledronate and tiludronate (**245**). These agents bind tightly to hydroxyapatite crystals and are retained on resorption surfaces. Local release of bisphosphonates occurs by acidification during the process of bone resorption to impair the osteoclasts' ability to resorb bone. In addition to their use in osteoporosis, bisphosphonates are also expected to be useful in the treatment of bone tumours.[371] Only recently, a selective oestrogen receptor modulator raloxifene (**74**) has been marketed

for prevention of postmenopausal osteoporosis. Recombinant human parathyroid hormone 1–34 is also approved for the treatment of osteoporosis. The parathyroid hormone treatment works by stimulating bone formation on all bone surfaces.

1.10   Summary

Drug discovery has been a continuously changing and evolving field of science over the years due to changing disease patterns, drug requirements and new targets and technologies.[372] More and more effective and safer treatments have been discovered. Although chemical and biological sciences have always played a major role in the discovery process, new scientific developments and technologies are altering the ways in which these sciences are applied to the discovery process. Advances in rapid DNA sequencing techniques have resulted in the discovery of the human genome sequence. Finding the disease-related genes, translating the gene sequences into biologically active proteins and evaluating their functions is likely to lead to new drug discovery targets based on new biochemical pathways. The genomic and proteomic studies may also lead to new therapeutic proteins and antibodies. Given the therapeutic success of the interferons, erythropoietin, GCSF, herceptin (trastuzumab), rituximab and many others, protein drugs are likely to make many additional therapeutic contributions.

Combinatorial library techniques and natural product libraries are providing large numbers of new compounds for screening. Automated high-throughput screening techniques are being developed continuously to test large numbers of available compounds in multiple screens. A combination of these two technologies along with the discovery of new target proteins (receptors, enzymes, etc.) has the potential to generate leads for various drug discovery programmes. However, before the leads can be taken seriously, it is essential to appropriately validate the target. Otherwise, the optimised leads are likely to fail in the later stages of development. In many cases where some treatments exist along with some knowledge about the causes of the disease, the need for the target validation and development of the relevant biological models is less stringent. The discovery of new medicines in these fields becomes a continuous process of identifying medicines that are more efficacious and convenient to administer in a larger number of patients and display the best possible toxicity profile.

The availability of leads along with advances in multiple parallel solid-phase synthetic and purification techniques would enable the lead optimisation procedure to be carried out in a relatively short period of time. The design strategies for lead optimisation are likely to be a combination of the types of approaches highlighted in the examples mentioned above. Structure–activity studies along with structural and modelling studies using cloned proteins (receptors, enzymes, etc.) are likely to make the lead optimisation procedure somewhat more rational. Availability of cloned receptor subtypes and various members of the enzyme classes in the early stages of the programme can be used to build selectivity in the receptor ligands and enzyme inhibitors. Better understanding of the signalling processes will enable the cellular processes to be controlled in a more efficient manner.

References

1. Myles DC. Novel biologically active natural and unnatural products. *Curr Opin Biotechnol* 2003;**14**:627–33.
2. Francois C, Hance AJ. Medical progress: HIV drug resistance. *N Engl J Med* 2004;**350**:1023–35.
3. Lee LM, Henderson DK. Emerging viral infections. *Curr Opin Infect Dis* 2001;**14**:467–80.
4. Crowley VEF, Yeo GSH, O'Rahilly S. Obesity therapy: altering the energy intake-and-expenditure balance sheet. *Nat. Rev Drug Discov* 2002;**1**: 276–86.
5. Clapham JC, Arch JRS, Tadayyon M. Anti-obesity drugs: a critical review of current therapies and future opportunities. *Pharmacol Ther* 2001;**89**:81–121.
6. Bray GA, Tartaglia LA. Medicinal strategies in the treatment of obesity. *Nature* 2000;**404**:672–7.
7. Flower R. Lifestyle drugs: pharmacology and the social agenda. *Trends Pharmacol Sci* 2004;**25**: 182–5.
8. Maitland K, Bejon P, Newton CRJC. Malaria. *Curr Opin Infect Dis* 2003;**16**:389–95.
9. Wiesner J, Ortmann R, Jomaa H, *et al*. New antimalarial drugs. *Angew Chem Int Ed Engl* 2003;**42**: 5274–93.
10. Moorthy VS, Good MF, Hill AVS. Malaria vaccine developments. *Lancet* 2004;**363**:150–156.
11. Blandin S, Levashina EA. Mosquito immune responses against malaria parasites. *Curr Opin Immunol* 2004;**16**:16–20.
12. Frieden TR, Sterling TR, Munsiff SS, *et al*. Tuberculosis. *Lancet* 2003;**362**:887–99.
13. Bames PF, Donald CM. Molecular epidemiology of tuberculosis. *N Engl J Med* 2003;**349**: 1149–56.
14. Britton WJ, Lockwood NJ. Leprosy. *Lancet* 2004;**363**: 1209–19.
15. Espinal MA, Laszlo A, Simonsen L, *et al*. Global trends in resistance to antituberculosis drugs. *N Engl J Med* 2001;**344**:1294–303.
16. Smolen JS, Steiner G. Therapeutic strategies for rheumatoid arthritis. *Nat Rev Drug Discov* 2003;**2**:473–88.
17. Goltzman D. Discoveries, drugs and skeletal disorders. *Nat Rev Drug Discov* 2002;**1**:784–96.

18. Henry G, Hosking D, Devogelaer J-P, *et al*. Ten years' experience with alendronate for osteoporosis in postmenopausal women. *N Engl J Med* 2004;**350**:1189–99.

19. Cochrane DJ, Jarvis B, Keating GM. Etoricoxib. *Drugs* 2002;**62**:2637–61.

20. Fenton C, Keating GM, Wagstaff AJ. Valdecoxib. *Drugs* 2004;**64**:1231–61.

21. Flower RJ. The development of COX-2 inhibitors. *Nat Rev Drug Discov* 2003;**2**:179–91.

22. FitzGerald GA. COX-2 and beyond: approaches to prostaglandin inhibition in human disease. *Nat Rev Drug Discov* 2003;**2**:879–90.

23. Stichtenoth DO, Frolich JC. The second generation of COX-2 inhibitors. What advantage do the newest offer? *Drugs* 2003;**63**:33–45.

24. Kurumbail RG, Kiefer JR, Marnett LJ. Cyclooxygenase enzymes: catalysis and inhibition. *Curr Opin Struct Biol* 2001;**11**:752–60.

25. Gupta RA, DuBois RN. Colorectal cancer prevention and treatment by inhibition of cyclooxygenase-2. *Nat Rev Cancer* 2001;**1**:11–21.

26. Dutta AS. Discovery of new medicines. In: Griffin JP, O'Grady J, eds. *Textbook of Pharmaceutical Medicine, 4th edn*. London: BMJ Books, 2002; 3–95.

27. Drews J. Drug discovery: a historical perspective. *Science* 2000;**287**:1960–64.

28. Olbe L, Carlsson E, Lindberg P. A proton-pump inhibitor expedition: the case histories of omeprazole and esomeprazole. *Nat Rev Drug Discov* 2003;**2**:132–9.

29. Dekel R, Morse C, Fass R. The role of proton pump inhibitors in gastro-oesophageal reflux disease. *Drugs* 2004;**64**:277–95.

30. Gillies PS, Dunn CJ. Pioglitazone. *Drugs* 2000;**60**: 333–43.

31. Clader JW. The discovery of ezetimibe: a view from outside the receptor. *J Med Chem* 2004; **47**:1–9.

32. Varghese JN. Development of neuraminidase inhibitors as anti-influenza virus drugs. *Drug Dev Res* 1999;**46**:176–96.

33. Langtry HD, Markham A. Sildenafil. *Drugs* 1999;**57**:967–89.

34. Tulp M, Bohlin L. Functional versus chemical diversity: is biodiversity important for drug discovery? *Trends Pharmacol Sci* 2002;**23**:225–31.

35. George SR, O'Dowd BF, Lee SP. G-protein-coupled receptor oligomerization and its potential for drug discovery. *Nat Rev Drug Discov* 2002;**1**: 808–20.

36. Pearce KH, Iannone MA, Simmons CA, *et al*. Discovery of novel nuclear receptor modulating ligands: an integral role for peptide interaction profiling. *Drug Discov Today* 2004;**9**:741–51.

37. Soudijn W, Wijngaarden IV, Ijzerman AP. Allosteric modulation of G protein-coupled receptors: perspectives and recent developments. *Drug Discov Today* 2004;**9**:752–8.

38. Kristiansen K. Molecular mechanisms of ligand binding, signalling, and regulation within the superfamily of G-protein-coupled receptors: molecular modeling and mutagenesis approaches to receptor structure and function. *Pharmacol Ther* 2004;**103**:21–80.

39. Hoyer D, Clarke DE, Fozard JR, *et al*. International union of pharmacology classification of receptors for 5-hydroxytryptamine (serotonin). *Pharmacol Rev* 1994;**46**:157–203.

40. Langlois M, Fischmeister R. 5-HT$_4$ receptor ligands: applications and new prospects. *J Med Chem* 2003;**46**:319–41.

41. Glennon RA. Higher-end serotonin receptors: 5-HT$_5$, 5-HT$_6$ and 5-HT$_7$. *J Med Chem* 2003;**46**: 2795–812.

42. Hedlund PB, Sutcliffe JG. Functional, molecular and pharmacological advances in 5-HT$_7$ receptor research. *Trends Pharmacol Sci* 2004;**25**:481–6.

43. Swainston T, Perry CM. Aripiprazole: a review of its use in schizophrenia and schizoaffective disorder. *Drugs* 2004;**64**:1715–36.

44. Witkin JM, Nelson DL. Selective histamine H$_3$ receptor antagonists for treatment of cognitive deficiencies and other disorders of the central nervous system. *Pharmacol Ther* 2004;**103**: 1–20.

45. Jablonowski JA, Grice CA, Chai W, *et al*. The first potent and selective non-imidazole human histamine H$_4$ receptor antagonist. *J Med Chem* 2003;**46**:3957–60.

46. Kitbunnadaj R, Zuiderveld OP, Christophe B, *et al*. Identification of 4-(1H-imidazol-4(5)-ylmethyl) pyridine (immethridine) as a novel, potent, and highly selective histamine H(3) receptor agonist. *J Med Chem* 2004;**47**:2414–17.

47. Wikberg JES. Melanocortin receptors: perspectives for novel drugs. *Eur J Pharmacol* 1999;**375**: 295–310.

48. Herpin TF, Yu G, Carlson KE, *et al*. Discovery of tyrosine-based potent and selective melanocortin-1 receptor small-molecule agonists with anti-inflammatory properties, *J Med Chem* 2003;**46**:1123–26.

49. Richardson TI, Ornstein PL, Briner K, *et al.* Synthesis and structure–activity relationships of novel arylpiperazines as potent and selective agonists of the melanocortin subtype-4 receptor. *J Med Chem* 2004;**47**:744–55.

50. Souers AJ, Virgillo AA, Rosenquist A, *et al.* Identification of a potent heterocyclic ligand to somatostatin receptor subtype-5 by the synthesis and screening of β-turn mimetic libraries. *J Am Chem Soc* 1999;**121**:1817–25.

51. Rohrer SP, Birzin ET, Mosley RT, *et al.* Rapid identification of subtype-selective agonists of the somatostatin receptor through combinatorial chemistry. *Science* 1998;**282**:737–40.

52. Weckbecker G, Lewis I, Albert R, *et al.* Opportunities in somatostatin research: biological, chemical and therapeutic aspects. *Nat Rev Drug Discov* 2003;**2**:999–1017.

53. Stadel JM, Wilson S, Bergsma DJ. Orphan G-protein-coupled receptors: a neglected opportunity for pioneer drug discovery. *Trends Pharmacol Sci* 1997;**18**:430–7.

54. Wilson S, Bergsma DJ, Chambers JK, *et al.* Orphan G-protein-coupled receptors – the next generation of drug targets. *Br J Pharmacol* 1998;**125**:1387–92.

55. McCormack MP, Rabbitts TH. Mechanisms of disease: activation of the T-cell oncogene LMO2 after gene therapy for X-linked severe combined immunodeficiency. *N Engl J Med* 2004;**350**:913–22.

56. Mhashilkar A, Chada S, Roth JA, *et al.* Gene therapy: therapeutic approaches and implications. *Biotechnol Adv* 2001;**19**:279–97.

57. Zhang YC, Atkinson MA. Gene therapy for type 1 diabetes: metabolism, immunity, islet cell preservation, and regeneration. *Curr Opin Endocrinol Diabetes* 2004;**11**:91–7.

58. Chan L, Fujimiya M, Kojima H. *In vivo* gene therapy for diabetes mellitus. *Trends Mol Med* 2003;**9**:430–5.

59. Wu L, Johnson M, Sato M. Transcriptionally targeted gene therapy to detect and treat cancer. *Trends Mol Med* 2003;**9**:421–9.

60. Lusis AJ. Genetic factors in cardiovascular disease, 10 questions. *Trends Cardiovasc Med* 2003;**13**:309–16.

61. Nelson KE, Paulsen IT, Heidelberg JF, *et al.* Status of genome projects for non-pathogenic bacteria and archaea. *Nat Biotechnol* 2000;**18**:1049–54.

62. Noble D. Will genomics revolutionise pharmaceutical R&D? *Trends Biotechnol* 2003;**21**:333–7.

63. Lander ES, Linton LM, Birren B, *et al.* Initial sequencing and analysis of the human genome, International human genome sequencing consortium. *Nature* 2001;**409**:860–921.

64. Venter JC, Adams MD, Myers EW, *et al.* The sequence of the human genome. *Science* 2001;**291**:1304–51.

65. Perna NT, Plunkett III G, Burland V, *et al.* Genome sequence of enterohaemorrhagic *Escherichia coli* O157:H7. *Nature* 2001;**409**:529–33.

66. Rosamond J, Allsop A. Harnessing the power of the genome in the search for new antibiotics. *Science* 2000;**287**:1973–76.

67. Beeley LJ, Duckworth M, Southan C. The impact of genomics on drug discovery. *Prog Med Chem* 2000;**37**:1–43.

68. Pennisi E. Rat genome off to an early start. *Science* 2000;**289**:1267–9.

69. Prosser H, Rastan S. Manipulation of the mouse genome: a multiple impact resource for drug discovery and development. *Trends Biotechnol* 2003;**21**:224–32.

70. Karlin S, Mrázek J, Gentles AJ. Genome comparisons and analysis. *Curr Opin Struct Biol* 2003;**13**:344–52.

71. Walther W, Stein U. Viral vectors for gene transfer: a review of their use in the treatment of human diseases. *Drugs* 2000;**60**:249–71.

72. Kay MA, Glorioso JC, Naldini L. Viral vectors for gene therapy: the art of turning infectious agents into vehicles of therapeutics. *Nat Med* 2001;**7**:33–40.

73. McTaggart S, Al-Rubeai M. Retroviral vectors for human gene delivery. *Biotechnol Adv* 2002;**20**:1–31.

74. Irvine AS, Trinder PKE, Laughton DL, *et al.* Efficient nonviral transfection of dendritic cells and their use for *in vivo* immunisation. *Nat Biotechnol* 2000;**18**:1273–8.

75. Gariepy J, Kawamura K. Vectorial delivery of macromolecules into cells using peptide-based vehicles. *Trends Biotechnol* 2001;**19**:21–8.

76. Rudolf U, Mohler H. Genetically modified animals in pharmacological research: future trends. *Eur J Pharmacol* 1999;**375**:327–37.

77. Zambrowicz BP, Turner CA, Sands AT. Predicting drug efficacy: knockouts model pipeline drugs of the pharmaceutical industry. *Curr Opin Pharmacol* 2003;**3**:563–70.

78. Zambrowicz BP, Sands AT. Knockouts model the 100 best-selling drugs – will they model the next 100? *Nat Rev Drug Discov* 2003;**2**:38–51.

79. Johnson JA. Pharmacogenetics: potential for individualized drug therapy through genetics. *Trends Genet* 2003;**19**:660–6.

80. McCarthy JM, Hilfiker R. The use of single-nucleotide polymorphism maps in pharmacogenomics. *Nat Biotechnol* 2000;**18**:505–8.

81. Suter L, Babiss LE, Wheeldon EB. Toxicogenomics in predictive toxicology in drug development. *Chem Biol* 2004;**11**:161–71.

82. Blackstock WP, Weir MP. Proteomics: quantitative and physical mapping of cellular proteins. *Trends Biotechnol* 1999;**17**:121–7.

83. Wang JH, Hewick RM. Proteomics in drug discovery. *Drug Discov Today* 1999;**4**:129–33.

84. Walgren JL, Thompson DC. Application of proteomic technologies in the drug development process. *Toxicol Lett* 2004;**149**:377–85.

85. Campbell SJ, Gold ND, Jackson RM, *et al.* Ligand binding: functional site location, similarity and docking. *Curr Opin Struct Biol* 2003;**13**:389–95.

86. Kinoshita K, Nakamura H. Protein informatics towards function identification. *Curr Opin Struct Biol* 2003;**13**:396–400.

87. Mayer TU. Chemical genetics: tailoring tools for cell biology. *Trends Cell Biol* 2003;**13**:270–7.

88. Jeffery DA, Bogyo M. Chemical proteomics and its application to drug discovery. *Curr Opin Biotechnol* 2003;**14**:87–95.

89. Marcotte EM. Computational genetics: finding protein function by nonhomology methods. *Curr Opin Struct Biol* 2000;**10**:359–65.

90. Qureshi EA, Cagney G. Large-scale functional analysis using peptide or protein arrays. *Nat Biotechnol* 2000;**18**:393–7.

91. Skolnick J, Fetrow JS, Kolinski A. Structural genomics and its importance for gene function analysis. *Nat Biotechnol* 2000;**18**:283–7.

92. Moult J, Melamud E. From fold to function. *Curr Opin Struct Biol* 2000;**10**:384–9.

93. Jones DT. Protein structure prediction in the postgenomic era. *Curr Opin Struct Biol* 2000;**10**:371–9.

94. Man O, Atarot T, Sadot A, *et al.* From subgenome analysis to protein structure. *Curr Opin Struct Biol* 2003;**13**:353–8.

95. Sali A, Kuriyan J. Challenges at the frontiers of structural biology. *Trends Cell Biol* 2000;**9**:M20–4.

96. Jeffery CJ. Moonlighting proteins: old proteins learning new tricks. *Trends Genet* 2003;**19**:415–17.

97. Johnstone RW, Ruefli AA, Smyth MJ. Multiple physiological functions for multidrug transporter P-glycoprotein. *Trends Biochem Sci* 2000;**25**:1–6.

98. Andrade MA, Sander C. Bioinformatics: from genome data to biological knowledge. *Curr Opin Biotechnol* 1997;**8**:675–83.

99. Geysen HM, Schoenen F, Wagner D, *et al.* Combinatorial compound libraries for drug discovery: an ongoing challenge. *Nat Rev Drug Discov* 2003;**2**:222–30.

100. Weaver DC. Applying data mining techniques to library design, lead generation and lead optimisation. *Curr Opin Chem Biol* 2004;**8**:264–70.

101. Lavastre O, Bonnette F, Gallard L. Parallel and combinatorial approaches for synthesis of ligands. *Curr Opin Chem Biol* 2004;**8**:311–18.

102. Di L, Kerns EH. Profiling drug-like properties in drug discovery. *Curr Opin Chem Biol* 2003;**7**:402–8.

103. Hann MM, Oprea TI. Pursuing the leadlikeness concept in pharmaceutical research. *Curr Opin Chem Biol* 2004;**8**:255–63.

104. Boldi AM. Libraries from natural product-like scaffolds. *Curr Opin Chem Biol* 2004;**8**:281–6.

105. Ortholand J-Y, Ganesan A. Natural products and combinatorial chemistry: back to the future. *Curr Opin Chem Biol* 2004;**8**:271–80.

106. Michels PC, Khmelnitsky YL, Dordick JS, *et al.* Combinatorial biocatalysis: a natural approach to drug discovery. *Trends Biotechnol* 1998;**16**:210–15.

107. Dolle RE. Comprehensive survey of chemical libraries yielding enzyme inhibitors, receptor agonists and antagonists, and other biologically active agents: 1992 through 1997. *Mol Divers* 1998;**3**:199–233.

108. Backes BJ, Harris JL, Leonetti F, *et al.* Synthesis of positional-scanning libraries of fluorogenic peptide substrates to define the extended substrate specificity of plasmin and thrombin. *Nat Biotechnol* 2000;**18**:187–93.

109. Walters WP, Ajay, Murcko MA. Recognising molecules with drug-like properties. *Curr Opin Chem Biol* 1999;**3**:384–7.

110. Lipinski CA, Lombardo F, Dominy BW, *et al.* Experimental and computational approaches to estimate solubility and permeability in drug discovery and development settings. *Adv Drug Deliv Rev* 1997;**23**:3–25.

111. Rishton GM. Reactive compounds and *in vitro* false positives in HTS. *Drug Discov Today* 1997;**2**:382–5.

112. Golebiowski A, Klopfenstein SR, Portlock DE. Lead compounds discovered from libraries. *Curr Opin Chem Biol* 2001;**5**:273–84.

113. Golebiowski A, Klopfenstein SR, Portlock DE. Lead compounds discovered from libraries: part 2. *Curr Opin Chem Biol* 2003;**7**:308–25.

114. Anderson AC. The process of structure-based drug design. *Chem Biol* 2003;**10**:787–97.

115. Joseph-McCarthy D. Computational approaches to structure-based ligand design. *Pharmacol Ther* 1999;**84**:179–91.

116. Ooms F. Molecular modelling and computer aided drug design. Examples of their application in medicinal chemistry. *Curr Med Chem* 2000;**7**:141–58.

117. Erlanson DA, McDowell RS, O'Brien T. Fragment-based drug discovery. *J Med Chem* 2004;**47**:3463–82.

118. Walters WP, Stahl MT, Murcko MA. Virtual screening – an overview. *Drug Discov Today* 1998;**3**:160–78.

119. Homans SW. NMR spectroscopy tools for structure-aided drug design. *Angew Chem Int Ed Engl* 2004;**43**:290–300.

120. Kuhn P, Wilson K, Patch MG, *et al.* The genesis of high-throughput structure-based drug discovery using protein crystallography. *Curr Opin Chem Biol* 2002;**6**:704–10.

121. Moore JM. NMR techniques for characterisation of ligand binding: utility for lead generation and optimisation in drug discovery. *Biopolymers (Pept Sci)* 1999;**51**:221–43.

122. Shuker SB, Hajduk PJ, Meadows RP, *et al.* Discovering high affinity ligands for proteins: SAR by NMR. *Science* 1996;**274**:1531–4.

123. Fejzo J, Lepre CA, Peng JW, *et al.* The SHAPES strategy: an NMR-based approach for lead generation in drug discovery. *Chem Biol* 1999;**6**:755–69.

124. Nienaber VL, Richardson PL, Klighofer V, *et al.* Discovering novel ligands for macromolecules using X-ray crystallographic screening. *Nat Biotechnol* 2000;**18**:1105–8.

125. Eddershaw PJ, Beresford AP, Bayliss MK. ADME/PK as part of a rational approach to drug discovery. *Drug Discov Today* 2000;**5**:409–14.

126. Kassel, DB. Applications of high-throughput ADME in drug discovery. *Curr Opin Chem Biol* 2004;**8**:339–45.

127. Rudin M. Molecular imaging in drug discovery and development. *Nat Rev Drug Discov* 2003;**2**:123–31.

128. Ugurbil K, Toth L, Kim D-S. How accurate is magnetic resonance imaging of brain function? *Trends Neurosci* 2003;**26**:108–14.

129. Hakumaki JM, Brindle KM. Techniques: visualizing apoptosis using nuclear magnetic resonance. *Trends Pharmacol Sci* 2003;**24**:146–9.

130. Gilman S. Medical progress: imaging the brain. *N Engl J Med* 1998;**338**:812–20, 889–98.

131. Wiebe LI. PET radiopharmaceuticals for metabolic imaging in oncology. *Inter Cong Ser* 2004;**1264**:53–76.

132. Aboagye EO, Price PM, Jones T. *In vivo* pharmacokinetics and pharmacodynamics in drug development using positron-emission tomography. *Drug Discov Today* 2001;**6**:293–302.

133. van Tinteren H, Hoekstra OS, Smit EF, *et al.* Effectiveness of positron emission tomography in the preoperative assessment of patients with suspected non-small-cell lung cancer: the PLUS multicentre randomised trial. *Lancet* 2002;**359**:1388–92.

134. Flamen P. Positron emission tomography in gastric and esophageal cancer. *Curr Opin Oncol* 2004;**16**:359–63.

135. Contag PR. Whole-animal cellular and molecular imaging to accelerate drug development. *Drug Discov Today* 2002;**7**:555–62.

136. Herschman HR. Micro-PET imaging and small animal models of disease. *Curr Opin Immunol* 2003;**15**:378–84.

137. Rees J. Advances in magnetic resonance imaging of brain tumours. *Curr Opin Neurol* 2003;**16**:643–50.

138. Honey G, Bullmore E. Human pharmacological MRI. *Trends Pharmacol Sci* 2004;**25**:366–74.

139. Dutta AS. *Small Peptides: Chemistry, Biology and Clinical Studies.* Amsterdam: Elsevier Science Publishers, 1993.

140. Dutta AS. Design and therapeutic potential of peptides. *Adv Drug Res* 1991;**21**:145–286.

141. Jordan VC. Antiestrogens and selective estrogen receptor modulators as multifunctional medicines. 1. Receptor interactions. *J Med Chem* 2003;**46**:883–908.

142. Jordan VC. Antiestrogens and selective estrogen receptor modulators as multifunctional medicines. 2. Clinical considerations and new agents. *J Med Chem* 2003;**46**:1081–100.

143. Jordan VC. Tamoxifen: a most unlikely pioneering medicine. *Nat Rev Drug Discov* 2003;**2**:205–13.

144. Watanabe N, Ikeno A, Minato H, *et al.* Discovery and preclinical characterisation of (+)-3-[4-(1-piperidinoethoxy)phenyl]spiro[indene-1,1'-indane]-5,5'-diol hydrochloride: a promising non-steroidal estrogen receptor agonist for hot flush. *J Med Chem* 2003;**46**:3961–4.

145. Johnston SRD, Dowsett M. Aromatase inhibitors for breast cancer: lessons from the laboratory. *Nat Rev Cancer* 2003;**3**:821–31.

146. Dutta AS. Luteinizing hormone-releasing hormone (LHRH) agonists. *Drugs Future* 1988;**13**:43–57.

147. Dutta AS. Luteinizing hormone-releasing hormone (LHRH) antagonists. *Drugs Future* 1988;**13**:761–87.

148. Dutta AS, Furr BJA, Hutchinson FG. The discovery and development of goserelin (Zoladex). *Pharma Med* 1993;**7**:9–28.

149. Dutta AS. Goserelin. *Drugs Today* 1987;**23**:545–51.

150. Weckbecker G, Lewis I, Albert R, *et al.* Opportunities in somatostatin research: biological, chemical and therapeutic aspects. *Nat Rev Drug Discov* 2003;**2**:999–1017.

151. Culler MD. Evolving concepts in the quest for advanced therapeutic analogues of somatostatin. *Dig Liver Dis* 2004;**36**(Supplement 1):S17–25.

152. Dasgupta P. Somatostatin analogues: multiple roles in cellular proliferation, neoplasia, and angiogenesis. *Pharmacol Ther* 2004;**102**:61–85.

153. Lamberts SWJ, van der Lely A-J, de Herder WW, *et al.* Drug therapy: octreotide. *N Engl J Med* 1996;**334**:246–54.

154. Zaman MA, Oparil S, Calhoun DA. Drugs targeting the renin–angiotensin–aldosterone system. *Nat Rev Drug Discov* 2002;**1**:621–36.

155. Schmidt B, Schieffer B. Angiotensin II AT1 receptor antagonists. Clinical implications of active metabolites. *J Med Chem* 2003;**46**:2261–70.

156. Moody TW, Jensen RT. Bombesin receptor antagonists. *Drugs Future* 1998;**23**:1305–15.

157. Meini S, Cucchi P, Bellucci F, *et al.* Site-directed mutagenesis at the human B_2 receptor and molecular modelling to define the pharmacophore of non-peptide bradykinin receptor antagonists. *Biochem Pharmacol* 2004;**67**:601–9.

158. Sawada Y, Kayakiri H, Abe Y, *et al.* A new class of nonpeptide bradykinin B2 receptor ligands, incorporating a 4-aminoquinoline framework. Identification of a key pharmacophore to determine species difference and agonist/antagonist profile. *J Med Chem* 2004;**47**:2667–77.

159. Herranz R. Cholecystokinin antagonists: pharmacological and therapeutic potential. *Med Res Rev* 2003;**23**:559–605.

160. Masaki T. Historical review: endothelin. *Trends Pharmacol Sci* 2004;**25**:219–24.

161. D'Orléans-Juste P, Labonte J, Bkaily G, *et al.* Function of the endothelin(B) receptor in cardiovascular physiology and pathophysiology. *Pharmacol Ther* 2002;**95**:221–38.

162. Ertl G. Endothelin receptor antagonists in heart failure. *Drugs* 2004;**64**:1029–40.

163. Remuzzi G, Perico N, Benigni A. New therapeutics that antagonise endothelin: promises and frustrations. *Nat Rev Drug Discov* 2002;**1**:986–1001.

164. Wu C, Decker ER, Blok N, *et al.* Discovery, modelling, and human pharmacokinetics of N-(2-acetyl-4,6-dimethylphenyl)-3-(3,4-dimethylisoxazol-5-ylsulfamoyl)-thiophene- 2-carboxamide (TBC3711), a second generation, ETA selective, and orally bioavailable endothelin antagonist. *J Med Chem* 2004;**47**:1969–86.

165. Vellard M. The enzyme as drug: application of enzymes as pharmaceuticals. *Curr Opin Biotechnol* 2003;**14**:444–50.

166. Schellinger PD, Kaste M, Hacke W. An update on thrombolytic therapy for acute stroke. *Curr Opin Neurol* 2004;**17**:69–77.

167. Banerjee A, Chisti Y, Banerjee UC. Streptokinase – a clinically useful thrombolytic agent. *Biotechnol Adv* 2004;**22**:287–307.

168. The ATLANTIS, ECASS and NINDS rt-PA Study Group Investigators. Association of outcome with early stroke treatment: pooled analysis of ATLANTIS, ECASS, and NINDS rt-PA stroke trials. *Lancet* 2004;**363**:768–74.

169. Benchenane K, López-Atalaya J-P, Fernández-Monreal M, *et al.* Equivocal roles of tissue-type plasminogen activator in stroke-induced injury. *Trends Neurosci* 2004;**27**:155–60.

170. Toombs CF. New directions in thrombolytic therapy. *Curr Opin Pharmacol* 2001;**1**:164–8.

171. Acharya KR, Sturrock ED, Riordan JF, *et al.* ACE revisited: a new target for structure-based drug design. *Nat Rev Drug Discov* 2003; **2**:891–902.

172. Burrell LM, Johnston CI, Tikellis C, *et al.* ACE2, a new regulator of the renin–angiotensin system. *Trends Endocrinol Metab* 2004;**15**:166–9.

173. Oudit GY, Crackower MA, Backx PH, *et al.* The role of ACE2 in cardiovascular physiology. *Trends Cardiovasc Med* 2003;**13**:93–101.

174. Abassi Z, Karram T, Ellaham S, *et al*. Implications of the natriuretic peptide system in the pathogenesis of heart failure: diagnostic and therapeutic importance. *Pharmacol Ther* 2004;**102**: 223–41.

175. Richards AM, Lainchbury JG, Troughton RW, *et al*. Clinical applications of B-type natriuretic peptides. *Trends Endocrinol Metabol* 2004;**15**: 170–4.

176. D'Souza SP, Davis M, Baxter GF. Autocrine and paracrine actions of natriuretic peptides in the heart. *Pharmacol Ther* 2004;**101**:113–29.

177. Tabrizchi R. Dual ACE and neutral endopeptidase inhibitors. *Drugs* 2003;**63**:2185–202.

178. Molinaro G, Rouleau J-L, Adam A. Vasopeptidase inhibitors: a new class of dual zinc metallopeptidase inhibitors for cardiorenal therapeutics. *Curr Opin Pharmacol* 2002;**2**:131–41.

179. Heath EI, Grochow LB. Clinical potential of matrix metalloprotease inhibitors in cancer therapy. *Drugs* 2000;**59**:1043–55.

180. Martel-Pelletier J, Welsch DJ, Pelletier JP. Metalloproteases and inhibitors in arthritic diseases. *Best Pract Res Clin Rheumatol* 2001;**15**: 805–29.

181. Bigg HF, Rowan AD. The inhibition of metalloproteinases as a therapeutic target in rheumatoid arthritis and osteoarthritis. *Curr Opin Pharmacol* 2001;**1**:314–20.

182. White RJ, Margolis PS, Trias J, *et al*. Targeting metalloenzymes: a strategy that works. *Curr Opin Pharmacol* 2003;**3**:502–7.

183. Auge F, Hornebeck W, Laronze J-Y. A novel strategy for designing specific gelatinase A inhibitors: potential use to control tumour progression. *Crit Rev Oncol/Hematol* 2004;**49**:277–82.

184. Supuran CT, Casini A, Scozzafava A. Protease inhibitors of the sulfonamide type: anticancer, anti-inflammatory, and antiviral agents. *Med Res Rev* 2003;**23**:535–58.

185. Diguarher TL, Chollet A-M, Bertrand M, *et al*. Stereospecific synthesis of 5-substituted 2-bisarylthiocyclopentane carboxylic acid as specific matrix metalloproteinases inhibitors. *J Med Chem* 2003;**46**:3840–52.

186. Lebon F, Ledecq M. Approaches to the design of effective HIV-1 protease inhibitors. *Curr Med Chem* 2000;**7**:455–77.

187. Goldsmith DR, Perry CM. Atazanavir. *Drugs* 2003;**63**:1679–93.

188. Derian CK, Maryanoff BE, Andrade-Gordon P, *et al*. Design and evaluation of potent peptide-mimetic PAR1 antagonists. *Drug Dev Res* 2003;**59**:355–66.

189. Huntington JA, Baglin TP. Targeting thrombin – rational drug design from natural mechanisms. *Trends Pharmacol Sci* 2003;**24**:589–95.

190. Desai UR. New antithrombin-based anticoagulants. *Med Res Rev* 2003;**24**: 151–81.

191. Bates SM, Ginsberg JS. Treatment of deep-vein thrombosis. *N Engl J Med* 2004;**351**:268–77.

192. Reiffel JA. Will direct thrombin inhibitors replace warfarin for preventing embolic events in atrial fibrillation? *Curr Opin Cardiol* 2004;**19**: 58–63.

193. Bell IM. Inhibitors of farnesyltransferase: a rational approach to cancer chemotherapy? *J Med Chem* 2004;**47**:1869–78.

194. Cox AD, Der CJ. Farnesyltransferase inhibitors: promises and realities. *Curr Opin Pharmacol* 2002;**2**:388–93.

195. Grandis JR, Sok JC. Signaling through the epidermal growth factor receptor during the development of malignancy. *Pharmacol Ther* 2004;**102**: 37–46.

196. Garratt AN, Ozcelik C, Birchmeier C. ErbB2 pathways in heart and neural diseases. *Trends Cardiovasc Med* 2003;**13**:80–6.

197. Levitzki A. PDGF receptor kinase inhibitors for the treatment of PDGF driven diseases. *Cytokine Growth Factor Rev* 2004;**15**:229–35.

198. Cross MJ, Dixelius J, Matsumoto T, *et al*. VEGF-receptor signal transduction. *Trends Biochem Sci* 2003;**28**:488–94.

199. Lambrechts D, Storkebaum E, Carmeliet P. VEGF: necessary to prevent motoneuron degeneration, sufficient to treat ALS? *Trends Mol Med* 2004;**10**:275–82.

200. Khurana R, Simons M. Insights from angiogenesis trials using fibroblast growth factor for advanced arteriosclerotic disease. *Trends Cardiovasc Med* 2003;**13**: 116–22.

201. Saklatvala J. The p38 MAP kinase as a therapeutic target in inflammatory disease. *Curr Opin Pharmacol* 2004;**4**:372–7.

202. Olson JM, Hallahan AR. p38 MAP kinase: a convergence point in cancer therapy. *Trends Mol Med* 2004;**10**:125–9.

203. English JM, Cobb MH. Pharmacological inhibitors of MAPK pathways. *Trends Pharmacol Sci* 2002;**23**:40–5.

204. Bogoyevitch MA, Boehm I, Oakley A, *et al*. Targeting the JNK MAPK cascade for inhibition: basic science and therapeutic potential.

Biochim Biophys Acta – Protein Proteomics 2004;**1697**: 89–101.

205. Tsai L-H, Lee M-S, Cruz J. Cdk5, a therapeutic target for Alzheimer's disease? *Biochim Biophys Acta – Proteins Proteomics* 2004;**1697**: 137–42.

206. Cruz JC, Tsai L-H. Cdk5 deregulation in the pathogenesis of Alzheimer's disease. *Trends Mol Med* 2004;**10**:452–8.

207. Smith PD, O'Hare MJ, Park DS. CDKs: taking on a role as mediators of dopaminergic loss in Parkinson's disease. *Trends Mol Med* 2004;**10**: 445–51.

208. Stewart ZA, Westfall MD, Pietenpol JA. Cell-cycle dysregulation and anticancer therapy. *Trends Pharmacol Sci* 2003;**24**:139–45.

209. Knockaert M, Greengard P, Meijer L. Pharmacological inhibitors of cyclin-dependent kinases. *Trends Pharmacol Sci* 2002;**23**:417–25.

210. Dai Y, Grant S. Cyclin-dependent kinase inhibitors. *Curr Opin Pharmacol* 2003;**3**:362–70.

211. Goedert M, Cohen P. GSK3 inhibitors: development and therapeutic potential. *Nat Rev Drug Discov* 2004;**3**:479–87.

212. Meijer L, Flajolet M, Greengard P. Pharmacological inhibitors of glycogen synthase kinase 3. *Trends Pharmacol Sci* 2004;**25**:471–80.

213. Jope RS, Johnson GVW. The glamour and gloom of glycogen synthase kinase-3. *Trends Biochem Sci* 2004;**29**:95–102.

214. Patel JD, Pasche B, Argiris A. Targeting non-small cell lung cancer with epidermal growth factor tyrosine kinase inhibitors: where do we stand, where do we go. *Crit Rev Oncol/Hematol* 2004;**50**: 175–86.

215. Craven RJ, Lightfoot H, Cance WG. A decade of tyrosine kinases: from gene discovery to therapeutics. *Surg Oncol* 2003;**12**:39–49.

216. Ciardiello F, De Vita F, Orditura M, *et al*. The role of EGFR inhibitors in nonsmall cell lung cancer. *Curr Opin Oncol* 2004;**16**:130–5.

217. Fabbro D, Ruetz S, Buchdunger E, *et al*. Protein kinases as targets for anticancer agents: from inhibitors to useful drugs. *Pharmacol Ther* 2002;**93**:79–98.

218. Dancey J, Sausville EA. Issues and progress with protein kinase inhibitors for cancer treatment. *Nat Rev Drug Discov* 2003;**2**:296–313.

219. Johnson LN, Moliner ED, Brown NR, *et al*. Structural studies with inhibitors of the cell cycle regulatory kinase cyclin-dependent protein kinase 2. *Pharmacol Ther* 2002;**93**:113–24.

220. Davies TG, Pratt DJ, Endicott JA, *et al*. Structure-based design of cyclin-dependent kinase inhibitors. *Pharmacol Ther* 2002;**93**:125–33.

221. Martinez A, Castro A, Dorronsoro I, *et al*. Glycogen synthase kinase 3 (GSK-3) inhibitors as new promising drugs for diabetes, neurodegeneration, cancer, and inflammation. *Med Res Rev* 2002, **22**:373–84.

222. Slamon DJ, Leyland-Jones B, Shak S, *et al*. Use of chemotherapy plus a monoclonal antibody against HER2 for metastatic breast cancer that overexpresses HER2. *N Engl J Med* 2001;**344**: 783–92.

223. Buchanan SG. Protein structure: discovering selective protein kinase inhibitors. *TARGETS* 2003;**2**:101–8.

224. Williams DH, Mitchell T. Latest developments in crystallography and structure-based design of protein kinase inhibitors as drug candidates. *Curr Opin Pharmacol* 2002;**2**:567–73.

225. Denny WA. Irreversible inhibitors of the erbB family of protein tyrosine kinases. *Pharmacol Ther* 2002;**93**:253–61.

226. Chen P, Doweyko AM, Norris D, *et al*. Imidazoquinoxaline Src-family kinase p56[Lck] inhibitors: SAR, QSAR, and the discovery of (S)-N-(2-chloro-6-methylphenyl)-2-(3-methyl-1-piperazinyl) imidazo [1,5-a]pyrido[3,2-e]pyrazin-6-amine (BMS-279700) as a potent and orally active inhibitor with excellent *in vivo* anti-inflammatory activity. *J Med Chem* 2004;**47**, 4517–29.

227. Harrington EA, Bebbibgton D, Moore J, *et al*. VX-680, a potent and selective small-molecule inhibitor of the Aurora kinases, suppresses tumour growth *in vivo*. *Nat Med* 2004;**3**:262–7.

228. Zhang Z-Y, Zhou B, Xie L. Modulation of protein kinase signaling by protein phosphatases and inhibitors. *Pharmacol Ther* 2002;**93**: 307–17.

229. Ishida A, Shigeri Y, Taniguchi T, *et al*. Protein phosphatases that regulate multifunctional Ca^{2+}/calmodulin-dependent protein kinases: from biochemistry to pharmacology. *Pharmacol Ther* 2003;**100**:291–305.

230. Umezawa K, Kawakami M, Watanabe T. Molecular design and biological activities of protein-tyrosine phosphatase inhibitors. *Pharmacol Ther* 2003;**99**:15–24.

231. Klumpp S, Krieglstein J. Serine/threonine protein phosphatases in apoptosis. *Curr Opin Pharmacol* 2002;**2**:458–62.

232. Cheon HG, Kim S-M, Yang S-D, *et al.* Discovery of a novel protein tyrosine phosphatase-1B inhibitor, KR61639: potential development as an antihyperglycemic agent. *Eur J Pharmacol* 2004; **485**:333–9.

233. Johnson TO, Ermolieff J, Jirousek MR. Protein tyrosine phosphatase 1B inhibitors for diabetes. *Nat Rev Drug Discov* 2002;**1**:696–709.

234. Shimaoka M, Springer TA. Therapeutic antagonists and conformational regulation of integrin function. *Nat Rev Drug Discov* 2003;**2**:703–16.

235. Gordon C, Tucker GC. Inhibitors of integrins. *Curr Opin Pharmacol* 2002;**2**:394–402.

236. Mousa SA. Anti-integrin as novel drug-discovery targets: potential therapeutic and diagnostic implications. *Curr Opin Chem Biol* 2002;**6**:534–41.

237. Patel SD, Chen CP, Bahna F, *et al.* Cadherin-mediated cell–cell adhesion: sticking together as a family. *Curr Opin Struct Biol* 2003;**13**:690–8.

238. George SJ, Dwivedi A. MMPs, cadherins, and cell proliferation. *Trends Cardiovasc Med* 2004;**14**:100–5.

239. Wang W, Borchardt RT, Wang B. Orally active peptidomimetic analogues that are glycoprotein IIb/IIIa antagonists. *Curr Med Chem* 2000;**7**:437–53.

240. Dooley M, Goa KL. Lamifiban. *Drugs* 1999;**57**:215–21.

241. Dooley M, Goa KL. Sibrafiban. *Drugs* 1999;**57**:225–30.

242. Dutta AS, Gormley JJ, Coath M, *et al.* Potent cyclic peptide inhibitors of VLA-4 (α4 β1 Integrin)-mediated cell adhesion. Discovery of compounds like cyclo(MePhe-Leu-Asp-Val-D-Arg-D-Arg) (ZD7349) compatible with depot formulation. *J Pept Sci* 2000;**6**:398–412.

243. Dutta AS, Crowther M, Gormley JJ, *et al.* Potent cyclic monomeric and dimeric peptide inhibitors of VLA-4 (α4β1 integrin)-mediated cell adhesion based on the Ile-Leu-Asp-Val tetrapeptide. *J Pept Sci* 2000;**6**:321–41.

244. Haworth D, Rees A, Dutta AS, *et al.* Anti-inflammatory activity of c(ILDV-NH(CH2)5CO), a novel, selective, cyclic peptide inhibitor of VLA-4-mediated cell adhesion. *Br J Pharmacol* 1999;**126**:1751–60.

245. Yusuf-Makagiansar H, Anderson ME, Yakovleva TV, *et al.* Inhibition of LFA-1/ ICAM-1 and VLA-4/VCAM-1 as a therapeutic approach to inflammation and autoimmune diseases. *Med Res Rev* 2002;**22**:146–67.

246. Yang GX, Hagmann WK. VLA-4 antagonists: potent inhibitors of lymphocyte migration. *Med Res Rev* 2003;**23**:369–92.

247. Arkin M, Wells JA. Small-molecule inhibitors of protein–protein interactions: progressing towards the dream. *Nat Rev Drug Discov* 2004;**3**:301–17.

248. David R, Owens DR. New horizons – alternative routes for insulin therapy. *Nat Rev Drug Discov* 2002;**1**:529–40.

249. Takacs L, Vazques-Abad M-D, Elliott EA. Therapeutic monoclonal antibodies. *Ann Rep Med Chem* 2001;**36**:237–46.

250. Sela M, Arnon R, Schechter B. Therapeutic vaccines: realities of today and hopes for the future. *Drug Discov Today* 2002;**7**:664–73.

251. Ladner RC, Sato AK, Gorzelany J, *et al.* Phage display-derived peptides as therapeutic alternatives to antibodies. *Drug Discov Today* 2004;**9**:525–9.

252. Crommelin DJA, Storm G, Verrijk R, *et al.* Shifting paradigm: biopharmaceuticals versus low molecular weight drugs. *Int J Pharm* 2003;**266**:3–16.

253. Harris JM, Chess RB. Effect of pegylation on pharmaceuticals. *Nat Rev Drug Discov* 2003;**2**:214–21.

254. Kaushansky K. Drug therapy: thrombopoietin. *N Engl J Med* 1998;**339**:746–54.

255. Goodnough LT, Monk TG, Andriole GL. Current concepts: erythropoietin therapy. *N Engl J Med* 1997;**336**:933–8.

256. Lane NE. Parathyroid hormone: evolving therapeutic concepts. *Curr Opin Rheumatol* 2004;**16**:457–63.

257. Fox J. Developments in parathyroid hormone and related peptides as bone-formation agents. *Curr Opin Pharmacol* 2002;**2**:338–44.

258. Cheer MC, Dunn CJ, Foster R. Tinzaparin sodium. A review of its pharmacology and clinical use in the prophylaxis and treatment of thromboembolic disease. *Drugs* 2004;**64**:1479–1502.

259. Leonardi CL, Powers JL, Matheson RT, *et al.* Etanercept as monotherapy in patients with psoriasis. *N Engl J Med* 2003;**349**:2014–22.

260. Culy CR, Keating GM. Etanercept. An updated review of its use in rheumatoid arthritis, psoriatic arthritis and juvenile rheumatoid arthritis. *Drugs* 2002;**62**:2493–537.

261. Cooper DA, Lange JMA. Peptide inhibitors of virus-cell fusion: enfuvirtide as a case study in

clinical discovery and development. *Lancet Infect Dis* 2004;**4**:426–36.

262. Dando TM, Perry CM. Enfuvirtide. *Drugs* 2003;**63**:2755–66.

263. Roskos LK, Davis CG, Schwab GM. The clinical pharmacology of therapeutic monoclonal antibodies. *Drug Dev Res* 2004;**61**:108–20.

264. Brekke OH, Sandlie I. Therapeutic antibodies for human diseases at the dawn of the twenty-first century. *Nat Rev Drug Discov* 2003;**2**:52–62.

265. Penichet ML, Morrison SL. Design and engineering human forms of monoclonal antibodies. *Drug Dev Res* 2004;**61**:121–36.

266. Harris RJ, Shire SJ, Winter C. Commercial manufacturing scale formulation and analytical characterisation of therapeutic recombinant antibodies. *Drug Dev Res* 2004;**61**:137–54.

267. Robonson MK, Weiner LM, Adams GP. Improving monoclonal antibodies for cancer therapy. *Drug Dev Res* 2004;**61**:172–87.

268. Trikha M, Yan L, Nakada MT. Monoclonal antibodies as therapeutics in oncology. *Curr Opin Biotechnol* 2002;**13**:609–14.

269. Taylor PC. Antibody therapy for rheumatoid arthritis. *Curr Opin Pharmacol* 2003;**3**:323–8.

270. Andreakos E, Taylor PC, Feldmann M. Monoclonal antibodies in immune and inflammatory diseases. *Curr Opin Biotechnol* 2002;**13**:615–20.

271. Torphy TJ, Li L, Griswold DE. Monoclonal antibodies as a strategy for pulmonary diseases. *Curr Opin Pharmacol* 2001;**1**:265–71.

272. Kufer P, Lutterbüse R, Baeuerle PA. A revival of bispecific antibodies. *Trends Biotechnol* 2004;**22**:238–44.

273. Presta L. Antibody engineering for therapeutics. *Curr Opin Struct Biol* 2003;**13**:519–25.

274. van Dijk MA, van de Winkel JGJ. Human antibodies as next generation therapeutics. *Curr Opin Chem Biol* 2001;**5**:368–74.

275. Brekke OH, Løset GA. New technologies in therapeutic antibody development. *Curr Opin Pharmacol* 2003;**3**:544–50.

276. Kellermann S-A, Green LL. Antibody discovery: the use of transgenic mice to generate human monoclonal antibodies for therapeutics. *Curr Opin Biotechnol* 2002;**13**:593–97.

277. Miller DH, Khan OA, Sheremata WA, *et al.* A controlled trial of natalizumab for relapsing multiple sclerosis. *N Engl J Med* 2003;**348**:15–23.

278. Lebwohl M, Tyring SK, Hamilton TK, *et al.* A novel targeted T-cell modulator, efalizumab, for plaque psoriasis. *N Engl J Med* 2003;**349**:2004–13.

279. Plosker GL. Rituximab. A review of its use in non-Hodgkin's lymphoma and chronic lymphocytic leukaemia. *Drugs* 2003;**63**:803–43.

280. Kazkaz H, Isenberg D. Anti B cell therapy (rituximab) in the treatment of autoimmune diseases. *Curr Opin Pharmacol* 2004;**4**:398–402.

281. Reynolds NA, Wagstaff AJ. Cetuximab in the treatment of metastatic colorectal cancer. *Drugs* 2004;**64**:109–18.

282. Starling N, Cunningham D. Monoclonal antibodies against vascular endothelial growth factor and epidermal growth factor receptor in advanced colorectal cancers: present and future directions. *Curr Opin Oncol* 2004;**16**:385–90.

283. Frampton JE, Wagstaff AJ. Alemtuzamab. *Drugs* 2003;**63**:1229–43.

284. Chapman TM, Keating GM. Basiliximab. A review of its use as induction therapy in renal transplantation. *Drugs* 2003;**63**:2803–35.

285. Ibbotson T, McGavin JK, Goa KL. Abciximab. An updated review of its therapeutic use in patients with ischaemic heart disease undergoing percutaneous coronary revascularisation. *Drugs* 2003;**63**:1121–63.

286. Damle NK, Frost P. Antibody-targeted chemotherapy with immunoconjugates of calicheamicin. *Curr Opin Pharmacol* 2003;**3**:386–90.

287. Perry CM, Scott LJ. Cefdinir. A review of its use in the management of mild-to-moderate bacterial infections. *Drugs* 2004;**64**:1433–64.

288. Zhanel GG, Walters M, Noreddin A, *et al.* The ketolides. A critical review. *Drugs* 2002;**62**:1771–804.

289. Wellington K, Noble S. Telithromycin. *Drugs* 2004;**64**:1683–94.

290. Bambeke FV, Laethem YV, Courvalin P, *et al.* Glycopeptide antibiotics – from conventional molecules to new derivatives. *Drugs* 2004;**64**:913–36.

291. Fenton C, Keating GM, Curran MP. Daptomycin, *Drugs* 2004;**64**:445–55.

292. Croom KF, Goa KL. Levofloxacin. A review of its use in the treatment of bacterial infections in the United States. *Drugs* 2003;**63**:2769–802.

293. Ohtsuo T, Aoki Y. N-myristoyltransferase inhibitors as potential antifungal drugs. *Drugs Future* 2003;**28**:143–52.

294. Jarvis B, Figgitt DP, Scott LJ. Micafungin. *Drugs* 2004;**64**:969–82.

295. Bang LM, Scott LJ. Emtricitabine. An antiretroviral agent for HIV infection. *Drugs* 2003;**63**:2413–24.

296. Chapman TM, McGavin JK, Noble S. Tenofovir disoproxil fumarate. *Drugs* 2003;**63**:1597–608.

297. Schmidt AC. Antiviral therapy for influenza. A clinical and economic comparative review. *Drugs* 2004;**64**:2031–46.

298. Carter BL, Ernst ME, Cohen JD. Hydrochlorothiazide versus chlorthalidone: evidence supporting their interchangeability. *Hypertension* 2004;**43**:4–9.

299. Bang LM, Chapman TM, Goa KL. Lercanidipine: a review of its efficacy in the management of hypertension. *Drugs* 2003;**63**:2449–72.

300. Wellington K, Scott LJ. Azelnidipine. *Drugs* 2003;**63**:2613–21.

301. Keam SJ, Goa KL. Fondaparinux sodium. *Drugs* 2002;**62**:1673–85.

302. Evans HC, Perry CM, Faulds D. Ximelagatran/ Melagatran. A review of its use in the prevention of venous thromboembolism in orthopaedic surgery. *Drugs* 2004;**64**:649–78.

303. Heart Protection Study Collaborative Group. Effects of cholesterol-lowering with simvastatin on stroke and other major vascular events in 20536 people with cerebrovascular disease or other high-risk conditions. *Lancet* 2004;**363**:757–67.

304. Topol EJ. Intensive statin therapy – a sea change in cardiovascular prevention. *N Engl J Med* 2004;**350**:1562–4.

305. Goff WL, Guerin M, Chapman JM. Pharmacological modulation of cholesteryl ester transfer protein, a new therapeutic target in atherogenic dyslipidemia. *Pharmacol Ther* 2004;**101**:17–38.

306. Brousseau ME, Schaefer EJ, Wolfe ML, *et al*. Effects of an inhibitor of cholesteryl ester transfer protein on HDL cholesterol. *N Engl J Med* 2004;**350**:1505–15.

307. Nourparvar A, Bulotta A, Di Mario U, *et al*. Novel strategies for the pharmacological management of type 2 diabetes. *Trends Pharmacol Sci* 2004;**25**:86–91.

308. Rendell M. The role of sulphonylureas in the management of type 2 diabetes mellitus. *Drugs* 2004;**64**:1339–58.

309. Diamant MD, Heine RJ. Thiazolidinediones in type 2 diabetes mellitus. Current clinical evidence. *Drugs* 2003;**63**:1373–405.

310. Hannele Y-J. Drug therapy: thiazolidinediones. *N Engl J Med* 2004;**351**:1106–18.

311. Rangwala SM, Lazar MA. Peroxisome proliferator-activated receptor in diabetes and metabolism. *Trends Pharmacol Sci* 2004;**25**:331–6.

312. Hsueh WA, Bruemmer D. Peroxisome proliferator-activated receptor-γ: implications for cardiovascular disease. *Hypertension* 2004;**43**:297–305.

313. Schiffrin EL, Amiri F, Benkirane K, *et al*. Peroxisome proliferator-activated receptors: vascular and cardiac effects in hypertension. *Hypertension* 2003;**42**:664–8.

314. Vosper H, Khoudoli GA, Graham TL, *et al*. Peroxisome proliferator-activated receptor agonists, hyperlipidaemia, and atherosclerosis. *Pharmacol Ther* 2002;**95**:47–62.

315. Robertson RP. Medical progress: islet transplantation as a treatment for diabetes – a work in progress. *N Engl J Med* 2004;**350**:694–705.

316. Hardikar AA. Generating new pancreas from old. *Trends Endocrinol Metabol* 2004;**15**:198–203.

317. Small CJ, Bloom SR. Gut hormones and the control of appetite. *Trends Endocrinol Metabol* 2004;**15**:259–63.

318. Chao CS, Sussel L. Ghrelin, insulin, and the pancreatic islet. *Curr Opin Endocrinol Diabetes* 2004;**11**:104–9.

319. Spira A, Ettinger DS. Drug therapy: multidisciplinary management of lung cancer. *N Engl J Med* 2004;**350**:379–92.

320. Ryan CJ, Small EJ. Advances in prostate cancer. *Curr Opin Oncol* 2004;**16**:242–6.

321. Li D, Xie K, Wolff R, *et al*. Pancreatic cancer. *Lancet* 2004;**363**:1049–57.

322. Gill S, Goldberg RM. First-line treatment strategies to improve survival in patients with advanced colorectal cancer. *Drugs* 2004;**64**:27–44.

323. Graham J, Muhsin M, Kirkpatrick P. Oxaliplatin. *Nat Rev Drug Discov* 2004;**3**:11–12.

324. Hall MD, Martin C, Ferguson DJP, *et al*. Comparative efficacy of novel platinum(IV) compounds with established chemotherapeutic drugs in solid tumour models. *Biochem Pharmacol* 2004;**67**:17–30.

325. Ho Y-P, Au-Yeung SCF, To KKW. Platinum-based anticancer agents: innovative design strategies and biological perspectives. *Med Res Rev* 2003;**23**:633–55.

326. Simpson D, Plosker GL. Paclitaxel as adjuvant or neoadjuvant therapy in early breast cancer. *Drugs* 2004;**64**:1839–47.

327. Larsen AK, Escargueil AE, Skladanowski A. Catalytic topoisomerase II inhibitors in cancer therapy. *Pharmacol Ther* 2003;**99**:167–81.

328. Subbaramaiah K, Dannenberg AJ. Cyclooxy-genase 2: a molecular target for cancer prevention and treatment. *Trends Pharmacol Sci* 2003;**24**:96–102.

329. Iniguez MA, Rodríguez A, Volpert OV, *et al.* Cyclooxygenase-2: a therapeutic target in angiogenesis. *Trends Mol Med* 2003;**9**:73–8.

330. Shiff SJ, Shivaprasad P, Santini DL. Cyclooxy-genase inhibitors: drugs for cancer prevention. *Curr Opin Pharmacol* 2003;**3**:352–61.

331. Lieb K, Zanarini MC, Schmahl C, *et al.* Borderline personality disorder. *Lancet* 2004;**364**:453–61.

332. Jenike MA. Obsessive-compulsive disorder. *N Engl J Med* 2004;**350**:259–65.

333. Cobb JP, O'Keefe GE. Injury research in the genomic era. *Lancet* 2004;**363**:2076–83.

334. Royo NC, Shimizu S, Schouten JW, *et al.* Pharmacology of traumatic brain injury. *Curr Opin Pharmacol* 2003;**3**:27–32.

335. Samii A, Nutt JG, Ransom BR. Parkinson's disease. *Lancet* 2004;**363**:1783–93.

336. Schloss P, Henn FA. New insights into the mechanisms of antidepressant therapy. *Pharmacol Ther* 2004;**102**:47–60.

337. Middlemiss DN, Price GW, Watson JM. Serotonergic targets in depression. *Curr Opin Pharmacol* 2002;**2**:18–22.

338. Mueser KT, McGurk SR. Schizophrenia. *Lancet* 2004;**363**:2063–72.

339. Belmaker RH. Medical progress: bipolar disorder. *N Engl J Med* 2004;**351**:476–86.

340. Avi A, Silberstein SD. The evolving management of migraine. *Curr Opin Neurol* 2003;**16**:341–5.

341. Kwan P, Sill GJ, Brodie MJ. The mechanisms of action of commonly used antiepileptic drugs. *Pharmacol Ther* 2002;**90**:21–34.

342. Loscher W. Current status and future directions in the pharmacotherapy of epilepsy. *Trends Pharmacol Sci* 2002;**23**:113–18.

343. Parihar MS, Hemnani T. Alzheimer's disease pathogenesis and therapeutic interventions. *J Clin Neurosci* 2004;**11**:456–67.

344. Cummings JL. Drug therapy: Alzheimer's disease. *N Engl J Med* 2004;**351**:56–67.

345. Grossberg GT. Cholinesterase inhibitors for the treatment of Alzheimer's disease: getting on and staying on. *Curr Ther Res* 2003;**64**:216–35.

346. Revel M. Interferon-β in the treatment of relapsing–remitting multiple sclerosis. *Pharmacol Ther* 2003;**100**:49–62.

347. Suhayl D-J. Glatiramer acetate (Copaxone) therapy for multiple sclerosis. *Pharmacol Ther* 2003;**98**:245–55.

348. UK MS Research Group, Zajicek J, Fox P, Sanders H, *et al.* Cannabinoids for treatment of spasticity and other symptoms related to multiple sclerosis (CAMS study): multicentre randomised placebo-controlled trial. *Lancet* 2003;**362**:1517–26.

349. Morrison KE. Therapies in amyotrophic lateral sclerosis – beyond riluzole. *Curr Opin Pharmacol* 2002;**2**:302–9.

350. LoGrasso P, McKelvy J. Advances in pain therapeutics. *Curr Opin Chem Biol* 2003;**7**:452–6.

351. Ballantyne JC, Mao J. Medical progress: opioid therapy for chronic pain. *N Engl J Med* 2003;**349**:1943–53.

352. Dickinson T, Lee K, Spanswick D, *et al.* Leading the charge – pioneering treatments in the fight against neuropathic pain. *Trends Pharmacol Sci* 2003;**24**:555–7.

353. Eguchi M. Recent advances in selective opioid receptor agonists and antagonists. *Med Res Rev* 2004;**24**:182–212.

354. George TP, O'Malley SS. Current pharmacological treatments for nicotine dependence. *Trends Pharmacol Sci* 2004;**25**:42–8.

355. Martin BR, Sim-Selley LJ, Selley DE. Signaling pathways involved in the development of cannabinoid tolerance. *Trends Pharmacol Sci* 2004;**25**:325–30.

356. Nestler EJ. Historical review: molecular and cellular mechanisms of opiate and cocaine addiction. *Trends Pharmacol Sci* 2004;**25**:210–18.

357. Hinz B, Brune K. Pain and osteoarthritis: new drugs and mechanisms. *Curr Opin Rheumatol* 2004;**16**:628–33.

358. Reynolds NA, Perry CM, Keating GM. Budesonide/formoterol in chronic obstructive pulmonary disease. *Drugs* 2004;**64**:431–41.

359. Klinkhoff A. Biological agents for rheumatoid arthritis. *Drugs* 2004;**64**:1267–83.

360. Olsen NJ, Stein CM. Drug therapy: new drugs for rheumatoid arthritis. *N Engl J Med* 2004;**350**:2167–79.

361. O'Dell JR. Drug therapy: therapeutic strategies for rheumatoid arthritis. *N Engl J Med* 2004;**350**:2591–602.

362. Dinarello CA. Therapeutic strategies to reduce IL-1 activity in treating local and systemic inflammation. *Curr Opin Pharmacol* 2004;**4**:378–85.

363. Sweeney SE, Firestein GS. Signal transduction in rheumatoid arthritis. *Curr Opin Rheumatol* 2004;**16**:231–7.

364. Berenbaum F. Signaling transduction: target in osteoarthritis. *Curr Opin Rheumatol* 2004;**16**: 616–22.

365. Saklatvala J. The p38 MAP kinase pathway as a therapeutic target in inflammatory disease. *Curr Opin Pharmacol* 2004;**4**:372–7.

366. Roshak AK, Callahan JF, Blake SM. Small-molecule inhibitors of NF-κB for the treatment of inflammatory joint disease. *Curr Opin Pharmacol* 2002;**2**:316–21.

367. Triadafilopoulos G. Gastroesophageal reflux. *Curr Opin Gastroenterol* 2004;**20**:369–74.

368. Gerhard R. Update in inflammatory bowel disease pathogenesis. *Curr Opin Gastroenterol* 2004;**20**: 311–17.

369. Brookes MJ, Green JRB. Maintenance of remission in Crohn's disease. Current and emerging therapeutic options. *Drugs* 2004;**64**:1069–89.

370. Panaccione R, Sandborn WJ. Medical therapy of Crohn disease. *Curr Opin Gastroenterol* 2004;**20**:351–9.

371. Heymann D, Ory B, Gouin F, *et al*. Bisphosphonates: new therapeutic agents for the treatment of bone tumors. *Trends Mol Med* 2004;**10**:337–43.

372. Dutta AS, Garner A. The pharmaceutical industry and research in 2020 and beyond. *Drug News Perspect* 2003;**16**:637–48.

CHAPTER 2

2

Pharmaceutical development

Gavin Halbert

2.1 Introduction

The current vogue in drug discovery is the identification and validation of a pharmacological target, followed by high-throughput screening to identify suitable chemical motifs or lead molecules that interact with the target. These molecules may be further refined by combinatorial or traditional medicinal chemistry approaches linked with computer modelling of the target site. This will provide a compound or series of compounds that is designed to elicit a maximal response from a specific target receptor in *in vitro* tests. At this stage, the candidate drug exists only as a powder in a 'test tube', or even maybe as a computer model, and is not in a state to benefit the ultimate end user, the patient. The drug is, therefore, formulated into a medicinal product that can be easily handled and administered by medical staff and patients. Such products may range from simple solutions through to transdermal patch delivery systems, the ultimate form depending on pharmacological, pharmaceutical and marketing considerations. All of these medicinal products or dosage forms will contain the drug plus a variety of additives or excipients whose role is to enhance product performance. It is, therefore, a general rule that patients are never administered a 'drug' *per se* but rather a medicinal product that contains the drug.

Pharmaceutical development of a medicinal product must retain the drug's promising *in vitro* pharmacological activity and provide a predictable *in vivo* response. The marketed product must be stable, correctly packaged, labelled and easily administered, preferably by self-administration. The product must also be economical to manufacture on a large scale by a method that ensures product quality. In addition, development and eventual production processes must comply with the regulatory requirements of proposed market countries, and all development studies must be performed to acceptable levels of quality assurance.

Pharmaceutical development involves multiple skills, processes and stages and is, therefore, a large undertaking requiring extensive resources. The earlier the pharmaceutical intervention occurs during development the better, to preclude, for example, the use of toxic solvents during manufacture or to employ computer models to determine potential bioavailability problems with candidate compounds. Changes introduced at later stages may necessitate costly retesting or delay product marketing and are best avoided. Development consists of several gross stages such as preformulation, formulation, toxicology and clinical trials, and, where possible, research is normally conducted in parallel in order to expedite the process. Because of drug diversity and the many possible approaches, there is no single optimum development model but the general stages presented in this chapter will be applied.

For the majority of drugs, the initial formulation will be an injectable solution for basic pharmacology, pharmacokinetic and toxicology studies in animals or man to confirm *in vitro* activity. Other more complex formulations will follow as the research and pharmaceutical development programmes progress. The eventual range and type of formulations produced for a single drug will depend on the drug's pharmacology and whether a local systemic action is required (Table 2.1). Some drugs can be administered by a variety of routes, resulting in several diverse formulations. Salbutamol, for example, is currently available in ten different formulations, excluding different doses and variations resulting from different manufacturers (Table 2.2).

2.2 Preformulation

Before product development studies are conducted, fundamental physicochemical information on the new chemical entity (NCE) or drug must be obtained.[1,2] This provides valuable data to guide future work and initiates a sequence of specification setting exercises that define the drug's boundaries for use. At early stages, only limited drug supplies will be available and there may be competition between continuing pharmacology and early *in vivo* testing and preformulation studies. The utilisation of material has to be balanced to ensure that adequate information is obtained to determine future progress. For example, chemical purity and stability are important in both pharmacology and preformulation studies.

2.2.1 Structure determination

After synthesis it is important to determine the drug's exact chemical structure. This will involve a variety of techniques such as mass spectrometry, nuclear magnetic resonance (H^1 and C^{13}), infrared and ultraviolet/visible spectrophotometry along with elemental analysis. This will confirm the medicinal chemist's proposed

structure and provide information useful in later stages such as analytical development.

2.2.2 Analytical development

An initial priority is to develop analytical methodology that detects the drug (main component), intermediate compounds carried over from synthesis and degradation products from chemical breakdown or instability. Paradoxically, these latter contaminants are of greater importance because their quantification, identification and control affect the quality of drug batches. In addition, chemical instability is more easily detected through an increased concentration of degradants than through decreased concentration of the main component. Methods are also required for quantification of other impurities such as residual solvents, catalyst residues and heavy-metal and microbial contamination. Further analytical tests will also be specified such as the general characteristics, colour, melting point, loss on drying and a basic identification method. The basic analysis of a new drug, therefore, necessitates the application of a full range of analytical techniques, all of which must be validated to a suitable level.[3]

Drug assays are usually conducted using a specific chromatography or separative technique such as high-performance (or pressure) liquid chromatography (HPLC)[4] or capillary zone electrophoresis (CZE).[5,6] These techniques ensure that the drug is separated from impurities and breakdown products, all of which can then be quantified. Development of these methods allows specifications to be set for the required percentage of the main component, usually 98–101% by weight, and limits for the tolerated level of impurities.[7] If required, identification of the impurities and degradants will also be conducted. A reference sample will be retained and used as a standard for subsequent analysis. Simple ultraviolet/visible spectrophotometric analysis may suffice for some experiments such as solubility testing.

It is common to find that early small-scale batches exhibit a higher or different purity or impurity profile to subsequent batches from

Table 2.1 Basic information on common routes of administration

Route	Advantages	Disadvantages	Product types
Parenteral suspensions[a] (injection)	Exact dose 100% compliance Suitable for unconscious patient Rapid onset, especially after intravenous administration	Painful Self-administration unusual Requires trained personnel	Solutions, emulsions, implants[a] Expensive production processes
Oral	Easy Convenient Acceptable Painless Self-administration possible	Inappropriate during vomiting Potential drug-stability problems Interactions with food Possible low availability Patient must be conscious	Solutions, syrups, suspensions, emulsions, powders, granules, capsules, tablets
Rectal	Avoids problems of stability in gastrointestinal tract No first-pass metabolism Useful if oral administration is not possible	Unpopular Inconvenient Erratic absorption Irritation	Suppositories, enemas (solutions, suspensions, emulsions), foams, ointments, creams
Buccal	Rapid onset of action No first-pass metabolism Dosage form recoverable Convenient	Taste Only suitable for low dose (high potency) drugs	Tablets, mouthwashes
Inhalation	Convenient Local or systemic effects No first-pass metabolism	Irritation Embarrassing Difficult technique	Gases, aerosols (solutions, suspensions), powders
Transdermal	Easy Convenient No first-pass metabolism Local or systemic effects	Irritation Potent drugs only Absorption affected by site of application Hard to administer	Solutions, lotions, sprays, gels, ointments, creams, powders, patches
Eye	Local action only	Inefficient Irritation Poor retention of solutions	Solutions, ointments, injections
Vaginal	Local or systemic effects (hormones) No first-pass metabolism	Inconvenient Erratic absorption Irritation	Creams, ointments, foams, tablets, pessaries

[a] Not for intravenous administration.

Table 2.2 Salbutamol preparations available in the United Kingdom

Route	Form	Product	Manufacturer	Strength
Parenteral	Solution	Injection	Non-proprietary	100 μg/mL
		Ventolin® injection	A&H	50 and 500 μg/mL
		Ventolin® intravenous infusion	A&H	1 mg/mL
Oral	Solution	—	Non-proprietary	2 mg/5 mL
	Syrup	Ventolin®	A&H	2 mg/5 mL
	Tablets	—	Non-proprietary[a]	2 and 4 mg
	Tablets (modified release)	Volmax®	A&H	4 and 8 mg
	Capsules (modified release)	Ventmax®	Trinity	4 and 8 mg
Inhalation	Metered dose inhaler	—	Non-proprietary[b]	100 μg/inhalation
		Aerolin® Autohaler	3M	100 μg/inhalation
		Easi-Breathe®	A&H	100 μg/inhalation
	Metered dose inhaler CFC free	—	Non-proprietary	100 μg/inhalation
		Airomir® Autohaler	3M	100 μg/inhalation
		Evohaler®	A&H	100 μg/inhalation
	Powder for inhalation	Ventodisks®	A&H	200 and 400 μg/inhalation
		Accuhaler®	A&H	200 μg/inhalation
		Rotacaps®	A&H	200 and 400 μg/inhalation
		Asmasal® Clickhaler®	Medeva	95 μg/inhalation
	Nebuliser	Solution	Non-proprietary[c]	1 and 2 mg/mL
		Nebules®	A&H	1 and 2 mg/mL
		Respirator solution	A&H	5 mg/mL

From British National Formulary 40, September 2000. Liquid, tablet and powder preparations contain salbutamol as the sulphate salt; aerosols contain the free base.

[a] Five manufacturer's preparations available.
[b] Six manufacturer's preparations available.
[c] Four manufacturer's preparations available.

large-scale production. As development progresses, the ability to synthesise the drug reproducibly must be determined so that impurity profiles are known and predictable and can be maintained within predetermined limits.

2.2.3   Salt form

The majority of NCEs synthesised are organic molecules of low molecular weight that are either weak acids or weak bases. There is, therefore, a choice between the free acid or base and a salt, with further complexity imposed by salt selection. The free acid or base does not normally possess an adequate aqueous solubility for the majority of applications and so salts are required. Since salt formation will occur during synthesis, the correct choice of salt at an early stage is critical. The non-steroidal anti-inflammatory drug fenoprofen is a derivative of 2-phenylpropionic

Table 2.3 Characteristics of fenoprofen salts

| Salt | Hydration | Form | Melting point (°C) | Aqueous solubility (mg/mL) | Weight change (%) Relative humidity (%) | | | | | |
					10	20	40	60	70	93
Free acid		O	40	0.05	—	—	—	—	—	—
K^+	Unknown	C	—	>200	Extremely hygroscopic					
Mg^{2+}	Dihydrate	—	—	>200	—	—	—	—	—	—
$Al(OH)^{2+}$	Dihydrate	A	—	0.1 0	0	—	0	—	—	0
Na^+	Anhydrous	A	—	>200	−0.5	+10.7	+12.5	—	+15.8	+36.5
Na^+	Dihydrate	C	80	>200	−11.4	+0.3	+0.4	—	+2.5	+9.3
Ca^{2+}	Anhydrous	A	—	2.5	+0.5	+1.7	+2.9	+3.7	—	+6.3
Ca^{2+}	Dihydrate	C	110	2.5	0	0	0	—	0	0

O, oil; C, crystalline; A, amorphous.

acid and the free acid exists as a viscous oil at room temperature.[8] The potassium salt was found to be hygroscopic, the magnesium salt did not crystallise and the aluminium salt was insoluble in water. Anhydrous sodium or calcium salts could not be obtained but the dihydrate salt was readily isolated. The sodium dihydrate was not stable and dehydrated at room temperature whereas the calcium dihydrate salt was stable up to 70°C (Table 2.3) and was therefore chosen for further development.

2.2.4 Chemical stability

The solid drug's chemical stability will be examined under a range of different storage conditions and over varying periods of time, using the stability indicating assays described above. Chemical degradation occurs through four main routes:

- hydrolysis resulting from the presence of H_2O, H^+ or OH^-
- oxidation
- photolysis
- catalysis by trace metals such as Fe^{2+}, Cu^{2+}.

Hydrolysis and oxidation are the two main routes of degradation for the majority of drugs. Harmonised guidelines are available for new drugs[9]

but these specify only two conditions: long-term testing at $25 \pm 2°C/60 \pm 5\%$ relative humidity and accelerated testing at $40 \pm 2°C/75 \pm 5\%$ relative humidity, which may not provide enough information to characterise degradation processes fully. To gain more information, testing at a range of temperatures from (depending upon stability) −80°C to 70°C, variable levels of relative humidity up to 90% and exposure to artificial or natural light (Table 2.4) may be conducted.[10] Elevated temperatures, humidity and light deliberately stress the drug and induce rapid degradation. Determination of the physical chemistry of the degradation process will allow the extrapolation of results from short tests under stressed condition to provide estimates of shelf life in ambient environments (Figure 2.1). This will provide basic information on the conditions, processes and packaging that can be used to manipulate and store the drug safely. For example, hygroscopic drugs may require packaging with a desiccant in containers that prevent moisture ingress.

Chemical stability studies will also be conducted on aqueous solutions of the drug at varying pHs and temperatures and in a variety of solvents, experiments that may be coupled with determination of solubility. This information is important for determining the shelf life

Table 2.4 Typical stress conditions used for stability testing

Test	Stress	Conditions
Solution, chemical stability	Heat and pH	pH 1, 3, 5, 7, 9, 11
Solution, chemical stability		Ambient and elevated temperature
Solution, chemical stability	Light	Ultraviolet and white light
	Oxidation	Sparging with oxygen
Solid, chemical stability	Heat and humidity	4°C, 25°C (60% and 75% RH), 30°C (70% RH), 40°C (75% RH), 50°C, 70°C
Solid, moisture uptake	Humidity	RH[a]: 30%, 45%, 60%, 75%, 90%
		Ambient temperature

RH, relative humidity
[a] Provided using saturated aqueous solutions of $MgBr_2$, KNO_2, NaBr, NaCl, KNO_3, respectively, or controlled humidity cabinets.

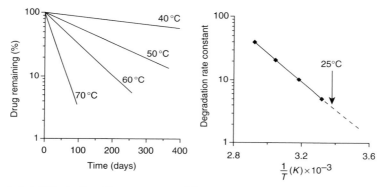

Fig. 2.1 Accelerated stability testing. The percentage of drug remaining at elevated temperatures with time is measured (left) and the rate constants for the degradation reaction calculated. Using the Arrhenius relationship, a plot of the log of the rate constant against the reciprocal of absolute temperature of measurement yields a straight line (right). Extrapolation of the line permits calculation of the rate constant at lower temperatures and the prediction of shelf life.

of stock solutions for pharmacology testing and analytical assays.

2.2.5 Physicochemical properties

The drug's physicochemical parameters are determined in order to provide essential information for interpreting subsequent studies and guiding formulation.[11] Solubility in aqueous media of differing composition (e.g. buffers, physiological saline) and pH will be determined, along with a range of biocompatible organic solvents (e.g. ethanol, propylene glycol,

polyethylene glycol). Solubility is important in the formulation of liquid dosage forms and is also a critical parameter controlling a drug's biopharmaceutical properties. For example, absorption from administration sites can only occur if the drug is in solution in the biological milieu at the absorption site. Intrinsic dissolution rates in aqueous media at various pH values will also be measured; the magnitude of this parameter is directly related to solubility. Dissolution is only important when it is the rate-limiting step in drug absorption and can arise if drug solubility is below 1 mg/mL in aqueous media at pH 7.0. The bioavailability of drugs with low aqueous solubility can be controlled by this parameter, which is itself affected by the surface area available for dissolution (see below). The drug's pKa will be measured because this also controls solubility in aqueous solutions. The partitioning of the drug between aqueous and organic solvents will be measured to determine the partition coefficient, although this parameter along with pKa can be assessed using computer programs.[12] This is useful for predicting drug absorption and distribution *in vivo* and for studies of structure–activity relationship, which may direct future synthesis.

2.2.6 Chiral properties

A large proportion of NCEs will have one or more chiral centres. Only single enantiomers can be used nowadays, whereas previously a racemic mixture would have been tested.[13] Different enantiomers produce different pharmacological responses, with one enantiomer usually being more active by at least an order of magnitude. There has been considerable debate on the administration of racemates versus the single active enantiomer or eutomer[14]; however, the current trend is to develop only the active optical isomer. The synthetic route employed will, if required, have to utilise chiral-specific reagents and catalysts or the compound will have to be purified after synthesis. With this type of compound, an additional specification or limit is required for the presence of the inactive enantiomer.[15]

2.2.7 Biopharmaceutical properties

Small-scale *in vitro* test systems may now be employed to assess biopharmaceutical properties or the drug's potential behaviour after *in vivo* administration. For example, drug penetration through monolayers of epithelial cells in tissue culture can be used to examine bioavailability.[16] The drug's metabolism can be studied *in vitro* using hepatic microsomes and potentially toxic metabolites identified before problems arise *in vivo*.[17] Although not absolute, these tests provide useful indicators of potential problem areas and may eliminate problematical drug candidates early.

2.2.8 Physical properties of the solid drug

Basic physical properties of the solid drug such as melting point, particle or crystal size, distribution, shape and possible polymorphic variations are important in determining the performance of solid dosage forms. These parameters have profound effects on the drug's behaviour and subsequent formulation and must be optimised. The bioavailability of drugs with low aqueous solubility and dissolution rate is inversely related to particle size distribution. For example, reduction of digoxin particle size from a diameter of 20–30 to 4 μm led to an increase in the rate and extent of absorption after oral administration.[18] For highly potent drugs, which may only form a small percentage of the formulation, a small particle size is essential to ensure homogeneity during mixing. Crystal shape will affect powder flow and mixing properties, and milling may be required to attain the desired characteristics. Crystal polymorphism can also have a profound effect on the bioavailability of solid dosage forms.[19] Chloramphenicol palmitate, for example, exists in three polymorphic forms: A, B and C. C is unstable under normal conditions; B is metastable and can be incorporated into dosage forms and A is the most stable polymorph. Orally polymorph A has zero bioavailability whereas B is absorbed, a difference attributable to the slower dissolution of A compared with B. The British Pharmacopoeia (1988) sets a limit of 10% on the content of polymorph A. Amorphous forms may also exist, which are usually more soluble and dissolve more rapidly than crystalline structures.[20]

The powder's flow properties are also important because they control the physical processes that are used to manipulate the material. Carrs's index, which is a measure of powder bulk density and angle of repose, provides information on flow properties, which are important when production utilises high-speed tableting machines.

Compression properties are important in determining the ability of the compound to form tablets with or without the presence of excipients.

2.2.9 Excipient compatibility

Successful formulation depends on the careful selection of excipients that do not interact with the drug or with each other.[21] This phenomenon can be investigated before formulation commences by studying drug–excipient mixtures using differential scanning calorimetry up to typical processing temperatures. This requires only small samples of drugs and is normally conducted with analysis in order to correlate any chemical degradation with known pathways. It can be used to screen a range of excipients. No interaction indicates stability, but the method is not absolute.

Preformulation testing provides a basic dossier on the compound and plays a significant role in identifying possible problems and suitable approaches to formulation. Such dossiers already exist for the common excipients.[22] The requirement for aqueous solubility is paramount and preformulation can identify salt forms that are appropriate for further development. Stability and solubility studies will indicate the feasibility of various types of formulation such as parenteral liquids and their probable shelf lives. Similar information can be garnered for solid products from the solid physical properties. By performing these studies on a series of candidate compounds, the optimum compound can be identified and further biological and chemical studies guided to provide the best results.

2.3   Formulation

The transformation of a drug into a medicinal product is a complex process that is controlled by a range of competing factors. The formulator must amalgamate the preformulation information and the clinical indication, which may suggest a particular route of administration (e.g. inhalation of salbutamol, Table 2.2), with toxicology and biopharmaceutical data determining the drug's required dose and frequency of administration. Dose is a major factor controlling the type of formulation and processing. Digoxin, for example, requires an oral dose of 125 μg, an amount too small to form a tablet on its own, so excipients are necessary; by contrast, a 500-mg paracetamol tablet requires minimal excipients in relation to the required dose. The regulatory requirements and local conditions of the proposed market countries also impinge on formulation. For example, the inclusion of alcohol may not be permitted in Muslim countries. Some excipients may also be excluded because of the incidence of adverse reactions[23] or insufficient data to warrant administration by a particular route. Different countries may demand varying specifications for product performance. For example, the test for antimicrobial preservative efficacy varies between European pharmacopoeias and the United States Pharmacopeia,[24] although attempts are being made to harmonise requirements (see International Conference on Harmonisation[7]). The formulation must therefore comply with the most stringent combination of regulations so that registration in all the proposed markets is possible. The formulation must also be suitable for rapid economical manufacture to provide a product of consistent performance and quality. The application of good pharmaceutical manufacturing practice (GMP)[25] during production will be useless unless similar quality principles are applied during formulation design. Even with all these strictures, there is still scope for variation in formulation: the pharmacopoeias, for example, provide standards for the drug content of tablets but do not state the excipients or processing to be used.

Formulation is an experimental stage in development to set specifications for the final product that will be sold and administered to patients. Studies must, therefore, be conducted to provide production limits for the product. A solution may require a specific pH for drug stability, for example, pH 7.0, so experiments will also be conducted at pH 6.5 and pH 7.5. If the drug is also stable at these two pH values, then the pH limits for the drug product can be set around the desired value of pH 7.0. Similar experiments will also be required with excipients to establish limits of variation in excipient properties that will not deleteriously affect product performance. An important element is that the formulation itself may alter the drug's biopharmaceutical behaviour, and *in vitro* and *in vivo* tests of formulation performance will be conducted to determine any relationship between formulation and response. For example, increasing compression pressure during tableting can alter disintegration and dissolution properties; *in vitro* dissolution tests can measure this effect and allow determination of compression pressure limits. Occasionally, the combination of drug, formulation and route of administration can lead to a product that produces adverse reactions, which are discovered only after administration to a large number of patients.[26] This is difficult to detect at an early stage but the formulator must be aware of this and aim for simple formulations that avoid potential problems.

The initial formulation for most drugs is to allow basic *in vivo* toxicology, pharmacology and biopharmaceutical assessments to be conducted. Aqueous solutions for injection are optimum for this application since the entire dose is administered at a single time point and the problem of bioavailability does not arise. It is important that these formulations are considered carefully, particularly for drugs that are poorly water soluble, because potentially useful compounds may be rejected inadvertently. These early formulations are also crucial because they set an *in vivo* benchmark for the drug's future performance.

2.3.1 Liquid formulations

Liquid formulations account for about 30% of products in the UK market and, because they are easy to swallow, are favoured for paediatric and geriatric use. An aqueous solution is the simplest formulation to produce, but more complex suspensions or emulsion systems will be required if the drug is poorly soluble. Liquid formulations can be administered by all routes and are probably the most versatile systems. Liquids are, however, bulky, difficult to transport and container breakage can result in catastrophic loss.

The ultimate aim is to provide the desired dose in a suitable liquid volume which, for oral products, is 5 mL.

Solution formulations require excipients to control their properties and improve performance, for example, buffers (such as citric acid) to adjust the pH, sugars or salts to alter the isotonicity of an injection or flavourings to enhance organoleptic properties. Non-sterile aqueous liquids are liable to microbial colonisation and, therefore, require the addition of antimicrobial preservatives. If the drug is poorly soluble, solubility can be enhanced by utilising co-solvents (e.g. ethanol, propylene glycol), altering the pH or the use of solubilised systems (e.g. surfactants). If the drug is insoluble in aqueous media, then non-aqueous media (e.g. soya bean oil) can be employed; however, these solvents are not suitable for intravenous administration.

A special requirement for parenteral or injectable formulations is that they must be sterile, apyrogenic and free from visible particulate contamination.[27] Current requirements are that a sterilisation decision tree[28] is followed and, if possible, sterilisation is conducted using a terminal sterilisation method, for example, autoclaving at 121°C for 15 min for aqueous liquids. This is a severe challenge to the drug's chemical stability, and studies must be conducted to ensure that degradation does not occur. Thermolabile compounds may be sterilised by filtration but this route has implications for large-scale production, which requires specialised facilities,[29] and testing.

Suspensions contain a solid drug as a disperse phase in a normally aqueous-based liquid and are termed either coarse (particles >1 μm diameter) or colloidal (particles <1 μm diameter). The particle size of chloramphenicol palmitate suspension, for example, should not exceed a diameter of 45 μm. Because suspension systems are physically unstable, the solid sedimenting and caking under gravity, the formulation must be designed to limit this phenomenon. Rapid sedimentation or caking will prevent the withdrawal of consistent doses. Typical excipients include wetting agents (e.g. surfactants), thickeners to reduce sedimentation speed (e.g. methylcellulose) and flocculating agents (e.g. electrolytes, polymers) to control the degree of interparticulate interaction, which leads to caking. Suspension stability is also determined by the drug's particle size, and limits will be required because small variations can induce physical instability if the formulation is not robust. Antimicrobial preservatives are necessary and flavours may be required, although, since the drug is not in solution, texture rather than taste could be a problem.

Emulsions are a two-phase system consisting of water and oil.[30] Two types are available: the oil-in-water emulsion, which has oil droplets dispersed in a continuous aqueous phase, and the water-in-oil emulsion, which has water droplets in a continuous oil phase. The former is the most common pharmaceutical presentation with the oil as the therapeutic agent, for example, liquid paraffin emulsion. An increasing use of emulsions is to solubilise water-insoluble drugs, particularly for intravenous administration. In this case, the oil is chosen for its ability to solubilise the drug and its compatibility with the route of administration. An oil-in-water emulsion is thermodynamically unstable and will tend to separate into two distinct liquid phases. The formulation must reduce the interfacial tension between the oil and water using emulsifying agents. Emulsifying agents can be natural (e.g. egg lecithin), synthetic (e.g. polysorbates) or semi-synthetic (e.g. methylcellulose), with the choice depending on the proposed application. Physical stability of the emulsion is paramount and the formulation must be designed to avoid coalescence by providing a large emulsifier layer around each droplet. Emulsions are particularly sensitive to adverse storage conditions such as changes in temperature and may require specialised storage. As with all aqueous-based preparations, an antimicrobial preservative will be required along with an antioxidant to prevent rancidification of the oil.

2.3.2 Semi-solid formulations

A diverse series of semi-solid formulations or vehicles exist and are normally employed for the topical application of drugs to the skin and mucous membranes in order to provide a local action. The drug can be either dissolved or suspended in the formulation, with the simplest system consisting of a single base, such as white soft paraffin, containing dissolved drug. More complex formulations consist of two-phase systems such as creams, which are oil-in-water emulsions, or ointments, which are anhydrous mixtures that can incorporate water to form water-in-oil emulsions. The emulsion systems have the same formulation constraints as the liquid formulations mentioned previously. Aqueous cream, for example, consists of emulsifying wax (cetostearyl alcohol and sodium lauryl sulphate in a ratio of 9 : 1), white soft paraffin and liquid paraffin dispersed in water.[31] When applied to skin, it 'vanishes' and is cosmetically acceptable, whereas white soft paraffin alone would form an occlusive hydrating layer. The vehicle can, therefore, have a marked effect on the response after application, and several of the systems can be used alone for their emollient and protective actions. To exert its effect, the drug must partition from the formulation into the skin, a process that is controlled by the drug's relative solubility in skin and formulation. The balance must favour partitioning into skin, and special derivatives of the drug may be required. The anti-inflammatory steroids are incorporated into creams and ointments as esters in order to increase skin penetration and effect. For example, hydrocortisone is rated as mild when applied topically whereas the butyrate ester is described as potent. Other excipients are also added to these systems, for example, antimicrobial preservatives, buffering agents and perfumes to improve cosmetic acceptability.

2.3.3 Solid formulations

Tablet formulations account for about 45% of the formulations marketed in the United Kingdom with capsules accounting for about 15%. These formulations have the advantage of providing the dose in a discrete unit form that is stable, easily produced, transported and, above all, easily administered. The tablet is favoured because it is marginally cheaper to produce and slightly more stable under in-use conditions. The simplest solid dosage form is the drug powder itself, a presentation mode that is still used for some antacid preparations. For modern drugs, the dose required is too small to be measured accurately by the patient and must therefore be presented preformed.

The tablet was introduced by Thomas Brockedon in 1843, and glyceryl trinitrate tablets appeared in the British Pharmacopoeia of 1885. Since that time, many variations have appeared but the basic process remains unchanged.[32] There are three main methods of tablet manufacture, with choice depending on the dose and the drug's physical properties such as compressibility and flow (Figure 2.2). A drug with a large dose (>100 mg) and good flow and compressibility properties may be directly compressed into a tablet after mixing with suitable excipients (Table 2.5).[33] Normally, however, the physical properties are not ideal and some form of pretreatment such as granulation is necessary.[34] In wet granulation, the drug is mixed with a diluent and then a solution of a polymeric binder is added during continuous mixing to form a wet powder mass. The mass is passed through a sieve with a mesh size of 1–2 mm to produce granules similar in nature to instant coffee. After drying in hot air and sieving to provide a homogeneous size, these granules are then further blended with a lubricant, disintegrant and maybe further diluents. The final granule mix

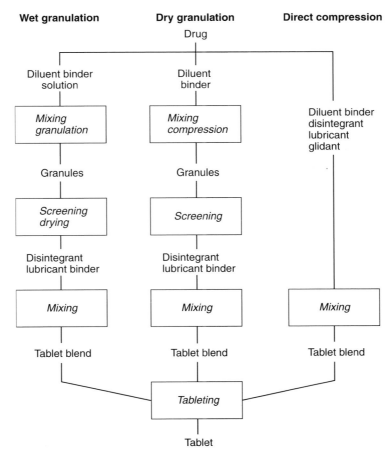

Fig. 2.2 The tablet production process. Process stages are shown in boxes.

Table 2.5 Tablet excipients

Excipient	Functions	Examples
Diluent	Bulking agent to adjust tablet weight and ameliorate poor bulk drug properties	Lactose, crystalline cellulose, dicalcium phosphate
Binder	Adhesive to bind together diluent and drug during granulation and compaction	Starch, cellulose derivatives, polyvinylpyrrolidone
Glidant	Aids powder flow properties during manufacture	Colloidal silica, starch
Lubricant	Prevents powder/tablets sticking to punches Aids punch movement	Stearic acid, magnesium stearate, sodium lauryl sulphate
Disintegrant	Aids tablet disintegration in aqueous environment	Starch, sodium starch glycollate, cross-linked polyvinylpyrrolidone
Coat	Physical protection of tablet Taste masking Control of drug release	Sugar, methylcellulose, cellulose acetate phthalate (for enteric coatings)

should flow easily and is fed into a die and then compressed between two punches to produce the tablet. If the drug is not stable in aqueous systems, granulation using solvents, such as isopropyl alcohol, is possible although difficult because of the volatile and flammable properties of the solvent. Thermolabile drugs can be granulated by compressing a drug–diluent–lubricant mix with rollers to produce large slugs of solid material. This can then be broken down into granule-sized pieces and treated as described above.

The basic tablet can be varied in many ways simply by altering the excipients used or by further treatment after production using coatings. The initial formulation is usually a simple rapidly disintegrating tablet, with modifications occurring only when further information is available. Dissolving tablets, for example, require water-soluble excipients; effervescent formulations utilise citric acid and sodium bicarbonate but require manufacture under dry conditions. A polymeric diluent without disintegrant produces a swelling tablet that will delay drug dissolution and provide a sustained release.

The traditional tablet coating is a sugar coat applied in stages. First the tablet surface is sealed to prevent the ingress of water, then a subcoat of an aqueous polymeric or sucrose solution is added to smooth the surface of the tablet. This can be repeated until the desired size and shape is achieved. Finally a coloured sugar coat is applied and wax polished, and the company logo may be printed on the tablets. This process is expensive and laborious and has largely been replaced by film coatings, which utilise a coat of a polymer dissolved in a suitable solvent.[35] The polymer characteristics can be modified by the addition of colours and plasticisers. The coat provides mechanical protection against chipping and also helps to mask the taste. The polymer coat can also be designed to provide a controlled release so that the tablet degrades only in the intestine (enteric coat) in order to protect either acid-labile drugs from the stomach or the stomach from irritant drugs. Unusual product specifications may be imposed by the marketing department in terms of tablet shape or colour. Usually this does not affect the tablet performance but may induce manufacturing problems and is difficult to blind when comparative clinical trials are performed. Specialised tablet formulations can be used for vaginal administration to achieve a localised effect.

Capsules consist of a gelatin shell, which may be either hard or soft, enclosing, respectively, powders or non-aqueous liquids. The most common type is the hard gelatin shell, consisting of two halves which are formed separately but loosely fitted together after production.[36] A free-flowing formulation that can be filled into the bottom half before the top is completely pushed home is required. Powder formulations must flow, and a suitable powder blend containing a diluent and glidant will be required. Similar excipients to those employed in tablet formulations can be used, but the properties required of the powder are different because of variations in the filling machines. Hygroscopic materials can induce problems by drying the gelatin shell, producing brittle capsules, or by drawing in water to soften the shell. Any flowing dry material can be placed into the hard shell, and a variation on powder blends is the spheronised formulation, which consists of small, granule-sized beads, which can be coated to control drug release. A novel technology for hard shell is the 'melt fill', which utilises a non-aqueous material, such as polyethylene glycol 6000, which is liquid at elevated temperatures but solidifies at room temperature after capsule filling. The drug is simply dissolved or suspended in the molten liquid, which reduces dust hazards normally associated with tablets or capsules. Soft gelatin capsules have to be formed at the point of fill from molten gelatin softened with glycerol or propylene glycol. The formulation is usually non-aqueous, for example, a fish oil or lipid–vitamin mixture, although molten gel fills similar to those described above can be used.[37]

2.3.4 Contemporary formulations

The introduction of novel materials, polymers and delivery techniques has allowed a range of formulations to be developed that provide greater control over drug delivery to the body than traditional formulations.[38,39] These formulations are designed for a specific drug, drug delivery system or therapeutic application, although several of them have generic uses. The basis is to provide a constant drug level either in the body or at the site of use, which will provide a constant effect rather than the variable drug levels associated with conventional formulations. Two basic types of controlled-release system exist: one contains a reservoir of drug, which is released via a rate-controlling membrane; the other entraps the drug in a matrix, which controls release by restricting drug diffusion out of the matrix.

The transdermal patch looks like a standard sticking plaster of 2–3 cm, which is applied to the skin (Figure 2.3). Several methods of controlling drug release are available. Membrane moderated patches consist of a drug reservoir enclosed by an impermeable backing material sealed on to a rate-limiting membrane covered with adhesive that sticks to the skin.[40] Drug is released into the skin through the rate-controlling membrane and is then absorbed systemically to exert its pharmacological effect. The rate of drug transfer through the skin is dependent on its properties and this system is only suitable for drugs that meet specific physicochemical criteria.[41] The drug must also be sufficiently active (low dose) because the quantity absorbed by this route is minimal. Ocusert® is a similar system for the prolonged release of drugs in the eye. A reservoir of pilocarpine is encased in a rate-limiting polymer membrane.[42] In the eye, pilocarpine diffuses through the membrane to deliver drug at a defined rate (20 or 40 µg/h) for periods of up to 1 week.

Spherical or pellet-based drug delivery formulations are possible, and range in diameter from millimetres down to nanometres. The larger systems are very useful for gastrointestinal administration,[43] especially where the system is enteric-coated to prevent drug release in the stomach. (The coating ensures that the tablet remains intact and does not disintegrate until it reaches the small intestine.) The passage of large enteric-coated tablets from the stomach is erratic, and pellet-based formulations of 1–2 mm diameter do not suffer from this problem.[44] Recent developments have extended this type of system to injectable (subcutaneous) formulations for labile peptide drugs that require a prolonged action, for example, goserelin and leuprorelin. These drugs cannot be

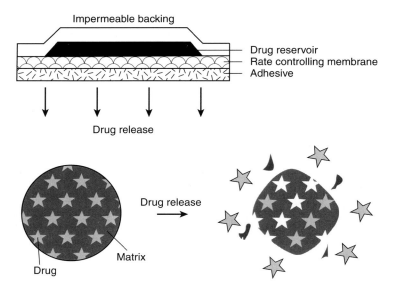

Fig. 2.3 Reservoir- (top) and matrix-based (bottom) drug delivery systems. The matrix system degrades during drug delivery, releasing the drug and matrix through either matrix erosion or degradation.

administered by the oral route, have very short plasma half-lives and would require repeated injections to be clinically effective. The drugs are, therefore, incorporated into the matrix of microspheres (tens of micrometres in diameter) of a biodegradable and biocompatible polymer (polylactide-co-glycolide).[45] The polymer degrades after injection, slowly releasing the drug to provide continuous therapy for between 1 and 3 months, depending on the formulation. Even smaller systems, such as nanoparticles,[46] are under investigation as drug delivery, and also drug targeting, systems and future developments to 'formulate' novel therapeutics, such as genes[47] and other biological molecules,[48–50] are undergoing concerted active research.

2.3.5 Packaging

The packaging of a medicinal product fulfils a variety of roles such as product presentation, identification, convenience and protection until administration or use. Selection of packaging requires a basic knowledge of packaging materials, the environmental conditions to which the product will be exposed and the characteristics of the formulation. Several types of packaging will be employed, the primary packaging around the

product, and secondary packaging such as a carton and subsequent transit cases. The following discussion concerns primary packaging.

The packaging must physically protect the product from the mechanical stresses of warehousing, handling and distribution. Mechanical stress may take a variety of forms, from impact through to vibration in transit and compression forces on stacking. The demands for mechanical protection will vary with product type: glass ampoules will require greater protection than plastic eye drop bottles, for example.

Other protection is required from environmental factors such as moisture, temperature changes, light, gases and biological agents such as micro-organisms and, importantly, humans. The global market for medicinal products requires that the products are stable over a wide range of temperatures ranging from subzero in polar regions, 15°C in temperate zones, up to 32°C in the tropics. Along with this temperature variation, relative humidity can vary from below 50% to up to 90%, a feature that the packaging should be able to resist if necessary. The majority of packaging materials (including plastics) is to some degree permeable to moisture and the type of closure employed, such as screw fittings, may also permit ingress of moisture. The susceptibility of the product to moisture and its hygroscopicity will have to be considered and may require packaging with a desiccant or the use of specialised strip packs using low permeability materials such as foil. Temperature fluctuations can lead to condensation of moisture on the product and, with liquids, formation of a condensate layer on top of the product. This latter problem is well known and can lead to microbiological spoilage as the condensate is preservative free. If the product is sensitive to photolysis, then opaque materials may be required. Most secondary packaging materials (e.g. cartons) do not transmit light, but in some cases, specialised primary packaging designed to limit light transmission is employed. The package must also prevent the entry of organisms; for example, packaging of sterile products must be absolutely micro-organism proof, hence the continued use of glass ampoules. For non-sterile products, the preservative provides some protection, but continual microbial challenge will diminish the efficacy of the preservative, and spoilage or disease transmission may occur.[51] Finally, the packaging material must not interact with the product either to adsorb substances from the product or to leach chemicals into the product. Plastics contain additives to enhance polymer performance. Polyvinyl chloride (PVC) may contain phthalate di-ester plasticiser, which can leach into infusion fluids from packaging.[52] Antimicrobial preservatives such as phenylmercuric acetate are known to partition into rubbers and plastics during storage, thus reducing the formulation concentration below effective antimicrobial levels.[53] A complication of modern packaging is the need for the application of security seals to protect against deliberate adulteration and maintain consumer confidence.

2.3.6 Stability testing

Once the optimal formulation and processing method have been determined and the most suitable packaging configuration decided, product stability tests may be commenced. The aim is to determine a shelf life and provide data that demonstrate the product's continued quality under the conditions of manufacture, storage,

distribution and usage. Since time is a major parameter in stability testing, a large amount of resources is involved in conducting stability tests, and mishaps can be costly. To ensure commercial returns on an NCE, it must be marketed when only limited stability testing of 1–2 years has been performed. Accelerated stability studies are therefore carried out where the product is deliberately stressed using elevated temperatures and humidity (Table 2.6).[10] Extrapolation of the results to ambient conditions allows the prediction of a shelf life or expiration date (Figure 2.1). The study should monitor all the product's characteristics that may be affected by storage and this normally means testing to the full release specifications. For example, products containing antimicrobial preservatives must meet the specifications of pharmacopoeial microbial challenge tests at all times during the proposed shelf life. Some tests that are not part of the release specification may also be conducted to provide greater information on product behaviour, such as dissolution testing in tablets. The regulatory authorities expect these data to be presented for at least three different batches of the product, using three different batches of active ingredient, in the final marketing packaging.[54] Also, the batches used should, if possible, be manufactured at the same scale as production batches.

One interesting feature of stability is that a product may have two shelf lives, one for the manufactured material and another for the reconstituted or opened pack. Methyl prednisolone sodium succinate lyophilised injection, for example, is stable for up to 3 years in the dry state but the reconstituted injection must be used within 12 h.

2.3.7 Scale-up and manufacture

The evolution and optimisation of a formulation is an experimental stage that will be conducted on small batches of the material. For a drug with a tablet weight of 250 mg, test batches would typically be 0.5–1 kg, providing up to 4000 tablets for analysis, performance testing and initial stability studies. Similar scales will be used in the optimisation of the product's packaging.

Table 2.6 Typical conditions and sampling profile for product stability tests

Sample time (months)	Storage conditions (temperature/relative humidity)							
	2–8°C		25°C/60%[a]		30°C/70%[a]		40°C/75%[a]	
	CT	Final	CT	Final	CT	Final	CT	Final
1	✓	✓	✓	✓	✓	✓	✓	✓
3	✓	✓	✓	✓	✓	✓	✓	✓
6	✓	✓	✓	✓	✓	✓	✓	✓
9	✓	✓	✓	✓	✓	✓		✓
12	✓	✓	✓	✓	✓	✓		✓
18	✓	✓	✓	✓	✓	✓		✓
24	✓	✓	✓	✓	✓	✓		✓
36		✓		✓		✓		
48		✓		✓		✓		
60		✓		✓				

The table shows one of a variety of possible test configurations; the EU requires at least 6 months of data before marketing. Clinical trial (CT) products do not require long shelf lives and therefore testing can be limited. For some thermolabile products, the temperature range may be lower, or testing at higher temperatures may be terminated quickly. A full analytical profile should be determined for all samples if possible.
✓, sample analysed.
[a] May also be conducted with light exposure.

The overall aim of pharmaceutical development is to transform the formulation into a product that can be manufactured on a large scale, which must be achieved without any deleterious alterations to the performance of the formulation. The complexity of scale-up is related to the proposed production batch size of the final product, typically around 2 million units, which for a 250-mg tablet is 500 kg of material. Additionally, the number of manufacturing sites to be employed must be considered, as ambient environmental conditions and equipment may vary, inducing variations in the final product. Several intermediate stages will be employed to gain experience with handling larger quantities of the formulation and ensure that no variations occur. Intermediate batches consuming 10–50 to 100 kg of material will be processed, and several problems may arise because of increases in batch size. Larger heating or mixing vessels have a smaller surface-to-volume ratio and may take longer to heat or cool, exposing the formulation to elevated temperatures and producing thermal degradation. Large-scale handling of powders in hoppers can induce separation of the constituents, leading to variation in tablet content during a production run. Development tablet machines produce about 100 tablets per minute, while a rotary tablet press (Figure 2.4) may produce up to 5000 tablets per minute. Regulatory authorities require that at least three full-scale production runs are conducted,[55] and that any of the processes employed, for example, sterilisation, are fully validated.[56] This will allow manufacturing personnel to gain familiarity with the product and ensure that product quality can be guaranteed before full production commences. The increasing level of product stocks that will be accumulated by this process can be employed in clinical trials and the latter batches may form part of the launch supplies.

Before the market launch of the product, regulatory authorities will inspect the production premises and processes to ensure that everything complies with the licence application and GMP.[25] GMP must be maintained throughout the production cycle, including, where required, suppliers and also the distribution chain. In fact,

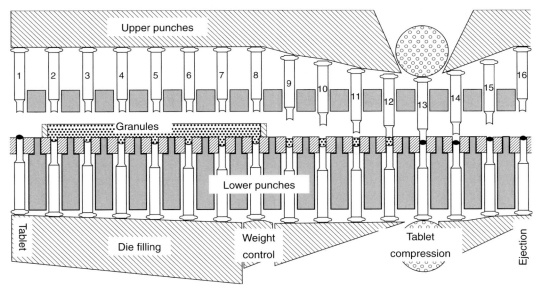

Fig. 2.4 A rotary tablet press. The punches and dies move in a circular manner around the die filling, weight control, compression and ejection stages. At positions 2–7, the bottom punch drops and the space created in the die is filled with granules flowing under gravity. The tablet weight is set at position 8 by raising the bottom punch to a set height and skimming off the excess granulate. The tablet is compressed between the top and the bottom punches at position 13 and then ejected by removing the top punch and raising the bottom punch in positions 14–1. In this example, a single tablet is produced for each cycle but some presses may have two cycles per rotation and multiple punches and dies, thus increasing production rate.

GMP (or its associated quality standards) should only end when the product is handed to the patient. At this stage, all control ceases.

Scale-up of drug synthesis will also be required, as initial manufacture will probably occur on a laboratory scale, providing only grams of material. The synthetic route may not be ideal for large-scale production and a new pathway may be required for the latter stages of development. Tests will have to be conducted to ensure that the active ingredient is not significantly different from the original material and that impurity levels are not increased. If different impurities arise from the new synthetic route, these will have to be studied.

2.3.8 Bioequivalence

Once a drug's patent protection has expired, it is common to find two or more products of the same strength and form produced by different manufacturers (see Table 2.2). This is a consequence of financial pressures to reduce prescribing costs and has led to the development of a burgeoning generic industry. Products marketed under approved or brand names are classed as chemically or pharmaceutically equivalent because they contain the same dose of the same drug. However, chemical equivalence does not guarantee that the products will behave identically when administered to the patient because they may contain different excipients and may have been produced by widely differing techniques. An early example of the problem of bioequivalence occurred with the antiepileptic drug phenytoin. In 1970, it was reported that a change in capsule diluent from calcium sulphate dihydrate to lactose produced phenytoin overdosage in patients receiving chemically equivalent capsules.[57] Bioequivalence arises from extravascular routes of administration (e.g. oral, intramuscular, rectal) where absorption occurs before the drug appears in the blood (Figure 2.5). Absorption has two

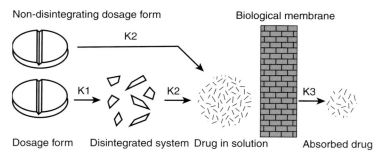

Fig. 2.5 Stages in drug absorption from an extravascular administration site (stomach, small intestine, intramuscular injection). Only drug in solution is absorbed. If the rate of dissolution (K2) is less than the rate of absorption (K3), then the rate at which the drug is released from the dosage form controls absorption. This permits modified or sustained-release formulations, but can also lead to bioequivalence problems.

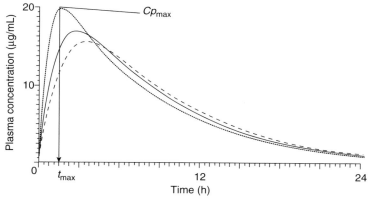

Fig. 2.6 Effect of variation in absorption rate on plasma drug concentration. The graph shows simulated plasma concentration–time curves for theophylline after oral administration, illustrating a 20% difference in Cp_{max} values resulting from variation in the absorption rate constant. Absorption rate constants: top curve 2.2 per h (Cp_{max} 20 μg/mL); middle curve 1.0 per h (Cp_{max} 18 μg/mL); bottom curve 0.7 per h. Note that t_{max} also changes. The established therapeutic concentration of theophyllin is 10–20 μg/mL. The most rapidly absorbed formulation produces the highest concentration and greatest chance of side effects. Also, the duration for which the plasma concentration is within the therapeutic range also varies. Pharmacokinetic parameters: dose, 400 mg: bioavailability, 0.8; volume of distribution, 29 L; half-life, 5.5 h.

important pharmacokinetic features: the extent of absorption and the rate of absorption.[58] The former is measured by comparing the area under the plasma concentration–time curve (AUC) after administration of the formulation with the AUC of an intravenous injection. Intravenous injection provides an extent of absorption of one since the entire dose reaches the blood or systemic circulation. The rate of absorption may be measured by determining the maximum plasma concentration, C_{max}, and the time taken to reach

C_{max}, t_{max}. The latter is a measure of the rate of absorption whereas the former is also dependent on the extent of absorption. Differences in either extent or rate of absorption can markedly alter the plasma concentration profile and produce different clinical effect (Figure 2.6).

There is a large literature on this subject, mainly concentrated in the field of oral products.[59] Bioequivalence is, however, a potential problem with other routes of administration such as transdermal, topical[60] and intramuscular routes. The prescriber and patient expect that chemically equivalent products are therapeutically equivalent and this requires the generic formulation to mimic the marketed product's *in vivo* behaviour. The arbiters of bioequivalence are the regulatory authorities, and the regulations of various countries are not identical.[60,61] In general, bioequivalence is demonstrated if the mean difference between two products is within ±20% at the 95% confidence level. This is a statistical requirement, which may require a large number of samples (e.g. volunteers), if the drug exhibits variable absorption and disposition pharmacokinetics. For drugs for which there is a small therapeutic window or low therapeutic index, the ±20% limit may be reduced. The preferred test method is an *in vivo* crossover study and, since this occurs in the development phase, necessitates the employment of volunteers. These studies are, therefore, expensive and animal experiments may be substituted, or *in vitro* experiments if they have been correlated with *in vivo* studies.

Bioequivalence problems arise only when the formulation is the rate-limiting step in drug absorption. All formulations should, therefore, be optimised to ensure maximal absorption equivalent to the administration of a solution, unless a controlled or sustained drug delivery is sought. In general, increasing formulation complexity and processing increases the risk of bioequivalence problems. Controlled-release preparations require proof of equivalence at steady state to already marketed rapid-release or sustained-release preparations. In addition, studies must prove the controlled-release characteristics claimed and rule out the possibility of 'dose dumping'. Other problems associated with alternative formulations can be the inclusion of new excipients that induce adverse reactions, or changes in patient preferences resulting from differences in product colour or presentation.

2.4 Clinical trial supplies

Initial clinical trials will be conducted early in the drug's development simply to evaluate the pharmacological response, perform pharmacokinetic studies or determine the maximum tolerated dose in humans.[62] The formulations administered in these early trials should be as close as possible to the eventually marketed product to avoid costly retesting. These trials present no problems, other than those of quality and stability since there is no element of deceit or blinding because both volunteer and physician are aware of the administered product. Subsequent Phase II, III and IV trials, however, may require blinding, particularly if some form of product comparison is undertaken. Blinding ensures that the patient (single blind) and maybe also the physician (double blind) do not know which treatment is administered[63] in order to eliminate any potential bias that may be introduced into the trial results. The trial protocol will be developed by the physician and the clinical research department of the sponsor; however, liaison with the pharmaceutical department should occur at an early stage to ensure that any proposed trial is pharmaceutically possible. The pharmaceutical challenge is to develop the appropriate manufacturing and packaging procedures that ensure the stability and quality of the trial supplies. In addition to this, blinding may be required by the clinical trial protocol. The simplest trial would be active product against matching placebo at a single dose level. Expanding the trial, for example, by using multiple dose levels or comparisons with competitors' products, increases the complexity of supplies and pharmaceutical demands. The level of complexity is also controlled by the types of formulations or products that are employed in the trial.

2.4.1 Blinding

Clinical trial supplies can be blinded using several techniques depending on the availability of resources and the consideration of competitor companies. The ideal situation is to produce a placebo or comparator product that looks and behaves in an identical fashion to its active test counterpart, for example, the same colour, weight, shape, size, markings, texture and taste. Colourless solutions or white tablets do not present a great problem, but if the drug is coloured, the placebo will have to match this. Production of in-house placebo formulations is relatively easy; however, if a competitor's product is involved, then difficulties can arise. The competitor can be asked to supply the drug in a form matching the product under test, but this may not always be possible for a variety of reasons. If a competitor's product cannot be matched, then it may be manipulated to eliminate differences between the two products. The ideal option is to reformulate the competitor's product to match the test product; however, great care must be taken to ensure that the two products (manipulated and original) are bioequivalent and exhibit the same stability, etc., as the original marketed product. Since this represents a new formulation, a great deal of time and effort would be required. To circumvent this, both products can be disguised, for example, by packaging small tablets in opaque, hard gelatin capsules or using rice paper cachets. Different tablets can be coated using either film or sugar coating to mask their distinguishing features and produce effectively similar products. Again, tests would be required to ensure that stability and bioequivalence was not compromised.

If products cannot be matched, for example, a tablet versus an aerosol, or if the above techniques are not possible, then blinding can be performed using the double-dummy technique, so-called because a matching placebo for both products is manufactured. The patient then has to administer two products at one time, only one of which contains the active drug (Figure 2.7). The advantage is that both products are used without manipulation, but it can be very confusing for the trial participants. In these cases, it is important that easily understood, explicit and comprehensive instructions are provided to the patient, possibly employing special packs to aid compliance. If different dose levels or dose escalations are required, then adaptations to the placebo and dummy techniques can be employed. For example, administration of three tablets three times daily would allow for doses ranging from nine placebo tablets through to nine

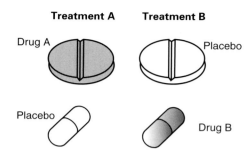

Fig. 2.7 The double-dummy technique. The patient always takes a tablet and a capsule. In treatment A, the tablet contains the active drug and the capsule contains the placebo. In treatment B, the capsule contains the active drug and the tablet contains the placebo.

active tablets daily. One drawback of complicated regimens is patient non-compliance or failure to take therapy as directed. This may have a capricious effect on trial results and a method to detect non-compliance should be employed, such as retrieval of the patient's supplies and determination of the number of doses administered. One feature of blinded clinical trials that has to be ascribed to human nature is the desire to break blinding, which may arise through a variety of routes. The active preparation will taste bitter, patients may prefer to crush or suck tablets before swallowing and the difference between placebo and active will be apparent.

2.4.2 Labelling of clinical trial materials

The United Kingdom Medicines Act 1968 regulations require that all medicinal products are properly labelled to certain minimum standards, but requirements vary from country to country. Clinical trial materials, however, cannot be labelled normally because if the trial is blind, nothing should reveal to the patient or physician the nature of the contents. The basic information on the label should provide the patient's name, study phase, study number, directions for use, any special warning or storage requirements, expiry date and the investigator's name and address, along with an indication that the drugs are 'for clinical trial use only'. The sponsoring company's name and address should also appear, together with a code that can be broken in the case of emergency to determine if the patient is receiving an active or placebo preparation.

2.4.3   Quality assurance of clinical trial supplies

European clinical trial products do not currently require manufacture to GMP; however, a new clinical trial directive is undergoing implementation and will necessitate the manufacture to GMP in licensed premises.

The manufacture and packaging of clinical trial supplies present interesting quality assurance problems. The manufacture of placebo products, for example, must include testing to ensure freedom from any contaminating active drug. The active products used must also be stability tested in the proposed packaging since specialist packaging will be employed to aid blinding and meet the requirements of the trial protocol. The packaging exercise requires an ordered approach to meet the protocol requirements, including randomisation schedules, crossover, labelling and blinding with placebo or dummy techniques. A double-dummy trial comparing two products at one dose level with a crossover would require the packaging of two sets of supplies, one with active A/placebo B and one with placebo A/active B. These would then have to be combined and labelled following the requirements of the randomisation schedule and crossover. If the trial involves two dose levels for A, then the initial packaging will require three sets of supplies. Protocols that require dosage changes during the trial necessitate the packaging of extra supplies for each patient that can be called on when required by the protocol. However, if it is performed, the supplies must all look identical. Hopefully the reader will realise that even simple trials can lead to incredible logistical problems in the provision of supplies. Once packaged, the supplies must be subjected to checking and quality control procedures, for example, analysis for the active substance, to ensure that the packaging is correct. Since the trial is dependent on the supplies, packaging and analytical documentation form an integral part of the quality assurance for the trial.

2.5   Conclusions

The process of pharmaceutical development is the transformation of the chemist's compound through the pharmacist's formulation and production of the product to become marketable merchandise. This long, involved process requires the input of large resources and a myriad of professional and technical expertise. Almost £3000 million[64] was spent on pharmaceutical research and development in the United Kingdom in 2000, with nominally about 60% spent on applied research and experimental development. The process consists of several distinct but overlapping and interlinked phases, which have a range of milestones to gauge progress: the initiation of preformulation studies, formulation of Phase I clinical trial products, commencement of Phase I trials in man, full-scale production runs and, eventually, market launch. Careful co-ordination throughout the process is necessary to ensure that the development of any adverse results is acted upon and decisions to either progress or drop the compound are taken before expenditure is excessive. Once a drug is marketed, the pharmaceutical development process continues with ongoing stability studies, post-marketing surveillance and the development of new formulations and therapeutic uses as clinical experience with the drug expands. A complaint procedure must be established and reported incidences investigated to ensure that the product performs in the field as expected. This chapter has presented the reader with only a surface veneer of information regarding the pharmaceutical development process; hopefully this will stimulate interest and further reading on this extensive subject.

Further Reading

Aulton ME, ed. *Pharmaceutics The Science of Dosage Form Development, 2nd edn.* London: Churchill Livingstone, 2002.

Cartwright AC, Matthews BR, eds. *International Pharmaceutical Product Registration: Aspects of Quality, Safety and Efficacy.* London: Ellis Horwood, 1994.

References

1. Wells JI, ed. *Pharmaceutical Preformulation: The Physicochemical Properties of Drug Substances.* Chichester: Ellis Horwood, 1988.
2. Carstensen JT. Preformulation. In: Carstensen JT, Rhodes CT, eds. *Drug Stability Principles and Practices, 3rd edn.* New York: Marcel Dekker, 2000; 237–60.
3. Anon. Text on validations of analytical procedures. In: *International Conference on Harmonisation of Technical Requirements for Registration of Pharmaceutical for Human Use,* 1994. http://www.ifpma.org/ich5q.html#Analytical.
4. Fong GW, Lam SK, eds. *HPLC in the Pharmaceutical Industry.* New York: Marcel Dekker, 1991.
5. Altria KD, Kelly MA, Clark BJ. Current applications in the analysis of pharmaceuticals by capillary electrophoresis. I. *Trends Anal Chem* 1998;**17**:204–14.
6. Altria KD, Kelly MA, Clark BJ. Current applications in the analysis of pharmaceuticals by capillary electrophoresis. II. *Trends Anal Chem* 1998;**17**:214–26.
7. Anon. Impurities in new drug substances (revised guideline) Q3AR. In: *International Conference on Harmonisation of Technical Requirements for Registration of Pharmaceutical for Human Use,* 1999. http://www.ifpma.org/ich5q.html#Impurity.
8. Hirsh CA, Messenger RJ, Brannon JL. Fenoprofen: drug form selection and preformulation stability studies. *J Pharm Sci* 1978;**67**:231–6.
9. Anon. Stability testing of new drugs and products. In: *International Conference on Harmonisation of Technical Requirements for Registration of Pharmaceutical for Human Use,* 2000. http://www.ifpma.org/ich5q.html#Stability.
10. Grimm W. A rational approach to stability testing and analytical development for NCE, drug substance, and drug products: marketed product stability testing. In: Carstensen JT, Rhodes CT, eds. *Drug Stability Principles and Practices, 3rd edn.* New York: Marcel Dekker, 2000;415–81.
11. Florence AT, Attwood D. *Physicochemical Principles of Pharmacy, 2nd edn.* London: MacMillan Press, 1988.
12. Ooms F. Molecular modeling and computer aided drug design. Examples of their applications in medicinal chemistry. *Curr Med Chem* 2000;**7**:141–58.
13. Cartwright AC. Introduction and history of pharmaceutical regulation. In: Cartwright AC, Matthews BR, eds. *Pharmaceutical Product Licensing. Requirements for Europe.* Chichester: Ellis Horwood, 1991;29–45.
14. Ariens EJ, Wuis EW, Veringa EJ. Stereoselectivity of bioactive xenobiotics: a pre-Pasteur attitude in medicinal chemistry, pharmacokinetics and clinical pharmacology. *Biochem Pharmacol* 1988;**37**: 9–18.
15. Fanali S, Aturki Z, Desiderio C. Enantioresolution of pharmaceutical compounds by capillary electrophoresis. Use of cyclodextrins and antibiotics. *Enantiomer* 1999;**4**:229–41.
16. Artursson P, Palm K, Luthman K. Caco-2 monolayers in experimental and theoretical predictions of drug transport. *Adv Drug Deliv Rev* 2001;**46**:27–43.
17. Li AP. Screening for human ADME/Tox drug properties in drug discovery. *Drug Discov Today* 2001;**6**:357–66.
18. Shaw TRD, Carless JE. The effect of particle size on the absorption of digoxin. *Eur J Clin Pharmacol* 1974;**7**:269.
19. Borka L. Review on crystal polymorphism of substances in the European Pharmacopeia. *Pharm Acta Helv* 1991;**66**:16–22.
20. Yu L. Amorphous pharmaceutical solids: preparation, characterization and stabilization. *Adv Drug Deliv Rev* 2001;**48**:27–42.
21. Crowley P, Martini L. Drug–excipient interactions. *Pharm Technol Europe* 2001;**13**:26–34.
22. Anon. *Handbook of Pharmaceutical Excipients.* London: Pharmaceutical Press, 1986.
23. Weiner M, Bernstein IL. *Adverse Reactions to Drug Formulation Agents. A Handbook of Excipients.* New York: Marcel Dekker, 1989.
24. Akers MJ, Taylor CJ. Official methods of preservative evaluation and testing. In: Denyer SP, Baird RM, eds. *Guide to Microbiological Control in Pharmaceuticals.* London: Ellis Horwood, 1990;292–303.
25. Anon. *Rules and Guidance for Pharmaceutical Manufacturers and Distributors.* London: The Stationery Office, 1997.
26. Florence AT, Salole EG. *Formulation Factors in Adverse Reactions.* London: Wright, 1990.
27. Groves MJ. *Parenteral Technology Manual, 2nd edn.* Buffalo Grove: Interpharm Press, 1989.
28. Morris JM. Sterilisation decision trees and implementation. *PDA J Pharm Science Technol* 1999;**54**: 64–8.
29. Walden MP. Clean rooms. In: Cole GC, ed. *Pharmaceutical Production Facilities.* Chichester: Ellis Horwood, 1990;79–126.

30. Eccleston GM. Emulsions. In: Swarbrick J, Boylan JC, eds. *Encyclopedia of Pharmaceutical Technology*. New York: Marcel Dekker, 1992; 137–88.

31. Eccleston GM. Properties of fatty alcohol mixed emulsifiers and emulsifying waxes. In: Florence AT, ed. *Materials used in Pharmaceutical Formulation*. Oxford: Blackwell Scientific Publications, 1984;124–56.

32. Lieberman HA, Lachman L. *Pharmaceutical Dosage Forms: Tablets, 2nd edn*. New York: Marcel Dekker, 1992.

33. Murray M, Laohavichien A, Habib W, *et al*. Effect of process variables on roller-compacted ibuprofen tablets. *Pharm Ind* 1998;**60**:257–62.

34. Keleb EI, Vermeire A, Vervaet C, *et al*. Cold extrusion as a continuous single-step granulation and tableting process. *Eur J Pharm Biopharm* 2001;**52**:359–68.

35. Rowe RC. Defects in film-coated tablets: aetiology and solutions. In: Ganderton D, Jones T, eds. *Advances in Pharmaceutical Sciences*. London: Academic Press, 1992;65–100.

36. Ridgway K, ed. *Hard Capsules Development and Technology*. London: Pharmaceutical Press, 1987.

37. Jimerson RF, Hom FS. Capsules, soft. In: Swarbrick J, Boylan JC, eds. *Encyclopedia of Pharmaceutical Technology*. New York: Marcel Dekker, 1990;269–84.

38. Kydonieus A, ed. *Treatise on Controlled Drug Delivery. Fundamentals, Optimization, Applications*. New York: Marcel Dekker, 1992.

39. Dressman JB, Ridout G, Guy RH. Delivery system technology. In: Hansch C, ed. *Biopharmaceutics*. Oxford: Pergamon Press, 1990;615–60.

40. Govil SK. Transdermal drug delivery devices. In: Tyle P, ed. *Drug Delivery Devices. Fundamentals and Applications*. New York: Marcel Dekker, 1988;386–419.

41. Walters KA. Transdermal drug delivery. In: Florence AT, Salole EG, eds. *Routes of Drug Administration*. London: Wright, 1990;78–136.

42. Mitra AK. Ophthalmic drug delivery devices. In: Tyle P, ed. *Drug Delivery Devices. Fundamentals and Applications*. New York: Marcel Dekker, 1988;455–70.

43. Ghebre-Sellassie I. *Multiparticulate Oral Drug Delivery*. New York: Marcel Dekker, 1994.

44. Wilson CG, Washington N. *Physiological Pharmaceutics: Biological Barriers to Drug Absorption, 2nd edn*. Chichester: Ellis Horwood, 2001.

45. Sharifi R, Ratanawong C, Jung A, *et al*. Therapeutic effects of leuprorelin microspheres in prostate cancer. *Adv Drug Deliv Rev* 1997;**28**: 121–38.

46. Kawashima Y. Preface nanoparticulate systems for improved drug delivery. *Adv Drug Deliv Rev* 2001;**47**:1–2.

47. Pouton CW, Seymour LW. Key issues in non-viral gene delivery. *Adv Drug Deliv Rev* 2001;**46**: 187–203.

48. Oussoren C, Storm G. Liposomes to target the lymphatics by subcutaneous administration. *Adv Drug Deliv Rev* 2001;**50**:143–56.

49. Harashima H, Kiwada H. The pharmacokinetics of liposomes in tumor targeting. *Adv Drug Deliv Rev* 1999;**40**:1–2.

50. Clark MA, Jepson MA, Hirst BH. Exploiting M cells for drug and vaccine delivery. *Adv Drug Deliv Rev* 2001;**50**:81–106.

51. Bloomfield SF. Microbial contamination: spoilage and hazard. In: Denyer S, Baird R, eds. *Guide to Microbiological Control in Pharmaceuticals*. Chichester: Ellis Horwood, 1990;29–52.

52. Boruchoff SA. Hypotension and cardiac arrest in rats after infusion of mono(2-ethylhexyl)phthalate (MEHP), a contaminant of stored blood. *N Engl J Med* 1987;**316**:1218–19.

53. Aspinall JA, Duffy TD, Saunders MB, *et al*. The effect of low density polyethylene containers on some hospital-manufactured eye drop formulations. 1. Sorption of phenyl mercuric acetate. *J Clin Hosp Pharm* 1980;**5**:21–9.

54. Cartwright AC. Stability data. In: Cartwright AC, Matthews BR, eds. *International Pharmaceutical Product Registration: Aspects of Quality, Safety and Efficacy*. Chichester: Ellis Horwood, 1994; 206–45.

55. Cartwright AC. New chemical active substance products: quality requirements. In: Cartwright AC, Matthews BR, eds. *Pharmaceutical Product Licensing. Requirements for Europe*. Chichester: Ellis Horwood, 1991;54–75.

56. Loftus BT, Nash RA, eds. *Pharmaceutical Process Validation*. New York: Marcel Dekker, 1984.

57. Bochner F. Factors involved in an outbreak of phenytoin intoxication. *J Neurol Sci* 1972;**16**:481.

58. Gibaldi M, Perrier D. *Pharmacokinetics, 2nd edn*. New York: Marcel Dekker, 1982.

59. Florence AT. Generic medicines: a question of quality. In: Wells FO, D'Arcy PF, Harron DWG, eds. *Medicines Responsible Prescribing*. Belfast: The Queen's University, 1992;63–83.

60. Rauws AG. Bioequivalence: a European Community regulatory perspective. In: Welling PG, Tse FLS, Dighe SV, eds. *Pharmaceutical Bioequivalence*. New York: Marcel Dekker, 1991; 419–42.

61. Dighe SV, Adams WP. Bioequivalence: a United States regulatory perspective. In: Welling PG, Tse FLS, Dighe SV, eds. *Pharmaceutical Bioequivalence*. New York: Marcel Dekker, 1991; 347–80.

62. Monkhouse DC, Rhodes CT. *Drug Products for Clinical Trials: An International Guide to Formulation, Production, Quality Control*. New York: Marcel Dekker, 1998.

63. Pocock SJ. *Clinical Trials*. Chichester: John Wiley & Sons, 1983.

64. Anon. *Facts and Statistics for the Pharmaceutical Industry*. London: The Association of the British Pharmaceutical Industry, 2001. http://www.abpi.org.uk/statistics.

CHAPTER 3

3

Preclinical safety testing

David J Tweats

3.1 Introduction

When developing a potential new pharmaceutical compound, the primary objectives are to demonstrate that under the conditions of therapy, the potential new drug is of constant chemical quality, is effective in a significant proportion of patients and is safe. Concerning safety, regulatory agencies need to be assured that the benefits of a new medicine outweigh the risks of therapy. Thus, toxicologists have to assist clinicians in determining the likely range of safe exposures to the new pharmaceutical and the possible consequences if these doses are exceeded. It is an advantage if biomarkers can be identified to indicate when safety limits have been breached, but before significant damage occurs. Such biomarkers allow monitoring of volunteers and patients in early controlled clinical trials to help identify safe exposures. Damage can include disruption of body systems and organs, resulting in lost or impaired function. Such damage can be reversible or irreversible; it may be observed after a single dose or it may be observed only after repeated and prolonged dosing; it may appear by degrees with slow onset or it may occur suddenly and precipitously. Toxicity can be observed in reproductive systems and/or in the developing embryo/foetus, while other changes can result in the formation of tumours. In humans, such tumours can develop decades after the initial exposure – there can be a long latent period. Tumours can result from damage to specific genes

involved in cell division (genotoxic carcinogens) or through a variety of mechanisms, such as prolonged hormonal disruption, which do not involve direct damage to genes (non-genotoxic). The risks to patients differ between these two types of mechanism in that genotoxic carcinogens are deemed to have no threshold for their effects, whereas most non-genotoxic carcinogens have an exposure threshold below which there is little risk, but risks increase once the threshold has been exceeded.

Clinicians and regulators need to be reassured that information concerning all of these different aspects is available to enable clinical trials to progress, and ultimately to support regulatory decisions on whether a new drug can be approved for marketing. Preclinical studies of potential new medicines were relatively superficial until several disasters had occurred: in particular, the thalidomide catastrophe in the 1960s, where exposure to this compound during early pregnancy resulted in limb deformities in developing embryos. Today there are national and international regulations that require manufacturers to provide information from a detailed package of preclinical studies. The timing and composition of these studies is linked to the type and extent of clinical trials that need to be supported. This section deals with requirements for initial studies in volunteers and patients.

Most regulatory toxicity studies are conducted in animals to identify possible hazards from which an assessment of risk to humans is made by extrapolation. Hazard in this context is regarded as the potential for a substance to cause harm, whereas risk is the likelihood that, under the conditions of use, it will cause harm. Comparison between the results of compound exposure in animals and man has shown that such extrapolations, although by no means perfect, are credible in most cases.[1,2] In an attempt to offset some species differences, regulatory agencies request studies in a rodent (usually the rat, although mice are required for specific studies) and a non-rodent. Dogs or non-human primates are most often used, although rabbits are required for particular reproductive toxicology studies. Other rodents and non-rodents may be selected if deemed more appropriate for studying a specific compound. This choice may be based on the results of comparative metabolism, where metabolism in a particular species may more closely resemble that seen or predicted in humans, or the desired pharmacology in a particular species may be more applicable to man than in other species. Often the rat and the dog have been the default, in the absence of data that would allow a more informed choice. However, it is hoped that the advent of new technologies, such as toxicogenomics (differential gene expression)[3]; toxicoproteomics (protein expression profiles)[4]; metabonomics or metabolomics (study of endogenous metabolites in body fluids and tissues using analytical techniques such as nuclear magnetic resonance, NMR)[5] together with characterisation of receptors and receptor distribution, will allow better informed selection of single relevant species in the future.

Adverse events affecting patients taking a medicine can occur with various degrees of frequency. For a serious adverse event, frequencies of greater than one patient affected per 10 000 treated or even one in 50 000 can be unacceptable. It is neither possible nor ethical to use animals in these sorts of numbers. In order to compensate for this, it is assumed that increasing the dose and prolonging the duration of exposure will improve both the sensitivity and predictivity of these tests. Thus, a 6-month study at higher doses gives a greater comfort level to regulatory authorities than a 1-month study at

lower doses. This is not necessarily based on scientific fact, and again it is hoped that the new tools described above, plus a greater knowledge of genetics, will allow the identification of early events induced by lower doses that will be predictive of toxic events in human populations and thus reduce the reliance on animal testing. Russell and Burch propounded the concept of the three Rs in relation to use of animals in research, that is, reduction of animal use, refinement of testing that requires fewer animals and replacement of animal studies by *in vitro* methods.[6] This concept is becoming more integrated into mainstream research as better tools are now available to allow this approach to become much more of a reality. A European regulatory law bans the use of animals if the required knowledge can be gained by other means.

3.1.1   The 'omic technologies'

A brief description of these emerging technologies is given below; the reader is referred to the referenced reviews for more details. A balanced view of the use of these technologies in toxicology is given in reference.[7] At present these techniques are not part of mandatory regulatory toxicology, but are being used increasingly to provide supplementary and supportive data alongside the required studies.

3.1.1.1   Toxicogenomics or transcriptomics

This technology allows the simultaneous monitoring of a small number to thousands of messenger RNAs (mRNAs) from cells and tissues. As mRNA expression can reflect the corresponding gene expression, this gives insight to what genes are being up-regulated in expression, down-regulated or whose expression is not changed following a given treatment or in a particular disease state. Thus, cells or tissues can be monitored before and after exposure to a toxin to determine the response of the cells to the toxin. From this information, patterns of gene expression or in rare cases single gene changes, can be linked to specific types of toxicity, for example, liver toxicity, kidney toxicity, etc., what tissues within an organ are involved in the toxicity or what mechanisms of toxicity are occurring, for example, oxidative stress, apoptosis, necrosis, etc.[8]

3.1.1.2 Toxicoproteomics

Compared to the genome, the proteome (the entire diverse protein content of a cell) is a far more dynamic system. Proteins undergo post-translational modifications such as phosphorylation, glycosylation and sulphation, as well as cleavage for specific proteins.[9] These alterations determine protein activity, localisation and turnover. All are subject to change following a toxic insult and, in some ways, the study of proteins holds more promise than the study of gene expression as the former is nearer to key activities in the cell.

Several techniques have been used to display protein profiles, for example, proteins can be separated by two-dimensional polyacrlamide gel electrophoresis (2D-PAGE). Differentially expressed or modified proteins associated with treatment may be identified by their absence or by the appearance of new spots on the gel followed by isoelectric focusing in the first dimension and molecular weight separation in the second. Proteins can be identified from historical data or by excising the spots followed by peptide cleavage and sequencing. Matrix-assisted laser desorption/ionisation (MALDI) mass spectrometry is being used increasingly to identify the spectrum of peptides.[10] Protein chips coated with specific surfaces to identify protein classes (Ciphergen's SELDI ProteinChip® system) are also of interest. This area is progressing fast, but technical challenges remain to identify important, low-abundance proteins that are often masked on gels by high-abundance proteins.[11]

3.1.1.3 Metabonomics

Metabonomics in the context of this chapter aims to define the status and changes of the endogenous metabolite profile in biofluids or tissues of animals or in *in vitro* systems in response to toxic insults. The most commonly applied methodology is ^{1}H NMR spectroscopy, which yields a spectrum describing all the relatively low molecular weight metabolites in studied materials.[12] Study of biological fluids, such as urine, is attractive as it is non-invasive and can allow real-time measurements to be made including those that can occur in recovery from a toxicity.

With all of these methods, understanding what is the 'normal' spectrum and also separating adaptive changes following changes in physiology due to, for example, dietary changes or diurnal changes, etc., from true toxicity-related changes, is paramount.[13]

3.1.1.4 Bioinformatics

All of the 'omic technologies described above produce huge amounts of data. The analysis of this data is a big challenge and requires complex statistical analysis to identify key changes through pattern recognition etc. In addition, large databases of historical data are needed to make the most of any findings. There are some major initiatives in progress (10 years to full delivery)[14] to allow the integration of the data from these technologies together with biological networks and traditional fields such as pathology and clinical chemistry, etc. If these projects are successful, they will revolutionise the field of preclinical safety.

3.1.2 The drug development process

The sequence of events in the modern drug development process is shown in Figure 3.1.

There is an increasing focus on trying to select more easily developable molecules at an early stage, so that the chance of failure at the very expensive later phases is minimised. Pharmaceutical companies therefore decide on which properties of a new molecule are key to faster development, for example, selection of soluble compounds to facilitate formulation. Amongst these is the selection of molecules with low or acceptable toxicity. Thus, a company may decide to develop high-throughput *in vitro* screens for cytotoxicity for use at the lead optimisation stage.

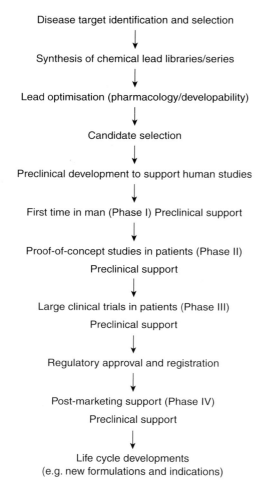

Disease target identification and selection

↓

Synthesis of chemical lead libraries/series

↓

Lead optimisation (pharmacology/developability)

↓

Candidate selection

↓

Preclinical development to support human studies

↓

First time in man (Phase I) Preclinical support

↓

Proof-of-concept studies in patients (Phase II)
Preclinical support

↓

Large clinical trials in patients (Phase III)
Preclinical support

↓

Regulatory approval and registration

↓

Post-marketing support (Phase IV)
Preclinical support

↓

Life cycle developments
(e.g. new formulations and indications)

Fig. 3.1 Drug development process.

Certainly by the 'candidate selection' stage, where there may be three or four possible candidates of which only one may go forward, there is a need for reassurance regarding toxicity to help in the selection process. Thus, companies may decide to screen for 'show-stopping' toxicities, for example, effects on cardiovascular parameters such as severe electrophysiology changes (see Section 3.2); genetic toxicity as well as a preliminary screen for whole animal toxicology in the rat or mouse, in which three doses may be tested in five animals per group, dosing for 2–7 days. This would be expected to flag up marked toxicities and allow ranking or elimination of specific candidates. The same compounds

would also go through screens in other preclinical functions – pharmacy, drug metabolism and pharmacokinetics, etc. – and the information pooled, along with the likely cost of manufacturing the compounds by the chemical synthesis routes identified. All of this information is considered in selecting a compound to go forward to the more regulatory defined activities, where the costs escalate rapidly and therefore the cost of failure of a compound becomes very significant.

The newer technologies (genomics, proteomics, etc.) also offer the possibility of developing specific screens for those compounds possessing undesirable toxicity (e.g. the ability to induce oxidative damage, mitochondrial toxicity, endocrine disruption), which can be used to filter out possible toxic compounds at an early stage. Molecular biology is also providing opportunities (e.g. antisense probes, knock-out mice, etc.) for exploring the receptors chosen as drug targets and discovering at an early stage whether changes in such targets result in toxicological liabilities (e.g. see Treinen et al.[15]).

3.1.3   Risk benefit

The regulatory toxicology programme (which supports clinical trials and registration of compounds) runs in parallel with the clinical programme. Single-dose studies in healthy volunteers (Phase I studies) require less toxicological support than multiple doses in sick patients. There are four phases in the clinical programme (see Box 3.1). As the programme progresses through the various phases, several things change:

1. The treated population changes from healthy volunteers in Phase I to sick patients in Phase II.
2. The duration of exposure to the drug can increase from a single dose in Phase I to prolonged repeated dosing for drugs being developed for chronic therapy.
3. Men are usually the volunteers in Phase I and women enter the programme typically in Phase II (unless a female-specific medicine is

being developed or there is an indication that
there may be important gender- specific effects).
4. The monitoring of volunteers/patients decreases through the programme. A volunteer will
stay in a clinic and will be very closely monitored
for any signs of toxicity, whereas a patient in a
Phase III trial may only be required to return to
their physician periodically.
5. The strict control on administration of a drug
often changes as it switches from the investigating physician to the patients. Thus, in
Phase I, the drug is administered by the physician
whereas in Phase III a patient may be sent home
with a pack of tablets with instructions to take
two a day.
6. The number of humans exposed gradually
increases.

The hazard to the population therefore
increases throughout the trial process as more
people are given greater cumulative amounts
of the drug in a less-controlled and monitored
manner. However, with each additional patient
treated, the clinical experience with the drug also
increases, providing a greater safety database in
the most relevant species, that is, man. The risk

to the individual should therefore decrease as the
clinical programme progresses.

It should be noted that the reliance on toxicity
data changes throughout clinical development.
The safety or comfort factor before initial dosing
in man is based largely on general toxicity in
animals, that is, single- or repeated-dose studies plus safety pharmacology studies measuring
pharmacologically mediated adverse effects on
vital systems, that is, respiratory, cardiovascular and central nervous systems and preliminary genetic toxicity studies. Human safety data
rapidly reduces the reliance on information based
on general toxicity studies in animals. This is not
the case, however, for the teratogenic or oncogenic potential of the drug, which will be based
on preclinical data for many years even after the
drug is marketed. This concept has been represented diagrammatically by Dr Michael Jackson
and is shown in Figure 3.2.

Box 3.2 shows the toxicity package typically
generated before a Phase I trial. These trials
are usually conducted in males, and thus do
not require formal reproductive toxicity studies.
In the United States, women can be included in
early trials without any animal reproductive toxicity if special precautions are taken to ensure that
pregnancy does not occur. A histopathological
assessment of the effects of the test compound
on the male reproductive tract is made in the
repeat-dose toxicity tests.

In a human volunteer study, there is obviously
no benefit to the individual except perhaps a
small financial gain. There is, of course, risk but
this is minimised by the small amounts of drug
that are administered and the careful monitoring
of the volunteer for any adverse signs caused by
the drug. Later in the programme, when treating
patients who are suffering from a disease, there is
a possible, but unproven, benefit that they may be
cured or symptoms may be alleviated. Obviously
for incurable, life-threatening conditions such as
AIDS and some cancers, a much higher level of
risk, that is, possible toxicity, is acceptable compared with other less serious conditions. This is
why some cancer chemotherapy, as well as being
highly toxic to dividing cells, may in itself be
carcinogenic.

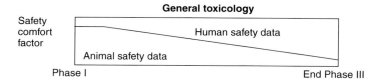

General toxicology

Safety
comfort
factor

Human safety data

Animal safety data

Phase I   End Phase III

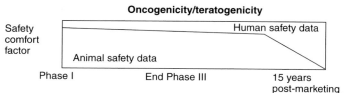

Oncogenicity/teratogenicity

Safety
comfort
factor

Human safety data

Animal safety data

Phase I   End Phase III   15 years
                                                             post-marketing

Fig. 3.2 Reliance on preclinical safety data (reproduced with kind permission of Dr Michael Jackson).

Box 3.2   **Basic package of data for Phase I trials**

- Safety pharmacology – indication of adverse pharmacologically mediated actions on central nervous, cardiovascular and respiratory systems
- Pharmacokinetics – preliminary studies on absorption, distribution, metabolism and excretion
- Acute toxicity – two species by two routes of administration (one is usually intravenous to ensure systemic exposure and the other is by the proposed clinical route). Usually an evaluation of the maximum repeatable dose (MRD) and possibly local irritancy
- Repeat-dose toxicity – rodent and non-rodent species are required. The duration of the test depends on the duration of clinical exposure but many companies conduct two 14-day studies before going into man. Studies should be done using the proposed clinical route
- Reproductive toxicology, usually embryo/foetal development studies in two species, is required in Europe and Japan if women of child-bearing potential are included. Not required in the United States for some early trials
- Mutagenicity – *in vitro* tests for mutagenicity and chromosome damage. Adapted from Scales[16]

The various safety studies, from those that are necessary to evaluate the risk of exposing the first human to those required by regulatory authorities in order to market a medicine, are considered below.

3.1.4   Good laboratory practice

It is important to ensure the quality and reliability of safety studies. This is normally assured by following the Good Laboratory Practice regulations.[17] Any deviation from this must be justified.

3.2   Preclinical Safety Pharmacology

3.2.1   Introduction

Once a compound, or a small series of compounds, has been identified as a potential development candidate, preclinical safety pharmacology studies are considered. These are single-dose studies in animals to determine whether the chosen candidates have pharmacological (as opposed to frank toxicological) side effects that would preclude or limit their therapeutic use. These studies can give an indication of potential safety margins and may also include interaction studies with other drugs. Safety pharmacology studies measure the pharmacodynamic actions of drug candidates on vital systems, that is, cardiovascular, respiratory and central nervous systems. There may be concerns that would extend such studies to other systems, for example, kidney, gastrointestinal tract, etc.

3.2.2   Regulatory guidelines

Although some regulatory guidelines for conducting safety pharmacology studies have been issued in the past (e.g. by the Japanese Ministry of Health and Welfare (MHW) in 1991), an International Conference on Harmonisation (ICH) guideline, was agreed upon in November 2000. This guideline replaces any previous guidance for safety pharmacology studies to register pharmaceuticals in the United States, European Union (EU) and Japan.

When deciding on the specific tests to perform on a new chemical entity, the following factors should be considered:

1. Mechanism of action, as adverse effects can be associated with desired effects, for example, antiarrhythmic agents can be proarrhythmic in some circumstances.
2. Class-specific effects, for example, disturbances of normal electrocardiogram (ECG) associated with many antipsychotics.
3. Ligand-binding or enzyme assay data suggesting a potential for adverse events.

3.2.3 General considerations

When selecting the relevant test models, factors to consider include the pharmacodynamic responses of the model (e.g. changes in blood pressure), pharmacokinetic profile (e.g. differences in adsorption, distribution, metabolism and elimination), species, strain, sex and age of the experimental animals, the susceptibility, sensitivity and reproducibility of the test system and available background data on the substance. *In vitro* systems, including isolated organs and tissues, cell cultures, cellular fragments, subcellular organelles, receptors, ion channels, etc., can also provide valuable information. These can identify potential problems and also help in defining mechanisms of effects seen *in vivo*.

In vivo studies are preferably carried out using unrestrained, unanaesthetised animals. Animals can be fitted with transmitters that allow data to be collected by telemetry. As for all animal studies, avoidance or minimisation of pain and discomfort is an important consideration. Information from the toxicological battery of studies, if they have been adequately designed to address safety pharmacology endpoints, can

result in reduction or elimination of separate safety pharmacology studies.

3.2.4 Experimental design

3.2.4.1 Controls
Appropriate controls should be used, for example, test systems exposed to the vehicle in which the test compound has been dissolved or suspended (negative control). The new ICH guideline also suggests that in some cases a compound known to have an adverse effect in a specific test system (positive control) should be used.

3.2.4.2 Route
In general, the expected clinical route of administration should be used when feasible. Regardless of route, exposure to the parent compound and its major metabolites should be similar or greater than that observed in humans. Because safety pharmacology studies are carried out before human studies are initiated, this may have to be inferred from information derived from *in vitro* studies, for example, with human hepatocytes and/or from information from similar compounds that have been used in humans. In some cases, early low-dose human studies may show that significant metabolites are formed in humans but were not formed in the animals used in safety pharmacology studies. In these circumstances, further studies will be needed in animals using isolated or chemically synthesised human metabolites.

3.2.4.3 Dose levels *in vivo*
It is necessary to define the dose–response relationship of any adverse effects observed. The onset and duration of effects should be measured. Because there are differences in sensitivity between species, the doses chosen need to exceed those used for therapy. The ICH guideline states that the highest dose tested should be a dose that produces moderate adverse effects, for example, dose-limiting pharmacodynamic effects or other toxicities. Such effects should not be so severe that they confound the interpretation of the results being sought. Safety pharmacology studies

are generally performed by administration of single doses rather than repeated dosing.

3.2.4.4   Dose levels *in vitro*

As for *in vivo* studies, it is necessary to establish a concentration–effect relationship. The upper limit of concentrations tested may be influenced by physicochemical properties of the test substance and other factors such as cytotoxicity.

3.2.5   Safety pharmacology core battery

As mentioned previously, the preliminary focus of safety pharmacology studies is to measure the effects of the test substance on the cardiovascular, respiratory and central nervous systems.

3.2.5.1   Central nervous system

The ICH guideline lists assessment of the effects of the test compound on motor activity, behavioural changes, co-ordination and sensory/motor reflex responses. A so-called functional observation battery[18] or Irwin's battery[19] will cover these parameters. Effects on body temperature should also be measured.

3.2.5.2   Cardiovascular system

The ICH guideline lists the assessment of effects on blood pressure, heart rate and ECG. *In vivo, in vitro* and/or *ex vivo* evaluations, including methods for electrical repolarisation and conductance abnormalities, should also be considered. These abnormalities can be associated with risks for fatal ventricular arrhythmias called Torsade de pointes.

In 1997, a regulatory 'points to consider' document was issued by the European Committee for Proprietary Medical Products (CPMP, now called the Committee for Medicinal Products for Human Use, CHMP) concerning this aspect (see EMEA/CHMP website for human medicines – safety, given in section titled 'Internet addresses for Regulatory Guidelines'). This document describes the use of *in vitro* and *ex vivo* test systems for measuring disturbances in electrophysiology. Some drugs can prolong the QT part of the ECG waveform. This is

due to interference or blockade of specific ion channels on conducting cells in the heart, which results in a prolongation of recovery of the ventricular muscle from electrical excitement (repolarisation). Most compounds inducing such effects interact with ion channels such as the potassium channel, disrupting the flow of electrical charge in and out of conducting tissues. Such effects are seen as indicating potential to induce Torsade de pointes.

An ICH draft guideline was issued in 2002 entitled 'ICH S7B, Note for Guidance on Safety Pharmacology Studies for assessing the Potential for Delayed Ventricular Repolarization (QT Interval Prolongation) by Human Pharmaceuticals', which reached preliminary agreement (step 2 of the ICH process) in 2004. This can be found at the Internet address given in section titled 'Internet addresses for Regulatory Guidelines', for CPMP (CHMP) guidelines. The core study required by the draft guidelines is an *in vivo* study in telemetred non-rodents to measure ECG changes in the presence of the test compound. This draft guideline also discusses the use of tests for changes in electrophysiology. For example, the guideline discusses the use of human ether-a-go-go related gene (hERG) potassium (IKr rectifier channel) models. These models use isolated cells (e.g. Chinese hamster ovary cells or human HEK293 cells) that contain cloned hERG genes.[20]

3.2.5.3   Respiratory system

The ICH guideline mentions measurements of airway resistance, airway compliance, tidal volume and blood gases.

3.2.5.4   Supplementary safety pharmacology studies

The core battery of studies should be carried out before a substance is administered to humans for the first time. Any follow up or supplementary safety pharmacology studies should be carried out if there is a cause for concern raised from the toxicological battery of tests and/or from studies in humans.

Novel centrally acting drugs may need to be tested for abuse potential. Primate self-administration tests may be used preclinic-ally to assess abuse potential. However, it should be borne in mind that regulatory authorities such as the Food and Drug Administration (FDA) of the United States give more weight to negative evidence of abuse potential from clinical assess-ment, for example, in experienced drug abusers, than to negative evidence from animal studies.

Investigation of potential adverse interactions with drugs likely to be co-prescribed with the test drug may also be required. A general-ised approach, such as the determination of effects on hepatic drug metabolising enzymes, may be sufficient, but in most cases, a number of drug-specific interaction studies will also be required.

The effects of the drug on the duration of loss of the righting reflex (sleeping time) in mice pre-treated with pentobarbital can be used as a broad screen for detecting effects on hepatic drug meta-bolism. At the relatively high dose used in this test, pentobarbital is a substrate for a large range of hepatic enzymes. Although sedative actions of drugs can increase sleeping time, unlike hepatic enzyme inhibitors, sedative drugs also potenti-ate loss of righting reflex induced by barbitone, which is excreted unchanged.

3.3 Single-dose Studies

Single-dose toxicity studies fall into two categor-ies: preliminary and definitive studies. Prelimin-ary studies are performed to provide an estimate of the maximum nonlethal dosage (MNLD) for use in definitive studies. Definitive studies are performed to evaluate effects that may result from acute exposure to the MNLD and predict effects of overdosage in man.

Single-dose studies are performed in two species, usually rat and mouse, by two routes of administration, usually intravenous, to ensure systemic exposure, and the proposed clin-ical route. Following the ICH guidance in November 1991,[21] non-rodent, single-dose tests are no longer required. If the proposed clinical route is intravenous, then one route is usually acceptable.

Single-dose studies may be performed early in a development programme. The information gained from these studies is rapidly superseded, in terms of its value for risk assessment, by repeat-dose studies.

The FDA allows single-dose human studies based on single-dose animal studies.[22] A rodent and non-rodent species are required and signs of major toxicity must be demonstrated. The study design is outlined in the publication by Munro and Mehta[23] and requires an observation period of 14 days after dosing.

3.3.1 Study design

3.3.1.1 Preliminary studies
Groups of four animals (two of each sex) are given a single dose of the test material. For oral dosing studies, animals are not deprived of food overnight before dosing. Groups are treated sequentially, the dosage for each stage being based on the response of the previous group, until the highest dose that does not cause deaths (MNLD) is determined. Animals killed for humane reasons are considered as drug-induced deaths. Animals are observed for 7 days, dur-ing which time clinical observations and body weights are recorded. At termination, anim-als undergo a full macroscopic examination and any unusual abnormalities are examined microscopically.

3.3.1.2 Definitive studies
Groups of 20 animals (10 of each sex) are dosed at the MNLD determined in the preliminary study. Control animals are included only when an unusual vehicle is present in the test for-mulation or if target organ toxicity is anticip-ated. Five animals of each sex are observed for 48 h and are then killed for autopsy to allow evaluation of early pathological changes. The remaining five animals of each sex are observed for 14 days before autopsy to eval-uate any delayed toxicity that may occur and to assess recovery from early onset changes. Clinical observations and body weight measure-ments are made during the observation period.

At termination, full macroscopic examination and microscopic examination of limited tissues (usually heart, lungs, liver, kidneys, spleen and any tissues related to route of administration tissues) are performed. Blood levels of the drug are not usually determined, as often an assay is still to be developed. Systemic exposure can be approximated, however, using a scaling model (see Section 3.8.3.5).

Only limited interpretation of the results of single-dose studies is possible. The MNLD can be determined and target organs can be identified. Frequently death can occur as a result of the exaggerated pharmacological action of the compound and often no target organ toxicity is seen in drug-induced deaths. Such studies do, however, give an indication of what may happen with massive acute overdosage in the clinic.

3.4   Repeat-dose Studies

The duration of repeat-dose studies for both clinical trials and marketing applications are given in Tables 3.1 and 3.2, which are taken from the ICH guideline on the timing of 'Non-Clinical Safety Studies for the Conduct of Human Clinical Trials for Pharmaceuticals', as amended in November 2000.

Repeat-dose toxicity studies should be performed in a rodent, typically the rat, and a non-rodent. The longer the duration of human exposure, the longer must be the duration of the toxicity studies. The ICH guideline indicates that for Phase I and Phase II studies, the clinical duration can equal the duration of the toxicity studies in all regions. This concords with the UK guidelines revised by the Medicines Control Agency (MCA) in December 1995.[24]

In Japan and the United States, the clinical duration for Phase I, II and III trials can equal the duration of toxicity studies (Table 3.1). In Europe, a more conservative approach is adopted as longer duration studies, equivalent to those expected for marketing, are needed for Phase III trials (Table 3.2).

The doses for the definitive repeat-dose studies are usually based on preliminary dose-escalating

studies. The design of such studies varies between companies. Spurling and Carey[25] have published a study design which allows the maximum amount of both toxicological and kinetic data to be obtained by using a minimum number of animals. The highly predictive nature of these MRD studies in assessing the outcome of longer duration studies is discussed by Scales.[26]

Toxicity studies usually follow this sequence: MRD, 2 weeks or 1 month, 3 or 6 months, and 9 or 12 months. The choice of duration usually depends on the length of the clinical trial to be supported. It should be noted that the ICH guideline for duration of non-rodent species (see note to Table 3.2) may allow the chronic non-rodent study to be limited to 9 months. In Europe, a 6-month non-rodent study is still acceptable to support chronic human therapy. In the United States, the FDA, in a Federal Register Notice referencing the ICH guideline, indicates that it will accept 6-month non-rodent studies (as the maximum required duration) for compounds given for short periods only, for example, drugs for migraine or erectile dysfunction. For compounds with novel pharmacology, those for osteoporosis, and drugs whose efficacy is measured by changes in surrogate markers (e.g. drugs for AIDS), 12-month non-rodent studies are required. Otherwise, 9-month studies will be acceptable.

The route of administration should be similar to that employed clinically. This is discussed in more detail in Section 3.5.1.

3.4.1   The MRD study

An MRD will be carried out for each species by each route of administration to be used in subsequent repeat-dose toxicity studies. It is usual to conduct an escalating-dose MRD study, in which increasingly larger dosages are administered to the same group of animals every 3–4 days until significant toxicity occurs. However, if local irritancy or target organ toxicity is likely to limit the dose, or if tolerance to repeated dosing is anticipated, a fixed-dose MRD study is more useful. The aims of both types of study

Table 3.1 Duration of repeated-dose toxicity studies to support Phase I and II trials in EU and Phase I, II and III trials in the United States and Japan[a]

Duration of clinical trials	Minimum duration of repeated-dose toxicity studies	
	Rodent species	Non-rodent species
Single dose	2–4 weeks[b]	2 weeks
Up to 2 weeks	2–4 weeks[b]	2 weeks
Up to 1 month	1 month	1 month
Up to 3 months	3 months	3 months
Up to 6 months	6 months	6 months[c]
>6 months	6 months	Chronic[c]

[a] In Japan, if there are no Phase II clinical trials of equivalent duration to the planned Phase III trials, conduct of longer duration toxicity studies should be considered, as given in Table 3.2.

[b] In the United States, as an alternative to 2-week studies, single-dose toxicity studies with extended examinations can support single-dose human trials.

[c] Data from 6 months of administration in non-rodents should be available before the initiation of clinical trials longer than 3 months. Alternatively, if applicable, data from a 9-month non-rodent study should be available before the treatment duration exceeds that which is supported by the available toxicity studies.

Table 3.2 Duration of repeated-dose toxicity studies to support Phase III trials in the EU and marketing in all regions[a]

Duration of clinical trials	Minimum duration of repeated-dose toxicity studies	
	Rodent species	Non-rodent species
Up to 2 weeks	1 month	1 month
Up to 1 month	3 months	3 months
Up to 3 months	6 months	3 months
>3 months	6 months	Chronic[b]

[a] The table also reflects the marketing recommendations in the three regions except that a chronic non-rodent study is recommended for clinical use >1 month.

[b] An ICH guideline entitled 'Duration of Chronic Toxicity Testing in Animals (Rodent and Non-Rodent Toxicity Testing)' indicates that a non-rodent study of 9 months may be acceptable in the United States, Japan and EU.

are to determine a profile of toxic effects, including target organ toxicity, and to evaluate pharmacokinetic parameters, that is, to determine evidence of absorption by measuring the time to reach (T_{max}) the maximum plasma concentration (C_{max}) and to provide an indication of exposure by the area under the plasma time concentration curve (AUC), the plasma elimination half-life ($T1/2$) and the minimum plasma concentration (C_{min}) after single and repeat doses. The pharmacokinetic determinations obviously depend on a suitable assay for the drug being available.

3.4.2 Definitive repeat-dose toxicity studies

The aims of these studies are to characterise any target organ toxicity identified in earlier studies, to determine any new target organs not seen in earlier studies and to check whether the pharmacokinetics determined in earlier studies are changed. Following the dosing period, a number of animals are often retained off dose to allow for observation of recovery from any toxic changes. This recovery period is usually 1 week for 14-day and 1-month studies and 2 weeks for studies of 3 months or more. The study design is outlined in Table 3.3.

Animals are usually dosed once daily during the dosing period. This may be increased to twice or three times a day to mimic human dosing or to create a kinetic profile in animals similar to that seen or predicted in humans. The low dosage is a small multiple of the estimated clinical dose (usually less than fivefold) based whenever possible on comparative kinetic data. The high dosage may be the MRD, the maximum non-irritant or minimally irritant dose, the maximum practicable dose (based on the physicochemical properties of the dose, but usually not less than 100 times the intended clinical dose) or the dose yielding a C_{max} or AUC at least 100 times that in man after a clinical dose or the dose at which these parameters become clearly non-linear. The intermediate dose is usually the geometric mean of the low and high dosages. If tolerance to repeat dosing is shown in the preliminary studies, an initial

period of dose incrementation may be required but should not normally exceed 1 week.

3.4.2.1 Study interpretation

The type of observations include those made in MRDs (i.e. clinical observations, body weight, pulse rate in dogs, haematology, clinical chemistry, urine analysis, plasma drug concentration, macroscopic and microscopic post-mortem examination) as well as ophthalmoscopy, electrocardiography (in dogs), organ weights and, in some laboratories, hearing tests. Although some types of toxicity may be obvious, more subtle changes may be difficult to separate from normal variation. Selection of suitable control groups for comparison with drug-treated animals is therefore vital, as is adequate pre-dose evaluation of various measurements.

Control animals usually receive a quantity of vehicle equal to the highest administered to the test groups. When the test material influences pH or toxicity of the dosing solution, and these properties are pertinent to the route of administration, the quantities of excipients administered to control animals may have to differ from those administered to the test animals; in such cases, it may be more important for test and control solutions to have the same physicochemical properties. Similarly, it may be necessary to administer qualitatively different excipients to the controls in order to keep the physical properties of test and control materials the same (e.g. in an intravenous study, if simple aqueous solutions of the test material are isotonic, the controls should receive physiological saline), and if the test material is administered without a vehicle, the controls are given water or are sham-treated. When the likely effects of a vehicle are unknown, two control groups, vehicle and negative (water, saline or sham-treated), should be included in the study. Statistical comparisons should initially be made against the vehicle control group.

Based on comparisons with an appropriate control group, abnormalities identified during the course of a study may require additional investigations to be undertaken to determine, if

Table 3.3 Study design for definitive repeat-dose studies – number of animals of each sex per group

Group no. and group name	1. Control	2. Low	3. Intermediate	4. High	Total number of animals
1-month toxicity study					
Rat	12(8)	12	12	12(8)	128
Dog	3(2)	3	3	3(2)	32
3-month toxicity study					
Rat	16(8)	16	16	16(8)	160
Dog	4(2)	4	4	4(2)	40
6-month toxicity study					
Rat	20(12)	· 20	20	20(12)	208
Dog	4(2)	4	4	4(2)	40
12-month toxicity study					
Dog	4(2)	4	4	4(2)	40

Numbers within parentheses represent animals retained after cessation of dosing for observation of recovery.

practicable, the significance, extent or mechanism of toxicity.

Statistical analysis is essential in order to gain an overview of the very extensive data collected during such studies and to highlight any underlying trends. This analysis also aids in determining the non-toxic effect level required by regulatory authorities.

Finally, any effects present at the end of the dosing period may be investigated during the following recovery period in which a proportion of the animals showing effects are retained undosed while recovery is monitored. Recovery periods of 2 weeks or 1 month are typical. These may not be sufficient to demonstrate complete recovery. However, signs of reversibility should be taken into account when making a risk assessment.

3.5 Oncogenicity Studies

Lifetime bioassays are conducted in animals to detect whether a compound can cause neoplastic changes. Neoplasms are caused by a tissue undergoing growth which is not under the normal control mechanisms of the body. Such growths are often referred to as tumours, but this is an imprecise term, which can be applied to any abnormal swelling. If the neoplasm closely resembles its tissue of origin and the growth is slow and does not spread to other tissues, it is a benign neoplasm. Neoplasms that grow quickly and invade other tissues and shed cells into blood or lymph vessels which lodge and grow at sites distant from the original neoplasm are termed malignant.

Lifetime bioassays are sometimes referred to as carcinogenicity studies. A carcinoma is a malignant neoplasm of epithelial cell origin, for example, adrenal adenocarcinoma; its benign counterpart is referred to as an adrenal adenoma. Malignant neoplasms, which arise from connective tissues are termed sarcomas, for example, fibrosarcoma. The benign counterpart of the malignant fibrosarcoma is a fibroma. Carcinogenicity studies imply to the purist that such studies are designed to detect carcinomas. Oncogenicity, on the other hand, refers to any neoplasm, benign or malignant, of either epithelial or connective tissue origin.

Oncogenicity studies, therefore, examine the ability of a material to produce neoplastic changes in a tissue or tissues. Short-term genotoxicity studies provide a good indicator of oncogenic potential as most oncogenic agents of concern cause damage to DNA or chromosomes. Normally, long-term, lifetime, animal studies are required to demonstrate the realisation of that potential and also to detect agents that cause neoplasms by an epigenetic (i.e. non-genotoxic) mechanism. Such epigenetic agents can act by a variety of mechanisms, including immunosuppression, chronic tissue injury, repeated receptor activation and by disturbing hormone homeostasis and thereby increasing cell turnover, which in turn increases the chance of developing a neoplasm.

In Europe,[27] oncogenicity studies will usually be required as part of the development of a pharmaceutical preparation in the following circumstances:

1. Where the substance would be used continuously for long periods (i.e. more than 6 months) or have a frequent intermittent use as may be expected in the treatment of chronic illness;
2. Where a substance has a chemical structure that suggests oncogenic potential;
3. Where a substance causes concern as a result of some specific aspects of its biological action (e.g. a therapeutic class of which several members have produced positive oncogenic results), its pattern of toxicity or long-term retention (of drug or metabolites) detected in previous studies: positive findings in genotoxicity studies.

Because of their size and duration and the corresponding costs involved, oncogenicity studies are usually conducted towards the end of the development of a pharmaceutical when clinical efficacy has been established and the majority of the toxicity studies have been completed. The requirements in the United States, Japan and Europe for clinical trials and marketing are compared in Table 3.4.

There is a continuing debate as to whether inbred or outbred strains of rodents should be used. In theory, inbred strains are preferable because a more accurate knowledge of background tumour incidence is available. It may be, however, that a particular inbred strain may metabolise the test material in a certain way or have a genetic resistance to the development of a specific tumour type. Usually outbred strains of rat or hamster are used, but occasionally inbred mice strains are included. An F1 hybrid mouse strain is frequently employed. In some circumstances outbred syrian hamsters may be the species of choice. The most important factor is to have a sound knowledge of the background incidence of tumours in the species or strain selected. This information complements the concurrent control data and provides information on the susceptibility of the strain to rare tumour types. Modifying factors, such as diet, cage density, etc., must be kept as constant as possible to enable correct interpretation of the results.[33,34]

The ICH guideline entitled 'Testing for Carcinogenicity of Pharmaceuticals' allows for a one-species carcinogenicity study plus alternative

Table 3.4 Regulatory requirements for oncogenicity studies

	Marketing	Clinical trials
United States	Recommended for drugs to be used for more than 3 months[28]	Only when there is cause for concern[29]
Japan	When there is cause for concern or when long-term clinical use is expected[30]	Recommended (but not always done) before Phase III for drugs according to market requirements criteria[31]
EU	When there is cause for concern or when long-term clinical use is expected[27]	Recommended as per marketing requirements[32] but not usually done before long-term clinical studies unless suspicions arise

in vivo tests such as rat initiator-promoter models, transgenic mouse assays (i.e. p53 +/− knockout mice: Tg.AC mice which carry an activated *v-Ha-ras* oncogene; ras H2 mice carrying a human *c-Ha-ras* oncogene and XPA mice which have lost a crucial DNA nucleotide excision repair gene), and neonatal rodent tests. The premise with these alternative oncogenicity assays is that the transgenic animals are predisposed to develop tumours without a lengthy latent period that is, induced tumours can appear in 6–9 months rather than up to the 2 years of the conventional assays. In addition animal group sizes are lower than for conventional studies, although at least one agency suggests that in addition to the transgenic animal groups, groups of wild-type animals should also be included in such studies to determine if tumours occur preferentially in the transgenic model.[35] These alternative oncogenicity studies have been undergoing evaluation for a number of years,[36] but it will be some time before they gain full regulatory acceptance internationally. There may be some instances, for example, where genotoxicity assessments are equivocal, when regulatory authorities may request data from a specific transgenic model to aid risk assessment. In the United States, FDA have requested some companies in these circumstances to provide data from the Syrian Hamster Embryo (SHE) transformation assay. In this assay pleuripotent cells are grown in culture. It is surmised that if a compound has tumorigenic potential it can induce these cells to lose the contact inhibition of normal cells such that they pile up on top of one another to form a flared colony or 'transformant'.[37] The use of this assay is controversial as scoring of transformants can be subjective, there is no unequivocal marker of transformation and the molecular mechanism of transformation is unknown.[38] If a compound is positive in this assay and a company wishes to progress with development, they have been required to provide data from a the P53 transgenic model, which is known to be sensitive to some genotoxic carcinogens. If such an assay is negative, companies have been allowed to proceed with development of the compound in question. If a relevant test compound has been found to be negative in the SHE assay, then development has been allowed without a P53 assay.

The rat will usually be the species of choice for the standard oncogenicity study because there is greater confidence in its predictivity for human carcinogenicity than the mouse or hamster. The species chosen, however, should be the most appropriate based on considerations such as pharmacology, repeated-dose toxicity, metabolism and toxicokinetics.

3.5.1 Route of administration

In general, the route of administration should be similar to the one used clinically.[39] Oral administration is the most widely used route of exposure, with the test material mixed in the diet, given in the drinking water or administered by gavage. Each route has its advantages and disadvantages.

Dietary and water administration rely on the administered mixture being palatable and stable in the formulation. Accurate administration is not possible, particularly if animals are multiply caged, and cross-contamination, especially from diet mixtures, may be a problem. The methods are relatively easy to use, however, with minimum resource being required, and more or less continual exposure to the material is guaranteed.

Administration by gavage ensures that each animal receives the correct dose but the method is labour-intensive and, depending on the kinetics involved, periods of 'drug holiday' may occur during the treatment period.

The other main route used for pharmaceutical preparations is inhalation using a 'head only' exposure system. Parenteral administration, although technically possible, is usually avoided because of the local irritant effects that can occur with repeated injection, particularly by the subcutaneous route. Topical administration is an option for materials intended for administration to the skin.

3.5.2 Dose selection

There has been, and continues to be, considerable debate about the selection of the high dose level for oncogenicity studies. European and Japanese regulatory guidelines have tended to accept the use of an arbitrary upper limit set at a multiple of 100 times the administered therapeutic dose. In the United States, the selection has been made on the basis of the MTD, a level that causes a moderate decrease in weight gain (not exceeding 10%). Literature has been produced regarding dose-selection procedures.[40] The ICH has issued a guideline entitled 'Dose Selection for Carcinogenicity Studies of Pharmaceuticals'.[41] In this document, the five following alternatives are suggested to determine the ceiling dose:

- MTD (which is still preferred by the FDA)
- Saturation of absorption (i.e. increased dose does not increase systemic exposure)
- The maximum feasible dose (e.g. 5% in the diet)
- Limiting pharmacodynamic effects (e.g. a dose which sedates the animals)
- A minimum of 25-fold AUC ratio when comparing that in rodents with that found when the drug is used clinically in man.

This guideline is a significant advance because it means that drugs of low toxicity will not have to be tested at the MTD. It is estimated that 15% of the drugs will be caught by the AUC criteria. The MTD, or equivalent, is determined on the basis of the results from a 90-day study, as well as palatability studies if the material is to be administered in the diet or drinking water. An addendum to this ICH guideline issued on 16 July 1997 (Addendum to 'Dose Selection for Carcinogenicity Studies of Pharmaceuticals'. Addition of a limit dose and related notes) indicates that a limit dose of 1500 mg/kg/day will usually be acceptable where there is no evidence for genotoxicity and where the maximum recommended human dose does not exceed 500 mg/day. The 1500 mg/kg/day limit will be acceptable if the animal exposure is at least an order of magnitude greater than the therapeutic human exposure.

It is agreed in this addendum that if a non-genotoxic drug induces tumours in rodents at doses above those producing a 25-fold exposure over humans, such a finding would not be considered likely to pose a relevant risk to humans.

However, concern would remain if a genotoxic compound induces tumours only at doses above 25-fold exposure over human exposure.

3.5.3 Group sizes

Typically group sizes of 50 animals per sex are used at each of three dose levels. A double-sized control group is commonly used, often split as two equal-sized groups. This is because:

1. Concurrent control information is the most important factor in the statistical analysis needed to confirm the presence of an oncogenic effect.
2. Splitting the control group gives information on naturally occurring variation in tumour incidence.

Additional animals will be required to provide pharmacokinetic information, especially in mouse studies where blood sampling sufficient for analysis usually requires the animal to be killed.

3.5.4 Conduct of study

Meticulous record-keeping systems are essential to cope with the immense amount of data generated in an oncogenicity study. Palpations to detect the onset of tumours and follow their duration are an essential part of the study conduct and are carried out with increasing frequency as the study progresses. Regular clinical observations are required to ensure that sick animals are identified, monitored and killed before they die naturally, thus preventing loss of important information through autolysis or cannibalism. A study losing more than 10% of animals through these causes is of questionable validity.

3.5.5 Duration of study

Carcinogenicity studies are usually carried out in rats for 24 months and in mice for 18 months. Although such durations meet guidelines issued by the Office for Economic Co-operation and Development, some authorities believe that these studies should be lifespan studies and would, therefore, expect to see a mortality of at least 50%. The maximum duration of study in the 1990 Japanese Guidelines for Toxicity Studies of Drugs Manual[30] is 130 weeks in rats and 104 weeks in mice and hamsters, even when mortality is low. The FDA statisticians impose a further requirement on such studies that for adequate analysis, at least 25 animals per sex, per group should survive to the end of the study. In addition, in order to prevent a carcinogenic effect being masked by toxicity, not more than 50% of the inter-current deaths in any group should be due to causes other than tumour formation.

Each sex can be terminated independently when survival is reduced to 50%. In order to meet all the restrictions outlined above, and because the longevity of the Sprague Dawley rat, particularly in the United States, is decreasing, many companies start with 60 or 70 animals per sex, per group.

3.5.6 Autopsy and microscopic examination

The importance of undertaking a careful detailed autopsy on each animal cannot be overemphasised. Organs should be sectioned in a standard manner. The pathologist should adopt a consistent nomenclature and a peer review of the slides has become an accepted part of Good Laboratory Practice.

3.5.7 Evaluation of results

The incidence of neoplasms is compared between the test and control groups for statistical significance and to detect whether there is a trend, that is, increasing incidence with higher doses. Such a comparison is made by tissue, so that all the neoplasms in the liver, for example, are compared between groups. Also, the total number of animals with single and multiple tumours is compared to see if there is a non-specific increase in tumour burden.

As well as comparing simple incidences, the time when the tumours were detected is taken into account. This is because a compound might not change the overall incidence of a particular type of tumour but it could cause it to develop in much younger animals and cause them to die earlier.[41]

The most important comparison is with concurrent control groups. However, there are occasions when it is necessary to use historical data, that is, information from control animals of the same strain on other studies. This is more relevant if the studies were conducted in the same laboratory under similar conditions and at the same time. The incidence of a particular neoplasm is often different between laboratories and may change with time. Historical data are most useful to get an idea of the variation in the background range of frequency and also to ascertain that rare tumour types can occur spontaneously.

Statistically, oncogenicity studies have a low sensitivity because of the small numbers of animals that are used.[42] However, complex statistical analysis, which should include a judgement on whether the tumour was the cause of death, duration to death and trend analysis can reveal valuable information about the risk to man of taking the product therapeutically.

3.6 Reproductive Toxicology

The assessment of a new pharmaceutical product for effects on reproduction must take into account that mammalian reproduction is a complex, cyclical process involving a number of stages, each complicated in themselves. The stages include

- Gametogenesis
- Fertilisation
- Implantation
- Embryogenesis; foetal growth
- Parturition
- Post-natal adaption
- Development and ageing.

These phases differ in duration depending on the species being considered.

3.6.1 Aims of studies

The two areas of the reproductive process that animal studies focus on are general reproductive effects and developmental effects.

3.6.1.1 General reproductive effects

Studies for general reproductive effects examine the possibility that agents may affect fertility, male or female, by specific pharmacological or biochemical means or by toxicity to a number of cell types, including gametes and their supporting cells. Some agents may alter the delicate hormone balance required for the mammalian reproductive process to maintain its cyclical progress. Others, often potent pharmacological agents, may result in loss of reproductive drive, for example, loss of libido, sexual dysfunction, etc.

Other agents, for example, cytotoxic drugs, target reproductive organs because of their ability to affect rapidly dividing cells, and to possibly induce damage to the genetic material.

Studies examining reproductive effects in animals are invariably lengthy and initially 'catch all'. An effect of reduced pregnancy rates in treated females having mated with treated males may be the result of a number of factors that would have to be examined methodically.

3.6.1.2 Developmental effects

The second, and more emotive, area of examination is developmental effects, where agents may induce abnormalities in the developing offspring. The difficulties in designing studies to detect these types of agents, commonly referred to as teratogens, are that interspecies response is often variable and the abnormalities induced invariably also occur spontaneously. Another confounding factor is that some abnormalities, for example, cardiovascular and behavioural defects, may only manifest themselves post-natally because of an increase in size or functional abnormalities of the offspring.

3.6.2 Types of studies

Before the ICH guidelines (see below), reproductive toxicity studies were divided into three segments which, in Europe,[43] were designed as follows:

Segment I: fertility and general reproductive performance study. This is an overall screening study,

covering the entire reproductive cycle of one generation, including the reproductive ability of the offspring of that generation. The test substance is only administered directly to the first (parental) generation and the test animal is usually the rat.

Females are dosed 14 days before mating (N.B. there are 5 days between ovulations) and through to lactation.

Previously, males were dosed 70 days before mating (N.B. the spermatogenic cycle is 50 days). However, recent studies in Japan have shown that almost all effects occur late in the cycle. Thus, dosing for 14 days before mating is deemed acceptable.[44]

Segment II: teratogenicity study. This concentrates on the most sensitive part of gestation, from the time of implantation until major organogenesis is complete. This is the period during which a test substance is most likely to cause malformation of the embryo. Exposure of the mother to the test substance is usually confined to this period. Conventionally, the study is conducted in rats and rabbits. Rabbits are intolerant to antibiotics and the mouse is an acceptable alternative in most cases.

Segment III: peri- and post-natal study. This concentrates on the late part of gestation, not covered by the teratogenicity study, on parturition and on the period of lactation. The study can be particularly useful in detecting subtle effects on the brain, which continues physical and functional development during the foetal and post-natal period, after dosing has ceased in the teratogenicity study. The test animal is usually the rat.

There were major differences in the protocol designs for rodent studies between Japanese and European studies. These were resolved by the ICH, which in 1993 published a guideline entitled 'Detection of Toxicity to Reproduction for Medicinal Products'.

The ICH guideline's 'preferred option' is a three-study design as follows:

Fertility and early embryonic development (rat). Provided no deleterious effects have been revealed by testicular histopathology assessment and testes weight measurements (ICH guideline,

'Toxicity to Male Fertility: An Addendum to the ICH Tripartite Guideline on Detection of Toxicity to Reproduction for Medicinal Products', as amended in November 2001) in a one-month repeat-dose study, a premating treatment interval of 2 weeks for both sexes can be used. The *treatment period requires justification*. Dosing should continue through mating and at least through implantation in the females.

If the short premating dosing interval is used, then the *in vivo* part of the study would take approximately 9 weeks compared with 32–35 weeks for a standard Segment I study.

Embryo-foetal development (rat and rabbit). This is a standard Segment II, teratogenicity study.

Pre- and post-natal development, including maternal function (rat). Females are exposed to the test substance from implantation to the end of lactation. F1 pups should be evaluated for post-natal development including fertility. The duration of the *in vivo* phase of this study would be approximately 20 weeks if F1 pregnant females are killed for caesarean section examination, 22–24 weeks if allowed to litter.

As an alternative to the 'preferred option', the ICH guideline allows flexibility in the choice of study designs, as long as the combination of studies chosen covers the complete reproductive cycle. This allows the toxicologist to design the reproductive toxicology package so that it is relevant to the compound class under test.

In addition to the above studies, a number of studies examining the pharmacokinetics of the test material need to be conducted to show whether the drug crosses the placenta, whether it is excreted in milk and whether pregnancy affects absorption, distribution, metabolism or excretion.

3.6.3 Timing of studies

Reproductive toxicity tests are not required to support Phase I clinical studies in men. Detailed histological evaluations of the male reproductive organs should be performed in the repeated-dose toxicity studies. Male fertility studies in the rodent, however, would be expected to support Phase III studies.

The FDA allows women to enter carefully controlled and monitored trials in which adequate contraceptive measures and pregnancy testing are performed without requiring results from animal reproductive toxicity tests. In Japan and Europe, because of the high level of concern regarding unintentional exposure of the developing embryo or foetus, an assessment of fertility in a rodent, and embryo/foetal development in a rodent or non-rodent are required if women of childbearing potential are to be included in a Phase I trial. The FDA would expect such results to support Phase II and Phase III studies.

The complete reproductive toxicity package, including the rodent peri- and post-natal studies, must be submitted with the marketing application.

3.6.4 Juvenile toxicity studies

Juvenile toxicity studies are recommended by both the Japanese and US regulatory agencies before inclusion of children in clinical trials. The studies are usually conducted in the offspring of untreated female rats (although juvenile dog studies have been requested for specific compounds), by giving test material directly to the pups. Dosing usually does not commence until 4 days *post partum*, because of technical difficulties, and is continued for 6 weeks. The survival and development of the offspring is monitored and full clinical chemistry, haematological and urine analyses are carried out. At autopsy, all major organs and tissues are retained and examined microscopically.

European agencies do not usually require such studies. It is unusual for paediatric trials to be conducted before there is considerable experience in adults, which is obviously more relevant for assessment of risk to children than are studies in juvenile rats.

3.6.5 Evaluation and interpretation of data

The following points should be considered when evaluating the data from reproductive toxicity studies.

3.6.5.1   Antifertility effects in males

The male rat has a large reserve of spermatozoa and it is difficult to detect antifertility effects by using pregnancy as an endpoint. This is because the ejaculate in rats contains over 1000-fold the number of sperm that will produce maximum fertility. In man the multiple is only 2–4 times and some studies have suggested that in certain Western populations, average human sperm counts appear to have declined over the past 50 years.[45] The rat's testes are also relatively about 40 times the size of man's. If antifertility effects are observed, it can be helpful to measure various sperm parameters (seminology) to help characterise effects.

3.6.5.2   Antifertility effects in females

These would be apparent on examination of the following parameters.

- Number of females failing to become pregnant (any likely contribution of the male to this effect should be eliminated by mating treated females with untreated males)
- Disruption of the oestrous cycle
- Increased incidence of pre-implantation loss (number of corpora lutea – number of implants *in utero*)
- Increased incidence of post-implantation loss (number of implants *in utero* – number of live foetuses).

3.6.5.3   Teratogenesis

Evaluation of the data should consider whether:

- There are any foetal abnormalities that have not been observed previously or only occur rarely.
- There is a significant increase in defects that occur spontaneously, especially without any significant maternal toxicity.

3.6.5.4   Post-natal effects

Parturition is a particularly stressful period for both the mother and the offspring. Delays or protraction of the process may have significant effects on data collected post-natally.

Parameters to consider are:

- Peri-natal survival of both dam and offspring

- Post-natal survival of offspring may be influenced by either underlying abnormalities, for example of the cardiovascular system, or as a result of poor lactation in the dam
- The function of vital senses should be evaluated in the offspring, for example, sight, hearing, balance, etc.
- Behavioural effects in the offspring can be evaluated by tests for locomotion, habituation, learning and memory.

3.7   Genotoxicity Testing

Genotoxicity refers to potentially harmful effects on genetic material (DNA), which may occur directly through the induction of permanent transmissible changes (mutations) in the amount or structure of the DNA within cells.[46] Such damage to DNA can occur at three levels.

1. *Gene (point) mutations* are changes in nucleotide sequence at one or a few coding segments (base pairs) within a gene. They can occur by base substitution (i.e. where one base in the DNA is replaced by another) or by frame-shift mutations (i.e. where there is addition or deletion of one or more bases, thus altering the sequence of bases in the DNA, which constitutes the reading frame).
2. *Chromosomal mutations* are recognised as morphological alterations in the gross structure of chromosomes, that is, they are structural aberrations which can be detected microscopically. Compounds which cause chromosome damage are called clastogens.
3. *Genomic mutations* are changes in the number of chromosomes in a genome, and are also called numerical aberrations. Loss or gain of chromosomes during cell division is called aneuploidy, and chemicals which cause this are called aneugens. It is possible to generate cells containing multiples of the whole chromosome set – these are polyploid cells. Both aneuploidy and polyploidy can result from damage to the mitotic spindle.

Many chemicals possess mutagenic properties, which present a potential hazard to future generations because mutations in germ cells of sexually reproducing organisms may be transmitted to the offspring. Furthermore, the relationship between mutational changes in DNA and carcinogenesis is strongly supported by the available evidence originating from research into the molecular biology of cancer, and the existence of cancer genes (oncogenes) and tumour suppressor genes. Consequently, the use of short-term genotoxicity tests as prescreens for carcinogen detection has grown over the past twenty years. Accumulation of mutagenic events is also associated with atherosclerosis, ageing processes, etc. There is a necessity to identify and limit the spread of chemicals with mutagenic properties in the environment, and therefore any new therapeutic substance, including new excipients, where a wide exposure can be anticipated, are screened for genotoxicity using testing procedures that detect both gene and chromosome damage, *in vitro* (e.g. using bacterial assays and mammalian cells in culture) and *in vivo* (using rodents).

In the pharmaceutical industry, it is usual to carry out genotoxicity screening at an early stage in the drug development programme. This is particularly so with regard to the use of *in vitro* assays. If problems concerning potential genotoxicity can be identified early, using bacterial genotoxicity tests for example, it may be possible to design a useful drug that is devoid of genotoxic properties by the consideration of structure–activity relationships. The *in vitro* tests require small amounts of compound and generate results quickly, making them particularly useful for such studies.

A harmonised three-test standard battery has been agreed[47] (Box 3.3) through the ICH process

and a new guideline issued (Genotoxicity: A Standard Battery for Genotoxicity Testing of Pharmaceuticals). The three-test battery will suffice for testing most new chemical entities. However, additional genotoxicity tests will be required in particular circumstances:

1. When testing antibacterial compounds where bacterially based mutation tests will be of limited value.
2. When 'structurally alerting' compounds (e.g. those possessing alkylating electrophilic centres) have given negative results in the standard battery.
3. When testing compounds that are not absorbed into the systemic circulation, where an all *in vitro* test battery may suffice.
4. When testing compounds that are completely novel in a unique structural class and are in a therapeutic class that would not normally be tested in chronic rodent oncogenicity assays.
5. to understand the mechanism of action for carcinogenic compounds that were negative in the standard battery, yet do not have a clear non-genotoxic mechanism of carcinogenicity.

Additional testing may include tests for DNA adducts (e.g. the ^{32}P-post-labelling assay[48]), DNA repair [e.g. the so-called COMET assay[49] or assays measuring unscheduled DNA synthesis (UDS)], mutation of transgenes *in vivo* in models such as the Mutamouse® and the Big Blue® mouse and rat,[50] etc., or simply the inclusion of both types of *in vitro* mammalian cell assay. Readers are referred to the guideline for further information. Products of biotechnology, for example, cytokines, monoclonal antibodies, etc., do not normally need to be screened for genotoxicity, unless impurities/contaminants or organic linker molecules cause concern (ICH guideline S6, Safety for Biotechnological Products). There is, however, some concern for growth factors that may induce high levels of proliferation in specific tissues, thus increasing the chance of spontaneous mutation in oncogenes and tumour suppressor genes.

Box 3.3   ICH harmonised test battery
- A test for gene mutation in bacteria
- An *in vitro* test with cytogenetic evaluation of chromosomal damage with mammalian cells OR an *in vitro* mouse lymphoma thymidine kinase± assay
- An *in vivo* test for chromosomal damage using rodent haematopoietic cells. ICH guideline, 'Genotoxicity: A Standard Battery for Genotoxicity Testing of Pharmaceuticals'

Before any human studies, results from two separate *in vitro* tests for mutation and chromosomal damage must be provided. The full test battery must be completed before initiation of Phase II trials.

For chemical intermediates it is also necessary to carry out bacterial genotoxicity tests for Health and Safety at Work labelling and classification purposes. Additional *in vitro* and *in vivo* assays of the type described for drugs are triggered as the tonnage manufactured per annum increases. The classification and labelling of intermediates in relation to their genotoxicity is important in ensuring that their safe manufacture, storage, transport, use and disposal can be accomplished.

Reactive chemicals are used to manufacture drugs and a proportion of these are genotoxic. A draft guideline has been issued by the Europe and CHMP that seeks to control patient exposure to most genotoxic contaminants to below a 'Threshold of Toxicological' concern of 1.5 μg/day. This is based on modelling data on known human carcinogens where such concentrations for specific compounds would not be expected to increase human cancer above 1 per 10^5 exposed individuals.[51]

3.7.1 Study design

Full study design details for the established regulatory tests for genotoxicity are given in the UKEMS volume on Basic Mutagenicity Tests.[52]

3.7.1.1 Bacterial tests for gene mutation
The most widely used *in vitro* assay is the reverse mutation assay for gene mutation using strains of *Salmonella typhimurium* and *Escherichia coli*, which are capable of detecting a wide variety of mutations. This assay measures reversion from histidine dependence to histidine independence for the *Salmonella* strains, and tryptophan dependence to independence for the *E. coli* strains and is carried out in both the presence and absence of an exogenous metabolic activation system (usually the post-mitochondrial fraction from the livers of rats treated with cytochrome P450 enzyme-inducing agents). In the test, bacteria are exposed to a range of concentrations of the chemical and plated onto minimal agar medium. After a suitable period of incubation at 37°C, the number of revertant colonies is counted and compared with the number of spontaneous revertants obtained in an untreated/solvent control culture.

3.7.1.2 Assays for chromosomal aberrations
The simplest and most sensitive assays for detecting clastogenic (i.e. chromosomal breaking) effects involve the use of mammalian cells. Cultures of established cell lines (e.g. Chinese hamster ovary) as well as primary cell cultures (e.g. human lymphocyte) may be used. After exposure to a range of chemical concentrations in the presence and absence of an appropriate metabolic activation system, the cell cultures are treated with a spindle inhibitor (e.g. vinblastine) to accumulate cells in a metaphase-like stage of mitosis. Cells are harvested at appropriate times and chromosome preparations are made, stained with DNA-specific dye and the metaphase cells are analysed under the microscope for chromosome abnormalities.

3.7.1.3 Mammalian cell tests for gene mutation
A variety of mammalian cell culture systems can be used to detect mutations induced by chemical substances. The L5178Y mouse lymphoma line, measuring mutation at the TK locus, is preferred. TK is an important enzyme involved in DNA synthesis. Cells are exposed to the test substance at various concentrations, in the presence and absence of a metabolic activation system, for a suitable period of time, and then subcultured to assess cytotoxicity and to allow phenotypic expression prior to mutant selection. Cells deficient in TK because of a forward mutation are resistant to the cytotoxic effects of pyrimidine analogues (antimetabolites), such as trifluorothymidine (TFT). This is because the antimetabolites cannot be incorporated into cellular nucleotides and kill the cell through inhibition of cellular metabolism. After treatment, cells are grown in a medium containing TFT; mutant cells can proliferate in the presence of TFT, whereas normal cells containing TK are killed. This allows the detection of an increase in mutant

cells after chemical treatment. Analysis of mutant colonies from this assay has shown that they can arise from a variety of genetic changes, including point mutation, large and small chromosomal deletions, recombination, etc.

3.7.1.4 Detection of chromosome damage in rodent bone marrow using the micronucleus test

The micronucleus test is a short-term mammalian *in vivo* assay for the detection of chromosomal damage or damage to the mitotic apparatus by chemicals. The basis of this assay is an increase in micronuclei in the polychromatic erythrocytes present within the bone marrow of treated animals when compared with the controls. The micronuclei, known to pathologists as the Howell–Jolly bodies, are formed from chromosomal fragments or whole chromosomes lagging in mitosis. When erythroblasts develop into erythrocytes, the main nucleus is expelled while the micronucleus may be retained within the cytoplasm, and is readily visualised. Animals are exposed to the test substance, usually a single dose, and 24 and 48 h after treatment, they are killed, the bone marrow is extracted and smear preparations are made. After suitable staining, the polychromatic erythrocytes are analysed under the microscope for micronucleus frequency. Following the issue in 1995 of the ICH guideline, 'Genotoxicity: Guidance on Specific Aspects of Regulatory Genotoxicity Tests for Pharmaceuticals', it is sufficient to use only male rats or mice for these tests, as long as no obvious difference in toxicity has been detected between the sexes.

3.7.1.5 UDS – *ex vivo* assay in rodent liver

This assay is normally carried out only if positive effects have been obtained in earlier *in vitro* tests. The UDS test measures the DNA repair synthesis which occurs after excision and removal of a stretch of DNA containing the region of damage, induced in hepatocytes of animals treated with the test chemicals. UDS is measured by the uptake of radioactively labelled nucleotide, usually tritium-labelled thymidine, into the DNA of the damaged hepatocytes. Animals, usually male rats, are treated with the test chemical, and

groups are killed 2–4 or 12–14 h after treatment. Suspensions of viable hepatocytes are prepared by liver perfusion, and these are cultured in the presence of tritium-labelled thymidine. The incorporation of radiolabel within the DNA is determined autoradiographically. The measurement of DNA damage serves as a surrogate for genetic alterations *in vivo*.

The ICH guideline requires that there must be proof of exposure of the target tissues to the test compound (and its metabolites) to validate the chosen *in vivo* assays.

The UK Department of Health Advisory Committee on Mutagens (COM) issued a new guideline document during 2000 on a strategy for testing chemicals for mutagenicity.[53] This document attempts to strengthen the detection of compounds that can induce changes in chromosome number, in particular aneugens. Such genotoxins are seen as contributing to human ill health, for example, foetal wastage, abnormal development and probably carcinogenesis. Aneugens can be detected by the mammalian cell assays cited in ICH guidelines, but newer techniques/tests may optimise detection. The COM guidelines cite the *in vitro* micronucleus test as an acceptable test in this regard. If aneugenicity is indicated, chromosome painting assays, centromeric staining, etc., can be used in confirmation.

3.7.2 Germ-cell tests

Because there is no good evidence that mutagens induce mutations exclusively in germ cells, it is not considered necessary to conduct germ-cell studies as part of the screening package. Such testing is only carried out if detailed risk assessment data is required (e.g. with anticancer drugs). The newer generation of *in vivo* tests using transgenic animals and also the comet assay has facilitated the study of genetic changes in germ cells and there is a resurgence of interest in this area.

3.7.3 Study interpretation

Guidance on the evaluation of genotoxicity data is given in the two ICH genotoxicity guidelines.

Comparative trials have shown that each genotoxicity test can generate both false negative

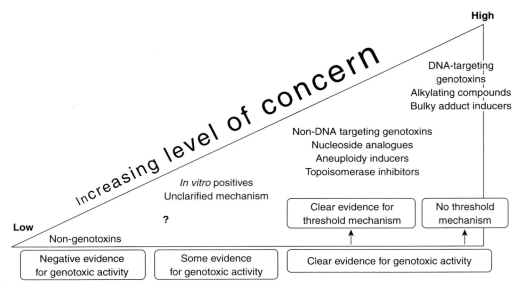

Fig. 3.3 Risk–benefit continuum for genotoxicity.

and false positive results in relation to predicting rodent carcinogenicity. Experimental conditions such as the limited capacity of *in vitro* metabolic activation systems can lead to false negative results in *in vitro* tests. Culture conditions (e.g. changes of pH, high osmolality, etc.) can lead to false positive results. The test battery approach is designed to reduce the risk of false negative results, while a positive result in any one *in vitro* assay does not necessarily mean that the test compound poses a genotoxic/carcinogenic hazard to humans.

For a compound that induces a biologically relevant positive result in one or more *in vitro* tests, an *in vivo* test, in addition to *in vivo* cytogenetic assay, using a tissue other than the bone marrow/peripheral blood, can provide further useful information. The target cells exposed *in vivo* and possibly the genetic endpoint measured *in vitro* guide the choice of this additional *in vivo* test. *In vivo* gene mutation assays using endogenous genes or transgenes in a variety of tissues in the rat and mouse are at various stages of development and have been used to help risk assessments, but there are still concerns regarding the lack of sensitivity of the current assays. Until such tests become improved, results from other *in vivo* tests for genotoxicity can be used.

(e.g. liver UDS assay), but the choice of assay should be scientifically justified.

If *in vivo* and *in vitro* test results do not agree, then the differences should be considered/explained, possibly following further studies on *in vitro/in vivo* metabolism, compound class information, etc. The final assessment of the genotoxic potential of a compound should take into account the totality of findings and compound class information, if available. Figure 3.3 (reproduced with kind permission of Lutz Müller) illustrates this strategy.[54]

3.8 Irritation and Sensitisation Testing

Topical drug preparations are applied for days or even weeks, cosmetics for a lifetime and skin contact is probably the most common form of exposure to industrial chemicals. Therefore, a knowledge of the cutaneous toxicity is important for an overall hazard assessment. Cutaneous toxicity or localised skin injury can be considered as a primary event, because the compound could be irritant or corrosive, or as a secondary immunologically mediated event causing a delayed hypersensitivity response.

The data obtained from irritation and sensitisation testing can be used for hazard assessment, thereby enabling safe handling precautions to be recommended, and as a basis for classification and labelling. Such studies also have to be performed to meet obligations of regulatory authorities for the clinical trials and marketing of drugs.

3.8.1 Irritancy

3.8.1.1 Skin

Primary irritant-contact dermatitis results from direct cytotoxicity produced on first contact. The cellular injury is characterised by two macroscopically visible events: a reddening of the skin (erythema) and accumulation of fluid (oedema). By observing or measuring these changes, one can estimate the extent of skin damage that has occurred. The most widely used single-exposure irritancy test is based on the Draize rabbit test.[55]

In this test, three rabbits are used to assess the irritancy potential following a single 4-h semi-occluded application, to intact rabbit skin, of 0.5 mL or 0.5 g of test material. The skin is observed 30–69 min and approximately 24, 48 and 72 h after patch removal. If irritation is persistent, additional observations can be carried out on days 7 and 14.

Scores for erythema and oedema at the 24 and 48-h readings are added together for the three rabbits (12 values) and divided by 6 to give the primary irritation index (PII). This index is used to classify the material from non-irritant (0), mild irritant (>0–2), moderate irritant (>2–>5) to severe irritant (>5).

There is some progress in developing alternative in vitro assays for some aspects of irritant potential.[56]

3.8.1.2 Eye

Toxic responses in the eye can result from direct topical ocular exposure of drugs from direct installation into the eye and also from dermal products which patients may accidentally get into their eyes. Until recently, the Draize rabbit eye test[55] using three rabbits has served as the major protocol to assess the irritancy potential of topically applied substances.

In the Draize test, a single dose of 0.1 mL or 0.1 g is introduced into the conjunctival sac of the right eye, the left eye acting as a control. The reactions of the conjunctivae, iris and cornea are scored for irritancy at approximately 1, 3, 8, 24, 48 and 72 h and again at 7 days after dosing. Test materials shown to be severe skin irritants or that are below pH 2 or above pH 11 are not tested but are assumed to be eye irritants.

The use of the Draize tests has been receiving attention for a number of years because of animal welfare considerations. Consequently, the modifications of the existing protocol and the development of alternative methods have been extensively examined by the cosmetic and chemical industry to reduce animal usage and the occurrence of severe reactions. One modification of this model uses reduced volumes of 0.01 mL and 0.01 g, which reduces severe reactions but does not compromise the predictive value of the test.

Several in vitro methods, including the hen's egg chorioallantoic membrane test (HET-CAM); the bovine cornea opacity and permeability assay (BCOP) and the isolated rabbit eye (IRE) test, have gained regulatory acceptance in Europe for the classification of severe eye irritants.[56] Many companies are using such techniques successfully to reduce in vivo testing during development.[57]

3.8.2 Immunotoxicology

3.8.2.1 Sensitisation

The interaction of a chemical (hapten) with epidermal proteins (carrier) can result in a hapten–carrier complex capable of activating skin-associated lymphoid tissue (sensitisation) and dissemination of antigen-specific T lymphocytes (induction). Subsequent encounter with the same or cross-reactive chemicals can result in the elicitation of a characteristic inflammatory skin reaction. The clinical condition is referred to as allergic contact dermatitis and is characterised by erythema, oedema, vesiculation and pruritus. Allergic contact sensitisation is, therefore, classed as a cell-mediated immunological response to chemicals that contact and penetrate the skin.

There are a number of models for detecting allergic contact dermatitis in guinea pigs. The maximisation test developed by Magnussun and Kligman[58] is the most widely used and employs both an intradermal and topical sensitisation phase, together with the non-specific stimulation of the immune system by the intradermal injection of Freund's complete adjuvant.

Approximately 54 animals are used in the test and the sensitisation response is classified by the percentage of animals showing a stronger response than that seen in the controls. The net response is classified from 0% for a non-sensitiser, up to 8% for a weak sensitiser and over 80% for an extreme sensitiser.

A negative result in this type of test indicates that the potential to sensitise is extremely low and that human exposure is unlikely to be attended by a significant incidence of sensitisation. Because the test can be overpredictive, some toxicologists recommend that a non-adjuvant test such as the Buehler test[59] should be used if a positive is obtained, to give a more realistic determination of the prevalence of human sensitisation. It should be remembered that contact sensitisation is a persistent condition; thus once sensitised to a chemical, an individual is at risk of dermatitis whenever exposed to the same or antigenically cross-reactive chemical, for example, nickel in jewellery.

Recent guidelines entitled 'Non-clinical Local Tolerance Testing of Medicinal Product' from the CPMP refer to the murine local lymph node assay as a method for the assessment of the induction phase of skin sensitisation. This method measures the ability of compounds to induce proliferative responses in skin-draining lymph nodes. This method uses fewer animals than alternative *in vivo* methods and reduces the trauma to which animals are potentially subjected.[60]

3.8.2.2   Immunosuppression

In appendix B of the CPMP Note for Guidance on Repeated Dose Toxicity (adopted October 2000), there is a request for an initial immunotoxicity screen (primarily for measuring immunosuppression). This consists of an assessment of haematology (i.e. differential cell counting),

lymphoid organ weights (i.e. thymus, spleen, draining and distant lymph nodes), microscopy of lymphoid tissue (i.e. as above plus Peyer's patches), bone marrow cellularity, distribution of lymphocyte subsets, and natural killer cell activity or primary antibody response of T-cells to antigen challenge (e.g. to sheep red blood cells) should be completed.

If the above investigations indicate that an effect has occurred, the document requests that further tests should be chosen from the following list, based on scientific justification:

- Delayed type hypersensitivity
- Mitogen- or antigen-stimulated lymphocyte proliferative response
- Macrophage function
- Primary antibody response to a T-cell antigen (if not already provided)
- *In vivo* models of host resistance, which are employed to detect increased susceptibility to infectious agents, and tumours, and may show the consequences of disturbed immune function.

The FDA has also issued a comprehensive, but different guideline to the EMEA/CHMP regulatory authorities and this topic was adopted as a topic for harmonisation by the ICH process in 2004.

3.8.3   Special routes

Ideally, toxicology studies should mimic, as near as possible, human exposure. Thus, both the route of administration and the exposure should, where possible, be similar to that in man. The classic route of administration in man is oral and thus most toxicology studies are conducted by the oral route. However, parenteral routes may be used either to mimic the clinical route or to ensure exposure. The administration of some medicines is directly on to highly differentiated surfaces such as the alveolar surface of the lungs or the skin. It is, therefore, important to assess the topical irritancy, absorption and subsequent systemic toxicity following such applications. It should be remembered that some compounds, for example, chlorinated hydrocarbons, may be more toxic when given by the inhalation route than when given orally or may directly affect the respiratory tract, for example, formaldehyde vapour.

Specialised studies may be conducted at any time during the development phase. If a special route is selected as the primary route of administration, then this route will be used throughout. Special routes used to supplement the main toxicology programme will usually be conducted before administration or exposure of man to the test material by the route equivalent to the special route. The duration of dosing recommended for the special routes in different species is presented in Table 3.5.

These studies generally follow the guidelines for conventional studies, for example, a control and three test groups receiving differing dosages. The designs are typically as follows.

3.8.3.1 Intramuscular

Varying concentrations of test material are injected into the muscle, using a constant dose volume to a maximum of 1 mL.

3.8.3.2 Inhalation

This can be subdivided into three routes:

1. *Intratracheal* – Small quantities, usually less than 1 mL, of varying concentrations of solutions or varying quantities of powder are placed or blown into the trachea of an anaesthetised animal using a cannula placed intratracheally.

2. *Intranasal* – Small quantities, usually <50 μL, of varying concentrations of solution or suspension of test material are placed into the nasal cavity by introduction through the external nares.

3. *Pulmonary* – Animals are placed in an exposure chamber, either whole body or snout only, or individually exposed via mask systems (dogs, primates and rabbits) and allowed to inhale an aerosol of known concentrations generated from a powder, solution, suspension or a vapour of the test material for periods of up to 23 h daily for durations approaching the animal's natural lifespan.

Typically exposure periods are 1 h daily, 7 days each week using snout-only systems for pharmaceutical products, or 6 h daily, 5 days each week using whole-body exposure systems for industrial chemicals.

Aerosols must be respirable, that is, have a mean aerodynamic diameter of less than 5 μm, to ensure that a reasonable proportion will penetrate the respiratory tract defence systems of the nasal passages and the mucociliary clearance mechanisms.

3.8.3.3 Topical

Test or control material is applied either onto or under an occlusive dressing to the abraded or unabraded shaved skin of animals. Wound

Table 3.5 Maximum duration of dosing by special routes recommended for different species

Route of exposure	Maximum dosing period (months)				
	Mouse	Rat	Dog	Marmoset	Rabbit
Intramuscular	Single	1	1	1	1
Inhalation	Life	Life	12	—	Life
Intratracheal	Single	Single	—	—	1
Intranasal	—	1	6	—	—
Topical	Life	Life	12	12	—
Intrarectal	—	—	1	—	1
Intra-arterial	—	—	—	—	Single[a]

[a]Required by Austrian Regulatory Authorities for injectable products.
Life – lifetime; Single–single dose only; — inappropriate or no experience.

Table 3.6 Multiplication factors for adjusting dosages (in mg/kg) to take account of differences in surface area: body weight ratios between species

From/to	Mouse	Rat	Marmoset	Dog	Man
Mouse (20 g)	1	$\frac{1}{2}$	$\frac{1}{3}$	$\frac{1}{6}$	$\frac{1}{12}$
Rat (150 g)	2	1	$\frac{2}{3}$	$\frac{1}{4}$	$\frac{1}{7}$
Marmoset (400 g)	3	$1\frac{1}{2}$	1	$\frac{1}{3}$	$\frac{1}{5}$
Dog (8 kg)	6	4	3	1	$\frac{1}{2}$
Man (60 kg)	12	7	5	2	1

healing can be assessed by applying large (e.g. 1 g/1 kg) topical doses of test material to an epithelial wound (e.g. an incision) and monitoring wound healing over a period of 14 days.

3.8.3.4 Intrarectal
This is usually done only in dogs. Different dosages are administered on standard sized suppositories (e.g. size 2 mL).

3.8.3.5 Intra-arterial
This is usually done only in rabbits. A single injection is made into the central artery of an ear. The contralateral ear artery is given the control material. This is to assess the effects of a subcutaneous or intravenous injection when it is accidentally injected into an artery, as drugs are rarely given by this route.

Absorption and systemic toxicity observed using special routes should be compared with the more usual intravenous or oral routes of administration to identify and assess the relevance of any significant differences observed. Plasma levels will obviously depend on the amount of drug absorbed. Higher systemic (i.e. circulating) levels of drug may help explain the differences in toxicity between routes. Corticosteroids, for example, are more toxic on the basis of administered dose when given by the inhalation compared with the oral route. It is the ratio of the AUC for the plasma concentration–time curve in the animal to that in man which constitutes the key element in predicting human toxicity.

If pharmacokinetic data are not available, an approximation can be given using a scaling factor which converts body weight to surface area. It was found by Freireich et al.[61] that toxicity of anticancer drugs between species equated to surface area. Using a scaling factor of $X^{0.66}$, where X is the body weight, converts milligrams of drug per kilogram of body weight to milligrams of drug to metre square of body surface, as shown in Table 3.6. The FDA[62] has recently indicated that a factor of $X^{0.75}$ may be more predictive for equating toxicity between species.

If oncogenicity studies have been conducted by the oral route and another clinical route is to be used in man, the need to repeat such studies should be assessed critically. Oncogenic potential is related to the concentration of the carcinogen at its site of action. Thus, if the oral route results in adequate exposure of the lung, there should be no need to perform additional inhalation oncogenicity studies. Inhalation studies of 1–3 months duration should be performed to assess possible local effects on respiratory tissue and also to gain pharmacokinetic data.

3.9 Animal Numbers, Costs and Ethics

Toxicity studies are costly in terms of both animals and resources, as indicated in Table 3.7. For a product developed for chronic oral therapy, approximately 4000 rats, 1300 mice, 100 rabbits, 50 guinea pigs and 160 dogs, a total of over 5000 animals, is used. If the foetuses and offspring from the reproductive toxicity studies are

Table 3.7 Toxicity studies – approximate cost, test material requirement and reporting times

Study type	Species	No. of animals[a]	Cost[b] (£ thousands)	Test material (Factor Q[c])	Report[d] (weeks)
Acute toxicity	Mouse	30	2	0.0006	6
	Rat	30	2	0.005	6
1-month toxicity	Rat	160	7	0.5	20
	Dog	32	85	4	18
3 months toxicity	Rat	160	100	1.8	22
	Dog	40	140	15	20
6 months toxicity	Rat	192	150	3.7	26
	Dog	40	190	30	24
12 months toxicity	Dog	40	280	60	24
ICH reproductive toxicity study	Rat	200 (1770)	70	1.13	36
Organogenesis	Rabbit	88 (440)	45	1.37	20
Peri-natal–post-natal	Rat	60 (1500)	80	0.35	20
90-day preliminary	Mouse	90	90	0.1	12
	Rat	90	90	1.0	12
Oncogenicity (gavage)	Mouse (80 weeks)	1100	600	5.4	48
	Rat (2 years)	600	600	33.7	48
Genetic toxicology					
Microbial			2.5	6	6
Mouse lymphoma			16	10	8
Human lymphocyte			16	10	12
Micronucleus	Rat	60	6	24	12

The figures are for study designs that meet worldwide regulatory requirements for pharmaceuticals. Variations that may be encountered are given in the notes.

[a] Numbers in parentheses are numbers of foetuses/offspring produced.

[b] Costs are approximate (as of 2002) and assume oral (gavage) administration and include costs of assay to confirm dose concentration and bioassay of pharmacokinetic samples. Significant variations for the same study design will be found between different contractors (±20%), different study designs (±25%) and different routes of administration (intravenous +25%, inhalation by snout only + 50–100%).

[c] The total quantity of test material required for the study, in grams, is given by the formula $Q \times$ sum of the dose levels in milligrams.

Example: A 6-month study of dog with dose levels of 100, 200 and 400 mg/kg requires 23.8 kg test material: that is, $34 \times (100 + 200 + 400)$ g.

Q takes into account, where appropriate, the inclusion in the study design of sufficient animals to study recovery and pharmacokinetics, the projected mean body weight of the animals over the study and a 20% contingency for unexpected losses, etc.

[d] Times given are for a QA audited report, from completion of the *in vivo* phase of the study, but excluding any recovery period. It is possible to reduce these times by one-third if given adequate priority.

included, the total doubles. However, the number of animals used in toxicity testing in the pharmaceutical industry compared with the total used is surprisingly low. It has recently been estimated this to be less than 7.5%. Pharmacological screening for drugs uses by far the greater proportion of animals.

The financial costs are also considerable. To complete the toxicology programme, an inhalation product would cost over £5 000 000 and with the most expeditious planning, would take 5 years to complete.

Is all this testing necessary? Retrospective studies show that the detection of clinically relevant toxicities by preclinical animal studies is high and useful, although it is by no means 100%.[2] In addition, fortunately, there has been no repeat of the scale of the thalidomide catastrophe of the 1960s. Most toxicologists agree that if one considers the list of studies required for regulatory approval, there is much room for rationalisation and cutting down on the full range of studies required, without compromising patient safety. There has been a tendency for Regulatory Authorities to increase the requirements for additional tests on largely theoretical grounds, where there is little or no clinical information to show that current methods do not describe the relevant toxicities adequately. Statistically, oncogenicity studies are very insensitive and as knowledge increases, it is becoming possible to argue that the large majority of genotoxic carcinogens are detectable by genotoxicity assays and non-genotoxic carcinogens by changes detected in repeat-dose toxicity studies, for example, hormonal imbalances, tissue-specific cell proliferation, etc.[63] It is hoped that the ICH process will continue to be a useful platform not only for a harmonisation of requirements but also for a complete rationalisation of the toxicity testing programme. Already ICH guidelines provide an opportunity to minimise animal use.[63] It has been estimated that the number of animals used in toxicology for registration of a 'standard' compound can be reduced by 50% (pre- and post-ICH).[64,65]

In the future, it is possible that the need for animal studies will be further minimised by the use of low and ultra-low dose studies in humans, where refinements in measuring such low doses[66] and the ability to measure and interpret toxicologically relevant changes by use of the 'omic technologies will increase over time.

Acknowledgements

David Scales wrote the early editions of this chapter and his insight and knowledge are gratefully acknowledged. Thanks also to Andrew Sullivan, Steve Damment, John Hyde, Malcolm Tucker, Mark Sutherland, David Gatehouse, Pete Sibley, David Alexander and Keith Capel-Edwards for their help, advice and input to the early editions. Finally thanks go to Ms Samantha Robertson and Ms Cassie Hill for their expertise in typing the original manuscript.

Internet addresses for regulatory guidelines

- ICH guidelines: http://www.ifpma.org/ich1.html
- CHMP guidelines: http://www.emea.eu.int/sitemap.htm
- UK COM guidance document: http://www.doh.gov.uk/com.htm

References

1. Zbinden G. Predictive value of animal studies in toxicology. CMR Annual Lecture, 1987.
2. Olson H, Betton G, Robinson D, *et al.* Concordance of the toxicity of pharmaceuticals in humans and in animals. *Regul Toxicol Pharmacol* 2000;**32**:36–67.
3. Pennie WD. Use of cDNA microarrays to probe and understand the toxicological consequences of altered gene expression. *Toxicol Lett* 2000;**112**: 473–7.
4. Steiner S, Wiltzman FW. Proteomics: applications and opportunities in preclinical drug development. *Electrophoresis* 2000;**21**:2099–104.
5. Robertson DG, Reily MD, Sigler RE, *et al.* Metabonomics: evaluation of nuclear magnetic resonance (NMR) and pattern recognition technology for rapid *in vivo* screening of liver and kidney toxicants. *Toxicol Sci* 2000;**57**:326–37.
6. Russell WMS, Burch RL. *The Principles of Humane Experimental Technique.* London: Methuen and Co Ltd, 1959.

7. Lynch A, Connelly J. Drug discovery and development: the toxicologist's view – non-clinical safety assessment. In: Martin R Wilkins, ed. *Experimental Therapeutics*. London: Martin Dunitz, 2003; 25–50.

8. Tugwood JD, Hollins LE, Cockerill MJ. Genomics and the search for novel biomarkers in toxicology. *Biomarkers* 2003;**8**:79–92.

9. Bandara LR, Kennedy S. Toxicoproteomics – a new preclinical tool. *Drug Discov Today* 2002;**7**:411–18.

10. Stapels MD, Barofsky DF. Complementary use of MALDI and ESI for the HPLC-MS/MS analysis of DNA-binding proteins. *Anal Chem* 2004;**76**: 5421–30.

11. Dare TO, Davies HA, Turton JA, *et al*. Application of surface-enhanced laser desorption/ionization technology to the detection and identification of urinary parvalbumin-alpha: a biomarker of compound-induced skeletal muscle toxicity in the rat. *Electrophoresis* 2002;**23**:3241–51.

12. Nicholson JK, Connelly J, Lindon JC, Holmes E. Metabonomics: a platform for studying drug toxicity and gene function. *Nat Rev Drug Discov* 2002;**1**:153–61.

13. Connor SC, Wu W, Sweatman BC, *et al*. Effects of feeding and body weight loss on the 1H-NMR-based urine metabolic profiles of male Wistar Han rats: implications for biomarker discovery. *Biomarkers* 2004;**9**:156–79.

14. Tong W, Cao X, Harris S, *et al*. ArrayTrack – supporting toxicogenomic research at the US Food and Drug Administration National Centre for Toxicological Research. *Environ Health Perspect* 2003;**111**:1819–26.

15. Treinen KA, Louden C, Dennis M-J. Developmental toxicity and toxicokinetics of two endothelin receptor antagonists in rats and rabbits. *Teratology* 1999;**59**:51–9.

16. Scales MDC. An introduction to regulatory toxicology for human medicines. *BIRA Journal* 1990;**9**:17–21.

17. Guide to the UK GLP Regulations 1999. Department of Health, The United Kingdom: Good Laboratory Practice Monitoring Authority, 2000; London: MHRA Publications.

18. Ross JF, Mattson JL, Fix AS. Expanded clinical observations in toxicity studies: historical perspectives and contemporary issues. *Regul Toxicol Pharmacol* 1998;**28**:17–26.

19. Irwin S. Comprehensive observational assessment. *Psychopharmacologia (Berl.)* 1968;**13**:222–57.

20. Witchel HJ, Milnes JT, Mitcheson JS, Nancox JC. Troubleshooting problems with *in vitro* screening of drugs for QT interval prolongation using HERG K$^+$ channels expressed in mammalian cell lines and Xenopus oocytes. *J Pharmacol Toxicol Methods* 2002;**48**:65–80.

21. Scales MDC. Implications of recommendations from the International Conference on Harmonisation (ICH) for the safety evaluation of new medicines involving animal studies for the pharmaceutical industry. *Adverse Drug React Toxicol Rev* 1992;**11**:5–12.

22. US FDA Docket No. 92 N-0136 (15 August 1996). *Single Dose Acute Toxicity Testing for Pharmaceuticals. Revised Guidance.*

23. Munro A, Mehta D. Are single-dose toxicology studies in animals adequate to support single doses of new drug in humans? *Clin Pharmacol Ther* 1996;**59**:258–64.

24. Medicines Control Agency. *Medicines Act* 1968. *Guidance Notes on Applications for Clinical Trial Exemptions & Clinical Trial Certificates*. Revised December 1995. London: HMSO, 1995.

25. Spurling NW, Carey PF. Dose selection for toxicity studies: a protocol for determining the maximum repeatable dose. *Hum Exp Toxicol* 1992;**11**:449–58.

26. Scales MDC. Relevance of preclinical testing to risk assessment. *BIRA J* 1990;**9**:11–14.

27. *The Rules Governing Medicinal Products in the European Communities*. Vol. III. *Guidelines on the Quality, Safety and Efficacy of Medicinal Products for Human Use*. Brussels: Office for Official Publications of the European Communities, 1989.

28. US Food and Drug Administration. *Federal Register. Draft for Comment* (14 April 1992). Rockville, MD: FDA, 1992.

29. Pharmaceutical Manufacturers Association. *Guidelines for the Assessment of Drug and Medical Device Safety in Animals*. Washington: Pharmaceutical Manufacturers Association, 1977.

30. *1990 Guidelines for Toxicity Studies of Drugs Manual*. Tokyo: Yakuji Nippo, 1990.

31. *General Guidelines (Draft) for Clinical Evaluation of New Pharmaceuticals*. Tokyo: Pharmaceutical Affairs Bureau of the Ministry of Health & Welfare, 1988.

32. CPMP. *Recommendations for the Development of Non-clinical Testing Strategies, Draft No. 7*. Brussels: Commission of the European Communities, 1990.

33. Roe FJC. Food and cancer. *J Hum Nutr* 1979;**33**: 405–15.

34. Peraino C, Fry RDM, Staffeldt E. Enhancement of spontaneous hepatic tumourigenesis in C3H mice by dietary phenobarbital. *J Natl Cancer Inst* 1973;**51**:1349–50.

35. CPMP/SWP/2592/04 Rev1. Conclusions and recommendations on the use of genetically modified animal models for carcinogenicity assessment. 2004.

36. Macdonald J, Freanch JE, Gerson RJ, *et al.* The utility of genetically modified mouse assays for identifying human carcinogens: a basic understanding and path forward. *Toxicol Sci* 2004;**77**: 188–94.

37. Custer L, Gibson DP, Aardema MJ, Le Boeuf RA. A refined protocol for conducting the low pH 6.7 Syrian hamster embryo (SHE) cell transformation assay. *Mutat Res* 2000;**455**:129–39.

38. Farmer P. Committee on Mutagenicity of Chemicals in Food, Consumer Products and the Environment ILSI/HESI research programme on alternative cancer models: results of Syrian hamster embryo cell transformation assay. International Life Sciences Institute/Health and Environmental Science Institute. *Toxicol Pathol* 2002;**30**:536–8.

39. IARC Working Group. *Monograph on the Evaluation of the Carcinogenic Risk of Chemicals to Humans. Suppl 2. Long Term and Short Term Screening Assays for Carcinogens: A Critical Appraisal.* Lyons: International Agency for Research on Cancer, 1980.

40. Robens JF, Piegorsch WW, Schveler RL. Methods in testing for carcinogenicity. In: Wallace Hayes A, ed. *Principles and Methods of Toxicology.* New York: Raven Press, 1989;79–107.

41. D'Arcy PF, Harron DWG. *Proceedings of the Third International Conference on Harmonisation,* Yokohama 1995. Belfast: Queen's University, 1996.

42. Peto R, Pike M, Day N, *et al.* Guidelines for simple sensitive significance tests for carcinogenic effects in long-term animal experiments. *IARC Monogr* 1980;(Suppl 2):311–426.

43. CPMP. Reproduction studies (October 1983). (Included in reference 12: Vol. III p. 99.)

44. Sakai T, Takahashi M, Mitsumori K, *et al.* Collaborative work to evaluate toxicity on male reproductive organs by 2-week repeated dose toxicity studies in rats. Overview of the studies. *J Toxicol Sci* 2000;**25**:1–21.

45. WHO. Report and Recommendations of a WHO International Workshop. Impact of the environment on reproductive health. *Dan Med Bull* 1990;**38**:425–6.

46. Tweats D, Gatehouse D. Mutagenicity. In: Ballantyne B, Marrs T, Syversen T, eds. *General and Applied Toxicology.* Basingstoke: MacMillan, 1999; 1017–78.

47. Müller L, Kikuchi Y, Probst G, *et al.* ICH – harmonisation guidances on genotoxicity testing of pharmaceuticals: evolution, reasoning and impact. *Mutat Res* 1999;**436**:195–225.

48. Reddy MV, Randerath K. Nuclease P1-mediated enhancement of sensitivity of ^{32}P-postlabelling test for structurally diverse DNA adducts. *Carcinogenesis* 1986;**1**:1543–51.

49. McGregor D, Anderson D. DNA damage and repair in mammalian cells *in vitro* and *in vivo* as indicators of exposure to carcinogens. In: McGregor DB, Rice JM, Venitt S, eds. *The Use of Short and Medium-Term Tests for Carcinogens and Data on Genetic Effects in Carcinogenic Hazard Evaluation.* IARC Scientific Publication No. 146. Lyon: IARC, 1999; 309–54.

50. Thybaud V, Dean S, Nohmi T, *et al.* In vivo transgenic mutation assays. *Mutat Res* 2003;**540**: 141–51.

51. Kroes R, Renwick AG, Cheeseman M, *et al.* Structure-based thresholds of toxicological concern (TTC): guidance for application to substances present at low levels in the diet. *Food Chem Toxicol* 2004;**42**:65–83.

52. Kirkland DJ, ed. *Basic Mutagenicity Tests.* Cambridge: Cambridge University Press, 1990.

53. UK Committee on Mutagens guidance document: http://www.doh.gov.uk/com.htm

54. Müller L. The significance of positive results in genotoxicity testing. In: D'Arcy PF, Harron DWG, eds. *Proceedings of the Fourth International Conference on Harmonisation,* Brussels, 1997. Belfast: Queen's University, 1998;253–9.

55. Draize JH, Woodward G, Calvery HO. Methods for the study of irritation and toxicity of substances applied to the skin and mucous membranes. *J Pharmacol Exp Ther* 1944;**83**:337–90.

56. Liebsch M, Spielmann H. Currently available *in vitro* methods used in regulatory toxicology. *Toxicol Lett* 2002;**127**:127–34.

57. Curren RD, Harbell JW. Ocular safety: a silent (*in vitro*) success story. *Altern Lab Anim* 2002;**2** (Suppl.):69–74.

58. Magnussun B, Kligman AM. The identification of contact allergens by animal assay. The guinea pig maximisation test. *J Invest Dermatol* 1969;**52**: 268–76.

59. Buehler EV. Delayed contact hypersensitivity in the guinea pig. *Arch Dermatol* 1965;**91**:171–5.

60. Kimber I. Skin sensitisation: immunological mechanisms and novel approaches to predictive testing. In: Balls M, Van Zeller A-M, Halder M, eds. *Proceedings of the Third World Congress on Alternatives and*

Animal Use in the Life Sciences. Progress in the Reduction, Refinement and Replacement of Animal Experimentation. Amsterdam: Elsevier, 2000; 613–21.

61. Freireich EJ, Gehan EA, Rail DP, *et al.* Quantitative comparison of toxicity of anticancer agents in mouse, rat, hamster, dog, monkey and man. *Cancer Chemother Rep* 1966;**50**:219–43.

62. Anderson C. Cholera epidemic traced to risk miscalculation. *Nature* 1991;**354**:255.

63. Monro AM, MacDonald JS. Evaluation of the carcinogenic potential of pharmaceuticals. Opportunities arising from the International Conference on Harmonisation. *Drug Saf* 1998;**18**:309–19.

64. Tweats DJ. A review of the reduction and refinement of regulatory studies for pharmaceuticals. In: Balls M, Van Zeller A-M, Halder M, eds. *Proceedings of the Third World Congress on Alternatives and Animal Use in the Life Sciences. Progress in the Reduction, Refinement and Replacement of Animal Experimentation.* Amsterdam: Elsevier, 2000; 783–91.

65. Lumley CE, Van Canteren H. Harmonisation of international toxicity testing guidelines for pharmaceuticals. Contribution to refinement and reduction in animal uses. *Eur Biomed Res Assoc Bull* 1997;November:4–9.

66. Lappin G, Garner RC. Big physics, small doses: the use of AMS and PET in human microdosing of development drugs. *Nat Rev Drug Discov* 2003;**2**:233–40.

4

Exploratory development

John Posner

4.1 Introduction

The term exploratory development (ED) can be defined as 'the first part of clinical drug development in which tolerability, pharmacokinetics and pharmacodynamic activity are defined in man and in which an early indication of therapeutic efficacy is often obtained'. A new molecular entity (NME) can be defined as 'an unlicensed new chemical or biological entity with activity in biological systems whose therapeutic potential is under investigation'. The overall aim of ED should be to select appropriate NMEs for full development (FD), that is, commitment to licence application and to reject those that will not make useful medicines, as early as possible.

Exploratory development begins with the identification of critical questions about an NME. Starting with preparation for the first administration to humans, studies in ED should be designed to provide answers to these questions. A small number of clinical pharmacology studies that have been well designed and conducted should go a long way to describing the profile of the drug, in particular providing information on the 'critical success factors'.

The objectives of the studies comprising ED are summarised in Box 4.1.

From the outset of ED, we aim to learn about the human pharmacology of an NME. Every attempt should be made to establish, as soon as possible, the range of drug doses that produce the desired effect, and the relationships between dose, plasma concentration and the magnitude of desired and undesired effects. If successful,

---

Box 4.1 Objectives of studies in exploratory development.
- To identify the relationship between dose and plasma (or other) concentrations – pharmacokinetics
- To define the shape and location of the dose/concentration/response curves for both desired and undesired effects – preliminary assessment of benefit/risk
- On the basis of these curves, to identify the range of dosage and concentrations producing maximum benefit with fewest undesirable effects.

---

much time and resource can be saved later in development because it should be possible to enter clinical trials with the clinically effective dose range.[1,2] The ratio of doses producing a particular undesired effect to that of the desired effect can be determined to provide a preliminary assessment of the therapeutic index. It is inappropriate to consider the incidence of adverse events without reference to the dose of drug, plasma concentrations and their variability, and both magnitude and variability of desired effects.

The terms proof of principle and proof of concept are used more or less synonymously and pertain to the criteria that must be fulfilled in human studies before an NME can be considered to be a candidate for FD. These are particularly useful terms when applied to a drug thought to act by a novel mechanism of action. For example, a drug may be the first known inhibitor of a particular enzyme or receptor and the proof of principle will be a demonstration that such inhibition results in a desired pharmacodynamic or clinical endpoint. The terms are perhaps less appropriate when the mechanism of action of the drug class to which the drug belongs is well established. In such cases, the critical issues relating to the specific NME may be the pharmacokinetic profile or comparison of therapeutic index with that of a competitor marketed product. Demonstration of such properties may be critical success factors for the drug but cannot really be considered proof of principle or concept.

The desired profile of a drug is usually easy to define since it is generic, that is, good efficacy, high oral bioavailability, once-daily dosing, low incidence of adverse reactions in the therapeutic range, no serious adverse reactions, etc., but drugs only occasionally turn out to fulfil such promise. From the point of view of drug development, it is more demanding but of much greater value to define the minimum acceptable profile (MAP), concentrating particularly on the critical success factors. Then, by comparing the actual profile, as revealed by ED, with the MAP, decisions can be made about the future of a project, that is, whether it is worth taking from ED into FD. The intention is that the findings in ED will predict the benefit : risk ratio that will be established in FD. FD should thus provide confirmation of the findings of ED, hopefully with few surprises and a low risk of failure late in development.

It is insufficient to define the MAP simply in terms of 'the drug works and seems to be safe'. The acceptable benefit : risk ratio will depend greatly on the seriousness of the target disease and the availability of other treatments.

For an agent that works by a novel mechanism of action and could be the first in class for treatment of a life-threatening disease the MAP will be quite different from that of a 'me too' for a non-serious condition. For the former, demonstration of clinical benefit despite troublesome side effects might be acceptable, whereas for the latter, success might perhaps depend on demonstration of a single advantageous property of the compound over its competitors, such as greater oral bioavailability or a longer duration of action. In general terms, there are three possible outcomes of ED, as summarised in Table 4.1.

To summarise, while there is always considerable uncertainty in ED and no decision will be infallible, the risk of selecting the wrong compounds for development can be minimised by identifying critical success factors and an MAP that will provide the basis for go/no-go decisions.

The term Phase I refers to studies in healthy volunteers or patients to determine the safety and tolerability, pharmacodynamic effects and the pharmacokinetics of an NME. The term is often used to imply studies performed in healthy volunteers, but early evaluation of cytotoxics, many biologicals and other drugs is performed in patients. Conversely, healthy volunteer studies are often performed throughout the drug development process. For example, studies of drug interactions and pharmacokinetics of new formulations are frequently conducted at a late stage in drug development, while clinical pharmacology studies to support new indications

Table 4.1 Outcomes of exploratory development

Outcome	Likely decision
Meets minimum acceptable profile (MAP)	Progress the drug into full development
Does not have the desired effect and does not meet MAP	Terminate the project
Has desired effect but does not meet MAP	Bring forward back-up compounds. May be suitable to use as probe in man to evaluate basis for drug action or to develop methodology to be applied to back-up compounds

and other line extensions may be performed years after the first licence is granted. Phase II refers to studies in patients with the target disease to determine tolerability, pharmacokinetics, with, if possible, preliminary evidence of the dose–response relationship and efficacy.

Thus, Phase I and at least part of Phase II are encompassed by ED. These terms provide a useful shorthand but are ambiguous and do not capture the exploratory nature of early drug development. They also suggest that the process is linear, whereas in practice the phases of drug development are often not well demarcated and different activities run concurrently. For these reasons, I shall not use these terms in this chapter.

4.2   Planning ED

4.2.1   The need for a regulatory strategy

If the purpose of ED is to generate data on which to base decisions about future development, the strategy for future registration of the drug needs to be well defined. It may seem premature to be discussing regulatory matters before the drug has been administered to humans but the plan for ED may look quite different depending on the target profile. Even if the design of the first one or two studies might not be affected, the data these studies generate will certainly be critical in deciding whether to continue or stop development, or change direction. For example, a molecule that has been shown to have both anticonvulsant and antinociceptive activity in animal models might be developed as an antiepileptic, an analgesic or both. The plan for ED will look quite different for these indications, and the MAP of pharmacokinetics and tolerability will probably differ substantially. Similarly, a molecule that is active in animal models of diabetes and obesity might be developed for either indication, or both. Again, the ED plan of studies and desired or acceptable outcomes will depend on the chosen indication. The strategy may seem relatively straightforward for an antibiotic with a long half-life in animals that would, if translated to man, give it a clinically meaningful advantage

over the competitors. However, even this needs careful definition of the MAP in terms of pharmacokinetics, spectrum of bacterial sensitivity, target diseases, tolerability and safety profiles by different routes of administration. There also has to be a clear understanding of the likely development times needed to achieve registration for different indications by different routes of administration and the impact on the drug's market potential.

4.2.2   Devising the plan

When starting to devise the plan, it is useful to consider a series of questions, shown in Box 4.2.

The timeline should of course be as short as possible and it may be possible to conduct some studies in parallel or at least with a stagger rather than sequentially; however, this must not be at the expense of the safety of the study subjects. Often there is no choice but to wait for the results of one study before starting the next. On the other hand, predefining the core data required for decision making, and making arrangements for rapid quality control and database lock, can substantially reduce the delays between studies.

Box 4.2   Questions to ask when devising the exploratory development plan

- What is the company's strategic goal for this new molecular entity (NME)?
- With a clear understanding of this goal, what is the minimum acceptable profile?
- Which features of this profile are known to be critical to the future of this NME?
- What findings would result in us stopping development?
- What information will expedite and optimise design of clinical trials if the compound progresses to full development (FD)?
- What is the minimum number of studies required to address these issues?
- How long will it take to carry out the studies and reach a decision milestone?
- What is the most appropriate population for each study – healthy volunteers or patients?

The ED plan should lead to one or more decision milestones at which an agreed body of information will be provided in a defined time. The plan may consist of as few as one or two studies in healthy volunteers, which will deliver in 6–9 months, or it may involve a complex series of studies in healthy volunteers and patients, which might take 2 years. Whatever is appropriate, the information available at the decision milestones should enable the company to compare the actual profile with the previously agreed MAP. The company will then be in a position to make a well-founded decision on whether to continue development with a much reduced risk of failure or whether to stop and concentrate precious resources elsewhere.

The first study commonly involves single ascending doses and the second study might involve repeated administration but the specific study objectives must be tailored to the strategic goals and provide clear information that will define the profile. For example, if it is critical that the absorption of an antiarrhythmic drug is not affected by prior ingestion of food, the effect of food on the bioavailability of the drug should be an objective that can be easily evaluated in the first study in humans. Or, if an antimigraine drug must be effective in doses that are devoid of sedative activity, tests of sedation, as well as spontaneous adverse event reporting, should be included in the first and subsequent studies. And, to take one of the examples mentioned in Section 4.2.1, the patient population, objectives and endpoints of the first study in patients for a drug targeted at diabetes will be quite different from those for a drug targeted at obesity, even if some of the patients may have both conditions.

4.2.3 Presentation of the plan

The ED plan is perhaps best composed of two parts:
• a brief summary of the project presented under the headings suggested in Box 4.3.
• a more detailed document providing the essential justification, scientific data and commercial information required to support the project, shown in Box 4.4.

Box 4.3 Summary of the exploratory development project plan
• Therapeutic indication and rationale for development
• Mechanism of action
• minimal acceptable profile
• Critical features of the profile for go/no-go decisions
• Information that will be generated in ED for milestone decisions
• List of proposed studies, with a brief outline of each
• Formulations and pharmaceutical material requirements
• Timeline, with critical path to milestone decisions

Box 4.4 Documentation to support the project plan
• Medical rationale for development – medical need, therapeutic target, current therapies available and their deficiencies
• Scientific rationale – mechanism of action, novelty, selectivity, potency, etc.
• Chemistry and pharmacy – synthetic route, physicochemical properties including stereochemistry, proposed formulation and route(s) of administration
• Safety – secondary pharmacology, toxicology
• Pharmacokinetics and metabolism – absorption, distribution, metabolism and excretion (ADME), including potential for interactions, polymorphisms of drug metabolising enzymes and exposures in man predicted from interspecies allometric scaling
• Pharmacodynamics – predicted effective concentrations in humans
• Time to registration with decision milestones
• Discussion of critical features of the minimal acceptable profile for go/no-go decisions
• Patent status
• Commercial assessment – competition, present and potential future size of market

---

An overview of the project plan, with timeline and delineated critical path, may be conveniently presented as a Gantt chart. A decision tree is another visual aid which can serve to clarify the critical information required for each milestone decision.

Although the ED plan should be carefully thought out and well defined, it must be recognised that it is not written in tablets of stone. The very scientific nature of ED means that there will be new, often unexpected, findings. Results of one or two doses administered to humans may show that assumptions were wrong and that the plan must be changed accordingly. For example, if a drug or one of its major metabolites is found to have a much longer half-life than predicted by preclinical studies, this is likely to affect not only the design of present and future studies but also the acceptable tolerability and safety profile and perhaps the commercial potential of the drug either favourably or adversely. The plan may have to be revised to take into account these considerations. Planning is therefore essential, but execution of the plan needs to be flexible and the plan may have to be modified considerably, even if the overall goals remain unchanged.

4.3 Requirements for Administration of a NME to Humans

4.3.1 Evidence of primary pharmacodynamic activity

Pharmacodynamics can be defined as 'the action of a drug on molecular or cellular targets or on the whole organism'. The decision to proceed with preclinical development of a compound should only be made after thorough characterisation of its pharmacodynamics in terms of dose–concentration–response relationships *in vitro* and *in vivo* in animals. The commitment to take a compound into man should not be taken lightly since very considerable resources are required to meet the demands of the safe and ethical administration of a NME to humans. No pharmaceutical company can afford to waste precious resources on projects that have little chance of success. By contrast, the cost of thorough evaluation of the mode of action and pharmacodynamic effects of a substance in relation to its desired therapeutic target is small. This is the scientific basis for all rational drug development today and is the information required for the design of the

first human pharmacology studies. It does not, however, preclude the possibility of serendipitous discoveries, which have played such an important part in drug discovery in the past.

4.3.2 Secondary pharmacodynamic activity and safety pharmacology

Characterisation of the activity of primary interest must be accompanied by an equally thorough evaluation of the pharmacology of the compound at other receptors and in other systems. Secondary pharmacodynamic activity refers to the pharmacology of a substance not related to its desired therapeutic target.[3] Studies of secondary pharmacodynamic activity may reveal desired or undesired properties. For example, a substance may be found to have the desired effect at sites or in systems other than the one first considered. On the other hand, non-selectivity may imply that the doses producing the desired therapeutic effect are likely to be accompanied by adverse effects. In addition to this secondary pharmacodynamic activity, a package of so-called safety pharmacology studies should be completed. As well as *in vitro* and *ex vivo* testing, these studies will generally include parenteral administration of high single doses of the compound and any major active metabolites to rodent and non-rodent species. These studies are at least as important as the formal toxicity studies for the initial selection of dosage in man. A typical safety pharmacology package is shown in Box 4.5. Such a safety package is not appropriate for biotechnology products.[4] A much reduced package may also be required for substances to be applied topically, which do, however, require specific studies of local irritancy, phototoxicity and photosensitivity.

4.3.3 Pharmacokinetics and drug metabolism

The physical properties and pharmacokinetic profile, with data on absorption, distribution, metabolism and excretion (ADME) in animals, form an essential part of the drug selection process since the desired pharmacokinetic profile

Box 4.5 Typical safety pharmacology package
- Receptor ligand and ion channel binding, enzyme assays, etc.
- Respiratory function
- Cardiovascular system – *in vitro* systems for potential to prolong QT interval, effects on heart and blood vessels, anaesthetised and conscious (reflexes intact) animals with effects on heart rate, blood pressure, ECG
- Autonomic nervous system
- Central nervous system – behavioural activity, sensory/motor responses and body temperature
- Bowel transit
- Other studies related to mechanism of action or target patient population for clinical trials

should be defined *ab initio*.[5] For example, if it is decided that a potential new antihypertensive drug is to have a half-life in humans of at least 15 h to permit once-daily administration, there really is no point in developing a compound that has a maximum half-life of 45 min in larger mammals. A potential antiarrhythmic, which is likely to have a low therapeutic index, requires consistent bioavailability; therefore, a compound that undergoes extensive first-pass metabolism or is absorbed poorly and inconsistently in animals is unlikely to be worth developing as an oral therapy to be taken over long periods. The potential value of a NME that is metabolised primarily by an enzyme exhibiting polymorphism in the general population, such as CYP2D6, needs to be carefully considered. Potent enzyme induction is another serious disadvantage which should be tested for in animals, and inhibition of cloned cytochrome P450 isozymes should be tested as part of a routine screen, since drug interactions with concomitant medications may be critical to the value of a new therapy.

The pharmacokinetics of a drug in rodents, dogs and primates are certainly of some predictive value to humans, although there can often be surprises. If there is good agreement between species, it is likely that humans will handle the drug in a similar fashion. Conversely, if the major clearance mechanism, metabolic or

renal elimination of unchanged drug or metabolite profile differ greatly between species, it is far more difficult to predict the pharmacokinetics in humans. Reliable predictions about metabolic clearance in humans can often be made using cloned human metabolic enzymes, human hepatocytes, microsomes or, if available, whole-liver slices.

When a compound undergoes metabolism, the pharmacokinetics of major metabolites, particularly those that have pharmacological activity or are responsible for toxicities, should be examined. A long half-life of a metabolite may result in accumulation long after the concentration of the parent molecule has reached steady state. Much of the evaluation of the pharmacokinetics and the rates and routes of metabolism will be studied in animals using radiolabelled drug, but should be supported by 'cold' assays.

4.3.4 Toxicology

This topic is covered comprehensively in Chapter 3 and the discussion here will be confined to a few salient points.

Physicians and other clinical scientists responsible for ED are unlikely to be expert in toxicology but they must be familiar with the preclinical safety requirements for human studies in general[6] and with the detailed toxicology of the NME under consideration. *The final responsibility for the decision whether and how to conduct the first study in man lies with the physician.* Toxicity findings that give cause for concern should always be discussed with the toxicologist even if they are considered to be unrelated to the drug. Explanation may suffice but if reassurance is inadequate, additional studies may be needed or it might be necessary to limit exposure in man until further information becomes available.

It should be appreciated that the objective of the toxicologist is to identify target organ toxicity whereas that of the clinical pharmacologist is to minimise risk and avoid significant toxic effects. Thus, the clinical pharmacologist needs to know:

1. The organs in which toxicity was demonstrated and any abnormalities in laboratory tests.

2. The maximum no observed (non-toxic) effect dose level (NOEL).

3. The maximum no observed adverse (toxic) effect dose level (NOAEL).

4. The toxicokinetics, in particular the peak concentrations (C_{max}) and exposure (AUC) to parent drug and any major metabolites at the NOAEL and at toxic doses in the animal species tested.

This information may affect selection criteria for the study population and the choice of tests in addition to routine safety monitoring, and will certainly determine the starting dose, range of doses, maximum exposure and dose increments to be studied. Pharmacokinetics in man may be quite different from those in animal species so that plasma and, if possible, tissue concentrations are generally more important than dose. One exception to this may be hepatotoxicity resulting from exposure of the liver to portal blood drug concentrations, when the oral dose administered to the animals may be more relevant than the systemic plasma concentrations, which reflect first-pass metabolism as well as absorption.

Before administration of a NME to man, a mutagenicity test in bacterial cells (Ames test), with and without metabolic activation, and tests for chromosomal aberrations in mammalian cells should be negative.[7] Any positive or equivocal results will require additional tests to be performed before proceeding to man. Studies of embryo–foetal toxicity should be performed before administration of a NME to women of reproductive potential. Studies of fertility, early embryonic development and pre- and post-natal development are not required at this stage of development; neither are carcinogenicity studies.

An additional consideration is the safety assessment of agents that will be used for challenge stimuli in the evaluation of pharmacodynamics. In some cases, there is a long history of uneventful clinical use of tests, for example, bronchial challenge with histamine and methacholine. If used in a similar manner, there may be no need to consider performing safety studies in animals prior to their application in ED. On the other hand, the use of agents that are much less well established and that have an unproven safety record must raise the question of whether appropriate toxicology and pharmacological safety assessments should be performed in animals.

4.3.5 Drug substance and pharmaceutical formulations

The size and quality of the batch of bulk chemical or biological material that will be formulated for the first study in man are critical to the expeditious transfer from animals to man. Required details of the drug substance are shown in Box 4.6. Wherever possible, the same batch that has been used for toxicology should be used for the human

---

Box 4.6 Pharmaceutical requirements for administration to humans

Drug substance

- Chemical structure
- Physical properties: appearance, solubilities, pH, pKa, etc.
- Details of the synthetic route
- Manufacturing process and controls
- Elucidation of structure
- Batch analysis
- Analytical procedures
- Stability data

Formulation

- Description and composition
- Manufacturing process and controls
- Contol of excipients
- Analytical methods
- Proof of structure, purity, proportions of impurities, identity of major impurities
- Stability of formulated as well as raw material
- Certificate of analysis giving date of manufacture, batch number, weight of material and range, dissolution characteristics, appearance excipients expiry data and assurance of compliance with good manufacturing practice
- Compatibility of injections with intravenous fluids and with plastics

studies. This avoids difficulties in attributing toxicity findings to different impurities or different proportions of the same impurities that are frequently encountered in early batches. Although the batch size may be limited, the amount of material required for the initial human studies is generally small compared with that used for toxicology.

It is always difficult to provide the pharmacist with sufficient information to facilitate manufacture of an optimal formulation. The dose range of interest is not known, and careful consideration should be given to selection of unit doses that will provide the greatest flexibility. Good communication is essential and adequate lead time must be allowed. Compounds with poor absorption are difficult to formulate and may take considerable time and resources. Repeated *in vitro* and *in vivo* testing in animals may be required before a satisfactory formulation is found.

All formulations for administration to humans must be prepared in compliance with good manufacturing practice (GMP) and the certificates of analysis must be provided. The European Clinical Trials Directive[8] requires that details of the formulations be provided to, and approved by, regulatory authorities and a 'qualified person' at the investigator site(s). In principle, the Directive has been in force throughout the EU since May 2004 though it has been implemented at various times in different member states. The Directive applies to healthy volunteer as well as patient studies. The requirements for pharmaceutical products for administration to humans are summarised in Box 4.6.

The need for placebos generally from the first human study onwards typically involves manufacture of dummy capsules or tablets, and if oral solutions or suspensions are to be used, these must be matched as closely as possible for taste, colour and appearance.

Consideration must also be given to agents that are intended to be used for challenge stimuli. Some may be available commercially for use in humans, others may not and considerable work may have to be done to obtain raw material of sufficient purity and stability, followed by

development and manufacture of an appropriate formulation.

4.4   Preparation for the first administration to man

4.4.1   The transfer from preclinical to clinical

The establishment of good working relationships between the preclinical scientists (chemists, immunologists, pharmacologists, toxicologists, drug metabolism, etc.) and the clinical scientists responsible for ED is of enormous value. This is sometimes hard to achieve when the different groups are separated geographically or a molecule is licensed in from another company or academic institution. However, it should be recognised that at this stage, the preclinical scientists generally have far more knowledge about the compound and of the related science than do the clinical scientists, and their contribution to the ED plan can be extremely valuable. On the other hand, the clinical pharmacologist has an important role to play in assessing the preclinical data. Consideration of the ED plan may reveal that studies additional to those planned may be required. Review of the toxicity, safety pharmacology and metabolism data acquired to date may raise concerns and indicate that further work is necessary.

Close cooperation for a year or more before the first administration to humans is likely to lead to a smooth transfer of the compound and the rapid movement of a compound out of preclinical into man. This lead time can be used to devise the ED plan, design the first studies and, when appropriate, to select and develop methodologies that will contribute to the drug's evaluation in man. This may include validation of pharmacodynamic measures to be used in the clinical pharmacology unit, assessment of various imaging techniques, development of bioanalytical methods. Not infrequently, the assays that were perfectly adequate to support preclinical work are insufficiently sensitive, specific or accurate to quantify the comparatively low concentrations of parent drug and major metabolites in humans. At the very least, assays require validation in human plasma and urine.

4.4.2   Preparation of the clinical investigator's brochure (IB)

The rate-limiting step, which usually defines when a NME can be transferred to clinical, is the subacute (usually 4 week) toxicology. While reports of these studies are being written, preparation of the key documents required for the first study in humans can begin. Once the toxicology reports are available, and are supportive of proceeding to man, the documentation can be completed. In addition to the protocol (see Section 4.4.3), and information for volunteers, with consent form, the IB needs to be prepared. It is usual for each of the preclinical disciplines to contribute sections to this document, but the clinical scientists need to ensure that the document is appropriate for a largely clinical readership. The outline content and format of the IB is provided in a guideline of the International Conference on Harmonisation (ICH) published by the European Medicines Agency.[9]

It should always be remembered that the IB is not a promotional document aimed at presenting the NME in its best light; on the contrary, it is intended to inform investigators and ethics committees about every aspect of the drug, to enable them to make wise judgements in the interest of study subjects, be they healthy volunteers or patients. The IB is necessarily a summary, but less than full disclosure of important information about the drug, whatever the source, is not acceptable and all documents should be referenced and made available on request.

The first edition of this important document will, of course, contain no clinical information, but the next edition should be produced immediately after completion of the first study in humans, with a summary of the findings. The principal investigator must become fully familiar with the IB when the protocol is being developed and, once finalised, both editions of the IB should

be submitted to the relevant independent ethics committee (IEC).

4.4.3   Aspects of the first protocol and ethics review

A protocol for the first and other early studies with a NME in man is similar to those for later studies in healthy volunteers and patients but has some particular features that are worth special consideration. The protocol should be written to satisfy not only the needs of regulatory authorities and personnel who will be involved in conduct of the study but also to facilitate the work of the IEC, which bears considerable responsibility in such cases. The nature of the scientific material contained in the protocol is often complex, highly specialised and quite unlike most protocols for clinical trials handled by such committees.

The emphasis is essentially on safety rather than ethics, although, of course, a study that does not minimise risk is also unethical. As well as a summary of the preclinical information, some comment and interpretation about its significance should be provided. The choice of starting dose and increments for dose escalation should be justified. The number of subjects and amount of data that will form the basis for a decision to escalate should be clearly stated, as should the criteria for stopping the escalation.

The clinical procedures that will be undertaken and intended doses may need to be revised after review of the first results. The protocol should therefore be written with some flexibility so that, for example, within a defined dose range, adjustments of dose can be made. Similarly, while the minimum interval between doses should be explicit, there should be an option to increase the proposed interval if the half-life is longer than expected. There should be some flexibility in timing of blood samples and urine collections, which may need to be changed in light of pharmacokinetic and pharmacodynamic data generated during the study, although the maximum number of samples and total blood volume to be sampled should be unchanged. On the other hand, this flexibility which is necessary for the smooth conduct of a 'first in man' study must not be taken to imply that ill-defined or vague objectives and procedures are acceptable and the IEC cannot and should not be expected to give *carte blanche*. Therefore, the basis for decisions and alternatives should be detailed carefully.

When the IEC meets to review the protocol, it is advisable for a senior toxicologist and the principal investigator to be available to answer questions if required. Of course, members of the committee may have access to any other company documents, such as toxicology reports, if they desire. More detail about the design of such studies is provided in Section 4.7.

Pharmaceutical companies frequently establish a committee of senior management to authorise the first study of a NME in humans, the review and approval generally being a prerequisite for submission to the external IEC. However, as stated in Section 4.3.4, the clinician responsible for the first study in humans must be personally satisfied that the preclinical data, relating to efficacy and safety, justify administration to man. A useful test is for the physician and other responsible personnel to ask themselves: 'Would I be prepared to volunteer for this study and would I be happy for a loved-one to do so?'

4.4.4 Request for clinical trial authorisation

The application for a clinical trial authorisation (CTA) for the first administration of a NME to man comprises the same elements as all other CTAs but, of course, there will be no clinical data. The regulatory authority known as the competent authority (CA) of the EU member state requires receipt of confirmation of the EU clinical trials database (EUDRACT) number, a covering letter, a completed application form, the protocol with all current amendments, the IB and a full Investigational Medicinal Product Dossier (IMPD) (see below). If the study is to be conducted in more than one member state, a list of CAs should be included. If the opinion of the IEC is available, it should be provided.

The IMPD should summarise the quality, manufacture and control of the IMP including chemical (drug substance), pharmaceutical (drug product) and biological data, derived from tests carried out to current standards of GMP, and the non-clinical pharmacology, pharmacokinetics and toxicology conducted to the standards of good laboratory practice (GLP). Assessors and reviewers prefer data presented as tables with a brief discussion of the most important results and any conclusions. The application should draw attention to, and justify any deviations from, the standards described in available guidelines. There should be sufficient detail in the summaries and tables for assessors to reach their own conclusions about the potential toxicity of the IMP and the safety of its use in the proposed study. The IMPD should include a section in which the data are integrated to provide an assessment of overall risk. Potential hazards should be identified and the safety margins based on the pre-clinical information and estimated exposure in humans over the proposed dose-range should be presented with measures that will be taken to monitor safety. There is rarely any prospect of benefit in a first study in man, with the possible exception of anticancer agents.

The suggested headings and arrangement of the document may be found in The Rules Governing Medicinal Products in the European Union Volume 2, Notice to Applicants Volume 2B Presentation and Content of the Dossier, Common Technical Document which can be accessed at the Commission website www.pharmacos.eudra.org. Information is also available at the European Medicines Agency website www.emea.eu.int.

4.5 Studies in Healthy Volunteers

4.5.1 What is a healthy (non-patient) volunteer?

In the report of the Royal College of Physicians on studies in healthy volunteers,[10] a healthy volunteer is described as 'an individual who is not known to suffer any significant illness relevant to the proposed study, who should be within the ordinary range of body measurements such as weight, and whose mental state is such that he is able to understand and give valid consent to the study'. In the Association of the British Pharmaceutical Industry (ABPI) guidelines for medical experiments in non-patient human volunteers,[11] it is stressed that the individual cannot be expected to derive therapeutic benefit from the proposed study. While these descriptions are correct, I would suggest that words like 'relevant to the proposed study' are too ambiguous and the definition should state unequivocally that a healthy volunteer must indeed be in good health. Perhaps a more satisfactory definition of a healthy or 'non-patient' volunteer (the word 'human' is superfluous) is as follows: 'An individual who is in good general health, not having any mental or physical disorder requiring regular or frequent medication and who is able to give valid informed consent to participation in a study'. Thus, a healthy young man taking an antibiotic for acne does not qualify but a woman taking an oral contraceptive does (unless specifically excluded by the protocol). Similarly, a migraine or hayfever sufferer who takes daily prophylactic medication is excluded but one who takes medication only at the time of infrequent acute attacks is acceptable, in principle. Obviously, individuals will not be able to participate if suffering from an acute attack or if they have taken medication within a period defined in the protocol.

Even with this somewhat stricter definition, there is room for discretion. A sportsman who takes an occasional puff of a bronchodilator for exercise-induced asthma but is otherwise asymptomatic may be considered eligible by some. Individuals who have undergone surgery for a congenital condition and are in excellent health may or may not be suitable. Thus, an asymptomatic patient with a hip prosthesis who is taking no medication may be acceptable whereas an equally healthy individual with a prosthetic heart valve should be excluded from a study involving a cannula because of the risk, however remote, of endocarditis. Clearly, whatever definition of a healthy volunteer is used, sensible clinical judgement is still required.

The use of healthy volunteers has revealed findings that are generally thought to be pathological but in fact are not associated with any adverse prognosis. For example, short runs of non-sustained ventricular tachycardia were found in 2% of healthy individuals with normal hearts on 24 h ambulatory ECG monitoring.[12] Microscopic haematuria is also a common finding. Epileptiform activity on EEG is found in subjects with no history of epilepsy. In addition, laboratory values will frequently fall outside the 'normal' range for the laboratory simply on the grounds of probability because of the statistical criteria used to define the normal range.

Although not of direct relevance to screening, it should also be recognised that some of the procedures to which a volunteer may be subjected can affect test results. Perhaps, the most important example of such findings is the rise in transaminases that occurs in some subjects resident in a clinical pharmacology unit for a week or more, possibly because of dietary factors. The importance of a placebo group to help distinguish between effects resulting from active drug and procedural-related abnormalities cannot be over emphasised.

Healthy volunteers can be of either sex, although early studies are mostly confined to men because results of reproductive toxicity are generally not available at the time. Companies are not usually prepared to incur the cost of a reproductive toxicology package before there is some confidence that the compound is a reasonable candidate for development. In the absence of such data, medicolegal and ethical considerations relating to the risk of causing embryo/foetal damage have deterred companies from including women in the first studies in humans. Men are also frequently favoured for later studies because of concerns over the inability to detect very early pregnancy and the possibility that the menstrual cycle or oral contraceptives may affect drug metabolism. Concerns that the results from studies conducted mainly in men may not be representative of both sexes are rarely justified because, unlike in the rat, there are few important sex-related differences in drug metabolism in humans.

For legal reasons, the lower age limit for volunteers is generally 18 years. The first studies with a new candidate drug are usually conducted in young healthy volunteers with an upper age limit of 35–40 years. The lower age limit for the elderly is usually 65 years but when specifically addressing tolerability, pharmacokinetics and pharmacodynamics in the elderly, a representative population should certainly include many subjects in their seventies or older.[13]

4.5.2 Why use healthy volunteers?

The decision to use healthy volunteers, a particular patient population or a combination of the two should be based on ethical, safety, scientific and practical grounds.

Some drugs are too toxic or produce effects that would be unacceptable in healthy volunteers. These include cytotoxic agents, neuromuscular blocking drugs, anaesthetics and many biological response modifiers, such as monoclonal antibodies, growth factors and interleukins. On the other hand, physicians responsible for patient care are, rightly, conservative about exposing their patients to unknown risks. Thus, asthmatics, who have hyperreactive airways, are far more likely to develop serious impairment of respiratory function because of bronchoconstriction from an inhaled material, drug or vehicle than are healthy volunteers. An elderly patient with an acute stroke is far more susceptible to the sedative effects of a NME than is a young healthy subject. Furthermore, the appropriate dose range to be studied can frequently be established in healthy subjects using biomarkers (see Section 4.6.3) so that exposure of patients to excessively high (or low) doses can be avoided. Of course, this does not imply that less caution is required when dosing healthy volunteers; it simply implies that the risks may be considerably reduced in this population.

In addition to the greater risk in patients, results in patients are frequently confounded by the effects of disease, concomitant medication, age and other variables. By contrast, healthy subjects are much more homogeneous and subjects are studied under standardised conditions. It is sometimes argued that healthy volunteers are not representative of the patient population and therefore that the studies are of less relevance. This argument fails to take the study objectives into account; some questions about a drug are much more easily answered by deliberately excluding sources of variation.

In addition to the scientific benefit to be gained from studies in healthy volunteers, there are a number of practical advantages.

- Healthy volunteers can generally be recruited much more rapidly than patients.
- Healthy volunteers are generally willing and able to make themselves available on scheduled study days so that groups of subjects can be studied together, thereby expediting the study and enabling efficient use of staff and laboratories.
- Clinical pharmacology studies are frequently very intensive, with a tight schedule of complex measurements, often requiring training and a high degree of co-operation from subjects. Young healthy volunteers are more suited to this type of study than most patients.

In summary, studies in healthy volunteers are an integral part of the development of most drugs because they are capable of rapidly providing a large amount of data that are not confounded by other variables and that can thereby expedite the subsequent evaluation of the drug in patients.

4.5.3 Source of healthy volunteers

The majority of healthy volunteer studies are conducted by contract research organisations (CROs), which recruit subjects from the general public by advertising and word of mouth. The composition of the volunteer database depends to some extent on the location, some being comprised mainly of students or the local residential population, others, particularly in large cities, having a preponderance of backpackers and temporary workers. The source of volunteers does have implications for safety, motivation and withdrawal rates. The more itinerant volunteers may not be available for follow-up and little may be known about their medical background. While the 'professional volunteer' is wholly inappropriate, a stable population of volunteers who understand what is involved and are well motivated and who have long-term medical screening records is highly desirable.

A few large pharmaceutical companies, mainly in Europe, run their own clinical pharmacology facilities, sometimes using company employees as volunteers. Such individuals often make excellent study subjects, being highly motivated and well informed, with medical screening records going back over several years. However, in such circumstances, it is essential that adequate safeguards and procedures are in place to ensure that performance reviews, career progression and other employment issues are quite separate from volunteer activities.

4.5.4 Facilities and staff

The minimum standards for the facilities in which clinical pharmacology studies should be conducted are described in ABPI guidelines.[14] Clearly, the same standards should apply to all organisations involved in conducting studies. In the United Kingdom, the Medicines and Healthcare products Regulatory Agency (MHRA) has instituted inspection of facilities and procedures, and a system of certification is in place.

Provision of adequate competent medical staff is essential for the safe and ethical conduct of studies in humans. Decisions about whether a volunteer fulfils the entry criteria for a healthy subject or should be withdrawn from a study, how to respond to an unexpected adverse event and when to discontinue a study can prove challenging to the most experienced physician. Similarly, research nurses need many organisational and other skills over and above those that they acquired during their basic clinical training. Scientific staff must be competent in the techniques that will provide the essential data. All must be properly briefed about what will be required of them during the course of a study, and must be fully familiar with local standard operating procedures (SOPs) in compliance with good clinical practice (GCP).

Non-clinical as well as clinical staff involved in conducting studies in humans, should be trained in basic life support with regular updates, preferably every 6 months, and medical and nursing staff should also receive training in advanced life support. Training records should be kept for each member of staff and practice emergency call sessions should be run frequently. Staff development is a subject beyond the scope of this text but it is worth emphasising the value of offering training for clinical research nurses in the medical and scientific aspects of their work, as well as expecting them to learn on the job under supervision. Motivation and performance will be greatly enhanced by staff who understand something of the science behind the compound being tested and the medical as well as commercial rationale for its development.

4.5.5 Recruitment procedures

Procedures for recruitment of volunteers vary slightly between organisations conducting healthy volunteer studies, but the checklist of procedures provided in Box 4.7 is generic.

Box 4.7   Volunteer recruitment procedures
- Provide brief information about study to potential volunteers
- Arrange to meet potential volunteers
- At meeting, provide written and oral information
- Check volunteer's understanding, giving ample opportunity for questions
- Check volunteer's willingness and obtain witnessed written consent
- Medical screen
- Obtain volunteer's permission to write to his or her doctor
- Check that the volunteer fulfils all entry criteria; review screening tests

---

Detailed written information, which generally constitutes part of the consent form, should not be provided to potential volunteers until ethics approval has been obtained. A checklist of the items that should be covered in the volunteer information is given in Box 4.8. Most importantly, the information should be provided in clear non-technical language.[15]

A copy of the study schedule and an oral explanation should complement the written

---

Box 4.8   Information for volunteers
- The rationale and objectives of the study, with some background information
- Information about the drug in animals and man, including possible adverse effects
- Dosages to be employed, comparison with dosage in animals and previous exposure in man, route of administration
- If appropriate, information about comparator drugs that may be used, including possible adverse effects
- What will be required of the volunteer, for example, number of study days and nights, insertion of cannulae, urine collections, follow-up blood samples
- Possible adverse effects of procedures
- Restrictions of, for example, food, caffeine, alcohol, smoking, driving or operating machinery, contraception
- Requirements for medical screening, including urine tests for pregnancy and drugs of abuse
- Arrangements for transport
- The right to withdraw at any time without prejudice
- The right to obtain more information
- Confidentiality of records, with access limited to study personnel and auditors
- The right to no-fault compensation
- Approval of the protocol by an ethics committee
- The honorarium that will be paid
- How to contact the physician or nurse out of hours

---

pharmacodynamic responses, a separate consent form should be provided for this purpose. If it is intended that a DNA sample be stored for future analysis, consent should be requested and it should be made clear that all data will be held in a format that will make it impossible to link the data to an identifiable individual. Subjects should be free to refuse or withdraw consent independent of their consent to participation in the study. In the event of a withdrawal, any samples taken should be destroyed.

The size of the honorarium should reflect the amount of *inconvenience* that the study causes to the participant, and not the perceived risk. It is best decided by relatively disinterested parties, such as a medical director in consultation with a senior research nurse. The sum must be submitted for IEC approval with the protocol and is non-negotiable.

The chance of a mishap occurring in a volunteer study is increased when little or nothing is known about the subject. It should be a precondition of acceptance of a volunteer into a study that he or she is registered with a general practitioner (GP) and that permission is given to contact the GP to inform them of the study and to seek confirmation that their patient is suitable to participate.[16] The information that can be obtained is vital to ensure that the volunteer is in good health; therefore, every attempt should be made to contact GPs including those of volunteers living abroad. Although communication about a patient between physicians is always confidential, the GPs may recommend that their patient does not participate without giving a specific reason; there is no obligation to do so and their opinion should generally be respected.

Another concern is that a volunteer may fail to disclose that they have recently participated in another trial or may even be currently doing so. To deal with this problem, efforts have been made on a voluntary basis to establish national databases that can cross-check volunteer participation. Of course, the value of such databases is dependent on the number of CROs, academic units and pharmaceutical companies who participate. In the United Kingdom, a database called TOPS (The Overvolunteering Prevention

information. Volunteers should be given every opportunity to ask questions and to obtain additional information. They should be encouraged to contact the study physician about any symptoms, however trivial, that occur between study occasions, particularly if they wish to take medication, such as analgesics, decongestants or antihistamines. A cooling-off period of at least 24 h should be allowed after provision of information to allow the volunteer to consider and have the opportunity to discuss with their partner, family or friends. Therefore, it may be inappropriate for consent and medical screening to follow immediately after an information session.

If volunteers are required to give specimens for genotyping for drug metabolising enzymes or for proteins that might be involved in

System) has been established and has succeeded in detecting volunteers who have participated less than 3 months prior to volunteering or even concurrently.[17]

A list of procedures comprising a medical screen is given in Box 4.9. Particular studies may require additional procedures, such as lung function tests, coagulation studies, exercise or 24 h ECG or a psychiatric interview.

Box 4.9   Medical screens
- Medical history
- Physical examination
- ECG, with report on intervals as well as rhythm and morphology
- Full blood count and plasma biochemistry
- Immunology for hepatitis B and C and HIV
- Urinalysis
- Screen for drugs of abuse
- Pregnancy tests for women of reproductive potential
- Other tests as appropriate, for example, tests of coagulation, respiratory function, cognition

---

4.5.6   Good clinical practice

The requirements of GCP, as described in the ICH guidelines,[18] are presented in Chapter 7 and will not be discussed further here. However, it is emphasised that the standards required of large clinical trials in patients apply equally to small clinical pharmacological studies in healthy subjects. Studies should be conducted in accordance with SOPs. Many SOPs will resemble those pertaining to later phase clinical trials, but some will be specific to healthy volunteer studies. Details of procedures not covered by SOPs should be specified in the protocol. Studies must be monitored by the sponsor or a representative; the monitor should not be one of the investigators so that monitoring visits and assessments can maintain objectivity.

4.5.7   Adverse reactions in volunteer studies

There are no accurate data that provide a comprehensive picture of the extent of healthy volunteer studies and hence of the incidence of adverse reactions. However, surveys and clinical series have been published from time to time. In 1984, the ABPI requested information from its member companies on their activities in this area.[19] Of the 43 companies that responded, 28 conducted in-house studies and all but two commissioned external work. In the in-house studies, there were 18,671 subject exposures to drugs. There were no deaths or life-threatening suspected reactions. The incidence of serious suspected reactions that might have been attributable to drug was 0.27 per 1000 subject exposures. Of the 8733 subject exposures in external studies, there was one death on which the inquest reported an open verdict and no life-threatening suspected reactions. The incidence of suspected serious reactions was 0.91 per 1000 subject exposures.

In another survey conducted by the clinical section of the British Pharmacological Society over a 1-year period from 1986 to 1987, 8163 healthy volunteers received drugs for research purposes.[20] Potentially life-threatening adverse effects were reported in 0.04% and moderately severe adverse effects in 0.55%, with no lasting sequelae. The three severe reactions were skin irritation and rash requiring hospitalisation, anaphylactic shock after an oral vaccine, and perforation of a duodenal ulcer after multiple-dose non-steroidal anti-inflammatory drug; all made a complete recovery. The results were similar to those reported in the earlier ABPI survey and the authors concluded that the risk involved in these studies is very small and that most of the moderately severe reactions are of the predictable kind, generally being attributable to the known pharmacological activity of the drug.

In a much larger survey of 93,399 subjects participating in non-therapeutic research in the United States,[21] 37 subjects were reported to be temporarily disabled and one to be permanently disabled. The latter was due to a stroke occurring 3 days after investigation, and its attributability is unknown.

In a report of two 5-year periods in a single centre in France, the incidence of adverse events in 1015 healthy volunteers was 13.7% in subjects receiving active drug and 7.9% in those receiving placebo.[22] Headache, diarrhoea and dyspepsia occurred in more than 10 per 1000. Three per cent of adverse events were rated severe but there were no deaths or life-threatening events. Some events, such as vasovagal attacks, were related to procedures rather than treatment.

All these studies indicate that the incidence of serious adverse events in such studies is very low and is comparable with the normal hazards of everyday life. Nevertheless, it must always be remembered that the volunteer is placing his or her welfare in the trust of the research physician, who therefore bears an enormous responsibility.

4.5.8 Insurance and compensation

These topics are covered at some length in the Report of the Royal College of Physicians[10] and the ABPI guidelines.[11] Essentially, the company must undertake to pay compensation to any volunteer who has suffered bodily injury as the result of participating in a study, without proof of negligence or evidence that a test drug or procedure failed to fulfil a reasonable expectation of safety. This contractual agreement should be stated in the consent form that the volunteer signs. Ethics committees should ensure that arrangements for such 'no-fault' compensation are in place. Regarding personal insurance, companies will not normally exclude cover for accidents occurring as the result of research, but volunteers are advised to seek clarification on this from their insurers, particularly when taking out a new policy.

4.6 Study Objectives in ED

The first and subsequent studies of a NME in humans should aim to obtain dose–concentration–response relationships for desired and undesired effects. These objectives may be summarised as follows:

- To investigate over a range of doses
- tolerability and safety
- pharmacokinetics
- pharmacodynamic activity.

4.6.1 Tolerability and safety

The word "tolerability" is perhaps a little clumsy but it describes accurately what is assessed, namely how well the drug is tolerated by those to whom it is administered. This last qualification is necessary because there are many instances in which a drug is better tolerated or less well tolerated by young healthy volunteers than by patients. For example, anxiolytics and tricyclic antidepressants are usually far better tolerated by patients with depression than by healthy volunteers. However, healthy volunteer studies generally provide useful information about tolerability even if it may under- or overestimate tolerability in patients. Many adverse reactions will be directly related to the known pharmacological activity of the drug and are therefore predictable.

The investigation of tolerability must cover a number of doses thought to be in the range required for therapeutic benefit. The relevance of these data can only be interpreted when they are related to plasma concentrations and, when appropriate, measurements of pharmacodynamic activity. Adverse reactions occurring at 10 times the therapeutic dose may not pose a problem; conversely, the absence of adverse reactions at one-tenth the therapeutic dose is of little relevance and, if misinterpreted, may give unfounded confidence. This may seem obvious but has important implications for study design that are frequently ignored (see Section 4.7).

"Tolerability" should not be confused with the term "tolerance", which describes the diminution in effects of a drug on prolonged exposure. Tolerance may be due to increased clearance because of autoinduction of the enzymes that metabolise the drug, such as occurs with some antiepileptic drugs, for example, carbamazepine. Tolerance may also result from altered pharmacodynamics, which is common with drugs acting on the CNS.

"Tolerability" should also be distinguished from "safety". A drug that causes mild sedation may be safe except to individuals undertaking certain activities that are affected adversely by sedation, for example, driving a car. On the other hand, a drug may be tolerated well in the short to medium term but may cause elevation of liver transaminases, suggesting that it is hepatotoxic. Similarly, a drug may be tolerated extremely well by healthy volunteers and by the vast majority of patients but may cause prolongation of the QT interval on ECG, which poses a significant risk of cardiac arrhythmias in susceptible patients. A preliminary assessment of safety may be obtained in repeat-dose studies in exploratory studies in healthy volunteers and patients, but it should be recognised that the chances of detecting an uncommon serious adverse event are remote because of the relatively small number of subjects exposed.

4.6.2 Pharmacokinetics

The pharmacokinetic information that can be obtained from the first study in man is dependent on the route of administration. When a drug is given intravenously, its bioavailability is 100%, and clearance and volume of distribution can be obtained in addition to half-life. Over a range of doses it can be established whether the area under the plasma concentration–time curve (AUC) increases in proportion to the dose and hence whether the kinetic parameters are independent of dose (see Figure 4.1). When a drug is administered orally, the half-life can still be determined, but only the apparent volume of distribution and clearance can be calculated because bioavailability is unknown. However, if the maximum concentration (C_{max}) and AUC increase proportionately with dose, and the half-life is constant, it can usually be assumed that clearance is independent of dose. If, on the other hand, the AUC does not increase in proportion to the dose, this could be the result of a change in bioavailability, clearance or both.

In addition to the pharmacokinetics of the drug, the first study in man can provide important information about its metabolites. If assay methodology has been developed, metabolites in plasma can be detected and the AUCs and half-lives determined. Further information can be obtained from assaying urine for drug and, if possible, metabolites. Renal clearance can be calculated over time intervals and the ratio of

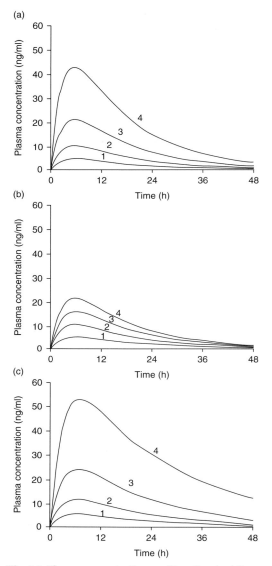

Fig. 4.1 Plasma concentration profiles after doubling doses showing (a) proportional increase with dose, (b) less than proportional increase with dose, (c) greater than proportional increase with dose.

renal to systemic clearance calculated so that the relative importance of renal and metabolic clearance can be assessed. The relative proportions of parent compound and identifiable metabolites will give an important, albeit incomplete, picture of how the drug is excreted in urine. The total amount of parent compound and metabolites measured in urine will give a minimum value for bioavailability of the drug. Early administration by both intravenous and oral routes can be extremely useful to ascertain the bioavailability and, if low, whether this is because of poor absorption or high first-pass metabolism.

It is a great mistake to think that the information obtained from such a study of pharmacokinetics is mainly the concern of pharmacokineticists. Pharmacokinetic data are essential for making rational decisions about the future development of a compound. At the simplest level, a half-life that is so short that the drug would have to be administered six times a day in order to maintain therapeutic benefit may be a good enough reason to discontinue development. A drug that has to be administered in very large doses to achieve adequate plasma concentrations, or fails to reach them at all because of poor or saturable absorption, is obviously unattractive. Large variability in bioavailability because of inconsistent absorption or extensive first-pass metabolism might constitute another reason for stopping development, particularly for a drug predicted to have a low therapeutic index. Saturation of clearance, mechanisms which, at the very least, will make dosing complicated, could result in unacceptable toxicity. The presence of a large number of metabolites may be undesirable, particularly if not all of them were detectable in the animal species used for toxicology so that additional toxicity studies might be required to support further work in humans. The presence of a major metabolite with pharmacological activity and a half-life much longer than the parent drug may be a useful way of extending the duration of action but its predicted accumulation on repeat dosing may pose a serious safety concern.

At the end of the first study in man, the pharmacokinetic profile should be compared with that desired for the compound. If reality compares unfavourably with the ideal, the unpleasant decision to discontinue development may have to be taken. Even if single-dose pharmacokinetics are acceptable, a further assessment will need to be made after repeat-dose administration of the drug since this may reveal plasma concentrations that do not match the predictions from single doses. For example, saturation of elimination resulting in higher than predicted steady-state concentrations, with associated toxicity, may make dosing too difficult for practical purposes. Conversely, autoinduction of metabolic enzymes, with resultant increased clearance, may occur, making it necessary to increase the dose over a period of weeks and also rendering the drug susceptible to interactions with other drugs and disease. Another consideration may be the accumulation of a metabolite that has a much longer half-life than that of the parent compound and which was perhaps undetectable after single doses. Some common reasons for stopping development on the basis of pharmacokinetic data are given in Box 4.10.

However, none of the reasons given for stopping development is applicable to all drugs. Thus, a short plasma half-life may be perfectly acceptable when the effect of the drug persists long after the drug has gone, for example, the effect of aspirin on platelet cyclooxygenase, or when only brief exposure is needed to obtain therapeutic benefit, for example, penicillin in pneumococcal pneumonia. Saturation of metabolism at high doses may be irrelevant if much lower doses are required for therapeutic benefit. Low bioavailability may not constitute a problem if the therapeutic index is high, for example,

---

Box 4.10 Some pharmacokinetic reasons for stopping development
- Half-life too short or too long
- Poor bioavailability
- Highly variable (often associated with poor) bioavailability with low therapeutic index
- Saturable clearance mechanisms producing non-linear kinetics
- Greatly increased clearance on repeat dosing because of autoinduction
- Multiple metabolites not covered by toxicity studies
- Active metabolite with half-life much longer than parent drug

propranolol or dosage can be readily adjusted to meet the needs of the individual patient, for example, oral morphine. The presence of multiple metabolites does not necessarily contraindicate proceeding; many useful lipophilic drugs undergo extensive metabolism. A persistent active metabolite may actually convert a drug that would have been unattractive into a very useful one; that, after all, is the principle of prodrugs. The point is that rational decisions can only be made if the information is actively sought and then matched against the desired profile.

Pharmacokinetics may also form the basis of a decision on the choice of compound from a series for development. It is not uncommon for a company to take three or four compounds of a series as far as the first study in man and to choose for development the compound that is most attractive from the pharmacokinetic point of view. Similarly, the development of achiral compounds rather than racemic mixtures is generally preferred and it may be necessary to establish whether stereoselective metabolism occurs in man and, if so, which enantiomer has the more desirable profile.

From the pharmacokinetics of single doses it is possible to simulate the expected accumulation and concentrations on reaching steady state that will occur on repeat dosing. However, it cannot be assumed that these predictions will hold, and repeat dosing studies in ED should generally include a comparison of pharmacokinetic profiles after the first dose and then at steady state, preferably after dosing for at least 10 days. An increase in clearance because of autoinduction will result in lower C_{max} and AUC and a shorter half-life than predicted. Conversely, saturation of metabolic enzymes at steady state may result in higher than predicted plasma drug concentrations. Accumulation of metabolites that were only present in low, perhaps undetectable, concentrations after single doses may be observed after repeat dosing.

4.6.3 Pharmacodynamics

The third major objective of ED studies in man is to evaluate pharmacodynamic effects that may

serve as biomarkers. A 'biomarker' is 'a characteristic that is objectively measured and evaluated as an indicator of a normal physiological process, pathogenic process or pharmacological response to a therapeutic intervention'. Such measures may be biomarkers of the desired effect of the drug (i.e. efficacy) or of undesired effects (i.e. toxicity). When a biomarker is not merely a measure of pharmacodynamic effect but is intended to substitute for a clinical endpoint, it may be called a 'surrogate endpoint'. The implication is that extensive study of the biomarker has generated sufficient confidence that linkage to a clinical endpoint has been established. A 'clinical endpoint' is defined as 'a characteristic or variable that measures how a patient feels, functions or survives'. When the validity of a surrogate endpoint is widely accepted, it may occasionally replace a clinical endpoint for registration purposes. Table 4.2 lists examples of established biomarkers that may be employed to assess the pharmacological properties of drugs in healthy volunteers.

As mentioned in the introduction to this chapter, decisions in ED will often depend on the dose–response curves for desired and undesired effects and hence, predictions about benefit : risk. It may be just as important to assess undesired as well as desired effects; such information can again be used as the basis for decisions on future development. For example, the decision to develop a new histamine H_1 antagonist, will depend on assessments of the dose–response curves for sedation and effect on the QT interval of the ECG, as well as demonstration of the dose–response for antagonism of weals and flares to intradermal histamine, or histamine bronchial challenge.

Imaging is used routinely to assess response to treatment in clinical practice and frequently contributes to efficacy end points in late-phase clinical trials. However, the contribution that ultrasound scanning, positron emission tomography (PET), single positron emission computed tomography (SPECT) and magnetic resonance imaging (MRI) can make to decision making early in clinical development is becoming increasingly recognised. For example,

Table 4.2 Examples of biomarkers of established utility in healthy volunteers

Activity	Biomarker	Drug class/activity
Enzyme activity	Serum ACE + renin, A-I, A-II	ACE inhibitor
ex vivo	Platelet MAO$_B$	Antiparkinsonian
	Neutrophil LO or urinary isoprostanes	Anti-inflammatory LO inhibitors
	Blood factor Xa	Anticoagulant
Physiological response without challenge	Psychomotor tests, for example, reaction time, tracking tasks, saccadic eye movements, body sway, EEG	Sedatives
	Tests of cognition	Cognitive enhancer
	Spirometry, flow–volume loops, plethysmography	Bronchodilators
	Vasodilatation by venous occlusion plethysmography, laser doppler	Vasodilators
	Acid secretion by gastric pH electrode	Gastric antisecretory drugs
	Gastrointestinal transit time by hydrogen breath test and radio-opaque markers	Gastrointestinal motility agents
Antagonism of response to challenge *in vivo* or *ex vivo*	Skin wheal and flare to i.d. histamine	H$_1$ antagonist
	Bronchoconstriction to inhaled histamine	
	Bronchoconstriction to inhaled leukotrienes	Leukotriene antagonist
	Late asthmatic response to inhaled antigen	Steroids, other anti-inflammatories
	Nasal airways resistance and cytology to inhaled antigen	Antiallergics
	Cytokine, stress hormone and vascular response to intravenous endotoxin	Immune modulators for shock and inflammation
	Vasoconstriction to angiotensin II	Angiotensin II antagonist
	Exercise-induced increase in heart rate	β blocker
	Blood pressure response to tyramine	MAO$_A$ inhibitor
	Ex vivo platelet aggregation	IIb/IIIa antagonists, NSAIDs
	Impairment of cognition to scopolamine	Cognitive enhancer
	Pain response to cold water	Opioid analgesic
	Gastric acid secretion to pentagastrin	H$_2$ antagonists, proton pump inhibitors
Immune response	Antibody response	Vaccine
	T cell responsiveness	Immunosuppressant

ACE, angiotensin-converting enzyme; A-I, A-II, angiotensin-I, II; H, histamine; LO, lipoxygenase; MAO, monoamine oxidase; NSAID, non-steroidal anti-inflammatory drug.

measurement of receptor occupancy using specific PET ligands to visualise cerebral receptors and enzymes (opioid, $5HT_{1A}$, $5HT_2$, dopamine D_2, muscarinic, nicotinic MAO_B) may prove a rapid and relatively simple means of selecting one or more doses for inclusion in clinical trials. This is likely to be of enormous value for trials of treatment of diseases in which group sizes can be extremely large, such as stroke and dementia.

Whenever possible, investigation of pharmacodynamics should be combined with pharmacokinetic measurements to establish the relationship between concentration and effect. Such relationships can be handled very simply or with modelling so that predictions can be made. This is discussed in Chapter 5.

The limitations of the use of biomarkers in healthy volunteers must be recognised. For example, although there have been attempts to simulate migraine headache in volunteers, to date none of these models can be considered adequate to serve as a surrogate endpoint. Patients with migraine are not difficult to recruit and are usually healthy apart from their migraine. In this case, it may be more appropriate to establish tolerability and pharmacokinetics in healthy volunteers and then to select a maximum well-tolerated dose with which to perform a small 'proof of principle' clinical trial in patients. This will need to be followed by larger trials to establish the dose–response relationship.

The value of biomarkers to establish the dose–response and concentration–response curves at the earliest stage of drug development cannot be overestimated. However, it should be recognised that the utility of any biomarker depends at least in part on the expertise of the experimentalists. Long before the study takes place a decision will need to be made about where the study will be placed and who precisely will perform the measurements. Whether assaying the concentrations of a hormone, performing respiratory function tests or measuring receptor occupancy with a PET ligand, adequate time must be allowed to assess the quality of data produced by a potential investigator or, if appropriate, whether to develop the technique in-house or in collaboration with an academic centre or CRO. Choice of an investigator must also take into account logistic concerns, such as availability of suitable subjects, capability of staff and access to particular equipment. All developmental methodology work must take place before its application to assessment of a NME so that results are sufficiently reliable as a basis for decisions about the NME.

Even if a technique is well established and the methodology has been used many times by the chosen investigator, it is usually worth including an active comparator in such studies. First and foremost, this acts as a verum – it is a concurrent control which verifies that the technique is capable of producing a positive result in that study, thereby avoiding the false negative conclusion. In addition, it will provide a measure with which the magnitude, duration and quality of responses obtained with the NME can be compared (i.e. a bioassay). The main exception to the use of an active comparator is the first study in humans in which formal statistical comparisons are rarely appropriate and the emphasis is on safety. Aspects of the design of the first study in humans will now be discussed.

4.7 Design of the First Study in Humans

The first study of a NME in man will inevitably involve an escalating-dose design, usually with single doses, although in oncology, repeat dosing is often more appropriate for ethical reasons. The choice of starting dose, increments, range and interval between occasions, number of subjects and use of placebo all need to be considered. Paramount is the safety of the subjects.

4.7.1 Choice of dose range

Factors that must be taken into account in selecting the dose range to be studied are listed in Box 4.11.

Knowledge of the concentration–response relationship and the nature of the pharmacodynamic responses and toxicity in animals are the

> **Box 4.11   Factors to be considered in selecting dose range for study in man.**
> - Maximum concentration (C_{max}) and exposure (AUC) in toxicity studies at NOAEL using the most sensitive species, based on the concentrations of drug unbound to plasma proteins (for which substantial corrections may be necessary if plasma protein binding in one or more species is above 95%)
> - The nature and severity of toxicity seen in animals – some findings are of more serious consequence than others
> - The range of doses and plasma concentrations that exhibited pharmacodynamic effects in animals, the nature of the effects, and the slope of the dose–response curve
> - The comparative disposition in different species and predicted exposure in humans, with particular attention to the presence of active metabolites with long half-lives
> - The range of doses and number of increments likely to be required in man

only sound basis for deciding on the starting dose and dosage increments to be used in man. This information needs to be interpreted and applied using common sense; application of formulae is not appropriate.

4.7.2   Magnitude of dose increments

It is quite usual to escalate the doses by doubling, which is consistent with the linear relationship between logarithm of the dose and response. However, if the slope of the dose–response curve is steep, doubling increments may be excessive, and for some drugs the relationship between dose (rather than log dose) and response is linear. Sometimes, it is preferred to start with a very low dose, examine the pharmacokinetics and then increase the dose four- to five-fold if appropriate. Once into the expected therapeutic range, increments should not generally be greater than doubling. Even when all this has been considered, the doses scheduled are only tentative and they may well need to be modified in the light of the first experience in man.

4.7.3   Should we dose to toxicity?

The choice of the top dose in a dose-escalating study may be difficult. The view is often expressed that dosing should continue to 'toxicity', that is, the dose should be escalated until intolerable adverse effects are experienced by one or more volunteers. Although an adequate definition is lacking, this suggests that the maximum tolerated dose (MTD) will be one increment below that toxic dose. There are certainly some drugs for which the therapeutic index is expected to be low and the putative therapeutic dose will be close to that which can just be tolerated. However, deliberate production of serious adverse events is never acceptable in healthy volunteers and usually unacceptable in patients, an exception in the latter case being haematological toxicity with cytotoxic chemotherapy. Therefore, for most ED studies of drugs with a low therapeutic index, it is of much greater relevance to determine a dose which produces some mild non-serious effects. The term minimum intolerated dose (MID)[23] has been applied to patients, and although the dose may be different, the term can equally be applied to healthy subjects. Examples of effects that determine the MID may be sedation, flushing, headache, loose stools or a small change in heart rate or blood pressure. Of no less importance is the dose below the MID, which may be defined as the maximum well-tolerated dose (MWTD). The MWTD is frequently used as the top dose in subsequent ED dose-range-finding studies in healthy volunteers and patients.

The 'dosing to toxicity' approach was adopted because investigators did not take the trouble to measure pharmacodynamic effects or even follow plasma drug concentrations during the course of a study. Many drugs have a reasonably high therapeutic index and for these it should be perfectly possible to stop the escalation at a predefined pharmacodynamic endpoint, such as maximum inhibition of a target enzyme. Similarly, the dose of an anti-infective agent devoid of pharmacological effects and with a high therapeutic index can usually be escalated to a particular plasma concentration that is greatly in excess of that predicted to be of therapeutic benefit from *in vitro* and perhaps *in vivo* animal studies.

4.7.4   Number of doses for individual subjects and interval between doses

It has been traditional in the United States to dose individual subjects just once, with a new cohort of subjects recruited for each dose level. In Europe first administration studies have more often involved dosing individuals at several if not all dose levels tested in a study.

If the number of dose increments expected is to be no greater than six, the study can often be conducted with a single group of volunteers, or with two groups dosed on alternate occasions. Such a design enables a set of pharmacokinetic as well as dynamic data to be obtained for each individual over a range of doses. Since intraindividual variation is generally much less than interindividual variation, it should be possible to make meaningful comparisons of pharmacokinetic parameters at each dose to establish whether the pharmacokinetics are independent of dose. With respect to pharmacodynamics, it is often possible to plot a dose–concentration–response for each individual.

An alternating group design is certainly preferred if the half-life of the drug or a metabolite is more than about 24 h. Thus, the first cohort might receive dose levels one, three and five (or placebo) and the second cohort dose levels two, four and six. This allows individual subjects to be dosed with a longer interval between doses, say 2 weeks, with dose escalation in the alternate cohort on the intervening weeks. However, drugs (or metabolites) with very long half-lives are best studied using a new cohort of volunteers for each dose.

Situations may arise when the dose range that has to be studied is very wide and the number of increments required to cover the range is large. It may then be advisable to use successive cohorts of volunteers so that the first cohort might receive dose levels 1–4, the second dose levels 4–7 and so on. Note that each cohort is introduced at the top dose level received by the preceding cohort, the overlap being necessary to avoid exposure of a naive subject to what might be a high dose.

Whichever design is preferred, the interval between dose escalations should be determined on grounds of safety, not convenience or availability of subjects. For drugs with half-lives of 2 or 3 h it may theoretically be possible to study the subjects two or three times in 1 week and thereby conclude the study quickly. However, analytical laboratories can rarely support such a short turnaround time and there is a limit to the time in which data can be collated and reviewed. Failure to obtain, scrutinise and evaluate all the data puts volunteers at unnecessary risk (see Section 4.8), as does inadequate time for follow-up safety assessments of subjects. For drugs or metabolites with long half-lives, clinical assessment and blood sampling for pharmacokinetics and clinical pathology may have to continue for many days or weeks before it is prudent to dose escalate, whether in the same or different individuals.

4.7.5   Use of placebo

In general, studies in ED should be placebo controlled, an exception being some pharmacokinetic studies, for example, bioavailability. In a dose-escalating design, it is obviously not possible to randomise or balance the order of doses, and there may be insufficient power to subject pharmacodynamic endpoints to statistical analysis; however, the advantages of a placebo group outweigh the disadvantages. It is not uncommon for a large number of trivial symptoms to be reported by volunteers and it may only be possible to interpret the significance of these when the incidence in the placebo and treated groups is compared. Substantial changes in vital signs, such as heart rate and blood pressure, occur in the course of a day, and a placebo is invaluable in distinguishing drug-induced effects from others. Similarly, it is not uncommon for some external factor such as an influenza epidemic, food poisoning, caffeine withdrawal or even a change in the weather to affect a study. Frequently, minor elevation of liver transaminases or lymphocytosis occur as the result of intercurrent viral infections. Liver transaminases also tend to rise with prolonged periods of incarceration in a study unit, probably because of diet, lack of exercise, or other lifestyle factors. A placebo group can be invaluable in deciding whether the problem is likely to be drug related.

4.7.6 Blinding

As far as possible, the study should be conducted under double-blind conditions. Sometimes, pharmacological effects, desired or undesired, tend to unblind the study but even in these circumstances the identity of treatment will be unknown to subjects and observers at the time of dosing and before onset of effects, thereby minimising bias. Specified personnel, such as the pharmacist, bioanalyst and pharmacokineticist, may need to know the treatment allocation code but this should not compromise the blinding of all other study personnel.

4.7.7 Parallel groups or crossover

If subjects are to receive more than one dose level of active drug, there are a number of ways in which subjects can be allocated to active drug (A) or placebo (P) but essentially they fall into two approaches.

1. Subjects are randomised to receive either A or P throughout the study, that is, parallel groups.
2. Subjects are randomised to receive A or P on different occasions in a crossover design.

Tables 4.3 and 4.4 show examples of parallel and crossover designs, with two alternating

Table 4.3 Parallel-study design with two alternating cohorts of eight subjects and a 6:2 randomisation to active drug (A) or placebo (P) – each subject receives either A on four occasions or P on four occasions

Subject	1	2	3	4	5	6	7	8	9	10	11	12	13	14	15	16
Dose 1	P	A	A	A	A	A	P	A								
Dose 2									A	P	A	P	A	A	A	A
Dose 3	P	A	A	A	A	A	P	A								
Dose 4									A	P	A	P	A	A	A	A
Dose 5	P	A	A	A	A	A	P	A								
Dose 6									A	P	A	P	A	A	A	A
Dose 7	P	A	A	A	A	A	P	A								
Dose 8									A	P	A	P	A	A	A	A

Table 4.4 Crossover study design with two alternating cohorts of eight subjects and a 6:2 restricted randomisation to active drug (A) or placebo (P) – each subject receives A on three occasions and P on one occasion

Subject	1	2	3	4	5	6	7	8	9	10	11	12	13	14	15	16
Dose 1	P	A	A	P	A	A	A	A								
Dose 2									A	P	A	A	A	A	P	A
Dose 3	A	P	A	A	A	P	A	A								
Dose 4									A	A	P	A	P	A	A	A
Dose 5	A	A	P	A	P	A	A	P								
Dose 6									P	A	A	A	A	P	A	A
Dose 7	A	A	A	A	A	A	P	A								
Dose 8									A	A	A	P	A	A	A	P

cohorts of eight subjects randomised to A or P in a dose-escalating design involving eight dose levels.

The advantages of a parallel-group design can be summarised as follows:

1. The design is simple and robust.
2. No doses are omitted so the full dose–response and linearity of pharmacokinetics can be established within individuals.

The disadvantages of a parallel-group design can be summarised as follows:

1. It can be very difficult to maintain the blind through the study because as soon as pharmacodynamic effects are observed both subjects and investigators will know whether an individual has been allocated to the active or placebo group for the remainder of the study.
2. Subjects cannot serve as their own placebo controls for intrasubject comparisons of pharmacodynamic effects, including adverse events.
3. Variability in intersubject data may obscure meaningful comparisons unless cohorts are large.
4. Only a proportion of subjects participating in the study receive active drug.

The advantages of a crossover design are as follows:

1. Maximum information is obtained from a comparatively small number of subjects.
2. Randomisation to A or P is different on every study day, therefore, it is comparatively easy to maintain the blind throughout the study.
3. Intrasubject variability in pharmacodynamics is generally much less than intersubject variability, allowing meaningful comparisons with placebo.

The disadvantage of a crossover design is as follows:

1. Individual subjects skip a dose level when they receive placebo so that no pharmacokinetic data are available for this subject/occasion and the subject is exposed to a large dose increment on the next occasion. This disadvantage can be avoided by administering every dose of A to each subject and in addition each subject receives placebo on one randomised occasion.

The problem with this modification is that after the first occasion, subjects are at different dose levels on any particular study day, making it difficult to obtain data from adequate numbers of subjects before dose escalation without using large cohorts.

4.7.8   Size of cohorts

The number of subjects per cohort needed for the initial study depends on several factors. If a well established pharmacodynamic measurement is to be used as an endpoint, it should be possible to calculate the number required to demonstrate significant differences from placebo by means of a power calculation based on variances in a previous study using this technique. However, analysis of the study is often limited to descriptive statistics such as mean and standard deviation, or even just recording the number of reports of a particular symptom, so that a formal power calculation is often inappropriate. There must be a balance between the minimum number on which it is reasonable to base decisions about dose escalation and the number of individuals it is reasonable to expose to a NME for the first time. To take the extremes, it is unwise to make decisions about tolerability and pharmacokinetics based on data from one or two subjects, although there are advocates of such a minimalist approach. Conversely, it is not justifiable to administer a single dose level to, say, 50 subjects at this early stage of ED. There is no simple answer to this, but in general the number lies between 6 and 20 subjects.

4.8   Minimising Risk

The principle governing all studies in humans is that of 'minimal risk', so that a healthy volunteer leaves a study in as good health as when he or she entered it. The Royal College of Physicians has stated that, 'A risk greater than minimal is not acceptable in a healthy volunteer study'.[8] A healthy volunteer stands to gain nothing directly from a new medication and the risk should therefore be negligible but it can never be reduced to zero. One must never be deluded into believing that a NME is going to be 'safe'. If all the toxicity studies are reassuring and the molecule belongs to a well-known class that has an exemplary safety record, the NME must still be treated with the greatest respect. Some of the ways in which risk can be minimised are mentioned below.

A comprehensive knowledge of all the preclinical information about a compound is an essential requirement for the safe conduct of the first study in man. Toxicology, metabolism, pharmacokinetics and pharmacodynamics are all important despite their limited predictive power for man. As explained above, the study design must take the findings into account.

The most carefully designed study and the most ethical protocol do not guarantee safety. A study that is not prepared and executed properly is likely to put volunteers at unnecessary risk. There must be sufficient staff to cover all practical aspects of the study. At least one nurse and a doctor should be present for dosing and for a specified period afterwards, usually at least a few hours. All staff should be thoroughly briefed by the investigator, the case report forms checked against the schedule, and every member of staff should know precisely what he or she will be doing during the course of a study day. The detailed schedule for each study day must also be optimal. For example, the design may require administration of intravenous infusions to six volunteers. It may be perfectly feasible to perform these on a single day but it is inadvisable to start all the infusions simultaneously. Drug-related adverse reactions would be likely to occur at the same time in all the subjects, which could be very difficult to manage and put subjects at unnecessary risk. Indeed, it may be wise to stop the study after the first significant adverse reaction has been seen and reconsider the dose, speed of administration or whether to proceed at all. For orally administered drugs with expected pharmacodynamic effects, it is wise to study two or three lead volunteers on 1 day before the remaining subjects receive the same dose on another day, or to keep the number of subjects studied at one time to no more than six, at least two of whom will receive placebo.

Interim reviews of the data are an essential requirement to minimise risk during dose-escalation studies. After each study day, or certainly after a predefined number of volunteers have received the next dose increment, the investigator, nurses, study physician and preferably one or two other experienced physicians who are not intimately involved with the study should meet to review the data. When the study is being conducted in a CRO, a sponsor company physician and a limited number of other personnel should participate by tele- or video-conference if not in person. A decision to stop, modify or continue dose escalation should be made jointly between the Principal Investigator at the CRO and the sponsor's physician. Such reviews should be conducted with maintenance of the double-blind and steps should be taken to avoid inadvertent unblinding, such as by coding of subject numbers. The data that should be reviewed are listed in Box 4.12.

It should be noted that pharmacokinetic data are included, which places a strain on the bioanalysts and laboratory facilities. However, with proper planning and adequate development time, preliminary but reasonably reliable data can usually be obtained within 2 or 3 days of receiving samples. Knowledge of maximum concentrations, dose proportionality of AUC and half-lives of the parent molecule and major metabolites greatly adds to making rational decisions about adverse events, times for sampling and measurements, the appropriate next dosage increment and the interval that should be allowed between study occasions.

Box 4.12   Interim safety review of data

- Overall progress: number of subjects, doses, etc.
- Adverse events: type, severity, duration, action taken, outcome, likelihood of attributability to study drug
- Pharmacodynamic measures
- Plasma concentrations, pharmacokinetics, any difficulties with assay methodology
- Laboratory data: blood and urine tests
- Procedures: any difficulties, compliance

Adverse events should be tabulated for easy inspection but the case report form should be available and all laboratory data such as blood counts, renal function and liver function tests should be inspected closely. The absence of obvious adverse events does not mean that all is well, and careful scrutiny of data by an experienced physician can often spot problems before they become troublesome. Not infrequently one or more volunteers become unwell during the course of a study, usually due to intercurrent viral infections, and decisions about postponement of study days and subject withdrawal follow-up can be made during these meetings. Data that are missing because of non-attendance of volunteers, for whatever reason, may lead to a delay in the study, with postponement of dose escalation until they have caught up.

The review requires that all the data be collated for presentation, which is a useful discipline. An opportunity is also provided for practical problems to be discussed and acted upon. All decisions should be documented and it is good practice for the sponsor to confirm the main outcome decision in writing to the CRO. Any significant modifications to the protocol will have to be put before the IEC before proceeding. The volunteers also need to be updated about any changes to the schedule and adverse events as the study unfolds. As always, a volunteer must be free to withdraw from a study at any stage.

The decision to halt a dose escalation is not always straightforward. There may have been adverse events that are not serious but that are disliked by the volunteers. While decisions about the future of a study must always be in the hands of the physicians; the investigator must listen carefully to the volunteers and nurses. When hitherto sensible and well-motivated volunteers begin to adopt a negative attitude to a study for whatever reason, it is usually time to stop.

4.9 Subsequent Studies in Healthy Volunteers

The limitations of the first study in man should be recognised. Even if the study has achieved all its objectives in terms of tolerability, pharmacokinetics and pharmacodynamics, the data will only be of a preliminary nature. It is then necessary to re-examine the provisional plan of exploratory studies and reconsider priorities and data, which require early verification in carefully designed, controlled studies. The design of subsequent studies cannot be discussed in detail here but the underlying principle is that the design must reflect the primary objectives, and these in turn are determined by the critical questions driving the ED plan. A few points about the design of commonly required studies are made in the next paragraphs.

4.9.1 Multiple doses

Frequently, information on tolerability and safety, and pharmacokinetics of multiple or repeat dosing for up to 14 days is the highest priority. A placebo-controlled, parallel-groups, dose-escalating design is generally appropriate, with each cohort receiving a single dose level or placebo for the defined duration. Typically, such a study would involve three or four dose levels, selected on the basis of results of the first study. If three dose levels were chosen to be studied, cohorts of 12 subjects might be randomised 9:3 A:P so that at the end of the study nine subjects will have received each dose level and nine will have received placebo. If biomarkers are to be employed to assess the relationships between dose, concentration and response, consideration should be given to use of a positive control as well. Plasma pharmacokinetic profiles should generally be obtained with the first dose and at the end of the dosing period with trough concentrations at selected times during the dosing period.

Many drugs active on the CNS will be subject to pharmacodynamic tolerance, that is, effects will diminish on repeat dosing despite maintenance of plasma concentrations. If development of tolerance is considered likely, consideration should be given to designing dose-escalation steps within each cohort with pharmacodynamic and pharmacodynamic assessments at some of these interim steps.

4.9.2 Pharmacodynamics

Study of single-dose pharmacodynamics of desired or adverse effects in healthy volunteers is best done using double-blind crossover designs, typically with three or four dose levels, placebo and active controls, randomised and balanced for order according to Latin squares. For studies in patients, multiple-limb crossover designs are less appropriate but crossover studies with single doses of A versus P are certainly feasible and, of course, parallel groups, single or repeat dosing are commonly employed designs.

4.9.3 Studies in the elderly

For a drug that will be used commonly in the elderly, it is important to obtain early information about tolerability and pharmacokinetics in this age group. Since glomerular filtration rate declines with age, exposure to drug is likely to be greatly increased in the elderly if the drug is eliminated primarily by the kidney. In the case of a high extraction drug, impairment of cardiac output in the elderly is likely to increase exposure because of reduced first-pass metabolism. Single- and multiple-dose studies in healthy elderly volunteers can provide extremely valuable information prior to exposure of patients in this age group, who are inevitably a vulnerable group and in whom many factors may confound results.

4.9.4 Drug and food interactions

If a drug is to be tested in patients who will inevitably be receiving other medications with which the NME is likely to interact, it may be important to design interaction studies in healthy volunteers early in ED. This is not merely a matter of whether dosage adjustment may be required. For example, the demonstrated ability of a NME to double the concentrations of a standard concomitant therapy due to inhibition of its metabolism may lead to a decision to stop development. The design of such studies will usually involve repeat dosing of one or both drugs to achieve steady-state concentrations. Potential interactions with drugs used commonly by the elderly, such as digoxin, antihypertensives and warfarin, need not be studied in the elderly but some of these studies may need to be done before exposing patients in clinical trials.[24]

A preliminary assessment of the effect of food on pharmacokinetics can generally be studied in a single-dose, two-arm, randomised, crossover design. Preliminary information can often be obtained by including a 'fed' occasion in the first, dose-escalating study. This will be insufficient for registration purposes, which require an adequately powered study performed with the final formulation, but the information should be sufficient to indicate whether there is need for restrictions on dosing relative to meals in repeat-dose studies in healthy volunteers and patient clinical trials.

4.9.5 Radiolabelled studies

Critical features of metabolism frequently require administration of radiolabelled material to man during ED. Such studies generally involve administration of single doses, with subsequent collection of excreta as well as blood sampling until virtually all drug has been eliminated. The clinical phase of such studies is generally not complex, but preparation for the study, with synthesis of the radioactive molecule and development of 'cold' assays of metabolites as well as parent molecule, may take many months. Such studies also require submission of applications with detailed dosage and radioactive exposure calculations for authorisation by external bodies such as the Administration of Radioactive Substances Advisory Committee (ARSAC) in the United Kingdom (www.advisorybodies.doh.gov.uk/ARSAC/).

4.10 Studies in Patients

The ED plan will enumerate which studies are to be performed in healthy volunteers and which in patients. As the first studies progress, the information generated needs to be constantly evaluated while still blinded, and, of course, on unblinding after database lock at the end of each study. The decision to proceed to the patient population should take into account how well the studies have actually achieved their objectives.

The first consideration, as always, will be safety; information that can be obtained more safely in healthy subjects, which may subsequently reduce risk to patients, should prompt a debate on whether it is wise to progress according to plan or whether an additional study should be performed in healthy subjects. Another option that may be considered is to proceed with the planned study in patients but to admit them to hospital or a clinical investigation unit for all or part of the dosing period. However, this might not be feasible because suitable facilities and staff are not available or because the anticipated rate of patient recruitment might be considered unacceptably slow.

Perhaps, the most frequent problem at this stage of ED is that the dose range of interest has not been adequately defined. If this can be achieved only in the target patient population there is no point in doing more studies in healthy subjects. If, on the other hand, an additional study using an established biomarker in healthy subjects would clarify the dose range of interest, thereby avoiding under- or overdosing and reducing the number of dose levels that need to be examined in the patient population, this option should be considered. While competition demands that drug development should proceed at a fast pace, companies frequently waste time in development because they fail to maximise the information they can obtain in ED. A delay of a few months to obtain critical data in ED may save a year or two of development time later on.

The use of biomarkers and surrogate endpoints in patients is well established in virtually all therapeutic areas. After all, blood pressure has been used as a surrogate for cardiovascular risk for many decades. Some other examples are given in Table 4.5.

An important qualification must be made. While a biomarker may be of proven value in establishing whether a drug has the desired effect in patients or healthy volunteers (see Section 4.6.3) and for evaluation of the dose–response relationship, a biomarker may not be a surrogate for the clinical endpoint.[25] Thus, suppression of testosterone after an initial rise will give an almost immediate endpoint for the effect of GnRH analogues in prostate cancer but the relationship breaks down later in the disease. Measures of blood glucose control are vital

Table 4.5 Examples of biomarkers of established utility in early drug evaluation in patients

Clinical endpoint	Biomarker	Drug class
Risk of cardiovascular events	LDL : HDL serum cholesterol	Statins
Complications of diabetes	FBG, HbA$_{1C}$, insulin sensitivity	Some oral antidiabetic agents
Relapse rate and disability in MS	Demyelination plaques on MRI scan	Various agents for MS
Frequency of epileptic fits	EEG photostimulation	Antiepileptics
Progression to AIDS	Serum viral mRNA	Anti-HIV drugs
Fracture rate in osteoporosis	Bone mineral density	Bisphosphonates, HRT, etc.
Progression of prostatic carcinoma	Serum PSA and testosterone	GnRH analogues

HDL, high-density lipoprotein; LDL, low-density lipoprotein; FBG, fasting blood glucose; HbA$_{1C}$, glycosylated haemoglobin A$_{1C}$; EEG, electroencephalography; HRT, hormone replacement therapy; PSA, prostate specific antigen; GnRH, gonadotrophin-releasing hormone.

for establishing dose–response in early studies of new oral agents for type 2 diabetes but they are not surrogates for the complications of the disease, despite the proven relationship between glycaemic control and complications. Furthermore, the benefit of some new, long-acting insulins appears to be the reduction in nocturnal hypoglycaemia with no effect on the traditional measures of glycaemia. Bone mineral density is inversely related to fracture rates in osteoporosis and is an end point for efficacy, but for regulatory purposes vertebral fracture rates constitute the primary outcome variable. An important exception is mRNA viral load in HIV-positive patients, which is accepted by regulatory authorities as a surrogate for a delay in progression to AIDS and survival.[26] Such a conservative approach may sometimes seem to place unnecessary demands on the pharmaceutical industry but there is precedent. Suppression of ventricular extrasystoles seemed at one time to be an obvious marker of efficacy of type Ic antiarrhythmic agents. The complete failure of this outcome to serve as a surrogate to predict the incidence of sudden death in patients with heart disease justifies the extremely cautious position of regulatory authorities in accepting surrogate endpoints for registration purposes.[27]

An interesting aspect of the use of biomarkers as surrogates is exemplified by the statins, which lower serum low-density lipoprotein cholesterol. It has recently been shown that their contribution to improved prognosis in patients with cardiovascular disease is not entirely due to lowering of cholesterol and may be related to anti-inflammatory activity. Thus, the apparently obvious surrogate turns out to be an inadequate biomarker for predicting outcome.

Of course, it is not always necessary to rely on biomarkers for rapid evaluation of dose–response relationships in ED. Thus, efficacy of new drugs is readily demonstrated in terms of the clinical endpoint for diseases, such as migraine, inflammatory pain, asthma, psoriasis, glaucoma and many others.

4.11 Outcomes of ED

As discussed in the introduction to this chapter, results of ED are intended to give a clear indication that the drug is a serious candidate for FD to product licence, or that it is not viable and development should be stopped forthwith. Sometimes it takes a little longer before the picture becomes clear but the aim should be to make a go/no-go decision at the earliest opportunity.

Overall, results of ED should impact on both the project itself and on the research programme from which additional compounds are actively being sought. Some common reasons for discontinuing a project and their possible impact on the research programme are shown in Table 4.6.

A more successful outcome of ED will usually commit the company to proceed with FD, usually on an international basis. If ED has achieved

---

Table 4.6 Discontinuation of a project and impact on basic research

Findings leading to project termination	Impact on research
Poor tolerability at effective concentrations	If due to specific compound, need back-up
	If a class effect, stop programme
Unsatisfactory pharmacokinetics or metabolism	May be possible to design a better molecule
Low potency	May be possible to design a more potent molecule
Low or absent efficacy	If principle disproved, stop programme

its objectives it should be possible to make use of the pharmacodynamic and pharmacokinetic information obtained to optimise the design of subsequent pivotal clinical trials. In particular, it should be possible to use dosage regimens that are rational and justifiable on scientific as well as commercial grounds. Active research programmes should proceed with the search for follow-up compounds.

References

1. The European Agency for the Evaluation of Medicinal Products. *ICH Tripartite Guideline. Dose–response Information to Support Drug Registration.* London: EMEA, 1994.
2. Schmidt R. Dose-finding studies in clinical drug development. *Eur J Clin Pharmacol* 1988;**34**:15–19.
3. The European Agency for the Evaluation of Medicinal Products. *ICH Topic S7 Safety Pharmacology Studies for Human Pharmaceuticals CPMP/ICH/539/00.* London: EMEA, 2000.
4. The European Agency for the Evaluation of Medicinal Products. *ICH Topic S6 Safety Studies for Biotechnological Products CPMP/ICH/302/95.* London: EMEA, 1995.
5. Center for Drug Evaluation and Research, US Food and Drug Administration. *Guidance for Industry, Drug Metabolism/Drug Interaction Studies in the Drug Development Process: Studies In Vitro.* Rockville, MD: FDA, 1997.
6. The European Agency for the Evaluation of Medicinal Products. *ICH Topic M3 Non-Clinical Safety Studies for the Conduct of Human Clinical Trials for Pharmaceuticals CPMP/ICH/286/95.* London: EMEA, 1995.
7. The European Agency for the Evaluation of Medicinal Products. *ICH Topic S2B Genotoxicity: A Standard Battery for Genotoxocity Testing of Pharmaceuticals CPMP/ICH/174/95.* London: EMEA, 1995.
8. Directive 2001/20/EC of the European Parliament and of the Council of 4 April 2001 on the approximation of the laws, regulations and administrative provisions of the member states relating to the implementation of good clinical practice in the conduct of clinical trials on medicinal products for human use. Eur-Lex. *Official Journal of the European Communities* 2001, L121 Vol. 44: 34–44. http://europa.eu.int/eur-lex/.
9. The European Agency for the Evaluation of Medicinal Products. *ICH Topic E6, 1996, Guideline for Good Clinical Practice Section 7.3 Content of the Investigator's Brochure.* London: EMEA, 1996.
10. Royal College of Physicians. Research on healthy volunteers. *J R Coll Physicians Lond* 1986;**20**:243–57.
11. The Association of the British Pharmaceutical Industry. *Guidelines for Medical Experiments in Non-patient Human Volunteers.* London: ABPI, 1988.
12. Stinson JC, Pears JS, Williams AJ, *et al.* Use of 24 h ambulatory ECG recordings in the assessment of new chemical entities in healthy volunteers. *Br J Clin Pharmacol* 1995;**39**:651–6.
13. Lacey JH, Mitchell-Heggs P, Montgomery D, *et al.* Guidelines for medical experiments on non-patient human volunteers over the age of 65 years. *J Pharm Med* 1991;**1**:281–8.
14. The Association of the British Pharmaceutical Industry. *Guidelines for the Facilities in Which Studies on Non-patient Volunteers are Conducted.* London: ABPI, 1989.
15. Jackson D, Richardson RG. Essential information to be given to volunteers and recorded in a protocol. *J Pharm Med* 1991;**2**:99–103.
16. Watson N, Wyld PJ. The importance of general practitioner information in selection of volunteers for clinical trials. *Br J Clin Pharmacol* 1992;**33**:197–9.
17. Boyce M, Nenthwich H, Melbourne W, *et al.* TOPS: the overvolunteering prevention system. *Br J Clin Pharmacol* 2003;**55**:418P–19P.
18. The European Agency for the Evaluation of Medicinal Products. *ICH Topic E6 Guideline for Good Clinical Practice CPMP/ICH/135/95.* London: EMEA, 1995.
19. Royle JM, Snell ES. Medical research on normal volunteers. *Br J Clin Pharmacol* 1986;**21**:548–9.
20. Orme M, Harry J, Routledge P, *et al.* Healthy volunteer studies in Great Britain: the results of a survey into 12 months activity in this field. *Br J Clin Pharmacol* 1989;**27**:125–33.
21. Carden PV, Dommel FW, Trumble RR. Subjects in non-therapeutic research. Survey of United States Department of Health, Education and Welfare. *N Engl J Med* 1976;**295**:650–4.
22. Sibille M, Deigat N, Janin A, *et al.* Adverse events in Phase I studies: a report in 1015 healthy volunteers. *Eur J Clin Pharmacol* 1998;**54**:13–20.
23. Cutler NR, Sramek J, Greenblatt DJ, *et al.* Defining the maximum tolerated dose: investigator, academic, industry and regulatory perspectives. *J Clin Pharmacol* 1997;**37**:767–83.

24. Committee for Proprietary Medicinal Products. *Note for Guidance on the Investigation of Drug Interactions EPMP/EWP/560/95*. London: CPMP, 1995.

25. Rolan P. The contribution of clinical pharmacology surrogates and models to drug development: a critical appraisal. *Br J Clin Pharmacol* 1997;**44**:219–25.

26. Deyton L. Importance of surrogate markers in evaluation of antiviral therapy for HIV infection. *JAMA* 1996;**276**:159–60.

27. Echt DS, Liebson PR, Mitchell B, *et al*. Mortality and morbidity of patients receiving encainide, flecainide or placebo: the Cardiac Arrhythmia Suppression Trial. *N Engl J Med* 1991;**324**:781–8.

5

Clinical pharmacokinetics

Paul Rolan and Valeria Molnar

5.1 Introduction

The term 'pharmacokinetics' refers to the time course of the passage of a drug and its metabolites through the body. It can be thought of as 'what the body does to the drug' in contrast to pharmacodynamics, which can be thought of as 'what the drug does to the body' (see Figure 5.1). The processes involved are absorption, distribution, metabolism and excretion and are defined in Box 5.1. Together, these processes play an important role in determining the duration and magnitude of both the desired and undesired pharmacodynamic effects of drugs.

It is not usually possible to measure the concentration of a drug at its sites of action. Plasma, which can be conveniently sampled, is generally used instead, but drug concentrations may be determined in other bodily fluids, such as saliva and cerebrospinal fluid, as well as, of course, the excreta, urine and faeces. There is often a relationship between plasma concentration and response, although this may sometimes be complex. Therefore, estimation of plasma concentrations, and how they are altered by the many factors that can affect drug handling, may be used to make predictions about dosage in the otherwise healthy individual and in the presence of organ failure or concomitant medications.

A growing appreciation of the predictive value of pharmacokinetics, together with a change in the attitude of regulatory authorities to the whole question of dosage, has led to increased importance of the clinical pharmacokinetics regulatory submission. It is no longer acceptable to register a dosage regimen based on a single empirically derived dose of proven efficacy and safety. Drug developers are now rightly required to demonstrate, wherever possible, that the optimum dose and frequency of dosing have been selected to give the greatest benefit for the least risk of adverse reactions. Regulatory authorities also require pharmacokinetic information to support

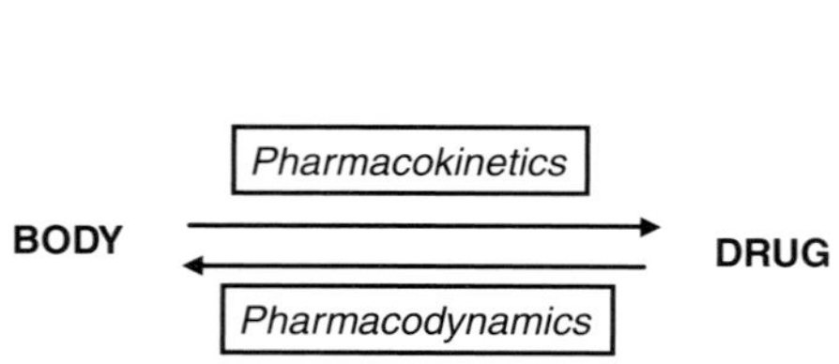

BODY ⇄ **DRUG**

Pharmacokinetics

Pharmacodynamics

- the study of the time course of a drug's passage through body fluids and tissues
- 'what the body does to the drug'

Fig. 5.1 Pharmacokinetics – definition.

Box 5.1   The pharmacokinetic processes

Absorption – the process of getting drug into the body (not necessarily the systemic circulation)

Distribution – the processes of distribution into fluids and tissues

Metabolism – the processes of changing the drug to another molecule

Excretion – the processes that remove drug from the body

Collectively these processes are referred to as ADME.

clinical data in order to make recommendations on how dosage should be modified for particular patient populations. The clinical significance of altered pharmacokinetics, and hence the requirement for dosage adjustment, will, to some extent, depend on the therapeutic index of the drug. Thus, while a clinical pharmacokinetics package forms a mandatory part of every regulatory submission for a systemically administered drug, a more comprehensive package will be generally required for drugs of low therapeutic index.

Although, like statistics, the details of pharmacokinetic analysis are best left to the experts, a pharmaceutical physician who is familiar with the basic concepts of how pharmacokinetic information contributes to a dossier will be able to interact more effectively with company colleagues and regulatory authority staff. It is the aim of this chapter to provide such a preliminary grounding.

5.2 Basic Concepts

The reader is referred to one of several texts giving detailed accounts of clinical pharmacokinetics.[1] However, an understanding of the basic concepts is essential in order to appreciate how pharmacokinetic data can provide insight into the physiological processes, which determine the time course of a drug in the body, and implications this has for the toxicity and therapeutic efficacy of drugs, particularly the new active substances in development.

5.2.1 Overview of the fate of administered drug

A drug can be administered directly into the vascular compartment or by an alternative route, such as orally. It can usually be assumed that the entire dose administered by the intravenous route reaches the systemic circulation. After oral administration, only a proportion may reach the systemic circulation because of incomplete *absorption* or because absorbed drug may be metabolised in the mucosa of the gastrointestinal tract or liver, a process known as *first-pass metabolism*. Once in the systemic circulation, the drug is transferred from the circulation to tissues and back again; this process is called *distribution*. Rates and extent of distribution to different tissues may depend on blood perfusion, diffusion, active transport and binding to plasma and tissue proteins. Also, once the drug is in the plasma, it can start to be removed, either by changing it to another molecule (*metabolism*) or by removal from the plasma in unchanged form (*excretion*) most frequently into urine, but sometimes bile or, more rarely, breath. Collectively, metabolism and excretion are known as *elimination*.

5.2.2 The plasma concentration–time curve

The effects of the processes listed above on the time course of the plasma concentration with time are as follows. Initially, as absorption starts, the plasma drug concentration rises. As soon as there is some drug in the plasma, distribution and elimination will start. Absorption will start to slow down as there is less drug to be absorbed. Eventually, the rate of drug going into the plasma from absorption will be equalled by the rate of drug leaving the plasma by distribution and elimination, so temporarily a plateau of maximum concentration is reached. Absorption continues to slow (as by now most of the drug has been absorbed) and the plasma concentration will continue to fall because of ongoing distribution and elimination. Often, elimination is slower than distribution resulting in an initial fast fall, mainly due to distribution and then a slower fall largely due to elimination.

Most physicians will be familiar with the basic shape of a plasma concentration–time curve following oral or intravenous administration, and they are likely to be familiar with, or at least readily understand, the simple terms that relate to this shape. Such terms – (1) maximum plasma concentration (C_{max}), (2) time to maximum plasma concentration (t_{max}), (3) area under the plasma concentration–time curve (AUC) and (4) half-life ($t_{1/2}$) – are illustrated in Figure 5.2.

(a)

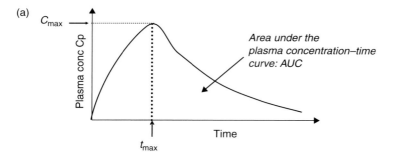

(b)

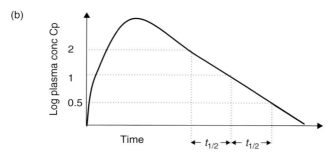

Fig. 5.2 Descriptive pharmacokinetic parameters: (a) plasma concentration–time plot and (b) semi-logarithmic plot.

5.2.3 Descriptive versus conceptual parameters

These simple descriptive terms can be used for any concentration–time profile, and do not require any conceptual understanding of how the drug is handled by the body. Although these terms are useful in designing a dosage regimen (as we shall see later), there is no way of understanding why two drugs dosed at the same nominal dose could have very differing values of C_{max} and half-life. To understand why the values are as they are, it is necessary to use a new set of parameters, which assist in the conceptual understanding of how the drug is handled by the body. The three most important parameters in this conceptual group – clearance (CL), bioavailability (F) and volume of distribution (V) (discussed in turn below) – are illustrated in Figure 5.3.

5.2.3.1 Clearance

Clearance is a measure of the body's ability to eliminate the drug substance from the plasma or blood by either metabolism or excretion. The main organs of clearance are the liver and the kidneys, although other organs can take part

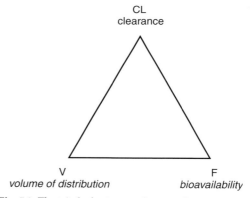

Fig. 5.3 The triad of primary pharmacokinetic parameters.

as well (gut, lung, peripheral tissues, etc.). Clearance is an important parameter because it is the property of a drug that determines the maintenance dosing rate needed to maintain a desired plasma concentration. Clearance can be defined in several ways, but the two most useful definitions are listed in Box 5.2.

When clearance is otherwise unspecified, the term 'clearance' is used to mean 'total plasma clearance', which is the sum of the individual

---

Box 5.2   Clearance – definitions and concepts
- Defined as 'rate of drug elimination divided by the plasma concentration'
- Equivalent to 'the volume of plasma completely cleared of drug per unit of time'
- Sum of metabolism and excretion
- Has units of flow (mL/min), which can be corrected for body weight (mL/min/kg)
- Total clearance is the sum of all organ clearances:

$$CL_{total} = CL_{renal} + CL_{hepatic} + CL \ldots$$

$$CL = Dose/AUC \text{ for intravenous drug}$$

$$CL = Bioavailable\ dose/AUC \text{ for all routes}$$

$$CL = F \times dose/AUC$$

- Note that there is *no* half-life term

---

organ clearances (hepatic clearance, renal clearance, etc.). Measuring or estimating individual organ clearances can be used to predict changes in drug handling under different physiological circumstances (as we shall see below). Given that one of the definitions of clearance is 'the volume of plasma completely cleared of drug in unit time', it can be readily seen that this is equal to the total plasma flow multiplied by the proportion of drug removed by the organ during the passage. This latter proportion defines the concept of 'extraction ratio' of an organ. If there is a high (>70%) extraction ratio across an organ, increasing the blood flow is likely to increase clearance. Conversely, when the extraction ratio is low (<30%), changes in blood flow are unlikely to change clearance because the eliminating capacity is not limited by the amount of drug being supplied.

5.2.3.1.1   Clearance units and range for values
As indicated in the definition, clearance has units of flow, for example, millilitres per minute or litres per hour; it can also be corrected for, say, body weight or body surface area. For drugs that undergo negligible renal elimination and are very stable metabolically, clearance values can be <1 mL/min. The maximum values for organ clearance approach total organ plasma or

blood flow. Hence, the maximum limit for hepatic clearance is about 1500 mL/min. Higher values for clearance would suggest that more than one organ is responsible for clearance or that the drug is metabolised in the plasma. For example, diamorphine has a systemic clearance of about 3000 mL/min because it is deacetylated in the plasma.

The kidney is a special case because, unlike with other organs, the amount of drug eliminated by that organ can be measured, in this case by measuring the amount of unchanged drug in urine. For all small molecules, the unbound drug in plasma is readily filtered at the glomerulus where the normal glomerular filtration rate (GFR) is about 120 mL/min. Hence, if the renal clearance of a drug is much higher than the GFR, then active tubular secretion must exist as a renal excretion pathway. This is important because, unlike filtration, which is a passive process, competition for tubular secretion, and hence the potential for clinically relevant drug interactions, can occur. Conversely, if the renal clearance is substantially lower than the filtered free drug clearance, then tubular reabsorption must be occurring. This raises the possibility of renal clearance being dependent on urinary flow rate or pH.

In addition to metabolism, the liver is also capable of secreting unchanged drug into the bile, sometimes against a high concentration gradient. This is also a form of hepatic clearance. An example of a drug that is almost exclusively eliminated by biliary secretion is the antimalarial drug atovaquone.

Whether a drug is eliminated largely unchanged in urine or primarily metabolised is a function of its physicochemical properties and its suitability as a substrate for metabolising enzymes. As a broad generalisation, hydrophilic (water-loving) drugs will be excreted in unchanged form in the urine while lipophilic (fat-loving) drugs will be primarily metabolised. The metabolites may subsequently be excreted via the kidneys.

For most drugs, clearance values for an individual subject are independent of dose. This would mean that, for example, when you double

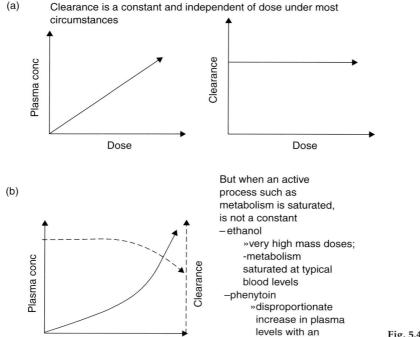

(a) Clearance is a constant and independent of dose under most circumstances

(b)

But when an active process such as metabolism is saturated, is not a constant
– ethanol
 »very high mass doses;
 -metabolism saturated at typical blood levels
–phenytoin
 »disproportionate increase in plasma levels with an increase in dose

Fig. 5.4 Clearance and dose-dependancy.

the dose, the plasma concentration is doubled (see Figure 5.4a). However, for some drugs, clearance may change with dose. This usually occurs when a drug is eliminated primarily by metabolism (and this is a saturable process) and the mass dose of the drug is high. For example, alcohol is a drug that is consumed in gram doses where the rate of metabolism is saturated after a small intake. A more clinically relevant example is phenytoin, where metabolism is saturated within the therapeutic dosage range (see Figure 5.4b). Terms used to describe this include 'non-linear kinetics', and this results in disproportionately high increases in plasma concentration when the dose is increased. Under such circumstances, clearance is concentration-dependent.

5.2.3.2 Bioavailability

Bioavailability is the other important conceptual pharmacokinetic parameter, in addition to clearance. The key concepts are summarised in Box 5.3. Bioavailability is defined as 'the proportion of an administered dose that reaches the systemic circulation'. It has no units and is

usually expressed as a percentage. Values range from 0% to 100%, and will be 100% or 'complete' for an intravenously administered drug. After oral administration, only a proportion of the drug may reach the systemic circulation because of incomplete absorption or because the absorbed drug may be metabolised in the gut wall or liver (first-pass metabolism). For orally administered drugs, bioavailability will be the product of the fraction of the dose absorbed into the body and the fraction of the dose that escapes gut and hepatic first-pass metabolism. For example, if a drug is 50% absorbed, but the absorbed dose undergoes 75% first-pass metabolism the bioavailability is $0.5 \times (1 - 0.75) = 12.5\%$. Examples of drugs with low bioavailability because of high first-pass metabolism include propranolol, verapamil and morphine.

As with clearance, the physicochemical properties of a drug can determine its absorption and hence affect bioavailability. Hydrophilic drugs may dissolve well in the gut lumen and hence cause few formulation problems, but cross cell membranes poorly and hence may be poorly

Box 5.3 Bioavailability definitions and concepts
- the proportion of an administered dose which reaches the *systemic circulation*
- no units – often expressed as %
- ranges between 0 and 100%
- is affected by
  - *absorption and*
  - *first-pass metabolism*
    - ≫ the proportion of an absorbed dose which escapes metabolism before it reaches the systemic circulation
    - ≫ therefore high (hepatic) clearance drugs will have low bioavailability
- usually calculated as AUC_{oral}/AUC_{iv}

absorbed, although there are some mechanisms of absorption of hydrophilic drugs between cells. In contrast, lipophilic drugs may dissolve poorly and hence cause formulation problems, but they may be well absorbed. These opposing constraints mean that very hydrophilic or very lipophilic drugs are often poorly bioavailable, and intermediate values are often sought by drug discovery to retain good bioavailability.

5.2.3.3   Volume of distribution
Volume of distribution is the third parameter to complete the triad of primary pharmacokinetic parameters. The key concepts are summarised in Box 5.4. Volume of distribution is defined as a proportionality constant relating the total amount of drug in the body to the plasma concentration. It is also sometimes described as the apparent 'volume' into which the drug distributes if all the drug in the body is at the same concentration as in plasma. Overall, the volume of distribution is a complicated concept and can be one of the most difficult to understand. It is also not a single parameter as the volumes of distribution can vary depending on when it is calculated following the dose. For example, it can be readily understood that shortly after an intravenous bolus, the volume of distribution may be quite small because the drug is still largely in the plasma compartment. However,

once steady state has been reached, the volume of distribution may be larger. In the terminal elimination phase, when tissues are loaded with drug and the plasma concentrations are being reduced by clearance, the volume can be even larger again.

It is rare for the volume of distribution to represent a real volume. The smallest possible distribution volumes will occur for drugs that are largely physically confined to the plasma compartment, for example, large, highly protein-bound drugs, such as some intravenous contrast agents. However, there is no upper limit to volume of distribution and it can be very much larger than body volume. Under such circumstances, one can conclude that the drug must be highly concentrated in at least one tissue. This may have important implications for therapeutic potential or for toxicity. For example, a lipophilic drug is likely to penetrate and be concentrated in the CNS, which may be desired or undesired.

The units of volume of distribution are those of volume (i.e. litres) and can be adjusted for, say, body weight. The two main uses of volume of distribution are in the calculation of loading doses for rapid onset of drug effect, and in understanding changes in half-life (see below).

5.2.3.4   Calculation of primary parameters
It is important to understand that the primary parameters clearance and volume of distribution can only be calculated following intravenous administration of the drug. This is because it is necessary to know the amount of drug that has reached the systemic circulation for these calculations. This is not known for a non-intravenous dose, unless one makes an estimate of bioavailability, for example, from urinary recovery of unchanged drug. Given the usefulness of knowing these primary parameters in being able to make physiological predictions about the drug, this is one reason why some regulatory authorities insist on having this information, which requires intravenous administration of the drug, even when there are no plans to administer the drug therapeutically intravenously.

Box 5.4   Volume of distribution – definition and concepts
- Defined as the amount of drug in the body divided by the plasma concentration
- Has units of volume (L) or can be corrected for body weight (L/kg)
- Minimum value is the plasma volume – large molecules that are confined to the plasma, and drugs that are highly protein-bound
- Maximum value is much larger than body volume:
  - Means that drug must be concentrated in tissue(s)
  - Means that drug probably crosses membranes
  - Drug is often lipophilic
- Usually calculated as terminal elimination slope × clearance
- Least useful of the three primary pharmacokinetic parameters

---

Box 5.5   Half-life – definition and concepts
- Time taken for plasma concentration to fall by 50%
- Determined by *both* volume of distribution *and* clearance
- $t_{1/2} = 0.7\ V/\text{CL}$
- Used in calculation of dosing regimens – the frequency of dosing is adjusted to keep the fluctuation of concentration between doses within acceptable limits
- Steady state is reached after 4–5 half-lives
- Time to reach 50% of steady state is one half-life ($t_{1/2}$)

Calculation of bioavailability requires a comparison of the AUcs following a non-intravenous and an intravenous dose, after correction for dose size. Without knowing the bioavailability, only 'apparent' clearance and volume of distribution can be calculated, and the ability to make predictions from these values is very limited.

5.2.3.5   Half-life

Physicians may be surprised to see that mention of half-life has been dealt with so late in this chapter, as it is likely to be the pharmacokinetic term most familiar to them. The key concepts are summarised in Box 5.5. As mentioned earlier, half-life is not only a primary pharmacokinetic parameter but is also one of the descriptive terms. Although many physicians will readily accept that changes in clearance will alter half-life, what is not quite so obvious is that half-life is equally determined by volume of distribution and in fact there is an equation relating these three terms:

$$t_{1/2} = 0.7\ V/\text{CL}$$

Thus, if we are comparing half-life values between two groups of patients, or in an individual before and after a potentially interacting drug, we cannot automatically assume that a prolonging of the half-life is the result of a reduction in clearance. This may be the case, but it is also possible that there are differences in the volume of distribution. Furthermore, if a drug has a long half-life it cannot be assumed to have a low clearance. For example, digoxin has a half-life of over a day but this is the result of a large volume of distribution because the drug is concentrated in tissues. In fact, its clearance is relatively high, and this is why measures to increase clearance (such as haemodialysis) are ineffective in removing a significant amount of drug from the body in cases of overdose, unless additional measures are taken to reduce volume of distribution, for example, digoxin antibodies.

The plasma elimination half-life can be determined from a semi-logarithmic plot of the plasma concentration–time plot (Figure 5.2b), following an intravenous dose, as the time taken for the plasma concentration to fall by 50%. The elimination half-life of some drugs is very short (seconds or minutes) whereas for others it may be very long (weeks).

The half-life determines the time it will take to achieve steady state and is useful for determining a dosing regimen. However, it does not give any clue to the processes involved in handling the drug, so that knowledge of the half-life alone cannot be used to make predictions about factors which are likely to affect the rate of elimination.

5.2.4 Predictions from pharmacokinetic parameters

Earlier we stressed the utility of being able to make predictions from knowledge of the primary pharmacokinetic parameters, and some examples have been given. A further example is as follows. Imagine we have undertaken a 'first-in-man' study where the drug has been given intravenously. Negligible amounts of unchanged drug were recovered in the urine, and the total plasma clearance was calculated to be 750 mL/min. Based on *in vitro* data, it is likely that the drug is metabolised. It is reasonable to assume that the total plasma clearance is likely to be largely due to hepatic clearance and hence we have a hepatic extraction ratio of about 50% (750/1500 mL/min). Already we can assume that the drug will have oral bioavailability no higher than 50% (because first-pass metabolism is likely to be about 50%) and that changes in hepatic blood flow and/or metabolising capacity will affect steady-state plasma concentrations. This is without having yet given an oral dose of the drug.

5.2.5 The use of pharmacokinetic information to design dosage regimens

An understanding of the pharmacokinetic properties of a drug is one of the major sources of information used in designing a dosing regimen.

1. The volume of distribution can be used to determine the size of the dose required to reach a desired target plasma concentration with the first dose, 'loading dose'.
2. Clearance will determine the maintenance dosing rate to maintain an average plasma concentration.
3. The half-life (i.e. both volume of distribution and clearance) will guide how the maintenance dosing rate should be divided in time to keep fluctuations in plasma concentration within acceptable limits.

However, there are other major factors in determining the dosing regimen, such as the nature of the concentration–response relationship for both efficacy and toxicity and commercial/compliance factors. There are additional reasons why caution should be applied in assuming an efficacy–time profile from a given plasma concentration–time profile. Some reasons why the time course of drug concentration and effect may differ are given in Table 5.1.

Furthermore, it should not be assumed that a constant plasma concentration is desirable. For example, aminoglycoside antibiotics are safer and more effective for systemic Gram-negative infection in immunocompetent individuals when given once daily rather than three times daily for the same total daily dose, despite a plasma half-life of less than 2 h. Secondly although traditionally pharmaceutical companies have tried to have the 'one-dose-for-all' approach for dose selection, this may be increasingly hard to maintain with the increasing amount of genetic and related information on an individual's capacity to handle and respond to a drug.

5.3 Bioavailability and Bioequivalence

Bioavailability and bioequivalence are related terms but they can be confused. Bioavailability as defined earlier is also known as *absolute bioavailability* and is simply the fraction of the administered dose that reaches the systemic circulation; it is therefore defined only in terms of the *extent* of drug absorption. However, in the Committee for Proprietary Medicinal Products (CPMP) guideline for the investigation of bioavailability and bioequivalence,[2] the former is defined as 'the rate and extent to which the active substance of therapeutic moiety is absorbed from a pharmaceutical form and becomes available at the site of action'. The reason that bioavailability has been defined in this way is because rate, as well as extent, is important when comparing the bioavailability of two pharmaceutical forms of an active substance to determine whether they are bioequivalent. Bioequivalence and comparative bioavailability are discussed later but absolute bioavailability will be described first.

Table 5.1 Factors that may cause the time courses of drug concentration and drug effect to differ

	Effect	Examples
Pharmacokinetic factors	Long time for tissue uptake	Plasma digoxin only correlates with effect >6 h after dose
	Drug trapped in tissues	Omeprazole, salmeterol: drug disappears from plasma but effect is long lasting
	Active metabolite(s)	Terfenadine: delay in onset of effect because it is mediated by a metabolite
Pharmacodynamic factors	Pharmacological tolerance	Benzodiazepines
	Threshold effects	Anticonvulsants
	Steepness of concentration–effect curve	LAAM – opioid for management of dependence – short duration of effect with high steepness
	The effect takes time to develop through a chain of effects, 'cascade effect'	Time course of onset of action of antidepressants and warfarin
	Irreversible effect	Selegiline (irreversible MAO_B inhibitor): short plasma half-life but effects last a week
Dosing factors	Drug concentration may be supramaximal due to high dose	Frusemide and penicillin, the effect is at its maximum throughout the dosing interval

5.3.1 Bioavailability

It would seem that when developing a drug that is intended purely for oral administration there would be no need to administer the drug intravenously. However, as mentioned above, the primary pharmacokinetic parameters cannot be determined without giving the drug intravenously. As drug regulators find these parameters helpful, they like to see this information.

It can be assumed that the bioavailability of an intravenous dose is 100% and a calculation of oral bioavailability can therefore be obtained by comparison of the AUCs after oral and intravenous administration, after correction for the exact dose:

$$F = \frac{\mathrm{AUC_{oral}}}{\mathrm{AUC_{iv}}} \times \frac{\mathrm{Dose_{iv}}}{\mathrm{Dose_{oral}}}$$

The AUCs can be obtained by administration of intravenous and oral formulations in a crossover study. It is important to use the exact dose rather

than nominal doses. The size of the intravenous dose should be reduced compared with the oral dose in proportion to the expected bioavailability so that the AUCs will be similar. This avoids assumptions about linear kinetics and maximises safety, since high plasma concentrations by the intravenous route are avoided. Similarly, it is appropriate to infuse the intravenous drug over a period comparable with the time to maximum concentration (t_{max}) after oral administration in order to avoid transient high peaks.

There may not be any intention to develop an intravenous formulation for therapeutic use but it will usually be necessary to produce one for the purposes of the study. For prodrugs (i.e. where the main pharmacological activity comes from a metabolite), the appropriate intravenous comparator is the active metabolite. There are, however, some drugs that cannot be administered by the intravenous route, either because it would not be safe or because it is not technically feasible to develop a suitable formulation. If there is a very high recovery of unchanged drug in urine, it may be possible to obtain a reasonable estimate of absolute bioavailability from oral administration. However, metabolites in urine cannot be assumed to derive from a drug that was bioavailable since they may have been formed in the gut by the action of intestinal bacteria, for example, and subsequently absorbed and excreted in urine. An alternative to intravenous administration is a reference oral solution; if this is not feasible, an oral suspension of standardised fine particle size may be the best option. Clearly these do not enable calculation of absolute bioavailability but might indicate whether the test formulation has less than optimal bioavailability. For a drug that exhibits high intraindividual as well as interindividual variability of clearance, or which has time-dependent kinetics, it may be useful to give the intravenous and oral formulations simultaneously. Drug administered by one route will need to be labelled with either a radioactive or stable isotope so that drugs administered by the two routes can be distinguished.

5.3.2 Bioequivalence

Two medicinal products containing the same active ingredients are therapeutically interchangeable if they produce the same clinical effect. However, assessment of clinical response would require a clinical trial for every new formulation, which is simply not feasible or justifiable. It is reasonable to assume that the effects of drug molecules, once they have reached the systemic circulation, should be independent of the formulation from which they came. Therefore, two products containing the same active ingredient can be regarded as bioequivalent if they produce the same plasma concentration–time profiles. This enables manufacturers to market a new formulation of a licensed product on the basis of bioequivalence rather than a full clinical package. Similarly, a generic formulation can be licensed with the only clinical study being a bioequivalence study. It should be recognised

that pharmacokinetic bioequivalence may not be a perfect surrogate for therapeutic equivalence since adverse reactions may differ because of biological effects of excipients. Furthermore, equivalent plasma concentrations may not imply indistinguishable clinical effects in the case of topical agents acting locally on the skin, lung, eye or within the gut lumen.

In contrast to the measurement of absolute bioavailability, for which only the extent of absorption is important, establishment of bioequivalence requires demonstration that the rates of absorption are also indistinguishable. This can be clinically important; for example, a capsule formulation of phenytoin produced higher and earlier peak plasma concentrations, which were associated with a higher incidence of adverse reactions although the extent of absorption was similar to the standard formulation.[3] Fortunately, a comparison of plasma AUCs is universally accepted as a valid means of comparing the extent of absorption, although there is little agreement as to the best measure of the rate. Since peak concentration (C_{max}) is obviously of great importance for many drugs, it is generally taken as the second important kinetic parameter for tests of comparative bioavailability or bioequivalence. Nevertheless, as mentioned earlier, as C_{max} occurs at a time after drug administration (t_{max}) when the rate of entry of drug into the plasma equals the rate of its removal, t_{max} is determined by the rate of distribution and elimination as well as the rate of absorption. t_{max} is also dependent on discrete sample times, in contrast to a continuous variable like concentration, and it, therefore, has less statistical power to reflect a real change in absorption rate.

Testing of bioequivalence is an area where drug regulatory authorities have produced extremely detailed and specific guidelines, not only on the design and conduct of the study but also on statistical analysis, sample analysis and drug sample retention. One reason for this is that manufacturers of generic medicines can obtain registration of a generic version of a drug of proven clinical safety and efficacy on the basis of a single bioequivalence study, without the need to perform clinical trials of safety or efficacy. Commercial pressures are clearly great and there have been a number of examples of misconduct, and a scandal involving gross fraud. The result is that the guidelines are extremely strict, and for products of high therapeutic index and excellent safety records, they seem excessive. However, there is little room for flexibility, and adherence to the guidelines is strongly recommended. Recently, the Food and Drug Administration (FDA) has proposed a classification of drug bioavailability which stratifies the need for a human study, depending on the physicochemical characteristics of the compound and its bioavailability. This has reduced the need for bioequivalence studies of minor changes in the formulation of well-absorbed drugs with the granting of a 'biowaiver'.[4] A reasonable approach to the problem is suggested as a series of questions, provided in Table 5.2.

Protein drugs also represent a special case. Unlike small molecules, two protein drugs with the same chemical formula (i.e. amino acid sequence) might have subtle changes in folding or in the sites of glycosylation which might affect function. Hence regulatory authorities do not, in general, accept pharmacokinetic bioequivalence to license 'generic' biopharmaceuticals. For such products, the concept of 'essential similarity' is proposed, which includes some relevant measure of drug effect, in addition to pharmacokinetics as well as extensive product characterisation. For example, there may be a complex relation with excipients which are not thought to be therapeutically active. An excellent review of this subject has been published.[5] Hence, in this complex area, expert advice will be required when reformulating a protein drug, and ideally the formulation should be optimised before the first human study so that all development continues with the one formulation.

In all this, it should be remembered that the role of regulatory authorities is to protect the public. For entirely justifiable reasons, they will apply very strict criteria to products with a low therapeutic index, non-linear kinetics or unfavourable physical properties. Digoxin, phenytoin and primidone provide notable examples of drugs where bioinequivalence issues have led to clinical problems.

5.4   Drug Interactions

5.4.1   Selection of studies

It is reasonable that data should be required to demonstrate whether the response of patients to a new active substance is likely to change or be changed by concomitant medication. However, there is clearly a huge number of potential drug combinations, and some rational selection is required. To assist with the selection of drug combinations for which data are required, the following seven questions at least should be asked.

What are the ADME characteristics of the drug? For drugs that are metabolised, there are a number of enzyme inhibitors and inducers which may potentially affect the same pathway. Selection of a drug interactions study at the level of hepatic metabolism is becoming much more rational

Table 5.2 Factors to be considered when deciding whether a new formulation requires a study to establish bioequivalence

Factors to be considered	Suggests study is required
Difference from reference	Substantial
Bioavailability	Low
Therapeutic index	Low
Kinetics	Non-linear
Dispersal/dissolution properties	Poor
Relationship to another drug	Other drug has known poor bioavailability or bioequivalence problems
Likely attitude of a regulatory authority in a commercially important territory	Authority has shown little flexibility in the past
Importance of drug to your portfolio	Commercially important drug

with the identification of a variety of isozymes of hepatic cytochrome P450 and the association of specific drug metabolising processors with each isozyme (see Section 5.4.3). Similarly, a drug that is mainly excreted in the urine, with a renal clearance much greater than GFR, is likely to be actively secreted by the renal tubule. If the drug is an organic acid, probenecid is likely to reduce its elimination; if it is basic, its renal clearance may be reduced by cimetidine.

Does the drug belong to a class of compounds known to interact with many other drugs? For example, drugs containing an imidazole ring, such as cimetidine and many antifungal agents, inhibit many reactions mediated by cytochrome P450. Therefore, a new compound of this chemical class is likely to behave similarly, and evaluation of its potential interactions will be required.

What is the therapeutic index of the drug? If the drug has a low therapeutic index, interactions are much more likely to have clinical consequences, so a variety of kinetic studies will be needed.

Is the drug likely to be co-prescribed with a drug of narrow therapeutic index? For example, a drug for angina, cardiac failure or an antiarrhythmic agent is likely to be co-prescribed with warfarin. If there is any evidence of enzyme induction or inhibition, a clinical study with warfarin may be required.

What are the chances of the drug being co-prescribed with a wide range of medicines? A drug that is to be given to young adults in single doses (e.g. for migraine) is far less likely to cause many clinically significant interactions than one that is intended for long-term administration, particularly in an elderly population that often receives several concomitant medications.

Pharmacodynamics. Although this chapter concentrates on clinical pharmacokinetics, it would be wrong to omit mention of pharmacodynamic interactions in a section on drug interactions. It is difficult to generalise, but drugs with marked pharmacological effects, particularly on the cardiovascular system and CNS are potentially subject to clinically important pharmacodynamic interactions.

Does the drug share a common mechanism of absorption or disposition with another likely co-prescribed drug? Two drugs that are intended to be co-administered might compete for active absorption or a common route of elimination.

5.4.2   Study design

There are several factors to take into account in the design of drug interaction studies.[6] Single-dose studies have been criticised but may be useful to exclude major effects. If an interaction is detected with single doses, it may be necessary to conduct a study at steady state, mimicking the dosage used in clinical practice to determine the true clinical consequences of interaction.

Whenever possible, interaction studies should not only be pharmacokinetic but should also include pharmacodynamic measurements in order to assess the likely clinical effect of an observed pharmacokinetic interaction. Furthermore, if possible, the design should go some way in explaining the mechanism of interaction. For example, measurement of a metabolite in plasma or urine may help to distinguish changes in elimination from changes in absorption as the reason for the change in AUC of the parent drug.

There are certain special cases which can seem difficult. For example, chronic full dosing of warfarin to volunteers has safety concerns, and the concentrations following a single standard dose can be regarded as sub-therapeutic. To address this, a design using a single large dose of warfarin has been shown to be reliable in detecting or excluding clinically significant interactions with warfarin.[7]

5.4.3   Enzyme induction and inhibition

Drugs that cause induction or inhibition of enzymes may affect the metabolism of concomitantly administered drugs, as well as of hormones and other endogenous substances. For this reason, such properties are considered undesirable, and sometimes they might constitute sufficient reason to discontinue drug development. At the very least, studies will be required to assess the magnitude of effect of likely interactions. Metabolic and toxicity studies in animals will usually provide the basis for suspicion, and studies in human liver slices, cultured hepatocytes and microsomal preparations can be extremely valuable in establishing metabolic pathways and the likelihood of enzyme induction or inhibition in man. There have been some important developments in this field in recent years and it is now possible to identify

• which cytochrome P450(s) is/are responsible for the metabolism of the test compound
• which cytochrome P450(s) is/are inhibited by relevant multiples of the therapeutic concentrations of the test compound.

These data will help predict other drugs which may affect the handling of the test drug and alternatively, concomitant medication for which the handling, and hence clinical response, may be altered by administration of the test drug. There is an increasingly extensive library of known inhibitors, inducers and substrates for each isozyme. This information can be used to predict which groups of drugs are unlikely to interact with the test drug, which can be justification for not performing the unnecessary studies. Unfortunately, extrapolation from the *in vitro* data is not perfect and hence *in vivo* data may be required with a likely concomitant medication of narrow therapeutic index.[8]

Once the *in vitro* screen has been performed, it is an increasingly common practice to use well-validated markers of each individual cytochrome P450 in order to make generalisations about the presence or lack of interactions of a certain group of compounds. Several reference probe compounds can even be given simultaneously using the 'cocktail' approach so that, for example, the presence or absence of an effect of the test compound on several cytochrome P450s can be studied conveniently in a single human study. This can be a powerful tool and can be very cost effective.[9]

One potentially serious consequence of enzyme induction relates to the oral contraceptive pill (OCP), which may be rendered ineffective by induction of its metabolism. The effect of a period of drug administration on circulating concentrations of the appropriate oestrogen and progestogens over the course of menstrual cycles may be examined in women taking the OCP, with additional non-hormonal precautions taken to avoid unwanted pregnancy.

Another approach is to investigate whether the drug causes *autoinduction* – whether its own clearance is increased by a period of drug administration compared with that after a single dose. This has implications for starting and maintaining dosage of the drug, as well as potentially for other drugs.

Environmental factors which may affect drug handling include changes in the diet (barbecued meat causes enzyme induction; grapefruit juice and some other fruit juices can inhibit cytochrome P450 3A4); the herb St John's wort causes significant enzyme induction; smoking (induction) and alcohol (acutely causes inhibition; chronically causes induction) and these substances must be avoided for a period before the study and until its completion. The duration of dosing with the test drug also needs some consideration. While enzyme inhibition may occur after a single dose, it may take 7–10 days for enzyme induction to fully develop as the new protein synthesis occurs.

5.4.4 Protein binding

Although at one time displacement from plasma protein binding sites was thought to be an important cause of clinically significant drug interactions, it is now recognised that it is only likely at the most to produce a temporary increase in drug effect in most drugs. It is only for a very few drugs that alterations in protein binding may be clinically important, and only following intravenous administration. For clinically significant drug interactions that have been attributed to displacement of plasma protein binding, alternative mechanisms, such as inhibition of metabolism, have been found to be responsible, for example, warfarin–phenylbutazone and tolbutamide–sulphonamide interactions. If the drug is highly protein-bound, screening *in vitro* for protein-binding displacement may help guide a search for suitable probe drugs to assess the clinical effect. However, displacement *in vitro* does not necessarily mean a clinically significant interaction *in vivo*. This subject and the implications for drug development have been reviewed elsewhere.[10]

5.5 The Elderly

The elderly, who for the purposes of drug regulation are generally defined as over 64 years of age, are a disproportionately large group of consumers of medicines. In the developed world, the proportion of the elderly in the population is increasing and will continue to do so for at least the next quarter of a century. Many drugs in development, such as those for ischaemic and degenerative diseases, are targeted almost exclusively at the elderly. It, therefore, becomes much more than a 'box-checking exercise' to evaluate both the dynamics and the kinetics of new active substances in this population.

Age-related differences in pharmacokinetics between the elderly and young are primarily due to

- diminished renal function
- altered proportions of body fat and water
- reduced cardiac output
- some degree of altered hepatic metabolism
- disease
- general debility
- concomitant medication.

For a drug that is to be developed for a disease that occurs mainly in the elderly, it is often advisable to evaluate tolerability and pharmacokinetics in healthy elderly volunteers before clinical trials in the patient population. Dosage may need to be reduced and particular care taken when the kidney is the major organ of elimination, which should be established in the healthy young before administration to the elderly. It should be remembered that the GFR in the healthy elderly with normal plasma creatinine and urea is generally much lower than that in the young. One reason why 'healthy elderly' studies have

attracted heavy criticism is that the carefully selected well-preserved subjects with normal ECGs, laboratory results and physical examinations do not really resemble the frail heterogeneous elderly population that they are meant to represent. This might result in a poor appreciation of the range of pharmacokinetic alterations in the elderly patient group[11]. It has been suggested in an FDA guideline[12] that the 'population approach' can be adopted to obtain information about pharmacokinetics in the elderly. Although this approach has a certain appeal, it also has serious drawbacks. This subject is discussed in Section 5.10.

5.6 Renal Impairment

As the kidney is one of the major organs of drug elimination, renal impairment is likely to affect the kinetics of many drugs. Although a wide range of processes (filtration, tubular secretion and active and passive tubular reabsorption) underlie renal drug handling, the overall renal clearance of drugs generally declines in parallel with GFR or creatinine clearance ('the intact nephron hypothesis'). However, the extent to which this affects total clearance depends on the proportion of renal clearance to total clearance. Pharmacokinetic studies in patients with renal impairment might, therefore, seem to be redundant for drugs that are cleared predominantly by non-renal processes, but experience has shown that studies may still be needed. For example, if a highly metabolised compound has a renally cleared metabolite with pharmacological activity, metabolite accumulation will occur if standard doses are given. Clinically significant effects resulting from an accumulation of an active metabolite from a highly metabolised drug include

- seizures produced by the accumulation of norpethidine after administration of pethidine
- toxicity from thiocyanate accumulation following administration of nitroprusside
- rash and allergy from accumulation of oxipurinol following administration of allopurinol

- narcosis due to morphine 6-glucuronide after administration of morphine.

Even when the major metabolite is inactive, clinically important pharmacokinetic changes for metabolised drugs may occur in patients with renal failure. The non-steroidal anti-inflammatory drugs that derive from propionic acid (e.g. ibuprofen, naproxen, ketoprofen, indoprofen and benoxaprofen) are metabolised to ester glucuronides in the liver. These are inactive and are normally rapidly eliminated by the kidney. However, when renal function is impaired, elimination of the glucuronide is delayed and plasma esterases convert the metabolite back into the parent compound, producing accumulation of the parent drug ('the futile cycle'). In the light of these examples, it is reasonable that if the drug is to be prescribed to patients with renal impairment, an appropriate study should be performed even for drugs which are highly metabolised.

A single-dose study is usually conducted before patients with chronic renal failure are included in clinical trials. The dose employed can be similar to that used for studies in subjects with normal renal function since C_{max} is unlikely to be increased greatly. The study of pharmacokinetics and tolerability at steady state may then be necessary, for which a lower dosage should be used if clearance was shown to be reduced in the initial study. When it is expected that renal disease will have only a modest effect on drug handling, it may be sufficient to compare the pharmacokinetics in a group of patients with advanced renal disease with those in healthy controls. However, when the kidney is the main organ of elimination, it would usually be necessary to examine the changes in kinetics in several groups of patients graded with respect to renal function. The effect of dialysis in patients with end-stage renal disease should also be investigated.

5.7   Liver Disease

As with renal impairment, a study in patients with liver disease is required to avoid a contraindication in this patient population. Unlike renal disease, there is no single clinical variable that can be used to predict reliably the extent of change of hepatic drug clearance of a given compound. However, the most widely used is the Child-Pugh classification,[13] which is based on several clinical and laboratory variables and has been useful in producing dosing information. In general, drug handling is more likely to be affected in advanced decompensated cirrhosis than when the disease is well compensated. Reactions mediated by mixed function oxidases (Phase 1) are thought to be affected earlier in the disease and to a greater extent than are large capacity conjugation (Phase 2) reactions. Alcohol further complicates the metabolic picture since it has a significant enzyme-inducing effect when taken chronically, but may acutely inhibit oxidative capacity when present in high concentrations.

In addition to changes in clearance, drug distribution may be altered in liver disease by the resulting low plasma protein concentrations and ascites. Intrahepatic and extrahepatic cholestasis are also likely to affect biliary transport of drugs, and studies in patients with these conditions may need to be considered for some drugs. Bioavailability may be increased by portal-systemic shunting allowing absorbed drug to escape first-pass metabolism. Pharmacodynamic changes that are not related directly to alterations in pharmacokinetics also occur in liver disease, for example, increased sensitivity to anticoagulants.

When designing a pharmacokinetic study in patients with liver disease, it is important to keep the target population for the disease indication in mind. Patients with severe liver disease are ill, and may not be likely to take medications for relatively minor illnesses. This is in contrast to patients with advanced renal failure, who may be otherwise relatively well. Given that the hepatic drug handling for a highly metabolised drug may be disturbed by advanced liver disease in a highly unpredictable manner (unlike in renal disease), it may be prudent to limit a study with the test drug to patients with relatively mild and compensated cirrhosis rather than decompensated cirrhosis, where marked changes and perhaps adverse clinical consequences could be expected. This restricted approach might be appropriate for a non-life-threatening indication (e.g. migraine), but for the treatment of Gram-negative sepsis it would be essential to study the kinetics and tolerability in advanced liver disease.

5.8 Disposition, Rates and Routes of Elimination of Drug

In the development of most new active substances, it is required to investigate the disposition of the compound and its metabolite(s) and their rates and routes of elimination. This is generally carried out with radiolabelled compound, usually [14]C. In the United Kingdom, approval of the Administration of Radioactive Substances Advisory Committee (ARSAC) is required for administration of radiolabelled compound to man. The purpose of the submission is to demonstrate that the dose of absorbed radiation is minimised by administration of the lowest dose that is consistent with meeting the objectives of the study. In general, the estimated absorbed radiation dose should be less than $500\,\mu Sv$, but higher amounts are permissible if they can be justified. The estimate is based on tissue distribution of radioactivity in animals and the pharmacokinetics in animals and man.

In addition to ARSAC approval, the protocol must also be approved by ethics committees in the normal manner for studies in man. The study should be conducted in between four and eight consenting subjects, in facilities where any spills of radiolabelled materials can be contained and monitored. Normally, subjects will be required to provide blood samples and to collect all excreta for a period determined by the known or estimated half-lives of the parent compound and metabolite. With cooperative subjects, recoveries of radioactivity should be close to 100%. Samples will be assayed for radioactivity and by cold chromatographic methods, and every attempt should be made to identify major metabolites

which may be revealed by radiochromatographic profiling.

The study should provide unique information on the plasma-concentration profiles of parent drug and metabolite. The rates and extended excretion in urine, faeces and, if appropriate, expired air can be defined.

Given the increasing public concern over radioactivity, it is becoming increasingly difficult to recruit adequate numbers of subjects to such studies. A new approach to undertaking these studies has recently become available. In conventional studies, drug-related material is detected by measuring the disintegration of [14]C. Accelerator mass spectrometry, in contrast, can count individual atoms of ^{14}C, and this can enable measurements of ^{14}C concentrations even when the dose is reduced by a thousand-fold or more compared with conventional studies. Such low doses may not require ARSAC approval or specific measures for dispensing of study drugs.[14]

5.9 Pharmacokinetic–Pharmacodynamic ('PK/PD') Modelling

As mentioned earlier in this chapter, there is usually a relationship between drug concentration and effects. Although the relationship might be simple, sometimes it is not obvious and may be complex. For example, since we are usually assaying plasma, time delay for the drug to reach the active site might obscure the underlying relationship between the effect and the concentration at the active site (which we usually cannot measure). Similar complications arise with the impact of active metabolites or the development of tolerance. However, data analytical tools, generally collectively referred to as 'PK/PD modelling' can be used to extract the underlying relationship.[15,16] If such a relationship is found, it is potentially very powerful as it enables extrapolation of the effect (which is often hard to measure) from plasma concentration (which is usually easier to measure). Dosing recommendation for special patient groups (e.g. children, organ impairment) may be based on such models. PK/PD analysis has been used to support the licensing of a dose which was not one of the doses tested in pivotal studies but an intermediate dose. The FDA has also stated that a 'well-characterised' PK/PD relationship might be the supporting evidence of efficacy additional to one clinical trial proposed under the Modernization Act.

5.10   Population Analysis

The usual way to examine the effect of a clinical variable (e.g. age, disease, concomitant medication, etc.) on the pharmacokinetics of a drug is to perform a small controlled study in which the experimental and control groups are homogeneous and closely matched and differ only in the variable of interest. This classic scientific method is well accepted by the scientific and regulatory communities and enables examination of a variable in a small group of subjects before including patients with that variable in a large clinical trial. However, there are some limitations with this approach. Perhaps the most important is that the small sample may not be truly representative of the population intended, as mentioned in Section 5.5 on the elderly. A summary of some of the advantages and difficulties of the traditional approach is given in Table 5.3.

An alternative method for searching for factors affecting variability in pharmacokinetics is the 'population approach'. This refers to a technique in which estimates of individual pharmacokinetic parameters are made from subjects from a potentially large population in which the PK and/or PD characteristics and the PK/PD relationship of a drug are investigated in a population of subjects, and the factors associated with between- and within-subject variability are sought. Such factors could include gender, age, race, smoking status, body weight, concomitant medications, genetics, abnormal liver function tests, etc. It is also possible to examine whether altered pharmacokinetics are associated with altered efficacy or safety, that is, making a population PK/PD model. Although this form of analysis can be performed within a single (usually large) trial, it is also particularly helpful to include the data from subjects in all trials, including small data-rich Phases I and II studies with the large but less data-rich Phase III studies. Such an analysis may be a powerful tool with which to justify an overall dosing regimen or a dosing recommendation for special patient groups, and is favoured by the FDA for this purpose.[17]

In order to appreciate the difference in approach, it is necessary to describe how pharmacokinetic analysis is traditionally performed. In a typical conventional pharmacokinetic study, a large number of samples is taken from a limited

Table 5.3 Advantages and difficulties of detailed pharmacokinetic studies in small groups of subjects – the traditional approach

Advantages	Difficulties
Well accepted	Not usually useful for 'screening'
Provides rich and high quality data	Frequent sampling is very difficult in patients in large clinical trials or in children
Can establish a causal link between altered pharmacokinetics and the variable of interest	Relationship between altered pharmacokinetics and clinical response may not be established
Early results from specific studies enable expansion of patient population in Phase 3 studies; not usually difficult to perform	Study sample usually does not represent the target population
Relatively straightforward and simple data analysis	Small sample may fail to elicit extremes of altered kinetics

number of subjects and pharmacokinetic parameters are calculated for each individual, with estimation of errors associated with these calculations. Average values of each parameter can then be calculated for the group.

By contrast, in the population approach, the raw data set that is analysed consists of concentration–time points (and other necessary data such as demographic information) taken from a large number (up to hundreds to thousands) of patients in Phase II and/or Phase III trials. The number of plasma samples per subject may be sparse but it is possible to estimate the individual pharmacokinetic characteristics of each subject and hence a measure of the mean parameters and their variability can be assessed. Relationships can be sought between patient characteristics (demographics, clinical status) and pharmacokinetic values is found, its consequence may be examined by looking for altered efficacy or safety which may not be possible in a traditional volunteer study. This might lead to demonstration of a therapeutic concentration range.

When planning to incorporate a population PK or PK/PD analysis, some extra resource is required, for example, to collect, transport and assay large numbers of samples (may be thousands), in studies where, traditionally, pharmacokinetic sampling had not been carried out in the past, for example, Phase III trials. For a meaningful analysis to be performed, the patient needs to be asked when the last dose (and perhaps one or two preceding ones) were taken in relation to the sample, and this is to be recorded in the case report form (CRF). How much dosing information is needed is governed by the pharmacokinetic characteristics of the drug. From a technical point of view, large databases need powerful computers and user-friendly software to avoid very time-consuming data analysis and to allow for the inclusion of Phase III data in the analysis. Even if these matters are resolved, the lack of experienced people with the necessary expertise, both at pharmaceutical companies and regulatory agencies, may be limiting.

The technique is powerful but it has to be remembered that demonstration of a statistical association does not necessarily imply causation. If a clinical variable is associated with altered pharmacokinetics, it might be necessary to perform a specific study to confirm or refute this, for example, a drug–drug interaction. The approach may not be appropriate to safely explore clinical variables that are likely to have a major effect on pharmacokinetics. For example, for a renally cleared drug which is likely to require a reduced dose in patients with renal failure, it may be necessary, for safety reasons, to perform a careful traditional pharmacokinetic study to determine the appropriate dosing regimen before these patients can be included in the main Phase II trials. The FDA has suggested that the population approach is a suitable method with which to explore the changes in pharmacokinetics in the elderly, but because age is often associated with altered pharmacokinetics, it is often necessary, again for safety reasons, to explore this before including elderly patients in the main efficacy studies using a standard dose. However, the results of a population analysis may eliminate the need for several smaller studies by answering questions relating to, for example, impact of age, concomitant medication or gender on the drugs pharmacokinetics or pharmacodynamics.

The decision to utilise a population approach should preferably be made early in the development of a drug to allow for the maximisation of its benefits. Preferably, data should be pooled starting with the early studies in healthy volunteers, and new data should be added to the database, data analysis carried out and the previous results challenged. By doing so, the knowledge of the drug will accumulate throughout the development of the drug, which will aid the developmental process by, for example, supporting the design of future studies and allowing timely scientific and strategic decision making based on all available information. The results of a population pharmacokinetic analysis may not be available until several months after the end of the main Phase III trials programme. This is likely to be around the time of the regulatory submission, and it is very late to find out about important clinical variables that affect handling of the drug. A way around this is to use only a part of the patient population from the Phase III trial(s) and to carry out the data analysis while the clinical programme is still ongoing. In this case careful consideration has to be placed on the issue of blinding and dispersion of results prior to finalisation of Phase III trial.

The population approach has found widespread application in all the phases of drug development and is generally perceived as beneficial for the development and approval of drugs.[18–23] With the accumulation of experience in this field, increased understanding and appreciation by drug developers combined with feedback from regulators, it may be expected that population analysis will be used increasingly in the future. At present the most appealing way forward appears to be a judicious mix of the traditional approach combined with population analysis in an interactive fashion, as data accumulate throughout the drug development process.

A summary of some of the advantages and difficulties of the population approach is given in Table 5.4.

5.11 The Rest of the Typical Clinical Pharmacokinetics Package

Box 5.6 lists the elements of a typical clinical pharmacokineticspackage for a systemically acting drug. Not all will be required for every submission, but omissions do need to be justified.

Topically administered drugs with local action, and sustained-release drugs are special cases that require a specialised approach.

5.12 The Ideal Drug from the Point of View of Pharmacokinetics

There are many examples of drugs which are successful in the marketplace but which have less than optimal pharmacokinetics. However, when a compound which has desirable pharmacokinetic characteristics is selected for clinical development, it can lead to a smoother clinical development programme, fewer regulatory concerns, a more straightforward datasheet and,

Table 5.4 Advantages and cautions/difficulties of the population approach

Advantages	Difficulties
Allows gathering of data in target population	Not widely understood and appreciated methodology
Can be used for screening for the effect of a large number of variables to identify factors important for variability and thus dosing	Can demonstrate correlation but not causation, for example, drug–drug interactions
Provides a tool to predict, for example, different dosing regimens and the PK of an individual from clinical/demographic data	Logistically challenging with large number of patients sampled, exact sample times and dosing history required
Possible to establish relationship among concentration, clinical response and adverse reactions using a large patient population	If data is obtained from the last Phase 3 trial, it may require late changes to the dossier or become rate limiting in submission
Limited sampling per patient makes the technique particularly appealing for studies in vulnerable patient groups, for example, the elderly and children	Technically difficult; complex software; limited number experienced operators

---

Box 5.6   The clinical pharmacokinetics regulatory submission
- Single-dose pharmacokinetics including relationship among dose and plasma concentration, absorption rate, total, metabolic and renal clearance, volume of distribution, elimination rate constant and half-life
- Multiple-dose pharmacokinetics
- Dose proportionately
- Absolute bioavailability by a given route
- Bioequivalence of any particular formulation compared with standard formulation used in clinical trials
- Identification and pharmacokinetics of major metabolites, often using radiolabelled drug
- Interactions with other drugs likely to be administered concomitantly, including enzyme induction and inhibition
- Pharmacokinetics in specific populations to demonstrate the effect of age and disease on kinetics, for example, young, elderly, patients with renal failure, liver disease, cardiac failure
- Effect of gender on pharmacokinetics
- Effect of food on drug absorption
- The relationship between pharmacokinetics and pharmacodynamic effects

---

Box 5.7   The ideal drug in terms of pharmacokinetics
- Intermediate lipophilicity/good hydrophilicity → good absorption
- Small (molecular weight <300) → good absorption
- Low clearance → good bioavailability and long half-life if this is important in the clinical situation
- Cleared by both renal and hepatic mechanisms so reduced capacity of one pathway (e.g. due to disease or drugs) will not lead to dramatic accumulation
- Not an inducer or inhibitor of cytochrome P450 enzyme → low drug interaction liability

---

ultimately, better clinical utility. In today's competitive marketplace, such characteristics may be key determinants of commercial success. A summary of some desirable pharmacokinetic characteristics, along with the reasons for those characteristics, is given in Box 5.7.

5.13   The Role of Pharmacokinetic Properties in Determining a Dosage Regimen

Determining the optimal dosing regimen for a new drug can be very difficult. However, considerable commercial superiority can be obtained by one drug over another by thoughtful selection of the dosing regimen, even if the two drugs have comparable pharmacokinetic and pharmacodynamic properties. Because pharmacokinetic properties of the drug determine the time course of plasma concentration, it is obvious

that this information will have some role in determining a dosing regimen. However, there are many other important types of information which are also relevant in determining a dosing regimen, and excessive reliance on pharmacokinetic properties alone can result in a sub-optimal dosing regimen. There is not space here for a full discussion of all of the factors that go into designing a dosing regimen, but a diagrammatic representation of the factors and their categories is presented in Figure 5.5.

5.14   Summary

Pharmacokinetics describes the absorption, distribution, metabolism and excretion of a drug by the body. Plasma concentration profiles, and in particular half-life, are important factors to consider in designing a dosage regimen. Calculation of primary pharmacokinetic parameters, such as clearance and volume of distribution, can provide insight into the physiological processes affecting plasma concentrations and enable some predictions to be made about the effects of age, disease and concomitant medication of these concentrations. The clinical pharmacokinetic regulatory package can, therefore, be assembled in a rational manner, providing sound support for the clinical trials regulatory submission. Increasingly a global model linking pharmacokinetics to pharmacodynamics is a source of competitive

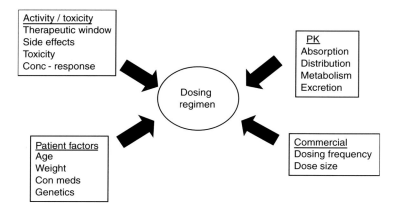

Adapted with permission from reference 1

Fig. 5.5 Factors affecting a dosage regimen. Adapted with permission from Rowland and Tozer (1995).[1]

advantage, allowing more rational dose selection, especially for special patient groups, and assisting regulatory review.

References

1. Rowland M, Tozer TN. *Clinical Pharmacokinetics: Concepts and Applications, 3rd edn.* Philadelphia: Lea and Febiger, 1995.
2. CPMP. *Note for Guidance on the Investigation of Bioavailability and Bioequivalence.* London: CPMP, 2000.
3. Neovonen PJ. Bioavailability of phenytoin: clinical pharmacokinetic and therapeutic implications. *Clin Pharmacokinet* 1979;**22**:247–53.
4. Food and Drug Administration (FDA). *Guidance for Industry. Waiver of In Vivo Bioavailability and Bioequivalence Studies for Immediate-release Solid Dosage Forms Based on a Biopharmaceutics Classification System.* Rockville, MD: FDA, 2000.
5. Schellekens H. Bioequivalence and the immunogenicity of biopharmaceuticals. *Nat Rev Drug Disc* 2002;**1**:457–62.
6. FDA Guidance for Industry. *In Vivo Metabolism/Drug Interaction Studies – Study Design, Data Analysis and Recommendations for Dosing and Labelling.* Rockville, MD: FDA, 1999.
7. Toon S, Hopkins KJ, Garstang FM, *et al.* Comparative effects of ranitidine and cimetidine on the pharmacokinetics and pharmacodynamics of warfarin. *Eur J Clin Pharmacol* 1987;**32**:165–72.
8. Tucker GT, Houston BJ, Huang S-M. Optimising drug development: strategies to assess drug metabolism/transporter interaction potential – towards a consensus. *Clin Pharmacol Ther* 2001;**70**:103–14.
9. Frye RF, Matzke GR, Adedoyin A, *et al.* Validation of the five-drug 'Pittsburg Cocktail' approach for assessment of selective regulation of drug-metabolising enzymes. *Eur J Clin Pharmacol* 1977;**62**:365–76.
10. Rolan PE. Plasma protein binding displacement interactions – why are they still regarded as clinically important? *Br J Clin Pharmacol* 1994;**37**:125–8.
11. Lacey JH, Mitchell-Heggs P, Montgomery D, *et al.* Guidelines for medical experiments on non-patient human volunteers over the age of 65 years. *J Pharm Med* 1991;**1**:281–8.
12. FDA Guidance for Industry. *Study of Drugs Likely to be Used in the Elderly.* Rockville, MD: FDA, 1989.
13. FDA Guidance for Industry. *Pharmacokinetics in Patients with Impaired Hepatic Function: Study Design, Data Analysis and Impact on Dosing and Labelling.* Rockville, MD: FDA, 1999.
14. www.xceleron.co.uk. Last accessed July 24, 2005
15. Colburn WA. Combined pharmacokinetic/pharmacodynamic (PK/PD) modelling. *J Clin Pharmacol* 1988;**28**:769–71.
16. Sheiner LB, Stanski DR, Vozeh S, *et al.* Simultaneous modelling of pharmacokinetics and pharmacodynamics: applications, to d-tubocurarine. *Clin Pharmacol Ther* 1979;**25**:358–71.
17. FDA Guidance for Industry. *Population Pharmacokinetics.* Rockville, MD: FDA, 1999.
18. Steimer JL, Vozeh S, Racine-Poon A, *et al.* The population approach: rationale, methods and applications in clinical pharmacology and

drug development (chapter 15). In: Welling PE, Balant LP, eds. *Handbook of Experimental Pharmacology*. Springer-Verlag: Berlin, 1994;110, 405–51.

19. Samara E, Granneman R. Role of population pharmacokinetics in drug development: a pharmaceutical perspective. *Clin Pharmacokinet* 1997;**4**:294–312.

20. Tett SE, Holford NHG, McLachlan AJ. Population pharmacokinetics and pharmacodynamics. An underutilized resource. *Drug Inf J* 1998;**32**:693–710.

21. Reigner B, Williams PE, Patel I, *et al*. An evaluation of the integration of pharmacokinetic and pharmacodynamics principles in clinical drug development. Experience within Hoffman La Roche. *Clin Pharmacokinet* 1997;**33**:142–52.

22. Minto C, Schnider T. Expanding clinical applications of population pharmacodynamic modeling. *Br J Clin Pharmacol* 1998;**46**:321–33

23. Sheiner LB, Steimer J-L. Pharmacokinetic/Pharmacodynamic modeling in drug development. *Annu Rev Pharmacol Toxicol* 2000;**40**:67–95.

CHAPTER 6

6 Purpose and design of clinical trials

Roger A Yates

6.1 Introduction

6.1.1 The clinical trial and pharmaceutical medicine

The discipline of pharmaceutical medicine has adopted the principal element in the scientific foundation of therapeutics – the controlled randomised clinical trial (RCT) – because new medicines must be proven to be therapeutically effective and safe before being licensed for prescription in clinical practice. Indeed, the precise regulatory requirements on evidence needed for a product licence (marketing authorisation) stimulated pharmaceutical companies to use existing principles and procedures for evaluating medicines and, more significantly, to develop and refine them. As a consequence, a high proportion of therapeutic research is nowadays sponsored by pharmaceutical companies and their staff who contribute greatly to the design, conduct, analysis and reporting of clinical trials. Pharmaceutical medicine not only adopted the clinical trial, but in many ways has developed it into the fundamental tool of drug evaluation.

6.1.2 Concept of the clinical trial

The concept of the clinical trial is relatively recent. The background to its development has been the increasing availability of more effective treatment modalities in the last 50 years or so. The main stimulus arose from the recognition of the possibility that by chance a patient's spontaneous improvement could coincide with the administration of a remedy and that this recovery could be attributed to the remedy when in fact the remedy was valueless. Therefore, some structured approach was necessary.

Efforts to evaluate different treatments began in the 1930s. The design of these early clinical trials leaned heavily on agricultural experiments, where randomisation had been employed to reduce bias by confounding factors (soil characteristics, moisture, sun, wind) and to reduce observer bias. This work by RA Fisher in the 1930s led many, including Sir Austin Bradford Hill, to adopt similar experimental designs in clinical trials. These really took on great importance in the 1940s and the 'British trial' evolved and was widely acknowledged as a template in clinical trial methodology.[1]

The other fundamental reason for organising clinical trials before a new medicine is licensed for widespread clinical use is that the effects of the medicine must be thoroughly assessed in patients with the illness that it is intended to treat. Because the response varies between individual patients and is affected by the situations in which the medicine is used, it is desirable to evaluate the medicine in groups of patients who represent a range of circumstances and to deduce from these trials the overall response.

The word 'control' means that the potential new medicine under investigation is compared with a 'control' group (see Section 6.6.7.4 for further discussion of control). The control may be placebo, no treatment, active control or different doses of the drug under investigation.

6.1.3 Types of clinical trial

All clinical trials should be conducted and analysed according to sound scientific principles, with due regard to ethical considerations, in order to achieve the trial objectives. Clinical trials as part of drug development aiming towards marketing authorisation must ask important questions and be designed to give answers that are as clear and unambiguous as possible. This is a tough challenge for an individual trial and more so for a complete clinical development programme.

There are a number of ways of classifying clinical trial designs. The most frequently used is according to the phases of clinical development. Clinical development is conventionally divided into four phases, which are a logical and progressive sequence within a continuously expanding process. Initial trials involve very few subjects observed closely under laboratory conditions and are followed by trials involving tens, hundreds and eventually thousands of patients as the licensing dossier is compiled. The concept underlying this classification is that results from each phase will inform the design of the next. The classical phases are:

Phase I. Clinical pharmacology in small numbers (tens) of healthy non-patient (or patient) volunteers to assess tolerability, preliminary safety, pharmacokinetics, and pharmacodynamics where practicable [i.e. biological effect using surrogate endpoints (see Section 6.6.5.1) or, rarely, therapeutic effect].

Phase II. Frequently divided into IIa and IIb:

IIa– clinical pharmacology in patients with the target disease (small numbers – tens to 200) to assess pharmacodynamics, pharmacokinetics and dose (or concentration)–effect responses for preliminary efficacy and safety, and to validate surrogate endpoints.

IIb– larger scale trials in patients (several hundreds) to formally assess the dose–response relationship and continue to expand the efficacy and safety databases.

Phase III. Formal therapeutic trials (randomised, controlled, in hundreds or thousands of patients) to determine efficacy and safety on a substantial scale; comparison with existing drugs; usually include two or more doses of test drugs; usually an international programme.

Phase IV. post-licensing studies in the target population, with widening of entry criteria to broaden experience in clinical practice; study objectives are typically surveillance for safety or further comparisons with other therapies. The results of such trials are more likely to be used for marketing purposes than in support of applications to regulatory authorities.

This can be further simplified to

- Phase I – does it do anything?
- Phase II – does it work?
- Phase III – how well does it work?
- Phase IV – look how well it works!

Although the logic and simplicity of these divisions is appealing, drug development is rarely as straightforward as this account implies. There are interactions, overlaps between phases and often redundancy in the process. The use of population pharmacokinetic screening to (1) more extensively investigate the plasma concentration–effect relationship, (2) establish the variability in dose–response across different age ranges, disease states and ethnic groups and (3) focus on sex differences has been integrated into Phases II and III of many clinical development programmes. These so-called 'population approaches' to assess variability in drug response and to refine the efficacy–safety relationships are complementing or replacing the 'special risk' group trials (see Section 6.5).

A complementary approach, and one geared more to the construction of a regulatory application, is to classify the trial according to its objectives.[2] Table 6.1 shows such a system; it will be appreciated that the types of study

Table 6.1 An approach to classifying clinical studies according to objective

Type of study	Objective of study	Study examples

Human pharmacology	Assess tolerability
	Define/describe PK and PD
		Dose tolerability studies
		Single and multiple dose
		  PK and/or PD studies –
		  some in special patient groups

	Explore drug metabolism and drug interactions Estimate activity	Drug interaction studies

Therapeutic exploratory	Explore use for the targeted
	  indication
		Earliest trials of relatively
		  short duration in
		  well-defined narrow study
		  subject populations, using
		  surrogate or pharmacological
		  endpoints or clinical
		  measures

	Estimate dosage for
	  subsequent studies
	Provide basis for confirmatory
	  study design, endpoints,
	  methodologies
		Dose–response exploration
		  studies

Therapeutic confirmatory	Demonstrate/confirm efficacy	Adequate, and well controlled studies to establish efficacy
	Establish safety profile	Randomised parallel dose–response studies

	Provide an adequate basis
	  for assessing the benefit:
	  risk relationship to
	  support licensing
		Clinical safety studies

	Establish dose–response
	  relationship
		Studies of mortality/
		  morbidity outcomes
		Large simple trials
		Comparative studies

Therapeutic use	Refine understanding of benefit:
	  risk relationship in
	  general or special
	  populations and/or
	  environments
		Comparative effectiveness
		  studies

	Identify less common
	  adverse reactions
		Studies of mortality/
		  morbidity outcomes

	Refine dosing recommendations	Studies of additional endpoints Large simple trials Pharmacoeconomic studies

PK, Pharmacokinetics; PD, pharmacodynamics.
Source: From Reference 2.

correspond approximately to Phases I, IIa, IIb and III. There has been an impetus for the manufacturer to include socioeconomic data in regulatory applications, because negotiations on the pricing of a new medicine, particularly its reimbursement, and the evolution of managed healthcare mean that, at the time of product launch, the manufacturer needs to have some evidence of the value of the product in terms of quality of life of the patients and for the patients' healthcare costs. Therefore, in the later stages of product development and extending into the immediate post-marketing period, clinical studies are likely to incorporate pharmacoeconomic measures as an integral feature. Other specific pharmacoeconomic studies may form a satellite programme starting before, and continuing after, marketing approval.

There is a continuous debate on which clinical studies provide the best evidence,[3] which, in turn, raises the question 'evidence for what?' In broad terms, evidence from clinical trials is required for five purposes:

1. To move a drug through a development programme.
2. To gain marketing authorization.
3. To guide treatment of individual patients.
4. To investigate specific aspects of the drug, for example, incidence of an adverse event.
5. To select one drug rather than another for addition to a therapeutic formulary and inform a health policy.

The debate about quality of evidence most frequently ranks large randomised controlled trials as the gold standard, at least for efficacy, with controlled observational studies in the middle, and uncontrolled studies and opinions at the bottom. The evaluation of therapeutic benefit and risk is, in fact, never ending because clinicians will subject marketed medicines to comparison with other existing or new medicines, and they will experiment with alternative dosage schedules and combined use with other treatments.

Clinicians are not necessarily convinced by one comparative clinical trial, even though it is scrupulously designed, conducted and analysed

and regulatory authorities require and expect specified numbers of RCTs (see Chapters 16, 17, 20–24). The controlled clinical trial aims to demonstrate that an observed effect is not the result of chance. But statisticians will argue among themselves about the representative validity of evidence in a population sample, and most will broadly agree that it is often equivocal. Added to this uncertainty, clinicians realise that the clinical trial adopts a specific framework of study, subject selection and assessment, which may be different from routine clinical practice. Therefore, one clinical trial is one piece of evidence on therapeutic value. The medical community will judge it, both formally, for example, by the National Institute for Clinical Excellence (NICE) in the United Kingdom issuing guidelines, and informally, to decide whether one treatment is more suitable than another for a particular type of subject (see Chapter 26).

It may be unreasonable to expect dramatic advances in a majority of patients with common but serious and multifactorial diseases such as cancer or heart disease. However even small treatment effects can be important in terms of their total impact on public health and should be sought. Thus, a classical dilemma is whether to run trials in a relatively small number of subjects predicted to have either a significant chance of responding to, or potentially benefit from, a given drug, or to expose a large number of study subjects knowing that only some will respond, but without being able to predict which individuals will respond. Advances in pharmacogenetics (see Section 6.4) are expected to assist in predicating individual subject responses. Amassing sufficient evidence to demonstrate small but valuable effects in wider populations from a number of trials uses the methods of systematic review[4]; analysing the accumulated results using appropriate statistical methods is termed meta-analysis (see Chapter 8).

The principles of a meta-analysis are that:

1. It should be comprehensive, that is, include data from all trials, published and unpublished.
2. Only RCTs should be analysed on the basis of 'intention to treat'.

3. The results should be determined using clearly defined disease-specific endpoints.

There are strong advocates and critics of meta-analysis as a concept. Arguments advanced against it are as follows:

1. An effect of reasonable size ought to be demonstrable in a single trial.
2. Different study designs cannot be pooled.
3. There is a lack of accessibility to all relevant studies.
4. There is a publication bias ('positive trials' studies are more likely to be published).

In the development of a new medicine the manufacturer controls the programme, and the structuring of the data from initial recording to electronic capture is decided by the sponsor. The meta-analysis of a series of clinical trials that share such commonality should be relatively easy. Rather than using a single study subject or a subgroup of study subjects as the unit of observation, collecting and merging data from the individual subjects can address not only the general benefits of a treatment, but the management of the individual subject.

Finally, a randomised comparative trial with one alternative marketed medicine can only address the choice between the two. Other comparative trials with other treatments build up a picture of overall therapeutic benefit and risk, and these trials may help to define groups of study subjects who differ in their response from the general population.

6.1.4   Controlled versus observational studies

A controlled clinical trial is an experiment and, as just mentioned, it deliberately alters the fabric of routine management of study subjects. It does so in two ways. First, it directs which treatment modality will be given to a particular subject, usually by randomised allocation without the doctor or subject knowing which treatment they will receive out of the two or three chosen for the trial. Therefore, a subject may not receive the conventional treatment that the clinician might otherwise have chosen. Second, the selection and

investigation of subjects distorts routine clinical practice by excluding some patients by virtue of certain characteristics, usually because of disease complications or other disorders or treatments that might make it difficult to distinguish the factor that really contributed to any improvement or deterioration. Thus, treatment allocation and definition of an appropriate patient population are fundamental features of the design of any comparative clinical trial.

However, once the product is generally available, it is important to identify if possible what is happening in routine medical practice and to do so without disturbing it. Ideally, one wants to look down as if from a helicopter and observe without intruding. More specifically, the decision to treat or not, and then the choice of treatment, must remain inviolate. The observational study is an important epidemiological (pharmacoepidemiological) tool and in pharmaceutical medicine it can provide unique surveillance of a medicine's actual usage compared with its recommended usage, its clinical efficacy and, in particular, its safety in those circumstances. The side effects can be distinguished from untoward effects of the disease being treated from effects of other concomitant disorders and of effects caused by other medicines taken by the subject by comparisons with data from other cohorts of subjects receiving one or more alternative remedies. Observational studies may be prospective (e.g. prescription event monitoring and cohort studies) as well as retrospective (see Chapter 15).

6.1.5   Global implications

Researchers in the pharmaceutical industry have realised that there are limits to the availability of economic and human resources in the development of new drugs. The costs of research and development can only be recovered if the whole global market is accessed. There are other advantages of conducting global studies. There may be a greater pool of suitable investigator sites and study subjects for a particular indication. The multicentre trial produces results faster by achieving quicker recruitment. It is also more likely to provide the critical power to the trial when trying to show small differences within acceptable confidence limits. These considerations have favoured design of multinational studies to generate one data set acceptable in all major territories as increasingly facilitated by the International Conference on Harmonisation (ICH) of Technical Requirements for the Registration of Pharmaceuticals for Human Use.[5]

6.1.6 Relevant guidelines

The procedures for assuring quality of clinical trials have evolved over the past 30 years, culminating in several published guidelines. There are three key documents – the GCP guidelines of the ICH, the Code of Federal Regulations (21 CFR) of the United States and the Declaration of Helsinki.[6–8]

Two other documents are relevant to clinical trials: the World Health Organisation (WHO) Guidelines for Good Clinical Practice for trials on pharmaceutical products,[9] still used for clinical trials in some parts of the world, and the new EU Clinical Trial Directive.[10]

The clinical trial process prescribed by these guidelines is the subject of Chapter 7.

6.2 Basic Ethical Considerations

The basic ethical questions raised by clinical research should never be underestimated. The pharmaceutical physician will need to be aware that failure, intentionally or because of misguided enthusiasm, to protect the health and well-being of each study subject can have very serious consequences. In an age where the medical profession is constantly under scrutiny, the drug industry is heavily criticised and the communication industry extremely active, mistakes in clinical trials are punished. Therefore, before a study is commenced, a review should be made that the scientific approach is current, the motivation is clear, the processes are unambiguous, and there should be sufficient data to judge the safety and effectiveness of the interventions proposed.

There needs to be a clear distinction between *medical research* and *medical practice*. In medical practice, the sole intention is to benefit the *individual* patient who is consulting the clinician; it is not to gain knowledge of general benefit, although such knowledge may incidentally emerge from the clinical experience gained. In medical research the primary intention is to advance knowledge so that patients in general may benefit in the future; the individual study subject participating in research may or may not benefit directly.

Medical research is not the same as a medical experiment or, for that matter, innovative treatment. Medical research is a systematic series of related and controlled investigations to establish facts, to create general knowledge and to deduce principles. One experiment will rarely achieve that level of understanding. On the other hand, a *medical experiment* is a single procedure chosen with the hope and expectation of succeeding and with the aim of seeing what happens. The medical experiment needs in turn to be distinguished from *innovative treatment*, where a clinician selects for an individual patient a treatment that is outside conventional medical practice. The sole motive for innovative treatment is choosing the best possible course of action in the particular and unique clinical circumstances of the patient's illness. Unfortunately, innovative treatment can masquerade as medical research, especially as doctors may apply the term loosely, and can evade the necessary constraints. If the purpose of the treatment is the acquisition of information for the benefit of future patients, especially if it is repeated, the treatment must be regarded as medical research and be subjected to the necessary controls. There is always a risk that a speculative new treatment or procedure will be adopted, especially where no treatment has previously been effective. This evasion of rigorous and critical testing can expose patients to suboptimal, valueless or even dangerous treatment.

Clinical trials can be divided into those that may result in some benefit to the participant, and those trials where no benefit can conceivably be expected. The most obvious example of the latter is the trial involving healthy non-patient subjects.

Such trials are frequently called non-therapeutic. Therapeutic studies are those from which the subject may derive benefit from exposure to the study drug. This is an oversimplification. For example, a Phase IIa dose-ranging study in study subjects with the target disease will include some doses which may be ineffective, or which prove to be too high. The design of the trial (e.g. crossover design) limits a therapeutic response within the confines of the study. Thus, therapeutic trials tend to occur in the later stages of clinical development at Phases III and IV. Consideration should be given to making an experimental medicine available to patients who have benefited from it in a clinical trial during the interval between the end of the trial and granting of a product licence.

Clearly, there is an ethical question as to whether the foreseeable risks and inconveniences to a study subject or patient participating in a clinical trial are outweighed by the anticipated benefits to that patient. Even more critical is the question of whether the risks being undertaken by the healthy volunteer are considered acceptable when the volunteer will not benefit medically.

Most people recognise the need for better medical treatments. However, there are many examples in modern history where the risks to the individual study subject have outweighed any benefit to either the subject or society. Society is rightly wary of medical research involving human study subjects.

6.2.1 Declaration of Helsinki

The principles of medical research are based on the Declaration of Helsinki. The general assemblies of the World Medical Association (WMA) have, since 1964, made recommendations for guiding physicians in clinical research involving human subjects. Although not legally binding, the Declaration forms the foundation of all other significant international documents on the ethical conduct of biomedical research.

The Helsinki Declaration covers all the important ethical considerations, such as the involvement of a qualified physician in any clinical

trial, putting the well-being of the study subject before science and society, the use of scientific principles in the design of the study, the need for informed consent and a review by an ethics review committee; in fact, all areas covered by the ICH GCP.

In October 2000, the latest revision of the Declaration of Helsinki[7] was approved by the WMA (see Appendix 1). The new version is very different from previous versions, with more detail on how clinical trials should be conducted. It requires that study subjects should have access to the best treatment identified by the study once the study has been completed. It also recommends that local participants in a study should be able to benefit from the study results, whether they are positive or negative. These principles were approved to avoid the exploitation of economically poor countries. In addition, the Declaration requires greater transparency regarding economic incentives involved in clinical research.

6.2.2 Peer review of proposed biomedical research

Modern medical research expects the proposed procedures and protocols of clinical trials to be submitted for peer review and that the human study subjects involved are provided with trial information before freely consenting to participate in that clinical trial.

Modern review boards or independent ethics committees (IECs) are required to act on behalf of the community in deciding whether the proposed research is justified on ethical grounds. They also act on behalf of members of the community in ensuring that there are sufficient safeguards to protect those individuals who directly participate in the research, and, for both the study subjects and those not directly participating, that confidentiality of participant's medical information will be maintained.

The independence of the review board is an essential feature. It is felt that those initiating and performing medical research should not be the sole judges of whether the research conforms to accepted codes of practice and, furthermore, that scientific or medical colleagues, if arbitrating alone, cannot be entirely independent, even though they are not directly involved. Researchers must recognise that fallibility in themselves and in others. Researchers may like to think that they fulfil their moral duty to other human beings, but ethical aspects can be easily overlooked, usually unwittingly, in enthusiasm for the aims of the studies or, more commonly, in commitment to the precise scientific design of the work planned. In the same way conviction that the study is justified might lead to understatement of risk, discomfort or inconvenience when inviting subjects to participate. Potential trial subjects may feel obliged, or occasionally pressured, to participate in studies. Trial processes should seek to minimise/avoid introducing any such feelings of obligation or pressure.

Today, an ethical review is an essential part of the biomedical research process. IECs provide ethical guidance on research protocols and ensure the protection of research participants. In the United States, similar bodies called institutional review boards (IRBs) have a similar role to that undertaken by IECs in the rest of the world.

In Europe generally, considerable variation in composition and in procedures occurs between IECs. Membership frequently depends on individuals who are willing to give their time without payment. Also, suitable members for this type of review board often have limited time. The new Clinical Trial Directive[10] should provide the incentive for greater uniformity. A single IEC will give an opinion on a multicentre study within 60 days.

6.2.3 Informed consent

The underlying principle is that subjects should only participate in a clinical trial if they agree to do so after they have fully understood the trial and its implications. In all studies, informed consent must be obtained from the subject or, where special situations occur, from his or her representative. How this is achieved depends on the study design, procedure and the country where the study is being conducted. Typically, it requires a four-stage process in which the signing of a form is the final stage. The stages are:

1. Verbal discussion between the investigator (or appropriate deputy) and the study subject.
2. Review by the study subject of the informed consent forms (ICF).
3. Time for the subject to consider what she or he has been told and read about the trial.
4. Signing of the ICF.

The structure of the ICF and more detail of the process of reaching informed consent are given in Chapter 7.

The whole process must have Ethics Committee approval before it is used.

6.2.3.1 Notification to the general practitioner

Where Phase II, III and IV studies are conducted in a hospital or contract research environment, it is strongly advisable to inform the subject's general practitioner (GP) in writing of the nature of the study and to obtain the GP's agreement, preferably in writing. This is essential for Phase I studies in non-patient volunteers, and it is routine practice in all Phase I clinical pharmacology units. However, increasingly, particularly in mainland Europe, study subjects will be found not to have a personal physician or, if they have, that their last visit to the physician could be a considerable time ago.

It is also advisable to tell the study subject that the GP will be informed about the clinical trial. Difficulties occur when the clinical trial is for an indication of a socially unacceptable condition such as a venereal disease. Rightly or wrongly, the subjects have fear that knowledge of the illness may not be safe with the 'family' doctor. In these exceptional circumstances, the IEC should decide whether the GP should be informed only with the agreement of the study subject.

6.2.3.2 Confidentiality

The actual name of the study subject should never appear on any documents relating to the clinical trial that leave the investigator's site and, as far as possible, the anonymity of the study subject must be maintained throughout any clinical trial.

All information generated during the course of the study with regard to the subject's state of health is confidential, and the subject's agreement must be obtained before disclosure of such information to a third party.

Normally, the study subject is informed both verbally and in the ICF that certain other individuals besides the investigator site staff will view his or her medical records. In clinical studies sponsored by pharmaceutical companies or institutions, the monitoring and quality assurance (QA) personnel from the sponsors and CROs, and inspectors from a regulatory agency will review the medical records of the study subject.

All the medical records of the subject should be available for comparison with the data recorded in the case report form (CRF). In the past, physicians have not allowed medical records to be available for the so-called 'source verification' by non-physicians since they felt that this broke the strict confidentiality of the study subject's medical records. However, frequent mistakes in transferring important clinical data to the CRF, the recruitment of subjects who do not meet the inclusion and exclusion criteria and the occasional blatant fraud has led to an insistence by sponsors and regulatory agencies for sponsor's review of study documentation. Indeed, verification of source data cannot take place without access to the medical records of the study subject by the sponsor's staff.

Modern clinical research requires considerable cooperation and partnership between the investigator, the sponsor and the regulatory authorities. In consequence, the investigator will need to treat certain 'outsiders' with the same amount of trust that is shown to nursing staff and fellow physicians. Violations of confidentiality of subjects are rare from sponsor staff and certainly no more frequent than that experienced from hospital staff.

6.2.4   The use of placebo

The new version of the Declaration of Helsinki (Edinburgh, 2000)[8] (see Appendix 1) has highlighted concerns in the use of placebos in clinical trials. The Declaration states in its twenty-ninth Ethical Principle that the 'effectiveness of a new method should be tested against that of the best current prophylactic, diagnostic, and therapeutic methods'. Although this principle does not rule out the use of placebo, IECs and some regulatory authorities are going to be more vigilant when a placebo treatment arm is used. At least one government agency (the FDA) believes that the placebo comparison is preferable to an active agent because it is a fixed and reliable reference point. However, in studies in which life-threatening disorders are being treated, comparisons will always be done with agents, if they exist, that may have a favourable effect on the disorder. The use of a placebo in clinical trials is discussed further in Section 6.6.7.5.

6.3   Compensation and Insurance

Should a study subject suffer any deterioration in health or well-being caused by participation in a study, the sponsors of the clinical research must provide appropriate compensation without regard to the question of legal liability. A statement to that effect should be present in the protocol. Frequently, the insurance policy of the sponsor includes the pharmaceutical company, clinical investigators and the institution where the clinical study is being undertaken.

There is considerable variation between countries concerning the type of insurance and compensation that is required for a clinical trial. These differences need to be considered before starting any multicentre clinical trials in different countries. Increasingly, the medical profession and some governments, particularly in Europe, are recommending moves towards no-fault compensation to reduce the huge costs of litigation.

In the United Kingdom, the information sheet provided to the consenting study subject in a clinical trial sponsored by a pharmaceutical company will usually contain a reference to the clinical trial compensation guidelines of the Association of the British Pharmaceutical Industry (ABPI).[11] It is not included in the information sheet of non-commercial studies. Study subjects taking part in clinical trials are not usually paid, unless it is a non-patient volunteer study. However, it may be necessary to compensate participants for out-of-pocket expenses such as travel, and this should be stated in the protocol and in the information sheet/ICF. Financial incentives for study subjects should not be the main reason for entering a study.

6.4 Pharmacogenetics

A good clinical trial is designed to take account of the variability in response (either efficacy or adverse event) that is expected when a new active drug is tested. This response depends on an individual's genetic make-up, and on a number of environmental factors, such as disease state, other drugs and age. The size of the trial and the selection of study subjects are carefully determined to reduce the variability in response to a minimum (i.e. to maximise the sensitivity of the trial) so that the trial endpoints can be determined with as much certainty as possible.

Pharmacogenetics is the study of the genetic differences among individuals with regard to clinical response to a particular drug, be that response efficacy or safety (adverse reaction). It is sometimes usually used interchangeably with, but is usefully distinguished from, pharmacogenomics, which is a broader term used to describe the 'commercial application of genomic technology in drug development and therapy'. Pharmacogenetics is not a new science; what is relatively recent is the advent of genomic technologies (in particular, rapid screening for specific gene polymorphisms and knowledge of genetic sequences of target genes, such as those coding for enzymes, ion channels and other receptor types involved in drug response) that have permitted the identification of polymorphisms in genes linked to drug effects and then to phenotypic responses.[12,13] This has led to the concept of 'the right medicine for the right study subject'. The use of pharmacogenetics in clinical trials has been introduced for certain drug development programmes in Phases I to III. These have been focused on drug disposition, pharmacodynamics and adverse drug reactions.[14,15] Significant advances have been made in the understanding of pharmacogenetics of drug metabolism enzymes, and a comprehensive listing of genetic polymorphisms influencing these enzymes that are of potential clinical relevance has been compiled. Significant examples that have implications for clinical trials include anti-HIV compounds that are potent inhibitors of metabolism mediated by cytochromes P450. Future trials may also need to take account of potential consequences of genetic polymorphisms in other pharmacokinetic processes. For example, in subjects who lack a functional protein (enzyme or transporter) the 'normal' doses of a given drug may evoke a different effect. In addition, or alternatively, such subjects may not be able to activate a prodrug or may not be able to metabolise drugs so efficiently. However, it must be stated that the current evidence for the clinical importance of genetically determined variability is not impressive; it is important to read the original source literature with a critical eye.[16] At present, knowledge of genotype alone cannot account for pharmacokinetic behaviour in most cases. The pharmacokinetic consequences of the activity of a polymorphic enzyme will also depend on, for example:

- Whether it mediates metabolism of the parent drug, primary metabolite or both
- The overall contribution of the affected pathway to clearance
- The relative capacity of alternative pathways of elimination
- The potency of active metabolites.

In turn, whether significant pharmacokinetic differences arising from the polymorphisms translate into relevant alterations in pharmacodynamics (and clinical efficacy) depends on the operating region of the concentration–response relationship, therapeutic index and utility, and whether kinetic variability is outweighed by variability in receptor sensitivity or number, or in the turnover of the natural receptor ligand.

An understanding of the pharmacogenetics of pharmacodynamics is probably less advanced than that of pharmacokinetics, but inherent variability in pharmacodynamics may be greater than in pharmacokinetics. In turn, whether pharmacokinetic–pharmacodynamic variability translates into clinically relevant differences in drug response depends on further clinical and operational issues, such as compliance, and doctor/patient perception of efficacy and side effects. To date, there are few solid examples, shown in replicated well-controlled trials, for associations between genotype or other nucleic-acid-derived data and pharmacodynamic responses to a drug.[17] Current thinking on the contribution of pharmacogenetics to dynamic responses (both efficacy and adverse events) has been assisted by classification of responses into type I and type II. Though not entirely separable, type I pharmacogenetics relates to genotype variants in pharmacological receptors and other processes that contribute to a disease or syndrome. Hence, unrecognised or undiagnosed disease heterogeneity provides one explanation for different drug responses. Type II pharmacogenetics represents genotypic variation that influences the response to a drug that is not related to the pathogenesis of the disease (i.e. to interindividual variability). Both types may contribute to a variable extent and to help explain variable responses to a drug in a multifactorial disease, such as essential hypertension or asthma.

The impact of these considerations on study subject selection, sample size and endpoint measures will need to figure in future clinical trial designs.

6.5   Studies in Special Groups

Studies in special groups pose ethical problems that are similar to those associated with studies in healthy young adult subjects.

Clinical trials may need to be conducted in certain study subject groups that are often either not included or are poorly represented in 'standard' clinical development programmes. These include children, the elderly and those with a quantified degree of renal or hepatic impairment and ethnic minorities. Moreover, it may be necessary to consider specific studies in women of childbearing age for drugs other than those specifically designed for them, such as

the oral contraceptive. Another consideration is the applicability of data generated from one ethnic group to the regulatory dossier for a country in which a different ethnic group predominates.

6.5.1   Paediatrics

The scientific basis for development and clinical usage of drugs for children, with some notable exceptions, lags sadly behind that in adults. There are a number of reasons for this, the most important of which are lack of commercial incentive, practical and ethical difficulties in trial conduct, and a historical perspective that children are 'small adults'. There are two significant consequences: first, there has been a lag phase before medicines with suitable indications used in adults become available for use in children. An example is treatments in asthma. Second, many drugs for prescribed for children are used either 'off label' or are licensed for another indication. However, the situation is rapidly improving, with publications, symposia and regulatory guidelines making their appearance.

In Europe, the adoption of the ICH EII guideline,[18] based on the existing EU CPMP guideline,[19] is in place. In the United States, the FDA introduced in 1997 the 'stick and carrot' legislation, whereby extra market exclusivity for 6 months for the whole product range is granted following an agreed and executed clinical trial programme in a paediatric population. The FDA also has stipulated under the Pediatric Rule (1998)[20] that a development plan for a new or marketed product will include a paediatric programme, unless the FDA specifically waives or defers studies. A carrot to encourage paediatric research is built into the 2005 PPRS in terms of increased research allowances (see Chapter 26).

An important step in the development of paediatric medicines has been the practical, if arbitrary, age and developmental categorisation as follows: preterm newborn infants, term newborn infants (0–27 days), infants and toddlers (28 days–23 months), children (2–11 years), adolescents (12–16 or 12–18 years, depending on the region). While studies may not be required in all age bands, and, indeed, it may be agreed that some bands are too wide for certain diseases, at least this approach gives a framework for a continuous clinical development programme in which the pharmacokinetic and pharmacodynamic characteristics can be related to physiological chronology.

The guidelines on development of paediatric medicines advise that the need for a paediatric component must be considered on the basis of the seriousness of the indication and the lack of satisfactory alternative therapies. It recognises three main categories:

1. Medicinal products for diseases predominantly or exclusively affecting paediatric patients – when a full development programme with the possible exception of initial safety and tolerability would be required at an early stage.
2. Serious or life-threatening diseases occurring in both adults and paediatric patients where there are currently no, or limited, therapeutic options – the paediatric component should be started early after initial proof of safety and of concept has been generated in adults, and the paediatric studies should form part of the marketing application.
3. For medicinal products intended to treat other diseases – studies in children would be less urgent and started only when results of adult Phase II/III trials were known to be reassuring. However, companies should have a clear plan, giving reasons for timing.

The types of trials to be undertaken demand a flexible approach, and depend on the seriousness of the disease, other therapeutic options and the pharmacokinetics at different ages. For example, if the disease process and efficacy endpoints are similar in adults and children, then an extrapolation from adult efficacy data, together with pharmacokinetic studies in the appropriate paediatric age range, together with safety studies, could form the basis of a successful application. Likewise, it may be possible to extrapolate efficacy from older to younger paediatric groups, with pharmacokinetic and safety studies in the relevant younger study subjects. Where there is no known correspondence between efficacy and

blood levels, then clinical or pharmacological effect studies in relevant age groups would be expected.

For novel indications or where the disease course and therapeutic outcome are likely to be different in adults and paediatric subjects, clinical efficacy studies would be needed. Other important considerations in studies of paediatric subjects are:

1. An appropriate formulation that is palatable.
2. Consideration of the volume of blood to be taken in a study of pharmacokinetics.
3. The need for monitoring long-term follow-up in post-marketing surveillance (PMS) and safety assessment of marketed medicines studies to determine effects of the drug on physical functions and development, such as bone maturation, growth and sexual development.

6.5.2 Ethnic factors in clinical trial development

The influence of ethnic factors on drug responses in clinical trials is important in two contexts. First, the regulatory application should contain data that is generated from subjects whose ethnic mix is in proportion to that in the population where the medicinal product will be used. Second, an applicant may wish that data generated in one country with one ethnic predominance should be used to gain marketing approval in another country where the ethnicity of the population is different.

The ethnic factors that may affect drug responses can be classified as intrinsic or extrinsic. Intrinsic factors are either genetically determined, such as polymorphisms in drug metabolism and genetic diseases that could influence response, or physiological and pathological, such as age, major organ function and diseases peculiar to the geographical region. Some intrinsic factors, such as height, weight, body surface area and receptor sensitivity, that govern kinetics and dynamics may be influenced by both mechanisms. Extrinsic factors (environmental) include climate, culture (educational status, socioeconomic factors), medical practice (especially other medicinal products) and differences in regulatory practice, methodologies (especially subjective endpoints, such as rating scales) and endpoint measures.

Factors, such as smoking, food habits and alcohol intake influence drug responses probably by both intrinsic and extrinsic mechanisms.

The scientific methodology for investigating the influence of ethnic factors on efficacy responses (with a few exceptions) is not well advanced. It is probably fair to say that too much anecdotal information has been put forward to suggest that ethnic differences exist. It is probable that ethnic differences are no more likely (and maybe less likely) to contribute to the variability in responses than are inherent differences in an unselected population drawn from a single ethnic population. However, as stated above, it would seem prudent to ensure that at least the major ethnic groups in whom the drug is to be used should be represented in a clinical development programme. Some properties of a medicinal product that might be sensitive to the effects of ethnic factors include: non-linear pharmacokinetics, a steep dose–response curve for efficacy and/or safety, a narrow therapeutic dose range, significant metabolism through a single pathway subject to polymorphism, low bioavailability, and the likelihood of multiple (and varying) co-medication.

Data predominantly generated in one ethnic group to be used for registration in another may be acceptable in their entirety, or 'bridging studies' may be required in the second ethnic population to determine if differences exist.[5]

The need for bridging studies depends on whether the medicine is 'ethnically sensitive' or 'insensitive' on the basis of the criteria discussed above. For example, if the product was metabolised through a route that displayed no genetic polymorphism, had a wide therapeutic index, a shallow dose–response curve and there were universally agreed endpoints to determine efficacy and safety, then no bridging studies would be needed.

Where the fate of a major development programme rests on foreign data, it is wise to discuss

their acceptability with the appropriate regulatory authorities at an early stage and to be guided by ICH topic E5.[5]

6.5.3 The elderly population

Many drugs will be used in elderly subjects, and certain diseases, for example, Alzheimer's disease, are associated with the ageing process. Clinical studies to test the efficacy and safety of medicinal products in elderly subjects need to take account of the following:

1. Will the drug be used predominantly or entirely in that age group?
2. How might age affect the pharmacokinetics or dynamic responses (tolerability and efficacy) of the drug under test?
3. To what extent can results be extrapolated from younger populations?
4. To what extent are the effects of age separable from those of deterioration in specific organ function (especially kidney and liver)?
5. Are there special ethical issues involved in the development of this drug?
6. Can some important questions concerning development and clinical use of this drug in the elderly be answered by a 'population screen' approach or will specific elderly study subject trials be required?

Definition of 'elderly' is arbitrary and it is obvious that chronological ageing does not necessarily correspond with physiological or pathological decline. As the populations of Western cultures are ageing, it is becoming increasingly recognised that experience of drug usage, either in preregistration or surveillance studies, in the frail and very elderly will become increasingly important. ICH guidelines on studies in geriatric patients[21] adopt 65 years and over as the cut-off point, but recognise that older age ranges should be studied. They also point out that it is important 'not to unnecessarily exclude study subjects with concomitant illnesses'. Again, this raises ethical dilemmas.

Trial endpoints need to be given particular consideration in the elderly. For example, health questionnaires that include practical outcomes, such as the ability to walk further or rise unaided from a chair, may be more appropriate in the elderly than measures of surrogate dynamic effects. Conversely declining intellectual function and attention span of the elderly (particularly if they have dementia) may make use of questionnaires and rating scales inappropriate for some trials. Correlations between changes in rating scale and clinical outcomes are particularly problematic in the elderly, and the duration of Phase III comparative efficacy studies needs careful consideration.

Another issue is whether to conduct Phase I safety and tolerability studies only in elderly subjects if the drug is specifically for use in that age group. It may be argued that it is unethical to conduct such studies in young healthy volunteers if such an age group will never receive the drug.

6.5.4 Patients with impaired hepatic or renal function

Consideration of the proposed indications for the candidate drug together with knowledge of its pharmacokinetics and metabolism in healthy volunteers will indicate whether specific studies in patients with impaired hepatic or renal function will be needed to be included in the Marketing Approval Application and NDA. Useful relevant guidelines are available on the FDA website[22] and it is advisable to discuss proposals with the relevant regulatory authorities. The topic is considered in more detail in Chapter 5.

6.6 Clinical Trial Design

6.6.1 General considerations

This section aims to provide sufficient information for the pharmaceutical physician to effectively prepare and support a clinical trial. However, clinical trials come in many forms and what is appropriate for a single-centre non-sponsored trial is totally inappropriate for a multicentre global study sponsored by a big pharmaceutical company or institution. Similarly, a Phase I non-patient volunteer study

is very different to a Phase IV study. The types and classification of individual clinical trials, and the purposes to which the results are put, have been broadly described in the introduction.

The principles should be the same for any clinical trial:

1. Achievement of the clinical study objectives should advance medical knowledge of a potential new drug or new or unproven use of a licensed one.
2. The design, conduct and analysis of the trial should comply with highest clinical, scientific and ethical principles.
3. Trial design should provide maximum possible protection for the study subject, with the involvement of all parties – the investigator, sponsor, IEC and the regulatory authorities.
4. There must be sufficient results from preclinical and human studies assessed by qualified experts indicating that the study drug and procedures are safe.
5. The study must not begin before it has been approved by all relevant authorities, such as an ethics committee and the regulatory authority.

6.6.2 Preparation for the clinical trial

Each individual clinical trial needs to 'stand alone' in the sense that each trial is set to answer specific questions, and that its objectives, design, conduct, results and conclusions are interpretable in their own right. The purpose should be clarified at the time the clinical development plan is formulated, when the clinical trial in question is put in the context of a series of human studies and clinical trials as part of an agreed strategy for evaluating a new medicine. This process of stating the reasons for conducting the trial is assisted by considering a series of questions.

1. What is the context of the proposed trial? For example, where does it fit into a drug development/research programme?
2. What data/decision is needed?
3. What use will be made of the results?

4. Is a specific trial required?
5. What hypothesis is being tested or what are the precise objectives?
6. Which trial design will deliver what is required?

Since most trials in clinical drug development are part of a series design, each needs to be considered on two levels. Included in the first level is an understanding of the context in which the trial will be conducted, extending through a series of steps to anticipating the outcome and deciding on consequential action. The second level of design is more focused and concentrates on selecting the optimal manner in which the trial will be conducted, choosing from various options in order to obtain the best plan.

This rest of this section will deal with design, both in the broader and narrower sense, although it will not be possible to give a detailed account of individual design strategies, for which the reader is referred to other excellent texts (see recommended reading list).

6.6.3 Preclinical investigations

The extensive investigations required before a study drug goes into man are discussed in Chapters 3 and 4. There is a requirement to provide the investigator in a Phase I study with as much information as possible concerning the probable pharmacokinetic and pharmacological profile of the study drug. The investigator will need to decide on the initial safe dose for the clinical trial and identify parameters for clinical monitoring of potential adverse effects. Later in development, the investigator will need to be satisfied that there is sufficient preclinical data to support the duration of dosing specified in long-term therapeutic trials and that the results of previous clinical trials support continued research with the drug.

6.6.4 Creating a hypothesis

A hypothesis is a proposition assumed for the sake of argument; it is a theory to be proved or disproved by experiment. In the context of the clinical trial, it is a statement of expected outcome to the study, which will provide a clear and interpretable answer to a realistic question. In that sense, hypothesis creation is about biological phenomena. Take, for example, the hypothesis that drug A will have a greater effect on blood pressure than will drug B. It is convenient to set about testing the hypothesis by assuming that the treatments are equally effective (or ineffective), as the case may be. This is the 'no difference' or null hypothesis. Thus, when two groups of study subjects have been treated, or each subject has had a course of each drug, as in a crossover study design, and it has been found that one drug produces improvement more frequently than the other, it is necessary to decide whether this difference is due to a real superiority of one drug over the other, or whether the result could have arisen by chance. This decision is reached by the application of tests of statistical significance. The correct significance test will establish how often a difference of the observed size would occur due to chance (random influences) if there were, in reality, no difference between the treatments. In a second example, the hypothesis might be to show that two drugs are equivalent or that one is not inferior to the other. A different set of statistics will be needed to test this hypothesis (see Section 6.6.7.6).

6.6.5 Selection of response variables

6.6.5.1 Efficacy endpoints
Efficacy variables are chosen according to the objectives of the trial. They may be the therapeutic effect itself (e.g. irradication of infection, healing of peptic ulcer) or a factor related to the therapeutic effect or some surrogate effect.

There is a considerable literature on surrogate endpoints.[23,24] From a practical point of view, the physician working in the pharmaceutical industry needs to be precise in the use of the surrogate endpoint.

The characteristics of an 'ideal' surrogate endpoint for use in Phase I–IV trials would depend on whether the emphasis is on the efficacy or the safety evaluation of the potential medicine.

The characteristics of an ideal surrogate efficacy endpoint include:

- Being an early stage in the biological process leading to therapeutic benefit
- A parameter that can be determined simply, repeatedly and reproducibly on different occasions and by different investigators
- Economically viable
- Acceptable degree of specificity and sensitivity
- Preferably non-invasive
- Applicable across a wide range of patients
- Sensitive to dose-related effects
- High predictive value for therapeutic or clinical endpoint.

The last point (i.e. a high level of validity) can only really be confirmed in Phase III or IV, when a sufficient number of study subjects have achieved a therapeutic response that can retrospectively be correlated with the change in surrogate marker. Thus surrogate markers, in this context, are most valuable for selecting second-in-class or follow-up drugs, when validity has already been tested with the first compound. This is a particularly important point and is often glossed over in debates with regulatory authorities as to whether a surrogate endpoint is an indication in its own right.

In the evaluation of pharmaceutical products, commonly used surrogate efficacy endpoints include:

1. Pharmacokinetic measurements, for example, plasma (serum) half-life, concentration–time curves of parent drug or active metabolite.
2. An *in vitro* or *ex vivo* measure of drug effect, for example, mean inhibitory concentration (MIC) of an antimicrobial against bacterial culture; inhibition of ADP-induced platelet aggregation with a fibrinogen receptor antagonist.
3. An *in vivo* marker of effect related to the pharmacology of the drug, for example, hypoglycaemic response to an antidiabetic agent; change in concentration of a 'serum marker of disease' such as C-reactive protein with antirheumatoid agents.
4. The *in vivo* antagonism by the potential drug to an exogenously administered agonist, for example, inhibition of weal and flare response to subcutaneous serotonin by 5-hydroxytryptamine $(5HT)_3$ antagonists; the inhibition by a leukotriene LTD_4 antagonist of bronchoconstriction induced by inhalation of LTD_4.
5. the investigational appearance of tissues or organs, for example, endoscopy findings of a peptic ulcer; the radiological appearance of joint erosions.

Surrogate endpoint data can be used for a number of purposes. These include:

1. 'Proof' of physiological–pharmacological effect.
2. determination of dose–response relationship prior to Phase III trials.
3. Confidence from Phase I and IIa trials that further evaluation of a pharmaceutical product is warranted.
4. Assistance in choosing among several compounds in the same biological or chemical class for progression to Phase II.
5. Yielding comparative effect or safety data between two drugs with a similar mechanism of action.
6. To register a drug for an indication.

In recent literature, the concept of surrogate endpoint has become inextricably linked to the term 'proof of principle' or 'proof of concept' study. There is nothing fundamentally new in this idea. It is an attempt by sponsors to design, execute and interpret 'small scale', preferably short-term trials at the exploratory phase of development in which a selected surrogate (or surrogates) is determined as the basis for a 'go/no-go' decision point for continuation or termination of a development programme. The overall objective is to reduce the increasing costs of clinical development, having recognised that the majority of novel substances that enter Phase I will not reach the marketplace. Only time will tell whether this new emphasis will be successful.

6.6.5.2 Safety endpoints

Safety variables are broadly of two kinds: those related to the unwanted pharmacological effects of the drug and those that are unpredictable.

The first require specific questions or investigations to be included in the trial at time points related to the pharmacodynamic and pharmacokinetic characteristics of the drug, for example, in vulnerable subject groups, such as the elderly or those with renal or hepatic disease, or during long-term studies when drug or metabolite accumulation might occur. It may be possible to measure surrogates for toxic effects such as QT interval for Torsades de Pointes. The characteristics of safety surrogates are similar to those of efficacy surrogates described in the previous section.

Non-specific safety questions are usually addressed in three ways:

1. A standard set of haematological and biochemical investigations is included before, during and after the trial. These investigations should be comprehensive, but not exhaustive, otherwise they will generate a large volume of data that will need processing and that may, by chance, throw up findings that are not related to drug effects.
2. Study subjects are asked about their response to treatment using an open question, such as 'How has the medicine suited you?'
3. An adverse event form should be provided by the sponsor, which will have clear instructions as to what constitutes minor, major and serious adverse events, how these are to be recorded, and what action is required as a consequence.

6.6.5.3   Subsidiary assessments
Clinical trials generate vast quantities of data, most of which are processed by the sponsor. Assessments should be kept to the minimum that is compatible with the safety and comfort of the subject. Highest priority needs to be given to assessment and recording of primary endpoints, as these will determine the main outcome of the study. The power calculation for sample size should be based on the primary critical endpoint. Quite frequently, trials have two or more evaluable endpoints. It must be stated clearly in the protocol whether the secondary endpoints are to be statistically evaluated, in which case power statements will need to be given, or are simply

descriptive. The temptation to include additional investigations, which is particularly easy when automated analyses are conducted in laboratories, should be avoided unless they add significantly to the trial. However, in long-term trials, it may be necessary to arrange extra visits at which critical trial data are not recorded but the subject is assessed for general well-being, tolerance of trial medication is confirmed (or otherwise) and to maintain good relationships between the doctor and study subjects and compliance with treatment.

6.6.6   Patient population in trials and in clinical practice

The indication (or indications) for which a new drug is designed is the prime determinant of the population in which it will be used in clinical practice. For some drugs, the indication is clear at the start of the clinical development programme, for example, a 'me-too' cyclooxygenase inhibitor or a novel delivery system for insulin. However, for many drugs, particularly those that interfere with one or more pathways in a complex series of biochemical or immunological steps, the final indication(s) may be less clear, for example, anti-TNF (tumour necrosis factor) agents. Furthermore, serendipity may come into play during the course of the trial programme, as was the case with the phosphodiesterase-4 inhibitors which are now in use for male erectile disorders, but were originally designed for the treatment of heart failure. Finally, if the aspirations of pharmacogenetics are realised (the right medicine for the right patient), then indications will be defined not just by disease, but also by population characteristics.

For the present and immediate future the general path of subject selection for clinical developmental trials will tend to follow the pattern of moving from highly selected and well-defined subject groups to an ever-broadening and less selected population, up to and beyond granting of a marketing authorisation. Inevitably, this will include study subjects who may or may not respond, but this knowledge must be balanced against the need to create a comprehensive safety database at the time of marketing.

6.6.6.1 Eligibility criteria

The defined population for the clinical trial will be chosen on the basis of a series of inclusion and exclusion criteria, which together constitute the eligibility criteria. Inclusion and exclusion criteria are of two kinds: general and specific. General criteria include age, sex, race, weight, previous medical history, previous and concurrent medication and status of major organ functions (e.g. hepatic and renal function). Specific inclusion criteria are of two kinds. The first set applies to trials testing therapeutic or surrogate endpoints. For example, in a trial of an antihypertensive drug, specific entry criteria for the level of systolic and diastolic blood pressure measured over a stated number of visits, in a particular position, and with a specific piece of apparatus, would be stated. The second set of specific inclusion criteria applies to trials of drugs in special groups, such as early phase studies in healthy normal volunteers to assess tolerability, safety and pharmacokinetics, or kinetic and metabolic studies in study subjects with renal or hepatic impairment in whom pharmacokinetics and therapeutic response may be different from that in other patients.

6.6.7 Choice of trial design

There is no generally accepted classification of trial design because each aspect of a design (e.g. dose ranging, blinding) can be used in combination with almost any other. It is simpler to describe the various design aspects from which one can select a combination that meet the trial objectives. Box 6.1 lists different aspects of trial design; pairings or groupings do not necessarily imply strict alternatives or mutual exclusion.

6.6.7.1 Pilot trials

There is no succinct and universally accepted definition of a pilot trial. It is usually open in design and small in scale. Its use sometimes implies some degree of uncertainty either about

---

> **Box 6.1 Aspects of clinical trial design**
> - Pilot/pivotal
> - Open/blind
> - Controlled/uncontrolled
> - Placebo/active comparator
> - Parallel/crossover/matched pairs
> - Dose–response/final dose/dose escalation
>
> - Dose–titration (response)
> - Concentration–responses

---

the safety (e.g. narrow therapeutic ratio) or efficacy of the medicine, or doubt about testing it in a particular context or indication. Pilot studies may examine feasibility (i.e. examine in one small-scale study the sense and practicability of testing a hypothesis so that large resources are not committed without some gain in confidence; for instance, the chosen endpoint may not be suitable or sufficiently sensitive). Pilot trials do not imply 'quick and dirty' research or a sloppy approach. They demand as much planning as other types of trial. They can be performed during any phase of drug evaluation, but are most frequent as a vanguard trial early on. Sometimes pilot studies lead to or are converted into definitive trials, and this possibility should be discussed with a statistician in advance of starting the pilot trial. Pilot trials can use many aspects of trial design: double blind, parallel or crossover.

6.6.7.2 Pivotal studies

Strictly speaking, pivotal (as with pilot) does not imply a particular design but rather the use to which the trial will be put. By convention, such trials will result in important decisions being made about the medicine (e.g. designing the dosage schedule or comparing it with a benchmark comparator) or a pivotal trial will be crucial in defining efficacy and safety. As such, the trial will be subjected to comprehensive QC and QA, and will attract a higher than usual degree of scrutiny by sponsors and regulators. Pivotal studies can occur at any phase in a drug development programme. In regulatory terms, the pivotal trials are those identified by the sponsor for the regulatory authority to judge the efficacy and safety of the drug.

6.6.7.3 Blindness

The term 'blind' refers to a lack of knowledge of the identity of the trial treatment. The aim of blinding is to avoid bias in trial execution and interpretation of results, and it is achieved by disguising the identity of the trial medications. The simplest method is to use formulations that look identical, which is frequently possible with tablets or capsules, but is more difficult for oral solutions that look and taste different. Alternatively, blinding can be achieved for the testing of two non-identical active comparators by the use of the 'double dummy' technique, whereby each active agent has a matched placebo and study subjects in each limb of the trial take two sets of tablets: one active and one placebo. Special considerations for blinding have to be given for studies involving suppositories, eye drops, skin patches or more esoteric treatments.

There are various levels of blinding, extending from open or open label (a term used by US investigators), where all concerned with the trial are aware of the identity of the trial medicine, to the other extreme of total blindness, in which everyone who interacts directly with the study subject or who comes into contact with the observations or data is unaware of treatment allocation; statisticians, efficacy review committees, pathologists and experts invited to interpret objective endpoint criteria are unaware of treatment identity. In between there are various combinations of blindness, for example, single blind (subject unaware, but physician informed) and double blind (both subject and investigator unaware of treatment allocation). The latter is most frequently used and it is generally regarded as generating the most reliable data for interpretation. Increasing levels of blindness bring increasing complexities, higher costs and longer time penalties to trials. The protocol author must bring common sense to bear on occasions. For example, when a drug and placebo are to be given intravenously and samples need to be made up fresh for each administration, is it really necessary for the pharmacist to be 'blind' to the preparation of the material? In multicentre trials in which mortality or significant morbidity is the endpoint, it is common practice to have a blinded 'efficacy endpoint' committee, but an unblinded 'safety review' committee.

There is much controversy over the use of open or open-label studies. It is a golden rule of clinical trial design that, wherever practicable and possible, open studies should not be conducted, but there are circumstances when they can or must be used (see Box 6.2).

Rules governing the unblinding of the trial must be given in the protocol. In the normal course of the trial, this occurs at the end of a stated period, although subjects may be maintained on 'open' observation for a further period of time. The 'breaking of the blind' is a serious matter, as it can spoil part or the whole of the trial. The occurrence of a major adverse event is the most frequent reason for unblinding and, in most circumstances, requires a discussion between sponsors and investigators.

Box 6.2 Use of open clinical trial design
1. Compassionate plea protocols – by definition, these must be open, and have the advantage to the subject of allowing early access to a potentially valuable medicine
2. Treatment IND (or non-US regulatory authority equivalent) – as in entry 1, the investigator takes the responsibility for the trial
3. Uncontrolled non-comparative studies
4. Phase I dose-ranging trials in subjects, as opposed to volunteers (e.g. in severely or terminally ill subjects)
5. Phase I pharmacokinetic trials
6. Phase II or III long-term continuation trials, particularly those following on a short-term double-blind efficacy trial, in order to increase subject exposure
7. Clinical trials in which it would be unethical to use a double-blind design
8. Some large, multicentre post-marketing surveillance studies, in which a comparison of the newly marketed drug and standard therapy is made

6.6.7.4 Controlled trial

The word 'controlled' in the context of clinical trial design has two meanings, one broad and one specific. In the broad sense, it relates to adherence to a tightly designed protocol in order to reduce the variability of factors and the biases that might influence the outcome. In the specific sense, control refers to the comparator treatment and/or 'population' used in the trial. By custom, the term 'controlled trial' has come to be equated with 'comparative trial'. Contrariwise, uncontrolled can mean a study which loosely adheres to entry criteria and procedures or, more specifically, to a design feature which does not include a comparator treatment or population group (non-comparative trial). Specific control groups are included in the clinical trial so that the medicine under test can be compared against a contemporary reference treatment. If no comparator control group is included, then the effect of the drug is compared with baseline or historical data. Sometimes comparisons are made with both baseline and comparator groups. The types of control groups used in clinical trials include:

- Concurrent placebo
- Concurrent active medication
- No treatment
- Different dose of the same medicine (dose-ranging studies)
- Concurrent use of usual or standardised care
- Historical comparison of data obtained from the same subjects on no therapy, the same therapy or different therapy
- Historical comparison of data obtained in other subjects on no, or some, different therapies.

The principle behind establishing a control group as opposed to a control treatment is the selection of a population as similar as possible to the group receiving the medicine under investigation. Whenever possible, a prospective rather than historical control should be used.

The choice of treatment control depends on a number of factors, including:

1. The phase of the drug development programme.

2. The specific objective of the trial (e.g. dose–response, comparison with active comparator).
3. The placebo response.
4. The ethical position of use of placebo or active drug in serious conditions, for example, epilepsy.
5. The availability, choice and applicability of active comparator.
6. The length of the study.

The major purpose of a control group is to allow discrimination of outcomes caused by the test treatment from outcomes caused by other factors, such as the natural progression of the disease, observer or subject expectation, or other treatments.

For further discussion on control groups and placebo in clinical trials, see Temple and Ellenburg.[25]

6.6.7.5 Placebo

A placebo is an inert medication (or procedure) that is used in conjunction with the double-blind technique to reduce bias in the population samples and in the treatment responses (subjective and objective). Placebo usage is useful to:

1. Distinguish the pharmacodynamic effects of a drug from the psychological effects of the act of medication and the circumstances surrounding it, for example, increased interest by the doctor, more frequent visits.
2. Distinguish drug effects from the fluctuations in disease that occur with time and from other external factors.
3. Avoid false positive or negative conclusions.

The value of the placebo-controlled trial in the early evaluation of a new potential medicine cannot be overemphasised. It is particularly valuable when there is no accepted standard therapy in common use. There are many examples of prescribed drugs in different therapeutic classes that have never been subjected to controlled placebo trials. Other scientific arguments in favour of the inclusion of placebo arms in trials include the following:

1. No standard medical treatment exists.
2. Standard medical treatment has been shown to be ineffective.

3. The drug under trial is innovative in terms of mechanism and/or administration.
4. The standard treatment is inappropriate as comparator (e.g. route of administration, choice of dose).
5. The response can only be measured by subjective endpoints.
6. A positive placebo response (particularly a large one) is well recognised in the condition to be treated.

There are a number of arguments against the use of placebo treatment that need to be considered.

1. It is unethical to withdraw an active treatment that is known to be beneficial, for example, in epilepsy and tuberculosis.
2. There is no suitable placebo available or it is impracticable to attempt a true placebo comparator group, for example, in a trial comparing an intravenous with an oral formulation.
3. Previous studies have convincingly defined the placebo response rate, and the study is designed to test dose–response or activity against a positive control.

Although some of these arguments against the use of a placebo involve questions of ethics, the use of a placebo treatment is often preferable to the continued use of treatments of unproven or dubious efficacy or safety. Some old remedies that are still in current use have never been subjected to a placebo-controlled trial, and the opportunity to include them in a placebo comparison may only be during the development of a new medicine.

Some disease states or trial conditions militate in favour of a high placebo response rate and lend support for the inclusion of placebo in a comparative trial. These include long treatment periods, previous treatments and response to them, innate characteristics of the study subjects (e.g. social class, educational level and personality type), influence of medical staff, environment and supervision during the trial, appearance and taste of trial drugs, and presence (or absence) of unwanted pharmacological effects.

Some conditions may permit the use of placebos for short periods (e.g. 2–6 weeks in chronic heart failure) but thereafter an active comparator would have to be introduced either routinely or on an 'as needed' basis.

The recent publication of the revised version of the Declaration of Helsinki[8] has in Section 29 the following statement:

The benefits, risks, burdens, and effectiveness of a new method should be tested against those of the best current prophylactic, diagnostic and therapeutic methods. This does not exclude the use of placebo, or no treatment, where no proven prophylactic, diagnostic or therapeutic method exists.

Section 29 was introduced to help protect people in poorer countries from being used as research subjects for the benefit of those in developed countries, when they themselves may derive no immediate or future advantage, for example, in the testing of new anti-HIV drugs. This is a laudable aim; however, such is the awe in which the Declaration is held that over-interpretation of it in order to challenge or even exclude the use of placebos in drug development in developed countries would have dire consequences for decision-making on drug safety and efficacy that would affect drug developers, regulatory authorities, healthcare professionals and patients. Among the many arguments in addition to those listed above for the retention of placebo-controlled studies in the right context as opposed to only active comparator trials are the following[26]:

1. Placebo-controlled trial of a new active medicinal product, if positive, means that the trial was capable of detecting a difference, and that the test treatment is, at least, more efficacious than placebo. This achieves two outcomes: provision of an internal validity check of the trial methods, and provision to regulatory authorities of a basis on which to judge the difference between a statistically significant but clinically inadequate effect that would probably lead to the drug not being licensed.
2. If only active comparator trials were available, then the trial objectives would have to be very precise from the beginning of a trials programme as to whether superiority, equivalence or non-inferiority is being tested.[27] Demonstration of

non-inferiority in turn depends on designing a trial with sufficient sensitivity, as it has to rely on indirect evidence that a trial is capable of showing a difference, without prior availability of placebo-controlled data[28] (see next section).

6.6.7.6 Comparator medicines

Active comparators are included to act as a 'benchmark' or 'gold standard' against which the new drug is to be compared. The selection of comparator depends on the specific objectives of the trial. The main considerations are as follows.

1. Is the comparison to test pharmacological or therapeutic effect?
2. What dose or doses will be chosen?
3. Will one active comparator serve for all countries in which the drug will be marketed?
4. Is it possible to 'blind' the study?
5. Is the active comparator the standard medication the study subjects will be receiving and how realistic is it to standardise dose and re-randomise into a clinical trial?

In practice in Phase II or III, the control or comparator group most frequently receives the medicine that is most widely prescribed, in a dose that has been established by regulatory approval and clinical experience to represent the optimal for that medical condition.

In some clinical disease states, a treatment regimen that has become the standard represents the best practice, and may involve three or more drugs with different mechanisms of action. The potential new medicine will need to be tested against a regimen of therapies rather than a single agent. It may still be feasible and ethical to conduct a placebo-controlled parallel-group study on top of the standard regimen, but there is an added level of complexity to this approach. For example, for patients who have survived an acute myocardial infarction, the treatment regimen may include aspirin, an angiotensin-converting enzyme inhibitor, a lipid-lowering drug and a fibrinogen receptor antagonist. Selection of study subjects and analysis of surrogate endpoints need to be carefully thought out.

There are three possible specific objectives for comparator trials: to show superiority, equivalence or non-inferiority of the new active substance. Each is governed by statistical and regulatory guidelines.[27–32]

Superiority trials of one active compound over another provide the second most convincing proof of efficacy after placebo-controlled studies. The usual reason for selecting this design rather than placebo has been alluded to already, that is, it is ethically unjustifiable to use a placebo; the other common, but less convincing, reason is to meet marketing requirements. The trial design must have the same key design features (e.g. primary variables, dose of comparator, entry criteria) as the previously conducted superiority trials in which the active comparator clearly demonstrated clinically relevant efficacy. A positive outcome depends on demonstrating that the 95% confidence interval of the observed treatment difference should be entirely to the right of the point of equivalence (see Figure 6.1).

There are two main categories of equivalence trial: bioequivalence and clinical equivalence. In the former, certain pharmacokinetic variables (C_{max}, AUC and $t_{1/2}$) of a new formulation have to fall within specific (and regulated) margins of the standard formulation of the same active entity (see Chapter 5). Proof of clinical equivalence can be much more difficult to demonstrate, but situations where it might be of interest are when the standard therapy has been shown to be beneficial but the innovative treatment is easier to use, has fewer side effects or is less costly. This study design may be of value when investigators seek to establish that a mechanistically related compound achieves clinical results similar to those of the standard therapy. The protocol must contain a clear statement that its objective is demonstration of clinical equivalence and the equivalence margins should be defined and justified. A positive outcome depends on demonstrating that the entire confidence interval of the result lies within the clinical limits defined in the protocol.

Non-inferiority trials are more common than equivalence trials in Phase III drug development. In these, the objective is to show that a new treatment is no less effective than existing treatment. It

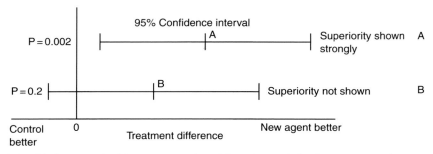

Fig. 6.1 Relationship between significance tests and confidence intervals for the comparison between a new treatment and control. The treatment differences A and B are in favour of the new treatment but superiority is shown only in A. In B, the outcome may meet criteria for equivalence or non-inferiority as defined in the protocol.

may be more effective or equivalent, but using the confidence interval approach, the only interest is in a possible difference in one direction. Design of such studies must include the key features described for superiority trials and definition of purpose and clinical equivalence as for clinical equivalence studies. A positive outcome depends on demonstrating that the lower confidence internal of the result lies above the lower limit of clinical equivalence defined in the protocol.

6.6.7.7 Parallel or crossover design

Most clinical trials for clinical drug development select two groups of study subjects. In a parallel design, subjects are randomly allocated to one of the two treatments and remain on it until the end of the trial. In a crossover design, every subject receives each treatment allocated in random order, changing over at a halfway point. In a parallel design the response of each group of subjects is compared with that in the other. The crossover design allows comparison of the effects of two (or more in complex trials) treatments in the entire study population.

The advantages and disadvantages of crossover and parallel-group designs have been subject to extensive debate, and are summarised in Table 6.2. Generally speaking, crossover designs are selected in the early phases of drug evaluation, particularly for the first dose-ranging trials in stable diseases. Parallel designs are frequently adopted for the definitive dose-ranging studies and for therapeutic efficacy trials.

Crossover designs are susceptible to carry-over effects, that is, the treatment effect from the first period has not worn off at the time of conducting the second period. Tests of analysis can detect carry-over effects, but it is too late then to modify the design. Similarly, period effects may confound the interpretation of cross-over studies, that is, the order in which one treatment occurs in a sequence compared with another influences the response to early treatment. Randomisation usually, but not always, precludes the effect.

6.6.7.8 Single-centre studies

There are considerable advantages in conducting single-centre studies in the early stages of the development of a new study drug. Most Phase I units using non-patient volunteers are single centres that have a population of volunteers, the expertise and the intensive monitoring required.[33]

The new EU Directive[10] now covers all such studies. This will almost certainly significantly change the previous situation, in which Phase I units were seldom subject to the regulatory scrutiny experienced by sites used at later stages of drug development. Some investigator-instigated research and non-commercial research failed to follow the GCP guideline and were not subject to the same Directives as those used in commercial research.

Single-centre studies are used where new devices are being developed. For example, the development of devices releasing local anaesthetic or analgesics will require various diverse

Table 6.2 Comparison of crossover and parallel designs in clinical studies

	Parallel	Crossover
Robust to trial violations (missed visits, missing data, etc.)	+	−
Variability of data obtained	Between-subject differences used to assess treatment differences: therefore, variability likely to be large	Within-subject differences used to assess treatment differences: therefore, variability likely to be smaller
Subject numbers	Large	Small
Disease condition	Stability desirable over course of trial, but design is tolerant of waxing and waning diseases	Stability mandatory; baseline at each crossing point must be similar
Carry-over effect	−	+
Period effect	−	+
Relevant effects of treatment should develop within the treatment period	Not essential	Yes

skills including engineering, surgery and pharmacology. A good reason for use of single centres is a requirement to investigate a particularly uncommon indication or for a specialised technique, and where there are sufficient appropriate subjects for meaningful analysis and sufficient experience and knowledge to minimise the risks to the study subjects.

6.6.7.9 Multicentre studies

Improvements in medical treatments have been substantial, so much so that benefits of recently introduced medicines over existing ones are smaller than when these standard treatments were originally developed and compared with remedies that existed then. The mean difference in some clinical efficacy endpoints between treatments may be less than 20%. This requires a large population sample in clinical trials in order to achieve sufficient power to detect a difference, if it really exists, with confidence. Most medical conditions (for instance, peptic ulcers) present rather infrequently at any single hospital centre and it would therefore be impossible for a single

centre to recruit 200 or 500 study subjects in a reasonable period of time. If instead one invites several investigating centres to recruit study subjects and to pool their findings, this constitutes a multicentre trial. Thus, one reason for conducting a multicentre trial is to increase efficiency. The advantages can be offset by differences in procedures, often resulting from differing interpretation of instructions. These mistakes, when coupled with other errors made in each centre, mean that the multicentre trial could turn out to be even less reliable than the single-centre trial in terms of quality of data.

It is therefore essential to incorporate procedures that will ensure not only that the clinical data are collected in a uniform and similar manner at each investigating centre but that they are also handled and analysed in an identical manner. Measures such as the use of compatible validated computer systems and similar databases will allow the merging of data. At each centre, critical efficacy data should be determined with identical procedures and, where appropriate, these should be specified in protocols and monitoring conventions. Standard operating procedures (SOPs) should be prepared to ensure that investigators at each site are carrying out the more common methodologies, such as blood pressure measurements, blood sampling, radiograph measurements, in a similar manner.

Obviously, it is desirable to use one centre for the central collection of data, but that requires sufficient resources and close liaison with the person(s) monitoring the trial. Pharmaceutical companies have learnt that it is simpler and more efficient if they became custodians of the data, using their own computing facilities for data capture and their monitoring staff to bring in high-quality records. The transfer of the data to the sponsor allows the pharmaceutical company to hold all the data electronically, not only data for a particular clinical trial but data from all the clinical trials relating to the development of a specific study drug. When regulatory submission takes place, agencies, such as the FDA, can 'interrogate' the clinical data in order to establish the validity of the analysis and interpretation. Computer-assisted new drug application (CANDA) is the frequent form of application in the United States. Without doubt, the use of paper applications will decrease in other regions of the world when global standards for the electronic transfer of regulatory information have been established[34] and computer systems are properly validated (see Section 7.5.4.1).

Multicentre trials have thrust pharmaceutical companies into the role of coordinating the design, conduct, analysis and reporting of all trials on a new medicine, and given them a real incentive and the resources to do so. In a similar manner some of the collaborative groups running large-scale intervention trials, which often span several countries and several thousand study subjects, adopt similar procedures. However, if the multicentre trial is being conducted independent of a pharmaceutical company or large institution, clinical data should not be analysed by each individual centre. The clinical data should be sent to one centre to be entered into a common computer database for analysis. If possible, the coding for the whole trial should be done by the same individual. It would also be

wise to employ sufficient expertise in statistical analysis of clinical trials and suitably trained computer staff, as well as a validated computer system.

6.6.7.10   Dose selection

In clinical practice, the optimal dose is the smallest that will result in the desired therapeutic response. Inherent within that statement is the concept of individualisation of dose for each given study subject, as it would not be unreasonable to expect considerable variation in response, depending on many factors such as body size, efficiency of the metabolising and excretory pathways, race, age, state of disease and so on (see Section 6.5). In practice, it is not possible for a sponsor to investigate more than a few doses, and frequently only one or two doses for registration of a given indication. It is often in clinical practice that adjustment (most frequently, downwards) to final regimens occur. The impact of pharmacogenetics on individual dose has yet to be shown.

6.6.7.10.1   Dose–response relationships, potency and efficacy

An understanding of the dose–response relationship is fundamental to successful clinical drug development and to therapeutic practice. The pharmacological effect of a drug is related to the concentration of the drug at its site of action – within certain limits, the higher the concentration, the greater the pharmacological effect. The relationship between the concentration of a drug at its site of action and the intensity of the pharmacological effect is called its dose–response curve. It often takes the shape illustrated in Figure 6.2, in which (by convention) the intensity of the response is plotted against the logarithm of the dose, giving a sigmoid curve.

The shape and position of the curve describes the potency of the drug. A steeply rising curve indicates that a small change in dose produces a large change in drug effect, for example, a loop diuretic. By contrast, the dose–response curve for the thiazide diuretics plateau at lower doses, and increasing the dose produces no additional diuretic effect.

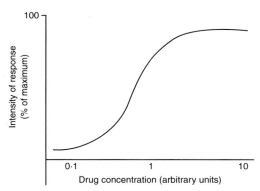

Fig. 6.2 The shape of most dose–(or concentration–) response curves is sigmoid in which the rate of rise of the response eventually flattens off despite increasing concentrations.

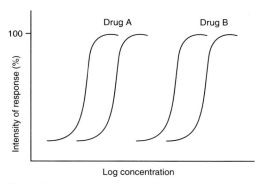

Fig. 6.3 Dose–response curves for two drugs A and B; B is less potent than A. The curves under A and B represent theorised positions of efficacy and toxicity relations. The distance between the individual pairs represents the therapeutic index.

The term *potency* is frequently used imprecisely and is often confused with efficacy. It is important to distinguish between the two when designing and interpreting clinical trial results. Potency is the amount of drug in relation to its effect. For example, if weight for drug A has a greater effect than drug B, then A is more potent than B, but the maximum therapeutic effect obtained may be similar for both the drugs. By increasing the amount of drug B, it may be possible to achieve the same response. Thus, the difference in weight of the drug that has to be administered has no clinical significance, unless it is high.

Pharmacological potency is a measure of the concentration of a drug at which it is effective. It refers to the strength of the response induced by occupancy of a receptor and has to be further qualified for agonists and antagonists.[35,36] Efficacy has both pharmacological and therapeutic definitions. Pharmacological efficacy refers to the strength of response induced by occupancy of a receptor by an agonist. It describes the way in which agonists vary in the response they produce, even when they occupy the same number of receptors.

Therapeutic efficacy, or effectiveness, is the ability of a drug to produce an effect, and refers to the maximum effect. Thus, if drug A produces a greater therapeutic effect than drug B, regardless of how much of drug B is given, then drug A has the higher therapeutic efficacy.

Drugs have both unwanted and wanted dose–response curves. The shape and position of the unwanted dose–response curve in relation to dose–response curve for the desired effect displays the relative toxicity of the drug. From a consideration of the relative positions of these two curves, the concept of the therapeutic index has arisen. This is the maximum tolerated dose divided by the minimum effective dose. In practice, such single doses can rarely be determined accurately and the index is never calculated this way in man; 'effective' doses are rarely available or determinable in sufficient subjects. However, the concept embodies a useful concept that is fundamental in comparing the usefulness of one drug with another, that is, its safety in relation to its efficacy. The concept is shown diagrammatically in Figure 6.3. Drugs with steep dose–response curves for efficacy and/or toxicity are relatively difficult to use in practice because small changes in dose can have dramatic clinical effects.

The application of the principles of dose–response relations to Phase II and III clinical trials focuses on the practical aspect of determining which doses will be selected for these trials and which will be taken forward to registration (see below). Each subject in a clinical trial will have his or her own efficacy and safety dose–response curve for a given drug. The shape and position of these curves will be determined by individual subject characteristics – age, gender, genetically

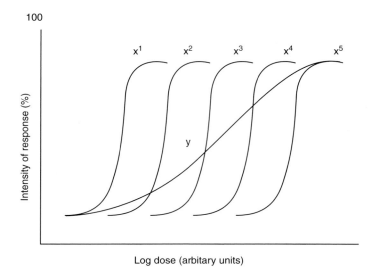

Fig. 6.4 X^1-X^5 are individual dose–response curves; Y is the average dose–response curve for the population.

determined metabolism and so on – so that the dose–response (or concentration–response) curve from each trial represents an average, with a measure of variability that describes that population. Figure 6.4 describes this schematically.

6.6.7.10.2 Dose titration and concentration–response designs

Dose titration studies involve starting study subjects at a predetermined dose, which is increased incrementally until the desired therapeutic effect is achieved. Interpretation of such studies is complicated by the difficulty in distinguishing between the effect of the dose increase and the increased duration of exposure – continued maintenance at a smaller dose may achieve the same effect. Dose titration studies for antihypertensives have received adverse criticism by FDA regulators because they have resulted in higher doses being recommended for clinical use in some instances. However, more recently, Sheiner and colleagues[37,38] have revived an interest in this design, taking account of the potential for period effects and period-by-dose interactions. They have suggested modification of the design (e.g. inclusion of a randomly assigned placebo arm for the duration of the study) and analysis (use of a parametric subject-specific dose–response model). Using complex dose–response models, they showed that dose titration designs could perform better overall than a parallel-group design for the model considered in the simulation, and slightly worse than a crossover design.

In a concentration–response design, subjects receive either a fixed dose (or dose range) of a medicine and their plasma concentrations are determined, usually at steady state, or various doses of a medicine are titrated until a predefined plasma concentration is achieved. In both designs, plasma concentrations are plotted against clinical response in order to determine if a relationship exists. These designs are only suitable for a selected group of drugs (e.g. short-acting intravenous anaesthetic agents); their application to a wider use is limited by the difficulties in extrapolating from plasma concentrations to effective oral dose.

These new designs are attracting considerable attention, but their place in standard dose–response studies has yet to be evaluated.

6.6.7.10.3 Dose schedules

Dose selection for exploratory studies requires knowledge of the pharmacology, toxicology, metabolism and kinetics in animals and man. This is discussed in detail in Chapter 4.

Dose selection for Phase II and III studies depends on a number of factors. These include:

1. The duration of action against the primary efficacy endpoint.

2. the pharmacokinetic characteristics of the parent compound and any active metabolites: in particular, the area under the concentration–time curve, clearance, plasma half-life and bioavailability of the formulation. On the basis of these data, it should be possible to decide on the dosing frequency for the study and the range of doses to be used. It is also possible to establish a relationship between the dynamic response and the plasma concentration of the drug (or metabolite).

3. The chances of detecting differences between intermediate doses based on the primary endpoint responses.

4. The number of study subjects (and centres) available for inclusion.

5. Whether a therapeutic or a surrogate endpoint is chosen as primary response measure.

By the end of a dose-ranging programme of studies, the sponsor should be able to define the following:

• The therapeutic dose range in the core population who will most frequently receive the drug
• The dose that is tolerated in the majority of the defined population
• The minimum effective dose(s)
• The maintenance dose range (when relevant)
• The therapeutic dose range in 'at-risk' groups, for example, the elderly, the hepatically impaired, etc.

6.6.7.11 Study subject compliance, tolerability and acceptability

Poor adherence to the schedule of taking the study medication will obviously confound interpretation of the efficacy and safety of the drug. There is usually good compliance in clinical pharmacology studies, especially those conducted in units where drugs are administered by the staff. However, in clinical research trials adherence to medication may be poorer.

Poor adherence to medication may be suspected from the assessment of compliance (e.g. tablet count, biological marker) or from a low efficacy response and/or low adverse event reporting rate. Poor compliance may result from a problem with the trial or with the medication. Features of trial design that lead to low compliance include frequent and inconvenient visits, poor relationship between the investigator and study subject and general lack of interest in the study. Problems with the medication can arise from poor acceptability (bad taste, pills too large or awkward in shape), complicated design regimen (too frequent, too many medications) or perceived or real adverse events (low tolerability). These issues can frequently be addressed in subsequent clinical trials and improvement in compliance can be expected.

During the course of the trial, compliance may be improved or assessed directly by:

1. Observing the subjects taking their medication.

2. Taking blood or urine or other biological samples to measure parent drug or metabolites.

3. Including in the medication a biological marker that is non-toxic, inert, chemically stable and easily detectable in biological fluids (such markers include riboflavin, phenol red and small quantities of digoxin).

4. making spot checks on the subjects at home.

Indirect methods to improve compliance include questioning the subject, assessing the biological response and making pill counts. The last method is not a reliable way of assessing compliance, although it is the most frequently used. It is easy to cheat, by throwing away pills or, worse, by taking a large number just prior to the clinic visit. The use of electronic counters in the cap of specially designed medicine bottles, which record the exact day and minute each time the container is opened, is possible. Obviously, it is no guarantee of ingestion, is expensive and could not easily be used in large trials. Subjects may obtain their clinical trial tablets from the pharmacist and not the investigator, and the former keeps a record of number dispensed and returned. There is some evidence that this improves compliance, as subjects seem reluctant to cheat a third party dispensing the drugs.

Assessment of compliance in a trial leads to the question as to whether the data generated from those who fail to comply should be included or excluded from analysis. The general principles that apply are that they should be excluded from Phase II (explanatory trial approach), but not from Phase III or IV trials. The reason for exclusion from Phase II is that these studies are designed to determine efficacy under well-defined eligibility criteria, and so non-compliers will dilute the efficacy response. Their data are usually included up to the point at which they discontinue, but the principle of 'last observation carried forward' should not be applied in the statistical analysis. However, the safety data from subjects up to the point of withdrawal must be included. The reason for including subjects in a Phase III trial is that the objective in these studies is to evaluate medicines under conditions that are close to clinical use in the target population. Under these circumstances, analysis is conducted on the 'intention to treat' principle, carrying forward the last observation to subsequent periods. Nevertheless, gross non-compliance throughout the trial by individual subjects warrants their exclusion. The rules governing the inclusion or exclusion of data from non-compliant subjects need to be determined during the protocol design phase.

The degree of study subject tolerability to a drug should be assessed in conjunction with the laboratory safety and efficacy data, so that an overall risk to benefit assessment can be made. Poorly tolerated drugs, however efficacious for use in self-limiting non-serious diseases, are unlikely to become successful medicines. On the other hand, study subjects with serious illnesses, such as active rheumatoid arthritis, are frequently quite prepared to put up with poorly tolerated drugs (e.g. intramuscular gold injections or intra-articular steroid injections) if efficacy is good and the alternatives are no more attractive.

6.6.8   Bias

Bias is the introduction of a systematic error or series of errors that distort the data obtained, and which may affect the analysis. Bias is distinct from random error that occurs by chance. During the design and execution phases of the trial, bias may occur in the selective sampling of subjects for the trial, in allocating the treatments, in measuring the critical endpoints and in recording safety and tolerability data. Bias may be introduced consciously or unconsciously by sponsor, investigator or study subject through a prejudice the individual may hold or through ignorance about one of these aspects in the trial design or execution.

Bias is best avoided by anticipation. Using prospective double-blind controlled trial designs incorporating stratification of subjects and randomisation of treatments rather than retrospective observational, cohort, case-controlled or uncontrolled designs will at least minimise the risk of bias. A statistician must be consulted during the protocol design stage, as many biases have a statistical basis that may not be obvious to those not trained in that discipline. Bias in execution of trial manoeuvres can be avoided by choosing objective rather than subjective assessments wherever possible, by employing validated instruments (such as questionnaires) and by using standardising techniques, for example, the questions about adverse events and the order of undertaking a series of tests. Digit preference is a recognised problem in recording numerical data, for example, in the recording of blood pressure; special instruments have been introduced to set the baseline at random so that the true recorded blood pressure is obtained by subtraction of this baseline from the observed reading.

Bias in subject selection may not be avoided simply by randomisation. Randomisation will avoid weighted allocation to one treatment regimen rather than another, but it will not avoid selection of the wrong kind of subject in the first place, which will subsequently affect the degree to which the data can be extrapolated. Thus, an investigator may have a preconceived idea about the safety of a drug or about its effectiveness in a particular subset of subjects who nonetheless meet the entry criteria. This prejudice may be avoided by stratification of subjects for defined risk factors before randomisation, so equal numbers will be allocated to the treatment regimens.

6.6.9 Sample size

A major decision is how many study subjects to recruit because this affects planning throughout the study. The sample size refers to the number of subjects who finish a trial, not to the number who enter it. The number required should be the minimum that will fulfil the objectives and test the hypothesis. For all trials, the required number of subjects is chosen on the basis of:

1. The magnitude of the effect expected on the primary efficacy endpoint – for between-group studies, the focus of interest is the level of difference that constitutes a clinically significant effect; note that this may not be the same as a statistically significant effect.

2. The variability of the measurement of the primary endpoints, that is, the mean and the standard deviation of this primary outcome measure.

3. The power or desired probability of detecting the treatment difference with a defined significance level – for most controlled trials, a power of 80% or 90% (0.8–0.9) is frequently chosen as adequate, although higher power is chosen for some studies.

The general rule is that the smaller the difference in effect to be detected between the two treatment groups, and the greater the variability in the measurement of the primary endpoint, the larger the sample size must be. Figure 6.5 gives an example of power curves, or statistical normogram,[36] that relate sample size to size of effect to be detected.

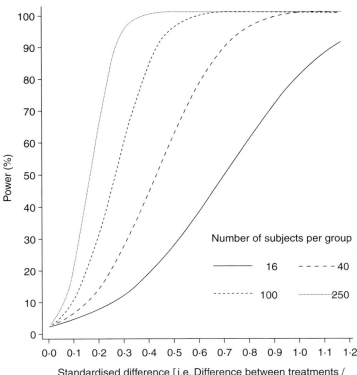

Number of subjects per group

——— 16   - - - - - 40

········ 100   ···········250

Standardised difference [i.e. Difference between treatments / standard deviation based on a two-sided test at the 0·05 level]

Fig. 6.5 Power curves: this is an illustrative method of defining the number of subjects required in a given study. In practice, the actual number would be calculated from standard equations. In this example, the curves are constructed for 16, 40, 100 and 250 subjects per group in a two-limb comparative trial. These graphs can give three pieces of information: the number of subjects that needs to be studied, given the power of the trial and the difference expected between the two treatments; the power of a trial, given the number of subjects included and the difference expected; the difference that can be detected between two groups of subjects of given number, with varying degrees of power.

Including too few subjects in a study can result in one or both of two kinds of error related to the efficacy endpoints.

1. Type I error finds a difference between treatments when in reality, none exists.
2. Type II error fails to find a difference between treatments when in reality they do differ, to an extent that might have clinical relevance.

The aim of any clinical trial is to have low risk of Type I and II errors and sufficient power to detect a difference between treatments, if it exists. Of the three factors in determining sample size, the power (probability of detecting a true difference) is arbitrarily chosen. The magnitude of the drug's effect can be estimated with more or less accuracy from previous experience with drugs of the same or similar action, and the variability of the measurements is often known from published experiments on the primary endpoint, with or without the drug. These data will, however, not be available for novel substances in a new class and frequently the sample size in the early phase of development has to be chosen on an arbitrary basis.

Many clinical trials designed to show a difference between the two drugs must be very large; for example, studies to detect improvement in mortality and morbidity after myocardial infarction or coronary artery bypass surgery involve tens of thousands of study subjects. These are major undertakings for the sponsors and require a determined commitment at the highest management levels. Conditions in which there is a high placebo response rate usually require large sample sizes, and while the literature may help in determining this placebo response rate, it often turns out to be quite different in a new trial.

In order to reduce the number of subjects on placebo in a clinical trial, some investigators employ an unequal randomisation technique, whereby fewer subjects receive placebo than receive active comparator. For example, the ratio of $1:2$, or $1:3$ may be chosen in a large clinical study. These designs are not considered acceptable by all statisticians

6.6.10   Statistical analysis of clinical trials

It is not the intention to give a detailed assessment of how to choose the correct statistical test and apply it for a given clinical study. (For this the reader is referred to Chapter 8.) Rather, some general guidelines to the use of statistical analysis will be provided.

6.6.10.1   Experimental error

Experimental errors are those inherent in the design or execution of the experiment; they are not due to bias, may be random or consistent, and may occur as a result of the instrumentation being used or in the calculation associated with the data they generate. Following GCP (see Chapter 7) will minimise errors in recording, transcribing, analysing or interpreting data.

6.6.10.2   Statistical analysis plan

The majority of studies designed and analysed by sponsors must have a significant input from a statistician. The protocol author and statistician will work together at the draft protocol stage and pay particular attention to the design strategy, avoidance of bias and the sample size. They will want to determine what size of effect they wish to observe in the trial, with what degree of statistical significance (usually at the 5% or 1% level) and with what degree of precision (usually at least 80% chance of detecting the defined useful target effect within narrow confidence intervals).

It is also necessary to decide how the primary endpoint variables will be analysed, what factors will be taken into account and how the result will be expressed. This most frequently involves analysis of variance or covariance. Predetermined comparisons of two or more treatments or doses can be made at specific time points, (e.g. each visit or selected visits) or may be assessed over time, giving an 'area under the time curve' analysis which will avoid multiple time-point analyses.

Criteria for use (or not) of data from patients who do not meet the protocol's inclusion criteria or who failed to provide complete data sets should ideally be defined before the study starts and definitely before the final analysis is initiated.

How the baseline measurement will be used in relation to the critical evaluable endpoints must be determined before analysis. Comparison of two or more treatments usually takes into account the differences between baseline values between treatment groups at the point of randomisation. The way in which the analysis will influence the report and publications needs to be decided, as some regulatory authorities have their own statistical criteria that need to be observed (e.g. for bioequivalence studies[27]).

If it is judged necessary to perform an interim analysis during the conduct of the study, the timing, purpose and possible consequences must be included in the protocol together with any necessary adjustments to the statistical approach to the final analysis.

The interpretation of the results from a clinical trial or series of trials denotes the process of discerning their clinical meaning or significance, or providing an explanation for the data under evaluation. The importance of interpretation lies both within the clinical trial and beyond it in the use to which the results will be put. Within the context of the trial itself, correct interpretation of the results will determine whether the objectives of the trial have been achieved and whether the hypothesis is proven. Interpretation beyond the immediate clinical trial concerns comparisons with other studies, extrapolation to different populations and the impact on medical practice.

6.6.10.3 Efficacy data

The efficacy endpoints defined in the protocol will be primary or secondary, and each of these may be a therapeutic or a surrogate endpoint. For each of these there is a statistical and a clinical interpretation of the results.

6.6.10.4 Statistical significance

The statistical significance relates strictly to the conditions under which the trial was conducted and will tell how often a difference of the observed size could occur by chance alone if there is, in reality, no difference between the treatments. The most widely accepted level of probability in therapeutic trials is set at 5%,

which indicates that if the no-difference or null hypothesis is true, a difference as large as that observed would occur only five times if the experiment were repeated 100 times. This is then acceptable as sufficient evidence that the null hypothesis is unlikely to be true (but not impossible); in other words, there is a real difference between the treatments. Any level of significance can be set for a given test; for example, at the 1% level, the chance of the null hypothesis being true would occur only once if the experiment were repeated 100 times. Such findings are generally said to be 'statistically highly significant' ($p = 0.01$) compared with 'statistically significant' ($p = 0.05$).

6.6.10.4.1 Confidence intervals

The statistical tests of significance determine whether an outcome could have occurred by chance. If the result of the test is that the observed difference is unlikely when there is truly no difference between treatments, it is necessary to know what degree of assurance or confidence can be placed in the power (or precision) of this estimate. For this, the confidence interval needs to be calculated. It reveals the precision of an estimate, showing the degree of uncertainty related to a result, whether or not it was statistically significant. For example, a result from a trial showing that a drug reduces systolic blood pressure by 2 mmHg may well be statistically significant, but it may be clinically meaningless. Doctors are interested in the size of the difference and the degree of assurance or confidence they can have in the precision (reproducibility) of this estimate. Confidence intervals are expressed as a range of values within which one can be 95% (or other chosen percentage) certain that the true value lies. The range may be broad, indicating uncertainty, or narrow, indicating a higher degree of certainty. Confidence intervals are thus extremely useful in the interpretation of small studies, as they show the degree of uncertainty related to a result whether or not it was statistically significant. Indeed, a finding of 'not statistically significant' can only be interpreted as meaning that there is no clinically useful difference, if the confidence

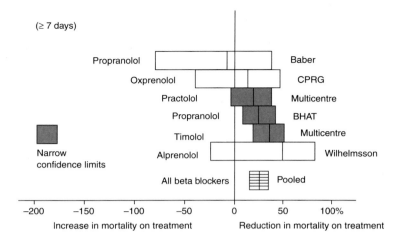

Fig. 6.6 Effect of beta blockers on post-infarction mortality. Difference in mortality rates is expressed as a percentage of control rate in six controlled trials of beta blockers (95% confidence intervals based on odds ratio consideration). Narrow confidence intervals are associated with the largest trials that are the major contributors to the pooled result.

interval of the result is also stated and is narrow. If the confidence interval is wide, a real difference may have been missed in a trial of a given size. Inevitably, this means that the sample size was too small[39] (see Figure 6.6).

The confidence intervals provide information on the likelihood of falling into Type I errors. However, the person interpreting the efficacy results must decide, as a guide for action, what target difference and what probability level (for either type of error) he or she will accept when using the results. The statistical significance test alone will not provide this information. It does not prove that a difference is due to one treatment being better than another (or not better); it merely provides the probabilities of the event. The significance findings and the interpretation of the position of the observed effect in relation to the zero point in the confidence interval can be combined to permit an interpretation of the clinical importance to be placed on the findings.

Although a 'statistically significant' result of observed differences between treated groups may be achieved (with narrow 95% confidence intervals which do not include zero), the difference observed may still be clinically unimportant. The setting of the target difference and achieving a narrow confidence interval about that difference will certainly help, but it is finally up to the clinical judgement of the sponsor and

investigator to decide on the clinical relevance of the finding.

6.6.11 Use and extrapolation of efficacy data

The effects of treatments on efficacy endpoints can be used for several different purposes. They may be used to set a new hypothesis in further clinical studies. This is particularly the case for unexpected findings, such as a negative result despite a well-conducted trial, or a positive result which is difficult to interpret, such as failing to show a difference between several doses of a drug, despite there being an overall difference compared with placebo. In Phase III, it is unusual for one clinical study to be conducted in isolation. Regulatory authorities usually require a minimum of two pivotal trials and the sponsors would probably undertake two studies in order to be sufficiently confident to proceed. These two pivotal trials are usually planned at the same time, but the results from one may be awaited in order to help design the second. The sponsor will wish to use the efficacy results from Phase II and III studies to make a therapeutic claim. The interpretation of the efficacy data will determine the target population for whom that claim is made, and while sponsors may wish this to be as wide as possible, the claim must reflect the trial population that has been studied. This will, of necessity, involve an interpretation of safety data in conjunction with efficacy results.

Once registration is granted, a new medicine will be compared both formally, within clinical trials, and informally, by clinical usage, with currently available medicines. Company representatives, both medical and commercial, will draw to the attention of potential prescribers the results of the major registration trials in published literature (sponsored or peer reviewed), in advertisements and at meetings. The key question for the individual physician with regard to the new drug will be 'How large a response in the most important efficacy variables is necessary to convince me that the new therapy is worth using in my patients?'. This will be supplemented by other questions relating to safety and, in turn, the risk:benefit ratio, the effects on quality of life, patient acceptance of the new medicine and costs of treatment. The wise clinical practitioner will scrutinise the results of the major efficacy trials and compare the study subject populations studied therein with his own patients. Because clinical trials.are designed to reduce the variability of response, early disappointments with new drugs used in medical practice frequently arise from circumstances outside the control of clinical studies. For example, usage in the home environment compared with hospital-based clinical trials or constant use of self-prescribed medications in clinical practice may confound interpretation of results if outside the clinical trial environment.

Recent publications on major clinical trials whose implications will involve a recommendation to change clinical practice have included summary statistics that quantify the risk of benefit or harm that may occur if the results of a given trial are strictly applied to an individual patient or to a representative cohort. Four simple calculations will enable the non-statistician to answer the simple question 'How much better would my chances be (in terms of a particular outcome) if I took this new medicine, than if I did not take it?'.[24] These calculations are: the relative risk reduction, the absolute risk reduction, the number needed to treat, and the odds ratio (see Box 6.3).

Box 6.3   Summarising benefit

Group	Outcome event		
	Yes	No	Total
Control group	a	b	$a+b$
Experimental group	c	d	$c+d$

Control event rate	= risk outcome event in control group, that is, $$\text{CER} = \frac{a}{a+b}$$
Experimental event rate	= risk of outcome event in experimental group, that is, $$\text{EER} = \frac{c}{c+d}$$
Relative risk reduction (RRR)	$$= \frac{\text{CER} - \text{EER}}{\text{CER}}$$
Absolute risk reduction (AAR)	= CER − EER
Number needed to treat (NNT)	= 1/AAR = 1/(CER − EER)
Odds ratio =	$$\frac{\text{(Odds of outcome event versus odds of no event) in experimental group}}{\text{(Odds of outcome event versus odds of no event) in control group}}$$

6.6.11.1   Interpretation of efficacy data at a healthcare level

Within the last 20 years or so, three major features of controlled clinical trials, in particular, have permitted significant advances in deciding whether treatments are of value or not: randomisation, systematic review and meta-analysis, and the concept of the large-scale, simple (to understand and conduct) randomised trial in areas where only moderate benefits can be expected.[40,41] All of these elements are likely to underpin future trials for purposes of regulation, pharmacoeconomics and healthcare policy. Yet there is no room for complacency or allowing standards to slip. Systematic reviews of some of the hundreds of thousands of trials published since 1948 are revealing that, in many trials, inadequate steps were taken to control biases, and insufficient numbers of participants were studied to yield reliable estimates of effects, that is, much effort, money and subject participation have been wasted. The pressure to give greater public access to types of, and results from, clinical trials is to be applauded on one hand, but the quality of those trials and their interpretation must be carefully investigated.

6.7 Sponsorship of Therapeutic Trials

The main sponsors of therapeutic trials are the pharmaceutical companies. Therapeutic trials are needed for regulatory approval of new medicinal products. Indeed, the manufacturer holds the investigational license and controls the supply of the trial medication. The medical department of the pharmaceutical company will be responsible for preparing a plan of development, which may be subject to alteration as the clinical data accumulates. The medical department will decide on the design and objectives of the clinical trial, prepare the protocol and select the comparative medicines and the investigators. Their decisions are crucial if the clinical data obtained are to convince the regulatory authorities to grant a marketing application.

The advent of a more active monitoring role by the sponsor and audits with the global framework of ICH GCP and other guidelines has significantly increased the quality of therapeutic trials sponsored by pharmaceutical companies. The new standards now also apply to trials conducted independently by individual clinicians.

Post-marketing trials of recently licensed medicines have been used as an opportunity for a pharmaceutical company to familiarise a doctor with a new product. Such studies have more to do with the marketing department of the pharmaceutical company than with serious research. Although regulatory authorities do not encourage such studies, there are undoubtedly several therapeutic issues, particularly related to safety, that remain to be answered at the time when a new medical product is licensed and marketed. Studies addressing these issues are termed PMS and safety assessment of marketed medicines (SAMM) studies and are usually carried out at the request of the regulatory authorities. Large sponsored clinical trials may be required for the investigation of post-marketing safety issues. The clinical trial should involve treatment of study subjects under normal clinical conditions rather than the more specialised environment of a clinical trial. In other cases, post-marketing clinical trials allow combination therapy or medico-economic benefits of the treatment to be evaluated (see Chapter 26). Whatever the nature of the trial, the principles spelt out in ICH GCP Chapter 2[6] still apply.

6.8 Ownership of Clinical Trial Data

In the past, various individuals and organisations have claimed to own the data produced from a clinical trial, including the state, the sponsor, the investigator and, in some cases, the patient or study subject. It is certainly true that with the advent of the EU Directive on Data Protection, the claim of ownership to his or her data by the patient or study subject has been strengthened. Unfortunately, there is no clear ownership of clinical data except that of society. Even then, society needs to respect the confidentiality and other wishes of individual subjects who have been clinical trial participants. Is there a difference in ownership between data produced from product-driven research to that produced in policy-driven therapeutic research?

In product-driven therapeutic research, the pharmaceutical company must satisfy the regulatory and government agencies as well as the prescribers that the new product is effective, safe and meets the qualities required of GMP. The institutions that will pay for the drug – an insurance company or a government health authority – will need to be convinced that the product is good value. In return, the pharmaceutical company may, at some time in the future, recoup sufficient profit to pay the shareholders but also to pay for the development of the product. In the past, pharmaceutical companies avoided their results being made available for inspection. The ownership of the clinical data was clearly that of the pharmaceutical company. However, the ever-increasing requirements of the regulatory authorities and the creation of inspectorates to enforce these requirements mean that the majority of pharmaceutical companies will provide all the data obtained from a clinical trial if requested by an appropriate authority. This has been reinforced by the new Declaration of Helsinki (Edinburgh 2000),[8] which requires the publication of both negative and positive results (Principle 27), and ICH GCP, where clinical trial reports need to be provided whether the clinical trials are completed or not.

Fundamental healthcare issues may also be involved in the situation of policy-driven therapeutic research. The future investment of society in health may require a large-scale national clinical trial to answer questions relating to the prevention of disease or premature death. This type of clinical trial will not simply relate to one manufacturer's product. As such, it is preferable that the trial is organised on a national level, not necessarily with the exclusion of the company(s) involved. An independent data-monitoring committee (IDMC) should oversee the clinical trial with as much support from the pharmaceutical company(s) as possible. The clinical data collected belongs to the state and should be treated with the same quality standards as any pharmaceutical company sponsored study.

6.9   The Final Report

ICH Guideline E3[42] describes how the clinical trial report should be prepared. The format should allow someone to repeat the trial, using an identical design and to re-analyse it or examine it more closely. The writing of the report ought to rest with those who contributed most to it in terms of design, conduct and analysis. Several authors may contribute to the writing of the report, covering the medical aspects, the statistics and interpretation. A medical writer may be involved in editing the contributions so

as to try to achieve uniformity of style and content. The pharmaceutical physician, either as the sponsor's medical input or as the investigator, should take particular interest in certain sections where his or her expertise will ensure that the correct medical terminology is used and that the interpretation is acceptable. The main findings of the study should be discussed in relation to the validity of the methods, the natural history of the disease and the subject population. The clinical relevance will need to be reviewed, and comparison of the study drug or treatment made with current practice. Limitations of the study, such as inconsistencies between measured parameters, protocol violations and target population, should be assessed.

Most clinical trials have problems, sometimes detected by inspection and audit. These can usually be resolved and, if so, the regulatory submission must include a full explanation of how they were dealt with. Therefore, an audit trail with all the data should be available, accompanied by a statement by QA confirming that the procedures have been audited.

Within the report, graphs should be consistent in format, for example, bar charts running vertically or horizontally but not both. The tables should be assembled in an identical format. Thus, the reader can easily read each of them and be equally comfortable when looking at an overall summary.

A target date for completion should always be set to ensure that any further developments are not held up by the lack of a report.

6.10   Regulatory Submissions

The submission must be formatted in a manner that is consistent with the requirements of the regulatory agency that will review the submission. The dossier may include 20 or more individual clinical trial reports. They should be uniform in format to assist the reader to assimilate evidence readily and to compare it between trials. The whole dossier should be one of accuracy, consistency and meticulous cross-referencing. Once again, the effort to reach these objectives must be made in the early planning stages.

The processes are changing for regulatory submissions. Three major drives are taking place or are about to take place:

1. Electronic submissions or CANDAs are being made instead of paper submission, particularly in the United States.
2. The development of electronic standards for the transfer of regulatory information.[34]
3. The publication of the organisation of the Common Technical Document.[43]

These changes mean that, very soon, submissions will be made globally using computer technology and with an identical dossier format. The advantages will be that the regulatory agencies will be able to interrogate the data, thereby avoiding delays in requesting responses from sponsors; the reviewers will have easy access to the whole submission, without the involvement of large amounts of paper; and there will be better consistency and quality in the reports because the format of the dossier will be clearly defined.

6.10.1   The expert report

When the new ICH Common Technical Document[43] is fully adopted, the pharmaceutical physician may be called upon to write an expert report or a clinical overview. It is essential that whoever writes the report or overview should have a good understanding of the trial. Inaccuracies are too frequent. The report is a comprehensive and critical review of the data submitted in the licence application and should not be more than 25 pages long (30 pages in the case of the clinical overview). The object of the report is to facilitate the review by the assessor and it should address the properties of safety and efficacy of the study drug, with cross-reference to the clinical study reports. The report will need to support the proposed labelling. It has several sections including: a problem statement (i.e. product development rationale), clinical pharmacology, clinical trials, conclusions and a reference list. In general, summaries of this nature should be in a linguistic style that is appropriate to a non-specialist, in clear simple English with repetition studiously avoided.

6.11   Publications

The dissemination of information to the scientific community is essential for the progress of research. Publications in scientific journals provide a key source of information. In the case of medical research, patients' lives may be at stake. There are other reasons for publication. Publication will provide prestige to the investigator, to the sponsor and to the institutions involved in the research. In addition, in some circumstances the published paper will be quoted in reference dictionaries and pharmacopoeia, in advertisements and other promotions. The pharmaceutical physician should take every opportunity to publish high-quality scientific papers, even if the findings are not sensational but provide useful additional information.

Publications must follow the journal style and therefore some rewriting of the final trial report will be required. The main problem is the provision of fewer data, usually in a summarised form, in a published paper. These amendments might be made by non-company authors or by editorial staff. The checking of these changes is crucial, as those making the changes have less knowledge of the database and may be prone to making mistakes. Proofreading must be thorough.

6.11.1   Authorship of publications

The basic principle accepted by biomedical editors is for authors to be responsible for those sections of the work performed by them. It follows that company staff should be authors. Indeed, it is important for readers to know their involvement. However, from time to time some company executives argue that their involvement might be construed as biasing the trial and therefore that they should be excluded. This attitude should be resisted as detrimental to the professional role and standing of the company staff and, potentially, to the quality of the resultant publication.

Some journals request that authors specify the individual contributions of authors to a paper, for example, original concept, statistical analysis and writer. They also insist on statements about sources of funding and competing interests.

These moves are welcome because they help to ascribe ownership and responsibility, and give a chance for more equal representation from commercial, academic and regulatory sources.

6.12   Conclusion

The controlled clinical trial is invaluable. It has been developed and refined so that it can offer reliable answers to most questions, but, like all tools, it is sometimes misused.

The therapeutic benefits and risks of a medicine, and therefore the choice of treatment for an individual patient, stem from evidence from a series of clinical trials. Taken together, these trials should reflect all likely therapeutic situations. From time to time, a particular problem arises that generates a new hypothesis. In order to obtain an answer to the specific question, we sometimes restrict the population sample to study subjects who do not possess a number of variables that may confound the outcome. In this manner, we move away from the realities of everyday clinical practice to an idealised, but artificial, environment. This is justifiable if the restriction is logical and if, with it, the hypothesis testing can be successfully completed. Otherwise, the issue may never be settled.

However, from time to time such restrictions on the population are perpetuated. The reasons may not be stated and even not recognised by many involved. This perpetuation of restriction may be an unthinking and even unwitting design feature, extended from the type of specific investigation to which we have just referred. On the other hand, the restriction may be deliberate in order to secure an early and clear-cut therapeutic outcome. Such distortion of therapeutic situations and practice can be misleading. Specific groups of study subjects may not be adequately studied, even though they will represent part of the target population once the medicine is approved for general use.

The development of new medicinal products for narrower indications in serious, and usually poorly understood, diseases, such as multiple sclerosis and motor neurone disease, have resulted in a closer approximation of study subjects selected for the controlled clinical trial to the patients encountered in clinical practice. Many of these products are biologically derived, and while efficacy in the two situations may be similar, longer and larger trials will be needed to fully appreciate adverse event profiles.

The impact of pharmacogenetics and pharmacoeconomics on clinical trial design, regulatory action and clinical usage is only just being appreciated. Technological advances that will make genetic approaches, in their broadest terms, possible are coming at a time when there is high pressure to contain the cost of drug treatment. The move by governments to widen the prescribing of medicines for patients to healthcare professionals other than doctors, and indeed to increase direct sales of medicines to patients is part of a cost containment drive. One can envisage a market in which the following access to medicines may be present:

1. Direct sales to patients or via pharmacists and other healthcare professionals.
2. Growth of the generic market as cheaper alternatives.
3. Continued but decreasing number of small molecules, which, in order to gain a place in Clinical usage, will have to satisfy increasingly stringent cost-effectiveness criteria.
4. Development of high technology products for select groups.

Regulatory authorities will have to respond to such a challenge by defining what kind of clinical trials will be pivotal to gain marketing authorisation. For example, for a new medicinal product indicated for a genotypically (or phenotypically) defined subgroup of patients with essential hypertension, how much study subject exposure for safety evaluation will be required? If the hypothesis of 'specific drug for specific disease/study subject' is valid in this example, how ethical will it be to conduct a placebo-controlled trial and how relevant is it to conduct a comparison with a non-specific active control?

These and other questions will challenge the selection of trial designs during drug development, but the principles described in this chapter will remain.

The next few years will witness a greater partnership between industry, regulatory authorities and universities. Attempts to harmonise the conduct of clinical trials between these three agencies is a positive move. Hopefully, the outcome will be the minimum necessary number of clinical trials, each of which will be designed well enough to make a contribution both to the evaluation of a particular drug development and eventually to the therapeutic armamentarium available for the patient's benefit.

References

1. Armitage P. Bradford Hill and the randomised controlled trial. *Pharm Med* 1992;**6**:23–7.
2. International Conference on Harmonisation of Technical Requirements of Pharmaceuticals for Human Use (ICH). *Topic E8 Note for Guidance on General Considerations for Clinical Trials, CPMP/ICH/291/95*. London: European Agency for the Evaluation of Medicinal Products, 1997.
3. Peto R, Baigent C. Trials: the next 50 years. *BMJ* 1998;**317**:1170–1.
4. Chalmers I, Altman DG. Meta-analysis in context. In: *Systematic Reviews in Healthcare*. London: BMJ Publishing, 1995.
5. International Conference on Harmonisation of Technical Requirements of Pharmaceuticals for Human Use (ICH). *Topic E5 Note for Guidance on Ethnic Factors in the Acceptability of Foreign Clinical Data, CPMP/ICH/289/95*. London: European Agency for the Evaluation of Medicinal Products, 1998.
6. International Conference on Harmonisation of Technical Requirements of Pharmaceuticals for Human Use (ICH). *Topic E6 Note for Guidance on Good Clinical Practice: Consolidated Guideline, CPMP/ICH/135/95*. London: European Agency for the Evaluation of Medicinal Products, 1996.
7. Food Drug Administration (FDA). *Protection of Human Subjects Code of Federal Regulations, Title 21, Part 50–55*. Washington: US Government Printing Office, 1997.
8. World Medical Association (WMA). Declaration of Helsinki, 52nd WMA General Assembly, Edinburgh, Scotland. Available at: http://www.wma.net/e/policy/17-c_e.html. Assessed 26 July, 2001.
9. World Health Organization (WHO). Technical Report Series, No. 850. *Annex 3 Guidelines for Good Clinical Practice* (GCP) *for Trials on Pharmaceutical Products*. Geneva, Switzerland: World Health Organization, 1995 (Modified 2000).
10. European Parliament. Directive 2001/20/EC of the European parliament and of the council of 04 April 2001 on the approximation of the laws, regulations and administrative provisions of the member states relating to the implementation of good clinical practice in the conduct of clinical trials on medicinal products for human use. *OJC* 2001; **121**:34–44.
11. Association of the British Pharmaceutical Industry. *Clinical Trial Compensation Guidelines, 418/94/6600M*. London: ABPI, 1994.
12. Roses AD. Pharmacogenetics and future drug development and delivery. *Lancet* 2000;**355**:1358–61.
13. Wolf CR, Smith G, Smith RL. Pharmacogenetics. *BMJ* 2000;**320**:987–90.
14. Pharmacogenetics Working Party Report. *Int J Pharm Med* 2001;**15**:59–100.
15. Meyer UA. Pharmacogenetics and adverse drug reactions. *Lancet* 2000;**356**:1667–71.
16. Dickins M, Tucker G. Drug disposition: to phenotype or genotype. *Int J Pharm Med* 2001;**15**:70–3.
17. Lindpaintner K, Foot E, Curlfield M, *et al.* Pharmacogenetics: focus on pharmacodynamics. *Int J Pharm Med* 2001;**15**:74–82.
18. International Conference on Harmonisation of Technical Requirements of Pharmaceuticals for Human Use (ICH). *Topic E11 Note for Guidance on Clinical Investigation of Medicinal Products in the Paediatric Population, CPMP/ICH/2711/99*. London: European Agency for the Evaluation of Medicinal Products, 1999 (Draft).
19. Committee for Proprietary Medicinal Products. *Note for Guidance on Clinical Investigation of Medicinal Products in Children, CPMP/EWP/462/95*. London: European Agency for the Evaluation of Medicinal Products, 1997.
20. Food and Drug Administration (FDA). Regulations requiring manufacturers to assess the safety and effectiveness of new drugs and biological products in pediatric patients. *Federal Register* 1998;**63**:632–72.
21. International Conference on Harmonisation of Technical Requirements of Pharmaceuticals for Human Use (ICH). *Topic E7 Note for Guidance on Studies to Support of Special Populations: Geriatrics,*

CPMP/ICH/379/95. London: European Agency for the Evaluation of Medicinal Products, 1994.

22. Pharmacokinetics in patients with impaired hepatic function; pharmacokinetics in patients with impaired renal function. @www.fda.gov/opacom/morechoices/industry/guidedc.htm

23. Rolan P. The contribution of clinical pharmacology surrogates and models to drug development – a clinical appraisal. *Br J Clin Pharmacol* 1997;**44**:219–25.

24. Greenhalgh T. *How to Read a Paper; The Basis of Evidence-based Medicine.* London: BMJ Publishing, 1997;93–5.

25. Temple R, Ellenburg SS. Placebo-controlled trials and active-control trials in the evaluation of new treatments. *Ann Int Med* 2000;**133**:455–63.

26. Lewis JA, Jonsson B, Kreutz G, *et al.* Placebo-controlled trials and the Declaration of Helsinki: Committee on Proprietary and Medicinal Products. *Br J Clin Pharmacol* 2001;**52**:223–9.

27. Committee for Proprietary Medicinal Products. *Note for Guidance on the investigation of Bioavailability and Bioequivalence, CPMP/EWP/QWP/1401/98.* London: European Agency for the Evaluation of Medicinal Products, 2000 (Draft).

28. International Conference on Harmonisation of Technical Requirements of Pharmaceuticals for Human Use (ICH). *Topic E10 Note for Guidance on Choice of Control Group in Clinical Trials, CPMP/ICH/364/96.* London: European Agency for the Evaluation of Medicinal Products, 2001.

29. Jones B, Jarvis P, Lewis JA, *et al.* Trial to assess equivalence: the importance of rigorous methods. *BMJ* 1996;**313**:36–9.

30. Lewis JA. Switching between superiority and non-inferiority. *Br J Clin Pharmacol* 2001;**52**: 223–80.

31. Senn SJ. *Cross-over, Sequential and Dose Finding Studies. Statistical Issues in Drug Development.* Chichester: John Wiley, 1997;237–9;257–64; 275–7.

32. International Conference on Harmonisation of Technical Requirements of Pharmaceuticals for Human Use (ICH). *Topic E9 Note for Guidance on Statistical Considerations in the Design of Clinical Trials, CPMP/ICH/363/96.* London: European Agency for the Evaluation of Medicinal Products, 1998.

33. Resuscitation Council (UK). *CPR Guidance for Clinical Practice and Training in Hospitals.* London: Resuscitation Council, 2001.

34. International Conference on Harmonisation of Technical Requirements of Pharmaceuticals for Human Use (ICH). *Topic M2 Electronic Standards for the Transfer of Regulatory Information* (Draft). Available at: http://www.ifpma.org/ich5e.html. Accessed 21 July 2001.

35. Baber NS. What does the investigator need to know about the drug? In: Cohen A, Posner J, eds. *A Guide to Clinical Drug Research.* London: Kluwer Academic, 1996;17–37.

36. Bowman WC, Rand M. *Textbook of Pharmacology, 2nd edn.* Oxford: Blackwell Scientific, 1980.

37. Sheiner LD, Hoshimoto Y, Beal SL. A simulation study comparing design for dose-ranging. *Stat Med* 1991;**10**:303–21.

38. Sheiner LD, Beal SL, Sambol NC. Study designs for dose ranging. *Clin Pharmacol Ther* 1989;**46**: 63–77.

39. Lewis JA, Ellis SH. A statistical appraisal of post-infarction in beta blocker trials. *BMJ* 1982;31–7.

40. Egger M, Davey Smith G, Altman DG, eds. *Systematic Reviews in Healthcare: Meta-analysis in Context, 2nd edn.* London: BMJ Books, 2001.

41. Chalmers I, Haynes B. Systematic reviews: reporting, updating, and correcting systematic reviews of the effects of healthcare. *BMJ* 1994;**309**:852–65.

42. International Conference on Harmonisation of Technical Requirements of Pharmaceuticals for Human Use (ICH). *Topic E3 Note for Guidance on Structure and Content of Clinical Study Reports, CPMP/ICH/137/95.* London: European Agency for the Evaluation of Medicinal Products, 1996.

43. International Conference on Harmonisation of Technical Requirements of Pharmaceuticals for Human Use (ICH). *Topic M4 Organisation of Common Technical Document for the Registration of Pharmaceuticals for Human Use, CPMP/ICH/2887/99.* London: European Agency for the Evaluation of Medicinal Products, 2000.

Recommended Reading

Friedman LM, Furberg CD, DeMets DL. *Fundamentals of Clinical Trials, 3rd edn.* New York: Springer-Verlag, 1998.

Laurence D, Bennett P, Brown M. *Clinical Pharmacology, 8th edn.* Sidcup, UK: Churchill Livingstone, 1997.

Rang HP, Dale MM, Ritter JM. *Pharmacology, 4th edn.* Sidcup, UK: Churchill Livingstone, 1999.

Senn S. *Statistical Issues in Drug Development.* Chichester, UK: John Wiley, 1997.

Spilker B. *Guide to Clinical Trials.* New York: Raven Press, 1991.

Useful Internet Addresses

British Pharmacopoeia	www.pharmacopoeia.org.uk
Centers for Disease Control	www.cdc.gov
Central Office for Research Ethics Committees (COREC)	www.corec.org.uk
Drug Information Association	www.diahome.org
European Drug Regulatory Affairs	www.eudra.org
European National Medicines Authorities	www.heads.medagencies.org
FDA	www.fda.gov
Food and Drug Law Institute (FDLI)	www.fdli.org
ICH	www.ifpma.org/ich1.html
Medicines and Healthcare products Regulatory Agency (MHRA)	www.mhra.gov.uk
National Institutes of Health	www.nih.gov
National Library of Medicine	www.nlm.nih.gov
Regulatory Affairs Professional Society (RAPS)	www.raps.org
Pharmaceutical Research Manufacturers Association	www.phrma.org
US Pharmacopeia	www.usp.org
World Health Organisation (WHO)	www.who.ch

CHAPTER 7

7

Conduct of clinical trials: good clinical practice

Roger A Yates

7.1 Introduction

This chapter is written primarily as a guide to running trials with new chemical entities during drug development. The principles described are also directly relevant to all other trials such as those comparing two or more licensed treatments (which may themselves be combinations) and research studies initiated and conducted in academic institutions without any support from the Pharmaceutical Industry. There will be some differences of detail in those other circumstances.

7.2 Good Clinical Practice

The procedures for assuring quality of clinical trials have evolved over the past 30 years, culminating in several published guidelines. There are three key good clinical practice (GCP) documents – the GCP guidelines of the International Conference on Harmonisation (ICH) of Technical Requirements for the Registration of Pharmaceuticals for Human Use, the Code of Federal Regulations (21 CFR) of the United States and the Declaration of Helsinki.[1–4] In today's global climate, the pharmaceutical physician should work to ICH GCP, of which the Declaration of Helsinki is the foundation.

Apart from a few minor differences, the FDA[5] has adopted the ICH GCP guidelines. The contents of the FDA Code of Regulations with reference to the protection of human subjects, institutional review boards and investigational new drug (IND) applications provide information for new study drugs that will need to be registered in the United States. Most potential new drugs will be marketed in the United States in order to reap a financial return.

Two other documents are relevant to clinical trials: the World Health Organisation (WHO) Guidelines for Good Clinical Practice for trials on pharmaceutical products,[6] still used for clinical trials in some parts of the world, and the new EU Clinical Trial Directive.[7]

7.2.1 Declaration of Helsinki

The principles of medical research are based on the Declaration of Helsinki. The general assemblies of the World Medical Association (WMA) have, since 1964, made recommendations for guiding physicians in clinical research involving human subjects. Although not legally binding, the Declaration forms the foundation of all other significant international documents on the ethical conduct of biomedical research.

The Helsinki Declaration covers all the important ethical considerations, such as the involvement of a qualified physician in any clinical trial, putting the well-being of the study subject before science and society, the use of scientific principles in the design of the study, the need for informed consent and a review by an ethics review committee; in fact, all areas covered by the ICH GCP.

In October 2000, the latest revision of the Declaration of Helsinki[4] was approved by the

WMA (see Appendix 1). The new version is very different from previous versions, with more detail on how clinical trials should be conducted. It requires that study subjects should have access to the best treatment identified by the study once the study has been completed. It also recommends that local participants in a study should be able to benefit from the study results, whether they are positive or negative. These principles were approved to avoid the exploitation of economically poor countries. In addition, the Declaration requires greater transparency regarding economic incentives involved in clinical research.

7.2.2   ICH GCP

In the 1950's, drug development experienced several events that gave weight to greater harmonisation within countries initially, and then, internationally. Earlier in the United States, a terrible mistake in the formulation of a children's syrup in the 1930s forced the American government to initiate the creation of a product authorisation system under the FDA. The thalidomide tragedy in Europe alerted many regulatory authorities to the dangers as well as the benefits of new synthetic drugs. Safety considerations in addition to efficacy became paramount in new drug treatments. With the public expectation for new drugs to be both safe and effective came an escalation of the cost of research, and an ever-increasing healthcare bill for governments.

Global harmonisation was felt to be an acceptable solution in reducing costs by avoiding unnecessary duplication of clinical trials in humans and by minimising the use of animal testing. Hence in 1990, drug regulatory authorities of the EU, Japan and the United States got together with representatives from the pharmaceutical industry to try to reach a consensus on the safety, quality and efficacy requirements for authorisation new medicinal products. This was the beginning of ICH.

At that time, the methodology for conducting clinical trials was very variable and there were a considerable number of guidelines from regions and countries relating to the conduct of clinical trials. Global directors of pharmaceutical companies would have a shelf full of the various versions of GCP guidelines, many of them country specific. With the advent of ICH GCP, a more uniform process of conducting clinical trials has been achieved globally. Many countries have modified the format of ICH GCP to the local conditions, but in general, the principles of ICH GCP have been observed.

7.2.3   EU Directive (2001/20/EC)

A new Directive[7] has been authorised by the EU to cover clinical trials undertaken in the EU. Each country has been required to adopt the Directive since 01 May 2004. Before the Directive was approved, there were variations between EU countries both in the legal requirements and, in some cases, the actual procedures adopted for conducting clinical trials, some countries adopting more vigorous ethical and scientific methodologies than others. For example, the GCP inspectorate in the United Kingdom had to be 'invited' to conduct most inspections since there was no legal basis for normal routine inspections. The Directive is designed to simplify and harmonise the administrative provisions governing trials and will apply to both commercial and non-commercial studies including healthy volunteer (Phase I) studies. Only non-interventional trials, where the assignment of the patient to a particular therapeutic strategy is not decided in advance by a protocol, are excluded from the scope of the Directive. In non-interventional trials, the treatment of the subject falls within current practice and the prescription of the medicine is clearly separate from the decision to include the subject in the study. No additional diagnostic or monitoring procedures will be applied to the subject.

The Directive covers:

- National authority approval
- Study subject benefit and risk
- The use of children and adults who are unable to give consent
- Establishment of ethics committees in each member country

- Establishment of inspectorates to verify GCP standards
- Setting up of a European database for all member states with clinical trial information (to limit unnecessary trials)
- Good manufacturing practices (GMPs) for study drugs and the provision for a manufacturing licence for investigational medicinal products (IMPs), and labelling requirements
- Pharmacovigilance standards
- Gene therapy trials and xenogenic cell therapy.

7.3   Preparation of Documentation for the Clinical Trial

7.3.1   The study master files

This term is generally used to denote the administration file kept for each trial and each investigation centre. Box 7.1 lists some of the documents that need to be present before a clinical trial starts. (See ICH GCP Chapter 8[1] for the full list.) Once the study has started, other documents will be added, including completed CRFs, ICFs and subjects' medical records and other documents directly involved in the study. Some documents have to be kept specifically at the sponsor's office or the controlling centre. Separate files will contain financial and budget-related documents.

7.3.1.1   The protocol

This document describes the objectives, design, methodology, statistical considerations and organisation of a trial. Other information should be present, such as the background and rationale, for the clinical trial. It is a document key to any clinical trial. There should be a logical approach to preparing a protocol (see Box 7.2).

7.3.1.2   Approach to construction of the protocol

Most pharmaceutical companies will have their own format for a protocol. Independent investigators will adopt their own or their institution's

format. All should follow the elements described in the ICH GCP guidelines (Chapter 6).[1]

Box 7.1   Study master files

- Investigator's brochure and all updates
- Signed protocol and amendments
- Sample of clinical record form (CRF)
- Copies of informed consent form (ICF) and all new versions that were given to subjects
- Copies of any other written documents to be given to subjects
- Copy of any advertisement for subject recruitment
- Financial agreement
- Signed agreement between involved parties – CRO, sponsor, investigator, institution
- Dated documentation of independent ethics committee (IEC) approval for:
  - Protocol and amendments
  - Information sheet/ICF and all versions given to subjects
  - Any other written documentation given to subjects
  - Advertisements
  - Details of subject compensation
  - Receipt of investigator's brochure (letters should clearly indicate what documents were received and when)
- Composition of IEC including professions and sex (signed and dated)
- Written procedures of IEC
- Statement that the IEC will work to ICH GCP
- Financial disclosure documents
- Regulatory authorities approval of study/investigator
- *Curriculum vitae* demonstrating that the site staff are qualified to do the study (signed and dated)
- *Curriculum vitae* for all monitoring staff demonstrating that they are trained to do their respective tasks[a]
- 'Normal' values/ranges for laboratory data – dated and signed by laboratory/investigator including updates
- Laboratory procedures – minimum methodology – dated and signed by laboratory/investigator
- Certification, accreditation or some other information, such as external quality assessment and internal quality control procedures, indicating

Box 7.1   Continued

that the laboratory is involved in producing quality data

- Sample of all labels used on study drugs[a]
- Shipping records for study drugs
- Receipts for the site receiving study drugs (signed by investigator and dated)
- Study drug accountability log at site
- Return shipping documents indicating what study drug went back to sponsor or destruction certificate indicating what was destroyed at site (once study has started)
- Instructions for handling study drug – may be in protocol or investigator's brochure
- Certificates of analysis for study drug (there should be clear indication that the study drug was prepared according to GMP)
- Decoding procedures for blinded studies
- Master randomisation list – to document the method of randomisation in the study population but *not* the actual codes[b]
- Study initiation monitoring report
- Monitoring reports[a]
- Site visitors log
- Subject screening log (if appropriate)
- Subject identification log[c]
- Subject enrolment log (if appropriate)
- Documentation in relation to CRF corrections
- Signature sheets for all staff involved in the study (including sponsor/CRO[a])
- Source documents[c]
- Signed and dated CRFs
- Form for recording the blood samples/tissue samples for special analysis (perhaps stored in fridge/freezer before dispatch)
- Notification documents and reports in relation to SAEs, etc. for sponsor, IECs and regulatory authorities
- Annual reports to IECs
- General communications, telephone messages, letters, etc. concerning the scientific conduct of the study
- Insurance/indemnity details
- Clinical study reports

[a] Normally only at the sponsor site
[b] Open codes identifying treatment of subjects in a blind study will only be with the statistician and/or supplier of study drug during the study
[c] Only at the investigator site

Box 7.2   The main contents of the protocol (ICH GCP Chapter 6)[1]

The following elements should be present:

- Front page (or following pages)
  Number (unique to protocol)
  Protocol study title
  Protocol identifying number
  Date and version of protocol
  Name and address of the sponsor or institution
  Name, title and address of the sponsor's medical expert for the trial
  Name, title, address of the investigator with his/her telephone number
  Monitor's address and telephone number of the pharmaceutical company
  Name and address of clinical laboratory and other institutions involved in study
- Signature page
  Signed by representatives of:
  Sponsor
  Statistician responsible for the statistical plan
  Investigator
- Summary
  Introduction
  Objectives
  Subject entry
  Treatments
  Study design
  Interventions and measurements
  Adverse events and laboratory safety tests
  Criteria for assessment
- Contents page
- Introduction
  Non-clinical studies with clinical significance
  Clinical trials relevant to the trial
  Known and potential risks
  Potential benefits
  Name and description of study drug
  Justification for the route and dosage
  Population to be treated
- Trial design
  Trial objectives and purpose
  Description of any primary and secondary endpoints
  Type of study, for example, double-blind, placebo-controlled, parallel- design
  Measures to avoid bias
  Description of treatment
  Duration of treatment
  Discontinuation criteria

Box 7.2   Continued
   Procedures for breaking of randomisation codes
   Identification of data to be recorded directly into CRF

- Subject selection
   Number of subjects
   Inclusion criteria
   Exclusion criteria
   Withdrawal criteria
- Trial treatments
   Study drug description, dosage and route, etc.
   Packaging and labelling of study drug
   Duration of treatment(s), follow-up
   Concurrent medication permitted
   Procedure for monitoring subject compliance
   Accountability procedures
- Assessment of efficacy
   Specification of efficacy parameters
   Methodology for assessing efficacy parameters
- Assessment of safety
   Specification of safety parameters
   Methodology of assessing safety parameters
   Handling of serious adverse events
   Handling of ordinary adverse events
   Procedure for breaking codes
   Type and duration of follow-up of adverse events
- Statistics
   Statistical analysis used and selection of subjects to be included
   Timing of any interim analysis
   Reason for sample size
   Power of clinical study
   Level of significance
   Criteria for termination of study
   Procedure for missing and unused data
   Reporting procedures for deviations from statistical plan
- Direct access to source data/documents
   All medical records available
- Quality control and assurance
   Role of monitor and site staff
   Audits
- Ethics
   Study approval
   Medical responsibilities
   Notification of general practitioner
   Consent
- Data handling and record keeping
   Distribution and storage

Box 7.2   Continued
   Monitoring procedures
- Financing and insurance
   Compensation
   Payment of subjects
- Publication policy
- Reference
   List of references to relevant literature
- Appendices

Frequently, the production of the protocol will involve 'cutting and pasting' from a previous protocol, which may or not define a similar study to that being written. Certain sections may be the same, but care needs to be taken to avoid specific information relating to some previous study suddenly appearing in the text of the new protocol.

Several individuals may be involved in preparing the protocol. In a pharmaceutical company, it is usually left to a senior member of the medical department to coordinate the contributions, which should include those of the pharmaceutical physician, the statistician and sometimes the senior investigator involved in the study. Input from the principal investigator at an early stage in the development of the protocol is important. He or she can often contribute on practicalities (e.g. selection of subjects) and primary endpoints. The protocols for independent studies may be prepared by the investigator but should always involve the advice of an experienced statistician familiar with clinical trials. Whether the protocol is for a commercially sponsored or an independent study, vigorous proof reading and review should take place. Reputable pharmaceutical companies will have protocol review boards with representatives from quality assurance (QA), data management as well as the pharmaceutical physician and statistician. A respected and disinterested colleague should review the protocols for independent studies.

When each new draft is produced, whether it is in development or considered final, each page must have 'footers' indicating the version and the date of preparation. This should prevent confusion about which draft is being reviewed or used and allow easy identification of any pages which become detached and mixed up with those from other versions. The final draft should be signed-off by a very senior representative of the medical department sponsoring the clinical trial, the statistician involved in the preparation of the protocol and, perhaps, the senior investigator or medical advisor specialising in the indication or procedure. These signatories are confirming that the content of the protocol is their professional responsibility. In addition, each individual investigator involved in the clinical trial will sign-off the so-called signature page present in each protocol, thereby agreeing to follow the protocol exactly.

Unfortunately, amendments to the approved protocol are frequent. These will require the same sign-off/approval of signatures as required for the original protocol. If the amendment has any impact on the clinical trial, either medically or statistically, it will need to be approved by an IEC.

The following questions must be answered before the final version of the protocol is ready:

1. Does the protocol make sense? It is recommended that someone other than a physician read the protocol. In the case where there are many investigator sites, the individuals reading the protocol may be tired and overworked! Also, laypersons such as those present on IECs will need to understand the document.
2. Is there a flow diagram of the essential elements of the study procedure?
3. Has the document been word processed? There should be no spelling mistakes, the contents page should match the pagination, and the presentation should be professional.
4. Is there a statement that the clinical trial will be conducted in compliance with the protocol, GCP and the applicable regulatory requirements?
5. Is there a clear description of what source data will be recorded directly into the CRF and what will be recorded in the medical records? Normally, the protocol identification number, the date of consent, the date of commencement of the study, the visit dates, the start and finish dates of the administration of study drug and/or treatment, concurrent medication, adverse events and

key efficacy parameters should be in the medical records. However, these items are the absolute minimum.
6. Are there clear instructions for reporting of adverse events and serious adverse events (SAEs)? There should be full instructions for the reporting of SAEs (including addresses and fax numbers), with time limits. It should be clear that these 'rules' also apply to SAEs that occur in subjects who have finished the study. All SAEs that come to the knowledge of the trialist should be reported unless the protocol provides guidance or time limit when the authors can justify that the occurrence of the SAE could not be related to the treatment received in the clinical trial. In a blinded study, there should be clear instructions on when and by whom the code for a particular study subject should be unblinded in an emergency.
7. Does the protocol state that personal medical data obtained from the clinical trial will be made available to monitors, auditors and inspectors from regulatory authorities?
8. Does the protocol clearly state that the study cannot begin without approval of the IEC or IRB? This section should describe the consent process and state when informed consent should be obtained.

7.3.1.3 The ICF
The ICF consists of two documents – the information sheet and the actual consent form. They must be considered as a pair of documents, not separate entities. Normally, a 'core' ICF should be present in the appendices. The core ICF may need modifications to comply with local regulations. It is the responsibility of the sponsor/institution, or in an independent study the investigator, to prepare an ICF that meets the requirements of ICH GCP[1] or any additional requirements of the local regulatory authority, and is only used after it has been approved by the relevant IEC.

The version number, date and page number (i.e. x of y pages) should be on each page. Without these features, new versions of the ICF can be mixed with old versions in the wrong page order in the 'bustle' of the investigator site.

Independent ethics committees and the institutional authorities often modify the core ICF. Local conditions, customs, interpretation of words and regulations may require some changes to the ICF. It may be acceptable to describe Alzheimer's disease as memory loss; however, removal of the section informing the study subject that other individuals besides the investigator will review his or her medical records is not acceptable since it is fundamental to ICH GCP.

The ICF should be written in a language that can be understood by the average study subject.[1,3,8] Simple words should be used wherever possible: for example, 'stop' instead of 'discontinue', 'avoid' instead of 'abstain' and 'cause' instead of 'induce'. Many study subjects will not understand technical words such as 'placebo' and 'erythema'. Measurements of volumes should be described in domestic measurement such as 'teaspoonful' rather than in millilitres. For therapeutic trials ICFs should include a description or mention of alternative procedures or courses of treatment.

There should be consistency between the possible adverse events described for the study drug in the protocol, investigator's brochure and ICF. Most countries have specific requirements for their ICF. It is essential that the requirements are known when the country-specific ICF is prepared. These examples could easily have changed by the time the reader is checking an ICF. In the United Kingdom, reference should be made to the ABPI (Association of the British Pharmaceutical Industry) Clinical Trial Compensation Guidelines.[9] In other countries, for example, Ireland, the study subject is allowed a specific length of time to decide whether to enter the study.

Mention has already been made of the new Directive on the protection of individuals when processing personal data and on the free movement of such data (Directive 95/46/EC).[10] At this time, the manner in which this Directive will be applied to data from clinical trials is still under review. However, the ICF needs to state the rights of the study subject. The subject will be told who controls the confidential data relating to him or herself, the purpose for which it is being collected

and who will receive the data. In addition, apart from reinforcing the confidentiality of the data, the subject will be told that they have a right of access to check that the data relating to them are correct.

If the ICF is to be translated into another language, then someone fluent in that language should do the translation. Expensive translation agencies often provide a grammatically correct translation but in archaic language. The translator should provide a translation certificate stating what was translated and when, and the translator's name, status and appropriate qualifications. The translator should state that the translation was carried out to his or her best ability, and the statement should be signed and dated. A different person should then translate the translated ICF back into the original language. The latter document will then provide confirmation that nothing was left out in the original translation.

7.3.1.3.1   *Obtaining informed consent*

Informed consent by the subject must be obtained before he or she participates in the clinical trial. Only in special circumstances when the subject is unable to give informed consent can other arrangements be made (see ICH GCP[1] chapter 4.8). In the simple protocol, a review by the investigator of the medical history of the subject will establish the subject's suitability to enter the study. The patient should be given sufficient time to read the information sheet, discuss any concerns with the investigator, personal physician, partner, family or friend before giving consent and entering the study (see Section 6.2.3). No invasive procedure (such as blood sampling or radiological examination) should be performed in deciding the suitability of a potential subject for the study until that subject has given written consent. In addition, no drug, even if it is known to be a placebo, should be administered to the subject before written consent is given, unless it is part of ongoing treatment of the subject for a previously established diagnosis. In some clinical trials there is a 'wash-out' period when the subject is not allowed to take his or her routine medication; again, this must not take place until the subject has given written consent. In the more complex protocols, guidance must be given as to when consent should be obtained. Some data may already have been acquired from routine medical procedures undertaken for that particular indication and it may be inappropriate to repeat the procedure, for example, radiological examination, after the subject has entered the trial. In volunteer non-patient studies there may be a separate protocol for conducting screening tests to establish the volunteer's suitability as a potential subject in Phase I studies. This protocol and its informed consent procedures must have Ethics Committee approval before it is used. Before a volunteer screened in this way enters a specific trial the consent process must be repeated with the trial specific information sheet/consent form.

In studies where subjects are mentally or physically unable to give proper consent, special arrangements will need to be made. Where appropriate, the ICF will be read to the subject in the presence of a witness, or consent will be provided by the next of kin or the subject's representatives. Studies in which the study subjects cannot provide informed consent will become more frequent as more difficult indications, for example, trauma, stroke, dementia and the handicapped or very young children, become the focus of clinical trials. The pharmaceutical physician should ensure that established mechanisms for consent are followed with agreement of the IEC and in compliance with ICH GCP chapter 4.8,[1] FDA Title 21 CFR Part 50 sections 24–27[3] and the EU Directive Articles 4 and 5[7].

7.3.1.4   Investigator's brochure

The investigator's brochure provides more detail than the protocol in relation to the background of the study, and should help to facilitate a better understanding of the rationale for the protocol and its key features. In an ideal world, the potential investigator will receive the investigator's brochure before deciding to participate in the study. The brochure should provide the investigator with sufficient information to decide if the proposed study is justified and, together with any published papers, allow the would-be investigator to answer any questions that arise from trial personnel at the site and the IEC. There will be contributions to the brochure from specialists, such as toxicologists and pharmacokineticists, and possibly from pharmacists if details of the study drug are included. A pharmaceutical physician should review this document carefully.

As more information becomes available concerning the study drug or treatment, new versions of the investigator's brochure should be prepared. Anything that might alter the perception of the trial and its risks, such as a serious finding, must be communicated in writing to the Investigators and relevant IECs. Subsequently, a new version of the investigator's brochure (or amended pages) should be distributed as soon as practical so that all concerned with the study have all the current relevant data. In any case, it is expected that a new version of the investigator's brochure will be prepared on an annual basis unless there is minimal new information. All documents should have the version number and date in the 'footer' to avoid confusion between different versions. Receipts will be required from the investigator when a new brochure is received, and old brochures should be recalled and accounted for. The investigator's brochure is a confidential document and its security should be entrusted to the principal investigator.

Reference should be made to ICH GCP Guidelines[1] when preparing an investigator's brochure. The recommended format includes the following elements: physical, chemical, pharmaceutical properties and formulations of the study drug; non-clinical pharmacology studies; pharmacokinetic and metabolism in animals; toxicology; effects on humans; summary of data and guidance for the investigator, which includes details of how to recognise and treat a possible overdose or adverse reaction caused by the study drug or treatment.

7.3.1.5   Case report forms

The CRF (sometimes known as the clinical record form) is the partner to the protocol and they should be prepared together. The CRF should be designed and printed in such a way that all information on each trial subject is collected in a sequence and manner dictated by the protocol. It also acts in part as a checklist. The data to be collected extend from the study subject's demographic data, to the endpoint measures and adverse events observed. In replying to a series of questions, the investigator will record the study subject's response, sometimes by marking prepared squares. For example, in a bronchitis study the squares will characterise the cough, its frequency, precipitating factors, and quantity and appearance of sputum. The CRF will contain objective measures (e.g. routine blood pressure readings and absence or presence of critical physical signs) and most endpoint measurements (for instance, peak expiratory flow readings). Most of these items may not be recorded in the medical records so the CRF is the only source of the data. The investigator or his or her co-investigators should sign that such items were correctly measured according to the protocol and accurately recorded in the CRF. CRFs should have accompanying explanatory and guidance notes to assist the investigating team, together with a summary of the trial activities, including the timing and key actions at each point (for instance, collection of a blood sample).

The protocol should clearly indicate the data that should be present in the medical records as well as in the CRF. For some types of source data, the CRF is accepted by regulatory agencies as the source document. However, much information will be transcribed from other original documents (e.g. radiological report, medical correspondence, laboratory results and the medical records).

Frequently, sections (sometimes known as modules) that have been used in other trials are collated together. This procedure has the advantage that ambiguities and mistakes found in other trials have been removed but, unless good quality control (QC) is in place, incurs the risk that sections that have no relevance to the present study will be left in. There should be 'field testing' of the CRF by colleagues and even investigators before the start of the study. The CRF must

be easy to understand, and the correct questions must be asked. The study statistician should be involved in the review of new CRFs to ensure that the questions asked meet the requirements of the statistical plan.

Depending on what will happen to the CRFs when they are completed, data managers should also be involved. The clinical data will need to be coded and then entered into a database before being further checked for completeness and correctness. The next step will be the analysis of the data. The manner of presentation of the data in the CRF will avoid some of the mistakes that can occur during data entry, particularly if it is entered manually rather than by electronic transfer.

Each page of the CRF should include investigator identification, study subject number, protocol number, subject initials, and visit and/or study day. All pages are numbered as x of y pages with the version and date of CRFs in a 'footer'. Each appropriate section requires the signature from the investigator and a final sign-off.

CRFs should be appropriate to the situations in which they are to be used. For example, in an endoscopy study, the site of lesions and other features can be recorded on a diagram. If study diary cards are used, they should be prepared at the same time as the CRF. The process for transfer of data from diary cards onto CRFs or directly into the trial database should be defined in advance. The preparation of the CRF will take time, particularly if guidance notes are interspersed with individual pages. The printer's proofs should be checked for accuracy before the printing is performed. The transfer of the final format to 'no carbon required (NCR)' paper in order to create immediate copies will prolong the process in preparing the CRF. NCR paper should be of high quality whatever the budget for the study, otherwise only the top copy will be readable.

7.3.1.6 Source documents
Source documents are original documents such as medical records, laboratory report sheets, subjects' diaries or evaluation checklists, pharmacy dispensing records, recorded data

from automated instruments, magnetic media and radiographs. In many cases, knowledge of the medical history contained in the medical records will decide whether the study subject meets the inclusion or exclusion criteria for the study.

The protocol should specify what should be recorded directly into the CRF and what will also be recorded in the medical records. The CRF will contain all the pertinent data associated specifically with the clinical trial but some will be repeated in the medical records, for example, the protocol identification number, date of consent, date of commencement of the study, key baseline medical findings, visit dates, start and finish dates of the study drug/placebo or treatment, concurrent medication, adverse events and key efficacy and any unscheduled or scheduled actions or interventions (such as escape medication). Additional information obtained from biopsy reports, radiographs and similar documents will provide confirmation that the data in the CRF are recorded correctly. Monitors, QA auditors and inspectors need to see all the medical records available to the investigator. It is not appropriate to create copies of data from CRFs or checklists derived from medical records and claim that these are source documents.

There are obvious benefits to any future consulting physician to know something of the medical history of a study subject, including any significant data obtained from a past clinical trial that might affect future medical care.

7.3.1.7 Storage of medical records
The investigator in the institution conducting the study should be aware of what happens to the medical records of study subjects who have participated in clinical trials. The medical authorities or the institution should have guidelines for the retention of records before they are changed into an electronic form by scanning, microfiched or destroyed. Usually when they are changed into another form, the medical records will be reviewed by administration staff and those items deemed not essential will be

removed and destroyed. The investigator should be aware that complete medical records will be required for any future inspection by a regulatory agency. The medical record for each participating subject should be labelled on the front, stating that the record should not be destroyed without consultation with the investigator or before a certain date. (For further information on length of storage of documents, see Section 7.5.4.7.) The routine medical record keeping procedures must be adequate to support running of the clinical trial, to GCP standards at each investigator site.

7.3.1.8 Study subject diary cards
These are small documents that form part of the source documents and are usually filled in by the subject during a study. They allow the subject to record on a daily basis any modest adverse event, for example, headache, that occurs while taking the new treatment or an efficacy parameter, such as a change in their medical condition. Again, care should be taken in the preparation of the diary so that it is 'user friendly'. It should record days and weeks, not dates, use domestic time, not the 24-h clock, and layman's terminology.

7.3.1.9 Alert card
The use of an alert card is not a specific regulatory requirement. However, in many clinical trials, it is appropriate that an alert card is given to subjects, particularly if they are outpatients. In an emergency, the alert card will identify that the subject is in a clinical trial and provide information on the nature of the clinical trial and whom to contact for information. The alert card should contain the sponsor's name and address (if appropriate), investigator's name, address and telephone number, with a 24-h contact number (the contact should have knowledge of the study and not just be an 'on-call' physician), the protocol number, the indication (perhaps modified to be more acceptable to the subject) and the subject's name and address and identification number.

7.3.1.10 Standard operating procedures

Standard operating procedures (SOPs) are detailed written instructions designed to achieve uniformity in the performance of a specific function. Many pharmaceutical companies, hospitals and institutions have documents which they call SOPs. SOPs may provide guidance that can be applied to any clinical trial. The manner that blood pressure is taken, the storage of clinical trial material, or contractual or budgeting processes and documents may also be subject to SOPs. The local IECs will have SOPs concerned with the review of protocols and other documents. There are also specific SOPs used by an investigator and by the sponsor providing details as to how to conduct a clinical trial and in some cases, specifically for a protocol. These types of SOPs can be used to support the maintenance of similar methodology in a global multicentre study, for example, unblinding procedures and the interpretation of data. Laboratories involved in the study should have SOPs defining maintenance, standardisation and use of their equipment and processes. SOPs should be written so that they can be of use to new or experienced staff both for training and for information. Forms, templates and checklists should be referenced in the SOPs and flow charts[11] should be used to illustrate the procedures being described. All SOPs should be reviewed and, if required, updated on a regular basis.

7.4 The Study Drug and its Documents

The time taken to prepare, pack and label medications in accordance with regulatory requirements can delay the start of clinical trials. Not so long ago, the care and attention devoted to the preparation of study drugs was far from stringent. However, the regulators pointed out that it was illogical that experimental products were not subject to the controls that would apply to the formulations of which they are the prototypes.[12] Nowadays, study drug material must be produced according to GMP.[13,14] A Certificate of Analysis and the documented

assurance that the material has been produced according to GMP are required. The New Clinical Trial Directive (2001/20/EC)[7] requires the issuing of manufacturing licences for IMPs and labelling requirements. Manufacture of the study material should start as early as possible. Foresight is not easy, particularly when a series of related trials using the same medicine is being planned and scheduled to start over perhaps a 2-year period. The enormity of and uncertainty in this task are self-evident.

7.4.1 Manufacture

Manufacture of the study drug may be by the pharmaceutical company sponsoring the clinical trial or may be contracted out. The primary and secondary manufacture of clinical trial medications requires a long run-in period, probably 6 months or longer. It is affected by other manufacturing commitments and the state of technical development of the study drug. A decision should be made as early as possible that the formulation being used in early studies could be used as the marketed formulation. In particular, delays will be encountered if several formulations are tried with different dissolution rates. In this situation, the extent and timing of the clinical response could vary between formulations. If such variation is potentially significant, a clinical comparison of the formulations (bioequivalence study[15]) may be required and, if the differences are marked, it could throw doubt on the medical meaning of the clinical trial(s) already performed.

The size of the order for clinical trial medication can be immense, equalling the order for start-up stock for the product when it is eventually launched. It is therefore a major undertaking if the whole requirement for the clinical development programme is ordered at one time; however, this is more efficient than placing smaller orders for supplies at irregular intervals. It is also sensible to anticipate the clinical-trial needs after the launch, when other comparative trials may be sponsored and independent investigators may ask for trial stocks.

7.4.2 Comparative medication

Apart from manufacturing placebo formulations, the company may need to approach the manufacturer of an already marketed product for clinical trial supplies if their medicine is chosen as a comparator. The precise requirements (such as similar size, colour and no identifying features) can be difficult to meet. Any approach may be met with some hesitation for valid reasons, but equally the reaction may be obstructive, asking for unreasonable access to information. It is customary to provide a copy of the protocol, or at the least an outline of it, with clear indication of the material needed and the timeframe for its supply.

Faced with difficulties in obtaining supplies directly from a rival manufacturer, the sponsoring company may decide to elect for a 'double-dummy' technique or to mask the identity of the marketed comparator and to simulate the appearance of the new medicine. In doing the latter, it must be realised that the absorption characteristics of the comparator might be changed (for instance, by a shellac coating) and it is essential that the bioavailability[15] of the modified and the original formulation is checked beforehand.

7.4.3 Presentation

The clinical trial material must be suitably packaged for the purposes of the trial, meeting the optimal pack size dictated by the period of medication and the intervals between visits when trial prescriptions are renewed. For instance, a built-in excess of tablets or capsules is customary, partly to meet a possible delay in renewing stocks of study drug, particularly in a long-term trial. Another reason for an excess of study drug is to provide the subject with a known amount of study drug that is more than they need. A count of the 'returns' will later reveal compliance, whereas if the number of tablets given was the exact requirement, the participant might be tempted to throw away those not taken, thus disguising their non-compliance.

The material must be appropriately labelled, giving a batch number and the medication code number. The latter must accord with the randomisation schedule. The necessary steps must be put in place and monitored in order to give the correct randomisation code for the study drug, comparator (if there is one) and placebo, and thereby ensure that each subject receives the correct allocation. Quality control (QC) steps in the packaging and labelling must be arranged and checked. The dosage instructions must be clear, and the identity of the investigator centre and of the sponsor given on the label. Where the study drug is being used in a blind study, it is essential to establish any differences between the test drug and the comparators in smell, appearance, consistency to touch and taste. Many blind studies have been unblinded by differences in such basic characteristics.

7.4.4 Shipping and importation

The transport of medication to the investigating centre, particularly if it is abroad, requires forward planning. In that instance, there will be a need for importation documents and if it is a research medication, waiving of custom's dues and certification, usually by an investigational licence, that its use has been approved.

The local company staff may be the recipients at the point of importation, often signing for and collecting the medication. Alternatively, the principal investigator may be the direct recipient. Local company staff will be able to provide the necessary documentation to give accreditation and clearance of the trial material and to advise on procedures and potential causes of delay. The registering and checking of these supplies at the investigating centre is important as all material received, used and returned must be accounted for. In the majority of investigator sites, the pharmacy will play an important part in the storage and accountability of the study material. In some countries (e.g. France), the local regulations insist that a pharmacist supervises the storage and allocation of the study drug. Occasionally, there is no pharmacy at the site or the investigator makes his or her own independent arrangements with the sponsor. In these circumstances, the investigator will be responsible for the practical arrangements of storing and administering the study drug without the involvement of a pharmacist.

The study drug should be stored in a secure facility free from pests and vermin, whether it is the hospital pharmacy or the consulting rooms at the investigator site. The environment where the study material is kept should be monitored and controlled for temperature and humidity.

7.4.5 Study drug documentation for the master files

Documentation should be available showing what is stored in the pharmacy or investigator's study drug cupboard, what has been administered to the subject and what has been returned in the form of leftover study drug or empty containers (see Box 7.3). In addition, there will

---

Box 7.3 Documents present in master files concerning the study drug(s)

• Document (may be in protocol or investigator's brochure) with full details of study drug including details of stability, method of destruction, etc.
• Certification of GMP compliance
• Certificate of analysis
• Dates, dosage and batch number(s) with expiry dates of study drug
• Shipping records
• Import licence (if appropriate)
• Study drug label(s)[a]
• Translation certificate of study drug label (if appropriate)[a]
• Receipt of study drug and decode documents signed and dated on receipt
• Documentation for relabelling
• Quality control documents for relabelling
• Drug dispensing log
• Returned study drug inventory forms (record of study drug returned to sponsor, etc.) with batch number and return date
• Certificate of destruction of study drug (if destroyed at site)
• Receipt for decode documents – in sealed containers when returned to supplier (at end of study)
• Master randomisation list in sealed envelope (if study still blind)[a]

[a] Usually present only in sponsor office

---

be other documents giving more details of the nature of the study drug, codes for unblinding subjects in a blind study in case of emergency, and, perhaps, import licences. These documents must be kept in the investigator and pharmacy master files and/or in the sponsor's or coordinator's office.

7.4.5.1 Shipping documents

The manufacturer of the study drug should provide a standard request form for the investigator or sponsor to use when ordering supplies. Well-designed forms help the person completing the form to provide critical information. Each shipment should be accompanied by a document listing the contents of the shipment. Particular attention should be given to the dates when the study drug was dispatched from the supplier and when it arrived at the study site. A long interlude implies that the study drug may have been stored in an unsuitable area on the way to the site (e.g. on a tropical airport runway in high summer). The investigator should acknowledge receipt of the shipment by completing a copy of the form and returning it to the supplier. There should be an indication of when the study drug reaches its expiry date. Ideally, the expiry date should be given on the label of the study drug.

Frequently, in early trials of a new study drug, the expiry date is extended as more stability data become available. Any additional labelling by the sponsor or by the investigator should be documented fully and, where possible, a second person should QC the process. The labelling should always meet the GMP regulations applicable in the location.

Unless there are specific instructions in the protocol to the contrary, there should be a clearly documented trail of the drugs supplies that came in, what was administered to the subjects and what was returned by the subject in terms of unused medication. Any relaxation of drug accountability, as is seen sometimes in a multicentre study of many thousand subjects, can cause problems in monitoring the correct formulations and dosages given to the subjects. The significance of the results in such a trial may then be called into question.

The amounts and dates of departure of the study drug from the pharmacy should match that of administration of the drug to the subject, unless the drug is being transferred to a hospital clinic for short-term storage. A similar procedure should take place if the study drug is being stored within the clinic, either all the time or temporarily. The investigator, pharmacist or their staff should always check any returned study drug. What is actually present in terms of number of capsules, tablets or pills in the returned containers from each individual study subject must be consistent with what is recorded in the CRFs, and on the dispensing and returns records. There should be destruction certificates if unused study drug has been destroyed by the pharmacy. Alternatively, there should be documentation that states clearly what was returned to the study drug supplier and acknowledgement from the supplier that they have received the unused drug.

7.4.5.2 Sealed codes used for unblinding a study subject

Sealed codes are usually sealed envelopes, 'advent' sheets or sealed label covers on the study drug containers that, when opened, will indicate which treatment the subject has been administered in a blind study. Their purpose is to provide the information the investigator needs for treating a subject for an SAE in an emergency. Only in a life-threatening situation (e.g. anaphylaxis) should the blind be broken by the investigator. Normally, the investigator should contact the sponsor for them to unblind the subject if necessary, thus improving the chances of maintaining the blinding of the whole study. There must be adequate arrangements to be able to unblind a subject in emergency outside the normal working day, and the sponsor or the investigator should provide a 24-h helpline that can provide the necessary information concerning a particular protocol.

The sealed codes should be provided with the study treatment, and a blinded study should not start until the sealed codes are available at the site. Investigators sometimes unblind their own study subjects out of curiosity when the study has been completed at their site. Investigators should be informed that this must not happen. All sealed (and unsealed) codes should be checked and returned to the supplier at the end of the study. Unblinding of a study should never take place until all the study subjects, including those subjects at other sites, have completed the study and then should only be done by the appointed statistician in a controlled manner – usually after the data have been checked and the database locked.

7.5 The Running of the Clinical Trial

7.5.1 Before the start of the study

7.5.1.1 Selection of the investigator

The selection of investigators is critical to the success of a clinical trial. Unless there are very special circumstances, the principal investigator should have previous experience of clinical trials and qualifications that reflect experience in the indication involved. Exceptions can be made when a study drug is being investigated in general practice. In this situation, not every practitioner will be trained to undertake clinical trials or have special knowledge of the disease being treated. The sponsors should overcome any deficiencies by providing training and good monitoring. However, many of the most relevant criteria of sufficient and suitable staff support, facilities and study subject population will be determined in the so-called prestudy visit (see Section 7.5.1.2).

The pharmaceutical physician may conduct his or her studies as an investigator or may be part of a sponsor organisation selecting investigators for a trial.

7.5.1.1.1 Considerations before becoming an investigator

The pharmaceutical physician who is in charge of an in-house clinical pharmacology unit or who holds an appropriate external clinical appointment will need to decide whether it is feasible for clinical trials to be carried out in his or her facilities. Similarly, the independent investigator should be honest with him/her self as to the practicalities needed before starting clinical research. The most important considerations are of time and resource. The physician should seek information about the sponsor: whether the reputation of the sponsor is known, both for adequate monitoring and support, and the use of user-friendly protocols and CRFs. The potential investigator should ask himself or herself about their motivation for doing the clinical trial. It is often financial, perhaps to provide additional funds for new equipment or staff, it may be scientific curiosity, or desire to improve patient treatment with a research drug, or it may be a desire to improve an individual's professional status by publication.

7.5.1.1.2 Considerations by the sponsor in selecting suitable investigators

There are various ways to select good investigators but none is foolproof. Investigators found to be satisfactory in previous studies may be selected. However, circumstances do change, supporting staff leave, enthusiasm wanes or other studies demand attention. The best investigator of a previous study, recruiting all study subjects requested and providing the cleanest clinical data, may fail in the next study.

There will often be a need for one or two opinion leaders to be involved in the study. They may have helped in the design of the study and contributed to the protocol and will contribute to any future publications. Their influence among their peers may help later to promote the use of the product. Often, but not always, they will wish to actively participate in the study although most of the clinical trial work at their site will be delegated to a more junior physician. It should never be assumed that an investigator with high professional standing in his or her field will necessarily be a good investigator. Often the opinion leader is called a 'principal investigator'. However, the term is often used loosely and can equally be applied to an investigator in charge of several co-investigators or subinvestigators at an individual site and having little influence on the design of the study.

Sometimes, pharmaceutical companies are familiar with suitable investigators in a therapeutic area with which they have previous experience. The opinion leaders themselves may know individuals suitable as investigators. Young investigators with some clinical trial experience may have suitable study subjects for a particular trial, and the ability and patience to cope with the considerable recording and documentation required in most clinical trials. However, recommendations that originate from the marketing department of pharmaceutical companies should be treated with caution. A physician who is a good customer for company products may not have the qualities required by an investigator.

There are now several commercial organisations that can provide a list of 'suitable' investigators for a particular indication. Any assumption that the individuals are in fact suitable should be based on an independent assessment. Assessment of suitability of a pharmaceutical physician as a principal investigator covers the same issues as selection of an external clinician – although some details will differ.

7.5.1.2 Prestudy visit

Experienced senior staff of the sponsor must always visit the investigator site before a new clinical trial starts, even if the investigator has been involved in previous studies. Most pharmaceutical companies have checklists and SOPs of the requirements of an investigator site. Key questions will need to be answered relating to staff support and the present workload of the site. The competence of the staff to conduct any procedures, the maintenance, calibration and QC of any equipment to be used, and whether other clinical trials demand too much resource are all questions that need answers. In addition, the facilities should be inspected to establish whether the site could store and securely archive the large amounts of documents and study drugs that will be present. The pharmacy may play a major role in the study and therefore the facility and the pharmacist should be visited.

Questions should always be asked about the site staff's understanding of GCP and whether the investigator appreciates the need for informed consent, ethical approval and the review of highly confidential documents by outsiders. Finally, the sponsor will need to explore the protocol with the investigator, which may be still in draft form at this stage. The investigator will need to know what will be required of him or her and the site staff, and whether the procedures in the protocol are acceptable to him or her. When the protocol is finalised, the investigator will need to follow the protocol exactly. Other interests (e.g. other clinical trials) of the investigator (see Section 7.5.1.1) at the site may interfere with any participation in the study and the site may not be able to provide sufficient suitable study subjects.

At the time of the prestudy visit, and certainly before any study subjects are recruited, other activities will need to take place. The medical management will need to select the laboratories to be used, and organise QA auditors to check any software houses involved in the production of software for the clinical trial. The software used [e.g. in electronic diaries or interactive voice response technology (IVRT)] will need to be audited to establish that validation procedures are in place. There should be plans for QA auditors to visit any plants involved in the distribution of the study drug. Only in very exceptional circumstances do the qualifications and experience of the pharmaceutical physician warrant their involvement in these exercises. He or she should understand that these activities need to be undertaken and the contribution that each activity will make to the study. Team cooperation at the sponsor site is essential for the future success of the study. However, the pharmaceutical physician will be involved if part of the clinical work is to be delegated to a CRO or a site management organisation (SMO), or they are part of a strategic team planning the clinical trial. Some of these entities are described below.

7.5.1.3 CROs and SMOs

There is a growing reliance by sponsors on contracting out part or all of the work of the clinical trial to a subcontractor. Manufacturers often find that they cannot organise every clinical trial that they require. The reasons are many, but commonly reflect limited staff resources, pressures of time, and inability to identify and organise investigators, especially into a collaborative group (for instance, general practitioners in one locality). In independent studies by investigators, additional expertise may be needed in statistical analysis or data management and similar areas. Subcontractors offer different services, from large CROs capable of conducting an international clinical trial with minimal contribution from the sponsor, specialised groups for data management, safety monitoring, auditing or a single consultant for statistical analysis or medical writing.

A recent development has been the emergence of SMOs which are really CROs involved at the sharp end of clinical trials, that is, the investigator site. Nearly half of all delays in clinical development occur with the setting up and initiation of studies at investigator sites. These delays result from obtaining IEC approval, study subject recruitment or the training of staff. Individual SMOs should be able to identify investigators capable of conducting the trial and with access to a large number of suitable study subjects. In addition, time can be saved by the sponsor by having a single contact for contract and budget negotiations, and having investigator sites familiar with GCP and the requirements of the local regulations. SMOs are usually regional or national business enterprises with one or more locations. Several varieties of SMOs exist, some specialising in particular indications perhaps attached to an institution focused on that indication, some providing support for independent investigators and some being totally independent business enterprises.

The pharmaceutical physician should be involved in the selection of CROs and SMOs. He or she is often best qualified to judge the professional competency of the physicians involved in any contractual work. There needs to be a clear understanding as to who will provide medical advice to the investigator and to the non-physicians in the clinical trial teams, who will be responsible for the assessment of the medical significance of adverse events, SAEs and safety issues in general and who will be conducting any medical coding. The responsibility for custody of the clinical data should be clearly defined at each stage from initial recordings to the final analysis. It is essential to define the roles and responsibilities of the sponsor, including the sponsor's medical expertise, those of the contracted organisation, as well as of the investigators, who will always have ultimate responsibility for their study subjects and their safety.

7.5.2 Technical considerations

Before a clinical trial starts, the use of technical aids such as IVRT, remote data entry and electronic diaries has to be considered. In Section 7.5.3.3, mention will be made of the use of electronic tracking system that provide status and monitoring reports. All these systems utilise computer systems that must be validated. Double and McKendry[16] described computer validation as the process which documents that a computer system reproducibly performs the functions it was designed to do. The document *Guidance for Industry – Computerised Systems used in Clinical Trials* published by the FDA in 1999[17] gives clear recommendations of what is required (also see Section 7.5.4.1).

7.5.2.1 Interactive voice response technology

The use of IVRT[18] can improve the efficiency of various procedures carried out at the investigator site. Investigators and their staff interact with the electronic technology by pressing the appropriate keys on their touchtone telephone in response to a recorded voice request. In a typical example, when a new subject is recruited to a clinical trial, the subject randomisation number can be allocated in return for demographic information, such as subject initials, eligibility criteria, age, sex and weight. In addition, IVRT can be used to track clinical trial material and ensure that the correct allocation of study drug is provided to each subject. Batches of study drug will be prepared in lots of two, three, four, etc. (e.g. placebo and

study drug; placebo, comparator and study drug; or placebo, comparator, study dose A and study drug dose B) – each lot ensuring that the ratio of subjects at a site receiving study drug, comparator and placebo is as defined in the protocol.

7.5.2.2 Remote data entry

Remote data entry is the process by which data are entered into a laptop or personal computer rather than onto a paper CRF. Normally, this process will take place at the investigator site. The computer screen provides a so-called electronic CRF (eCRF), which, like the paper CRF, will require a series of answers or parameters to be recorded. The system provides screen prompts and checks. These remind the investigator to complete responses and can immediately draw attention to any inconsistency between responses. Not all the data can be recorded directly into the eCRF and, as with the paper CRF, key elements will still need to be recorded in the study subject records.

The internet provides a modern solution for the transmission of data to the sponsor office. Web browsers provide a point-and-click interface that allows data to be downloaded to a remote server. Monitors can review the data from the sponsor's office and instruct the investigator in any corrections required. This procedure has the potential to provide higher quality data through earlier interventions. In addition, analogue signals from physiological parameters, such as ECG and blood pressure monitors, can be routinely downloaded onto the internet and transferred for remote analysis, before the findings are entered into the clinical trial database. Security of the internet has been an issue but can be better ensured with the use of electronic signatures and encrypted data transmission.

7.5.2.3 Electronic subject diaries

Paper subject diaries are notoriously poor in their legibility, completeness and accuracy. Electronic diaries are small, portable devices that can present text and graphics to the subject. They allow the subject to record and store responses, which can be time-stamped for each entry made.

The data can then be downloaded directly into the clinical trial database. The main drawbacks include the need for training the subject in the diary's use, possible errors in local time settings and the logistics of distribution, maintenance and recovery of the diaries.

7.5.2.4 Clinical laboratories

Traditionally, the local hospital pathology department was used to provide laboratory safety data for clinical trials. Increasingly, sponsors are using central laboratories to which some or all the laboratory samples for a multicentre study are sent. Central laboratories provide standard methodology, which reduces variation between investigator sites and provides a single and well-established reference range. In addition, all the laboratory results can be transferred electronically to the main database, thus avoiding the opportunities for mistakes to occur in the manual copying of data from the laboratory report sheet onto the CRF and then into a database.

However, there are drawbacks as well as advantages. Clinical trials for certain intensive care indications, for example, trauma and acute myocardial infarction, will require frequent monitoring of certain laboratory parameters, and the use of quick results as provided by a local laboratory is essential. In other situations, investigators will sometimes obtain laboratory data from two sources – local and central – of the same sample. This may be due to poor training but frequently reflects the investigator's mistrust of data from an unfamiliar and perhaps foreign central laboratory. The protocol must be very clear about which results will be used in any safety analysis. The regulatory authorities will not accept an arbitrary selection based on favourable or unfavourable results that may bias any future safety analysis. Some laboratory parameters of the samples, for example, mean cell volume, prothombin time and microbiology, may need to be measured quickly at the local laboratory. Blood samples for the estimation of drug or metabolite levels may need to be analysed quickly, before degradation takes place. In addition, the central laboratory

selected may be in a different part of the country or even in another continent and samples will need to be sent by courier.

A good central laboratory will provide adequate packaging and arrange the courier service. The International Air Transport Association (IATA) regulations for the transport of biological samples across national borders need to be observed. Most blood samples will fall into risk group II (moderate individual risk, limited community risk). Further information can be obtained from the IATA website (www.iata.org). Staff responsible for the packaging of the samples for dispatch will require appropriate recognised training.

7.5.2.5 Training of the investigator and site staff

The competence of the investigator and the site team is clearly the responsibility of the institution or employing authority, and at a practical level, of the investigator. The sponsor cannot train them on the medical, scientific or technical aspects of procedures related to study subject investigation or care. The sponsor, the institution or the independent investigator will need to ensure that the basic procedures required in the clinical trial are explained. At a practical level, all staff involved in a clinical trial will be required to undergo training in both the basic principles of ICH GCP and in the key elements of the specific clinical trial. Inspectors from regulatory agencies will expect fully documented training. Each member of the clinical management team should participate in a relevant long-term training programme. The training of site staff will be carried out at initial visits to the site and at investigator meetings.

7.5.2.6 Investigator meetings

Pharmaceutical physicians should view investigator meetings as an important part of the process of meeting investigators, obtaining expert advice on trial design, learning about problems before they occur and contributing to smooth running of the trial.

Investigator meetings can be single-centre or multicentre meetings and may have global representation. Meetings should be attended by the investigators, their staff and key individuals from the sponsors. They should always occur before a study starts and before a clinical trial commences at a particular site. Sometimes, investigator meetings take place during a study to update investigator site staff and train new investigators to the study. They should include sections relating to GCP and safety aspects, drug accountability and administration, recording of data and a detailed review of the protocol. If the actual meeting is well structured and planned, it is an opportunity to ensure uniformity of procedures and the resolution of any misunderstandings.

7.5.2.7 Ethics committee application

Since the implementation of the EU Directive in 2004, a new Central Office for Research Ethics Committees (COREC) has been established to streamline the work of research IECs in the United Kingdom. Briefly, applications are made centrally and considered at the recognised research ethics committee covering the area in which the chief investigator works with input on site-specific issues from ethics committees covering other involved trial centres. The chief investigator is responsible for the application via COREC to conduct the clinical study at his or her site and for the appropriate supporting documents [mandatory requirements are the application form, protocol, chief investigator's *curriculum vitae*, patient information sheet and consent form and evidence of indemnity for non-National Health Service (NHS) sponsored studies]. The sponsoring company should provide assistance in obtaining approval via COREC and in preparing supporting documentation for the chief investigator. Decisions on valid applications are delivered within 60 days. A full description of the process and necessary forms is available on-line from COREC.[19]

The chief investigator is also responsible (with support from the sponsor) for notifying the IEC of any new safety information and of any protocol amendments that will require approval. Annual or more frequent reports of the progress of the study and any safety issues, including SAEs, will need to be provided.

7.5.2.8 Regulatory approval

Clinical trials must be approved by the appropriate government agency before they start. The new European Directive (2001/20/EC)[7] has almost standardised the process of regulatory approval within the EU. Briefly, the sponsor obtains a EudraCT trial number and then applies to the relevant competent authority by submitting the necessary application form along with supporting documentation (particularly EudraCT number, protocol and patient information and consent forms, investigators brochure, IMP dossier, relevant preclinical pharmacological and toxicological data and a risk assessment). Full details are available at the European Clinical Trials Database website (eurdact.emea.eu.int). In the United States, an IND application is made to the FDA using Forms 1571 and 1572, the latter giving details of the investigators, facilities, and IEC(s).[20]

7.5.2.9 Budgets and contracts

Responsibilities must be clearly defined.[21]

7.5.2.9.1 The budget

The budget must be set, the means of payment agreed and contractual arrangements for premature trial termination decided. In addition, the legal contract should include payments, if any, when a study subject drops out or when it is impossible to evaluate an individual subject (e.g. protocol violations by an investigator, such as recruitment of subjects who do not meet the inclusion criteria – which are an indication for extra clarification of protocol requirements). There should be a clear understanding of the costs and expenses that the site's institution or hospital will absorb and what the sponsor will pay for either directly or indirectly.

It is essential to have a written contract with the institution. In preparing it, one must identify other supporting services (for instance, laboratory investigations and the use of the pharmacy) that are effectively subcontracted by the clinical investigators, but are sometimes omitted as recipients even within their own institution. It is helpful to try to separate the cost of materials and equipment hire from the cost of the services provided by staff. In some cases, the institution where the investigator site is situated will demand a 'handling charge' for handling the contract and dealing with the invoices. This may cover some or all the salaries of the site staff, the use of the facilities and equipment and disposable supplies. Many larger pharmaceutical companies now utilise a contracts manager aided by someone skilled in purchase negotiations to manage trial costs. In all financial matters concerning clinical trials, all costs and expenses must be clearly recorded.

7.5.2.9.2   The contract

The contractual basis should be outlined in a 'letter of agreement'. In addition to the undertakings relating to the particular trial, some standard provisions should be included either in the contract, in the protocol or in both. These include an indemnity statement, a study subject compensation statement, an inspection/audit understanding and a publication statement. The investigators' responsibilities under ICH GCP guidelines and related procedures should be identified. Often most of these can be simply listed and it is recommended that industry-agreed procedures (for instance, ABPI guidelines[9]) are adopted and quoted as these are widely accepted.

7.5.2.10   Financial disclosure

Globally, there is concern that biased results could be produced from studies conducted by investigators who own shares or other financial benefits in the pharmaceutical company sponsoring their trials. The Declaration of Helsinki (2000) requires that 'sources of funding, institutional affiliations and possible conflicts of interest should be declared in any publication'. All studies conducted on products that are likely to be part of a submission to the US FDA require the sponsor to make a disclosure of financial holdings of the investigators that participate in all studies. Any significant payments (US$25 000)

that could influence the outcome of the trial, proprietary interest in the product under study or significant equity interests (excess of US$50 000) need to be declared by the investigator.[22]

Before commencing a study, the investigator should make a financial disclosure. Most future products will need to benefit from the potential sales of the US market. Even when there is a considerable financial interest in the success of the product, the financial disclosure will not necessarily rule out the investigator's role in the study totally. Most inspectorates are more interested in what is not declared than what is.

7.5.3   During the study

7.5.3.1   Study subject recruitment

In the past, the recruitment of study subjects had been highly dependent on the activities of the investigator and the study subjects who were attending his or her clinic. Recommendation of a study subject by the treating physician is still the preferred method for recruiting study subjects. However, advertisements for suitable study subjects are being used increasingly. These may be placed on notice boards in clinics, in the local press and on television and radio. The most recent development has been the use of the Internet, particularly for studies where recruitment is difficult.

However, tempting it is for the pharmaceutical physician, the investigators and the sponsors to use advertising, they should be aware that there are certain guidelines and regulations[23] to observe before embarking on any advertisement for a clinical trial.

An IEC should review the advertisement or the recording of the proposed video or audio message before it is publicised. Only limited information should be presented – the name and address of the clinical investigator, the purpose of the research and, in summary form, the eligibility criteria for the study, a precise description of any benefits to the subject, the time or other commitment required by the subject, the location of the research and the person to contact for information. No claims should be made, either explicitly or implicitly, that the drug or device is safe or effective for the indication.

Terms such as 'new drug', 'new medication' or 'new treatment' should not be used without an explanation that the study drug or treatment is experimental. Advertisements should not promise 'free medical treatment' when the intent is not to charge for taking part in the investigation. The key aspect is that subjects should not enter clinical trials purely because they cannot afford to obtain medical treatment for their illness.

7.5.3.2 Collection of the data

The expertise of the pharmaceutical physician when employed by a sponsor will be used to support the clinical trial team in four main areas during a clinical trial.

1. He or she will be required to support the monitoring staff and understand their function at the site. In particular, he or she may be required to give medical interpretation when inclusion and exclusion criteria are considered.
2. He or she will be required to review, understand the importance of, and respond appropriately to adverse events and SAEs. He or she will be required to have an overview of new safety issues.
3. He or she will be required to interpret the significance of the laboratory data in relation to the study drug.
4. He or she may be required to support the coding of medical terms before the clinical data are analysed.

7.5.3.3 Monitoring visits

One of the advantages of working with a large institution or pharmaceutical company is that the clinical trial should be properly monitored. Investigators conducting independent studies should be aware that a study nurse or another physician does not replace the role of the independent monitor or clinical research associate. The clinical trial monitor acts as a QC supervisor, usually covering several centres involved in the same trial, and so achieving uniformity in the checking and in the remedial actions taken. The monitor will help in the interpretation

of the protocol or relay procedural instructions, which can reduce misunderstandings, and help to create uniformity across all investigating sites. The monitors are required to carry out source data verification, that is, to compare individual subject's medical records and other supporting documents with what is recorded in the CRF and to check that the information in the CRF is complete, accurate and legible. Omissions such as concomitant drug treatment or development of a concurrent illness should be corrected. In addition, all missing visits and subjects failing to complete the study, and the reason for each failure, must be recorded. Informed consent documentation and the documents present in the master file at the site should be checked.

Both ICH GCP and the FDA require the monitor 'to assure adequate protection of the rights of human subjects involved in clinical investigations and the quality and integrity of the resulting data'. The investigator and the site staff will have primary responsibility for these aspects of clinical research. The regulatory inspectorates have, on numerous occasions, observed failures in both consent and ethical approval procedures, and in data recording, when there has been no, or inadequate, monitoring.

After each visit to the site, the monitor is required to record the errors and the remedial action in the visit report. These visit reports may be reviewed by the regulatory authorities. Repetitive errors will be highlighted in the monitoring reports, along with the status of each subject recruited at the site. In some pharmaceutical companies, the information in the report is recorded on an electronic tracking system. The system will provide rapid updates on the progress at a particular investigator site. These updates, together with others from other investigator sites, allow rapid assessment of the progress and status of the whole trial. Errors found in the CRF or in documentation in the files are recorded in a convenient manner, usually by tabulation in 'error logs'. These list the corrections required from the investigator and provide indicators where improvements are required. Efforts to produce high-quality, so-called 'clean' CRFs at the site will be rewarded later when preparing the clinical trial database for analysis. Any queries and corrections that occur once the CRF has left the site will require the correction to be approved and signed-off by the investigator.

The clinical trial monitor is a temporary member of the site team. A good monitor will conduct scheduled visits, and the investigator and the site staff should provide sufficient time to answer questions and correct data in the CRF that has been transferred incorrectly from source documents. Common errors are omitting negative answers and signatures. The monitor will need space to work and should be provided with requested documentation, including medical records, for review.

7.5.3.4   Use of the Independent Data-monitoring Committee

The pharmaceutical physician may be asked to serve on an Independent Data-monitoring Committee (IDMC). It is an independent committee that may be established to assess at intervals the progress of clinical trials, with respect to the safety data, and critical efficacy endpoints. The members of the committee are mainly physicians who have the power to recommend the continuation, modification or stopping of a clinical trial. When working with a 'blind' study, some of the members may sometimes be unblinded and great care needs to be taken not to unblind the other members. Another use for IDMC is to provide an independent pool of experts to evaluate a particular parameter of efficacy in a multicentre study, such as the size of a growth in a radiograph. This provides some degree of uniformity when many different physicians and specialists at individual sites are measuring many radiographs.

7.5.3.5   Adverse events and reactions

There is considerable confusion in the use of terminology in this area. Edwards and Aronson[24] proposed the following definition. An adverse drug reaction is 'an appreciably harmful or unpleasant reaction, resulting from an intervention related to the use of a medicinal product, which predicts hazard from future administration and warrants prevention or specific treatment, or alteration of the dosage regimen, or withdrawal of the product'.

An adverse effect is an all-encompassing term, which includes all unwanted effects, making no assumptions about mechanism, evoking no ambiguity and avoiding the risk of misclassification. But it is an adverse outcome that can be attributed to some action of a drug. 'Adverse reaction' and 'adverse effects' are interchangeable terms, except the former is seen from the point of view of the subject and the latter from the point of view of the drug.

An adverse event is an adverse outcome that occurs while a study subject is taking a drug, but is not necessarily attributable to it. It is important to distinguish between event and reaction. In clinical trials, this acknowledges that it is not always possible to ascribe causality.

7.5.3.5.1   Types of adverse drug reaction

There are several classifications of adverse reactions, but the most commonly employed define two principal kinds (A and B) and three subordinate classes (C, D and E).

1. Type A (augmented) reactions are due to the pharmacological effect of the drug, often in exaggerated form. They are dose related, predictable, and they can occur in anyone.

2. Type B (bizarre) reactions occur only in some people and are not part of the known pharmacology of the drug. They are not dose related and are the result of unusual interaction of the study subject with the drug. These effects may be predictable where the mechanism is known (e.g. the genetic polymorphism associated with some hepatic metabolising enzymes) or unpredictable (e.g. due to immunological processes).

3. Type C (continuous) reactions are due to long-term use of the drug (e.g. analgesic nephropathy or peripheral neuropathy with reverse transcriptase inhibitors).

4. Type D (delayed) reactions are teratogenic or carcinogenic responses.

5. Type E (end-of-use) reactions occur with rebound withdrawal phenomena.

Recently, a Type F has been added: unexpected failure of therapy.

Table 7.1 Number of patients that need to be studied to give a good chance of detecting adverse events

Expected incidence of adverse reaction	Required number of patients for event		
	1 event	2 events	3 events
1 in 100	300	480	650
1 in 200	600	960	1 300
1 in 1 100	3 000	4 800	6 500
1 in 2 000	6 000	9 600	13 000
1 in 10 000	30 000	48 000	65 000

Source: Council for the International Organisations for Medical Science. *Safety Requirements for the First Use of New Drugs and Diagnostic Agents in Man.* Geneva: CIOMS (WHO) 1983.

In Phase I and II studies, Type A reactions are by far the most frequent. Type B are rare, which is fortunate as some can be serious or even fatal. Table 7.1 shows the number of subjects that need to be studied to give a good chance (95%) of detecting an adverse event when there is no background incidence. The problem is many orders of magnitude worse if the adverse reaction closely resembles spontaneous disease that has a background incidence in the trial population.

7.5.3.6 Reporting adverse events and establishing causality

An adverse event or experience (as in the preceding section) is defined as 'any undesirable experience occurring to a subject whether or not considered related to the investigational product(s)'. Sponsors will have their own set of definitions and SOPs governing reporting of adverse events. The following account is generally applicable to most situations.

Adverse events can be described as serious or non-serious. The ICH GCP[1,24] classifies an event as serious if it has one or more of the following characteristics:

- Is fatal
- Is life threatening

- Results in persistent or significant disability/incapacity
- Requires hospitalisation or prolongation of hospitalisation
- Is associated with a congenital abnormality/birth defect.

The investigator has the responsibility to notify the sponsor immediately that he or she has knowledge of an SAE. Where applicable, the IEC and relevant authorities should also be informed either by the sponsor or by the investigator. This will allow the appropriate measures to be taken to safeguard the study subjects. Although the timeframes below provide more time than originally was required by regulatory authorities (e.g. the FDA), the reporting of SAEs, whether considered alarming or not, should have priority over most other activities in a clinical trial. The ICH guidelines[25] (Topic 2A) states that certain SAEs may be sufficiently alarming so as to require very rapid notification to the sponsors and appropriate authorities. Fatal or life-threatening unexpected SAEs require notification by telephone or fax within seven calendar days by the sponsor or investigator to the authorities. The telephone or fax report must be followed by a hardcopy report within a further eight calendar days. The report must include an assessment of the importance and implication of the findings, including relevant experience with the same or similar entities. All other serious unexpected SAEs that are not fatal or life threatening must be reported as soon as possible but within no more than 15 calendar days.

Establishing a cause–effect relationship between an adverse event and the use of a drug is a serious and difficult problem. Karch and Lasagna[26] proposed degrees of certainty for attributing an adverse event to a drug, as shown in Box 7.4. With this kind of classification in mind, how can a sponsor (or anyone else interested) assess whether an adverse event is associated with a particular medicine? Broadly, there are two approaches – global introspection and use of algorithms. Both rely on the application of logic to the set of circumstances presented. Global introspection is most frequently used and

> **Box 7.4 Karch and Lasagna's[26] proposed degrees of certainty for attributing an adverse event to a drug**
>
> • Definite. Time sequence from taking drug is reasonable. Event corresponds to what is known about the drug. Event ceases on stopping drug. Event returns on restarting drug.
> • Probable. Time sequence reasonable. Corresponds to what is known of the drug. Ceases on stopping drug. Not reasonably explained by subject's disease.
> • Possible. Time sequence reasonable. Does not correspond to what is known of the drug. Could not be reasonably explained by the subject's disease.
> • Conditional. Time sequence reasonable. Does correspond to what is known of the drug. Could not be reasonably explained by the subject's disease.
> • Doubtful. Event not meeting the above criteria.

involves one or more experts considering the factors associated with the medicine and the institution. The main factors to consider are:

1. Previous experience with the medicine and background incidence of reaction in this disease group.
2. The study subject's medical history, for example, more frequent in the elderly and hepatic and renally impaired; previous exposure to the medicine and presence of other disease.
3. The characteristics of the adverse event, for example, timing of event, plasma concentration of parent drug and metabolites, laboratory tests.
4. Effects of rechallenge, dechallenge and response to treatment.
5. Alternative explanations of adverse event, for example, other therapies.

The risk of rechallenge has to be very carefully considered. Its use will depend on the severity of the reaction, availability of a specific antidote, ease and speed of reversing the effect and the subject's willingness to be exposed for a second time. Rechallenge is not infrequently undertaken in Phase I studies when an exaggerated response (Type A reaction) occurs and a smaller dose can

be used. IEC approval must be obtained and consideration given to the use of active drug and placebo in a randomised double-blind administration.

7.5.3.7 Determining clinical significance of an adverse event

If an adverse event has been causally linked to the use of the drug in the trial, the sponsor, usually in conjunction with the investigator, will need to decide on the clinical relevance of the event and the action that needs to be taken. The issue is important to:

• The individual subject
• The rest of the subjects in the trial
• Those about to receive the drug in the clinical development programme
• The overall future of the drug.

The clinical significance (in both the narrow and wider context) of the adverse event will be determined by considering the following factors.

• How serious is the event?
• Will it reverse spontaneously and completely?
• What specific therapy is available?
• Are particular groups of subjects at risk and should clinical usage be restricted?
• Are there any clinical or investigational factors that could predict who may develop the adverse event?
• What is the benefit:risk ratio?
• Is the drug a novel medicine in an otherwise poorly treated and severe disease?
• Are alternative medicines toxic?

These deliberations may result in several outcomes. Clinical development may continue as planned, but additional vigilance with more frequent visits and special tests may be added. The dose may be reduced or certain 'at-risk' subjects may be excluded from further trials. The drug may proceed to registration, but the authorities may stipulate that a post-marketing surveillance study be conducted. The drug may even be withdrawn from further clinical development.

7.5.3.7.1   Council for International Organization of Medical Science (CIOMS)

CIOMS is associated with safety, providing various forms such as the form normally used to report SAEs (CIOMS I) but also many other types of forms, for example, CIOMS II for the international reporting of periodic drug-safety update reports. The council is active as a medium for international discussion on safety and bioethics (see Chapter 15).

7.5.3.7.2   Laboratory safety data

When the CRFs arrive at the data manager's office, questions will arise relating to laboratory safety data. Queries may occur at the investigator site and advice can be requested from the pharmaceutical physician associated with the clinical trial in the sponsor company.

There are several different kinds of laboratory safety data that require interpretation. These include routine screening for study subject selection, diagnostic evaluation of the subject, identification of risk factors, monitoring the progress of the disease or treatment, detection of adverse reactions, determination of appropriate dosages for certain 'at-risk' subject groups (e.g. those with renal impairment).

In general, the interpretation of laboratory safety data is undertaken for the following reasons:

1. To identify trends in the data, even if the individual or mean values lie entirely within the 'normal' reference ranges. Delta checking generates 'flags' that appear in a laboratory result printout for a parameter indicating inconsistency with previous results. The laboratory equipment has to be programmed so that significant changes will be flagged. They could indicate change in the subject's condition or a wrong specimen or reagent.
2. To identify predictable or unpredictable laboratory abnormalities, which may need particular attention in further studies.
3. To identify abnormal values in an individual study subject.
4. To identify groups who are potentially at high risk.

5. To establish a 'denominator' for any problems that may occur in this or subsequent studies.

7.5.3.7.3   References ranges and sources of error

The trends in data or individual abnormal values are only interpretable if the reference values are known and the test is reliable. Reference ranges usually refer to the mean value and two standard deviations on either side of the mean. Thus 95% of a sample population who are free of disease will fall inside this range, with 2.5% above and 2.5% below. The sponsor should know the source of subjects who provide this normal range, and most laboratories periodically update their ranges of reference values to reflect the population they serve. Reliability indicates that the test is consistent over time and a reliable test correlates highly with successive measures.

An individual study subject with one or more abnormal safety values in a trial may have responded adversely to the drug, but other causes should be sought. These include concurrent and intermittent illnesses, concurrent medications, alcohol or drug abuse and progress of the disease. The careful follow-up of the subject with repeated laboratory tests during and after treatment will usually resolve whether the observations are attributable to the drug.

Some changes in laboratory values in groups of subjects, but remaining within the normal range, are more difficult to interpret. Seeking similar trend patterns in concurrent or subsequent clinical trials may help to confirm or dispel beliefs about attributing the abnormal findings to the drug. A not so infrequent finding of this kind is a transient rise in liver transaminases or creatine kinase, but usually a careful history and follow- up investigations will determine whether the enzyme changes are, for example, due to an acute viral infection or an exposure to the drug.

Laboratory safety data can be erroneous, and this must always be considered when abnormalities are reported. There are numerous sources of error, which may be related to the study subject (e.g. self-medication, certain foods, undue exercise), sample collection technique, storage and transport, the analytical technique used

Table 7.2 Sources of error in laboratory values

Reason for error	Possible result
Slow separation of blood	Increase in plasma potassium, phosphate, total acid phosphate, lactate dehydrogenase, hydroxy butyrate dehydrogenase, and aspartate aminotransferase
Haemolysis of blood during venesection, prolonged venous stasis	Increased calcium, thyroxine, total protein, lipids and subfractions
Infusion in same arm as sampling	Increased electrolyte and glucose levels, dilution of all other parameters
Thawed samples	Low glucose and protein and loss of plasma enzyme activities
Inaccurately timed urine collection	Erratic clearance data
Palpation of bladder and prostate catherisation	Rise in tartrate-labile acid phosphate
Glucose not in fluoride bottle	Low glucose
Incorrect container for blood	EDTA or oxalate cause low calcium with high sodium and potassium

(e.g. high variability, inappropriate reference ranges, interfering substance in the sample) or to the report (e.g. transcription errors). Some of the sources of error are listed in Table 7.2. When there is doubt about the validity of the test, it should be repeated and, if necessary, at a different laboratory.

7.5.3.7.4 *Action taken in response to abnormal findings*

Individual study subjects may have to be withdrawn from the trial if abnormalities in laboratory safety data are confirmed and considered serious. Trends in laboratory findings in certain groups, for example, the elderly, or in all study subjects may result in additional investigations being requested in subsequent clinical trials, for example, measurement of hepatic transaminases. Further clinical trials will provide information as to how well the study drug is tolerated and whether the benefits revealed by laboratory safety and efficacy data outweigh the overall risk.

7.5.4 Data management

The assembling of clinical trial data before analysis constitutes a major workload, dictated by the quantity and the quality of the data. If the quality is poor, the process is extended by remedial steps going all the way back to the investigator site. Therefore, all the preceding efforts to bring high-quality data from investigators are amply justified by the resources and time actually saved during the data management process. Computerised systems are essential for handling the quantity of the data, and for future interrogation. Organisations and pharmaceutical companies are still inclined to create separate databases for each trial, using different machines, different codes and different locations (for instance, different countries). In the drive to save time and money, it is essential to avoid this situation. IT specialists will reassure that, with a little programming, the merging of such data from many trials will be easy, but still problems frequently occur.

Two elements are features of modern data management: a validated computer system and highly professional specialist staff. Non-validated computer systems are unacceptable. The FDA documents 'Computerised Systems Used in Clinical Trials'[17] and the 21 CRF 11 Regulations[27] should be followed when processing clinical data in any computer system, even if the results will never be required to be used in any US regulatory application. All indications suggest that the principles in these documents should be adopted globally for clinical trial work. Specialist staff should be responsible for handling of the clinical data. Nowadays, data management is a recognised discipline with professional associations and university courses. Trained programmers and statisticians support them. Any temptation to avoid the use of trained staff and instead relying on secretaries, investigator site monitors or nurses could prolong the time of processing and may endanger the integrity of the results.

7.5.4.1 Computer systems in clinical trials

Because the use of computer systems in data management is so important, it is appropriate to have a basic understanding of what is required for a validated computer system. In simple terms, certain features distinguish a validated computer system from a non-validated system. The computer system has to be developed, implemented, operated and maintained in a controlled manner, from the design stage to its decommissioning. Each stage will need to be fully documented. Written functional specifications should be available. In many cases, the computer systems will be off-the-shelf commercially available systems and the vendor will need to have evidence that the product has been developed in a controlled environment. Often the QA personnel from an organisation using the particular system will visit the vendor to try to establish that accepted validation practices are being followed. They may be allowed to see the test results that must exist of the development and installation.

When any new software or hardware is used in the data management centre, so-called end-user testing should be undertaken. Also, if changes are made to the system or perhaps new versions of software introduced, then additional testing may be required and certainly the alterations or maintenance documented. There will be a need for written guidance documents, for example, SOPs relating to the use of the system, proper backup of data and, most importantly, security to prevent unauthorised individuals entering the system and changing data. Finally, all staff using the system need to be trained in its use.

7.5.4.2 The process

The system shown in Figure 7.1 reflects the process undertaken in many data management

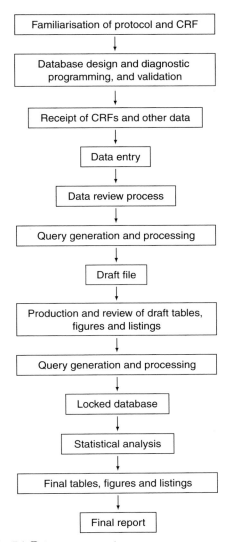

Fig. 7.1 Data management process.

groups. Although the positions of some of the stages such as data entry and query generation may vary, as in the case of electronic data capture at the investigator site, the activities will be similar for all data management. The clinical data may arrive in various forms at the data management centre. CRFs can arrive by fax, post or courier, central laboratory data by email or by diskette, scans by courier, assessments by an expert panel via courier, ECG and Holter data by courier or post, etc. It is therefore essential that proper tracking systems are in place.

The data manager will need to liaise with the programming and statistical individuals to decide the structure of the database. The requirement of interim analyses may impact on the processes and is of major significance if a clinical trial is blinded. Separate staff will be needed for the interim analysis if the regular staff are to remain blinded for the final analysis. Other considerations include the coding of the data and the dictionaries to be used, when and how the SAE/adverse event data will be incorporated into the structure and how much of the cleaning of the data will be done electronically (i.e. diagnostic programming). If data entry is performed in several centres (for instance, different countries) the standards must be identical. A centrally based validation group will monitor that these standards are being maintained and will identify early any persistent problems so that these can be avoided everywhere. Once the majority of data have been prepared as draft tables, figures and listings, and the final review has been carried out, the database is 'locked'. Only by a controlled and fully documented process should the database be unlocked to allow changes to be made. Inevitably, 'late' SAEs will cause additions to be made to the 'unlocked' database.

7.5.4.3 Coding

The process of coding was originally used to refer to 'data entry'. Coding was required because the old databases had little storage and by the selection of a corresponding code (numeric, alphabetic or alphanumeric) to the word or phrase of medical terminology, the database storage space could be conserved and searches of the database were possible. With modern sophisticated databases, storage should not be a problem. However, the use of coding does allow more advanced medical terminologies to be used and facilitates data search and manipulation. It also provides reproducibility and standardisation. Many large data management groups have professionals who concentrate solely on coding. These personnel are usually medically trained

and have a thorough understanding of the coding dictionaries. An important factor of having one central team performing the coding means that the coding is standardised and the clinical database is held in a central and uniform manner.

The pharmaceutical physician will have a role in ensuring that the coding has been carried out correctly. His or her medical training could easily be required to confirm some of the coding. Specific clinical data could be lost or misrepresented because a particular disease or adverse event was coded too generally. The opposite of this problem is coding that is too specific. A term can be coded in a way that fails to describe the disease or event because there is not enough flexibility in the coding. This can also cause problems when the clinical study report is written and when safety clinical data are being interpreted. Translation can cause problems during the coding process; it is important that the translation is done by a trained translator.

There is a plethora of medical terminologies available but the Medical Dictionary for Regulatory Activities (MedDRA)[28] has been adopted by the ICH as the standard medical terminology for regulatory communication.

7.5.4.4 Audit and data trails

A fundamental principle of GCP is that the data recorded in the CRF or in any of the accompanying documentation, for example, copies of diary cards, cannot be changed without the agreement in writing of the investigator. Changes due to errors or missing data will have to be made to the computer files to produce 'clean data files' (files free of known errors). These changes should be noted on the original CRFs or in error logs on to which written amendments are added, signed and dated by the investigator. Many individuals, including senior pharmaceutical physicians, have wanted to alter data on CRFs because 'they know the data are wrong'. However, an unauthorised change to any data supplied by the investigator is unacceptable. Once a 'clean file' is declared, any subsequent changes must be justified and authorised. Modern computer systems can provide a record of all the changes (i.e. audit trail) that have been made, by whom and why, a feature that could be required at any future regulatory inspection. Any changes, for instance, to a classification of study subjects, must be justified and agreed by all concerned. Another important series of steps is extraction of data and, in a similar manner, a 'data trail' should be established, showing how data were manipulated to create tables, graphs and data sets or lists for statistical analysis. It is crucial that the manner in which these were structured (i.e. rules applied, identifiers of data sets) is recorded so that they can be reproduced later, for instance, when more data from other trials are available. The statisticians will rightly ask questions about the database, essentially seeking assurance on the points outlined above. Their analysis can only be judged to be correct if it truly reflects the original CRF data. Understandably, the statisticians' confidence in the data presented to them is of paramount concern and their questioning of data should be regarded as legitimate.

7.5.4.5   Statistical analysis

Before the study starts, at the stage of the clinical trial design and the preparation of the protocol, a qualified statistician must be consulted and a statistical analysis plan produced. A summary of this plan will be included in the protocol but usually a more detailed document of the plan is prepared. The qualified statistician will have experience of clinical trials and ideally should be a chartered statistician or equivalent. It is essential that the statistical analysis described at the beginning of the study is used at the end of the study or reasons documented as to why it has been changed. Frequently, the results of the analysis are not as expected. It is tempting for some research workers to 'massage' the data with statistics in an attempt to produce the results that they would like. The treatment of missing data, data for subjects who did not meet inclusion criteria and should therefore have been excluded, and missing critical or secondary endpoint data feature frequently in many revised plans. In addition, when there are protocol changes, the

impact on the original plan is often underrated. The ICH has produced a number of guidance documents.[29–31]

7.5.4.6   Data integrity

The institution, pharmaceutical company or independent investigator carry considerable responsibility as custodian of trial data and is potentially exposed to charges of bias, of suppression or even of alteration of data. Data may be modified in order to correct errors but all changes must be tracked. QC and assurance steps must be part of the process – not only carried out but also recorded (see Section 7.7).

7.5.4.7   The end of the study

The closing down of the clinical trial at the site after the last visit of the last study subject has finished and all the CRFs are completed is an important part of the clinical trial. The process of archiving the documentation, both at the site and at the sponsor office, needs to take place – ideally as soon as possible after the end of the clinical phase of the study. The effort required to do this well is very much less than that which will be required if deficiencies are identified later – particularly if that occurs during a regulatory authority inspection!

The clinical trial monitor should visit the investigator site and ensure that the appropriate arrangements have been made to archive, and officially close down the site. These documents will include nearly all the documents in the investigator's master file, the investigator's copies of the CRF and any records that are in the pharmacy associated with the study. The monitor will advise the investigator to try to prevent the medical records of the study subjects from being deleted or lost and check that all randomisation codes have been returned from blind studies without being opened except in a recorded emergency. Study drug, returned from subject use or unused, will be destroyed or sent back to the supplier. The final safety report will be sent to the IEC.

The investigator may wish to archive the site's documents at the site or may wish the sponsor to supply space. In this case, the documents should be sealed so that there is no opportunity for anyone but the investigator to see these documents. All the documents at the sponsor's office, whether paper or electronic, should also be archived.

The length of time required to archive the documents is at least 2 years after the last approval of the marketing application or any contemplated marketing application, or at least 2 years after the formal discontinuation of clinical development (ICH GCP 5.5.11).[1] These requirements make long-term planning for archiving difficult because usually one does not know what the status of the study drug will be in 6 months' time, and certainly not in 2 or 3 years.

7.5.4.8 Regulatory inspections and QA audits

The new European Directive (2001/20/EC)[7] has reinforced the need for European agencies, as well as those of the United States and Japan, to conduct inspections of clinical trials. Sponsors, mindful of the implications of failed inspections, are carrying out audits by their QA units to try to ensure that standards at a particular site meet the regulatory requirements of GCP, and of any future regulatory inspection. Frequently, the inspections will occur 2 or more years after the end of the study.

Inspectors will visit the investigator site and may possibly wish to visit the sponsor's office. They will review the documentation of the study file (see Box 7.1). Approval documents of the IEC will be compared with any amendments made to the protocol or to the subject's information sheet/ICF. Consent forms for the study subjects will be inspected to establish who actually gave consent and whether this was before entry into the clinical study. A thorough source data verification of the CRF with the source documents, including the medical records, will be undertaken. Documentation relating to drug accountability will be matched with each subject's CRF. The facilities will be reviewed and the site staff interviewed. Further information can be obtained from

FDA guidance manuals.[32,33] Frequent questions asked include:

- The whereabouts of original documents if only photocopies are available.
- Is there sufficient source documentation to indicate that the study subject existed?
- Is the medical condition suffered by the subject appropriate for the study?
- Did the subject attend all the visits or otherwise?
- Who collected the trial data and was this appropriate?

In a similar manner, QA departments and consultants paid for by the sponsor will conduct audits of investigator sites. Again, as with the clinical trial monitor, there may be some annoyance among the investigator and his staff that some person, who may not be a physician, should be appointed by the sponsor to review the clinical trial documentation at the site.

7.6 Preparation of the Clinical Report

7.6.1 General considerations

The purpose of a clinical trial is to gain new knowledge that adds something to existing evidence and so it may, together with other trials, influence therapeutic decisions. If the knowledge is not written down, then it is unlikely to be known by more than a few individuals. This section concentrates on the technical requirements of a clinical trial report for the registration of a pharmaceutical product. However, readers would be well advised to use the recommendations of ICH Guidelines E3[34,35] on the preparation of such a report.

Extensive tables of data will accompany the regulatory application so that the regulators can run an independent analysis. In contrast, only limited data are published in journals. The editor and the reviewer, when provided with the scientific paper to be published, are seldom provided with adequate data to allow a detailed critique. For the manufacturer, the findings from clinical trials form the basis of what is said about the efficacy, safety and quality of a new medicine when applying for a marketing licence and when persuading doctors to use the medicine. Whether the report is of a small academic investigation or part of the research for a future commercial product, its preparation justifies care and attention.

The ICH GCP requires that all clinical trials involving human subjects should be reported, even if only one study subject is involved (ICH GCP 5.22).[1] This is another protective wall, along with ethical approval and informed consent, against unapproved and sloppy experimentation on humans.

7.7 Quality Management

The final principle of ICH GCP states that 'systems with procedures that assure the quality of every aspect of the trial should be implemented' (ICH GCP 2.13).[1] The word 'quality' is often misunderstood, although freely used when referring to processes and documentation in clinical trials. It should mean that a degree or standard of excellence has been reached particularly because the health of study subjects is at stake. Some regulatory authorities, such as the FDA, require evidence the reliability and completeness of the data to support a quality claim. They conduct inspections of the investigator site and critically interrogate the clinical data collected. Regulatory frameworks, such as ICH GCP, have been established for all research destined to support the licensing of new medicines.

The GCP guidelines have not always been fully applied to other biomedical research, such as some independent studies on marketed products initiated by clinicians without support from the manufacturer. The training that clinicians, scientists and technicians receive from company-based staff before and during a sponsored clinical trial adds considerably to the quality standards.

In Europe, the new EU Clinical Trial Directive[7] requires all, non-commercial and commercial, clinical trials to be conducted to the GCP standard.

In some pharmaceutical companies and institutions, the principles of total quality management (TQM)[36] or philosophies associated with

European Foundation for Quality Management (EFQM)[37] have been adopted. Schemes designed to encourage the involvement of factory workers in quality management do not always lend themselves successfully to clinical trial management. A more precise and, in many cases, a more vigorous approach is the series of quality management standards and guidelines called ISO 9000.[38] Sweeney[39] has provided details of how the original versions of ISO 9000 standards could be applied to clinical trials. However, all these quality systems can provide only a limited foundation. Independent reviewers, auditors from QA groups and inspectors from regulatory agencies must reinforce the quality systems.

7.7.1 QC and QA

Many scientists confuse the terms QC and QA. In terms of clinical trials, there is a very real difference. QC is the operational techniques and activities undertaken by all participants to verify that the quality requirements of the clinical trial have been fulfilled whereas QA verifies that the QC has satisfied these requirements. In other words, QC is where the data recorded is checked with source documents, and that measurements and procedures followed are those described in SOPs and the protocol. QA is where independent individuals establish that QC is in place and report any deficiencies without bias.

7.7.1.1 Quality control

Quality control should be present at all phases of a clinical trial whether in the preparation, during or in the analysis of the clinical data and writing of the clinical trial report. The clinician has been perceived as harbouring hesitation in using QC in clinical research, perhaps, due to a fear of finding mistakes in processes that reflect on clinical professionalism, a lack of time or in some unfortunate cases, arrogance that nothing could be wrong. This has resulted in the drug industry recruiting non-medical scientists to independently monitor the activities occurring at the site. At the investigator site, the investigator and his or her staff will have essential tasks and responsibilities, which if not scrupulously followed might alter the outcome of the trial. The site needs to have the right subject, with the right disease, who is receiving the right treatment in the right dose at the right time. The next requirements are the right observations made correctly, recorded accurately and checked as being complete. The objective measurements (such as blood pressure, peak expiratory flow, gastric emptying times, skin thickness, reaction times) can be defined, sometimes calibrated and the reproducibility of repeated measurements validated. Any variability should be related to physiological or other factors (for instance, diurnal changes, food intake, exercise, anxiety). Subjective endpoints have to some extent been structured and validated (for instance, anxiety or depression rating scales) and the training of staff in their consistent use in multicentre trials is essential before the study starts. All these observations will be recorded in CRFs and in many cases in the medical records of the subject.

7.7.1.2 The role of the clinical trial nurse or coordinator

Many investigator sites employ part- or full-time nurses to support the clinical trials. Nurses should never be considered to be an extravagance, because without them, the onus of administration and QC is solely on the investigator. The clinical trial nurse can help the investigator in many ways, but two of the most important are ensuring that the CRF reflects what is present in the source documents, such as essential events of the medical history of the subject, and close liaison with the sponsor's monitor.

7.7.1.3 Quality assurance

All clinical trials should be subjected to QA, either by an in-house department or by external consultants. QA is defined as 'all those planned and systematic actions that are established to ensure that the trial is performed and the data generated, documented (recorded), and reported in compliance with GCP and the applicable regulatory requirements(s)' (ICH GCP 1·46).[1] Those persons

undertaking QA should have sufficient independence of the clinical trial and its management to report any deficiencies without bias. QA will conduct audits to establish whether QC has taken place, whether SOPs are being followed and that the quality systems in place will provide accurate and correct clinical data to GCP standards. The word 'audit' is often used for various QA and QC functions. However, some QA experts prefer not to use the word 'audit' when operations are carried out by QC individuals because of the danger that the QC process is confused with that of QA. If a regulatory authority conducts an audit, it is usually called an 'inspection'.

Quality assurance has many other functions. As mentioned, QA should be part of the review board for new protocols and the associated documents, but in addition, individuals from the QA department will conduct audits of investigator site. The clinical data that have so laboriously been obtained may be of a high quality but the manner in which they are processed and analysed can reduce the quality and create numerous problems. The QA auditors should audit the processes of the data management, statistics and safety reporting groups on a regular basis.[40] The clinical study report should also be audited. One would hope that vigorous QC processes are in place, but these processes can vary depending on the availability of suitable QC individuals and the frequent pressure to meet timelines.

Increasingly, the QA department conducts audits of systems and processes in the general organisation and management of the clinical department, any contracted research organisation and vendor. The regulatory agencies will expect all functions in the clinical trial that are subcontracted to meet the requirements of GCP. For example, the central laboratory, the software house that provides the programming for the electronic diary used in a particular study and the contract archives used to store documentation from a clinical trial need to be audited. Often the QA department will provide a supporting function in the preparation and revision of SOPs and in the training of staff involved in clinical trials.

7.7.2 Fraud/misconduct

The FDA defines fraud as the deliberate reporting of false or misleading data or the withholding of reportable data. Although the agency has used the word 'fraud', in the United States the word usually implies injury or damage to victims and therefore the word 'misconduct' is preferred. Fraud in clinical research may be a rare phenomenon[41] but no one really knows how many cases are undetected or not reported. In the United Kingdom, a pharmaceutical company reporting an investigator for fraud may experience a backlash from the local professional and lay community before the full facts become known. The motives of a fraudulent investigator may be financial gain or professional promotion, trying to produce results either too quickly or too precisely. In some cases, work overload or mental illness provide a backdrop to the crime.

The fraudulent investigator may add data where the original are missing, possibly not wanting to admit that they forgot to obtain or record them or that they lost them (for instance, broken blood sample tube). Serious cases involve falsification of subject data where study subjects do not exist or were not actually recruited. Ethical approval and consent documentation are 'created' at the site.[41–43]

Certain quality management measures already outlined, and summarised in Table 7.3, will reduce the opportunities for fraud.

Fraud should be contained with regular monitoring, an active QA unit and an increasing role for inspectors from the regulatory agencies. Statisticians should routinely scrutinise demographic

Table 7.3 Methods of detecting fraud

Method	Comment
Verify if the original source data match that which is recorded and reported	Importance of sufficient source documents, for example, medical records, radiographs and laboratory results
Do the data fit together with time?	Do visit dates match collection of samples? Are the values consistent?
Check reasons for missing records	Missing records should be explained, correspondence files should confirm explanation
Can you read the erasures? Are the results too good to be true?	No whiteout; erasures can be read; 'perfect' results on paper without wear and tear should be checked
Establish who is recording the data	Is the investigator signing-off the CRF? Is the delegation of roles of staff being followed? Consent forms should contain more than one handwriting style
Do the data look real?	There should be some deviation in the data and erratic data points. Check, variation with other sites using biostatistics
Is the site meeting expectations or does it appear 'too efficient' to have achieved all the work?	Can all the work be done in the timeframe allowed with the facilities and equipment available?

differences in the subjects recruited at one centre compared with other centres, clustering of laboratory data, and variations in data to establish both the scientific significance of the results and also whether the data of a particular site need investigation for fraud.[42]

As soon as fraud is suspected, a series of steps needs to be followed which have been thought out and written down as an SOP before any clinical research commenced. Where possible, additional evidence should be obtained, usually by the use of a competent QA auditor. In the meantime, only the minimum key individuals should be made aware of the problem until sufficient evidence has been obtained to establish the truth. The appropriate authorities such as the national drug industry organisation and the regulatory authorities should be informed if fraud has taken place. Sometimes, other sponsors will have reported additional evidence that fraud is taking place at a particular site. The site will need to be closed if study subjects are still being recruited and a full explanation provided to the authorities. Any clinical data collected will need to be reviewed and a decision made as to whether any of the data can be included in an analysis. To a pharmaceutical physician, fraud is never an easy situation. It usually involves a professional colleague and there is always the worry that the established facts have been misinterpreted. However, a fraudulent individual cannot be tolerated in modern clinical research.

Fraud is not limited to the investigator and his or her staff. Staff of pharmaceutical companies and institutions may alter CRFs, modify data sets, alter tables, suppress reported side effects or bias written reports. The detection of such activities, inside or outside an institution, by investigators or company staff relies on others in the same team recognising that something is suspicious. Double checking of data by colleagues and authentication of those data is the best deterrent to misconduct.

7.8   Conclusion

The perception that the impact of GCP and the new EU Directive will lead to bureaucracy and the stifling of investigator-instigated and non-commercial research is a pessimistic view. An improvement in the quality of the data and greater respect for the study subject should provide ample benefit over any disadvantages, especially if the regulators are receptive to the ever-changing climate of research. The regulatory authorities will continue to issue guidelines for the registration of drugs, but sponsors must be prepared to take the decision on their interpretation after due consultation. There is no evidence that the investment in manpower and other resources necessary to execute clinical programmes will decrease, and the use of specialist contract organisations in all areas – trial monitoring, data handling, report writing and consultancy – is likely to continue. As companies strive harder for shorter, surer paths to regulatory approval, the well-conceived, well-executed and correctly interpreted clinical trial will continue to be pivotal.

References

1. International Conference on Harmonisation (ICH) of Technical Requirements of Pharmaceuticals for Human Use. *Topic E6 Note for Guidance on Good Clinical Practice: Consolidated Guideline, CPMP/ICH/135/95*. London: European Agency for the Evaluation of Medicinal Products, 1996.

2. Food Drug Administration (FDA). International conference on harmonisation, good clinical practice: consolidated guidelines. *Federal Register* 1997;**62**:25692–709.

3. Food Drug Administration (FDA) *Protection of Human Subjects Code of Federal Regulations, Title 21, Part 50–55*. Washington: US Government Printing Office, 1997.

4. World Medical Association (WMA). Declaration of Helsinki, 52nd WMA General Assembly, Edinburgh, Scotland. Available at: http://www.wma.net/e/policy/17-c_e.html. Assessed 26 June 2001.

5. European Agency for the Evaluation of Medicinal Products. *Explanatory Note and Comments to the ICH Harmonised Tripartite Guideline E6: Note for Guidance on Good Clinical Practice, CPMP/768/97*. London: European Agency for the Evaluation of Medicinal Products, 1997

6. World Health Organization (WHO). *Technical Report Series, No. 850. Annex 3 Guidelines for Good*

Clinical Practice (GCP) for Trials on Pharmaceutical Products. Geneva, Switzerland: World Health Organization, 1995 (modified 2000).

7. European Parliament. Directive 2001/20/EC of the European parliament and of the council of 04 April 2001 on the approximation of the laws, regulations and administrative provisions of the member states relating to the implementation of good clinical practice in the conduct of clinical trials on medicinal products for human use. *OJC* 2001;**121**:34–44.

8. Hochhauser M. The informed consent form: document development and evaluation. *Drug Inf J* 2000;**34**:1309–17.

9. Association of the British Pharmaceutical Industry. *Clinical Trial Compensation Guidelines*, 418/94/6600M. London: ABPI, 1994.

10. European Parliament. Directive 95/46/EC of the European parliament and of the council of 24 October 1995 on the protection of individuals with regard to the processing of personal data and on the free movement of such data. *OJC* 1995;**281**:31–50.

11. Doclo RJ. Improving SOP writing with process mapping. *Appl Clin Trials* 2000; **9**:62–70.

12. European Commission. *Revision of Annex 13 to the European Guide to Good Manufacturing Practice.* Brussels: Directorate-General Office, 1996 (new draft 2001).

13. Commission of the European Communities. The rules governing medicinal products in the EC. In: *Good Manufacturing Practice for Medicinal Products.* Luxembourg: Commission Office for Official Publications of the EC, 1992.

14. Food and Drug Administration (FDA). *Current Good Manufacturing Practice in Manufacturing, Processing, Packaging or Holding of Drugs; General. Code of Federal Regulations 210, 211.* Washington DC: National Archives and Records Administration, 1997.

15. Committee for Proprietary Medicinal Products. *Note for Guidance on the Investigation of Bioavailability and Bioequivalence, CPMP/EWP/QWP/1401/98.* London: European Agency for the Evaluation of Medicinal Products, 2000 (Draft).

16. Double ME, McKendry M. *Computer Validation Compliance.* Buffalo Grove, IL: Interpharm, 1994.

17. Food and Drug Administration (FDA). *Guidance for Industry – Computerised Systems Used in Clinical Trials.* Rockville, MD: Division of Compliance Policy, 1999.

18. O'Shea K. Interactive voice response technology. *Appl Clin Trials* 1998;**7**:30–4.

19. Department of Health (UK). *Governance Arrangements for NHS Research Ethics Committee.* London: Central Office for Research Ethics Committees (COREC), 2001.

20. Food and Drug Administration (FDA). *Investigational New Drug Application. 21 Code of Federal Regulations Part 312.* Washington DC: National Archives and Records Administration, 1998.

21. Tarantowski R. Writing a clinical trial budget. *Appl Clin Trials* 1996;**5**:26–40.

22. Food and Drug Administration (FDA). Financial disclosure by clinical investigators. Title 21 Code of Federal Regulations Parts 54, 312, 314, 320, 330, 601, 807. *Federal Register* 1998;**63**:5233–54.

23. Food and Drug Administration (FDA). Recruiting study subjects. In: *Guidance for Institutional Review Boards and Clinical Investigators Section in Information Sheets.* Rockville, MD: Office of the Associated Commissioner for Health Affairs, 1998 (update)

24. Edwards RI, Aronson JK. Adverse drug reactions: definitions, diagnosis and management. *Lancet* 2000;**356**:1255–9.

25. International Conference on Harmonisation (ICH) of Technical Requirements of Pharmaceuticals for Human Use. *Topic 2A Note for Guidance on Clinical Safety Data Management: Definitions and Standards for Expedited Teporting, CPMP/ICH/377/95.* London: European Agency for the Evaluation of Medicinal Products, 1994.

26. Karch FE, Lasagna MD. Adverse drug reaction. *JAMA* 1975;**234**:1236–41.

27. Food and Drug Administration (FDA). Code of Federal Regulations Title 21, Part 11, electronic records and electronic signatures. *Federal Register* 1997;**62**:13, 430–66.

28. International Conference on Harmonisation (ICH) of Technical Requirements of Pharmaceuticals for Human Use. *Topic M1 Medical Terminology* (Draft). Available at: http://www.ifpma.org/ich5e.html. Accessed 21 July 2001.

29. International Conference on Harmonisation (ICH) of Technical Requirements of Pharmaceuticals for Human Use. *Topic E10 Note for Guidance on Choice of Control Group in Clinical Trials, CPMP/ICH/364/96.* London: European Agency for the Evaluation of Medicinal Products, 2001.

30. International Conference on Harmonisation (ICH) of Technical Requirements of Pharmaceuticals for Human Use. *Topic E9 Note for Guidance on Statistical Considerations in the Design of Clinical Trials, CPMP/ICH/363/96.* London: European Agency for the Evaluation of Medicinal Products, 1998.

31. International Conference on Harmonisation (ICH) of Technical Requirements of Pharmaceuticals for Human Use. *Topic E4 Note for Guidance on Dose–Response Information to Support Drug Registration, CPMP/ICH/378/95.* London: European Agency for the Evaluation of Medicinal Products, 1994.

32. Food and Drug Administration (FDA). *Compliance Program Guidance Manual (7348-811) Clinical Investigators.* Rockville, MD: Division of Compliance Policy, 1999.

33. Food and Drug Administration (FDA). *Compliance Program Guidance Manual (7348.810) Sponsors, Contract Research Organisations and Monitors.* Rockville, MD: Division of Compliance Policy, 1999.

34. International Conference on Harmonisation (ICH) of Technical Requirements of Pharmaceuticals for Human Use. *Topic E3 Note for Guidance on Structure and Content of Clinical Study Reports, CPMP/ICH/137/95.* London: European Agency for the Evaluation of Medicinal Products, 1996.

35. International Conference on Harmonisation (ICH) of Technical Requirements of Pharmaceuticals for Human Use. *Topic M4 Organisation of Common Technical Document for the Registration of Pharmaceuticals for Human Use, CPMP/ICH/2887/99.* London: European Agency for the Evaluation of Medicinal Products, 2000.

36. Feigenbaum AV. *Total Quality Control.* New York: McGraw-Hill, 1951.

37. European Foundation for Quality Management. The Excellence Model. Brussels: European Foundation for Quality Management. Available at: http://www.efqm.org.html. Accessed 21 July 2001.

38. International Standards Organisation. *International Standard ISO 9001, Quality Systems – Model for Quality Assurance in Design, Development, Production, Installation and Servicing.* Geneva, Switzerland: International Standards Organisation, 1994.

39. Sweeney F. Merging GCP and ISO 9000 requirements – a source of synergy in quality management of clinical research. *Drug Inf J* 1994;**28**: 1097–104.

40. Campbell H, Sweatman J. Quality assurance and clinical data management. In: Rondel RK, Varley SA, Webb CF, eds. *Clinical Data Management, 2nd edn.* Chichester, UK: John Wiley, 2000;123–41.

41. Buyse M, George SL, Evans S, *et al.* The role of biostatistics in the prevention, detection and treatment of fraud in clinical trials. *Stat Med* 1999;**18**:3435–51.

42. Mackintosh DR, Zepp VJ. Detection of negligence, fraud and other bad faith efforts during field auditing of clinical trial sites. *Drug Inf J* 1996;**30**:645–53.

43. Lock S, ed. *Fraud and Misconduct in Medical Research, 2nd edn.* London: BMJ Publishing, 1996.

Recommended Reading

Friedman LM, Furberg CD, DeMets DL. *Fundamentals of Clinical Trials, 3rd edn.* New York: Springer-Verlag, 1998.

Senn S. *Statistical Issues in Drug Development.* Chichester, UK: John Wiley, 1997.

Spilker B. *Guide to Clinical Trials.* New York: Raven Press, 1991.

Useful Internet Addresses

British Pharmacopoeia	www.pharmacopoeia.org.uk
Centers for Disease Control	www.cdc.gov
Central Office for Research Ethics Committees (COREC)	www.corec.org.uk
Drug Information Association	www.diahome.org
European Drug Regulatory Affairs	www.eudra.org
European National Medicines Authorities	www.heads.medagencies.org
FDA	www.fda.gov
Food and Drug Law Institute (FDLI)	www.fdli.org
ICH	www.ifpma.org/ich1.html
Medicines and Healthcare Products Regulatory Agency (MHRA)	www.mhra.gov.uk
National Institutes of Health	www.nih.gov
National Library of Medicine	www.nlm.nih.gov
Regulatory Affairs Professional Society (RAPS)	www.raps.org
Pharmaceutical Research Manufacturers Association	www.phrma.org
US Pharmacopeia	www.usp.org
World Health Organisation (WHO)	www.who.ch

CHAPTER 8

8

Medical statistics

Andrew P Grieve

8.1 Introduction

The rapid accrual of biomedical information has led to considerable interest both in the notion of evidence-based medicine and also in the history of the use of quantitative evidence in medicine. Tröhler[1] has shown that the origins of a quantitative approach to medicine can be traced back to the eighteenth century in Britain and was a movement begun by physicians who believed that there was a need to move to an empirical approach to medicine and away from the systemic-pathophysiological approach of antiquity.

Today, statistics is a necessary and important link in the interdisciplinary chain of drug discovery and development. There is no part of the drug development process where statistics does not have a place: from screening chemicals for activity in drug discovery, through all phases of clinical development, through pharmaceutical development and manufacturing, to the forecasting of the potential sales of a new drug. In all of these contexts statisticians and statistics are involved in helping scientists understand the size of effects relative to considerable variability, whether it is biological variability, in the animal or human case, or seasonal variability when it comes to forecasting sales of an antihistamine. In this chapter, we concentrate on the application of statistics to clinical research.

8.2 Probability

The basis of all statistical inference is probability and in order to understand properly such ideas such as confidence intervals and significance tests, a basic understanding of probability is necessary.

8.2.1 What is probability?

What does it mean to say 'the probability of heads is half when a coin is tossed'? It simply means that if we were to toss the coin a very large number of times, heads would occur approximately half of the time. If we were to toss the coin 1000 times we would expect to get about 500 heads, not exactly 500 heads, but about 500 heads. Of course, if we were to toss the coin only twice, there is no guarantee that heads will occur only once. If we were to toss the coin four times, there is no guarantee that heads will occur twice. So what can we say about the distribution of likely outcomes in this latter case? How likely is it that we might get three heads and a single tail? We can determine how likely different outcomes are by enumeration. Table 8.1 gives the possible outcomes from tossing a coin four times.

Allowing for the order of the occurrences of heads and tails, we can readily determine the probability of given outcomes. For example, the probability of getting three heads and one tail can be seen to be $\frac{4}{16} = 0.25$.

As a second example, the chance of getting a one or two from throwing a fair die is $\frac{1}{3}$. What is the likely outcome if the fair die is tossed 10 times? Enumeration could again be used to determine the probability of zero, one, two, etc., occurrences of one or two. As a result of the process the distribution of outcomes is shown in Figure 8.1 from which it is determined that

Table 8.1 Enumeration of the results of tossing a coin four times

Number of Heads					
0	**1**	**2**	**3**	**4**	
TTTT	TTTH	TTHH	THHH	HHHH	
	TTHT	THTH	HTHH		
	THTT	THHT	HHTH		
	HTTT	HTTH	HHHT		
		HTHT			
		HHTT			
Total 1	4	6	4	1	16

the most likely outcome is three out of 10 with a probability of just over one quarter; the probability of getting zero occurrences is approximately one in 60; there is a very small probability of getting eight or more occurrences.

The distribution illustrated in Figure 8.1 is an example of what is called a sampling distribution and it will be important when we come to consider statistical tests.

8.2.2 Inductive probability

The sampling distribution determined in the previous section is an example of a deductive use of probability. Given that the probability of an occurrence of a one or two is known, we were able to deduce the probability of the outcomes that could arise if the die was tossed 10 times. In medical research, however we do not know what the true probability (response probability) is. Ours is the reverse problem, we observe a response rate, for example, 23 out of 80 patients respond positively to a given treatment, and want to infer what the true population response rate is. The requirement is to be able to make inductive probability statements.

To illustrate, consider the following information about asymptomatic women participating in breast screening given by Gigerenzer.[2]

1. The probability of any woman having breast cancer is 0.8% (less than one in 100);

2. if a woman has breast cancer the probability of a positive mammogram is 90%;

3. if a woman does not have breast cancer the probability of a positive mammogram is 7%.

Suppose that a woman has a positive mammogram. What is the probability that she in fact has breast cancer? To solve this problem statisticians use Bayes' Theorem, a theorem in conditional probability introduced by the non-conformist minister the Reverend Thomas Bayes in 1763.[3] Gigerenzer explains how Bayes' theorem works by converting the problem into 'natural frequencies'.

If there are 100 000 asymptomatic patients in the population, then 800 will have breast cancer (0.8%–**1**). Of these, 720 (90%–**2**) will have a positive mammogram. The remaining 99 200 women do not have breast cancer, but 6944 (7%–**3**) will nonetheless have a positive mammogram. Therefore, in total 7664 women will have a positive mammogram, of which 720 would in reality have breast cancer. Thus the probability that a woman with a positive mammogram has breast cancer is 720/7644 = 9.4%.

While the use of Bayes' Theorem in this context is not generally controversial its use more generally in medical and clinical research has not always been positively received.[4] It is not the scope of the present chapter to illustrate the use of Bayesian statistics in a more general context and interested readers should read the excellent introduction to the use of Bayesian methods in health-care evaluation provided by Spiegelhalter et al.[5]

8.3 Scales of Measurement and Clinical Endpoints

When you can measure what you are speaking about, and express it in numbers, you know something about it; but when you cannot measure it, when you cannot express it in numbers, your knowledge is of a meagre and unsatisfactory kind: it may be the beginning of knowledge, but you have scarcely, in your thoughts, advanced to the stage of science. [Sir William Thomson (Lord Kelvin). Lecture to the Institution of Civil Engineers (May 3, 1883). In *Popular Lectures and Addresses*,

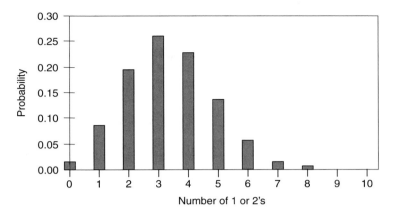

Fig. 8.1 Distribution of the number of one or two's out of 10.

Vol. 1, London & New York: Macmillan and Co., 1891; 80.]

The movement towards quantification in medicine required the development of measures of clinical effect. When assessing the effectiveness of his approach to removing bladder stones, the lithotomist William Cheselden measured the impact on mortality by determining the proportion of patients who died.[1] Similarly when measuring the pain relief of a treatment for migraine headache we need to define and measure pain. In whatever circumstances we are researching heart disease, depression, etc., we have to measure the severity and extent of the disease. From a statistical perspective, what is important is the scale of measurement. Statisticians generally recognise three types of scale: qualitative, ordinal and quantitative.

8.3.1 Qualitative data

The simplest form of qualitative data is *binary data* in which there are only two possible values, for example, death/survival; or success/failure each of which needs to be defined within a specified time interval; has pain relief been achieved within two hours of treatment, success – or not, failure. This form of data is extremely common in medical research and yet it ignores the possibility of gradation, success may not be total but only partial and yet not be total failure. These considerations lead naturally to the concept of *ordered categorical* or *ordinal* data.

As its name implies, the defining property of ordinal data is that there is a natural ranking in the outcome. For example, the pain associated with migraine headache is often measured on a 4-point ordinal scale: absent, mild, moderate or severe, wherein the pain being absent is better than experiencing a mild pain, is better than experiencing a moderate pain, is better than experiencing a severe pain. Often the categories are assigned a numerical value: 0 = absent, 1 = mild, 2 = moderate and 3 = severe, but care needs to be taken in the interpretation of such numbers since they do not comprise a true numerical scale. Thus, the difference between absent and mild is not necessarily equivalent to the difference between mild and moderate.

8.3.2 Quantitative data

There are two main types of quantitative data: discrete and continuous. Discrete quantitative data usually come about by the counting of numbers of events. Examples of this form of data are the number of asthma attacks, the numbers of rescue tablets taken, the number of relapse events, etc. There are two types of continuous quantitative data defined by, whether there is a true zero point of the scale or not. If there is such a zero point the scale is a ratio scale, otherwise it is an interval scale. Examples of the former are height, weight or volume, etc, while a typical example of the latter is temperature in which the origin is essentially arbitrary – 0°F is not equivalent to 0°C. In practice this distinction has no impact on the statistical analysis of data and the same techniques are applied to data from both ratio and interval scales.

8.3.3 Measurement and endpoints

It is important when choosing a particular measurement scale to answer a number of questions. Is the choice that is made of clinical relevance? How is the endpoint to be measured? Can we measure the clinical endpoint directly, or must we choose an indirect approach? Is the choice that is made sensitive enough to measure real treatment effects? Having collected the information how are we to analyse it? Some of these issues are illustrated in the following sections.

8.3.3.1 Responder rates

Increasingly clinical researchers ask questions like: what proportion of patients responds to treatment A? Do a greater proportion of patients respond to active treatment rather than placebo? In these circumstances, the endpoints tend not to be directly measured but are derived from other measurements. For example, suppose we are interested in measuring the reduction in blood pressure following treatment, in particular the primary interest is in determining the proportion of patients who experience a reduction of at

least 15 mmHg – defining such improvement as being a response. Figure 8.2 show data from 100 patients with the responder cut-point also being displayed. We can determine from the distribution that 73% of patients are classified as responders. Alternatively, we can fit a mathematical distribution to the data and estimate the rate from properties of the distribution. From the data in Figure 8.2 we can estimate the arithmetic mean of the data as well as the standard deviation – these are defined in Sections 8.4.1.1 and 8.4.1.2 – giving values of 26.8 mmHg and 10 mmHg. If the data can be assumed to follow a normal distribution then we can estimate that 76% of the distribution will lie below −15 mmHg.

The first point to be made is that if we can use a mathematical distribution to estimate the responder rate, it is more efficient than to count the number of observations meeting the condition. Such efficiency gains mean that using the distribution we will need fewer patients to estimate the rate to the same degree of accuracy. Senn[6] reports that the former approach can give rise to sample sizes 40% higher than using the original measurements. Intuitively this is reasonable because the use of a cut-point essentially says that we can distinguish between a reduction of 14.9 mmHg and 15.1 mmHg, whereas in reality those two measurements are essentially equivalent in terms

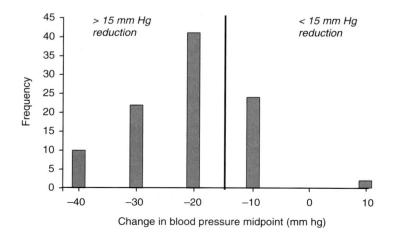

Fig. 8.2 Distribution of change in blood pressure (mmHg).

of the information they provide about the benefit of a treatment. Secondly, the choice of the cut-point is itself arbitrary. Why should a reduction of 15 mmHg be anymore important than any other? In his article, Senn strongly criticises this approach. However, it is widely used and does have its own supporters.[7]

8.3.3.2 Biomarkers and surrogate endpoints

In clinical trials intended to provide sufficient evidence for marketing approval of drugs, what is most important is to collect unequivocal evidence of a positive risk–benefit profile relative to an active comparator or placebo. For diseases that are life-threatening or those associated with severe morbidity, it is preferable that the primary endpoint is of clinical relevance, examples being mortality, a measurement of the patient's quality of life, such as relief of disease-related symptoms, improvement in ability to carry out normal activities or reduced hospitalization time. Unfortunately such trials may need to be very large; consequently they tend to have a long duration, and can be extremely costly.

In such circumstances there is an inevitable desire to find alternative, surrogate endpoints that allow the length and size of clinical trials to be considerably reduced.[8] A common approach has been to utlilise endpoints that are correlated with the outcome of primary interest. Minimally, all that this may require is that patients who experience some benefit on the surrogate tend to experience benefit on the clinically meaningful endpoint. While such an approach may be useful to demonstrate biological activity, in general it is not sufficient to make a reliable demonstration that a treatment will also positively impact the true clinical endpoint. As Fleming and DeMets[9] note 'a correlate does not a surrogate make'. What is required is that the effect of treatment on the biomarker correlates well with that on the final endpoint, so that a valid surrogate endpoint allows correct inference to be drawn regarding the effect of an intervention on the true clinical endpoint of interest.

Many statistical approaches have been proposed to ensure the validity of surrogates. The seminal work of Prentice[10] that focused on hypothesis testing has been followed by estimation-based methods such as Buyse and Molenberghs,[11–14] which aim to quantify the degree of validity of a surrogate.

There are many examples of biomarkers, which have been used as surrogates[9] in prominent clinical trials that have been subsequently found to be inadequate, illustrating the difficulty in identifying a surrogate endpoint. One notable scenario is that of a biomarker that responds to therapy and is highly predictive of survival, but does not predict the effect of treatment on survival. The use of CD4+ counts in HIV trials is an example of such a biomarker.[15,16]

Temple[17] has argued that there may be problems in correctly assessing the risk–benefit profile of a drug on the basis of findings on a surrogate. This may be the case, if the relationship between the biomarker and the clinical endpoint is coincidental or co-related by a third factor. Furthermore, favourable or unfavourable drug effects may remain undetected by the surrogate.[18]

Finally, there are time issues associated with biomarkers and surrogates. Biomarkers may be better predictors of short-term treatment effects than long-term effects[19] and therefore we need to be specific about the timing of outcome assessment when evaluating a biomarker. A distinction is drawn by Hughes et al.[20] between a concurrent surrogate, measured during the same time period as the clinical endpoint and an intermediate surrogate, which explains the effect of treatment on a clinical endpoint at some future time point.

8.3.3.3 Rating scales

In Section 8.3.1 we introduced the idea of a simple ordinal rating scale such as the 4-point scale for a migraine headache: absent, mild, moderate, severe. Another simple approach to measurement is the so-called visual analogue scale (VAS). The VAS is simply a line – normally 100 mm long – the ends of which are associated with descriptions of opposite extremes of the disease.

For example, in the treatment of depression the descriptions might be:

'Couldn't be feeling better' and 'Couldn't be more depressed'. The patient marks on the line, where his/her current experience of depression falls.

The advantage of this approach over a simple ordinal scale is that it has the characteristics of a continuous scale, and hence more sensitive methods can be used and potentially at least will result in smaller sizes. However, there are questions that are often raised concerning this approach.

• Can patients understand what they are supposed to do?
• If patients rate themselves on a VAS scale on two occasions when their disease is stable, will they provide similar results?
• Do patients use the scale in a similar way (Grieve[21])?

All the evidence available in the literature suggests that in general these concerns should not preclude the use of VAS scales in clinical studies.

In some diseases a simple ordinal scale or a VAS scale cannot describe the full spectrum of the disease. There are many examples of this including depression and erectile dysfunction. Measurement in such circumstances involves the use of multiple ordinal rating scales, often termed items. A patient is scored on each item and the summation of the scores on the individual items represents an overall assessment of the severity of the patient's disease status at the time of measurement. Considerable amounts of work have to be done to ensure the validity of these complex scales, including investigations of their reproducibility and sensitivity to measuring treatment effects. It may also be important in international trials to assess to what extent there is cross-cultural uniformity in the use and understanding of the scales. Complex statistical techniques such as principal components analysis and factor analysis are used as part of this process and one of the issues that need to be addressed is whether the individual items should be given equal weighting.

The use of these multiple rating scales is an attempt to develop a simple representation of what may be an extremely complex construct. Part of the statistical developments of these scales will be to identify so-called sub-domains of the disease, for example, physical, emotional and sexual. The identification of these subdomains will require close collaboration between the statistician and the clinical researcher in the interpretation of the results.

8.4   Basic Statistical Principles

There are two principal forms of statistics: descriptive and inferential. The purpose of descriptive statistics is to give a description of the data that have been collected, whether from a clinical trial, epidemiological investigation or survey. Inferential statistics is aimed at making probability-based statements about hypotheses, parameters of populations, etc.

8.4.1   Descriptive statistics

A major part of descriptive statistics is the use of graphical methods to represent data. It is not the scope of this chapter to cover graphical methods; however it is good statistical practice to produce a visual summary of data. In the following sections we concentrate on summary statistics that describe important aspects of data.

8.4.1.1   Measures of location and central tendency

The idea behind measures of location and central tendency is contained within the notion of the average. There are predominantly three summary statistics that are commonly used for describing this aspect of a set of data: the arithmetic mean – normally shortened to the mean, the mode and the median.

1. The mean of a set of values is determined by dividing the sum of the values by the number of values. It is mostly utilised for quantitative data, but if applied to binary that has been coded 0 or 1, the mean is the proportion or rate with the given characteristic.

2. The median is the typical value. It is the midpoint of the values when arranged in ascending

order and has 50% of the values above it and 50% below it. The median can be used for both quantitative and ordinal data. If there are an even number of values and therefore strictly no middle value, the average of the two middle values is taken.

3. The mode is the most commonly occurring value and can be used for qualitative, ordinal as well as quantitative data.

The data listed below and displayed in Figure 8.3 are random measurements of blood glucose (mmol/L) taken from 40 first year medical students.[22]

2.2	2.9	3.3 3.3 3.3
3.4 3.4 3.4	3.6 3.6 3.6	3.7 3.7
	3.6	
3.8 3.8 3.8	3.9	4.0 4.0 4.0
4.1 4.1 4.1	4.2	4.3
4.4 4.4 4.4	4.5	4.6
4.7 4.7 4.7	4.8	4.9 4.9
5.0	5.1	6.0

The arithmetic mean is:

$$\frac{2.2 + 2.9 + \cdots + 5.1 + 6.0}{40} = \frac{162.2}{40}$$

$$= 4.055 \text{ mmol/L}$$

As there are 40 values the median is determined by the average of the 20th and 21st values. Since these are both 4.0 the median is 4.0 mmol/L. The value 3.6 mmol/L occurs four times, more than any other, so 3.6 mmol/L is the modal value.

The three summary statistics are displayed in Figure 8.3. Clearly, for this data the mean and median are similar, and this is true for any distribution of values that is symmetric, which is the case here. The mode is somewhat removed from both the mean and median. In fact, the mode is not often used as a summary of data because it records only the most frequent value, and this may be far from the centre of the distribution. A second difficulty with the mode is that there can be more than one mode in a sample. For example, had one of the values 3.6 been instead 3.5, there would have been eight distinct modal values: 3.3, 3.4, 3.6, 3.8, 4.0, 4.1, 4.4 and 4.7 mmol/L.

The median does not use the actual numerical values; rather it used their relative magnitudes. The median remains unaffected by extreme values far out into the tails of the distribution. For example, had the value 6.0 mmol/L been 16.0 mmol/L the median value would have remained unchanged at 4.0 mmol/L.

The mean uses the most information from the sample, relying as it does on the actual numerical values. It is the most commonly used measure of location and therefore can be misused. For example, we have noted that it is inappropriate to use it for ordered categorical data such as: 0 = absent, 1 = mild, 2 = moderate, 3 = severe since in taking an average the implicit assumption is being made that a change from absent to mild is identical to a

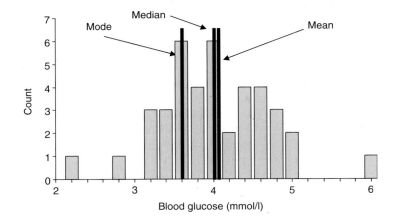

Fig. 8.3 Distribution of blood glucose levels from 40 students.

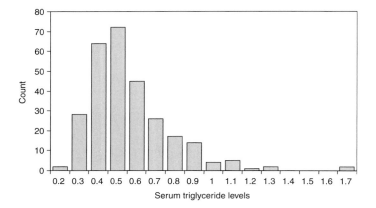

Fig. 8.4 Distribution of serum triglyceride levels from cord blood of 282 babies.

change from moderate to severe. The arithmetic mean is also sensitive to discrepant values. For a sample in which the value 6.0 mmol/L is replaced by 16.0 mmol/L, the mean changes from 4.055 mmol/L to 4.305 mmol/L. For this reason, the mean should not be used when data are asymmetric.

Figure 8.4 shows serum triglyceride level in cord blood from 282 babies.[22] Clearly, these data are not symmetric. The arithmetic mean is 0.506 units, while the median is 0.460 units. Bland[22] has shown that the logarithms of the data are remarkably symmetric and under such conditions, a more appropriate measure of location is the geometric mean, which can be calculated in two steps. First, the data are log-transformed and the arithmetic mean of the log-transformed data is calculated. Second, the arithmetic mean is back transformed using an exponential function to give the geometric mean. For the triglyceride data, the arithmetic mean of the log-transformed data is −0.761, and the corresponding geometric mean is 0.467 units, which is considerably closer to the median.

A final measure of location is the harmonic mean. This is rarely used explicitly although again it may be implicitly used. For example, when considering the analysis of heart rate data, many statisticians would recommend that the reciprocal of the heart rate be analysed rather than the heart rate itself. Again, this has to do with an attempt to make the distribution of the transformed variable be more symmetric. The

resulting variable is the duration of a heartbeat. If the arithmetic mean of the durations is determined and the reciprocal of this value taken, the resulting summary is the harmonic mean of the original heart rate data.

8.4.1.2 Measures of variability

In the previous section, we covered different summary measures for the location of a set of data. Measures of location on their own are not sufficient to characterise data. We also need to be able to measure the variability in data, a measure that indicates to what extent individual measurements differ from one another.

The simplest such measure is the range measuring the interval between the smallest and largest values in the sample. Although simple, it has the disadvantage that it tends to increase with sample size, since in larger samples we are increasingly likely to see extreme values. For the blood glucose data the range is $6.0 - 2.2 = 3.8$ mmol/L.

A second, simple measure of variability is the inter-quartile range that is the interval between the upper and lower quartiles. The upper quartile of a set of data is that value that is less than 25% of the data and greater than 75%; similarly, the lower quartile is the value that is greater than 25% of the data and less than 75%. For the blood glucose data the lower quartile is 3.6 mmol/L and the upper quartile 4.55 mmol/L, giving an inter-quartile range of 0.95 mmol/L.

Like the median, neither of these ranges accounts for the numerical values of all the data only their relative magnitudes. The standard deviation, which is the square root of the variance, accounts for the individual magnitudes and is a measure of the average squared-deviation of individual values from the sample mean. If the individual values are denoted by $y_i, i = 1, \ldots, n$ and the sample mean by $\bar{y}$, then the sample variance is

$$\frac{\sum_{i=11}^{n} (y_i - \bar{y})^2}{n}$$

from which the standard deviation is directly

$$s = \sqrt{\frac{\sum_{i=11}^{n} (y_i - \bar{y})^2}{n}}$$

It is usual to replace the n in the denominator by $(n - 1)$ so that the resulting estimate of the population value is unbiased.

For the blood glucose data the variance is 0.488 and the standard deviation 0.698.

The measures we have considered have been to do with the sample and while this may be of interest in its own right, more often we will be interested in understanding the variability not of the sample, but of a statistic based on the sample. In order to think about the variability of a statistic we need to consider again the sampling distribution of a statistic in just the way we did in Section 2.1.

To illustrate the point we can conduct a sampling experiment. Suppose that the 40 blood glucose measurements in Figure 8.3 comprised the total population of values. A sampling experiment can be carried out by randomly selecting values from the original 40, calculating their mean and repeating the process for a given number of times. Concretely we took 40 random samples of size 10 from the population of blood glucose values. This gives us 40 sample means that are not equal to one another, so like the original measurements they show random variability. There a very large number of ways of choosing 10 values from 40, and the 40 that have been chosen are a random sample from the so-called sampling distribution of the mean.

In Figure 8.5 we display both the population histogram as well as the histogram of sample means, and clearly these distributions differ. Since the 40 values are themselves a

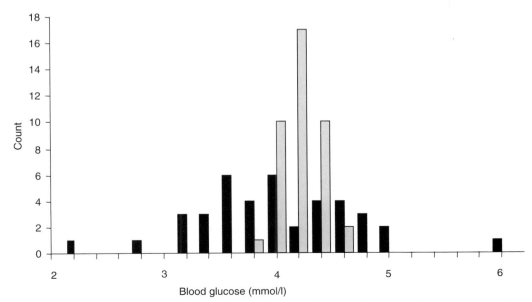

Fig. 8.5 Comparison of population histogram and sampling distribution of the mean of blood glucose levels.

random sample from a distribution, we can determine certain characteristics of the distribution, for example, the sample mean and standard deviation. The mean of the means is 4.102 mmol/L and the standard deviation is 0.177 mmol/L. The original population mean was 4.055 mmol/L so that the mean of the sampling distribution is reasonably close to it. In contrast, the standard deviation of the population was 0.698 mmol/L and that is considerably larger than the standard deviation from the sampling distribution. This result mirrors intuition since we would expect sampling means to be less variable than the individual population values. The standard deviation of this sampling distribution is known as the standard error of the mean. For the original 40 blood glucose level values the standard of the mean is $0.698/\sqrt{40} = 0.110$.

This example shows that the standard deviation of the sampling distribution is less than that of the population. In fact, this reduction in the variability is related to the sample size used to calculate the sample means. For example, if we repeat the sampling experiment, but this time based on 15 rather than 10 random samples, the resulting standard deviation of the sampling is 0.159, and on 25 random samples it is 0.081. The precise relationship between the population standard deviation σ and the standard error of the mean is:

$$\text{s.e.(mean)} = \frac{\sigma}{\sqrt{n}}$$

The difference between these two concepts, the population standard deviation and the standard error of the mean, is important and we will return to it when considering confidence intervals.

8.4.2 Inferential statistics

Historically, the role of statistics in biomedical research has been largely to test hypotheses. More recently, there has been a move to supplant hypothesis tests from their dominant position by confidence intervals. This move has been endorsed by The International Committee of Medical Journal Editors and climaxed with the publication, under the auspices of the British

Medical Journal of *Statistics with Confidence*.[23] Hypothesis tests and p-values continue to be, and will continue to be of importance; this review of medical statistics covers all three.

8.4.2.1 Confidence intervals

The estimation of a parameter alone is not sufficient since a single estimate tells us nothing about how accurate the estimate is. The main purpose of confidence intervals is to indicate the precision, or imprecision, of the estimated statistic as representing the population values. The confidence interval will give us a range of values within which we can have a chosen confidence of it containing the population value. The degree of confidence usually presented is 95%.

When estimating a population mean, the 95% confidence interval is approximately given by

$$\bar{y} \pm 1.96 \times s/\sqrt{n} \text{(sample mean} \pm 1.96$$
$$\times \text{standard error of the mean).}$$

Applying this to the blood glucose level data for which we know that the sample mean is 4.055 mmol/L and the standard error is 0.110 mmol/L, the 95% confidence limits are approximately $4.055 \pm 1.96 \times 0.110 = 3.84$–$4.13$ mmol/L.

One question that is often asked of statisticians is: in what sense can we be 95% confident that the population mean lies within the limits 3.84 and 4.13? To answer the question we can again conduct a sampling experiment as follows. Suppose that the 40 blood glucose measurements in Figure 8.3 comprised the total population of values. For random sample of size 10 from the populations of blood glucose values determine the sample mean, standard error and the corresponding 95% confidence interval. Repeat the process 100 times. The results of such an experiment are shown in Figure 8.6.

In this figure, each individual confidence interval has been drawn as a vertical straight line joining the lower and upper limits. The horizontal line is positioned at the value 4.055 mmol/L – the population mean. This gives us 40 sample means that are not equal to one another, so they on their own like the original measurement show random

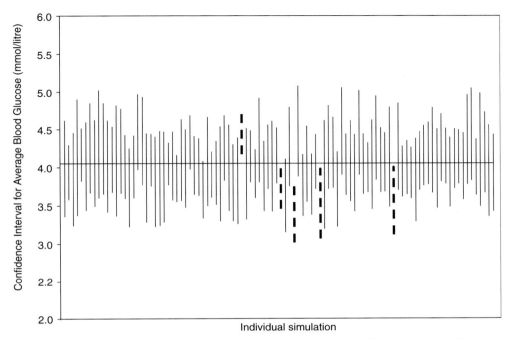

Fig. 8.6 Confidence intervals from 100 samples of size 10 from the population of blood glucose levels.

variability. There a very large number of ways of choosing 10 values from 40, and the 40 that have been chosen are a random sample from the so-called sampling distribution of the mean. Clearly most of the 100 intervals include the population mean value. In fact, 95 of the 100 include the population value, while five of them, indicated by the dashed lines, do not. This demonstrates the basis of confidence in a confidence interval. It is a confidence based on the idea that if we repeat sampling from a population a large number of times and each time determine the confidence interval, then in 95% of the cases the interval will include the population value and in 5% of cases it will not.

From the formula for a confidence interval, its width is determined by three parameters: the sample size, population variability and the degree of confidence. Plainly, if the sample size is increased then we have seen the standard error will be reduced and hence the width of the interval will also be reduced. If we can reduce the variability of the characteristic being studied then we can again reduce the standard error and hence reduce the width. The reduction of variability is not always simple since part of variability is natural, biological variability. However, there is also a component of variability that is dependent on the measurement process. For example, when measuring blood pressure we can attempt to reduce variability by: consistently measuring the blood pressure while sitting after a period of rest; taking the measurement at the same time of day; ensure the measurement is taken by the same nurse or doctor; make use of an automatic sphygmomanometer. Finally, by increasing the degree of confidence – say to 99% from 95% – the width of the interval will be increased.

8.4.2.2 Hypothesis tests, tests of significance and *p*-values

So far we have concentrated on estimation and confidence intervals. Often, however, researchers will be interested in testing specific hypotheses. The vehicle that is used to test hypotheses is generally the significance test. We will illustrate the

Table 8.2 30-min post-inhalation urinary salbutamol excretion (% inhaled dose) in nine subjects following inhalation of 4×100 mg salbutamol using a metered-dose inhaler (MDI) and a dry powder inhaler (DISK)

Voluteer	MDI	DISK	Difference	+/−
1	0.70	0.85	−0.15	−
2	0.26	0.80	−0.54	−
3	1.18	0.92	0.26	+
4	1.32	3.45	−2.13	−
5	0.37	3.85	−3.48	−
6	2.18	4.96	−2.78	−
7	2.62	2.11	0.51	+
8	0.85	1.97	−1.12	−
9	1.27	2.47	−1.20	−
Mean	1.19	2.38	−1.18	

concepts behind significance tests using the data in Table 8.2.

The data in Table 8.2 are taken from a study reported by Hindle et al.,[24] the purpose of which was to determine whether a new dry powder inhaler (DISK) was equivalent to a traditional metered-dose inhaler (MDI) in its ability to deliver doses of a bronchodilator to the lungs of volunteers. The data are the percentages of an inhaled dose of salbutamol recovered in a urine sample taken 30 min post-inhalation for each method of delivery in nine volunteers. A measure of treatment effect is the difference in percentages within volunteers, shown in the fourth column. Of these differences seven are negative and two are positive (fifth column) and the question we need to answer is how likely is it that if there is no difference between the inhalers, we would see this degree of imbalance between negatives and positives?

The significance test requires us to specify:

1. A null hypothesis to be tested – defining that there is no difference between the treatments.
2. The null hypothesis is tested against an alternative hypothesis – that defines how the treatments may differ. This will be important

when considering sample sizing and power in Section 8.5.8. This difference can be in either direction, giving rise to one-sided and two-sided tests.
3. A test statistic – a measure of how much the data depart from the null hypothesis.

If there were truly no difference between the inhalers then we would expect that any individual difference is as likely to be negative as it is to be positive. In other words, in these circumstances the probability of a negative is $\frac{1}{2}$. The null hypothesis then will be

$$\text{Probability(MDI} > \text{DISK)}$$
$$= \text{Probability(MDI} < \text{DISK)} = 0.5$$

This is precisely the situation considered in Section 8.2.1 where we considered the distribution of heads and tails from the toss of a coin 10 times. As there, we can determine the sampling distribution of the number of negatives as shown in Figure 8.7. From the Figure we can see that the probability of achieving exactly seven negatives out of nine is approximately 0.07. This probability is not the p-value. The p-value is the probability that a value of the test statistic as large, or larger than that seen in the study would occur by chance if there were no difference in the treatments. For this example, the p-value is the probability of observing either seven, eight or nine negatives out of nine and this is approximately 0.09. This is a one-sided p-value. If we are interested in alternatives in both directions, we have to consider values as far from the expected number in the other direction. The expected number of negatives is 4.5 and it is clear from Figure 8.7 that the distribution is symmetric about this value and therefore in the other direction, we will be interested in zero, one or two negatives out of nine and this has the same probability 0.09. The two-sided p-value is the sum of theses two values giving a value of 0.18.

How is the p-value to be interpreted? On one level, it can be interpreted as a measure of how likely is it that pure random variation would give the magnitude of differences seen in the study. If the p-value is small then it can be argued that, all other things being equal, it is unlikely that the differences could be due to chance variation

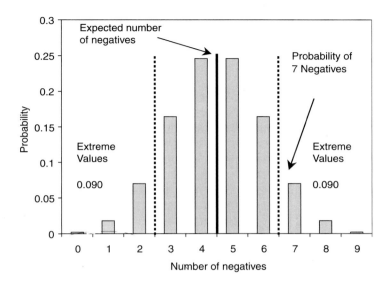

Fig. 8.7 Distribution of the number of negatives out of nine given the null hypothesis is true.

alone. Standardly a value of 0.05 is often used as a cut-point to determine whether the p-value is small or not. If the p-value is smaller than 0.05 then we could 'reject the null hypothesis', or state the treatments are statistically different. If we strictly follow this rule, then if we were to carry out 100 studies in circumstances in which there was no true difference between the treatments then we would expect, by chance, five times out of these 100 to conclude that the null hypothesis was false. Making a decision to reject a true null hypothesis is termed an error of the first kind, and the probability of such an error under the null hypothesis is called the type-I error, significance level or false positive rate.

The test of significance that we used as an illustration utilised only the sign of the differences – whether it was negative or positive. Generally, the actual differences are used. If we think about the differences themselves then if there were no difference between the treatments we would expect the average difference to be zero. This defines the null hypothesis. The sample mean of the differences divided by its standard error, is the test statistic and a large value of this statistic would indicate that there is likely to be a difference between the treatments.

The data in Table 8.2 give a sample mean difference of -1.181 percentage units with a standard error of 0.459 giving a test-statistic of $-1.181/0.459 = -2.573$. This should be compared to a so-called student's t-distribution which tells us that – given a suitable tabulation of values – that the p-value for a difference as large or larger than the average difference seen here is 0.0165 for a one-sided test or 0.0330 for a two-sided test.

8.5 Issues in Design

The medical statistician's role in regard to the investigation should be that of obstetrician, rather than morbid anatomist, for it is unfair to expect him to extract scientific knowledge by performing a kind of mathematical post mortem upon the numerical remains of a badly planned study. [Green FHK, Principle Medical Officer, Medical Research Council, *The Lancet*, 1954; **ii**: 1084–1091.]

Many of the important statistical aspects of clinical trials design are dealt with in detail in Chapter 6 of this volume (Nigel Baber and John Sweatman) and so here only specific statistical aspects are discussed.

The prospect facing us before we conduct a clinical trial is that:

1. We want to collect data concerning the efficacy and safety of a new treatment regime.

2. We want to test hypotheses concerning the drug that are of interest to us.

3. We want to convince the regulators as to the results.

4. We want to convince the prescribers as to the value of the drug.

An important aspect of achieving this is that in the protocol we say what we are going to do; in the statistical analysis plan, developed before the data are collected, we implement what we said we were going to do and carry it through to the statistical analysis itself; finally in the study report we verify that we did what we said we were going to do. Many of the problems associated with the running of clinical trials would be minimised if clinical researchers followed this simple recipe. This is no more than Good Clinical Practice,[25] or thought of in another way it is similar to Total Quality Management, which recognises that it is preferable to build quality into a product than to try and correct its output. Critical to much of this is a careful understanding of the aims and objectives of the clinical trial.

8.5.1 Study aims and objectives

A key figure in the development of clinical trials methodology in the 20th century was Sir Austin Bradford Hill. In his *Principles of Medical Statistics*[26] which first appeared as a series of articles in *The Lancet* and was subsequently published as a book, he described the clinical trial as being 'a carefully, and ethically, designed experiment with the aim of answering some precisely framed question'. It is notable that this definition talks of a question, not questions. To illustrate he describes an early trial of streptomycin in which the object was 'to measure the effect of the drug on respiratory tuberculosis'. He points out is that this objective is too vague. Questions that need to be answered are:

- Which aspects of the illness are important?
  a. the minimal lesions on acquisition
  b. the advanced, progressive disease with poor prognosis
  c. the chronic, relatively inactive state

- Since speed of recovery depends on age, we need to specify more closely the age groups to be included.

Greater precision is required in the objectives. We need to have

- A defined population
- Defined endpoints
- Relatively few questions to be answered.

As Hill pointed out: 'it would of course be possible deliberately to incorporate more and different groups (of patients) in a trial, but to start out without thought and with all and sundry included, with the hope that the results can somehow be sorted out statistically in the end is to court disaster'. In essence, simplicity is to be admired.

The need for clarity in the objectives of a study is also addressed in drug regulations. Here are four examples:

1. Is a difference sought or is equivalence the objective? International conference of harmonisation (ICH E9[27]) makes it clear that 'it is vital that the protocol of a trial, designed to demonstrate equivalence or non-inferiority contains a clear statement that this is its explicit intention' (ICH E9, Section 3.3.2). In the past if a trial failed to show that a new treatment gave benefit compared to a standard, it was commonplace to claim that the new treatment was therefore as effective as the standard. Such an argument is no longer acceptable as will be discussed in Section 8.5.6.

2. Is there a specific subgroup of patients of extra interest? In this case ICH E9 states, 'any claim of treatment efficacy (or lack thereof) or safety based solely on exploratory subgroup analyses are unlikely to be acceptable' (ICH E9, Section 5.7).

3. Is one specific treatment comparison important? ' ... any aspects of multiplicity ... should be identified in the protocol; adjustment should always be considered. ... an explanation of why adjustment is not thought necessary should be set out in the analysis plan.' (ICH E9, Section 5.6)

4. Is one variable more important than others? 'Redefinition of the primary variable after unblinding will almost always be unacceptable, since the biases this introduces are difficult to assess' (ICH E9, Section 2.2.2)

The issue covered in the second and third examples relate to elevating the type-I error as we carry out more and more individual tests. There are three circumstances in which this may occur:

1. Multiple comparisons – in which comparisons are made amongst more than two treatments.
2. Multiple endpoints – in which two treatments compared with many endpoints.
3. Multiple looks at the data – examples of which are interim analyses and subgroups.

To illustrate the problem in subgroups, suppose we separately compare treatments in both males and females. Then we have the following possibilities:

		Females	
		Type-I error (α)	**No type-I error ($1 - \alpha$)**
Males	Type-I error (α)	α^2	$\alpha(1 - \alpha)$
	No type-I error($1 - \alpha$)	$\alpha(1 - \alpha)$	$(1 - \alpha)^2$

From which we can determine the probability of at least one type-I error as

$$\alpha^2 + \alpha(1 - \alpha) + \alpha(1 - \alpha) = 2\alpha - \alpha^2$$

$$= \alpha(2 - \alpha) > \alpha$$

If we are using a standard 5% type-I error then this probability $= 0.05(2 - 0.05) = 0.0975$ which is almost twice the pre-specified value. As the number of subgroups is increased, this probability grows as is shown in Table 8.3 and this provides the caution that ICH E9 expresses about subgroup analyses.

To illustrate how the type-I error may be elevated by using interim analysis we conduct a sampling experiment. The data below are 50 values of the Ritchie Index, a measurement of joint

Table 8.3 Impact of multiple subgroup testing on the overall probability of at least one type-I error

Number of subgroups	Probability of at least one type-I error
2	0.0975
3	0.1426
4	0.1855
5	0.2262
6	0.2649
7	0.3017
8	0.3366
9	0.3598
10	0.4013

stiffness in patients with rheumatoid arthritis taken from a study reported by Barnes et al.[28] The values were obtained during the study run in a pre-treatment phase.

14	9	8	9	1	20	3	3	2	4
2	3	6	1	2	11	16	24	16	21
19	22	33	12	12	12	19	10	33	2
19	40	1	20	1	2	4	7	9	4
9	6	14	8	27	10	27	7	24	21

The mean of these data is 12.18 units and the standard deviation is 9.69 units. Let us suppose that we wish to test the null hypothesis that the population mean is 12.18, in other words the null hypothesis is true. Suppose also that we can conduct the study in one of the two ways. In the first, we take a random sample of 20 subjects from the population and test the hypothesis at the 5% level at the end of the trial. In the second, we plan to take a maximum of 20 patients from the population, but allow ourselves the option of testing after 10 patients, again at the 5% level, and if the result were significant stopping the trial, otherwise continuing to the end at which point a second 5% level test would be conducted. The sampling experiment consists as before of randomly sampling from the population under each design and then repeating the process a large number of times, in this case 100 times.

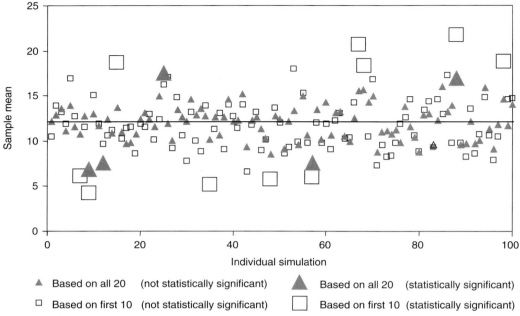

Fig. 8.8 Results of a simulation experiment comparing a design with analyses after 10 and 20 patients, and a design with a single analysis after 20 patients.

The results of the simulation are shown in Figure 8.8. In this figure, we see that in the first design in which there is one analysis after 20 patients, there are five cases where we would falsely declare a significant result and this is consistent with a 5% level of significance. On the other hand, if we were to test at the interim, and if not significant continue to the end, we find that there are in total 12 cases where we would falsely conclude significance. In other words by repeating the test the false positive rate is increased. In 1969 Armitage et al.[29] investigated issues associated with multiple tests of accumulating data. Their work led directly to the development of group sequential designs and the use of stopping rules initially by Pocock in 1977,[30] O'Brien–Fleming in 1979[31] and the α-spending function of Lan and DeMets in 1983.[32]

There are two potential solutions to this problem. First, we can pre-specify a single test (group) on the primary endpoint at a single point in time, much in line with Hill's views. Or, we can attempt a statistical solution based on adjusting the type-I error for the individual tests.

The group sequential tests are such a statistical solution to the repeated testing case. For multiple subgroups, we can use the so-called Bonferonni[33] correction. In the case of two subgroups this requires us to test each individual subgroup at a type-I error of 0.0253 leading to a probability of making at least one type-I error of 0.05 as required.

8.5.2   Explanatory/pragmatic trials

As we have seen in many ways, good research is characterised by studies that address a well-defined question. There are essentially two types of questions to be answered: explanatory and pragmatic, a distinction originally drawn by Schwartz et al.[34] Explanatory studies focus on mechanisms looking for a potential benefit by adhering to laboratory conditions, and can be thought of as proof-of-concept studies. They tend to be scientific in nature, concentrating on furthering scientific knowledge. Pragmatic studies, on the other hand, assess whether such potential can be realised in a more realistic setting, first in phase-III confirmatory trials and then ultimately in phase IV or post-marketing trials. They are more likely to be 'technological' in nature with the aim of providing clinically relevant recommendations for treating patients. The distinction between these two types of trials is crucial since it has direct influence on the designs, conduct, analysis and interpretation of the results of the studies. Many studies attempt to answer both type of questions simultaneously but care should be taken in recognising and acknowledging this: 'The protocol should make a clear distinction between the aspects of a trial which will be used for confirmatory proof and the aspects which will provide the basis for explanatory analysis' (ICH E9 Section 2.1.3).

To illustrate how explanatory and pragmatic trials differ from one another we look in turn at subjects, treatments and delivery, outcome measures, conduct and analysis.

8.5.2.1 Subjects

Subjects in an explanatory study are more likely to be high-risk patients in whom a high response can be anticipated, for example, because of a good history of treatment compliance. The population of patients will tend to be relatively homogeneous, controlled by tight inclusion/exclusion criteria and hence the sample size will tend to be relatively small. In contrast, pragmatic studies are more likely to have a much wider inclusion criteria, to ensure representation from the target population. As a consequence, the patients will tend to be more heterogeneous leading to larger sample sizes.

8.5.2.2 Treatment and delivery

In explanatory studies, there is a tendency to compare a new treatment to placebo and to rigidly adhere to single doses of the new treatment in anticipation of maximising treatment compliance. On the other hand, pragmatic studies are more likely to compare the new treatment with the best available alternative and to use a more flexible attitude to dosing, for example, including the possibility of individual dose titration. The delivery of treatment is likely to mimic real-life usage.

8.5.2.3 Outcome measures

In explanatory trials, endpoints are likely to be objective, possiblly surrogate, and may be chosen to maximise the sensitivity to detect treatment differences. In contrast, endpoints in pragmatic trials will tend to be more patient-centred including, for example, survival and quality of life.

8.5.2.4 Conduct

The conduct of explanatory trials will include close monitoring of the study in an attempt to ensure strict adherence to the protocol. There is likely to be exhaustive recording of data. In contrast, the conduct of pragmatic trials will tend to mirror real life. There will be attempts to minimise data recording, but there is likely to be exhaustive follow-up of all patients.

8.5.2.5 Analysis

In explanatory trials, we are likely to exclude both protocol violators and treatment non-compliers. The objective behind these exclusions is to increase the efficiency. However the exclusions may give rise to bias and hence to compromise the results if too many patients are excluded. Such an analysis population is termed as completers, or per protocol, population. In pragmatic trials, we generally include all patients using the intention-to-treat (ITT) principle.

8.5.2.6 Intention-to-treat (ITT)

The purpose of utilising an ITT analysis population is to minimise the bias that can occur by excluding patients who do not complete a trial. The late Prof Ken McRae illustrated the concept using the following simple example.

A physician believes that fell-running is the best treatment following a myocardial infarction. He decides to test this by sending patients to run up Ben Nevis. Of the 25 patients who complete the course (of treatment), all 25 survived for at least 10 years. However, before concluding that fell-running is the best treatment, we should not forget the 25 who refused to the treatment, the 25 who were lost on Ben Nevis and the 25 who dies while running.

There are many different definitions of an ITT population tailored to specific diseases or trial designs. Amongst these are the following:

• All randomised patients (in the groups to which they were randomised)
• All randomised patients (correctly allocated)
• All randomised patients with at least one dose of study drug,
• All randomised patients with at least one dose of study drug and at least one observation of the efficacy variable after baseline.

Whichever definition is to be used it must be defined in the protocol.

One issue that is important to determine is how missing data will be handled in an ITT analysis. ITT was largely developed in clinical trials in which the major endpoints were events, mortality, infarctions, etc. In such studies it is possible to follow-up on patients who withdraw from treatment and determine whether the event has occurred or not and indeed in such trials every effort should be made to do this. For other types of data, for example, a pain scale other approaches are necessary.

Very often, a last-observation-carried-forward analysis is carried out in which the last available observation in any patient is used.

8.5.3   Choice of endpoint

It was noted in Section 8.3.3 that in choosing the primary endpoint to be used in a study there are a number of questions that need to be considered:

• Which aspects of the disease are we interested in measuring?

• Of the potential endpoints:
  a. are they clinically meaningful?
  b. are they relevant to patients?
  c. How is each measured? Can they be measured directly?
  d. Are they sensitive to treatment?
• How do we analyse what we have measured?

To illustrate how there can be a strong link between the endpoint of the method of analysis we consider the case of binary data in the next section.

8.5.3.1   Defining the endpoint for binary data

The data in Table 8.4 have been extracted from an investigation reported by Miranda-Filho *et al.*[35] who compared the treatment of tetanus by the intrathecal route with the standard intramuscular route. The primary endpoints of the study were disease progression and death and we concentrate here on the former.

Any inferences about the difference between the effects of the two treatments that may be made upon such data are the observed rates, or proportions of deteriorations by the intrathecal route. In this example, amongst those treated by the intrathecal route $22/58 = 0.379$ of patients deteriorated, and the corresponding control rate is $37/60 = 0.617$. The observed rates are estimates of the population incidence rates, π_t for the test treatment and π_C for the controls. Any representation of differences between the treatments will be based upon these population rates and the estimated measure of the treatment effect will be reported with an associated 95% confidence interval and/or p-value.

Table 8.4 Incidence of deterioration and death in patients treated for tetanus by the intrathecal and intramuscular routes

	Treatment	Deteriorated	Stable/Improved	Total
Disease deterioration	Intrathecal	22	36	58
	Intramuscular	37	23	60
	Treatment	**Died**	**Survived**	**Total**
Mortality	Intrathecal	4	54	58
	Intramuscular	10	50	60

Typically statisticians use one of the three approaches to represent treatment differences for such data: absolute rate reduction (ARR), relative risk (RR) and the odds ratio (OR).

In the first approach we look at the difference between rates $\delta = \pi_C - \pi_t$. For this tetanus data, the estimated ARR is $0.617 - 0.379 = 0.238$, indicating that the intrathecal route reduces the rate of deterioration by approximately 24%. The 95% confidence interval associated with this estimate is 0.0621–0.4127 and because the interval does not contain zero the p-value is less than 0.05.

In the case of RR, we look at the ratio of the rates: $\phi = \pi_C/\pi_t$. For the tetanus data, the estimated RR is $0.617/0.379 = 1.63$, in other words the risk of becoming infected with typhoid among controls is approximately twice that among those inoculated. The 95% confidence interval for the estimated RR is 1.35–2.03, and again because the interval excludes the null value, in this case one, the p-value is less than 0.05.

Finally, the OR is defined as: $\theta = \pi_C(1 - \pi_t)/[\pi_t(1 - \pi_C)]$. For the tetanus data the estimated OR is $0.617 \times 0.621/(0.383 \times 0.379) = 2.63$ and its associated 95% confidence interval is 1.25–5.53 once again indicating a p-value of less than 0.05.

In Table 8.5, we compare the response rates for the two primary endpoints – disease deterioration and mortality for the Hindle *et al.* study. What is interesting is that for the mortality endpoint ARR shows less deviation from the null than in the case of disease deterioration, while the converse holds for the RR. This is often regarded as a major defect of the RR as a measure of treatment effect, in that it does

not take account of baseline, or control risk. In fact, there are examples in which the converse is true, increased ARR but reduced RR. The choice between the measures cannot, or should not be based, upon such differences but upon the relevance of absolute or relative effects.

There is considerable evidence that the form in which data is reported has an impact on the understanding of the results, and on the decisions, which are taken on the basis of the data.[36–45] For example, Misselbrook and Armstrong[42] report the results of an investigation in which hypertensive and matched non-hypertensive patients were offered treatment for chronic mild hypertension. They were provided information of the positive impact of the offered treatment on the likelihood of their suffering a future stroke. The information was presented in different formats, including RR and ARR. When the information of the benefit of treatment was given in the form of RR, 92% percent of patients responded that they would accept treatment. In contrast, when the same information was presented in the form of ARR only 75% patients reported that they would accept treatment. The confusion is not restricted to patients. Forrow *et al.*[39] report the results of a study in which physicians reported they were more likely to treat both hypertension and hypercholesterolemia when data were presented in the form of RR rather than ARR.

Laupacis *et al.* introduced the number needed to treat (NNT) into the medical literature[46] as an easily understood and useful measure of treatment effect for clinical trials in which the main outcome variable is binary. It has been argued that the NNT is more easily

Table 8.5 Incidence of deterioration and death in patients treated for tetanus by the intrathecal and intramuscular routes

Endpoint	Rates		Summary measures	
	Intrathecal	Intramuscular	ARR	RR
Disease deterioration	0.617	0.379	0.238	1.626
Mortality	0.161	0.063	0.092	2.339

understood by practising physicians than more statistically-based measures. Mathematically the definition of the NNT is extremely simple as it is just the reciprocal of the ARR:

$$\text{NNT} = \frac{1}{\text{ARR}} = \frac{1}{\pi_C - \pi_t}$$

Conventionally, this is interpreted as meaning that if NNT patients are treated with each treatment, one additional patient will benefit from being treated with the new treatment compared to the control. Applying this definition to the mortality data from the Hindle *et al.* study gives an NNT of $1/(0.161-0.063) = 10.83$. Conventionally this is interpreted as meaning that approximately 11 patients need to be treated intrathecally to save one life.

Since its inception the NNT has been widely used not only to report the results of individual clinical trials, but more particularly in the evidence-based medicine world to report the results of systematic reviews, or meta-analyses (see Section 8.6). Its use by the evidence-based medicine fraternity has led to the NNT being incorporated into a number of treatment guidelines. Three of four recent clinical practice guidelines issued by the Australian and New Zealand College of Psychiatrists used the NNT in summarising results.[47–49] Despite its popularity with clinicians, not all statisticians have been as supportive.[50,51]

8.5.4 Prevention of bias

As pointed out in ICH E9 'the most important design techniques for avoiding bias in clinical trials are blinding and randomisation, and these should be a normal feature of most controlled clinical trials intended to be included in a marketing application'. The avoidance of bias is absolutely crucial if the interpretation of the results of a clinical trial is to be valid. We noted in Section 8.4.2.2 that the logic of significance test is that 'all other things being equal' a small p-value would allow us to conclude that there was a significant difference between the

treatments. The meaning of the phrase 'all other things being equal' is that the only differences between the patients in the treatment groups are the treatments that the patients receive. Randomisation and blinding provide us with the means to ensure this.

8.5.4.1 Randomisation

Why do we randomise? Randomisation is a procedure based on a chance allocation of subjects to treatments. Its purpose is to produce groups of patients comparable, or balanced, with respect to factors that may influence outcome apart from the treatments themselves thus allowing us to make a strong causal connection between the treatments and their different outcomes. What is important here is to realise that randomisation protects us not only against imbalance with respect to important known prognostic factors but also against imbalance with respect to the unknown, possibly unmeasured factors. While many people would argue that the justly famous Medical Research Council study of streptomycin for the treatment of tuberculosis[52] was the first trial to use randomisation, this is not the case.[53,54] Indeed the notion of balance was known to be important in the 18th century.[1]

A second reason for randomisation is that from a statistical perspective it ensures the validity of the standards approaches to statistical inference, t-tests, analysis of variance (ANOVA), etc.

8.5.4.1.1 *Unrestricted randomisation*

The simplest form of randomisation is unrestricted randomisation. Suppose we need to randomise 12 patients to two treatments A and B and that, we have access to a table of random numbers (e.g. Table A in Campbell and Machin[55]). Choosing randomly the 21st row and fourth block the next 12 random numbers in this table are 316427816281. If even numbers are assigned to A and odd numbers to B, then the randomisation which is generated is: BBAAABABAAAB giving seven A's and five B's. Although unrestricted randomisation is in principle simple it doesn't guarantee that there are equal number of patients per treatment group, as here.

8.5.4.1.2 Blocked randomisation

If using blocked randomisation, we ensure balance between treatments within a block of patients. Suppose for example, we again wish to randomise the two treatments A and B to 12 patients in blocks of size four. Then within each block of four patients, treatments are randomly allocated to patients to ensure that two patients receive both A and B. For example:

Block		
2	1	3
AABB	ABBA	BABA

The advantages of blocked randomisation are that it protects against time effects, by which it is meant that if the characteristics of the patients entered into the study change, blocking protects you against lack of balance. Secondly, in multicentre trials it reduces the risk of serious imbalance with respect to the numbers of patients allocated to each treatment. The disadvantages are that the last treatments allocated in each block may become known if there is the possibility of functional unblinding through known properties of the treatments. Secondly, it is practically implemented with only a small number of stratification factors (see Section 8.5.4.1.3). The first disadvantage can be mitigated by making the block size long enough to avoid predictability or having block length – four, six or eight for example – and secondly by making investigators blind to block length.

8.5.4.1.3 Multicentre studies and stratified randomisation

In multicentre trials, it is usual to use a separate randomisation procedure within each centre to ensure that there is balance – or at least near balance within each centre. In such circumstances ICH E9 (Section 2.3.2) recommends that the randomisation be performed centrally, with several blocks allocated to each centre. This procedure is a simple form of stratified randomisation.

A second, important, use of stratified randomisation is in those cases where it is known that a particular set of variables are, or are believed to be, important prognostically. It is desirable in such cases to ensure balanced allocation within each combination of the levels of these prognostic variables that can lead to enhanced efficiency in comparing treatments. As a simple illustration, suppose that gender and age are important, and that the strata for the latter are defined by: <40, 40–59, >60 years. Within each combination of the strata, a separate randomisation list, perhaps based on blocks, is prepared to give:

Strata		Blocks		
Sex	Age	1	2	3
F	<40	AABB	BABA	ABBA
F	40–59	BAAB	AABB	BBAA
F	>60	BBAA	AABB	AABB
M	<40	ABBA	BABA	BBAA
M	40–59	BABA	BABA	AABB
M	>60	ABBA	BAAB	ABAB

The advantages of stratified randomisation are (1) to minimise the chance of accidental bias with respect to important factors; (2) increase the precision with which the treatments are compared and the power (Section 8.5.7) to detect treatment differences; (3) to make the trial results more convincing by being able to demonstrate the balance with respect to the important factors. As far as disadvantages go, the need for central randomisation may slow the process of randomisation for an individual patient, although computer systems make this less of an issue than was previously the case. Secondly, there is always a danger that misclassification of patients to strata can occur and this is only found out later leading to a danger of increased imbalance. Thirdly, while there are improvements to precision and power, the gains are limited. Finally while stratified randomisation can reduce bias and imbalance, there is a school of thought that suggest that post stratification, for example, Analysis of Covariance (ANCOVA) can reduce bias.

8.5.4.1.4   Dynamic randomisation – minimisation

When there are a large number of prognostic variables to account for, it may be practically difficult to implement a fully stratified randomisation scheme. The reason being that with a large number of factors there are even more individual stratum combinations and therefore there will be very few patients in many of the combinations. In such circumstances the method of dynamic allocation, or minimisation, has been recommended.

Minimisation is based on the idea of biasing the treatment allocation so as to minimise the total imbalance between treatments according to some criterion.

To illustrate, consider the case shown in Table 8.6. This shows the current balance of individual prognostic factors in a hypothetical study with three prognostic factors run in three centres. So far 50 patients have been randomised to each treatment. Suppose that the next patient has following characteristics:

Disease severity   – moderate
Age   – < 55
Length of Illness   – ≥ 10
Centre   – 2

Table 8.6 Balance of four prognostic factors in a hypothetical trial after 50 patients have been randomised

Factor	Level	No. on each treatment	
		A	B
Disease severity	Moderate	30	31
	Severe	20	19
Age	< 55	18	17
	≥ 55	32	33
Length of illness	< 10 yrs	21	22
	≥ 10 yrs	29	28
Centre	1	19	21
	2	8	7
	3	23	22

For each treatment, we add together the numbers corresponding to the characteristics of the next patient to give:

Treatment A : $30 + 18 + 29 + 8 = 85$

Treatment B : $31 + 17 + 28 + 7 = 83$.

Minimisation then favours B since this has the smallest total. There are two ways of favouring B. One is to bias the allocation probability in favour of B, for example, B has an 80% chance of being chosen, and A a 20% chance. The other approach – deterministic minimisation, allocates B with 100% chance.

The main advantages of minimisation are that it achieves good balance on prognostic factors and thereby increases efficiency. However, it has been criticised, particularly deterministic minimisation, for not guaranteeing the underlying randomness assumed by the statistical methods used to analyse the data. A second disadvantage is that because minimisation is a dynamic process it uses information on subjects already entered to allocate to future patients. Since these patients may be in other centres the process is usually carried out by a centralised system using the internet, fax or telephone.

8.5.4.1.5   Ethical issues and randomisation

There are ethical issues with randomisation. There are two types of ethics which are associated with human, medical research – individual and collective ethics.[56,57] Individual ethics recognises the primacy of the individual and is aimed at doing what is best for the subjects in the current trial. In contrast, collective ethics is aimed at doing what is best for all future patients who will benefit from the results of the current trial. Clearly, there is a tension between these two principles that is recognised in the declaration of Helsinki, which comes down on the side of the individual:

'Concern for the interests of the subject must always prevail over the interest of science and society.' (World Medical Association[58])

Many have argued that concerns for the individual intuitively lead to the use of adaptive designs in which randomisation is biased towards the more successful treatment or treatments. One type of adaptive design is the randomised-play-the-winner (RPW) design. Such designs are often described in terms of the following urn model. At the start of the trial, an urn contains α balls, each of two colours, white and red, representing the two treatments, A and B respectively. When a patient requires treatment, a ball is selected at random from the urn and subsequently replaced. If it is white then the patient is allocated to A, if red to B. When the response of a previously allocated patient becomes available, the content of the urn is updated in the following way. If the patient was located to treatment t, either A or B, and responded positively, β balls of colour t and γ balls of colour s (the complement of t) are added to the urn. On the other hand, if the patient was located to treatment t, and responded negatively β balls of colour s and γ balls of colour t are added to the urn. In time, the urn will contain a higher proportion of the more successful treatment.

Despite their ethical appeal, RPW designs have rarely been used in medical research in general, or drug development in particular. This may be due to the negative impact of a study reported by Bartlett et al.[59] This trial was in newborn babies with severe respiratory failure and compared extra corporeal membrane oxygenation (ECMO) with a standard ventilator. The endpoint was survival and given that it was anticipated there would be a major benefit of ECMO, it was decided to run it as an RPW(1,1,1). It resulted in the following sequence of allocation and data (S: success, F: failure):

Patient number												
Treatment	1	2	3	4	5	6	7	8	9	10	11	12
ECMO	S		S	S	S	S	S	S	S		S	S
Standard		F										

The study was stopped after the result from the 12th patient was known because the statistical analysis showed that there was significant evidence favouring ECMO. These results generated controversy, first about the appropriate statistical analysis of such data, and second about the wisdom of definitely concluding benefit in favour of ECMO when only one patient was treated with the standard. This latter issue could have been addressed either by increasing the number of balls in the urn initially, for example, by using an RPW(10,1,1), which would have slowed down the imbalance in favour of ECMO, or by using a randomised block of say 10 patients before an urn model was used and in which the initial ratio of coloured balls is determined by the results of the randomised block.

However, there is a counter argument.[60] In the ECMO trial, after the result of the nineth patient became known the RPW design requires that the patients be randomised to ECMO compared to the standard ventilator in the ratio $9:1$. Clayton argues that if the one treatment is so much superior to the other that 90% of patients are allocated to it, it is unethical to withhold it from the remaining 10%. If we accept that argument, is it also true if the ratio is $8:1$? or $7:1$? How much information is sufficient to make us, ethically, refuse to randomise patients? Such questions are not simple.

8.5.4.2   Blinding

The primary purpose of blinding is to minimise any conscious, or unconscious bias, in the conduct of a clinical trial. Such biases may arise through allocation, through assessment of treatment effects by physician, the attitude of the patient knowing that they are receiving a particular treatment, decisions made by the physician as to the cause of adverse events, withdrawal of treatment, etc. All of these may be influenced by knowledge of the treatment. The purpose of blinding is to prevent the identification of treatments until such time as there is no longer a possibility of bias.

There are generally three levels of blindness:

- Double blind: in which neither the patient nor any clinical staff involved in the management and assessment of the patient are aware of the treatment.

• Single-blind: in which the patient alone is unaware of the treatment
• Open-label: in which both the patient and physician are open to the treatment. In these trials, it is often sensible to have the assessment of the patient be handled by a physician who is blind, even if the treating physician and the patient are open.

There is an ethical imperative, despite blinding, to protect the patient from harm. Therefore, it is most important that a system is developed to allow the blind to be broken in circumstances, for example, when a patient suffers a serious adverse reaction. The study protocol should describe those conditions under which the blind may be broken and the system itself should allow the breaking of the blind in a single patient, rather than the whole study.

8.5.5 Control groups

Often statisticians are asked to consider the use of control data other than those arising from contemporaneous randomised controls and more often than not, they reply that such use is inappropriate. What are the alternatives that need to be considered and why are they not appropriate?

8.5.5.1 Concurrent, non-randomised controls

A trial is conducted in which a physician decides to allocate some patients to a new treatment, and other patients he treats with what until now has been his first choice of treatment. He monitors the changes in all the patients over time and at a predetermined time compares the results from the two groups of patients. A difference is found. In order to be confident that the observed difference is real, the physician needs to assume that the patients in the two groups are essentially identical in respect to all important factors that are important to the disease and its prognosis. Unfortunately, without randomisation we cannot be sure that such an assumption is valid. As we noted in Section 8.5.4.1 the strength of

randomisation is that it protects against biases unconscious or conscious.

8.5.5.2 The patient as their own control

There are two circumstances in which patients act as their own control: crossover designs and pre-test, post-test designs.

8.5.5.2.1 Crossover designs

The essential feature of a crossover design is that each patient receives at least two of the treatments under consideration. In the simplest two-period two-treatment crossover, with treatments A and B, patients are allocated to one of the treatment sequence AB. As is often the case the most succinct statement of advantages and disadvantages of crossover design is to be found in Hill.

In some instances it may be better to design the trial so that each patient provides his own control – by having various treatments in turn. This is known as a "crossover" trial . . .. By such means we may sometimes make the comparison more sensitive since we have eliminated the variability that must exist between patients treated at the same stage of the disease in question (so far as can be judged). We have done so, however, at the expense of introducing as a factor the variability within patients from one time to another, i.e. we may be giving the patient treatment A and treatment B at different stages of the disease. [Hill AB, Principles of Medical Statistics.]

The primary advantage of such a design is that the patient being his/her own control increases the precision of the treatment comparisons because they are made within patients rather than between patients. This has important ethical and economic consequences. Ethical, in that we would want to minimise the number of patients who receive the less efficacious treatments; economic, because the use of fewer patients will reduce the costs. Such advantages might suggest that crossover designs should be the design of choice if not for three disadvantages. First, crossover designs because they last approximately twice as long as parallel group designs may be more prone to patient withdrawal. Second, they are only applicable in stable, chronic diseases where patients would be expected to return to their pre-treatment severity after a short period without treatment. Finally, and most importantly, if the effect of treatment is not confined to the period in which it is applied – so-called carry-over, or if the treatment effect differs from period to period, estimates of treatment effects may be biased.

This latter disadvantage led the crossover design to be described as 'not the design of choice in clinical trials, where unequivocal evidence of treatment effects is required'.[61] Over the last 25 years, many statisticians have been more positive about the place of the crossover design in clinical research.[62,63]

Of course, the control in a crossover design is not contemporaneous because it occurs within different treatment periods. Nonetheless, such trials are randomised and the effect of differential period effects can be allowed for in the analysis and does not give rise to bias in treatment estimates.

8.5.5.2.2 Pre-test/Post-test designs

In a pre-test/post-test design, each individual subject is measured on two occasions separated by the same treatment and the difference between the two measurements, appropriately averaged across subjects is an estimate of the effect of treatment. In order for this to be a valid measure of the treatment intervention, we need two assumptions. First, there is no change in the experimental conditions, an example would be that in estimating a treatment for hay fever the pollen count remains constant over the period of the experiment. Second, there is no natural progression of the disease over time, an example would be the treatment of a common cold that might be expected to improve within 4 or 5 days without treatment.

This second assumption is equivalent to an assumption that there is no 'regression-to-the-mean'.[64] Regression-to-the-mean is a phenomenon originally reported in 1885 by Galton[65] who showed that the children of tall parents tend to be shorter than their parents, and conversely children of shorter parents tend to be taller than their parents. This is of importance in the context of clinical research because patients are chosen to participate in a clinical trial because they have

in some sense extreme values. As an example, high blood pressure is a surrogate for coronary artery disease and patients entered into a study to reduce blood pressure will have high values, in expectation that it can be lowered.

Changes seen after treatment may not be due to the treatment alone because untreated patients will generally improve because of regression-to-the-mean. There is therefore a need to disentangle the treatment effect from regression-to-the-mean. In order to this we need concurrent randomised controls.

8.5.5.2.3 Historical controls

Since many clinical trials are conducted in the same diseases, with the same control treatments there is an obvious desire to make the most use of this potentially valuable information. Can we compare the results of a new treatment in a group of patients with a group of control patients extracted from a historical database? For example, suppose we are testing a new treatment for migraine headache and 60% of patients improve in the first 2 h post-treatment, compared to 30% in a group of historical control patients treated who had been treated with the current 'gold standard'. Are we able to conclude that the new treatment is preferable to the 'gold standard'?

In order to be able to sustain this conclusion we need to assure ourselves that the groups are essentially similar in every respect but treatment. They need to be similar with respect to their demographic profiles; similar with respect to disease severities; there should have been no changes to the way patients are treated – no new standard method for handling patients apart from a pharmacological intervention. To assure all of these is difficult since we can only investigate characteristics that are measured. As we have already remarked, randomisation protects against lack of balance with respect to all characteristics, measured or not.

8.5.6 Active control groups

In active control trials, there is a natural tendency to believe that if we show no statistical difference between a new treatment and active control then we are justified in concluding that the treatments are equivalent. To illustrate consider the data below taken from a report of 1904 by Pearson[66] on prevention of typhoid by inoculation.

Treatment	Infected	Not infected	Total
Inoculated (I)	7 (25.0%)	21	28
Not inoculated (NI)	3 (23.1%)	10	13

A test of the null hypothesis that the rates of infection are equal – $H_0 \times \pi_I/\pi_{NI} = 1$ gives a p-value of 0.894 using a chi-squared test. There is therefore no statistical evidence of a difference between the treatments and one is unable to reject the null hypothesis. However, the contrary statement is not true that therefore the treatments are the same. As Altman and Bland succinctly put it, 'absence of evidence is not evidence of absence'.[67] The individual estimated infection rates are $\pi_I = 0.250$ and $\pi_{NI} = 0.231$ that gives an estimated RR of $0.250/0.231 = 1.083$ with an associated 95% confidence interval of 0.332–3.532. In other words, inoculation can potentially reduce the infection by a factor of three, or increase it by a factor of three with the implication that we are not justified in claiming that the treatments are equivalent.

Consider a second example. A surgeon devises a new method of carrying out a surgical procedure and pilots the technique in 10 patients of which none suffer a post-operative infection. Can he claim therefore that the new technique is safe? The answer again is no because in this case the upper end of the 95% confidence for the true infection rate is 0–26 % so that infection rate could be as high as one in four. (Hanley and Lippman-Hand[68] developed a simple approximation for the 95% confidence for cases in which the observed data are of the form 0 out of n. They show that approximately the interval is 0–3/n %. This is known as the rule of three.

In order that we can claim equivalence of treatments, specially designed studies need to be conducted.

8.5.6.1 Equivalence and non-inferiority studies

What was missing in the previous section was a definition of what is meant by equivalence. Since it is unlikely that two treatments will have exactly the same effect we will need to consider how big a difference between the treatments would 'force' us to choose one in preference to the other. In the typhoid example there was a difference in rates of 1.9% and we may well believe that such a small difference would justify us in claiming that the treatment effects were the same. But had the difference been 5% would we still have thought them to be the same? Or 10? There will be a difference, say $\delta\%$, for which we are no longer prepared to accept the equivalence of the treatments. This is the so-called equivalence boundary. If we want then to have a high degree of confidence that two treatments are equivalent it is logical to require that an appropriately chosen confidence interval (say 95%) for the treatment differences should have its extremes within the boundaries of equivalence.

In Figure 8.9, we illustrate various cases that can arise from studies intended to show equivalence and the relationship between significance in the traditional sense and clinical significance as determined by the confidence interval and the boundaries of equivalence. In case (A), the 95% confidence interval includes both the null hypothesis of no difference and is within the boundaries of equivalence and from both a statistical and clinical perspective there is no evidence of a difference between the treatments. In case (B), in contrast, the confidence interval is still within the boundaries, but does include the null hypothesis, so from a statistical perspective there is a difference between the treatments but it is not clinically relevant. Case (C) shows both statistical and clinical significance, as the confidence interval lies outside the equivalence boundaries and therefore cannot include the null hypothesis. In the final case, (D), the confidence interval includes

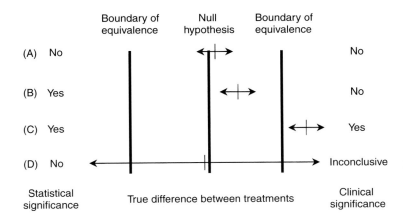

Fig. 8.9 Relationship between statistical and clinical significance in clinical equivalence studies.

the null hypothesis but its extremities lie outside the boundaries of equivalence, so that statistically there is no difference, but clinically the result is equivocal.

If in Figure 8.9 a positive difference between treatments were indicative of a benefit for the test treatment then case (C) would indicate significant superiority of the new treatment. In such circumstances, we would not wish to conclude that only the treatments were not equivalent. In such circumstances, we can use a single boundary and such studies are called non-inferiority studies in which the objective is to show that the new treatment is no more than a small amount worse than the standard. The conduct of the inference remains similar: if the confidence interval is to the right of the non-inferiority boundary, we can conclude that the new treatment is non-inferior to the standard.

There are a number of issues in using such studies to achieve marketing authorisation. First, there needs to be a justification of the boundaries. How can we be sure that the choice of δ is appropriate? Second, has an appropriate choice comparator been made? Is the dose of the comparator appropriate? Is the population of patients appropriate? Third, while for superiority trials it is generally accepted that the appropriate analysis population is an ITT population, it has been argued that for equivalence and non-inferiority studies that the as per protocol population also has a role to play. Finally we need to be sure that an equivalence or non-inferiority study is

capable of showing a difference between treatments, should one exist. This is termed assay sensitivity. The difficulty here is that in superiority trials the achievement of statistical significance is by definition proof of capability while in equivalence or non-inferiority studies there is no equivalence proof of capability from within the study itself. Many of these issues are discussed in ICH E10[69] and Jones et al.[70]

8.5.7 Choice of analysis

The appropriate choice of analysis depends on many of the issues that we have already considered. For example

1. The study objective – is it to show that the treatments are different or that they are different by no more than a small amount (Section 8.5.6.1).
2. The scale of measurement – quantitative compared to qualitative (Section 8.3).
3. The endpoint itself (Section 8.5.3.1).

In studies in which there are important prognostic factors accounting for them as part of the analysis can be important in increasing the precision with which treatment effects can be estimated. Such analyses generally involve the use of an analysis of covariance (ANCOVA) type of approach.

To illustrate ANCOVA we consider the data in Table 8.7 taken from a study reported by Rikkers et al.[71] that compared the effect of two types

Table 8.7 Pre- post-operation MRUS values in a randomised trial of splenorenal shunts

Control operation		New operation	
Pre-treatment	Post-treatment	Pre-treatment	Post-treatment
34	16	51	48
40	36	35	55
34	16	66	60
36	18	40	35
38	32	39	36
32	14	46	43
44	20	52	46
50	43	42	54
60	45		
63	67		
50	36		
42	34		
43	32		

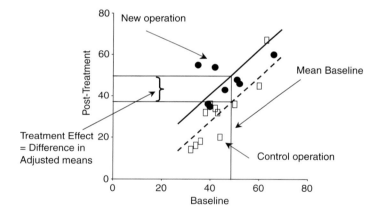

Fig. 8.10 Illustration of analysis of covariance using data from Rikkers *et al.*, 1978.

of splenorenal shunts in the treatment of cirrhotic patients. The primary measurement was the maximum rate of urea synthesis (MRUS) measured both pre- and post-treatment. The basic question here is: how do we interpret treatment effects in the light of potential differences in baseline severity? One simple approach is to take the difference between pre- and post-treatment measurements and to analyse these. Statistically it is more appropriate to use ANCOVA, a technique that provides a mathematical adjustment of the treatment to allow for baseline imbalance in severity.

Figure 8.10 illustrates how ANCOVA works for the MRUS data. In this figure, we have plotted the post-treatment MRUS values against the pre-treatment values with the treatment groups being separately identified. A linear regression line is determined for each treatment group, assuming that there is a common slope. Then, for any value of the pre-treatment the vertical separation of these two lines is an estimate of the treatment differences in post-treatment values adjusted for a common baseline value. For these data the pre-treatment adjusted estimate of the treatment difference is −12.8 with an associated

95% confidence interval $(-21.1 : -4.5)$. Had the treatments been compared without this adjustment the treatment difference would have been estimated as -15.7 with associated confidence interval $(-28.0 : -3.3)$. This latter interval is almost 50% larger than the adjusted interval indicating that ANCOVA has resulted in a more precise treatment estimate.

8.5.8 Sample size and power calculations

In Section 8.4.2.2 we encountered the concept of the type- I error that was defined as rejecting the null hypothesis when it is true. When considering how to sample size a study we need to consider a second type of error – the type-II error. The relationship between this second error and the null hypothesis is illustrated in the Table below.

		H_0 True	H_0 False
Decision	Accept H_0	✓	Type-ll error
	Reject H_0	Type-ll error	✓

We see that in contrast to the type-I error, the type-II error is defined as occurring when accepting the null hypothesis if it is false. The power of a test is defined to be the probability of detecting a true difference and is equal to $1 -$ probability (type-II error). The type-II error and power depend upon the type-I error, the sample size, the clinically relevant difference (CRD) that we are interested in detecting and the expected variability. Where do these values come from?

1. Type-I error – this is preset and usually takes the value of either 0.05 or 0.01;
2. The CRD, as its name implies, needs to be relevant; an example might be a drop in 15 mmHg in diastolic blood pressure;
3. An estimate of the population variability may be obtained from a pilot study, a literature meta-analysis (see Section 8.6) or phase I/II studies.

In most cases we will be interested in determining the sample size for a given type-II error, which is typically fixed at values of 0.1 or 0.2.

Many sample size determinations take the form

$$n = \frac{2\sigma^2}{\text{CRD}^2} \times f(\alpha, \beta)$$

where n is the number of patients in each group, σ is the population variability, CRD is as above, α is the type-I error, β is the type-II error and $f(\alpha, \beta)$ is a function that depends upon the cumulative normal distribution function and takes the form:

		β			
		0.05	0.1	0.2	0.5
α	0.1	10.8	8.6	6.2	2.7
	0.05	13.0	10.5	7.9	3.8
	0.02	15.8	13.0	10.0	5.4
	0.01	17.8	14.9	11.7	6.6

What is clear form this formula and the tabulated values of $f(\alpha, \beta)$ are that:

1. Sample size will increase if the type-I and type-II errors, α and β, are stricter in the sense that they are smaller,
2. If σ is large, sample size will be large; this is related to the relationship between sample size and a reduced standard error, which was dealt with in Section 8.4.1.2.
3. If the clinically relevant difference is large the sample size will be small.

To illustrate the use of the formula suppose we are designing a trial to compare treatments for the reduction of blood pressure. We determine that a clinically relevant difference is 5 mmHg and that the between-patient standard deviation σ is 10 mmHg. A type-I error is set at 0.05 and the type-II error at 0.20. Then the required sample size, per group, is

$$n = \frac{2 \times 10^2}{5^2} \times 7.9 = 63.2 \sim 64$$

There are a number of ways to sample size a trial. The scientific approach is

- to specify what we are interested in detecting – the CRD
- determine the likely variability – σ
- decide what probabilities of type-I and type-II error we can tolerate

- determine the sample size

and this is the approach illustrated above.

The resource planning approach is

- To specify the likely budget and thence the sample size
- Determine the likely variability – σ
- Decide what probabilities of type-I and type-II error we can tolerate
- Determine the minimum difference that is detectable.

The argument against this approach is that this minimum difference may be clinically unrealistic and hence the true power will be much less than specified and this can be regarded as unethical, since patients are being exposed to a new therapy when there is little likelihood of a successful outcome. There is evidence that many studies are underpowered at the planning stage. Freiman *et al.*[72] investigated 71 'negative' taken principally from the *New England Journal of Medicine, The Lancet* and the *Journal of the American Medical Association.* They restricted their attention to studies with a binary outcome and for which there was a clear statement of lack of statistical significance. For 67/71 (94%) of the studies, they determined that there was >10% type-II error of missing a 25% therapeutic improvement; 50/71 (70%) there was a >10% type-II error of missing a 50% therapeutic improvement.

There are of course practical considerations in clinical research. We may find patient recruitment difficult in single centre studies and this is one of the major drivers to multicentre and multinational trials. Alternatively, we may need to relax the inclusion/exclusion criteria or lengthen the recruitment period. Unfortunately, while each of these may indeed increase the supply of patients they may also lead to increased variability that in turn will require more patients. A second issue is the size of the CRD which, if it is too small, will require a large number of patients. In such circumstances we may need to consider the use of surrogate endpoints (Section 8.3.3.2). Finally, the standard deviation may be large and this can have a considerable impact on the sample size – for example, a doubling of the standard deviation leads to a four times increase in the

sample size. The issues concerning components of variability in Section 8.4.2.1 are relevant here.

It is generally the case that when more complex statistical analysis strategies and designs are under consideration, standard sample size calculations are inadequate to cover them. In such circumstances simulation is often used to determine the type-I and type-II errors of the proposed studies for a given sample size.

8.6   Meta-analysis and Summaries

Meta-analysis is the practice of using statistical methods to combine and quantify the outcomes of a series of studies in a single, pooled analysis. The ideas of meta-analysis are not new. One of the first recognisable meta-analyses is due to Pearson[66] in a paper in 1904 in which he provided an overview of the results of inoculating British soldiers against typhoid. In the 1930s the idea of combining results from independent experiments arose both in physics, for example, Birge[73] and in agricultural research, for example Cochran[74] and Yates and Cochran.[75] In Contrast, the term itself did not appear until 1976 when Glass first coined It.[76] In all of these contexts a meta-analysis or, as it is sometimes also termed an overview, can be seen to be a retrospective analysis of studies that have already been conducted.

In simple terms, meta-analysis is the practice of using statistical methods to combine and quantify the outcomes of a series of studies in a single, pooled analysis. What is crucial in this definition is the emphasis on the use of statistical methods. In most biomedical research, the scientific review has a lengthy history and is still widely used. However, insofar that it does not utilise statistical methods for pooling results, and tends to summarise more in qualitative rather than quantitative terms it cannot be regarded as meta-analysis.

Many of the published meta-analyses in clinical research have been as a result of the extraction of a summary data from published sources, for example, death rates in the treatment of patients after a myocardial infarction. For such studies, much of the research interest has been centred on issues surrounding the appropriateness of the statistical techniques and on the methods that should be used to reduce the almost inevitable bias associated with meta-analyses. In the case of the former, the issues relate to the use of fixed effect or random effect models and whether the treatment effect may be assumed to be homogenous across studies. For the latter, one needs to consider problems associated with publication bias, selection bias, size bias and the premature termination of studies because of a positive result in an interim analysis.

More recently, there has been evidence that the results from meta-analyses are not always confirmed by very large randomised studies and it has been argued that meta-analyses based on individual patient data provide a much more reliable method of combining data from similar studies. In particular basing meta-analysis on individual data is the best method for looking at subgroups of patients and for incorporating prognostics variables and other important covariates. In the context of drug development, such individual data are almost always available and this leads to the possibility of a planned series of trials that can be subjected to a meta-analysis of the raw data.

8.6.1 Uses of meta-analysis and their strengths and weaknesses

It is useful to make a distinction between the exploratory and confirmatory uses of meta-analyses.

8.6.1.1 Exploratory use of meta-analysis
There are a number of uses to which meta-analyses can be put in an exploratory mode.

First, they can be used to generate hypotheses. Because of their nature when data are extracted from the literature across diverse study protocols meta-analyses can be extremely useful in generating hypotheses particularly concerning subgroups of patients. In this sense their use mirrors one potential objective of a population pharmacokinetic study that may be to determine interesting covariates, which influence drug

absorption and elimination. Second, they can generate data that can subsequently be used to help plan new studies. When designing new studies we need to have some idea not only of the level of effect that we may see in the study but also some idea of the likely variability. Meta-analyses can be an invaluable source of such data. Third, they can be used to judge the consistency of results across different settings. Fourth, they can be used to appropriately present result from a series of studies. Finally they can help in increasing the precision of treatment estimates; this can be important in its own right or again in the context of study planning.

8.6.1.2 Confirmatory use of meta-analysis
It might be hoped that a meta-analysis of small studies could in some way replace the registration requirement of two individual, positive, pivotal phase III studies supporting a drug's registration. It seems that this is unlikely to be satisfactory in the classical sense of a meta-analysis in which data is extracted from the literature. However, it is possible to envisage circumstances in which a planned meta-analysis as part of drug development program could be acceptable. For example, suppose that the treatment of recurrence of a condition within a fixed time period is a secondary endpoint in a drug development program and that recurrence occurs in, say, only a small proportion of patients. Studies sized for the primary endpoint would be too small for the secondary endpoint but a planned meta-analysis over a number of similar studies would be feasible. A second use might be in terms of supporting a claim based upon one or two studies.

8.6.1.3 Weaknesses of meta-analysis
There are two major types of weaknesses associated with meta-analysis. Bias and heterogeneity. When planning a clinical trial every effort is made to minimise the impact of bias on the results. For example, clinicians and patients are kept unaware of the treatment being used for each individual patient, so-called double-blind studies and patients are randomly allocated to a treatment. However, in meta-analysis there

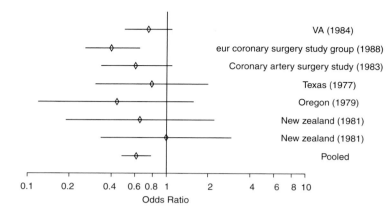

VA (1984)
eur coronary surgery study group (1988)
Coronary artery surgery study (1983)
Texas (1977)
Oregon (1979)
New zealand (1981)
New zealand (1981)
Pooled

Fig. 8.11 Meta-analysis of mortality following coronary bypPass surgery in the study reported by Yusuf *et al.*, 1994.

is the potential for the re-introduction of bias as an issue. For example, there is a tendency that only positive studies are published and that negative studies remain unpublished. This so-called publication bias can lead to an overestimation of the true effect of a drug if it remains unknown. There are graphical techniques, for example, the 'funnel plot' that endeavour to identify when publication bias is occurring (Light and Pillemer[77]). A similar problem is selection bias that can occur if, not all published trials are used in the meta-analysis. Both of these biases should be addressed in the planning phase of the meta-analysis, before data have been collected. In studies in which interim analyses are performed, biased treatment estimates may arise if the study is terminated early and account needs to be taken of this in combining this information with other studies. These bias issues are unlikely to be as important in a drug-development program because the sponsor will be able to exercise a far greater degree of control than in a classical meta-analysis.

8.6.1.4   An example of a meta-analysis
Coronary artery bypass surgery has been used for more than 30 years to treat ischaemic heart disease, but the evidence for its efficacy to reduce mortality in individual studies has been varied. Some studies have questioned whether bypass surgery while undoubtedly improving quality of

life, has any impact on increasing life expectancy. A meta-analysis reported in *The Lancet* in 1994[78] combined the evidence from seven trials comparing bypass surgery with medical treatment. It estimated that 5 years after treatment the mortality rate in bypass patients was 10.2%, while in the medically treated group the corresponding rate was 15.8%. The advantage was maintained at 7 and 10 years after treatment.

The Figure 8.11 illustrates the result of the meta-analysis using the odds ratio as an endpoint. Values of the odds ratio less than one indicate a reduction of mortality in favour of bypass surgery, greater than one in favour of medical therapy. What is clear here is that while only one of the seven studies showed any significant evidence of benefit for surgery, all but one of them showed an excess mortality in the medical treatment group. The pooled estimate of the odds ratio clearly shows a benefit in favor of bypass surgery.

References

1. Tröhler U. *To Improve the Evidence of Medicine: the 18th Century Origins of a Critical Approach.* Edinburgh: Royal College of Physicians of Edinburgh, 2000.

2. Gigerenzer G. *Reckoning with Risk: Learning to Live with Uncertainty.* London: Allan Lane The Penguin Press, 2002.

3. Bayes T. An essay towards solving a problem in the doctrine of chances. *Philosophical Transactions of the Royal Society* 1763;**53**:370–418.

4. Feinstein, AR. Clinical biostatistics. XXXIX. The haze of Bayes, the aerial palaces of decision analysis, and the computerized Ouija board. *Clin Pharmacolg Ther* 1977;**21**:482–96.

5. Spiegelhalter DJ, Abrams KR, Myles JP. *Bayesian Approaches to Clinical Trials & Health-Care Evaluation*. Chichester: John Wiley and Sons, 2003.

6. Senn S. Disappointing dichotomies. *Pharma Stat* 2003; **2**:239–40.

7. Lewis JA. In defence of the dichotomy. *Pharm Stat* 2004; **3**:77–9.

8. The Biomarker Definitions Working Group. Biomarkers and surrogate endpoints: preferred definitions and conceptual framework. *Clin Pharmaco Ther* 2001;**69**:89–95.

9. Fleming TR, DeMets DL. Surrogate endpoints in clinical trials: are we being misled? *Ann Intern Med* 1996;**125**:605–13.

10. Prentice RL. Surrogate endpoints in clinical trials: definition and operational criteria. *Stat Med* 1989;**8**:431–40.

11. Buyse M, Molenberghs G, Burzykowski T, *et al.* Statistical validation of surrogate endpoints: problems and proposals. *Drug Inf J* 2000;**34**: 447–54.

12. Buyse M, Molenberghs G. Criteria for the validation of surrogate endpoints in randomized experiments. *Biometrics* 1998;**54**:1014–29.

13. Buyse M, Molenberghs G, Burzykowski T, *et al.* The validation of surrogate endpoints in meta-analyses of randomized experiments. *Biostatistics* 2000;**1**:49–67.

14. Molenberghs G, Geys H, Buyse M. Evaluation of surrogate endpoints in randomized experiments with mixed discrete and continuous outcomes. *Stat Med* 2001;**20**:3023–38.

15. Tsiatis AA, DeGruttola V, Wulfsohn MS. Modeling the relationship of survival to longitudinal data measured with error. Applications to survival and CD4 counts in patients with AIDS. *J Am Stat Assoc* 1995;**90**:27–37.

16. Ellenberg SS. Surrogate markers in AIDS and cancer trials – discussion. *Stat Med* 1994;**13**: 1437–40.

17. Temple RJ. A regulatory authority's opinion about surrogate endpoints. In: Nimmo WS, Tucker GT, eds. *Clinical Measurement in Drug Evaluation*, New York: Wiley, 1995;1–22.

18. Lesko LJ, Atkinson AJJ. Use of biomarkers and surrogate endpoints in drug development and regulatory decision making: criteria, validation, strategies. *Annu Rev Pharmacol Toxicol* 2001;**41**:347–66.

19. Albert JM, Ioannidis JPA, Reichelderfer P, *et al.* Statistical issues for HIV surrogate endpoints: point/counterpoint. *Stat Med* 1998;**17**:2435–62.

20. Hughes MD, DeGruttola V, Welles SL. Evaluating surrogate markers. *J Acquir Immune Defic Synd Hum Retrovirol* 1995;**10**:S1–S8.

21. Grieve AP. Do statisticians count? A personal view. *Pharm Stat* 2002;**1**:35–43.

22. Bland M. *An Introduction to Medical Statistics.* Oxford: Oxford University Press, 1987.

23. Altman DG, Machin D, Bryant TN, Gardner MJ, eds. *Statistics with Confidence, 2nd edn.* BMJ Books, London, 2000.

24. Hindle M, Newton DAG, Chrystyn H Dry powder inhalers are bioequivalent to metered-dose inhalers. *Chest* 1995; **107**:629–33.

25. International Conference of Harmonisation. E6: Guideline for Good Clinical Practice, 1996. http://www.emea.eu.int/pdfs/human/ich/013595en.pdf, Accessed January 2005.

26. Hill AB. *Principles of Medical Statistics, 11th edn.* Edinburg: Livingstone, 1984.

27. International Conference of Harmonisation. E9: Statistical Principles for Clinical Trials, 1998. http://www.emea.eu.int/pdfs/human/ich/036396en.pdf, Accessed January 2005.

28. Barnes CG, Berry H, Carter ME, *et al.* Diclofenac sodium (Volarol®) and indomethacin: a multicentre comparative study in rheumatoid arthritis and osteoarthritis. *Rheumatol and Rehabil* 1979; Supplement **2**:135–46.

29. Armitage P, McPherson CK, Rowe BC. Repeated significance tests on accumulating data. *J R Stat Soc [Ser A]* 1969; **132**:235–44.

30. Pocock SJ. Group sequential methods in the design and analysis of clinical trials. *Biometrika* 1977; **64**:191–99.

31. O'Brien PC, Fleming TR. A multiple testing procedure for clinical trials. *Biometrics* 1979; **35**:549–56.

32. Lan KKG, DeMets DL. Discrete sequential boundaries for clinical trials. *Biometrika* 1983; **70**: 659–63.

33. Perneger TV. What's wrong with the Bonferonni adjustments. *Br Med J* 1998; **316**:1236–8.

34. Schwartz D, Flamant R, Lellouch J. *Clinical Trials.* London: Academic Press, (translated by MJR Healy), 1980.

35. Miranda-Filho D, Ximese R, Barone A, *et al.* Randomised controlled trial of tetanus treatment with antitetanus immunoglobulin by the intrathecal or intramuscular route. *Br Med J* 2004; **328**: 615–8.

36. Bobbio M, Demichelis B, Giustetto, G. Completeness of reporting trial results: effect on physicians' willingness to prescribe. *The Lancet* 1994; **343**: 1209–121.

37. Bucher HC, Weinbacher M, Gyr K. Influence of method of reporting study results on decision of physicians to prescribe drugs to lower cholesterol concentration. *Br Med J* 1994; **309**:761–4.

38. Fahey T, Griffiths S, Peters TJ. Evidence based purchasing: understanding results of clinical trials and systematic reviews. *Br Med J* 1995; **311**:1056–9.

39. Forrow L, Taylor W, Arnold RM. Absolutely relative: How research results are summarized can effect treatment decisions. *Am J Med* 1992; **92**:121–4.

40. Hoffrage U, Lindsay S, Hertwig R, *et al.* Communicating statistical information. *Science* 2000; **290**:2261–2.

41. Malenka DJ, Baron JA, Johansen S, Wahrenberger JW, Ross JM. The framing effect of relative and absolute risk. *J Gen Intern Med* 1993; **8**:543–8.

42. Misselbrook D, Armstrong D. Patients' responses to risk information about the benefits of treating hypertension. *Br J Gen Hypertension* 2001; **51**: 276–9.

43. Moriarty PM. Using both 'relative risk reduction' and 'number needed to treat' in evaluating primary and secondary clinical trials of lipid reduction. *Am J Cardiol* 2001; **87**:1206–8.

44. Naylor CD, Chen E, Strauss B. Measured enthusiasm: does the method of reporting trial results alter perceptions of therapeutic effectiveness. *Ann Intern Med* 1992; **117**:916–21.

45. Sheridan SL, Pignone, M. Numeracy and the medical student's ability to interpret data. *Eff Clin Pract* 2002; **5**:35–40.

46. Laupacis A, Sackett DL, Roberts RS. An assessment of clinically useful measures of the consequence of treatment. *N Engl J Med* 1988; **318**:1728–1733.

47. Royal Australian and New Zealand College of Psychiatrists Clinical Practice Guidelines Team for Panic Disorder and Agoraphobia (2003). Australian and New Zealand clinical practice guidelines for the treatment of panic disorder and agoraphobia. *Australian and New Zealand Journal of Psychiatry* 2003; **37**:641–656.

48. Royal Australian and New Zealand College of Psychiatrists Clinical Practice Guidelines Team for Depression (2004). Australian and New Zealand clinical practice guidelines for the treatment of depression. *Australian and New Zealand Journal of Psychiatry* 2004; **38**:389–407.

49. Royal Australian and New Zealand College of Psychiatrists Clinical Practice Guidelines Team for Schizophrenia and Related Disorders (2005). Australian and New Zealand clinical practice guidelines for the treatment of schizophrenia and related disorders. *Australian and New Zealand Journal of Psychiatry* 2005; **39**:1–30.

50. Hutton JA. Number needed to treat: properties and problems (with discussion). *J R Stat Soc [Ser A]* 2000; **163**:403–19.

51. Grieve AP. The number needed to treat: a useful measure or a case of the emperor's new clothes. *Pharm Stat* 2003; **2**:87–102.

52. Medical Research Council Streptomycin in Tuberculosis Trials Committee. Streptomycin treatment for pulmonary tuberculosis. *Br Med J* 1948;**ii**:769–82.

53. Chalmers, I. Why transition from alternation to randomisation in clinical trials was made. *Br Med J* 1999; **319**:1372.

54. Chalmers I. Comparing like with like: some historical milestones in the evolution of methods to create unbiased comparison groups in therapeutic experiments. *Int J Epidemiol* 2001; **30**: 1158–64.

55. Campbell MJ and Machin D. *Medical Statistics: a Commonplace Approach.* London: Wiley & Sons, 1993.

56. Palmer CR, Rosenberger WF. Ethics and practice: alternative designs for phase III randomised clinical trials. *Control Clin Trials* 1999; **20**:172–86.

57. Palmer CR. Ethics, data-dependent designs, and the strategy of clinical trials: time to start learning-as-we-go? *Stat Methods Med Res* 2002; **11**: 381–402.

58. World Medical Association. *52nd Assembly, Declaration of Helsinki: Ethical Principles for Medical Research Involving Human Subjects.* Edinburgh: World Medical Association, Inc., 2000.

59. Bartlett RH, Roloff DW, Cornell RG, *et al.* Extracorporeal circulation in neonatal respiratory failure: a prospective randomised trial. *Paediatrics* 1985; **76**:479–87.

60. Clayton DG. Ethically optimised designs. *Br J Clin Pharmacol* 1982;**13**:469–480.

61. Food and Drug Administration. A report on the two-period crossover design and its applicability in trials of clinical effectiveness. *Minutes of*

the Biometric and epidemiology Methodology Advisory Committee (BEMAC) Meeting, 1977.

62. Senn SJ. *Crossover Trials in Clinical Research* London: Wiley, 1983.

63. Jones B and Kenward MG. *Design and Analysis of Cross-Over Trials* London: Chapman-Hall, 1989.

64. Bland M, Altman DG. Regression towards the mean. *Br Med J* 1994; **308**:1499.

65. Galton, F. Regression towards mediocrity in hereditary stature. *J Anthropol Inst* 1885; **15**:246–63.

66. Pearson K. Report of certain enteric fever inoculation statistics. *Br Med J* 1904; **3**:1243–46.

67. Altman DG, Bland JM. Absence of evidence is not evidence of absence. *Br Med J 1995; 311*:485.

68. Hanley JA, Lippman-Hand A. If nothing goes wrong is everything all right? Interpreting zero numerators. *J Am Med Assoc* 1983; **249**: 1743–45.

69. International Conference of Harmonisation. E10: Choice of Control Group and Related Issues in Clinical Trials. http://www.emea.eu.int/pdfs/human/ich/036496en.pdf, Accessed January 2005.

70. Jones B, Jarvis P, Lewis JA *et al*. Trials to assess equivalence: the importance of rigorous methods. *Br Med J* 1996; **313**:36–9.

71. Rikkers LF, Rudman D, Galambos JT, *et al*. A randomized, controlled trial of the distal splenoral shunt. *Ann Surg* 1978; **188**:271–82.

72. Freiman JA, Chalmers TC, Smith HJ, *et al*. The importance of beta, the type II error and sample size in the design and interpretation of the randomized control trial. Survey of 71 'negative' trials. *N Engl J of Med* 1978; **299**:690–4.

73. Birge RT. The calculation of errors by the method of least squares. *Physical Review* 1932; **40**:207–27.

74. Cochran WG. Problems arising in the analysis of a series of similar experiments. *J R Stat Soc* 1937; *(Supplement)* **4**:102–18.

75. Yates F and Cochran WG. The analysis of groups of experiments. *J Agric Sci* 1936; **28**:556–80.

76. Glass GV. Primary, secondary and meta-analysis. *Educ Res* 1976; **5**:3–8,

77. Light RJ and Pillemer DB. *Summing Up: the Science of Reviewing Research*. Cambridge, Mass: Harvard University Press, 1984.

78. Yusuf S, Zucker D, Peduzzi P, *et al*. Effect of coronary artery bypass graft surgery on survival: overview of 10 year results from randomised trials by the Coronary Artery Bypass Graft Trialists Collaboration. *The Lancet* 1994; **344**: 563–70.

CHAPTER 9

9

Development of medicines: full development

Alan G Davies and Peter D Stonier

9.1 Introduction

Full drug development involves management of the whole project from early proof of concept to post-launch activities. The very large financial and human resource costs associated with scale up of a development project from early phase work through to Phase III and launch in major markets require that the risks associated with the investment are managed appropriately.

Nevertheless, rapid progress through Phase III development will allow a longer effective patent life, which will increase the commercial return on a new medicine. In recent years, this factor alone has been a major driver for large pharmaceutical companies to project manage their product portfolios more efficiently.

The changing nature of the pharmaceutical industry, with increasing numbers of small companies whose survival depends on rapid registration and successful marketing of one drug candidate, means that additional risks, such as intellectual property rights, shareholder return, and contractual and legal relationships, are part of the risk associated with the investment. Management of business risk, which is outside the scope of this chapter, has been identified as a significant problem for small companies.[1]

9.2 Background

Total drug development costs are huge and continue to increase over time. In 2003, development costs of 68 randomly selected new drugs were US$403 million each (year 2000 dollars).[2] Capitalising out-of-pocket costs to the point of marketing approval at a real discount rate of 11% yields a total pre-approval cost estimate of US$802 million for each new medicine (year 2000 dollars) and the costs have increased at an annual rate of 7.4% above general price inflation.[2] The majority of drug development costs are in Phase III development: these include not only the clinical trial programme itself, but significant associated regulatory and manufacturing scale-up costs.

The long-forecasted consolidation in the pharmaceutical industry happened in the 1990s, and has paused in the mid-2000s. The impact of this consolidation was demonstrated by an increase in product failures and increased trial cancellations in 1999 and 2000. However, during 2001, Phase III activity increased again, albeit by a small increase of 1.8% (to 385 projects) compared with 2000, and this activity has continued to increase to 404 projects in 2004. *Pharmaprojects* in mid-2004[3] was reporting on 32 775 drug candidates with 1654 active companies researching 7368 drugs currently in active R&D in 218 therapy areas.

9.2.1 Senior management perspective

Taking into account all marketing and development failures, cost calculations demonstrate that companies have to develop more 'blockbuster' products with annual sales over US$1 billion if they are to maintain historical rates of returns to shareholders, or they must cut significantly the development costs. Thus, the focus of management is increasingly on the high costs of Phase III programmes, and there is a need to reduce risks and costs in Phase III by:

1. Aggressive portfolio management in early phases of development.
2. Life-cycle management, including risk management.
3. Continued spending on local trials after submission to fill gaps in the development programme, such as paediatric or geriatric subjects in Phases IIIb and IV.

The biotechnology explosion has also finally arrived. Globally, the total number of companies working on pharmaceutical R&D continues to rise and in May 2004, 656 companies were working on only one or two compounds.[4] The number of companies with one product in development, which is a useful proxy for biotechnology-driven or emerging pharmaceutical companies, has increased each year from 212 in 1998 to 373 in 2001 and 656 in 2004. Moreover, the top 25 pharmaceutical companies have a significant proportion of R&D drugs in development that are licensed, typically from smaller pharmaceutical companies or research laboratories.[4]

Ranked by total numbers of drugs in R&D, the top five companies are GlaxoSmithKline (188 drugs in development), Pfizer (154), Roche (135), Johnson & Johnson (134) and Aventis (123). Of the 188 R&D drugs that GlaxoSmithKline has in development, 112 (60%) are their own drugs, Pfizer has 90 (58%), Roche 78 (58%), Johnson & Johnson 86 (64%) and Aventis 123 (63%).[4]

This changing picture of full drug development means that the largest pharmaceutical companies are now having to be adept at intellectual property protection, legal and contractual development and co-marketing agreements, as well as accelerated drug development. The single product companies must also be skilled at managing their cash flow, relationships with their shareholders and the market place in which they need to thrive.

Recovery of costs by successful marketing of products is essential in order to maximise shareholder return. As R&D costs continue to increase by between 8% and 11% per annum, and sales turnover increases by between 5% and 7% per annum, R&D takes up an increasing proportion of the pharmaceutical budget, and for the largest pharmaceutical companies it is about 17% of turnover.

Clearly, there is a limit to how much the research costs can increase and companies are beginning to think in new ways about how to manage their R&D costs. There is an increase in the number of alliances and partnerships with academic groups, small biotechnology companies and healthcare providers who, it is hoped, will provide the entrepreneurial drug development skills that large pharmaceutical companies are currently unable to generate internally. Networks, modelled on successes such as cancer,[5] and involvement of patient groups will continue to increase in importance.

The International Conference on Harmonisation (ICH), the EU Clinical Trials Directive (2001/20/EC) and the draft GCP (Good Clinical Practice) Directive (issued on 1 July 2004) provide a more unified standard for clinical trials and also facilitate mutual acceptance by the regulatory authorities in Europe, Japan and the United States. Development of the guidelines and, in the European Union, the Directives have allowed companies to streamline their drug development programmes by mandating a more uniform approach through the European Union. Consequently, the approach is probably better driven from the head office rather than at a country or company subsidiary level, especially as regulatory convergence develops within Europe.

9.3 Taking Products into Later Development Phase

9.3.1 Clinical perspective

This chapter focuses on the clinical development of new medicines. This is an area where companies can plan and control much more of their activity. As more drug development projects are terminated at Phase II, companies have to be careful that the Phase II studies are particularly well designed to avoid the likelihood of a Type II error. This means that the studies do not miss a significant clinical difference or advantage for the product. Clarity of thought and detailed design considerations for Phase II studies are increasingly important in drug development. The use of external advisory boards can be especially helpful, and it can be useful to include drug development and regulatory specialists on advisory boards together with the more traditional academic staff members.

If the area of endeavour is crowded there will be significant competition for patient recruitment to clinical trials. Currently, these therapy areas include diabetes, oncology and cardiovascular medicine, and it may become necessary to seek patients outside Western Europe and the United States. Investigator fees are rising and competition for patients is helping to increase fees in these geographical areas and also in some areas of Central and Eastern Europe. However, even significant investigator fees may not be sufficient to encourage recruitment if there is little investigator excitement about the product. Investigators are keen to work on innovative products and may well seek increased fees to support other academic work if the product is not particularly exciting for them.

The likely effectiveness of the product, derived from the preclinical and early clinical work, will determine study design, complexity and size. It is a mistake to try to answer too many questions in a single study, despite the apparent commercial attractiveness of such a strategy. A study overburdened by many secondary objectives is more likely to fail when the design is implemented in many centres worldwide. What seems a good idea in head office can often be hard to implement in the clinic. Statistical advice is vital, and statisticians offer excellent opinions about the utility of complex study designs.

The expected adverse event profile will also determine the study design. A drug for which the prescription is to be initiated in a tertiary referral clinic by leading experts in the field, such as many oncological compounds, will have a different safety profile compared with a product which will be widely used across many different specialties in primary and secondary care. Characterisation of the risk–benefit profile is an important consideration in study design.

Consideration needs to be given to suitable clinical endpoints. It can be tempting, because of cost and speed of development, to use surrogate endpoints in a pivotal study. A surrogate endpoint is defined as an endpoint that is intended to relate to a clinically important outcome but does not, in itself, measure clinical benefit. A surrogate endpoint should be used as a primary endpoint when appropriate, for example, when the surrogate endpoint is reasonably likely to, or is well known to, predict clinical outcome. However, great care needs to be taken in basing a pivotal and full development programme on the use of surrogate endpoints. Typically, these endpoints are used in early development and discussion with the regulatory authorities is advised before using such endpoints in a full development programme. The use of surrogate markers is discussed in the *ICH Guideline E8: General Considerations for Clinical Trials*. The guideline makes the point that these markers are most often useful in exploratory therapeutic trials in well-defined narrow patient groups.

9.3.2   Regulatory perspective

The regulatory authorities are increasingly welcoming informal or formal discussions about drug development programmes. There are differences in approach between the European Medicines Evaluation Agency (EMEA) and the US Food and Drug Administration (FDA), and it is wise to take regulatory advice before contacting the agencies. The FDA tends to require a formalistic approach to the development programme. This can have strengths in that the programme direction is clear, but it can be rather limiting in terms of defining a mandatory series of trials and a particular development strategy. Nevertheless, it can be particularly useful if the development programme is likely to be in a new area of medicine or is unusual in any way.

The National Institute for Clinical Excellence (NICE) was set up in 1999 as a Special Health Authority for England and Wales. Its role is to provide patients, health professionals and the public with authoritative, robust and reliable guidance/guidelines on current 'best practice'. The guidance covers individual health technologies following appraisal and guidelines are developed relating to the clinical management of specific conditions. In practice, the pharmaceutical industry has tended to see NICE as an additional 'fourth' hurdle acting after the Medicines and Healthcare Products Regulatory Agency (MHRA) or EMEA has approved the quality, safety and efficacy of a new product. Consideration has to be given in any development programme to applications to NICE and other bodies throughout the world, and companies may need to consider special and additional studies to meet any objections these bodies may have in allowing a product to be satisfactorily commercialised.

The common technical document (CTD) (ICH M4)[6] is now a requirement. The CTD is the agreed common format for the preparation of a well-structured application to the regulatory authorities and has had an impact on all organisations as database integration and electronic submissions become more common.

The ICH has played an important role in establishing guidelines for drug development. Although these are only guidelines and are not legal documents, companies would have to justify deviations from the guidelines in any application for approval. The World Health Organisation (WHO) has recently stated that it expects the ICH guidelines to be adopted in non-ICH countries eventually. Based on the ICH, the European Union has recently developed a new system (Directive 2001/20/EC) of clinical trial regulation which is in the process of being transposed into national law in each Member State. This will have the effect of making failure to comply with the 'GCP Directive', for example, a criminal offence.

The EU Clinical Trials Directive (2001/20/EC) and associated guidelines and Directives (such as the Good Clinical Practice Directive: draft issued on 1 July 2004) should allow regulatory convergence over time in Europe. The guidelines provide benefits for clinical trial subjects: they are protected during studies, and they can be confident that the studies are based on good science. The Trials Directive is associated with a large number of guidance and other Directives. These include the following guidance: Competent Authority Submission, Ethics Submission, EU Clinical Trials Database, EU Suspected Unexpected Serious Adverse Reactions (SUSARs) database, Adverse Reaction Reporting, Revised Annex 13, Qualification of Inspectors for GMP Inspection and two Directives: 2003/94/EC (the 'GMP Directive') and the draft 'GCP Directive'. All the key principles applying to the new system are mentioned in 2001/20/EC. These include: legal representation, compliance with GCP, obligations to regulatory authorities, obligations to ethics committees, compliance with CMP, EU database of clinical trials, pharmacovigilance, and GMP and GCP inspections.

As always, increased regulation has resulted in increased costs, offset slightly by an increase in standardisation of procedures across regions of the world. There are new databases to master, including the European Database of Clinical Trials – EudrACT, and a new pharmacovigilance database for SUSARs; responsibility for both of these lies with the EMEA. At the time of writing, the revised practices are new and unfamiliar. In time, these new relationships with competent authorities, ethics committees, EudrACT and SUSAR databases and the need for legal representation will become easier and more routine. The value of regulatory convergence will then become more apparent.

9.3.3 Commercial perspective

Apart from the traditional costs associated with commercial development, the costs of selling and marketing the product will require evaluation. Decisions have to be made about whether the product will be sold by the company's own sales force or licensed to partners in some markets. Such discussions are beyond the scope of this chapter.

The company franchise in a particular area of therapeutic endeavour may be enhanced or compromised by active patient groups. There is increasing pressure to place more development and clinical trial information in the public domain. For example, in the United Kingdom, the pharmaceutical industry trade association, the Association of the British Pharmaceutical Industry (ABPI), has agreed to develop a register of Phase III trials conducted in the United Kingdom, 3 months after drug approval in a major market – which might not be the United Kingdom. Patients will therefore be in a position to seek entry into trials and may demand this from their physicians.

The development of AZT (Retrovir®, zidovudine), by Wellcome (now GlaxoSmithKline) is an interesting example of patient power. Patient groups obtained copies of early phase drug development protocols and some subjects demanded to be placed into these clinical trials for HIV/AIDS. The scrutiny of the protocols by patient groups resulted in improvements in clinical trial designs and the political pressure exerted by these groups ensured that the drug regulatory process became more politicised. This resulted in more rapid approval of drugs by some regulatory authorities and also pushed forward discussions about surrogate markers. It is probable that AZT did not fully meet the established principles of safety and efficacy when it was approved, and further development was required after approval. Whether this approach was beneficial to the entire community of AIDS patients remains debatable.

Other patient groups in areas as diverse as osteoporosis research, dementia and oncology, have learnt from the AIDS patient groups about the power of politics in medicine, and these groups will have an increasing impact on drug development. Some of this impact will be positive but some is likely to be negative and may encourage a too rapid assessment of drug efficacy and safety by the authorities. Indeed, there is evidence of increased product withdrawal by the FDA. Eleven products have been withdrawn between 1997 and mid-2001, compared with eight product withdrawals in the previous

10 years. Whether this is a result of more rapid early development, a more rapid assessment process or simply due to bad luck is open to conjecture. However, it is clear that a product withdrawal in either late-phase development or early post-marketing can have a devastating effect on a company's share price as a result of the expected decrease in revenue and the potential for poor public relations. Within a day of announcing the withdrawal of rofecoxib (Vioxx®), more than £14 billion was wiped from Merck's stock market value, equivalent to a quarter of its worth and the share price plunged to an 8-year low.[7]

The market potential of a drug or device is clearly critical in determining the desirability of proceeding into later phase development. An increasing number of programmes are stopped at Phase II because it is not economical for the company to develop these products. DiMasi[8] in 2001 estimated that, compared with the 1981–6 period, where 29.8% of products were terminated because of economic reasons, between 1987 and 1992 the number of terminations was 33.8% and that this upward trend has continued.

Likely shifts in demographic factors and prescribing mean that drugs for the elderly, such as therapies for Alzheimer's disease or osteoporosis, are increasingly attractive as targets for drug development. Oncological drugs and drugs for chronic diseases also continue to be important for companies' financial health.

The political environment continues to be important. All governments want to constrain healthcare costs, and an easy target is prescription drug costs. This is not necessarily the most sensible target, as improving health service management may have as important an effect on the national purse. Nonetheless, there is a continuing downwards pressure on healthcare prescribing.

9.3.4 Exit strategy

Most pharmaceutical companies cannot market products by themselves in all countries of the world. This may be because, for example, there is no subsidiary in the relevant country, or because the sales forces' other commitments mean that this drug cannot be adequately marketed in one particular market. For whatever reason, all development programmes must consider an exit strategy for the product in each market. Are there to be co-licensing, co-marketing or other agreements? Is the drug to be licensed out in other markets? Such discussion is beyond the scope of this chapter, but involves important considerations for any full drug development programme.

9.4 Preparing the Plan

9.4.1 Structure of the plan

The candidate drug has passed the early development hurdles. In particular, the early preclinical toxicology and commercial environments are suitable. Care must be taken regarding any intellectual property concerns, and that preliminary drug supply and manufacturing forecasts look favourable. Early evaluation and planning will take about 12 months to execute, being a complex process with many interactions and requiring the integration of many different processes. Typically, and best practice for the development of such a plan, this requires a relatively senior project manager or development scientist to take primary responsibility and ownership of the project. The 'owner' must have the authority to obtain the necessary information from different departments within the organisation and from external suppliers.

The plan will eventually prescribe a likely filing date for a marketing authorisation application (MAA) (product licence). This date is vital and when the plan becomes public information, any slippage in the date is likely to impact on the share price of the company. Accordingly, senior members of the company must be confident that the date can be met. There will always be pressure to bring the date forward but this has a cost in resources, and risks damaging credibility with investors if the accelerated timelines cannot be met.

Thus, a sequential plan is safe, cost-effective in terms of resources and manageable by most organisations. Unfortunately, such a plan has a cost in terms of unacceptable delays to

shareholders. In the early 1990s, there was a vogue for massively parallel plans which ran many activities simultaneously in order to address and bring forward 'stop-go' decisions and filing dates. Stop-go decisions were made aggressively and the plans were continually examined to review ways to bring the filing date forward. Such plans are now less common. The principal reason cited by organisations is that such plans throw many of the company resources onto a single product. If the product fails in late stage development, other candidate compounds will have been neglected. Such plans are therefore a significant gamble for even well-resourced and capitalised organisations. If they fail, a gap appears in a company's product pipeline, with serious consequences for the well-being of the organisation.

More recently, a trend within companies has been to accelerate development plans without utilising a significant part of the company's resources on any one product. Thus, it may be necessary to outsource some of the development work, but this ensures a more even pattern of portfolio management, which has benefits for the organisation. The efforts of the pharmaceutical industry have begun to be beneficial to the industry. In general, approval success rates and times increased in the first half of the 1990s to levels not seen since the 1970s[9] (see Tables 9.1 and 9.2). Table 9.2 shows the trends in investigational new drug (IND) filings for four new chemical entity (NCE) approval phases.[9]

Table 9.1 Percentage of new drug applications (NDAs) approved by period of submission[9]

Period of NDA submission	Percentage of NDAs approved
1963–9	94.6
1970–4	88.5
1975–9	88.5
1980–4	76.2
1985–9	78.9
1990–4	86.1

Table 9.2 Years from 'first-into-man' studies to NDA submission and from submission to approval by period of submission and FDA priority rating[9]

Period of NDA submission	FDA priority rating	Years from 'first-into-man' to NDA submission	Years from NDA submission to approval
1963–75	Standard	3.7	2.2
	Priority	5.7	2.2
1976–85	Standard	7.4	3.1
	Priority	8.6	2.1
1986–95	Standard	8.1	3.0
	Priority	11.2	2.0
1996–9	Standard	8.1	1.6
	Priority	7.2	1.0

Clinical development and US approval phases by FDA therapeutic rating (priority or standard) show that priority times have decreased and standard times have been stable since 1970s. In 2004, the mean approval time is cited to be 90.3 months (7.5 years),[10] so US approval times have stabilised again.

Quite how the plan is reviewed depends on the organisation, the therapeutic class and regulatory priority rating. Large organisations will review on a 12-monthly cycle the overall shape of the drug development portfolio for, say, the next 10 years, the near-term portfolio and resource requirements, say over 3 years, and closely review the detailed plan for the next 12 months. This allows the company to define the next 12 months in terms of budget and resource, and the next 3 and 10 years in some detail to establish if there are likely to be gaps in the portfolio 10 years hence that can be filled by in-licensing of compounds. Such a strategic review is vital for the successful integration of new compounds into the company. Furthermore, such a review allows integration of a registration package, which will be acceptable to most major markets, into a single dossier. This avoids fragmentation of the clinical development programme. Duplication of activities is minimised and the major, pivotal, Phase III studies and analysis are performed only once and then integrated. Knowledge of the compound

and likely questions from the regulatory authorities from the major markets can be centralised. This saves time and resources.

Smaller companies and venture capital funded organisations are likely to be focused on a single compound, its analogues, metabolites and differing formulations. Without the luxury of a 10-year strategic development plan, such organisations are naturally tightly focused on the success of their product. Within these companies, pressure to bring the filing date forward can be intense and if the date is missed this can have serious consequences for the market capitalisation of the company.

9.4.2 Therapeutic targets

Clinical success rates and attrition rates by phase of clinical trial for new drugs are important indicators of how effectively companies are utilising drug development resources. The proficiency with which this is done reflects a complex set of regulatory, economic and company-specific factors. Success rates differ by therapeutic class, and typically vary from about 28% success rate for an anti-infective compound to 12% for respiratory drugs.[9] Table 9.3 shows the details.

It is mandatory to ensure that the therapeutic target is appropriate and commercially attractive, and to define the required product performance

Table 9.3 Current and maximum possible success rate by therapeutic class with INDs first filed from 1981 to 1992[9]

Therapeutic class	NCE	Approved NCE	Open NCE[a]	Current success rate (%)[a]	Maximum success rate (%)[b]
Analgesic/anaesthetic	49	10	4	20.4	28.6
Anti-infective	57	16	3	28.1	33.3
Anti-neoplastic	38	6	6	15.8	31.6
Cardiovascular	120	21	6	17.5	22.5
Central nervous system	110	16	14	14.5	27.3
Endocrine	33	6	4	18.2	30.3
Gastrointestinal	15	3	2	20.0	33.3
Immunological	13	2	0	15.4	15.4
Respiratory	25	3	0	12.0	12.0
Other/miscellaneous	43	3	4	7.0	16.3

[a] As of 31 December 1999.
[b] Assumes all open NCEs will eventually be approved.

to ensure successful marketing. These activities demand close cooperation between discovery, development and marketing departments before embarking on a full development plan. In the treatment of herpes zoster infection, for example, there is a precedent using the speed of crusting of the vesicular lesions as a marker for the efficacy of drug treatment, with significantly more rapid crusting, associated with the active agent, permitting registration. This is hardly of major relevance to the clinical situation as a beneficial effect on the disappearance of vesicles is of minor consequence to the patient who has a painful condition. The important clinical question is the effect of treatment on pain acutely, and in the longer term, in the prevention of post-herpetic neuralgia. This creates an interesting dilemma. Should the primary clinical endpoint be crusting of lesions, given that this approach will undoubtedly result in more rapid execution of studies and therefore faster registration, or should it address the real medical issue, that is, pain, an area where the clinical evaluation of the efficacy of treatment will be more complex? The responsible clinical decision is to measure both endpoints, but the implications for marketing must be understood.

The use of the different therapeutic targets, and the implication for the organisation, surrounds competitive advantage. What may be a minor clinical advantage for a new compound can sometimes be converted into a significant commercial lever that will facilitate marketing. Many companies use the draft Summary of Product Characteristics (SPC) to establish needs and wants, allowing a useful dialogue between the drug development and marketing groups.

Draft labelling and a draft SPC are produced at the beginning of the development process and these embody the features that the marketing group regards as minimal to ensure commercial success ('needs'). These needs must be tempered by input from medical and development to ensure that the requirements are realistic. The draft would also include features that are perceived to have significant advantages over competitor agents ('wants') and those that would provide useful talking points ('nice to have').

It is always tempting to design a minimalist programme of studies, that is, the minimum required to obtain registration for a given indication, but this approach may not even address the 'needs', particularly in an area where there is relative satisfaction with available therapy and therefore intense competitor activity. For example, the development of a non-steroidal anti-inflammatory drug may include studies in relatively small numbers of patients, aiming to demonstrate less gastrointestinal blood loss than that associated with an established comparator. In such a competitive area this is likely to be insufficient without demonstrating that this translates into real clinical benefit compared with the comparator, for example, reducing the incidence of major gastrointestinal blood loss requiring transfusion. A large-scale clinical study such as this may not therefore be required for registration but would be required for launch in order to demonstrate to clinicians the place of a new agent in a crowded therapeutic area.

During this process, it is necessary to establish that the marketing 'wants' are indeed achievable. For example, there may be a need for an adequate therapy for delayed nausea and vomiting associated with chemotherapy. Clinicians may state that this is a clinical need. Depending on the current therapies and the early profile of the candidate drug, a good estimation of the drug's likely effectiveness in the indication can be made. However, if there are already therapies in later development or in the market place which partially address the clinical need, it might require significant therapeutic endeavour, usually through late Phases III and IV clinical trials, to establish the product in the market place. It is therefore important to identify the place of an individual drug in the therapeutic armamentarium.

The prescriber will base a decision on a consideration of the relative risk–benefit, whereas the regulator will consider the drug entirely on its own merits and will tend to assess the efficacy, safety and quality of a drug in its own right. A relative judgement is straightforward in an area of high unmet medical need, when there is simply a consideration of whether it is better to have the disease treated or untreated, but much more difficult and subtle in an area where drug treatment is already available. The complexity of the decision tends to increase with an increasing number of treatment options and

under these circumstances the prescriber will be more inclined to consider the options for the individual patient. For example, when treating hypertension in a middle-aged man the first choice may be a beta blocker. The choice of which beta blocker may depend on (1) whether the particular drug has been shown to have any primary or secondary role in preventing myocardial infarction, its effect on cholesterol and its propensity to affect adversely the peripheral vasculature; (2) whether it limits exercise tolerance or (3) whether it has undesirable effects in a patient with asthma. It is therefore important to mirror this thought process when considering the market support programme and also to take account of preclinical data that may point to establishing clinical differentiation from a competitor. Studies examining such endpoints are always attractive to marketing departments.

The use of surrogate markers is always attractive. They allow drug development timelines to be shortened and may allow particular marketing angles to be pursued, for example, a cholesterol-lowering effect in a cardiovascular agent. Regulators are increasingly likely to question the use of surrogate markers for large-scale pivotal Phase III studies. Typically, at least one clinical endpoint trial is necessary. Such a trial is large and costly and it may take a considerable time to enrol and follow-up subjects in the study. The large cardiovascular intervention and survival studies are examples of such studies.

Regulators may require specific studies to address specific questions, for example, use of the drug in the elderly, in children or other at-risk populations. Design of these studies needs detailed consideration: the subjects might be difficult to recruit, and comparative or placebo studies may be complex, potentially unethical or unduly expensive in terms of time and resources. Drug development expertise, as well as good support from the biostatistical and biometrics groups, is vital. The ICH guidelines can be particularly helpful when conducting clinical trials in special populations. Sometimes, of course, the guidelines are ambiguous at best.

9.4.3 Safety

About 20% of new drugs will fail because of safety concerns.[9] Nevertheless, with a clinical development programme involving an average of about 4500 patients (see below), the potential prescriber of a new drug is faced with the absence of a large amount of safety data. The safety profile of a drug will develop over time as adverse reactions occur spontaneously in a normal clinical setting. While there is no substitute for spontaneous reporting in the identification of rare side effects, it is important to consider whether useful safety information can be generated soon after launch.

In this context, a decision on whether post-marketing surveillance studies should be built into the development programme must be taken. Such an observational study may signal the occurrence of adverse events or alternatively it may signal and quantify the frequency of adverse events. At this point in the life cycle of a new medicine, post-marketing surveillance is likely to involve cohort observational studies of 10–20 000 patients. The value of these studies is likely to be three-fold:

1. To generate safety data during use of a drug in routine clinical practice, to enable a comparison to be made of the safety profile in an uncontrolled population and the controlled clinical trial population.
2. To provide safety data in a defined group incompletely covered in the registration package, for example, the elderly.
3. To enlarge the 'formal' safety database and thereby act as an insurance policy to address problems occurring at a later stage in a drug's evolution.

The possibility for such studies will depend on the disease, disease frequency and whether the prescribing setting is in primary or secondary care. The value of these studies is likely to be greatest if data are generated as soon as possible after launch, and plans for implementation must occur well in advance of submission of the regulatory dossier. Such studies might also be a condition of registration.

Post-marketing (Phase IV) studies also generate safety data, but qualitatively these are likely to be similar to those collected during the preregistration phase. In Western Europe, larger Phase IV studies that have the evaluation of clinical safety as a primary objective have been embraced by the Post-Authorisation Safety Assessment (PASS) or Safety Assessment of Marketed Medicines (SAMM) guidelines, which have superseded previous guidelines on post-marketing surveillance and which are incorporated into the EMEA pharmacovigilance guidelines.

In recent years, there has been a growth in the field of mega-studies, usually clinical outcome studies involving 5000–25 000 patients, with a simple primary endpoint such as mortality and a number of secondary morbidity endpoints. The potential for studies of this magnitude to throw up less frequent side effects than those seen in the preregistration programme is clear.

9.5 The Detailed Clinical Development Plan

In this section, we consider the requirements for the clinical programme leading to global registration, as well as other studies that will form part of the overall programme. Scheduling is covered elsewhere in this volume, but it must be emphasised that each activity in the clinical study programme has to be identified and an appropriate order determined. A realistic estimate of timing can thus be made and, when the sequence and timing of events has been determined, the critical path can be established. This is the chain of essential events that must be accomplished to achieve a particular goal; clearly, a change to one of these events has a fundamental effect on development time.

As with any plan, well-defined milestones and checkpoints must be incorporated and subsequent activity should not proceed until these have been achieved. The plan must always be sufficiently detailed to identify supporting activities, such as toxicological studies, that must be completed to allow development to continue without interruption. Many of these activities can, and should, run in parallel.

9.5.1 Number of patients

Although there are no fixed rules in devising the Phase III programme, the more subjects admitted the better in terms of a safety evaluation, but it must be kept in mind that ethical considerations demand that only sufficient patients to meet the scientific criteria of study endpoints should be randomised. For example, for a disease-modifying drug for rheumatoid arthritis, approval has been granted on a database of up to about 6000 subjects. On the other hand, a novel immunosuppressant agent has been granted an approval with fewer than 2000 subjects. Based on their experience, however, Blake and Ratcliffe suggested that about 3000 patients per indication is average for an NDA in 1991.[11] The Tufts Institute in 2001 suggested that about 4500 subjects is average for an NDA.[9] These two numbers are consistent with an annual compound increase in numbers of about 7%. Others have suggested that about 100 patient-years experience is satisfactory for some established drugs for well-understood disease areas, such as new formulations of insulin. Much also depends on the additional supportive data that can be included in the application.

The number of subjects is likely to vary depending on the degree of unmet medical need and the seriousness of the disease indication. It is likely that a drug shown to be effective in treating stroke, a condition with a high mortality and morbidity where no effective treatment is available, will require a database of fewer than 3000 patients. Conversely, an anxiolytic, used to treat a non-life threatening condition where effective treatments already exist, may require a much larger database. However, 4500 patients represent a reasonable working total.

9.5.2 Number of studies

Having established the number of patients to be included in the preregistration clinical programme, it is important to consider how these will be distributed and hence how many studies are required. This is very variable. The Tufts Institute reported that, for biopharmaceuticals,

there were on average only 12 studies and 1014 subjects per NDA compared with 37 studies and 4478 subjects for a conventional pharmaceutical NDA.[12]

Generally speaking, the FDA will require placebo-controlled studies wherever possible to demonstrate efficacy at the dose to be marketed and these are termed pivotal studies. Pivotal studies do not have to be placebo controlled, however, and in some areas, such as depression, the ICH guidelines suggest a three-arm study, with both an active comparator and a placebo control. The Declaration of Helsinki, revised in 2000, suggested that in some disease areas, placebo-controlled studies are to be examined very carefully for their ethical content. This includes areas where conventional best therapy is generally acceptable. In this case, great care needs to be taken with the choice of active comparator.

It is widely accepted that two placebo-controlled pivotal studies are necessary, although it is not clear whether this is a mandatory regulation in the FDA or EMEA regulations. There is, however, a certain insurance in this approach as studies, even of drugs that are effective, can occasionally fail to show a statistically positive result if the treated population somehow deviates from the norm or if the placebo response is unexpectedly increased. In Europe the use of an active comparator in a pivotal study is more common.

Sample sizes for clinical trials are discussed more fully elsewhere in this book and should be established in discussion with a statistician. Sample sizes should, however, be sufficient to be 90% certain of detecting a statistically significant difference between treatments, based on a set of predetermined primary variables. This means that trials utilising an active control will generally be considerably larger than placebo-controlled studies, in order to exclude a Type II statistical error (i.e. the failure to demonstrate a difference where one exists). Thus, in areas where a substantial safety database is required, for example, hypertension, it may be appropriate to have in the programme a preponderance of studies using a positive control.

The increasing use of active comparator studies has meant that more studies are being powered on a 'non-inferiority' basis. It is essential to discuss such designs with statisticians. Other novel designs, for example, initial open-label therapy followed by a randomised treatment arm following disease exacerbation, are becoming more common. These novel designs must be discussed with a statistician and with the regulatory authorities before expensive mistakes are made.

Conversely, if demonstration of efficacy is more critical than establishing safety, for example, in Alzheimer's disease, then placebo-controlled studies are appropriate. Although the studies may include fewer patients, the number of studies may be approximately the same as for a hypertension programme.

It is eminently sensible to aim to have the smallest number of studies in the dossier as this makes data management and analysis less complex and therefore less time consuming. It is inevitable, however, that some studies which are not universally necessary will find their way into the core dossier. In France, for example, pricing is inextricably linked to technical approval and, when granting a price, the authorities make reference to an already available treatment wherever possible. It would therefore be virtually impossible to obtain pricing approval unless a comparative study with a reference drug had been undertaken. As pricing approval is the immediate step after technical approval, the 'pricing study' needs to begin at the same time as the core registration studies; hence, it becomes part of the regulatory dossier.

While it is desirable to avoid duplicating activity, there will undoubtedly be some duplication of studies in the clinical programme given the foregoing discussion. It is important nevertheless to ensure that *ad hoc* studies do not find their way into the plan by default. The importance of studies designed to demonstrate competitive advantage has been mentioned and while data from many of these studies may not find their way into the regulatory dossier, the studies are, nevertheless, part of the overall clinical programme. Under these circumstances,

there is little point in allowing duplication of comparator drugs between studies. For example, there is a considerable variety of drugs for the treatment of depression, ranging from the old tricyclic compounds, such as amitriptyline and imipramine, to the more recent and less toxic compounds, such as the selective monoamine and serotonin re-uptake inhibitors. In between, there is a host of antidepressant drugs with distinguishing properties; some are sedative, while others have anxiolytic activity. The most widely used drug will also vary from country to country. This situation, therefore, presents an opportunity to implement an international programme to test the new agent against a variety of competitors in order to tease out differences and provide data that may be required to support registration and that will also be of major use at the time of launch and subsequent marketing in individual countries. Care must be taken at head office that local studies do not jeopardise the overall regulatory and marketing plan, as embodied in the draft SPC. A study in which the drug dosage is halved for local marketing reasons might have the potential to undermine the whole regulatory package unless there are clear medical reasons for such a study.

Finally, in addition to studies that may be included to address potential regulatory questions, it is important to consider whether 'in-filling' is needed. In an attempt to speed drug development, a high-risk strategy is to take the decision to enter full development as early as possible. This may mean that many elements of the Phase IIb programme are not carried out sequentially and one strategy, for example, is to carry out formal dose-ranging studies as part of the large-scale Phase IIa efficacy and safety programme. 'In-filling' can be used to describe any study that forms part of the essential regulatory package that is not conducted in conventional Phases I–III sequence.

9.5.3 Duration of treatment

In Europe, a drug that is likely to be administered long term will require a minimum of 100 patients treated for 1 year to gain approval. This will vary, however, depending on the circumstances. It is likely that a new antihypertensive agent will require significantly more long-term experience than this before a licence is granted, whereas a drug that is effective in treating gastric cancer may require less. It is important to remember that data generated as a result of long-term administration will be required to support registration applications for drugs used to treat recurrent diseases, such as peptic ulcer, as well as chronic diseases, such as hypertension.

Most Phase III studies in a chronic disease will require 1 year of therapy. Most oncology studies will require 12-months' survival data.

9.5.4 Dose

The FDA demands, at opposite ends of the dose range, a dose that demonstrates efficacy but is associated with side effects and a dose that is largely ineffective. A range of doses may be studied within these limits, with the aim of identifying a dose that is both effective and tolerable. In Europe, there is greater scope to justify the choice of dose in a particular set of clinical circumstances. Choice of dose should also take account of further development for new indications, for example, an antihypertensive drug may also be effective in treating angina or heart failure but the dose is likely to differ significantly.

9.5.5 Patient categories

It is important to include all age ranges that are of clinical importance. Development of an anti-asthma drug, for example, should include a programme of evaluation in children as well as adults because they will form a significant portion of the database and risk–benefit considerations will be different. Development of an anti-arthritis compound, on the other hand, will be undertaken predominantly in older patients and particularly detailed information on efficacy and safety in the elderly will be required.

This raises the important question of 'what is elderly?'. In the average regulatory dossier, the majority of patients are likely to be less than 75 years old, yet population demographics point to the increasing importance of the 'older elderly' – those aged more than 75 years. Abernethy reports, reassuringly, that there is little or no evidence to date to suggest that the toxicity of any drug is unique to the elderly and therefore it follows that the 'older elderly' are probably not a discrete group.[13] It would appear prudent, however, in a clinical situation where a drug is likely to be taken by large numbers of patients in this category for there to be an appropriate evaluation of the risks and benefits. This may not need to form part of the regulatory package but data could be generated by a cohort observational study as part of a post-marketing surveillance programme.

The FDA Modernisation Act of 1997 (FDAMA) included a number of elements that have increased the number of studies being performed on children. This was largely successful at increasing data on paediatric studies in the United States and has been now replaced by the Best Pharmaceuticals for Children Act, 4 January 2002 (Public Law No. 107–109). The European Commission has released (29 September 2004) proposed regulations that aim at promoting medicines for children which draw heavily on the successful FDA model. The regulations will probably be transposed into law in individual Member States in 2006. This means that all development plans will have to actively consider paediatric studies in the future.

9.5.6 Coexisting medical conditions/concomitant drug interactions

It is important to ensure adequate collection of data in patients who have coexisting medical conditions in whom drug elimination may be reduced, particularly those with hepatic or renal impairment, as lower doses are likely to be required in these patients. It is also important to investigate potential drug interactions both clinically and pharmacologically, particularly for drugs prescribed for conditions that are likely to coexist, and specific clinical pharmacology studies must be built into the programme. For example, it is necessary to determine the effect of a new antihypertensive agent co-prescribed with an angiotensin converting enzyme (ACE) inhibitor, nitrate, calcium channel blocker, beta blocker and diuretic, in terms of both drug interactions and potentiation of antihypertensive effect. Interaction via an effect on the cytochrome P450 system must also be investigated should there be any suggestion from preclinical data that this may occur.

9.5.7 Dosage form

Is the dosage form to be used for large-scale development, and hence is commercialisation the same as that used for earlier phase studies and is the choice underpinned by an appropriate toxicology work-up? It is common for the dosage form to change during the course of the development process. Early studies may be carried out using liquid or capsule preparations because of the ease of formulation. Almost invariably, the marketed formulation will be different and it is important to ensure that inclusion in the regulatory dossier of data obtained using the early formulations can be justified by appropriate bioavailability studies, which may be required as part of the full preregistration plan. It is highly desirable, however, that the full development programme, which will generate the largest amount of data for the registration file, utilises the formulation to be marketed in order that safety and efficacy data can be amalgamated. Phase III studies should be undertaken with the intended market formulation.

It is important to consider the impact of different formulations. The requirements for an inhaled drug, for example, will be quite different from the requirements for the same drug given orally.

Is the development of two formulations to proceed in parallel or sequentially? The size of the programme may be doubled if a second formulation is aimed at a different target group. On the other hand, it may be more cost-effective to carry out a larger programme than to come back at a later date. For example, in the development of a new agent to treat inflammatory bowel disease it may be inappropriate to use an orally active formulation in a patient with disease confined to the distal end of the large bowel. While this situation may account for a relatively small proportion of patients, it is nevertheless desirable to have a range of formulations suitable for use by all patients. Under these circumstances, it would substantially increase the cost of the programme to study these patients at a later date, given that during the screening process to identify patients suitable for inclusion in a trial of oral medication, these patients would be identified and would not be included in the study. The length of time taken to gather data on the major formulation is unlikely to be increased as there is no competition for patients, but gathering data on the secondary formulation represents an increase in workload. The trade-off is therefore an increase in workload versus a more cost-effective and clinically comprehensive programme.

9.5.8 Clinical trial supplies

This is a crucial area and one which should be given maximum attention during the planning process, as the length of time required to ensure adequate clinical trial supplies can never be underestimated. Inadequacy of clinical trial supplies can be a reason for delay in the execution of a clinical development programme. The Clinical Trials Directive (2001/20/EC), GMP Directive (2003/94/EC) and Annex 13 Guidance allow verification of compliance with GMP as well as GCP. Investigational medicinal products (IMPs) have to be manufactured to a standard 'at least equivalent to' EU GMP. This relates to the finished dosage form and not just the active pharmaceutical. Placebo has to be manufactured to GMP as well. GMP codes vary across the world and specific steps must be taken to ensure that EU GMP standards are met. In practice, this relates mostly to drug manufactured in the United States, as there is no Mutual Recognition Agreement between the United States and the EU GMP. A qualified person (QP) release is required for each batch of all IMPs and this might be especially difficult to achieve for active comparator products.

The explanation for delay is likely to be three-fold.

1. Insufficient information is provided to colleagues in pharmaceutical development early enough, so that insufficient compound has been synthesised and manufactured according to the relevant GMP standards.

2. Insufficient time is allowed for packaging and distribution. Clinical trials packaging is becoming increasingly complex, particularly when a drug that may be for a second-line treatment is being tested. For example, it would be unethical to stop an ACE inhibitor and diuretic in a patient with heart failure, therefore, administration of a new drug will be against this backdrop. In order to maintain double-blind conditions, it will be necessary to employ a double-dummy technique; therefore, a minimum of four different agents per patient must be packaged: the ACE inhibitor, diuretic, new agent and placebo. The situation can be hugely complex as, for example, the testing of a new anti-Parkinsonian agent, where packaging of more than a dozen tablets per patient per day may be necessary. Complexity is further increased if the trial is international and dosage instructions have to be supplied in a number of languages. Despite this, drug supplies have to be distributed to a number of different countries, each of which requires different documentation to satisfy local customs regulations. It is hardly surprising that this aspect of the clinical development plan sometimes does not receive the attention it warrants. The use of an interactive voice randomisation system (IVRS) becomes increasingly useful as the study design becomes more complex. IVRS also allows scarce drug supplies to be rapidly dispatched to the appropriate site.

3. Insufficient time is allowed to obtain supplies of comparator drugs. Companies are notoriously bureaucratic, or even obstructive, in dealing with requests for supplies of active drug and placebo; it therefore pays to start negotiations early. Protocols involving comparator drugs from other companies must be targeted for early drafting, particularly if they are on the critical path, as the approval process is likely to be prolonged. If adequate time is allowed then it is always possible, even if there is a refusal to supply active drug and placebo, to extract the active substance from a marketed formulation, reformulate, demonstrate bioequivalence with the approved formulation and manufacture sufficient supplies for the clinical programme, together with matching placebo. This is clearly much less efficient than negotiating successfully with another company.

9.5.9 Length of the programme

The importance of taking a long-term strategic view when designing the full development programme has already been stressed, but clearly it is impossible to plan in detail studies which may or may not start some years in the future. The most crucial timing in the programme is the point at which the clinical cut-off will occur to permit compilation of the clinical section of the registration dossier. From this point, the timing of submission of the dossier can be predicted and hence the timing of regulatory approval and launch. It is thus important to be able to estimate with some degree of accuracy the length of time necessary to achieve the goal of clinical cut-off and to ensure that the major pivotal studies will be finished at that point. This fact mandates that the pivotal studies should receive high priority in the execution of the plan.

As anyone involved in the conduct of clinical trial knows, it is notoriously difficult to estimate the length of time it will take to recruit patients into a study. Formal inclusion and exclusion criteria can severely restrict the number of patients suitable for a trial, even when common conditions are being studied. An additional and common complication is the 'overoptimistic investigator syndrome'.

It is becoming increasingly common to conduct fairly rigorous feasibility studies to determine the likelihood of patient and investigator recruitment in different countries. A complicating factor is competing studies. This is particularly so in areas of great scientific endeavour, such as oncology. It is not uncommon for large oncology centres to be running more than 50 different studies. Competition for patients can be intense.

In more recent years, in an attempt to overcome these problems, it has become fashionable to include more centres than what may be necessary in a study on the basis that some will be successful at recruiting whereas others will not. All, of course, have to be assessed to ensure that they can operate within the principles of GCP. It is important to be realistic in estimating the speed at which recruitment will occur and even in common disease areas, it is often unreasonable to expect centres to recruit at the rate of more than 1–2 patients per month. Nevertheless, the geographical distribution of clinical research is of major commercial concern because involvement of influential clinicians in the evaluation of a product is vital. It necessarily follows that involvement of influential clinicians in potentially large markets is of prime importance. Studies should, therefore, be conducted in these areas as first choice. However, this mandates willingness on behalf of the investigator to participate in pivotal studies and to meet development deadlines, which, of course, assumes the existence of an appropriate patient population and facilities for the conduct of the study.

A further factor that will affect the speed at which the clinical programme can proceed is the human resource committed to the programme. There are some activities, however, that will not be affected by manipulation of resources, such as the 'in-life' phase of a 2-year carcinogenicity study. On the other hand, reporting time for the study can be reduced if more resource is applied. Various models for predicting resource allocation exist but none is particularly reliable. While trial monitors and data handlers may be a resource dedicated to one programme, physicians and statisticians invariably have a range of commitments and will therefore be called upon to deal with unexpected problems, which cannot be taken into account in the planning process. Blake and Ratcliffe[11] have generated a model describing drug development, running either sequentially or in parallel. For reasons that have already been considered, the former

situation generally does not exist because of time constraints, although it makes more efficient use of human resources. Blake and Ratcliffe estimated that for an average NDA of about 3000 patients, with studies proceeding in parallel, it is necessary to recruit around 200 centres. Clearly, for an NDA that requires an average of about 4500 subjects, these numbers should be extrapolated upwards. Blake and Ratcliffe estimated that the programme would require the dedicated tie-in of 25–30 staff, of whom three-quarters would be trial monitors and data processors and the remainder physicians and statisticians. This gives some idea of the level of resource commitment required to discharge a successful programme and some notion of the continued commitment of resource to market support studies.

9.5.10   Data management

In many companies, data collection, handling and analysis constitute a major bottleneck and are a source of irritation to investigators and frustration to commercial colleagues. The process of data collection begins with the protocol, which must be clear and unambiguous. If it is confusing in English it will be more so in a foreign language. There must be a flow diagram. The practical parts of the protocol, that is, those in daily use during the running of a trial, should be separate from the remainder and in a form allowing easy reference. If the protocol facilitates the study it will reduce error and hence rework.

The case report form (CRF) should be unambiguous and simple to use. Its completion should minimise the need for text. CRFs should consist of three modules. One module is common for all trials (laboratory data, etc.), one is common for all trials in the clinical programme for a given compound and one is specific to the study in question. In this way, data handlers become familiar with the forms and can therefore manage a larger number with fewer mistakes. A mechanism should be in existence to ensure that the clinician completes the CRF adequately.

Recently, significant efforts have been made in most organisations to reduce the time from last patient out to final report. As always, a balance must be struck between satisfactory resource utilisation and cost. Most companies are now looking at an 8–12-week period from the last patient out to final report. The most significant delay is in resolving final data queries at study sites and this depends principally on the clinical research associate monitoring schedules and the availability of study personnel at the study site. It should be the objective of every trial monitor to produce a complete set of clean data within 1–2 weeks of the last patient completing the trial, with the target of closing the database and initiating the analysis and statistical reporting of the primary variables with the minimum of delay. Data are of little value unless they are analysed and reported; indeed, data left in an office may be potentially dangerous.

To simplify the process, it is important that a single database is developed for the whole programme. This is particularly relevant to the production of safety data, not only in the interests of efficiency but also so that any safety issues will be recognised as they arise. If a particular set of adverse events is suggested by preclinical toxicology then they should be flagged in the database so that the monitors' attention is drawn to them.

9.5.11   Cost

The full clinical development plan will be a major expense, so has to be costed accurately and conducted as economically as possible. The conduct of clinical trials is being increasingly seen by investigators as a business, and grants to investigators are the largest out-of-pocket expense incurred in the clinical development phase. It is estimated that drug development costs about US$403 million per drug, on average, as per prices in 2000,[2] but this includes manufacturing and all on-costs, rather than just the drug development programme.

9.5.12   Technology

Although superficially attractive, there has not been the widespread adoption of technology that

many have predicted for the past 15 years. The use of electronic data capture (EDC) remains in its infancy. There are many suppliers, and most companies have conducted studies with EDC. However, the difficulties in training investigators and ensuring consistent technological support 24 h a day, 365 days a year, in many different countries remain formidable. As internet access improves, electronic diaries may become more widely used for some particular types of studies, such as asthma and diabetes, where patients are accustomed to keeping diaries in any event.

Electronic medical records are not yet useful for significant clinical development research.

9.6   Executing the Plan

There can be no substitute for excellent planning and this is why a substantial portion of this chapter has been devoted to a consideration of the important elements of the clinical development programme. There needs to be a clear and concise map of activities leading to compilation of the clinical section of the regulatory dossier and beyond. However, good the programme is, there will be a successful outcome only if it is executed in an efficient and timely manner. The important factors are:

- Selection of sites
- Prioritisation of trials
- Quality control
- Quality assurance
- Use of contract research organisations (CROs)
- Training – technical and process
- Communication
- Process improvement.

9.6.1   Selection of sites

Reference to the principles of GCP has been made; only investigational centres whose personnel and facilities are capable of working to GCP should be selected to participate in the programme. The selection of an investigator is a balance between value for money and desirability of having a particular individual working within the programme.

9.6.2   Prioritisation

The importance of identifying pivotal studies and studies on the critical path was discussed in a previous section. It is important that these studies are given the highest priority both in execution and reporting and that provision is made to identify early if there are problems recruiting patients so that appropriate remedial action can be taken. The studies of longest duration should be started first.

9.6.3   Quality assurance

While quality assurance of data is rightly demanded by the FDA and EMEA, it increasingly forms an integral part of other aspects in the execution of clinical trials. Investigators must understand that this is part of the process of participating in a study and must expect to be audited and the quality of their data recording be monitored. Most companies now have a quality assurance function which, for management reasons, reports outside the clinical organisation. This function can also be outsourced.

9.6.4   Quality control

One of the measures of the quality of the preregistration clinical programme is the total time from the decision to enter full development to the first regulatory approval in a major market. It is also important to monitor quality in other ways. One option is to assess the frequency with which predetermined milestones are achieved. More subtly, quality can be assessed by examining the number of incomplete, inaccurate or indecipherable CRFs that are returned or the number of protocol amendments made which are not based on new information. Milestones may still be achieved when quality is poor, that is, when there is inefficiency, but this means that they were wrongly established and can be improved if efficiency improves.

9.6.5   Contract research organisations

In a discussion on the allocation of resource and analysis of workload, the decision on whether to engage a CRO for an element of the programme should be taken during the planning stage. It is important to remember that a CRO has to be managed and this can be as much as 5–10% of the company resource that would otherwise be directly involved in carrying out the programme. It is important that the objectives for the CRO are clear and that the scope of the task involved, including cost and milestones, is agreed by both parties before any contractual commitment. It must also be remembered that the CRO has to be audited and quality assured.

Contract research organisations are likely to be more efficient, and on occasion can be faster than the company. A balance has to be struck between the outsourcing costs, internal costs (which are often underestimated) and the management requirements and skill sets of the CRO and internal staff.

9.6.6   Training

It is obvious that appropriate technical training should be provided for anybody joining a development programme, and staff already working on the programme should be encouraged to keep abreast of developments in the therapeutic area. Equally important is process training to ensure that the principles of GCP are fully understood and applied, and that internal processes in the form of standard operating procedures (SOPs) are fully documented and understood. The process, and hence the SOPs, will need to satisfy all those customers and providers who will contribute to the development programme and ensure that the many tasks involved will be performed once and only once to avoid waste. The ability of all staff to work to SOPs and therefore work between countries and disciplines with a degree of consistency is paramount in executing a successful programme and this ability should be tested by regular audit. This is a particular advantage in times of stress when personnel may become interchangeable.

9.6.7 Communication

All personnel involved in the programme should have the same level of knowledge of progress and this can only be achieved using a computer-based clinical trials management system, which must be constantly and accurately updated. The central monitors who have an overview of the programme must initiate remedial action, should recruitment – especially into pivotal studies – be less than anticipated. Equally, information concerning adverse reactions should be disseminated promptly so that investigators can be kept closely informed and enjoy a uniform level of knowledge. Finally, in order to develop and foster teamwork, regular meetings involving internal and external staff must be arranged so that a two-way exchange of information can occur and problems solved.

9.6.8 Process improvement

The importance of documenting internal processes in the form of SOPs has already been mentioned. Any activity forming part of the development plan is a process. Each SOP should be looked on as a dynamic document and opportunities for improving each process should be sought continually. For example, the time that elapses between the last patient completing a clinical trial and production of the statistical report is an activity very much on the critical path.

This activity or process can be broken down into its smallest components, each of these examined carefully for opportunities to reduce cycle time, and pieced together again, with the objective of producing a significantly quicker time overall. The implications in terms of total development time are huge and yet many companies are not attempting to harness the benefits that process improvements can bring by establishing formal process improvement initiatives.

Acknowledgements

We are indebted to Dai Rowley-Jones and Paul A Nicholson, who authored this chapter in the third edition of this textbook, for their leadership and the free use of their material when preparing this chapter.

References

1. Arthur Anderson. *Managing Risk, Building Value. Risk Management in the UK Life Sciences.* London: Arthur Anderson, 2001.
2. DiMasi JA, Hansen RW, Grabowski HG, *et al.* The price of innovation: new estimates of drug development costs. *J Health Econ* 2003;**22**:151–85.
3. Pharmaprojects Website: http://www.pjbpubs.com/pharmaprojects/index.htm accessed 17 October 2004.
4. Pharmaprojects. *2004 Annual Review.* Richmond, Surrey: PJB Publications, 2004.
5. Watts G. Negotiating research priorities. *Brit Med J* 2004;**329**:704.
6. Committee for Proprietary Medicinal Products. *ICH M4. Common Technical Document for the Registration of Pharmaceuticals for Human Use – Organisation CTD, CPMP/ICH/2887/99.* London: CPMP, 1999.
7. Debashis S. Merck withdraws arthritis drug worldwide. *Brit Med J* 2004;**329**:816
8. DiMasi JA. Risks in new drug development: approval success rates for investigational drugs. *Clin Pharmacol Ther* 2001; **69**:297–307.
9. DiMasi JA. New drug development in the United States from 1963 to 1999. *Clin Pharmacol Ther* 2001; **69**:286–96.
10. DiMasi JA, Grabowski HG, Vernon J. R&D costs and returns by therapeutic category. *Drug Inf J* 2004; **38**:211–23.
11. Blake P, Ratcliffe MJ. Can we accelerate drug development? *Drug Inf J* 1991;**25**:13–18.
12. Tufts Center for the Study of Drug Development. *Outlook 2001.* Boston, MA: Tufts Center, 2001.
13. Abernethy, DR. Research challenges, new drug development, preclinical and clinical trials in the ageing population. *Drug Safety* 1990;**5**:71–4.

PART II

Medical department issues

CHAPTER 10

10 The medical department

Darrall L Higson
(with revisions by PD Stonier)

10.1 Introduction

Medical departments can be large, as in the headquarters of a multinational company, or small, as in one of its subsidiary operating companies. There are probably as many ways of organising a medical department as there are companies. Although there may be national, cultural and regulatory differences between countries, which further complicate their construction, the influence of the European Union, through the introduction of guidelines and directives, is leading to medical departments across Europe operating in similar ways. No matter how they are organised, there are certain responsibilities that all medical departments should accept.

This chapter outlines these areas of responsibility and the key players who are needed to fulfil these. It also describes how, by working in cross-functional teams, the members of the medical department contribute to the process of product development.

10.2 The Role of the Medical Department

The common objective of all pharmaceutical companies is to discover, develop and market safe and effective medicines that will bring benefits to patients and consumers and result in profitable returns to the company. In this process it is important that, at all stages in the life cycle of a pharmaceutical product, the needs and interests of those who will receive these medicines should be paramount.

To this end, the major areas of responsibility for the medical department are to:

1. Act as the medical conscience of the company.
2. Ensure adherence to relevant legal requirements and guidelines.
3. Provide a medical perspective to product development.
4. Provide the medical input to the servicing and support of marketed products throughout their life cycle.
5. Provide general as well as specialised medical expertise, as required.
6. Act as the company's expert interface with all sectors of the medical profession.

How these responsibilities are shared among the members of a medical department will become apparent from the descriptions of the various roles in Section 10.3. The degree to which the medical department is usually involved in what is traditionally described as the four phases of clinical development will also be outlined.

There exist guidelines and regulations, described elsewhere in this book, to control:

1. The conduct of clinical evaluation during the development of a new product.
2. The regulatory process which allows the product to be marketed.
3. The way in which the product can be promoted.

Beyond these guidelines, the medical department has the important role of keeping the company aware, at all times, of the needs of patients and of the medical and allied professions. It is therefore important that there should be medical input to a company's strategy by having the head of the medical department, usually in the role of medical director, as a member of the senior management team. The development of pharmaceutical medicine into a specialty, as described in Section 10.3.1, has strengthened the role of the pharmaceutical physician, who is qualified not only to provide medical expertise but also, through the tradition of the Hippocratic Oath, to represent the needs and interests of patients. While the pharmaceutical physician remains bound by the requirements of good medical practice, as laid down in the United Kingdom by the General Medical Council,[1] recently specific guidance has also been provided in a report produced by the Faculty of Pharmaceutical Medicine.[2]

10.3   Who are the Key Players in the Medical Department?

The medical department is usually headed by a senior pharmaceutical physician (the medical director), who is supported by a team consisting of other physicians, graduates and administrative staff. The non-medical graduates are normally pharmacists or life scientists and, in addition to providing informed scientific input, may look after some administrative areas. In some companies they, rather than the physicians, may be responsible for staff management, thus allowing the physicians to concentrate on their advisory roles.

In a modern, progressive company, members of the medical department can expect to play an important role at all stages in a product's life cycle. Working with commercial colleagues from the earliest planning stages, their specialist skills and expertise help the team to drive the development process down the right path from earliest clinical development to product marketing and beyond.

Key players from the medical department are likely to be as follows, although not every company will place all these specialists within the medical department:

- Pharmaceutical physicians
- Clinical research scientists (CRSs)
- Statisticians and data managers
- Medical information scientists/scientific advisers
- Regulatory executives
- Drug safety/pharmacovigilance scientists
- Pharmacoeconomics advisers.

In whatever way it is organised, the medical department will of course need the support of the human resources department as well as administrative and secretarial services. Thus, while it is not possible to propose any specific organisational structure for a medical department, the organogram presented in Figure 10.1 reflects the issues that need to be considered when deciding on the preferred organisation within the company.

Let us now consider what each player brings to the process of product development.

10.3.1   The pharmaceutical physician

Currently, there are few, if any, specific requirements for medically qualified approval, for example, final approval of promotional material.[3] It is possible for a small organisation to meet these requirements by employing physicians on a part-time advisory basis; so it might be reasonable to wonder why a medical department needs physicians at all. In the United Kingdom over 700 physicians are employed full time in the pharmaceutical industry, so it is evident that companies see them having a wider role. Although the legal and regulatory requirement for medical signatories may be limited, the internal policies of many companies require that certain matters can only be conducted or approved by a registered medical practitioner. For example, standard operating procedures (SOPs) might require a medical signatory on clinical trial protocols and amendments, clinical

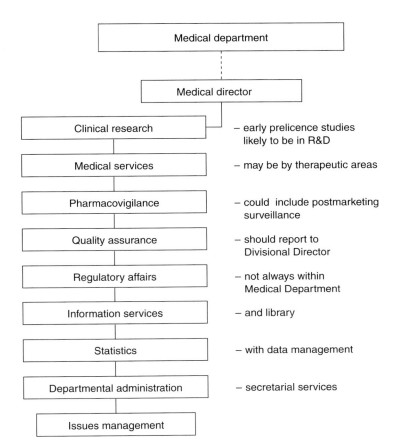

Fig. 10.1 Organogram of the preferred organisation of the medical department.

study reports, clinical investigators' brochures, 'Dear Doctor' letters and 'named patient' supplies of medicines. At least one physician would also be a member of a company's safety board, making decisions about all aspects of drug development, from its first introduction into man to major medical decisions about safety issues, such as batch recalls and product withdrawal.

It is expected that, before entering the industry, the physician has acquired a good base of medical knowledge and broad clinical experience. However, pharmaceutical physicians are not usually employed for their clinical expertise because although some retain honorary clinical posts, with the consent of their employing companies, this is rarely sufficient for them to remain clinical 'experts' and clinical advice is best sought from current full-time clinicians. On the other

hand, it is possible for a pharmaceutical physician to become an internationally recognised expert on clinical research in a particular therapeutic area and, through this clinical contact, to have valuable access to key opinion leaders.

There are certain personal attributes over and above a medical degree and clinical experience that make for a successful pharmaceutical physician. To be valued, the pharmaceutical physician must be able to provide insight into the clinical benefit, and hence the commercial potential, of a compound at any stage in its development. He or she must also have the planning skills to realise that potential, and an ability to communicate at all levels, both inside and outside the company. If the medical department is to act as the company's medical conscience (see Section 10.2), it will need to have a medically qualified and suitably experienced person on its staff.

Most physicians in the pharmaceutical industry work in one of three main areas, which correspond to the well-defined phases through which a drug passes in its clinical evaluation, namely:

- Clinical pharmacology
- Clinical research
- Medical services or medical affairs.

The ratio of pharmaceutical physicians in each area is approximately 1 : 4 : 8. In some small companies, a physician's responsibilities may extend across more than one of these areas. In larger companies, clinical pharmacology is likely to be the responsibility of the research part of a company, while the medical-services function resides within local operating companies.

In recent years, an increasing proportion of early clinical research involving healthy volunteers (Phase I), and falling under the responsibility of the clinical pharmacologist, is conducted in clinical research units as part of the contract research sector working with, but outside, the pharmaceutical companies.

Historically, the medical department's involvement in clinical research was in late-stage (Phase IV) studies for local market needs. Nowadays, although pre-licence clinical studies are most likely still driven by the research part of the company, the medical departments of local operating companies will probably coordinate these early international clinical studies in their own countries. As a result clinical research now tends to be much more integrated, with good clinical practice (GCP) being applied to all phases, both pre- and post-marketing approval. Similarly, Phase IV or post-marketing studies tend to be international as registration and marketing strategies become pan-European. The pharmaceutical physician has an important role in determining the therapy area and product strategy well before product launch, and this requires close liaison with colleagues in research and development.

To be effective, the pharmaceutical physician in the medical department has to recognise both the clinical needs of patients and the commercial needs of the company. Commercial colleagues look for constructive advice on how to fulfil these needs while operating within ethical and legal constraints. Such advice would include providing insight into the decision-making processes of clinical colleagues.

The specialty of pharmaceutical medicine and the concept of the pharmaceutical physician have developed in the last 40 years from the role of 'medical adviser in the pharmaceutical industry'. In the United Kingdom this development led, in 1989, to the foundation of the Faculty of Pharmaceutical Medicine within the Royal Colleges of Physicians. From this, Europewide recognition of pharmaceutical medicine as a specialty is slowly becoming a reality. Legal and regulatory changes are also driving a requirement for specialist registration and accreditation.

The pharmaceutical physician provides a medical direction to marketing strategy and ensures that product literature and promotional material are legal and factually accurate. This is an important contribution to the medical department's role as 'medical conscience', as discussed in Section 10.2. Medical input remains necessary to the servicing and support of marketed products throughout their life cycle.

Such support can involve responding to complaints about promotional activities, which may come from other companies or external agencies such as, in the United Kingdom, the Prescription Medicines Code of Practice Authority. A medically qualified person should certainly have overall responsibility for clinical drug safety issues (see Section 10.3.6). Pharmaceutical physicians are usually involved in the training of sales representatives. In addition, a good pharmaceutical physician can be a credible ambassador for the company when lecturing to external audiences or dealing with the communication media.

The medical director is, of course, not only a senior pharmaceutical physician but a senior manager and needs to be fully conversant with all the issues facing the company and understand all the principles and procedures which govern its operation. Nowadays, this will include personnel issues, such as awareness of the laws related to employment. Without this broad understanding, the medical director will not be able to lead the activities of the medical department in a way that is optimal for the organisation while maintaining all the required professional and ethical standards.

10.3.2 The CRS

The CRS is involved in all aspects of clinical trials from planning and design through initiation and monitoring and on to report writing and publication. The medical department is likely to be involved in organising late pre-licence or post-licence clinical studies, with healthy volunteer and perhaps even early patient (Phase IIa) studies, to proof of concept stage, being the responsibility of the research part of the company. In the past, some studies in support of marketed products have come within the remit of the marketing department. The introduction of GCP across all stages of patient studies has meant that this is no longer practicable. The primary objective of Phase III studies is to contribute to the dossier for marketing authorisation, which, once approved, is a watershed in a product's life. This will establish the initial profile of the product. In addition, there is a need to incorporate economic parameters into late Phase (IIIb) trials, as well as to broaden patient populations so that they more accurately reflect the real world. For successful marketing, clinical trials will be needed very shortly after product launch to further define the product profile, any additional claims that can be made about it and the treatment options. In certain therapeutic classes there may also be opportunities to switch some form of the product to a non-prescription classification. The studies needed to obtain the data to satisfy all these requirements will need to be planned, and probably started, before the first marketing authorisation. It is clear, therefore, that those involved in each set of trials need to collaborate closely.

The organisational structure for clinical research depends on such factors as size and whether the department is within headquarters or a local operating company. The transition through the phases of clinical research needs to be smooth and the decision-making process behind the research clear and well communicated. In larger companies, the responsibilities of clinical scientists may be divided into therapy areas. Alternatively, monitoring responsibilities may be divided geographically, especially in the case of field-based staff.

Given the uncertainty of clinical research, one major asset of any CRS is flexibility. If this is combined with an aptitude for self-motivation, as well as team working, then the individual should be well qualified for the task.

The introduction of GCP has accelerated the need for quality control and quality assurance, particularly in the field of clinical research. Quality control is carried out by the staff who are responsible for the particular activity, working to SOPs that cover all the tasks under scrutiny. SOPs not only need to be written but must also be updated regularly. Quality assurance is the process which seeks to confirm that SOPs have been observed; this is accomplished by the process of auditing. Internal audit departments should be under a separate management from the medical department. Regular audits can not only assure external bodies, such as regulatory authorities, that proper procedures have been followed, but also serve to deter those rare attempts at fraud on the part of clinical investigators, which occasionally become evident.[4]

In most companies today, it is likely at some time that CRSs within a company will collaborate with counterparts within contract research organisations (CROs). CROs range from small, often specialised groups, to large multinational companies. The services offered cover virtually every facet of clinical research, as well as of the regulatory process necessary for obtaining a marketing authorisation. CROs provide a flexible resource to cope with peaks of activity without the need to employ additional staff. As well as contracting projects out to them, it is possible to take staff on 'secondment' from a CRO for a set period of time. These arrangements can work very well but there may be some disadvantages. For example, an in-house clinical research team will probably be more familiar with the company's products and, through closer relations with the sales force, have greater commercial awareness. In addition, while clinical investigators may see CRO staff as representing the pharmaceutical company, the company is unlikely to have direct control over their day-to-day activities. Finally, by using a CRO, there is less opportunity to develop professional relationships between clinicians and the company.

Agreements drawn up between companies should include not only financial arrangements, but should also define SOPs and methods of monitoring and auditing. In the United Kingdom, the Association of Independent Clinical Research Contractors (AICRC) was founded in 1988 to help ensure high standards. Its members agree to operate to the standards and practices set out in the AICRC code and undergo regular independent inspections to ensure that they do.

10.3.3   The statistician

The role of the statistician in clinical development has, in recent years, expanded from the traditional role of providing advice on patient numbers and data analysis. Nowadays, statisticians are likely to have input not just to individual studies but across entire development programmes. By providing general statistical advice they can completely change the design of studies and later provide not only the analysis, but also valuable advice on how to interpret the results and use them appropriately. Such advice may be equally valuable in relation to the results from published studies used in support of promotional claims. It is essential to have a sound statistical rationale behind a clinical research project if it is to stand up to scrutiny by regulatory agencies and ethics committees.

10.3.4   The data manager

The data manager needs to work closely with the CRS, the statistician and the pharmaceutical physician to design reliable and practical methods of capturing and storing data gathered in clinical trials. Whether this data is recorded on the traditional case record form (CRF) or by means of computer-based technology, such as remote data entry, the data manager must ensure that the method used is investigator-friendly. If it is not, it will lead to erroneous data, which no amount of statistical analysis can repair. Confidentiality and anonymity in pooled data are important and the source of the data must be kept secure.

Time invested by both the data manager and statistician in designing the structure of the database should also reap rewards at the analysis stage. In addition, a good-quality database is essential if the study is to pass the auditing process.

10.3.5   The medical information scientist

Within the medical department there may be two types of information support. There will be medical information scientists, who provide the external 'scientific service', now required by Article 13 of Directive 92/28/EEC (on advertising) of the Council of the European Communities. In addition, there may be those, sometimes called 'scientific advisers', who provide specialised information support to a product or therapy area within the company. Many medical information scientists are qualified pharmacists.

Requests for information about a company's products come from many sources, both inside and outside the company. Hospital information pharmacists, often on behalf of hospital doctors, are the most frequent source of enquiries, but community pharmacists and individual clinicians may also contact the company. Sometimes, a suspected adverse drug reaction lies behind the enquiry and the medical information scientist should be trained to recognise this. The adverse event report can then be passed to the company's pharmacovigilance department in order to initiate documentation, follow-up and appropriate reporting to regulatory authorities. Other sources of enquiries are nursing staff, consumer groups, the media and, increasingly, patients and other members of the public. Companies offer an out-of-hours emergency enquiry service for both product information and emergency enquiries arising from clinical trials.

In the United Kingdom, until recent years, the provision of information in response to enquiries from members of the public was not allowed, and individuals were referred to their medical practitioner. However, as the provision of information about medicines directly to the public has increased through such innovations as patient pack inserts and greater access to the internet, so a better informed public now demands greater involvement in their own clinical management. This demand is likely to be fuelled further as an increasing number of medicines are reclassified from prescription only medicine ('POM') to over-the-counter ('P'). Consequently, it is now accepted that members of the public can be provided with factual answers to questions about their medicines, which can include copies of a product's summary of product characteristics (SPC), European public assessment reports and package leaflets, all of which may be published on the internet. The medical information scientist is trained to respect the principle that, like a pharmacist, in providing such information they must not come between a patient and their doctor and, when appropriate, should encourage the enquirer to seek medical advice.

10.3.6 The scientific adviser

In larger companies, this role has evolved from the medical information service. The scientific adviser is the product or therapy area expert, who is custodian of all the information related to their specialist field. The scientific adviser is a key member on cross-functional teams with commercial and medical colleagues and will work with advertising agencies on the creation of a product's promotional platform.

10.3.7 The regulatory executive

The regulatory department may be part of the medical department or the research function,

or report directly to the head of the company. Wherever it is placed, the role of regulatory executive is crucial to the success of the company. The regulatory executive defines the pharmaceutical, toxicological and clinical data required to prove the quality, safety profile and efficacy of a product and to obtain a medically and commercially favourable marketing authorisation (product licence), as ultimately reflected in its SPC. This includes defining the appropriate regulatory strategy to achieve rapid product development and registration. Since this advice will need to be given several years before the submission is made, this requires the regulatory executive to be completely up to date not only with national, European and international regulations and guidelines but also with their own national regulatory authority's thinking. To this end, strong and effective working relationships need to be built up with regulators. The regulatory executive also needs to keep the company informed of the potential impact of any proposed changes to regulations and, if necessary, provide comment on these to the regulatory authorities via the appropriate trade associations.

It is often not appreciated how much work is required to ensure that the marketing authorisations are kept up to date through being renewed and amended as necessary. Similarly, it may not be realised that a 'simple' variation to a product licence, such as a small change in the amount of excipient, will require the submission of a variation document to the authorities.

Other responsibilities include applications for regulatory approval of clinical trials and ensuring that promotional material for a product is in line with its licence.

10.3.8 The drug safety/pharmacovigilance scientist

Effective handling of all information relating to drug safety is one of the most important responsibilities, if not *the* most important responsibility, of the medical department. The size of a company and the volume of work will dictate whether the responsibility for monitoring drug safety resides with members of staff who have other responsibilities for the various compounds, or with a specialised drug surveillance group.

Every company is required by European law to have a nominated person responsible for pharmacovigilance (Council Regulation EEC 2309/93 Article 23). They are not required to be a physician but must have access to one.

The most important task relating to drug safety monitoring is the timely processing of spontaneously reported suspected adverse drug reactions relating to marketed products as well as adverse events reported in clinical trials of both pre-licensed drugs and marketed products. Timelines for passing such reports to national and international regulatory authorities are closely regulated. The reason for such defined timelines is that if any reports of suspected adverse reactions could lead to changes in the regulatory status of a product, they need to be received as soon as is practicable.

Clearly, therefore, those involved in drug safety monitoring need to liase closely with both clinical research and medical information scientists. In addition, those responsible for clinical drug safety must undertake periodic safety update reports (PSURs) at predetermined intervals, in accordance with current International Conference on Harmonisation (ICH) guidelines. Such routine analyses can identify new safety signals as soon as they become detectable.

Other activities that fall within the area of post-marketing surveillance require input from, if not handling by, those responsible for clinical drug safety. These may include observational (non-interventional) studies, which may be retrospective or prospective, and other projects specifically designed to investigate a safety issue.

Overall responsibility for clinical safety matters must rest with a senior pharmaceutical physician who will be able to provide appropriate professional opinion and advice.

10.3.9 The pharmacoeconomics adviser

It is no longer sufficient to show that a drug is effective and well tolerated. With healthcare costs rising, it is necessary to provide economic measurements of the benefits that a new drug can provide. Such comparisons will need to include not only measurements against competitor drugs but also against other medical interventions. The science of pharmacoeconomics has arisen in response to this challenge and, as a member of the medical department team, the pharmacoeconomics adviser, like the statistician, should be involved in the early stages of clinical development planning.

10.4 Team Working

It is clear from looking at their roles that, to work effectively, members of the medical department need to interact not only with other members of the department but also with colleagues in other departments, such as commercial, legal and communications. An effective medical department is one that fulfills the major responsibilities described in Section 10.2 in a creative and constructive way. If successful, commercial colleagues will perceive the medical department as having the role of a facilitator rather than a policeman. Commercial and medical staff can facilitate the work of each other on a daily basis. For example, a sales representative may put a doctor interested in clinical research directly in contact with a company's clinical research manager. Conversely, a doctor who has developed a favourable view of a company from working as a clinical investigator may be more disposed to granting interviews to sales representatives from that company. It is a powerful asset to a company that pharmaceutical physicians have unique channels of access to clinicians that are not afforded to commercial colleagues.

Many companies have found that bringing the different contributors together in cross-functional teams can produce synergistic results. For example, a team responsible for ensuring the successful launch of a newly licensed product might include a product/marketing manager, a pharmaceutical physician, a clinical trial scientist, a scientific adviser, a market researcher, an advertising agency representative, a financial manager and a senior member of the sales team. They may invite other members of the team, such as lawyers and public relations, as required. By sharing commonly agreed objectives, the members of the team are encouraged to work together to achieve the same goal.

Similarly, clinical trial strategy teams bring together CRSs with statisticians, data managers, regulatory executives, pharmaceutical physicians and marketing managers to discuss the clinical data that is needed, and the timescales and costs, to achieve specific commercial objectives.

Another area requiring a pooling of expertise is issues management. Pharmaceutical companies must be geared to respond quickly and appropriately when faced with external issues, which are often medical issues, such as drug safety. A core team, whose individual roles are clear, needs to be prepared to deal with such situations.

The principal elements of issues management relate to anticipating an issue wherever possible, identifying and documenting the true facts of the case, preparing reasoned arguments and answers to potential questions, and training in facing the press, media and public to debate the issue.

The facts of the case and 'question and answer' documents should be prepared. Key members of such a team are therefore the medical director, or a designate, senior managers who are able to quickly implement actions, a legal adviser if appropriate, and a member of the public relations/communications department, who knows how to communicate the team's outputs effectively.

Training for media appearances, and regular 'refreshers', are essential for anyone who might be required to represent the company.

Professional guidance enables individuals to make best use of the media in communicating the factual messages relating to a particular issue.

Similarly, staff required to give presentations, particularly outside the company, should undertake training in presentation skills if they are to be successful ambassadors of the company.

The professionalism of any presenter is thrown into question when they appear to have little enthusiasm for the subject or empathy for the audience and cannot communicate clearly, either verbally or by means of audiovisual aids.

10.5 Summary

It is clear that while the medical department can be seen to be a team in itself, its members play on many other different teams. A successful medical department is one that is contributing to the commercial success of the company while maintaining the highest professional and ethical standards.

References

General Medical Council. *Good Medical Practice*, 3rd edn. London: 2001.

Ethics Subcommittee Report. Guiding principles; ethics and pharmaceutical medicine. *Int J Pharm Med* 2000;**14**:163–71.

Prescription Medicines Code of Practice Authority. *Code of Practice for the Pharmaceutical Industry 2003, Clause 14.1.* London: PMCPA, 2003.

Lock S, Wells F, Farthing M, eds. *Fraud and Misconduct in Biomedical Research*, 3rd edn. London: BMJ Books, 2001.

CHAPTER 11

11

Medical marketing

John H Young

11.1 Introduction

It was over 20 years ago, but I can still remember vividly my first exposure to pharmaceutical marketing. I had joined Merck Sharp & Dohme one week earlier and as my boss was away, I was sent to represent the medical group at a planning meeting for the launch of a new non-steroidal. I had spent part of my hospital training in rheumatology and was confident that I could hold my own at the meeting.

How wrong I was! The meeting launched off into areas that I had never been exposed to before; the competition, market segments, inventory, formulation issues, public relations campaigns, opinion leader development. It was clear to me that I was out of my depth and I had better learn about marketing and production as quickly as possible, and certainly before the next planning meeting. This was nothing like a hospital ward round!

These days we are all much more aware of the power of marketing and the importance of brands and brand image, but it is still true that most physicians entering the industry will only have a passing knowledge of marketing.

Most of the chapters in this textbook focus on the various aspects of the research, development and licensing of pharmaceuticals. Physicians and non-medical scientists working in departments other than sales and marketing do, however, require some understanding of marketing. The depth of the knowledge that they require will vary depending upon their role. The requirements of, for example, someone working in a Phase I clinical pharmacology unit will be vastly different from a physician working as a medical advisor alongside sales and marketing colleagues.

As it is beyond the scope of this book, in this chapter I have given a brief overview of pharmaceutical marketing. Physicians working as medical advisers will need a much more work-detailed understanding of the subject but this will be acquired as part of their training and through their work experience.

This chapter is written from a UK perspective and readers in countries outside the United Kingdom will need to make allowances for this. Some specific points may not be relevant to your country but in general, the principles apply to most healthcare systems.

11.2 Pharmaceutical Market

The world pharmaceutical market is buoyant and grew in 2003 by 16.6% to a total of just over $414 billion[1] (Figure 11.1). However, the market is not a single market but is made up of a number of therapeutic segments. The largest 12 segments make up 50% of the total market[1] and are shown in Figure 11.2. The largest group of products on a worldwide basis used to be antibiotics but are now cardiovascular drugs. All therapeutic segments showed significant growth in 2003, the largest growth (over 20%) being seen

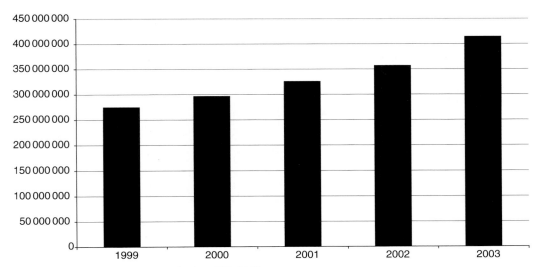

Fig. 11.1 Worldwide pharmaceutical sales, 1999–2003.

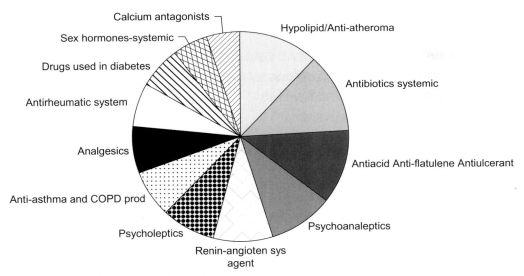

Fig. 11.2 Worldwide pharmaceutical sales for 2003 by therapeutic agent.

in hypolipidaemics, psycholeptics, anti-asthma and COPD products (Figure 11.3).

The United Kingdom spends less on medicines per head than almost any other western country[2] (Figure 11.4). In addition, the United Kingdom is very conservative and it takes a very long time for UK prescribers to take up a new product. General practitioners (GPs) in the United Kingdom are often described as profligate in their prescribing but in reality it is not so.[3] For all therapeutic classes there is a relatively slow pattern of uptake. Change in the prescribing pattern of physicians in the United Kingdom is much slower than in other western countries. Conversely this does mean however that once a drug becomes established in the United Kingdom, doctors are

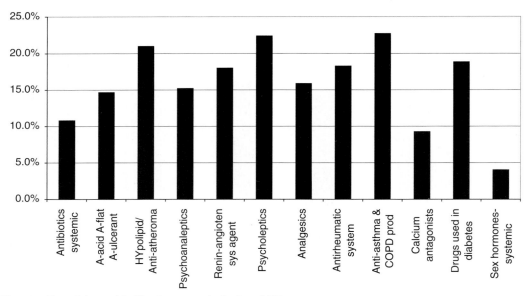

Fig. 11.3 Growth in worldwide pharmaceutical sales – 2003.

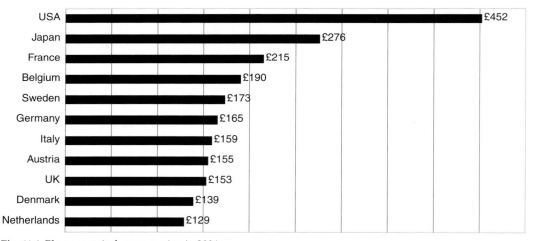

Fig. 11.4 Pharmaceutical consumption in 2004.

much more reluctant to switch to alternative therapies.

The pharmaceutical market is highly complex; there are a large number of therapeutic areas, differences in the ways countries use medicines and many companies competing in the market place. Unlike most other global industries the pharmaceutical industry is highly fragmented and even the biggest companies such as Pfizer or Glaxo SmithKline (GSK) are not involved in all therapeutic segments. Pfizer has a market share in the United Kingdom of approximately 14% but is involved in only a limited number of therapeutic areas. Companies tend to have a presence in a certain range of therapeutic areas, usually referred to as 'franchises'. The ability to dominate a franchise is often a key factor in remaining successful. I will return to the question of franchises later in the chapter.

11.3 Strategic Planning

The importance of marketing in the success of a product cannot be underestimated. A marketing plan that is well thought out, executed, constantly revised and updated is just as important for the success of a new drug as is a well designed and executed clinical plan. With Industry estimates of £350 million and 10–12 years to bring a product to the market the need for active cooperation between the marketing and clinical development groups cannot be over-emphasised.

In the past, it was not unusual for the clinical research group and marketing not to interact until a product was within 2 years to 18 months of launch. This paradigm is no longer viable. For a product to be successful, it is vital that personnel from R&D work collaboratively with their marketing colleagues on the product from the time of discovery right through the product life cycle until patent expiry.

The given wisdom in marketing circles is that the first 6 months following the launch of a new product are the most important. If the marketing strategy is wrong, no matter how good the product, it will fail to meet its sales potential. Re-launching a product after a failed first launch is possible, but difficult and only a few products are successfully re-launched.

When contemplating developing a new product there are a number of alternative strategies a company could take. Each choice is a balance between the risks of the product getting to the marketplace and how successful it will be commercially, once it gets there.

The area of greatest potential, but also greatest risk, is when there is a condition for which a biological target has been identified, but no proven product has yet been developed for it.

At a slightly lower risk is to develop a compound for a condition where therapeutic agents have been identified and proof of concept-studies completed, which validate the approach. In such circumstances, it would be possible to develop a new compound and also be relatively early to market it in that therapeutic field.

At lower risk scientifically, but at higher risk commercially, is the development of so called 'me too' compounds. Here the target is well known and compounds are already established in the market. If the new compound being considered offers significant advantages over those already in the market, it can be very successful. The compound may have better pharmacokinetics, better tolerability or be more selective. Perhaps the best example of how a compound coming late into an established class can be successful is the beta-1 antagonist, Tenormin (Atenolol), which became the most widely prescribed beta-blocker in the United Kingdom.

A company may embark on one or all of the above strategies depending upon the mix of products it has in its portfolio. Such a decision cannot be taken in isolation and needs joint agreement of the R&D and marketing groups. Once a project is underway, the desired product claim structure must be established and the clinical and marketing plans built on those claims. Clinical development often does not go completely according to plan and the regulatory claims may need to be modified as clinical development progresses. In such an eventuality, the marketing plans will need to be changed and updated accordingly.

11.4 Customers

To be successful in this highly competitive market place, there are a number of elements that need to be considered when formulating a marketing plan. The strategy and tactics proposed will vary depending upon the stage a product is in its life cycle. The plan would, for example, be markedly different for a product not yet launched to one that is near to the end of its patent life. One of the fundamental elements of any marketing plan must be an understanding of the customer.

The aim of marketing is to meet and satisfy target customers' needs and wants. Understanding customers' behaviour is, however, never simple. Customers may say one thing and do another.

In this respect, the pharmaceutical market is like any other and doctors may and often do, say one thing and do another. In one respect, however, the pharmaceutical market is unique in that the end user of the product (the patient) for the most part leaves the choice of medicine to his physician.

Increasingly the patient is becoming more involved in this choice. This is particularly true in the United States where the patient may bear a large part, if not all, of the cost of the drug. In Europe where the cost is partly or entirely borne by the State or the patient's insurance, involvement of the patient though is less is now increasing.

The definition of 'the customer' is thus complex in the pharmaceutical market. One might assume that the physician who prescribes the medicine is the customer. It is true that he or she is still probably the key customer, but the situation is far from clear. Nowadays the prescriber does not operate in a vacuum and is heavily influenced by a number of external factors (Figure 11.5).

All these different stakeholders in the prescribing process will need to be considered in

a company's promotional strategy. All have markedly different agendas that needs to be addressed in the marketing plans. The relative importance of these customers need to be established, and then a number of questions need to be asked including:

• What do we wish to achieve?
• What are the customers' needs?
• What behavioural changes are we expecting?
• What is the best medium to deliver the message?

Hospital specialists have an important influence in prescribing but since the majority of patients are treated in general practice, this is where the bulk of prescribing occurs. For this reason, the GP remains the main focus for the industry. However, the recent changes in the UK healthcare system have changed the relative importance of the GP as a customer. In the United Kingdom, reforms in the National Health Service (NHS) and the increase of Primary Care Organisations (PCOs) have changed the GP's role. Some GPs are affected more than others

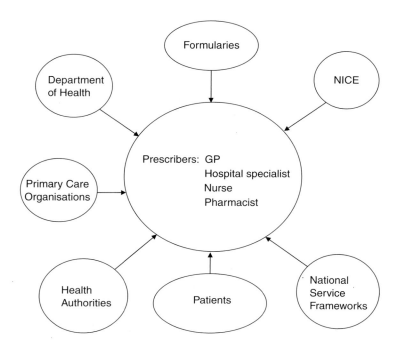

Fig. 11.5 Factors that influence prescribing behaviour.

by these changes and it is important for a company to be aware of how GPs are reacting to the pressures put on them.

To this end, most companies have developed data bases that are constantly updated by the sales representatives as they come into contact with customers. A company must build relationships with all the stakeholders in the prescribing process and keep updating the data on these individuals. Detailed knowledge of what customers are doing and saying is important to the staff at headquarters as they track and evaluate sales and promotional strategies. It is also useful in ensuring that promotional campaigns are targeted accurately and resources are not wasted.

11.5 Market Research and Market Intelligence

We have seen above how companies update their intelligence on prescribers and other stakeholders via representatives but this is only one piece of a wider collection of data on how the market is reacting. Not only is it important to know what prescribers are thinking and doing but it is important also to track the competition.

Most companies will purchase a range of datasets from a variety of commercial companies who specialise in collecting and collating such data. The sources of information are wide and varied and includes panels of GPs and specialists who record what they are prescribing and for what indication, to information from wholesalers and pharmacists. Companies will also sponsor individual market research studies with questionnaires and face-to-face interviews with individual panels of doctors or focus groups.

To be successful in the pharmaceutical market it is vital that data on how your product is progressing and what the competition is doing is constantly updated and evaluated. It is also important to keep track of what might be occurring in alternative fields, which may have an impact on the market. A new surgical technique or new medical device may be introduced that completely alters the way a disease is managed.

It is important therefore not to be too focused on other pharmaceutical competitors, but to keep one's definition of the competition as wide as feasible.

One of the most critical times, where accurate competitor intelligence is needed is when a company is considering developing a new product. With a development time of around 10 years, as much information as possible needs to be gathered about competitor activity before a decision to commit to the development of a new product can be made.

In the past, such considerations were of less importance and companies 30 years ago could look to 5–10 years of exclusivity in a therapeutic area before a competitor in the same therapeutic class entered the marketplace. Now that gap is down in some cases to a few months. Not only that but the third entrant may also be only months behind[4] (Figure 11.6).

When developing the Phase III programme for a new drug, accurate competitor intelligence and a detailed knowledge of the drugs used, or that will be in use at the time of launch, is required and needs to be built into the clinical plan. In many therapeutic areas, there is increasing harmonisation between countries in the major drugs used, but it is possible that in certain countries one particular product may dominate the market. Whether or not to incorporate that product into the Phase III programme or to address the question in the Phase IV programme needs to be thought through. In an ideal world, data will be available for comparing your new product against the leading competitor in the major markets at the time of launch. However, financial or time pressures may limit the scope of the Phase III programme, in which case the Phase IV studies will need to fill the gaps.

11.6 Promotion

How do companies go about the process of disseminating information about their products? As discussed above, it is now common place for marketing to become involved early in the development phase of a compound. One of the earliest elements in a promotional campaign, and should

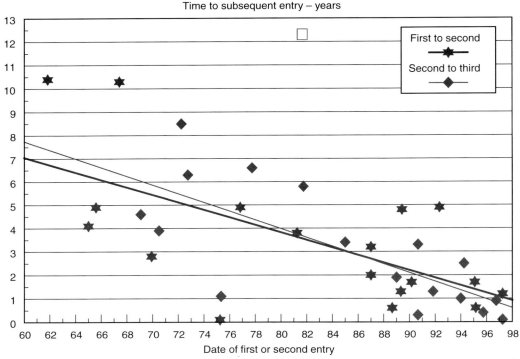

Fig. 11.6 Therapeutic exclusivity – the time before second and third competitors enter a market is decreasing.[4]

be established well before launch, is a public relations (PRs) programme. Once a product is under clinical development this is announced to the financial press and financial analysts. Companies have obligations to their shareholders and the financial markets to disclose information that may have an effect on the share price. Analysts' briefings have, therefore, a dual role of informing the financial community about drugs under development but also raising their profile to a wider audience. If the compound is sufficiently novel such financial information may well spill over into the general press or television. This PR media campaign early in development is valuable in creating awareness of the product and creating demand with respect to the physicians. Clinical trial publications and their dissemination will also be part of a PR campaign to increase awareness of the product and its potential benefits to patients and prescribers. At the time of launch, symposia will be organised to further

increase the exposure of the new therapeutic agent to prescribers. One approach is to arrange company-sponsored symposia as satellites to regional or international medical meetings. It is important that such symposia are of a high scientific standard if they are to attract the interest of physicians and avoid criticism for being promotional. Typically, a symposium would open with a keynote presentation on the current knowledge of the disease under discussion, the programme then going on to review current treatment options and studies showing how the new therapeutic agent fits into management of the condition. It is important that keynote speakers must be independent authorities and thus help to facilitate a lively conclusion to the programme with an unbiased and open discussion of the merits and limitations of the new product and suggestions for further studies. The venue for the meeting should be chosen carefully. A university or academic facility is preferable but it may well be that a hotel is more convenient or offers better conference facilities. Care should be taken to ensure that the scientific content of the meeting takes precedence over the facilities and level of hospitality.

Finally, at launch and beyond, plans need to be in place for journal advertising and detailing of the product to doctors by sales representatives. As noted above, the customer base of pharmaceuticals is complex and the needs of individual customers differ. For GPs and specialists, information about the product will be via advertising, representative detailing and mailings. For NHS staff such as those working in Health Authorities or within PCOs, the information will need to be more focused on cost effectiveness and service provision. For practice nurses, the emphasis will be on educational materials and practical aspects of the product's use. Disease awareness programmes for patients will be developed where appropriate.

The main customer remains the physician. GPs gain information about new products from a variety of sources including their peers and hospital colleagues. Although advertisements in medical journals are an important element in building awareness among prescribers they are not usually the basis on which physicians will start prescribing a new compound.

Hospital specialists will readily start to prescribe a new product if they are convinced of its safety and efficacy, provided it is for use in their own specialty. They are much less ready to try a new compound if it is outside their area of expertise. A cardiologist, for example, would be much less likely to try a new anti-ulcer drug than an antihypertensive until first discussing it with a gastroenterologist colleague.

General practitioners by the very nature of their job will initiate new drugs in many different therapeutic areas. Here they will be guided by what the local hospital specialists are recommending and by discussion with their peers. Detailing by company representatives is a significant factor in influencing prescribing behaviour and the information delivered by the representatives is seen to be valuable by both the hospital specialists and GPs.[5]

11.7 Medical Information

One further element to consider when discussing increasing the awareness of a product is the use of the medical information department. This is not and must not be promotion in the marketing sense, but the provision of accurate and upto date scientific data about the company's products can be valuable in establishing and maintaining the company's image. If a company is known by prescribers as providing an excellent scientific service then its image and reputation will be enhanced. A strong positive company image can only be of assistance to the company's representatives when dealing face to face with customers.

To ensure that the information given out in response to enquiries is comprehensive and as upto date as possible most companies have a worldwide-computerised system. The data that supports the individual statements in the summary of products characteristics (SPCs) are collated and fully referenced and are used to respond to enquiries from prescribers and pharmacists. Often the question may not be readily answered and a response entails a detailed literature search. Having completed the search, it makes sense to share that dataset and response with other subsidiaries around the world. Headquarters staff will check and validate the response generated from the search and once validated it is then made available to other subsidiaries. This avoids duplication of effort and ensures consistency of responses across the globe. Critics of the industry quite rightly look for evidence of dual standards between the United States and Europe and less developed parts of the world. Linking medical information departments around the world and sharing information with all parties ensures that a company is delivering a consistent message.

11.8 Brands

When a new drug comes to the market it will have a series of properties outlined in the SPC including indications, dosage form, precautions, frequency of dosing, contraindications and side effect profile. All these features collectively establish the product in the marketplace and form the basis of the 'brand'. The creation of a strong brand image is fundamental to advertising and this is as true for pharmaceuticals as for any other product. For example, the Mercedes badge is instantly recognisable and carries with it a collection of tangible and intangible benefits of the company. Marketing is concerned with perception and a successful brand will be perceived by the consumer as having unique benefits, which meet their needs.

Prescribers form opinions and beliefs about drugs in the same way as they do about consumer products. Shaping their perceptions and the creation of a strong positive brand image is key to differentiating the product from the competition and to success in the marketplace. Companies go to great lengths to build the brand image of their products and endeavour to achieve consistency of brand messages on a global basis. Over time in the product's life cycle, new indications and formulations will be developed and introduced to strengthen the brand image and further differentiate the product.

11.9   Patients

Except in the United States of America and New Zealand, where direct to consumer (DTC) advertising of prescription medicines is allowed, companies are not allowed to communicate directly with patients. The Association of the Pharmaceutical Industry (ABPI) Code of Practice has been relaxed a little in this area in recent years and companies can now communicate in a very limited fashion with the general public. Clause 20.2 of the Code allows the provision of non-promotional information either in response to a direct enquiry from an individual or via press conferences, press announcements, lectures and media reports, public relations activities and the like.

Over the last few years, there have been a number of initiatives by companies in the United Kingdom to carry out disease awareness programmes but again these have not discussed prescription medicines explicitly.

There has been a debate at the European level over relaxing DTC advertising in a limited number of therapeutic areas. At the time of writing this chapter these suggested changes have been shelved and there are no plans to allow even limited DTC within the EU.

In the Government's White Paper (*Saving Lives: Our Healthier Nation*) published in July 1999 plans were set out for an Expert Patients progamme. The concept being that patients, especially those with a chronic illness, would be best placed to cope with their disease. The old doctor/patient relationship where the doctor knows best is changing and the Government is encouraging patients to have a more active role in their disease management.

The concept of the Expert Patient is evolving and companies need to be aware of these changes and the challenges and opportunities that they pose. Patients demanding the best and not being satisfied with second best can only be a valuable asset to companies introducing innovative new therapies.

11.10   Franchises

Earlier in the chapter, we saw that the pharmaceutical market is not one market but is composed of a number of highly diverse segments.

Some companies dominate specific fields and the ability to build and defend their franchise within a market segment seems to be one of the important features that single out successful companies. It takes years, if not decades, to build a franchise and, once built, companies will do all they can to maintain their position within a given field. Because they have been in a field for a while, companies would have established relationships with their customers, especially local or international opinion leaders. This group of physicians will work on the early development trials for a new product, will act as experts at the time of regulatory approval, publish papers on the product and discuss its use and its place in management of the disease in question at global conferences.

The long-term relationship that form the basis of a franchise mean that physicians in a particular field tend to work with a selected group of companies that they know and trust. This creates a barrier to entry into a given market for a new competitor. A new entrant may chose to enter it alone and a large pharmaceutical company will have the resources to break into a market, but a small start-up or biotech company may chose to form an alliance with an established player. Equally, large pharmaceutical companies with an established franchise and facing patent expiries may wish to licence in compounds in its field of expertise to maintain their market position. Such a strategy may not always be successful. Glaxo had a dominant position in gastrointestinal disease in the late 80s to mid 90s with Zantac, but when the patent on Zantac was lost and no follow-up compound materialised, either coming from internal research or licensed in, its franchise and influence evaporated very quickly. This was one of the reasons why Glaxo merged with Wellcome in the mid 90s.

Glaxo SmithKline has been more successful though, in building and maintaining its franchise in the asthma market. This is partly because not only has it brought new compounds to market at regular intervals but also because of its investment in delivery technology. A large part of asthma prescribing is for drugs delivered to the lung via inhaler devices. Investment in delivery technology has meant that GSK has maintained market dominance long after the patents on certain products have expired. Developing new delivery devices is not easy and physicians and patients tend to remain loyal to devices they know and find easy to use. This mix of product and delivery device has created significant barriers to new entrants into the inhaler market.

11.11 Patent Expiry and Generics

A pharmaceutical product has a limited life cycle and once the patent expires, generic competitors rapidly enter the market. There are a number of strategies that companies can adopt to try to extend patent life. These include line extensions, reformulations, combination products or switching to over-the-counter (OTC) sales. In the United States, but at this point not the European

Union, a 6 months extension of exclusivity may be granted if studies are performed demonstrating safety and efficacy in a paediatric population. In the European Union the problem of off-label use in paediatrics has been recognised by the Commission and a proposal is now in draft form to introduce new legislation in 2006.

Where it is not possible to reformulate or develop combination products, the response in the marketplace to the loss of a patent can be very dramatic. In the United Kingdom particularly and also to an increasing extent in the United States, generic competitor entry and penetration of the market can be very swift. In other European countries there tends to be much more brand loyalty and the penetration of the market by generic competitors is much slower. An example of how rapidly the market in the United Kingdom can change following patent loss is given by Innovace (Enalapril)[1] (Figure 11.7) where, within a few months, prescription volumes for the branded product had fallen to a fraction of their pre-patent loss level.

11.12 Demonstrating the Benefits of Medicine

The clinical trial programme of a new compound through Phases I, II and III is concerned with collecting sufficient data to pass the regulatory hurdles regarding safety and efficacy. In the present climate, the possession of a product licence demonstrating efficacy may not be enough to satisfy the market in terms of clinical effectiveness. In many markets, including the United Kingdom by way of the National Institute of Clinical Excellence (NICE) (discussed below), clinical effectiveness must first be demonstrated but then, this effectiveness must be balanced against its associated costs.

A stream of publications demonstrating clinical efficacy are important to keep the product in the physician's mind and form the basis of promotional claims. More may be needed, however, if the product is to succeed in the marketplace. Decisions need to be made on whether sufficient data exists for modelling of clinical effectiveness

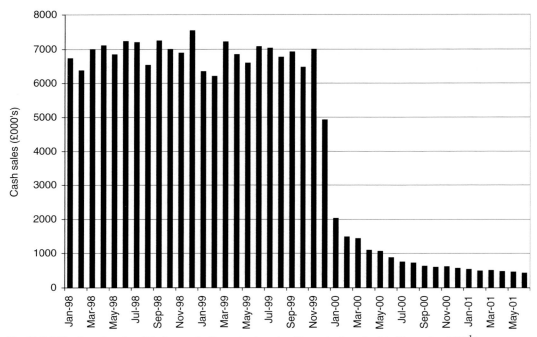

Fig. 11.7 UK sales of enalapril before and after patent expiry (the patent expired in December 1999[1]).

or whether an outcome study needs to be performed. In certain therapeutic areas it may be possible to 'piggy back' some cost and quality of life questions onto the Phase III programme without making the study too complex.

In other therapeutic areas, such an approach in Phase III may not be feasible. This is particularly true for conditions where the endpoint in Phase III is a surrogate for the endpoint of interest to physicians and payers. Examples would include hypertension, hypercholesterolemia or HIV infection.

Outcome studies looking for a hard clinical endpoint, such as death or myocardial infarction or gastrointestinal bleed, are often long, large and very expensive to perform. If the result of the trial is positive they can, however, transform a product's performance in the marketplace. One of the best examples to illustrate this point is Zocor (Simvastatin) following the Scandinavian Simvastatin Survival Study (4S).[6] In the late 80s and early 90s there was great controversy surrounding the effectiveness of cholesterol lowering drugs. The feeling

among leading cardiologists and general physicians was that although high cholesterol was a risk factor for heart disease, there was no evidence that lowering cholesterol was of any benefit. Some experts considered that cholesterol lowering might well be harmful and associated with an increased risk of developing cancer. There were calls in the medical press for the use of lipid lowering drugs to be restricted.[7]

The publication of the 4S study in 1994 transformed the debate. The study demonstrated unequivocally that cholesterol, lowered total as well as cardiovascular mortality with no increased risk of cancer. Cardiologists, who as a group, were previously sceptical of the value of cholesterol lowering, became strong advocates of a change in public health policy. As Professor Oliver wrote in the British Medical Journal in 1995 'Lower patient's cholesterol now – trial evidence shows clear benefits from secondary prevention'.[8] As noted previously, UK physicians are remarkably conservative, and largely follow the principles of evidence-based medicine. When the evidence is presented to them they do, however, react, which can be clearly demonstrated (Figure 11.8). Prescribing levels for Simvastatin were fairly flat prior to the 4S study but increased rapidly post publication. The drug went on to be the most widely prescribed product in the United Kingdom before it lost its patent in mid 2003.

11.13 NICE

In 1999, the government established the National Institute for Clinical Effectiveness (NICE) as a special Health Authority. When introduced the government's objectives behind NICE were to encourage the faster uptake of effective new treatments, to promote more equitable access to treatments and to improve the use of NHS resources. In one sense, industry welcomed the introduction of NICE in that the United Kingdom has one of the slowest uptakes of innovative therapies across Europe, they have among the highest rates of cancer and heart disease and 'post code' prescribing persists. The industry, however, remains concerned about the impact NICE will have on the pharmaceutical industry in the United Kingdom. Industry's concern is that far from encouraging faster uptake of medicines as the government has suggested, the reverse will be the case. This would have a negative impact on the United Kingdom as location for clinical research and investment. NICE has transformed the UK marketing landscape and companies need to build the capability to respond to an appraisal of one of its compounds. The NICE website (www.nice.org.uk) gives guidance on the elements and the timing of technology appraisals. There are four main elements of a technology appraisal and given below is a summary of the components of these subsections:

1. Introduction
    a. epidemiology
    b. development of the technology
    c. problem definition
2. Clinical effectiveness
    a. inclusion and exclusion criteria for studies used in the submission

b. comparisons
    c. clinical data
3. Cost effectiveness
    a. resource use and costs
    b. discounting
    c. dealing with uncertainty
4. Wider implications of the technology for the NHS
    a. budget impact
    b. service impact
    c. consideration of equity.

A large proportion of the technology appraisals so far performed by NICE on pharmaceuticals have been on products recently introduced into the marketplace. This has created difficulties for manufacturers trying to answer the questions posed by the appraisal. For most compounds, at the time of launch it is very unlikely that outcome studies will have been completed that allow accurate cost effectiveness calculations to be performed. The emphasis in Phase III is on clinical efficacy and safety to satisfy the requirements of the regulatory authorities. In most cases, it is impossible (and probably unethical) to perform 'pragmatic' studies on the general population until safety and efficacy have been satisfactorily demonstrated in a tightly defined trial population.

The only alternative open to manufactures faced with a technology appraisal soon after launch is to base their cost effectiveness argument on computer modelling. This is far from satisfactory but it is the best that can be done in the circumstances.

Although NICE is a UK (strictly England and Wales) institution, many countries already have or are establishing bodies that for evaluating the clinical effectiveness of new compounds. My comments on the need for outcome studies to potential changes to Phase III programmes and computer modelling are equally applicable in such countries.

One additional element that needs to be built into a company's plans for NICE is how to handle the uncertainty in the marketplace when an appraisal is announced and then performed by NICE. Once an appraisal of a compound has been

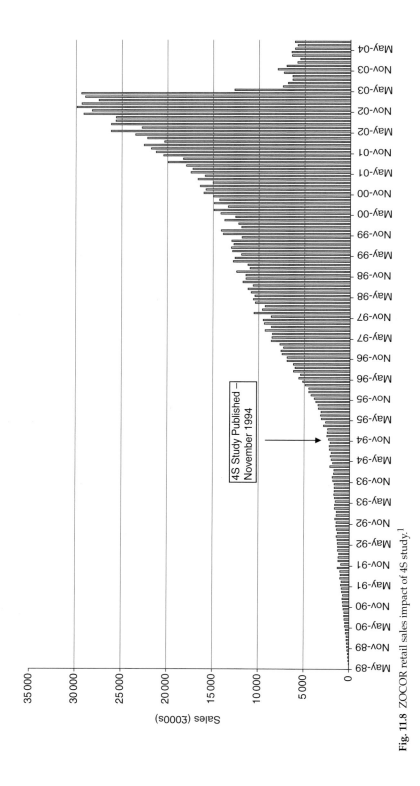

Fig. 11.8 ZOCOR retail sales impact of 4S study.[1]

announced and the timetable for the appraisal made public by NICE there is a tendency for prescribers and NHS bodies to adopt a 'wait and see' approach to the prescribing of the new medicine. If strategies are not introduced to overcome this hurdle, to initiation and use of the product, then it will languish largely unused for a couple of years while the appraisal process unfolds.

11.14   Conclusions

For many physicians and non-clinical scientists working in industry, particularly in early clinical development, their involvement with marketing will be peripheral to their roles. For those in medical advisory roles it will be central. My comments below are addressed more to those in an advisory role.

Conduct a literature search and collate publications on benefits and disadvantages of current treatment. As soon as possible, write a review of the proven and potential benefits of the new product for education of internal staff and possibly for publication.

Make a list of potential questions including: mechanism of action, safety profile, use in paediatric and elderly populations, benefit or lack of benefit in pregnancy. Write standard answers to these questions to ensure that the response to questions from physicians, pharmacists, government agency physicians and research workers represents the best currently available scientific and medical opinion and provides a response that is consistent throughout the world.

Prepare lecture notes for presentation at national and international symposia. Prepare lecture notes too for educational purposes within the company including presentations to the sales representatives.

Identify the essential information which the patient will want to know and which the patient needs to know and prepare a patient information leaflet.

Pay meticulous attention to proposed promotional literature, making sure it is consistent with the product licence and obtain legal approval of the proposed literature from your corporate legal department in writing.

If you have any doubts over the validity of the statements or consider there is the possibility for an independent reader to misinterpret any proposed promotional statement, refer the piece to the relevant internal consultant, for example, safety assessment. If you reject the proposed literature, ensure you have adequate supportive documentation and quote it in your formal response with copies to appropriate colleagues including legal counsel.

The issue of any promotional material that is not in accord with the MA, is inconsistent with labelling approved by the regulatory authority and is misleading is a criminal offence under the Medicines Act (1968) and carries financial penalties and potential for a custodial sentence. Conviction of such an offence usually leads to erasure from the Medical Register by the General Medical Council (GMC).

Medical marketing is a balancing act between the commercial interests of the Company and the responsibility as the voice of ethics for the Company.[9] However, in the final analysis it is your responsibility as the Medical Advisor to ensure that the interests of and benefit to the health of the patient take precedence over all other considerations.

References

1. Data from International Medical Statistics, reproduced with permission.
2. Association of the British Pharmaceutical Industry. *PHARMA Facts and Figures*. London: ABPI, 2000.
3. Emery P, Hawkey CJ, Moore A. Prescribing in the UK. *Lancet* 2001;**357**:809.
4. MSD, data on file.
5. Jones MI, Greenfield SM, Bradley CP. Prescribing new drugs: qualitative study of influences on consultants and general practitioners. *BMJ* 2001;**323**:378–81.
6. Scandinavian Simvastatin Survival Study Group. Randomised trial of cholesterol lowering in 4444 patients with coronary heart disease;

the Scandinavian Simvastatin Survival Study (4S). *Lancet* 1994;**344**:1383–9.

7. Davey Smith G, Pekkanen J, Marmot MG, *et al.* Lowering cholesterol concentrations and mortality. *BMJ* 1990;**301**:552.

8. Oliver M, Poole-Wilson P, Shepherd J. Should there be a moratorium on the use of cholesterol lowering drugs? *BMJ* 1992;**304**:431–4.

9. Holden P. The role of the Medical Department. *Pharmaceutical Times* November 1992;12.

CHAPTER 12

12 Information and promotion

D Michael Humphreys

Promise, large promise, is the soul of an advertisement.

Samuel Johnson (1709–84)

12.1 Introduction

Information is defined as 'the act of informing or communicating knowledge' and as 'news or advice communicated by word or writing'.[1] All pharmaceutical companies are expected to provide detailed information regarding all aspects of their medicinal products, including devices and diagnostic agents, either statutorily upon request by means of the summary of product characteristics (SPC) or in response to questions from healthcare professionals. In addition, they are required to provide essential information about the product or material used in the promotion or advertising of the product.

Promotion can be defined as 'the mechanism or mechanisms by which any purveyor of goods or services may seek to influence prospective purchasers or consumers in the purchasing or consuming of those goods or services'. I.H. Harrison, in his magnum opus *The Law on Medicines: a Comprehensive Guide*,[2] states that the aims of advertising are to draw the attention of the public, or a section of the public, to the availability and utility of a product or service, thus creating a demand for it, and to keep the product or service in the public eye so as to maintain or increase its market share. The Medicines Act 1968,[3] together with its detailed regulations, comprehensively controls the manufacture, packaging, labelling, distribution and promotion of medicines for both human and animal use in the United Kingdom. The Act also replaced a variety of controls that had been legislated over the previous century.

By its existence, the Medicines Act recognises the right of the pharmaceutical industry to advertise and promote its products, and by the standard provisions for product licences, it is possible to control product advertising in an appropriate way, thereby ensuring that adequate information is given, misleading information is prevented and that safety is promoted. As with the advertising and promotion of non-medical products, voluntary codes of practice have been developed, and pharmaceutical companies have agreed to observe these provisions that include the *British Code of Advertising Practice*,[4] the Proprietary Association of Great Britain (PAGB) *Code of Standards of Advertising Practice for Over-the-Counter Medicines*,[5] the Independent Television Commission[6] and the Radio Authority[7] Codes, and the Association of the British Pharmaceutical Industry (ABPI) Code of Practice for the Pharmaceutical Industry[8] applicable to human prescription medicines. The ABPI Code of Practice is the most relevant document relating to this chapter, representing as it does an act of self-discipline with regard to maintaining appropriate standards of marketing conduct. This document has lately been revised to provide more explanation

At the present time two relatively recent and relevant Statutory Instruments are available on www.hmso.gov.uk. These are the Medicines (Advertising and Monitoring of Advertising) Amendment Regulations 1999 and the Control of Misleading Advertisements (Amendment) Regulations 2000.

and greater clarity for those called upon to abide by its content.[9]

While information may be used in both promotional and non-promotional settings, it is important to understand that promotional activities and the provision of information regarding prescription medicines are targeted largely at professionals qualified in the provision of healthcare, usually doctors and pharmacists, and not at the consumers (i.e. the patients), for whom, in any case, such advertisements are prohibited. The insertion of a third party, the prescriber, between the purveyor and the consumer is unique to the pharmaceutical industry and arises in respect of prescription medicines. Promotion to the public direct is, however, permitted specifically in respect of pharmacy- or P-classified and general sales list (GSL) classified medicines, which may be sold over the counter. Increasingly patients, members of the public and patient associations are seeking information on medicines directly from the manufacturers, and companies have learned to provide such information within the provisions of the ABPI Code of Practice and without infringing the Act or intervening in the doctor–patient relationship.

The EU has approved Council Directive No. 92/28/EEC[10] (of 31 March 1992, now consolidated as Articles 86 to 100 of Directive 2001/83/EC) on the advertising of medicinal products for human use, thus bringing Member States into line with common requirements and standards. The UK regulations have been amended to comply with the Directive. The Directive, Part IV of the UK Medicines Act 1968 as amended by the Advertising Regulations, and the ABPI Code of Practice for the Pharmaceutical Industry are broadly in line with one another. The commentary below on promotion relates primarily to the United Kingdom. While there have been some moves towards the international harmonisation of controls on promotion, these have had only a limited effect, despite the fact that in Europe, Member States all comply with Directive 92/28.

The European Federation of Pharmaceutical Industries' Associations (EFPIA) has produced the European Code of Practice for the Promotion of Medicines.[11] Each EFPIA member association has to adopt the European Code or incorporate its requirements into its own code. Each association also has to establish a committee, which includes independent members, to deal with complaints. The European Code incorporates the provisions of the EU Advertising Directive. Total harmonisation has not been achieved, however, because individual associations can add additional requirements of their own and because the European Code is not sufficiently specific in certain areas. For example, while advertisements have to include essential information compatible with the SPC, neither the Advertising Directive nor the European Code spells out what comprises the essential information although this is covered by the 1999 Guideline on Summary of Product Characteristics.[24]

On a wider basis, the International Federation of Pharmaceutical Manufacturers' Associations (IFPMA) has produced the IFPMA Code of Pharmaceutical Marketing Practices.[12] Originally developed as a model code, it is now primarily used to control promotion in developing countries that do not have adequate controls of their own. Associations in the countries in which the head offices of companies are domiciled are responsible, in conjunction with IFPMA itself, for dealing with any complaints about the promotional activities of those companies in developing countries. The IFPMA Code has been revised to bring it into line with the World Health Organization's ethical criteria for medicinal drug promotion and is available on the Intranet.

The situation in each country regarding the control of promotion is thus unique, varying as to both the requirements and the method of control, the latter varying from the United Kingdom, where enforcement is largely by self-regulation, to the United States, where enforcement is largely the responsibility of the Food and Drug Administration (FDA). However, each association belonging to the IFPMA has to have a code that incorporates at least the requirements of the IFPMA Code of Pharmaceutical Marketing Practices, and this helps to ensure the attainment of a reasonable standard in most countries.

12.2   Legislation, Controls and Codes and their Enforcement

12.2.1   Legal controls

There is extensive legislation in the United Kingdom on advertising. Some of this legislation applies to all advertising, such as The Control of Misleading Advertisement Regulations 1988,[13] and some is specific to the advertising of medicines. This section will concentrate on the Medicines Act 1968 and a number of statutory instruments amending the Act, which together form the principal legal controls over pharmaceutical advertising. These include statutory instrument (SI) numbers 1994/1932, 1994/1933, 1994/3144, 1996/1552 and 1999/267. These regulations implement Directive 92/28/EC.

12.2.1.1   The Medicines Act 1968 and regulations

Part VI of the Medicines Act 1968, entitled 'Promotion of Sales of Medicinal Products', deals with the advertising of medicines and includes a number of specific provisions relating to the promotion of medicines to medical and dental practitioners. The general provisions can be summarised as follows: it is an offence to issue a false or misleading advertisement or to make a false or misleading representation about a medicinal product; it is also an offence to issue an advertisement or make a representation on an unauthorised indication, for example an indication not covered by the product licence for the medicine, and it is taken as implicit in these provisions that promotion of a product may not take place prior to being granted a licence authorising its sales or supply. SI 1999/267,[14] amending the Medicines Act, with respect to advertising and monitoring of advertising, now specifically establishes three general principles, under section 3A.

1. No person shall issue an advertisement relating to a relevant medicinal product unless that advertisement complies with the particulars listed in the SPC characteristics.
2. No person shall issue an advertisement relating to a relevant medicinal product unless that advertisement encourages the rational use of that product by presenting it objectively and without exaggerating its properties.
3. No person shall issue a misleading advertisement relating to a relevant medicinal product.

The licensing authority is empowered under Part VI of the Act to require copies of advertisements issued within the past 12 months to be submitted to it. There are also a number of enabling provisions under Part IV under which regulations may be made to further control the advertising of medicines.

Specific provisions within Part IV of the Act require an SPC to be supplied when promoting a medicine to persons qualified to prescribe or supply. The Act specifies that the SPC must be supplied at the time, or within the previous 15 months, of sending or delivering an advertisement or making a representation. Separate regulations under the Medicines Act apply to journal advertising, requiring an SPC to have been provided within the previous 15 months or for there to be a prominent statement in the advertisement that an SPC is available on request. The *ABPI Data Sheet Compendium*,[15] which is published every 15 months and is distributed to all practising doctors and to pharmacies, contains data sheets and SPCs of products currently marketed. This allows companies to meet their legal obligations to provide an SPC every 15 months. Where the SPC/data sheet for a marketed medicine is not in the Compendium, it must be provided separately. It is also a requirement under the Act that all advertising or representations on medicines to the medical and dental professions must not be inconsistent with the SPC for the medicine.

The most important regulations relating to pharmaceutical advertising are The Medicines (Advertising) Regulations 1994[16] (SI 1994/1932, as amended), which covers advertising to both the public and health professionals. In relation to health professionals, the Regulations cover the information that must be included in advertisements, making special provision for audio–visual advertisements, abbreviated advertisements and promotional aids. The regulations also cover the supply of free samples, the activities and training of medical representatives and the provision of inducements and hospitality. They prohibit the advertising of any medicine in respect of which no product licence is in force. All of these matters are dealt with similarly in the Code of Practice for the Pharmaceutical Industry, although in many areas the Code goes into much greater detail and provisions cover areas not included in the regulations. The regulations also implement the relevant EU Directives, including 92/98 EC, 65/65 EC and 92/73 EC.

12.2.1.2 Enforcement

The Medicines (Monitoring of Advertising) Regulations 1994[17] (SI 1994/1933, as amended) set out the ways in which the requirements for advertisements are to be enforced. Civil remedies have been introduced for the first time under which it will be possible for the Medicines Control Agency, now renamed the Medicines and Healthcare products Regulatory Agency (MHRA) to seek an injunction to prevent the publication or further publication of a particular advertisement. An important feature of the new regulations is that if the MHRA receives a complaint about promotion, then it can, with the agreement of the complainant, refer it for adjudication to a self-regulatory body, such as the Prescription Medicines Code of Practice Authority (PMCPA), particularly where the complaint does not involve a breach of legislation.

These powers do not affect the availability of criminal proceedings as a means of enforcement because any breach of The Medicines (Advertising) Regulations 1994 is a criminal offence. A feature is that not only can advertisers be subject to criminal proceedings but also health professionals who solicit or accept any prohibited gift, pecuniary advantage or hospitality, etc. In practice, the licensing authority through its administrative arm, the MHRA, has not used prosecution through the courts as the primary means of enforcing the Provisions of the Medicines Act and the Regulations. Only one major pharmaceutical company has been prosecuted in the courts for issuing a misleading advertisement for a prescription-only medicine (POM). On that

occasion, both the company and its medical director who had authorised the offending advertisement were prosecuted. The threat of a possible prosecution in the courts is thus a powerful sanction. In most circumstances the parties concerned, being the MHRA and the pharmaceutical company whose advertising is challenged, will strive to seek common ground over an issue in order to avoid recourse to the courts. The licensing authority also has considerable powers under The Medicines (Standard Provisions for Licences and Certificates) Regulation 1971[18] in relation to advertising, which has been amended and extended by SI 1999/267, which also amends SI 1994/1933. Under these regulations, the licensing authority may require the licence holder to furnish particulars of any advertisement it proposes to issue, including the contents and form of the proposed advertisement, the means, medium and media by which it will be issued and the time and manner of such issue. The licensing authority may stop a licence holder from issuing or reissuing an advertisement, or require an advertisement to be modified, or require certain precautions or warnings to be included in it in order to meet the objectives specified in the Medicines Act. These objectives exist in order to ensure that accurate information is given about a medicine, to prevent the giving of misleading information and to promote safety in relation to such products.

The MHRA takes a particular interest in the advertising of new chemical entities and those medicines subject to the black triangle symbol, which require special reporting of adverse events. In addition to monitoring advertising and taking up matters with companies where the MHRA considers there are problems in the advertising of a medicine, it also receives and acts on complaints about the advertising of medicines. This is separate from complaints dealt with under the self-regulatory systems discussed below. Companies have reported that on occasion they have been required to submit advertising to the MHRA for vetting prior to use and/or for certain warning statements to be included in material, for periods of up to 1 year. The MHRA may request submission of advertising material for scrutiny prior to issue for reasons such as: new licence, new indication, POM to P switch or previous breach.

As indicated above (see Section 12.2.1.1), the Medicines (Monitoring of Advertising) Regulations 1994 (SI 1994/1933) will allow the MHRA to refer to a self-regulatory body, such as the PMCPA, a complaint which it receives about promotion, if the complainant agrees. Guidance on advertising and promotion has been issued recently by the MHRA (MHRA Guidance Note No. 23).[19]

12.2.2 Self-regulation

Although there is extensive legislation on the promotion or advertising of medicines, the principal method of control in both the prescription and over-the-counter (OTC) medicine sectors is through the self-regulatory codes established and operated by the pharmaceutical industry. These are the PAGB Code of Standards of Advertising Practice for Over-the-Counter Medicines, which governs the advertising of OTC medicines to the general public, and the ABPI Code of Practice for the Pharmaceutical Industry. The latter code of practice will be considered in detail.

12.2.2.1   ABPI Code of Practice
The ABPI is the trade association that represents the manufacturers of prescription medicines. Formed in 1930, it now represents some 80 companies, which produce over 80% of the medicines supplied to the National Health Service (NHS). The ABPI has had a code of practice since 1958, the Code of Practice for the Pharmaceutical Industry, which governs the promotion of medicines to health professionals, and has operated a system whereby complaints made about the advertising of prescription medicines are taken up and considered under the Code. It is a condition of membership of the ABPI to abide by the Code of Practice. In addition, some 70 companies that are not members of the ABPI have given their formal agreement to abide by the Code and to accept the jurisdiction of the PMCPA over complaints made under the Code. Thus, the Code

is accepted by almost all pharmaceutical companies operating in the prescription medicines market in the United Kingdom.

The edition of the Code issued in 1994 further modified the substantially rewritten 1993 edition, which was the first major revision of the Code of Practice since 1978. At that time, it was revised following a series of negotiations with the Department of Health which led to the introduction of detailed regulations on pharmaceutical advertising to the medical and dental professions under the Medicines Act. The review of the Code of Practice and the complaints system that gave rise to the 1993 Edition of the Code was prompted by a number of factors, the most important of which were the changing circumstances of promotion under the reformed NHS, the advent of a European Code of Practice[11] and the EU Directive on pharmaceutical advertising referred to above (see Section 12.2.1.1). Further revisions of the Code have been issued in 1998 and 2001, of which the latter includes for the first time clauses relating to the internet and, most recently, in 2003.

The Code applies to the promotion of medicines to UK health professionals and to appropriate administrative staff in hospitals and health authorities and the like, and to information made available about those medicines to the general public. The Code does not apply to the promotion of OTC medicines (defined as those medicines primarily promoted to the general public rather than health professionals) except in certain circumstances; namely, when they are promoted to a health professional with a view to the writing of a prescription rather than simply recommending the purchase of the medicine by the patient.

The definition of promotion under the Code is broad and is designed to encompass any activity undertaken by a pharmaceutical company or with its authority that promotes the prescription, supply, sales or administration of its medicines. Within that definition, there are a number of exclusions from the scope of the Code such as 'trade practices' and 'trade advertisements'. The content of data sheets and SPCs is also excluded from the scope of the Code, as they are documents viewed as being agreed as part of the licensing process for medicines. The Code reflects the legal requirements and extends well beyond them. The Code itself was drawn up in consultation with the MHRA, the British Medical Association and the Royal Pharmaceutical Society of Great Britain.

The principal requirements of the Code can be summarised as follows:

All promotion must be in accordance with the product licence and the SPC or data sheet. It must be accurate, balanced, fair, unambiguous and objective and based on an up-to-date evaluation of all the evidence. It must not mislead either directly or by implication. All information, claims and comparisons must be capable of substantiation with such substantiation being provided promptly on request by members of the health professions and administrative staff in hospitals and health authorities. Promotion must never be disguised. It must recognise the special nature of medicines, the professional standing of the recipients and the canons of good taste. Certain obligatory information, 'the prescribing information', must be included in all promotion, with exemptions for abbreviated advertisements, which must meet certain special requirements and promotional aids in certain circumstances.

These provisions relate directly to the legal requirements under the Medicines (Advertising) Regulations 1994 discussed above (see Section 12.2.1.1). Standards for the conduct and training of company representatives are defined under the Code, together with those for acceptable gifts and the provision of hospitality by the pharmaceutical industry at meetings and other occasions. (These requirements are discussed in further detail in Sections 12.3.1.5 and 12.3.1.6.)

The advertising of a POM to members of the general public is prohibited under the Code and under the law. Information on medicines may, however, be made available to the general public either directly or indirectly, as long as certain principles are observed.

Numerous other detailed provisions exist in the Code, for example, dealing with the use of the word 'safe', the provision of prescribing information on audio–visual material, the number of pages permitted in a journal advertisement and, most recently, the internet (see Section 12.3.1.4).

Any practical application of the Code requires careful attention to the details contained in the Code, and the accompanying supplementary information is intended to clarify the requirements and to draw attention to particular problems that may occur.

12.2.2.2 Enforcement of the Code

Enforcement of the Code rests in the first instance with the pharmaceutical companies themselves. All promotional material is required to be examined and certified by two signatories – one a doctor and the other an appropriately qualified senior executive – that, in the belief of the signatories, the material is in accordance with the relevant advertising regulations and the Code of Practice, is not inconsistent with the product licence or data sheet, and is a fair and truthful presentation of the facts regarding the medicine. Such certificates must be retained for a defined period, together with information on the data and method of dissemination and details as to whom the material is addressed. The names of signatories are submitted to the MHRA and the PMCPA. Signatories take personal responsibility for the material they authorise and may be held personally accountable for that material under the law.

Complaints about pharmaceutical advertising made under the ABPI Code of Practice are taken up by the PMCPA. The PMCPA was established by the ABPI as from 1 January 1993 to administer the ABPI Code of Practice and consists of a director, secretary and deputy secretary. The authority is responsible for the provision of advice, guidance, conciliation and training on the Code of Practice, as well as for the operation of the complaints procedure. It is also responsible for scrutinising journal advertising on a regular basis.

Complaints submitted under the Code of Practice are considered in the first instance by the Code of Practice Panel, which comprises the Director, Secretary, Deputy Secretary and Executive Officer of the Code of Practice Authority, acting with the assistance of independent expert advisers. Both the complainant and the respondent company may appeal to the Code of Practice Appeal Board against rulings made by the Panel. The Code of Practice Appeal Board is chaired by an independent, legally qualified chairman and includes representatives of the pharmaceutical industry within the United Kingdom as well as independent members from outside the industry. Details of its composition appear in the PMCPA: Constitution and Procedure, which appears with the Code of Practice.

The Appeal Board has a dual role, acting over the activities of the Code of Practice Panel and the PMCPA as both an appeal body and as a supervisory body. All complaints received by the Authority and all rulings by the Code of Practice Panel are reported to the Appeal Board, thus ensuring independent scrutiny from outside the pharmaceutical industry of both the authority's and the panel's activities by the independent members and independent chairman of the Appeal Board. Where promotional material or activities are ruled in breach of the Code, the company concerned must cease to use the material or cease the activity in question forthwith and provide a written undertaking to that effect. Reports on all cases under the Code of Practice are also published, naming companies ruled in breach of the code. These reports receive wide coverage, particularly in the pharmaceutical press and occasionally find their way into the lay press.

The Code of Practice Appeal Board may also require a company ruled in breach to take steps to recover items distributed in connection with the promotion of a medicine. A variety of additional sanctions are available to the ABPI Board of Management following receipt of a report from the Appeal Board. The ABPI Board of Management can reprimand a company and publish details of that reprimand, require an audit to be carried out by the Code of Practice Authority of the company's procedures in relation to the Code and, following that audit, decide whether to impose a requirement on the company to improve its procedures in relation to the code. The ABPI Board of Management can also require a company to publish a corrective statement and, in extreme

examples, can suspend or expel members from the ABPI. In the case of a non-member company, the board can remove that company from the list of non-member companies that have agreed to comply with the code and would then advise the MHRA that responsibility for that company will no longer be accepted under the code.

All members of the ABPI are required to pay an annual Code of Practice levy in addition to the ABPI subscription, to assist in funding the Code of Practice Authority. Certain administrative charges, payable by both members and non-members of the Association, may be levied by the Code of Practice Authority in relation to complaints under the Code of Practice. These charges are akin to costs awarded in civil cases in the courts. The charges are based on the number of matters ruled in a case. The number of matters that will attract an administrative charge is determined by the Director of the Code of Practice Authority. The charges are fixed at two levels. The level that applies is determined on the basis of whether the final ruling in a case is made by the Code of Practice Panel or, on appeal, by the Code of Practice Appeal Board. The charges are paid either by the company ruled in breach of the code or, where there is a rule of no breach of the code, by the complainant where the complainant is a pharmaceutical company. Complainants from outside the industry are not required to pay any charge, whatever the outcome.

The current level of complaints runs at more than 120 per annum, with some 50% of complaints coming from members of the health professions, mainly doctors and pharmacists. Pharmaceutical companies are the other major group of complainants and are responsible for approximately 50% of complaints. Companies are now encouraged to attempt to settle intercompany disputes over advertising material without recourse to the formal complaints procedure. It has become apparent that there is now quite a substantial level of contact between competitor companies challenging or seeking substantiation of claims in each other's advertising. Comparisons between products are, not surprisingly, a fruitful source of complaint between competitors. Criticisms of pharmaceutical advertising or promotional activities in the public domain, whether in the medical, pharmaceutical or lay press or on radio or television, are also routinely taken up and dealt with as complaints under the Code of Practice. Provision also exists for the Code of Practice Panel and the Code of Practice Appeal Board to take up possible breaches of the Code in promotional material that has been brought before the Panel or Appeal Board, which were not raised by the complainant in a case.

The PMCPA also carries out a routine scrutiny of journal advertising under which advertisements are checked for compliance with the code on straightforward matters. Where potential breaches of the code are identified, these are taken up with the company concerned. Only where the matter raised under scrutiny cannot be settled between the Authority and the company is it then referred through to the Panel and the Appeal Board for a formal ruling.

12.2.2.3 Complaints under the Code and their management

It is undoubtedly difficult for pharmaceutical physicians, even up to the level of medical director, to have an all-seeing eye as to the perceptions that may prevail in the minds of the recipients of promotional material. What may be entirely clear to the 'informed' approver of material may be entirely unclear in the mind of the 'uninformed' or even 'informed' recipient. After all, if the recipient is misled, no defence is possible that says that material is not misleading. It really is essential for the approver of promotional material to stand back and say to him/herself 'Is what we say capable of misleading or being misunderstood?'. As an Appeals Board member, I would say that at least half the complaints that come to the PMCPA relate to Clauses 7.2, 7.3, 7.4 and 7.10 of the Code. These relate to accuracy, balance, fairness, objectivity, lack of ambiguity and the full reflection of the total and up-to-date evidence; comparisons must be carefully and appropriately presented; information claims or comparisons must be capable of substantiation. So often defences presented by companies are ill-prepared and

irrelevant when sent to the PMCPA, although a better job is generally done for the appeal. Occasionally, on appeal, the defendants have failed to understand why they have been found in breach. In creating and approving promotional material, the advice is simple. Ask yourself some simple questions. Do the data support the claim? Is what is being said capable of misleading or being misunderstood? Are we taking data out of context or, worse, are we citing an outcome that was not a prespecified and a statistically valid outcome of the trial? It is surprising how often seasoned people in long-established companies get this wrong.

One also has to learn as a medical director that unwillingness to respond intelligently to a complaint, be it from industry or a healthcare professional, will lead ultimately to being found in breach by the PMCPA and, in the absence of perception and understanding, to a hearing before the Appeals Board. The procedures demand significant and costly staff and management time. Inter-company complaints are likely to provoke retaliation. Cherished marketing claims will be given up only under duress. It is sometimes surprising to see how careless the response to the PMCPA can be, which then has to be followed by serious effort to convince the Appeals Board that the initial judgement was either incorrect or unreasonable.

The majority of the remaining complaints coming to the PMCPA and the Appeals Board relate to hospitality, travel and meetings, to the promotion of unlicensed indications – generally elements of disease that are not specified in the product licence – and the conduct of medical representatives and/or not maintaining high standards. With respect to the first, the best advice to both recipients of invitations and to sponsors arises from two questions. One: 'Would you wish these arrangements to be known by colleagues and the public at large?'. The second relates to the balance of education and hospitality: 'Does the educational content of the meeting outweigh the hospitality offered?'. The latter demands the greatest judgement on behalf of those preparing such meetings and, again, ultimately comes back to whether one could be criticised for what is being offered. The conduct of medical representatives and/or the maintenance of high standards are frequently contentious since facts are often lacking and opinion is prevalent. However, there have frequently been cases where management control is lacking and individuals have grossly abused their position. It is difficult for the pharmaceutical physician to manage such situations but, as in so many other aspects, good collaboration with marketing colleagues will ensure that such excesses are at least reduced to a minimum.

Breaches of Clause 2, that of bringing the industry into disrepute, often appear contentious and are usually defended by companies. Again, the verdict often depends entirely on the evidence. However, often the company representatives defending such a change seem blind to the implications of their advocacy, forgetting that a little humility, regret or clear evidence of intention to improve can often work in their favour. Being found in breach of an undertaking not to repeat a Breach of the Code will almost invariably lead to a finding of breach of Clause 2. Guidance on the use of Clause 2 and on appeal procedures have recently (2003) been published in the Code of Practice Review.

Finally, one can only advise those who are called upon to generate, review and approve promotional materials to stand back sometimes and think objectively about how the recipient of promotion will think about what is said or written. Certainly one's best chance of avoiding being found in breach of the code lies in doing this and also in using Joan Barnard's excellent little book *The Code in Practice*, recently reprinted.[20]

12.2.2.4   Other codes

The advertising of medicines to the general public is controlled mainly through the PAGB Code of Standards of Advertising Practice for Over-the-Counter Medicines.[5] Under this Code, members of the PAGB, the trade association representing the manufacturers of medicines advertised direct to the consumer, submit their advertising material to the PAGB for clearance before use. Packaging, labels and leaflet copy is now submitted to the MHRA for approval.

Complaints about the advertising of medicines to the general public are considered by the Advertising Standards Authority under The British Code of Advertising Practice,[4] except for television and radio advertising of which complaints are considered by the Independent Television Commission[6] and the Radio Authority[7] under their own code of practice. The PAGB has also now established a code of practice[21] to cover the advertising of OTC medicines to health professionals and the retail trade, with a view to recommending their purchase by members of the public. This was an area of advertising not hitherto covered by either the ABPI Code or the PAGB Code of Standards of Advertising Practice for Over-the-Counter Medicines. The PAGB operates a complaints system under this Code whereby it will take up and consider complaints made about such advertising. The PAGB does not vet such advertising material before use. Finally, there is a separate code[22] governing the promotion of medicines for use in animals, administered by the National Office of Animal Health (NOAH), which represents the manufacturers of veterinary medicines. This code is not considered further in this chapter.

12.3 Marketing, Advertising and Promotion of Prescription Medicines

Physicians working for, or under contract to, pharmaceutical companies selling medicinal products including medicines, vaccines, medical or surgical devices and diagnostic agents, will find themselves working alongside an industrial discipline that appears alien to their undergraduate teaching, their subsequent postgraduate training and clinical or non-clinical practice. It comes as something of a shock to realise that sales and marketing departments and colleagues within a company expect service and support, not only from the whole medical department, but also from the individual physicians who may be assigned to provide medical advice in respect of particular products that are currently being promoted. The demand for that service is usually directly related to the need for the commercial success of that product or products in the medical market place. There is a commercial emphasis and pressure on what the pharmaceutical physician is being asked and paid to do.

It is therefore important not only to retain a sense of proportion about the needs of the selling departments but also to understand that in providing a professional service, one may assist one's colleagues to maximise the benefit of the product when it is prescribed by clinicians for the management or investigation of disease. In fact, one is not hired as a policeman but as a trained professional adviser who can encourage, guide and, to an extent, manage the methods used by the marketing departments in bringing a good medicinal product to the attention of the prescribing physician. Once one comes to understand the subtlety of this medico-marketing interface, one comes to realise how the medical department can and, indeed is, under an obligation to think positively about the process, without feeling that ethical or professional instincts are being compromised. As reforms within the NHS change the commercial understanding of NHS doctors, this element will become less 'alien' as time goes by. General practitioners and doctors in private practice have been well aware of the importance of a business-like or commercial approach to their practices for many years. Because this aspect of pharmaceutical medicine may be difficult to comprehend on joining the pharmaceutical industry as a medical adviser, it is essential that the more experienced, for example, the medical director or medically qualified department heads, provide support, advice and training about these matters to the young physician on entry to the medical department. It is also essential that there is an open dialogue between medicine and marketing, so that areas where there may be contention or disagreement are thoroughly discussed before positions are taken, costs are incurred and complaints, particularly external, are received. Indeed, marketing colleagues are usually extremely grateful for good ideas that are medically acceptable in promotional terms and especially so when careful review of the data allows the strong support

of claims or advantages for a particular product. Thus, it is in part the job of the medical adviser to conduct such careful review, often with his or her statistician colleagues. One has almost invariably found that when marketing and medicine sit down together with blank paper and just a few ideas, a dialogue begins, which leads to good promotional material that is ethically acceptable and non-contentious. One's colleagues are best advised to consult the relevant Medical Adviser early in the process, rather than coming along with a prepared draft of what the Product Manager wants to say, which the Medical Adviser is then expected to edit to meet the Code of Practice.

It has to be clearly understood that the creation of ethical promotional material is a team exercise, the key players being the product manager, the product physician and the regulatory affairs department. A competent review of the data relevant to the claims being made for the product, together with a reading for compliance with the product licence and the ABPI Code of Practice, are the minimum needs in the generation of material intended for promotional use. The final document then has to be 'approvable' by the company's senior executives, usually the medical director or senior medical colleagues and possibly the marketing director. The names of these approving persons are lodged with the MHRA and the Code of Practice Authority as the responsible and official signatories. The managing director is also involved since any breach of the Code and/or the advertising section of the Medicines Act will, of necessity, be notified to the senior company executive. Practising physicians contracting to provide part-time medical support and advice to companies marketing medicines, are well advised not only to understand the obligations under the code that they are taking on, but also to ensure that they receive training on the Code of Practice.

12.3.1 Methods of promotion

12.3.1.1 Verbal promotion
The time-honoured and traditional method of verbal promotion is performed by company

sales representatives, who visit the prescribing doctors at their surgeries or institutions and present information about the company's medicinal products. Often the sales representative will work from printed or prepared material (see below) but the essence of the exercise is a dialogue between representative and physician as to the relative merits of the product. The representative will present the advantages, if any, of the product and will seek to ascertain whether the doctor has patients for whom the medicine might be indicated, perhaps whose disease may be inadequately controlled by a product the doctor is already prescribing. Often the representative is trying to persuade the physician that if he or she tries the medicine being promoted in an inadequately controlled patient, then the physician will think well of the product and use it the next time a patient with the same disease presents. The representative also has a golden opportunity to educate the doctor, since few doctors have an all-embracing personal formulary in their minds and, equally, few are able to read all the scientific literature. Thus, a well-trained and well-informed representative can be invaluable in discreetly and tactfully informing the potential prescriber of information, he does not know.

The pharmaceutical physician has an important role to play in the training of representatives, who are required to have gained significant expertise with respect to their products and the manner in which they are promoted. The ABPI requires of member companies that all medical representatives are professionally trained under the Code of Practice, and are required to pass an examination set by the ABPI within 2 years. The pharmaceutical physician will generally be asked to teach representatives sufficient understanding of the diseases (and their conventional treatment) to which the company's products are relevant. He or she will be familiar with the clinical data for the product(s), and the published and unpublished reports and manuscripts, and can therefore teach the representatives about the issues that are important for the proper discussion of the product characteristics when the representative meets the prescribing physician.

Finally, the representative must learn the details of the product licence and thus know how, when promoting the product, to avoid being in breach of either the Medicines Act or the ABPI Code of Practice, which is written specifically to assist company personnel in promoting products to prescribers in an appropriate manner.

While the style and personality of the sales representative and the knowledge he/she has absorbed are fundamental in promoting a product successfully, it is evident that the pharmaceutical physician has an important role in informing, guiding and advising medical representatives so that their verbal promotion is informed and appropriate.

Usually, the content of verbal promotion varies according to whether the recipient is a general practitioner or a hospital consultant or specialist. The former tend to prefer clear messages about the possible merits and disadvantages of particular products in conditions that are commonly treated in general practice. 'Blinding with science' is not likely to gain significant numbers of adherents since time is at a premium. The hospital physician or specialist will be very familiar with the literature regarding key medicines in his or her speciality and is likely to want a more sophisticated approach from verbal promotion. Both increasingly wish to know the likely costs in relation to benefit. The pharmaceutical physician will therefore assist his or her sales colleagues substantially in providing them with comprehensive information regarding the characteristics of the company's ethical medicinal products.

12.3.1.2 Written, printed and documentary promotion

Pharmaceutical companies have recourse to all the art of sophisticated advertising, promotion, public relations and specialist agencies, as well as having their own trained marketing professionals. Consequently written, documentary and published promotional items are usually reviewed and scrutinised by the company medical advisers for conformity with the known data and the ABPI Code of Practice, while the regulatory affairs professionals usually ensure conformity with the product licence. A pharmaceutical physician is obliged to 'sign off' written and published promotional material before it can be made available to prescribing doctors.

Promotional material is expensive to produce. No company wants to distribute poor-quality material and style, format and appearance are important. The company therefore relies on its medical staff to ensure that the content is appropriate for the promotional purpose. The exercise is time consuming and complex to conduct, and companies are advised to have a standard operating procedure (SOP) that covers the generation and approval of all ethical promotional material of whatever type. This should be written and approved by the Medical Director, together with experienced colleagues who know the relevant parts of the Medicines Act and the Code of Practice and who hold positions of authority within the company (see below). The document should also have the approval of the marketing and managing directors since it is the procedures and the performance that will be judged by the MHRA and the PMCPA. Ultimately, in the event of serious breach of the Medicines Act, the company and the responsible medical signatory could be prosecuted. These are potent incentives for the pharmaceutical physician to 'get it right' and to ensure that Marketing also gets it right.

Written and published items constitute the majority of the pharmaceutical physician's workload in terms of promotional materials since these are generally left with prescribing doctors, as both sources of information and reminders about the product. Reviewing these is time consuming and demands a practised eye. Pieces vary from lengthy detail aids, in which a full profile of the medicine is presented, to abbreviated advertisements, simple 'mailers' or promotional letters, and reminders – small items that can be used in day to day practice such as sticky labels, note pads, pens, coffee mugs, wall charts, drug interaction discs – to large advertisements that appear in the medical and paramedical press. For all items, there are both general and specific rules. Thus, if breaches of the Act or the Code are to be avoided, it is essential that pharmaceutical physicians come to understand, can interpret

and are trained in the application of these rules. It should be noted that the PMCPA is most willing to provide training and guidance with respect to promotional material.

Published data and company 'data on file' provide the main support for much of the printed promotional material. Pharmaceutical physicians must be able to understand and interpret the data available and then be able to advise on how those data may be incorporated into promotional copy without loss of context or being open to misunderstanding or charges of being misleading. One must also be able to anticipate the unexpected reaction of the reader. A claim or highlighted item may be perfectly clear to the writer but may be interpreted quite differently by the reader. There are practising physicians and pharmacists who take a particular interest in the way that pharmaceutical companies promote their products and who may appear to 'specialise' in ensuring that the industry obeys the rules.[23] These are individuals who often publicly criticise promotional copy. However, most physicians are fair minded about promotion, and complaints are generally made by doctors who feel that companies are overstating their case or are taking unfair advantage. The generating or reviewing medical adviser must have an eye for these possibilities before the printed material has been disseminated, usually at significant company expense.

Finally, it should be understood by pharmaceutical physicians that marketing and medical staff from competitor companies are also highly sensitive to promotional material from a competitor in a field where they may have a similar product. Complaints about printed promotional material and promotional behaviour are not infrequent between companies. Again, 'breaking the rules' or taking unfair advantage is also resented by one's colleagues in other companies, and complaints will arise. Tactical intercompany complaints have diminished since the ABPI made adverse comments about this practice to managing directors. The recent revisions of the Code of Practice complaints procedures are intended to ensure that inter-company complaints are well founded and are not simply 'tactical'.

Many companies publish newspapers providing information and commentary on conferences or congresses on large-scale trials, using academic or senior clinical opinion, or interviews that may be relevant to particular therapeutic areas. Pharmaceutical physicians must be aware of the pitfalls that can arise as a result of such publications. One must work on the principle that all printed material that is generated, sponsored or distributed by, or on behalf of, the marketing department of a pharmaceutical company, or which contains promotional claims for a medicinal product, must be reviewed for format, content and style according to the local procedures governing the approval of ethical promotional material. Only then can one avoid falling into the trap of condoning inappropriate or even illegal promotional copy. One should also be aware of the external opinions that may be stated so as to avoid the possibility of the company being drawn into a breach of the code by citation of known but contentious opinion.

12.3.1.3 Audio–visual promotion

The modern era has seen the arrival of both audiocassette and video film recording as well as CD-ROM, as a potent means of promotion. Clinicians can be interviewed readily and many enjoy performing with this medium, seeing it as a form of teaching. Actors are readily hired for the quality of their voices in doing introductions, link pieces, voiceovers and even conducting the actual promotion. Such items are treated no differently from any of the more conventional forms of promotional material and it is essential for the pharmaceutical physician to review carefully the script *in toto* and then to listen to the audio tape or watch the film, in order to see that items have not been promoted overzealously or inappropriately edited or taken out of the context intended by the speaker. It is good practice to ensure that invited clinical or scientific speakers review and approve the use of their own text and also that the pharmaceutical physician ensures that his clinical colleagues do not inadvertently breach the rules. The finished item should then be signed off as a whole according to local SOP or routine procedure.

Scientific congresses often attract television, radio or newspaper journalists interested in new medical discoveries or the financial performance of companies. Pharmaceutical physicians must be cautious when being interviewed because what they say may be construed as promotion in the eyes or ears of a third party. Pharmaceutical physicians likely to find themselves in this position should be media trained in order to minimise the risk inherent in the on-the-spot interview. Equally, companies may find that the material gained at such meetings is interesting from a promotional point of view. Interviews can be bought through recording companies. It is important that these items, too, are assessed and formally approved before being used by the marketing department.

12.3.1.4 The internet

The internet represents the best new method of disseminating information since the invention of the printing press, and with it come opportunities for commerce, advertising and promotion. It cannot therefore be a surprise that the pharmaceutical industry has come to see the internet as offering tremendous opportunities for its medicinal products. It would appear, equally, that the regulatory authorities, accustomed to seeing the traditional methods of sales and promotion contained within the boundaries of national jurisdiction, have viewed the transnational availability of the internet with concern. The situation is not made easier by the differing legislation in the European Union and many other countries, where direct-to-customer advertising is not permitted, whereas it is permitted in the United States. As the century has turned, it would seem that the concerns may or may not be diminishing. Just as the FDA remains able to inspect and enforce in the United States for material that originates there, so authorities and codes of marketing practice have been able to accommodate the internet under exactly the same principles as with other materials. In part, companies have continued to target their promotion to healthcare professionals and even in the United States, promotion to the patient or their relatives appears to be responsible and informative from examples that I have seen. In Europe, US internet advertising has become tolerable, only because there is no legislation to enable action over statements that the content of the advertisement is not relevant to patients outside the United States. Throughout, companies appear to have understood, and authorities to have acknowledged, that the provision of information about medical conditions, scientific results about medicinal treatments and medicines themselves, to patients, relatives and carers, as well as healthcare professionals, is not only not harmful but desirable. It is clear that the MHRA supports the supply of balanced informative material and it is noteworthy that the majority of pharmaceutical company websites contain SPCs, European Public Assessment Reports (EPARs) and patient information leaflets (PILs) as their sources of information. The caveat remains and is being respected by all parties that such information shall not be promotional. It is interesting that, despite the huge growth of information on the internet about diseases and their management, there have been only two contested cases before the Code of Practice Appeals Board. Both were found to be for the complainant but neither related to fundamental dissatisfaction with the principle of provision, but merely a failure to perceive a lapse into promotion in respect of a single statement in an early page of a huge website in one case, and in the other, a technical argument as to where in an e-advertisement, the generic name of the product should be located. The answers were already in the Code of Practice, and, in fact, the content of the specific website information and of the e-advertisement was otherwise of excellent quality.

Further modifications to advertising, Articles 86–100 of the EU Pharmaceutical Legislation Review 2001, now consolidated,[10] do not even mention the internet. Should the proposals be accepted, the term 'advertising of medicinal products' will in future include the phrase 'awareness of the availability' of such products. This will, by implication, include the internet. The MHRA has published advice on advertising on the internet[19] which states unequivocally that there is an ongoing debate in Europe on the acceptability of the advertising of medicines on the internet. 'Therefore, until this is concluded, the MHRA considers that advertisements for prescription only medicines are acceptable only on websites whose nature and content is directed at health professionals'. The MHRA has produced no formal comment or guidance with regard to information that may be posted on the internet. It is for companies to ensure that in providing information they avoid breaches of the medicines legislation and the Code of Practice.

12.3.1.5   Meetings and conferences

Many scientific meetings and congresses are financed, in large measure, by the pharmaceutical industry and could not occur without such sponsorship. The large international and national learned medical societies could not afford to hold their annual meetings without the assistance of companies. The industry naturally expects a return on its investment, and promotional stands and exhibits are commonplace at conferences of all sizes. Clinicians are, rightly, expected and encouraged to visit a sponsor's stand or exhibit, and companies make full use of the opportunities thus presented for promotion of their medicinal products. Companies also sponsor individual attendance at such meetings, which, in the main, are extremely well run and provide a level of medical education, debate and information that cannot readily occur elsewhere. Regulatory and consumer bodies concur as to the importance of such meetings where research workers can meet and exchange ideas and younger doctors can be readily educated. The pharmaceutical physician provides valuable support to his or her marketing colleagues by being available to discuss product information and data, either on the stand or during breaks from the scientific sessions. He or she can also bring clinicians to the stand to meet marketing people or to use the facilities and services provided by the company, including on-line literature search facilities, reprints, promotional material, etc., and even tea, coffee or soft drinks. All of these activities support product promotion, are legitimate and merely need care and attention to see that the rules are adhered to. The majority of companies work ethically on these occasions and the symbiotic atmosphere is both visible and cordial. One has to be aware that product licences may differ from country to country and some products may not be licensed in some countries. Accordingly, it is important that clinicians exposed to promotion of products at international congresses are not misled as to the regulatory status of a particular product. One should therefore indicate when promotional material dispensed on such occasions is not appropriate for the country of the recipient. Avoiding being misleading is again the principal aim and, furthermore, it is important that laws pertaining to the host country are observed.

12.3.1.6 Promotional gifts and prizes

The rules regarding promotional gifts are clearly dealt with in the ABPI Code of Practice. Gifts to prescribers are not forbidden but must conform to certain sensible rules. They should not cost the donor more than £6 excluding VAT and they must have some relevance to the practice of medicine. Gifts should not be so prominent that they put the recipient under obligation, and doctors do not wish to find the Inland Revenue taking an interest in such matters. One's marketing colleagues, whose job it is to create a rationale for a particular promotional gift and its relevance to medical practice and the pharmaceutical physician, in approving such an item, must be alert as to what is reasonable. Would a 'reasonable' individual perceive the appropriate nature of such a gift upon hearing a simple explanation? If the explanation is prolonged or obtuse then it is better to point out the probable inappropriate nature of the gift. Marketing staff will understand a judgement if they are aware that a gift might not pass the scrutiny of the Code of Practice Panel or Appeal Board should it be complained about. The Code of Practice does not prevent the provision of medical and educational goods and services that will enhance patient care or benefit the NHS if their provision is not connected with promotion.

Competitions have also become fashionable as a means of promotion of products. Advice should be given by the medical adviser regarding both the nature of the competition, which must be a proper test of skill, and the suitability of the prizes, as for promotional gifts. A promotional prize must not cost the donor more than £100 excluding VAT.

12.3.1.7 Promotional hospitality

Hospitality provided for the medical, scientific and caring professions can cause great contention, and the company can find itself in considerable difficulties if it gets this wrong. Complaints arise when hospitality is clearly inappropriate. How can the pharmaceutical physician ensure that he or she judges propriety correctly and then advises the company accordingly? It is not just those who have not been invited who may complain but also recipients of hospitality whose consciences are pricked or embarrassed by excess. Again, the rules are clear: inappropriate cost, the presence of spouses when the company is paying, and inappropriate venues all constitute breaches of the Code as well as common sense. Pharmaceutical physicians must use a sensible measure of judgement whether advising the company or when personally entertaining clinical or scientific guests. One only has to think about one's own expense allowance, as a rule. Managing directors (and chief accountants), and the code, expect that a reasonable attitude will prevail. The value of the entertainment or hospitality should not exceed the value of the purpose of meeting and should not be so lavish that it induces an obligation or distraction from an ethical position. Equally, one's guests are often persons of substance and inappropriate hospitality in the reverse direction (i.e. poor quality) is not appreciated. The medical or scientific purpose of a meeting at a time or occasion when hospitality is offered or arranged should always be more important than the hospitality itself, which should always be subordinate to the occasion. For example, the ABPI Code of Practice in its recent revisions very clearly specifies, in relation to representatives' activities, sporting occasions are inappropriate venues to which to invite guests who are directly involved with the provision of healthcare.

12.3.1.8 Sponsorship

Companies, through either the marketing department, Medical Grants Committees or the medical department, are regularly and frequently approached for the provision of financial support or sponsorship. This varies widely from charitable appeals to learned societies to individuals seeking to travel to meetings, or sponsorship or a salary or a position abroad. Young physicians want financial support or supplies of drugs for personal research, and medical students ask for help with the costs of student electives in faraway places. Most companies have a budget for such sponsorship although it has become increasingly difficult to afford salaries. Clearly, in deciding whether to accede to requests of this type, pharmaceutical industry managers, including the medical director, have to regard this as a form of investment which is therefore promotional, whether it is of the company's name or products. Thus, judgements and recommendations have to be made.

12.3.1.9 Samples and postmarketing trials

Companies frequently wish to assist the prescribing doctor in gaining familiarity with a medicinal product by making samples available. Free goods or bonus stock provided to pharmacists and to others are neither samples, nor are 'starter packs', which are small packs provided to allow a doctor to initiate treatment in an emergency situation. Samples provide an opportunity for promotion. However, the ABPI Code of Practice lays down strict rules as to how and on what scale samples may be provided. In particular, samples may only be supplied in response to a specific request from a health professional, who must sign and date any request card. No more than 10 samples of a particular product may be given to a particular recipient in the course of a year. By the same token 'seeding' trials are not permitted simply to give the physician a chance to use the medicine.

Phase IV trials, like trials in Phases I–III, must be genuine investigations that are properly conducted and the data analysed. Free drug may not be given to doctors solely for them to use as they think fit. The restrictions do, however, reduce the chances for physicians to assess the new medicine personally and thus to form a rounded view of the product. The argument must therefore rest on clinical and scientific merit.

Free drug must, however, be made available for Phase IV trials approved by the Ethics Committees.

12.3.1.10 Services to doctors and patients

The provision of services to doctors and, indirectly, to patients is an accepted form of promotion. Many responsible companies provide information and specific services that can be made available to patients by the treating physicians or nurses. Such services create a favourable impression of a company and its products in the minds of doctor, health professional and patient. For example, a videograph on the correct procedures for operating a nebuliser can be made available to patients through the doctor or the asthma nurse by the manufacturers of a nebuliser solution. This helps with branding or product preference by the doctor and patient. Similarly, funding practice nurses to be trained in the clinic management of asthma or hyperlipidaemia helps to ensure that the patient is referred by the trained nurse to the doctor for treatment. Because such activities are provided by companies wishing to promote the use of the products, they are classified as promotional activity. Recently the PMCPA and the Appeals Board have become concerned that the identification of patients with particular diagnoses or already receiving specific treatments has become possible when company representatives have been given access to practice databases for reasons purporting to be diagnostic review and therapeutic management by the practitioners. Such activity is unacceptable and will be censured most strongly by the PMCPA and by the Appeals Board. Confidential data simply must not be known to third parties. The Code of Practice and Medicines Act prohibit the advertising of prescription medicines to the public (i.e. patients) and therefore services provided in this manner that bring companies into contact with patients must not constitute advertising for such products. An up-to-date review of what constitutes acceptable practice with respect to the provision of goods and services has been published under the auspices of the Code of Practice.[24]

12.3.1.11 Market research

Market research is mentioned here only to point out that such activity is permissible, must follow certain guidelines[25] and may not be disguised promotion. Indeed, promotional activities of all types may not be disguised as to their true intent.

12.4 Information

It is mandatory that pharmaceutical companies should have a scientific service which is responsible for information about medicines that they market. Council Directive 92/28/EEC[10] (the advertising directive) states this clearly. Prescribers and qualified suppliers of medicines must have access to neutral and objective information about products that are available and companies have accepted that an information service department is a necessary and responsible facility. These are usually staffed and managed by qualified pharmacists, information scientists and nurses and, in general, should form part of the company's medical department so that impartial advice is provided. Such a service can only be maintained provided that the professional staff so employed are trained in information database searching and have access to the major external scientific literature databases as well as the company's product database. The information services department may also administer the company's product safety database, handling spontaneously reported adverse events, which may or may not be related to the company's product, and having access to the MHRA's anonymised database of reported adverse events and reactions. This will need careful management since most companies also have a drug safety department that expects to manage the data entry for spontaneously reported adverse events. However, interdepartmental interaction may be wise since the information services department may also be handling technical complaints that may include or even disguise adverse reactions (ADROIT).

Information regarding medicinal products is available to health service professionals from a variety of external and independent sources. These include:

- *The Drug and Therapeutics Bulletin*
- *Prescribers' Journal (now discontinued)*
- *The British National Formulary*
- *The Monthly Index of Medical Specialities (MIMS)*
- *The Medicines Resource Centre (MeReC)*
- *The Drug Information Service*
- *The MHRA*
- *Bandolier.*

Their functions, orientation and scope are well summarised in *Medicines: Responsible Prescribing*[26] and will not be repeated here. Rather we shall confine ourselves to considering the scale and scope of medicinal product information generated and normally provided either mandatorily or on demand by pharmaceutical companies.

12.4.1 Summary of product characteristics

This is the name of what we used to know simply as the data sheet, or colloquially as the package insert. The SPC is the document that must be submitted in draft by companies to the MHRA/Reference Member State/European Medicines Evaluation Agency upon application for a marketing authorisation and, once approved, must then be provided to prescribers or suppliers of medicines, either with the product or at the time of promotion or within the previous 15 months of promotion of the product, written or verbal. The SPC includes the prescribing information for the product and represents the product licence approval for the medicine (see Section 12.2.1.1). It is the definitive statement between the competent authority and the company and, more importantly, is becoming the common basis of communication between the competent authorities of all member states. The content can only be changed with the approval of the originating competent authority and/or all member states.

The sequence of particulars on the SPC is listed in Box 12.1, but for amplification the reader is referred to the Note for Guidance of the CPMP Working Party.[27]

The MHRA has already addressed the relationship between the SPC and the data sheet and how the latter is superseded by the former. Additional guidance has been released recently regarding the content and format and the presentation of 'undesirable effects' and has been adopted for updated or new SPC in future in the European Union.[28] This is aimed at providing

---

Box 12.1   The sequence of particulars on the SPC

1. The name of the medicinal product
2. Qualitative and quantitative composition
3. Pharmaceutical form
4. Clinical particulars
   4.1 Therapeutic indications
   4.2 Posology and method of administration
   4.3 Contraindications
   4.4 Special warnings and special precautions for use
   4.5 Interaction with other medications and other forms of interaction
   4.6 Pregnancy and lactation
   4.7 Effects on ability to drive and use machines
   4.8 Undesirable effects
   4.9 Overdose
5. Pharmacological properties
   5.1 Pharmacodynamic properties
   5.2 Pharmacokinetic properties
   5.3 Preclinical safety data
6. Pharmaceutical particulars
   6.1 List of excipients
   6.2 Incompatibilities
   6.3 Shelf life
   6.4 Special precautions for storage
   6.5 Nature and contents of container
   6.6 Instructions for use/handling
   6.7 Name of, style and permanent address or registered place of business of the holder of the marketing authorisation

---

the prescriber with information on the likely frequencies of adverse reactions.

12.4.2   Patient information leaflets and labelling

Originally, the information given to patients was that given verbally by the doctor when prescribing a medicine, reinforced by the instructions transferred from the prescription to a label, which was then stuck on the medicine container. The implication was that it was not necessary for the patient to understand what his or her problem entailed but merely that he or she should follow the dosing instructions. Inevitably, the information given to the patient was highly variable. In 1984, mechanically printed labels were required and in 1987, the Guide to Cautionary and Advisory Labels for Dispensed Medicine became a matter of professional conduct. Professor George's work with an experimental patient information leaflet (PIL) led to the conclusion that patients exposed to such a leaflet were better informed, although he could not conclude that they took medicines as instructed or were more compliant. Following substantial consultation with regulatory, consumer and medical bodies, a working party set up by the ABPI was able to define a series of recommendations regarding the content of PIL, including minimum requirements, together with procedures for the review and approval of the leaflets. Council Directive 92/27/EEC[29] came into force in March 1992 and deals with the labelling of medicinal products for human use and leaflets inserted in the packaging. The Directive deals first with the particulars required either on the outer packaging or, if none, on the immediate packaging of the product, and second, with the contents of the user package leaflet. Mockup packaging and the draft package leaflet are to be submitted for approval by the approving authority. Statutory Instrument 1994/3144[30] adopted the Directive into UK legislation from January 1995, providing comprehensive regulations regarding marketing authorisations, etc., for medicines for human use. Labelling and package leaflet information is now (from January 1999) assessed according to the guideline on the readability of the label and package leaflet of medicinal products for human use,[31] the intention being to apply standards to the requirements for eligible, comprehensible and indelible information, its content and its format. The Guideline represents a determined effort to ensure that patients can understand the medical content of the information given. It is recognised in the introduction that companies will have queries specific to individual products and that the Agency will expect to offer advice on the drafting of PIL.

The labelling requirements are more straightforward. Products currently licensed will continue to be subject to the existing regulations until their next licensing renewal. The Homeopathic Directive requires that homeopathic products obtaining a full product licence shall become relevant medicinal products for the purposes of labelling and leaflets regulation. Routes for leaflet/labelling approval within the agency are clearly shown according to whether a change of product licence is involved. In the future PIL will be subject to the readability requirements of the European Union.[31]

Labelling requirements are relatively simple to adopt, with guidance given on legibility, print size or type, concertina and foldout labels/leaflets, the non-use of packaging inner services, changes to approved labelling and carton labelling on self-medication products. The information to be included on the label is set out with additional guidance on areas of particular difficulty. These include:

- Product name
- Form and strength
- Contents
- Excipients
- Special warnings
- Expiry date
- Storage and disposal warnings
- Product licence holder's name and address.

Exemptions from labelling requirements are given.

With respect to leaflets, all information given must be approved by the Agency with final versions being sent on confirmation. Leaflets must not be promotional and must be consistent with the product licence, which will be the source document for assessment of the PIL. The information required is given, together with extensive footnotes in the guidance prepared by the Agency. Areas of interpretation where difficulties may arise are as follows.

- Excipients, E numbers and brand names
- Licence holder and manufacturer's name and address
- Indications, contraindications, warnings, precautions and side effects
- 'Roll-up' warnings
- Dosage and method of administration
- Action to take in the case of overdose.

It is fair to say that dialogue needs to continue between the Agency and the pharmaceutical industry regarding the terminology that the requirement of 'ALL contraindications, warnings, precautions and side-effects' will mandate and its usefulness in informing patients. The question of 'roll-up' warnings remains a subject for discussion, as does a debate about the difference between adverse events and adverse reactions.

While English is the only MHRA-approved language, other language versions may be used upon certification of identical content. Symbols, pictograms and educational material are also discussed. The MHRA guidance and appendices are essential reading for those required to write PILs, generally members of the medical department.

12.4.3 Information services department

In general, the provision of product information is the responsibility of the medical department in so far as the information sought and provided is non-promotional in nature. Companies vary in how such a department may be integrated within a medical division but the principles underlying the provision of such a service are relatively constant. The qualifications of those who should provide medical product information are, as may be expected, are based on medicine, nursing, pharmacy or information science. The company physicians and pharmacists are best placed to give prescribing advice regarding the company's medicinal products and will have the product development database readily available to them. Information science is a discipline of specialist nature. The discipline has arisen because medical and scientific databases have become so enormous that searching them for specific information has become a science in its own right. Information scientists will either have a scientific qualification from a college or university and then learn information science as postgraduate training or, increasingly, will have taken a specific undergraduate course in information science at a recognised institution. The Institute of Information Technology and, more specifically, the Association of Information Officers in the Pharmaceutical Industry provide support to information scientists in the industry.

Information services departments often have a dual role in that they can provide not only medical product information to external enquirers but also provide scientific information internally within the company to those planning and designing clinical trials and developing product strategies and promotional material. Logically, the company library will be managed by the information services department, as will with the archives of published and unpublished reports relating to the company's medical products. Other aspects that may be managed by an information department or in collaboration with a drug safety department may include spontaneous reports of adverse events or reactions associated with the use of the company's medicinal products, access to the MHRA's adverse reaction reporting database and control of the company's clinical trials data and patient-related archive. This requires information technology with which to manage the flow and storage of documents related to the conduct of the clinical trials conducted by the company in support of its medical product development programmes, since both internal quality assurance

and external regulatory audit will need to be satisfied upon inspection of the clinical trials archive.

The term 'Medical Services', often itself a department or section of the Medical Division, includes and implies the provision of medical product information to those seeking information. All companies are familiar with the volume of day-to-day contact by telephone and letter from hospital and retail pharmacists and from prescribing physicians, directly or through the sales representative field force. In the United Kingdom, a moderate-sized pharmaceutical company can expect to receive several thousand telephone calls per annum. Questions posed may relate to the chemistry or pharmacy of the product, its use in conjunction with other medicines, its use in patients with severe organ dysfunction or in poor health or even its use in ways that are not covered by the SPC (see Section 12.4.3.1). A doctor or pharmacist using a medicine with which he or she is relatively unfamiliar may want to know about the risk of side-effects in particular circumstances or conversely, upon encountering a particular side-effect or adverse event, whether the event has been recorded previously. Almost any question can arise and many are asked repeatedly. Product physicians and pharmacists become not only adept at responding readily and comprehensively to such questions but also acquire a substantial knowledge of their products as a result. All companies view the provision of such information as an important ethical responsibility. Few companies wish to be complained of for poor performance in this respect. After all, their reputations are at stake.

Finally, since some of the questions posed to information services departments are of medicolegal importance, for example, prescribing advice or adverse event reporting and/or management and liability, information scientists will normally seek the support or advice of the company physician or pharmacist and even the legal department, in providing a response. The company physician or pharmacist should always be prepared to respond personally to the health service professional who is making the enquiry, especially at the request of a non-medical colleague.

12.4.3.1   Information on the unlicensed use of medicines

Medicines are often used for indications for which they do not have a product licence, either because data exist showing the medicine to be beneficial or because clinical trials in new indications are still being conducted. It is quite clear in both the medicines legislation and the ABPI Code of Practice that no medicine may be promoted for an indication for which a product licence has not been obtained. However, the medicines legislation accepts, pragmatically, that doctors may prescribe any substance that they believe may be of benefit to their patients while remaining professionally responsible for the judgement in doing so. The ABPI has published notes for guidance on the supply of unlicensed medicines[32] and the *Drug and Therapeutics Bulletin*[33] has published advice for prescribers regarding the unlicensed use of medicines. The industry, while also endeavouring to behave in an ethical fashion with respect to unlicensed use of its marketed compounds according to the legislation, has traditionally made available experimental drugs for patients whose condition is not responding to currently available medication. There has been a mood prevailing to inhibit doctors from prescribing medicines unlicensed in a particular indication by threatening them with an unquantifiable risk of liability for side-effects. This has had more to do with reducing the cost of medicines than to do with a real risk. Management of prescribing in this respect has become more practical with the advent of evidence-based medicine and the concept of systematic review, for example, the Cochrane Library. In general, companies have always been willing to make experimental drugs available where a real need has been demonstrated and the government has benefited from the generosity, even if promotionally orientated, of the pharmaceutical industry in making medicines available for such patients. Accordingly, there is an obligation upon companies not only to provide published information regarding the investigation of their medicinal products in unlicensed or experimental indications but also to be able to provide medical advice on how to use such compounds and under what circumstances. Information pharmacists and product physicians can, in our experience, invariably provide such information as is at their disposal without in any sense being thought to be promotional in doing so. It is important that senior medical management is on hand to assist junior professional colleagues in providing responsible and unbiased information.

12.4.3.2   Formulary packs and product monographs

It is an unfortunate fact that editors of peer-reviewed journals simply do not have the space to publish all the data that pharmaceutical companies have at their disposal in obtaining product licences, particularly when editors, as at present, are demanding the publication of negative trials and even refusing to publish trials unless they are managed independently of the sponsors by academic physicians and scientists. Equally, companies are criticised for subscribing to journal supplements or for paying to have clinical data reported in journals that operate for that purpose. Yet, when a new product is launched commercially, it is almost invariable that much of the company's database, while reported to the MHRA, is not published in medical journals that are read by the majority of prescribing physicians. The *Drug and Therapeutics Bulletin* has, on occasion, made judgements on the basis of small and statistically invalid studies in preference to listening to a company's professional staff when reviewing a manuscript. Fortunately, the MHRA and the Committee on Safety of Medicines (CSM) are more pragmatic in reviewing the totality of a product database in reaching a view as to whether a product should be licensed and made available for prescription.

Recognising the problem about the publication of data, most companies are willing to make 'data on file' available to physicians or pharmacists that ask for it, and therefore quote such data in their product information. As part of the service to their marketing colleagues, medical staff are happy to write reviews, summaries and monographs about products they have researched and know well. These documents form part of the impartial and unbiased database that companies are more than willing to make available on a non-promotional basis and are increasingly expected to provide. After all, it should be obvious to all that company medical and scientific professional staff are glad to report data for publication that they have generated and of which they have a right to feel proud.

Increasingly with the advent of drug formularies and formulary committees, companies will recognise that the ultimate hurdle is not registration of a medicinal product but acceptance and inclusion in a hospital or general practice formulary. Comparative efficacy and safety of medicines, while not required for regulatory purposes, have become part of development programmes and cost–benefit and cost–effectiveness data are increasingly expected and available. Minds are becoming focused by the need today to provide clinical and cost–effectiveness data to the National Institute for Clinical Excellence (NICE), which will then report independently. Company professional staff will become adept advocates of products they have helped to develop by writing review articles that are factual but also aimed at persuading a formulary committee to agree to include that product or product range. In cost-conscious times, it will be the articulate and thoughtful advocate who prevails, but the data will also have to be good enough!

12.4.3.3   Meetings and conferences (see also Section 12.3.1.5)

Meetings and conferences undoubtedly perform a dual purpose, being both promotional in nature as well as permitting the interchange of unbiased scientific information. If pharmaceutical companies did not provide substantial sponsorship to such meetings at both national and international level, such meetings would not occur. However, critics of pharmaceutical industry sponsorship tend to see only the opportunities for promotion provided by such events. As with all such

opportunities, it is important for both physicians and pharmaceutical companies to be reasonable. Learned societies cannot expect to have meetings funded without allowing companies to promote their products. With reasonable rules, neither expects to be exploited and both expect to benefit. It is recognised by the European Union in the drafting of the requirements of the EU Advertising Directives that without industry sponsorship of scientific meetings and attendance by doctors at such meetings, the medical community would be less well informed. In my experience, the quality of data presented as such meetings from studies that have been sponsored by companies is outstanding. None of us would wish to have poorly conducted studies reported at major international congresses. We are open to criticism by our scientific colleagues on a much too public basis.

As a pharmaceutical physician, one has to be alert to the modern methods of publication of information that, by virtue of industry sponsorship, then becomes promotional in nature. One is wise to review material, both written and verbal, that is to be disseminated as information or 'a service to medicine'. The rules require that such items report the data fairly and without bias and that if made available in support of a product as information or promotion, the relevant rules are observed (see below Section 12.5). Companies have been found in breach of the Code of Practice when so-called 'independent' speakers of known opinion have been used too frequently in support of a product.

12.4.4   Promotional information

All information supplied through a pharmaceutical company's marketing department will be regarded as promotional in nature. After all, the information would not be disseminated unless it was designed to increase the consumption of the medicinal product in question. Information can only be regarded as non-promotional, if its dissemination is supervised by the medical department and is clearly scientific and factual in nature. Even then, it should be clearly understood that information sent out by the medical department can be subject to and considered under the Code of Practice. The concept of 'promotional information' can be readily controlled and be acceptable to prescribers as unbiased information when it has been seen to be subject to medical department review and approval in the same way that promotional material is reviewed and approved. Indeed, one would advise that when scientific information is to be used on a promotional basis, for example, a scientific article or medical report, it should be clear that it is being used with the support of the medical department's review process.

12.5 Procedural Aspects Relating to Information and Promotion

Promotional activity and the dissemination of information are so closely linked that it is hard to see where one ends and the other begins. In the modern era, where many pairs of eyes are on the industry's activities, eager to criticise and to control, the only real option for companies is to conform to the rules and to play fair. I would suggest that since companies act by SOPs for their conduct of clinical trials, so it makes sense to have an SOP for the preparation and approval of ethical promotional material. If one does not create written procedures to cover the multiple steps in the preparation and approval of promotional copy, mistakes can be made and complaints may follow.

There are two stages inherent in developing promotional material: generation and approval. The creative part involves a number of individuals: the product manager, who should coordinate the exercise, the product physician, who will review the clinical data that will be referred to, the regulatory affairs professional, who should see that the material conforms with the product licence and finally a reviewer, whose knowledge of the ABPI Code of Practice is such that errors or omissions under the Code can be rectified. It is essential that all of these individuals consider the materially carefully, agree about the contents and are in accord that it can be recommended to the official signatories. While the marketing department has the right to expect that the medical department will interpret the data to permit the maximum exploitation permissible, the medical department must stand up firmly in opposing claims or statements that the data simply do not support. All of those involved in the creation of promotional material must be alert to possible misinterpretations or over interpretations that may be put upon claims and statements by the company, as well as that the material must not mislead. Protection is conferred by having several persons review and comment on what is being written; this can be documented if the process of creating the material follows a routine procedure. The procedure, whatever it is, must not be bypassed in the interests of haste, expediency or a printer's deadline, and the excessive pressure to agree must be withstood. Usually the product physician and the regulatory affairs professional have many other concurrent activities and while they must accord the reading of promotional material and its references a priority, equally they should not be pressured into agreeing with material without due time to consider it. Up to 48 h would seem a minimum for the physician to read and consider the promotional material and the accompanying referenced documents. When the regulator is involved, the MHRA allows five working days. Simple mailers may be easy to do, a new detail aid or videograph may be time consuming to get right. It is important for the product managers to use their medical and scientific counterparts effectively. One finds that the maximum of prior discussion and consultation as to what the marketing department wishes to say is valuable in avoiding mistakes. When a cherished idea is committed to paper in the absence of prior discussion, it becomes much more contentious when the medical or regulatory affairs professionals cannot agree to it. My advice is therefore to work out the steps that ought to be included, write them down as a formal procedure and then operate by that SOP.

The approvers or official signatories must also review the material and fit into the SOP. The creators may often be younger and less experienced, and the seasoned eye frequently has useful comment to make. No one should, in my view, approve a piece in the absence of agreement and consensus between the creators. If there is a dissension, it is my practice to refuse to 'sign off' on the piece until the creators have reached agreement that the piece is appropriate. One should not, in my view, adopt the position of referee between dissenting parties. If there is a disagreement about the use of words or the meaning of data, there is likely to be something wrong with the material. The approvers should send it back to the creators to resolve.

A further document that medical directors might consider writing for the benefit of their own and their marketing colleagues is an SOP or, perhaps more appropriately, a set of guidelines regarding the dissemination of promotional and non-promotional information. Again, it is important to distinguish between the two. When information is sent out from the medical department, it is usually deemed to be non-promotional and it is important if companies wish to have a trustworthy reputation that the information is truly non-promotional and factual. Information that is sent out from the marketing department is promotional by definition, irrespective of whether it is factually correct, even if not in a promotional format. Since the dissemination of information may be considered promotional and/or non-promotional, it will be useful to have either an SOP (more difficult to write) or a set of guidelines as to how information shall be provided. It is important to understand that all information sent out by the company may be subject to the ABPI Code of Practice.

It is up to individual companies via their managing, marketing and medical directors, as to how formally they wish to proceed with respect to promotional material and the dissemination of information. As a working medical director with a clear remit from the managing director to avoid complaints regarding the promotion of medicinal products, one can only state that it is very helpful to colleagues, both medical and marketing, to have an SOP and appropriate guidelines in the management of promotion and information, both of which could become key elements in the successful sales of medicinal products.

References

1. *Webster's Complete Dictionary of the English Language*. London: George Bell and Sons, 1883.
2. Harrison IH. *The Law on Medicines: a Comprehensive Guide*. Lancaster: MTP Press, 1986.
3. The Medicines Act. London: HMSO, 1968.
4. Committee of Advertising Practice. *The British Code of Advertising Practice*. London: Committee of Advertising Practice, 1988.
5. The Proprietary Association of Great Britain. *Code of Standards of Advertising Practice for Over-the-Counter Medicines*. London: PAGB, 1986.
6. Independent Television Commission. *Code of Advertising Standards and Practice*. London: ICT, 1998.
7. Radio Authority. *Code of Advertising Standards and Practice and Programme Sponsorship*. London: Radio Authority, 1991.
8. Association of the British Pharmaceutical Industry. *Code of Practice for the Pharmaceutical Industry*. London: ABPI, 1994.
9. Association of the British Pharmaceutical Industry. *Code of Practice for the Pharmaceutical Industry*. London: ABPI, 2003.
10. Council Directive 92/28/EEC of 31 March 1992. *Official Journal of the European Communities*. 1992; L113/13–18.
11. European Federation of Pharmaceutical Industries' Associations. *European Code of Practice for the Promotion of Medicines, 2nd edn*. Brussels: EFPIA, 1992.
12. International Federation of Pharmaceutical Manufacturers' Associations. *Code of Pharmaceutical Marketing Practice*. Geneva: IFPMA, 1993.
13. The Control of Misleading Advertisements Regulations (No. 915). London: HMSO, 1988.
14. The Medicines (Advertising and Monitoring of Advertising) Amendment Regulations 1999 (1999 No. 267). London: HMSO, 1999.
15. *Medicines Compendium, 2002*. London: Pharmaceutical Press, 2002.
16. The Medicines (Advertising) Regulations 1994 (1994 No. 1932). London: HMSO, 1994.
17. The Medicines (Monitoring of Advertising) Regulations 1994 (1994 No. 1933). London: HMSO, 1994.
18. The Medicines (Standard Provisions for Licences and Certificates) Regulations 1971 (1971 No. 972), as amended. London: HMSO, 1971.
19. Medicines Control Agency. *Advertising and Promotion of Medicines in the UK* (MHRA Guidance Note No. 23). London: MHRA, 1999.

20. Barnard J. *The Code in Practice*. London: J. Barnard Publishing, 2001.

21. The Proprietary Association of Great Britain. *Code of Practice for Advertising Over-the-Counter Medicines to Health Professionals and the Retail Trade*. London: PAGB, 1992.

22. National Office of Animal Health. *Code of Practice for the Promotion of Animal Medicines*. Enfield: NOAH, 1987.

23. Herxheimer A, Collier J. Promotion by the British Pharmaceutical Industry, 1983–8; a critical analysis of self regulation. *BMJ* 1990;**300**: 307–11.

24. *Code of Practice for the Pharmaceutical Industry (Clause 18.1) 2001*. London: ABPI, 2001.

25. Association of the British Pharmaceutical Industry/ British Pharmaceutical Market Research Group. *Guidelines on Pharmaceutical Market Research Practice*. London: ABPI, 1992.

26. Wells FO, ed. *Medicines: Responsible Prescribing*. Belfast: Queen's University, 1992.

27. Committee for Proprietary Medicinal Products Operational Working Party. *Note for Guidance.* *Document 111/916/90-EN*. Commission for the European Communities. London: EMEA 1990.

28. Medicines Control Agency. *Guidelines on the Summary of Product Characteristics (SPC) for Human Medicinal Products. Version 3, March 2001*. London: MHRA, 2001.

29. Council Directive 92/27/EEC of 31st March 1992. *Official Journal of the European Communities.* L1113/912.

30. The Medicines for Human Use (Marketing Authorisations, etc.) Regulations 1994 (No. 3144). London: HMSO, 1994.

31. *A Guideline on the Readability of the Label and Package Leaflet of Medicinal Products for Human Use*. Brussels: EFPIA, 1998.

32. Association of the British Pharmaceutical Industry. *The Supply of Unlicensed Medicines*. London: APBI, 1990.

33. Consumers Association. Prescribing unlicensed drugs or using drugs for unlicensed indications. *Drug and Therapeutics Bulletin* 1992;**30**:97–9.

34. Guideline on Summary of Product Characteristics. E.C. Notice to Applicants Dec. 1999.

CHAPTER 13

13 The supply of unlicensed medicines for particular patient use

Amanda Wearing and John O' Grady

The use by the medical profession of medicines with no current marketing authorisation and of authorised medicines outside the terms of their marketing authorisation raises various regulatory issues. Leaving aside use in a clinical trial, such products are also used to treat the particular clinical needs of individual patients. This is known variously as 'named patient', 'particular patient' or 'compassionate use' supply. The first of these terms is misleading, because there has never been any requirement to identify a particular patient and for the purposes of this chapter the term 'particular patient supply' is used instead.

Supply on a particular patient basis encompasses various categories of unauthorised use of medicinal products. A product may be unauthorised because it has been specially formulated for use; it may be at the clinical trial stage of development, but be requested by doctors for use outside a trial; it may have been authorised previously and then withdrawn from the market for commercial reasons, or because of safety, efficacy or quality concerns; or it may be authorised currently, but for a different indication or patient population, or in a different country.

This chapter describes the regulatory framework covering the supply of medicinal products on a particular patient basis. This framework is the outcome of the balancing by the regulators of two important but conflicting principles. On the one hand, there is the need to ensure that patients are not exposed to any unnecessary risks, hence the extensive legal framework regulating the placing on the market of medicinal products.

On the other hand, there is the desire to respect the clinical freedom of medical practitioners to determine the most appropriate treatment for their patients.

13.1 Legal Framework

13.1.1 EC law

13.1.1.1 Directive 2001/83/EC

There is only limited EC legislation dealing with the supply of medicinal products for particular patient use and there were no relevant provisions prior to 1989. Article 6.1 of Directive 2001/83/EC (previously article 3 of Directive 65/65/EEC) sets out the general rule that a medicinal product must have a marketing authorisation before being placed on the market. However, article 5, which repeats wording introduced by Directive 89/341/EEC, provides an exception from this general rule:

A Member State may, in accordance with legislation in force and to fulfil special needs, exclude from the provisions of this Directive medicinal products supplied in response to a *bona fide* unsolicited order formulated in accordance with the specifications of an authorised health professional and for use by his individual patients on his direct personal responsibility.

This provision allows Member States if they wish (there is no obligation to do so) to make national arrangements for the supply of unlicensed medicines for particular use, but only in the very limited circumstances specified by the Directive.

13.1.1.2 Volume 9 of Notice to Applicants

The only other reference at a European level appears in Volume 9 (Pharmacovigilance) of the Notice to Applicants issued by the European Commission. The Notice to Applicants does not have the force of law, but represents best practise. Paragraph 1.3.4 states:

Compassionate or named patient use of a drug should be strictly controlled by the company responsible for providing the drug and should ideally be the subject of a protocol. The protocol should ensure that the patient is registered and adequately informed about the nature of the medicine and that both the prescriber and the patient are provided with the available information on the properties of the medicine with the aim of maximising the likelihood of safe use. The protocol should encourage the prescriber to report any adverse reactions suspected of being related to use of the medicine to the company, and to the competent authority where required on a national basis. Companies should continuously monitor the balance of benefits and risks of drugs used under such conditions and follow the requirements for reporting to the appropriate competent authorities.

13.1.1.3 Regulation 726/2004/EC

Recently, changes have been made to the rules governing the centralised authorisation procedure. For the first time, there are specific provisions dealing with what the legislation calls 'compassionate use'. These are set out in article 83 of Regulation 726/204/EC.[1]

Article 83.1 states that Member States may make a medicinal product falling within the scope of the centralised procedure available for compassionate use.

Article 83.2 defines 'compassionate use' as meaning:

Making a medicinal product [falling within the scope of the Regulation] available for compassionate use reasons to a group of patients with a chronically or seriously debilitating disease or whose disease is considered to be life-threatening, and who cannot be treated satisfactorily by an authorised medicinal product. The medicinal product concerned must either be the subject of an application for a [centralised] marketing authorisation . . . or must be undergoing clinical trials.

If a Member State 'makes use of the possibility provided for in paragraph 1', it is obliged to notify the European Medicines Agency under article 83.3.

Where compassionate use is envisaged, article 83.4 states that the Committee for Medicinal Products for Human Use (acting on behalf of the agency) may, after consulting the manufacturer or applicant, adopt opinions on various matters. The matters to be covered are the conditions for use, the conditions for distribution and the patients targeted. The opinions must be updated on a regular basis.

Article 83.5 requires Member States to 'take account' of any available opinions.

Under article 83.6, the agency is required to keep and update list of such opinions and publish that list on its website.

Article 83.6 also states that Articles 24(1) and 25 (which set out adverse reaction reporting requirements for centrally authorised products) will apply to products supplied for compassionate use.

Article 83.7 makes it clear that the fact that an opinion has been obtained from the committee will not affect the civil or criminal liability of a manufacturer or an applicant.

The legislation makes specific provision for the time between authorisation and placing on the market. In some Member States, where it is necessary to obtain approval for reimbursement, this may entail a delay of some months. During this time, where a compassionate-use programme has previously been set up, article 84.8 states that 'the applicant shall ensure that patients taking part also have access to the new medicinal product'.

Finally, article 84.9 states that the operation of this article is without prejudice to the operation of the clinical trials Directive 211/20/EC and the national provisions for compassionate use in article 5 of Directive 2001/83/EC.

There is nothing in the final version of this article relating to costs. Early drafts of this article had proposed that supply should be free of charge, but this was removed and the position is therefore that companies may charge for such supplies.

There are a number of general points to note. First, the article seems to be broader in scope than article 5 of Directive 2001/83/EC, since what is envisaged is a properly coordinated, pro-active approach to use of the product (rather than a passive system relying on requests from individual doctors). Second, the provision only applies to a small category of products. For products not falling within the scope of the cent-ralised procedure, the national rules will remain and there will be no harmonisation of the con-ditions of supply in individual Member States. Third, it is not clear how the procedure will be applied as a matter of practice. The wording leaves open a number of questions on how Mem-ber States will operate this provision and, at the time of going into press, no guidance had been issued at either a national or a European level.

13.1.2　UK law prior to 1 January 1995

The UK legislation has for many years permitted particular patient supply in specified circum-stances.

The original provisions date back to the early 1970s. Under section 7(2) of the Medicines Act 1968, it was necessary to hold a product licence in order to sell, supply, export or import a medi-cinal product; to procure those activities; or for the manufacture or assembly of the product. However, various exemptions from the licens-ing requirements, including those relating to particular patient supply, were provided for in the act and in related statutory instruments. The most important exemptions were contained in sections 9 and 13 of the act, the Medi-cines (Exemption from Licences) (Special and Transitional Cases) Order 1971,[2] the Medicines (Exemption from Licences) (Special Cases and Miscellaneous Provisions) Order 1972[3] and the Medicines (Exemptions from Licences) (Import-ation) Order 1984.[4]

13.1.3　1995 onwards

Significant changes to the legal basis for the exemptions, rather than to their scope, were introduced by the Medicines for Human Use (Marketing Authorisations Etc.) Regulations 1994,[5] which came into force on 1 January 1995. These regulations disapply much of the

Medicines Act for 'relevant medicinal products', including section 7 (and consequently all exemp-tions relating to section 7). Relevant medicinal products are defined in the 1994 Regulations as those medicinal products for human use to the provisions of Directive 2001/83/EC apply. This broad definition includes most medicinal products. The exceptions are medicinal products for clinical trial use, products prepared in a pharmacy in accordance with a pharmacopoeial formula for direct supply to a patient, intermedi-ate products, registered homoeopathic products, non-industrially produced herbal remedies and some products which are not medicinal products within the meaning of the Directive, but which by order have been made subject to control under the Medicines Act 1968. For products desig-nated under such an order, the old provisions on particular patient supply are still applicable. In practice, there are very few such products.

Regulation 3(1) of the 1994 Regulations states that no medicinal product may be placed on the market or distributed by way of wholesale dealing, unless it has a marketing authorisation. This replaces the product licence requirement in section 7 of the act. The exemptions to this requirement are provided for by regulation 3(2) and Schedule 1 to the regulations. They permit supply for individual patients and also enable practitioners to hold limited supplies of stocks of unauthorised medicines. The provisions apply equally to doctors and dentists.

13.2　Scope of Exemption

The supply of unlicensed medicinal products for individual patients is governed by paragraph 1 of Schedule 1 to the regulations. The text fol-lows the wording of the Directive quite closely, although curiously it omits any reference to the requirement 'to fulfil special needs':

Regulations 3(1) shall not apply to a relevant medicinal product supplied in response to a *bona fide* unsolicited order, formulated in accordance with the specification of a doctor or dentist and for use by his individual patients on his direct personal responsibility, but such supply shall be subject to the conditions specified in paragraph 2.

The conditions specified in paragraph 2 are:

a. the product is supplied to a doctor or dentist, or for use in a registered pharmacy, hospital or health centre under the supervision of a pharmacist, in accordance with paragraph 1;

b. no advertisement relating to the product is issued with a view to being seen generally by the public in the United Kingdom, no such advertisement, by means of any catalogue, price list or circular letter, is issued by any person involved in the manufacture, sale or supply of the product, and the sale or supply is in response to a *bona fide* unsolicited order;

c. the manufacture and assembly of the product is carried out under conditions which ensure that the product is of the character required by, and meets the specifications of, the doctor or dentist;

d. written records of manufacture and assembly are made, maintained and kept available for inspection by the licensing and enforcement authorities;

e. the product is manufactured, assembled, or imported into the EU by the holder of the authorisation referred to in Article 40 of Directive 2001/83/EC [for products manufactured or assembled in the EU, a manufacturer's authorisation; for products imported in finished form into the EU, a wholesale dealer's (importation) licence];

f. the product is distributed by way of wholesale dealing by the holder of a wholesale dealer's licence.

Paragraph 3 extends the exemption to the supply of product for limited stocks, subject to a number of conditions:

1.

a. the medicinal product is specially prepared by a doctor or dentist, or to his order, for administration to one or more patients of his. Where that doctor or dentist is a member of a practice group working together to provide general medical or dental services, the proposed recipients can be the patients of any other doctor or dentist in that group; or

b. the manufacture/assembly of such stocks is procured by a registered pharmacy, a hospital or health centre, where this is done by, or under, the supervision of a pharmacist;

2. the product is manufactured and assembled by the holder of the appropriate licence (see above);

3. only limited stocks of such products are held: no more than 5 L of fluid and 2.5 kg of solid of all such products per doctor or dentist.

Paragraph 4 sets out an exemption in certain circumstances for medicinal products not requiring a prescription for sale or supply, which are prepared by, or under, the supervision of a pharmacist and are sold or supplied to a person exclusively for use by him in the course of his business for the purpose of administration to one or more persons.

Paragraph 5 contains an exemption for radiopharmaceuticals prepared from an authorised kit, generator or precursor in respect of which there is a marketing authorisation in force, subject to certain conditions.[6]

Paragraph 6 requires any person selling or supplying a relevant medicinal product to maintain, for a period of at least 5 years, records showing:

a. the source from which that person obtained the product;

b. the person to whom, and the date on which, the sale or supply was made;

c. the quantity of each sale or supply;

d. the batch number of the product sold or supplied; and

e. details of any suspected adverse reaction to the product sold or supplied of which he is aware. This does not require suppliers to search the literature for reports concerning the substance, however.

Paragraph 7 requires that person to notify the licensing authority of any such suspected serious adverse reaction and to make available for inspection at all reasonable times the records referred to in the previous paragraph.

13.3 Particular Issues

13.3.1 Advertising

Paragraph 2(b) of the schedule makes it clear that no advertisement or representation may be issued to encourage the sale or supply of medicinal products for particular patient use. Sale or supply must be in response to a *bona fide* unsolicited order from the doctor. While the paragraph prohibits issuing catalogues, price lists and circulars referring to relevant medicinal products, it does not prohibit the advertising of a special manufacturing facility, provided no specific products are mentioned. A manufacturer may also respond to an enquiry as to whether or not a particular product could be supplied.

This raises the question of whether the schedule prevents the supplier from giving the doctor at the time of supply purely factual, technical information on the use of that product. Since the rationale for particular patient supply is that the doctor has requested the product on his own accord and is acting on his direct personal responsibility, it would seem reasonable to assume that he is familiar with its use and should not need any further information. On the other hand, particularly where there is known to be significant risks associated with the use of the product, it may be prudent to issue safety information to minimise the product liability exposure of the supplier. As noted above, the provision of such information is also recommended by the European Commission in Volume 9 of its Notice to Applicants. It seems unlikely that the Medicines and Healthcare Products Regulatory Agency would consider this to be advertising, although no formal guidance has been issued on this point. If a company does decide to provide such information, it must ensure that the wording cannot be said to be an invitation to the doctor to order further supplies of the product, since that would arguably amount to soliciting subsequent orders in breach of the regulations.

In addition to the specific prohibitions set out in the regulations, companies should also have in mind the more general provisions against the advertising of unauthorised medicinal products. It is a criminal offence under Regulation 3(1) of the Medicines (Advertising) Regulations 1994[7] to issue an advertisement for a relevant medicinal product in respect of which there is no marketing authorisation in force, and under Regulation 3A, to issue an advertisement which does not comply with the particulars listed in the summary of product characteristics. These regulations implement Directive 92/28/EEC on the advertising of medicinal products for human use (now Title VIII of Directive 2001/83/EC). Corresponding restrictions upon the availability of promotional materials also appear in the ABPI Code of Practice.

13.3.2 Quantity

The regulations do not expressly impose any limit on the amount of medicinal product which the company may supply for use by the doctor's individual patients under paragraph 1 of the schedule. In view of the specific provisions upon stock set out in paragraph 3 (a total of 5 L of fluid and 2.5 kg of solid of all such products per doctor or dentist), it is likely that supply under paragraph 1 should be limited to a reasonable course of treatment for a specific patient for whom the doctor is prescribing the product. Companies should always be suspicious of large orders from doctors and enquire why such large quantities are being sought.

13.3.3 Doctor's specification

Supply must be 'formulated in accordance with the specification' of a doctor or dentist. Strictly, this means that the product should be made up, or imported, in accordance with the doctor's specification and must not be manufactured in advance of any order being received, unless that product is already on the market in a country from which it is being sourced. As a matter of practice, it is rarely the case that a product is formulated in response to a detailed specification provided by a doctor.

13.3.4 Special needs

Directive 2001/83/EC requires supply to be to 'fulfill special needs'. Curiously, this condition is omitted from paragraph 1 of Schedule 1 to the UK regulations and it is necessary to consider whether this omission has any significance. The prevailing view is that the regulations should be interpreted in a manner consistent with the Directive and that the exemption should only be available where there is no equivalent product containing the same active ingredient already authorised and on the market in the United Kingdom. This view has recently been endorsed in the Guidance Note issued by the Medicines and Healthcare Products Regulatory Agency.[8]

It is then necessary to review the meaning of 'special needs'. It is difficult to see how such needs can exist where there is a licensed version of the product on the market for the physician to use. However tempting it may be for medical institutions to save costs by requesting an unlicensed version of a licensed product, economic needs will never be special needs in this context. This accords with the rationale underlying the Directive, which requires only authorised medicinal products to be placed on the market unless exceptional circumstances apply.

The more difficult question arises where the product to be manufactured differs in some way from the licensed version. The Guidance Note issued by the Medicines and Healthcare Products Regulatory Agency states that unlicensed products which are the 'pharmaceutical equivalent' of available licensed medicinal products will not be permitted. A medicinal product will be regarded as a 'pharmaceutical equivalent' where it contains the same amount of the same active substance, in the same dosage form, and it 'meets the same or comparable standards considered in the light of the clinical needs of the patient at the time of use of the product'. In the light of this guidance, a different formulation of an authorised substance (e.g. for children or the elderly, or those with an allergy to a particular excipient) would probably satisfy the principle of fulfilling special needs.

13.3.5 Manufacture overseas

The Medicines (Exemption from Licences) (Importation) Order 1984 set out additional conditions to be complied with in the case of unauthorised medicinal products imported for particular patient supply but, as noted above, that order was disapplied by the 1994

Regulations. There were no provisions in the 1994 Regulations to parallel the 1984 Order and consequently the controls on imported unlicensed products were reduced to the level of those on products manufactured in the United Kingdom. This was clearly the result of an oversight and additional controls were reinstated in February 1999 by the Medicines (Standard Provisions for Licences and Certificates) Amendment Regulations 1999.[9]

The regulations introduce a number of amendments into Schedule 3 (standard provisions for wholesale dealer's licences) of the Medicines (Standard Provisions for Licences and Certificates) Regulations 1971.[10] The 1999 Regulations reproduce the relevant wording from the Directive (including the reference to 'special needs'). Supply of an 'exempt imported product' falling within the scope of this wording is only permitted provided certain conditions are complied with:

a. at least 28 days prior to each importation, the licence holder must give written notice to the licensing authority, together with certain specified details relating to the product, the quantity to be imported and the manufacturer/assembler/supplier;

b. if, within 28 days of acknowledgement of receipt of the notice by the licensing authority, it notifies the licence holder that the product should not be imported, the licence holder must comply with this notification; if, within this period, he has received notification that the product may be imported, he may proceed with the importation;

c. in addition to the usual record-keeping requirements for wholesale dealers, the authorisation holder must keep records of the batch number of the product and of any adverse reaction of which he becomes aware;

d. the licence holder may import on each occasion no more than what is sufficient for 25 single administrations or for 25 courses of treatment not exceeding 3 months; he must not import more than the quantity referred to in the notice;

e. the licence holder must inform the licensing authority forthwith of any matter coming to his attention which might reasonably cause the authority to believe that the product can no longer be regarded as safe for administration to human beings or as of satisfactory quality for such administration; the licence holder must cease importation or supply if he receives a written notice from the licensing authority requiring cessation;

f. the licence holder must not issue any advertisement, catalogue, price list or circular, or make any representations, relating to the exempt imported product.

13.3.6 Controlled drugs

Where the medicinal product in question is a controlled drug within the Misuse of Drugs legislation,[11] additional controls will apply. Drugs are classified in various schedules according to their perceived risk of harm. In the case of most of the products covered by the legislation, it will be necessary to obtain a licence from the home office in order to import the product from another country.

13.3.7 Patients ordering products over the internet

Where a patient orders a product for his own use direct from a supplier in another country, that will not normally be caught by the rules on particular patient supply, since the product will not be 'placed on the market'. However, it is possible that the supplier of that product (which is likely to be a prescription-only medicine) will be committing an offence in the country in which it operates, particularly if it has advertised the product or supplied it otherwise, than in response to a prescription.

13.3.8 Labelling

Confusion remains on the rules covering the labelling of unauthorised medicines. Special provisions were contained in Regulation 11 of the Medicines (Labelling) Regulations 1976.[12] The Medicines for Human Use (Marketing Authorisations Etc.) Regulations 1994 disapplied the 1976 provisions, but did not introduce replacement provisions for medicinal products without a marketing authorisation. In the absence of further legislation on this point, many companies are continuing to label their products in compliance with Regulation 11 of the 1976 Regulations on a voluntary basis.

13.3.9 Charging for supply

The regulations do not deal with this point. Companies may charge doctors for products supplied to them on a particular patient basis. There are no general Department of Health restrictions on the levels of price or price increase, as the Pharmaceutical Price Regulation Scheme only governs products with a marketing authorisation.

13.3.10 Other types of authorisations

The schedule only provides exemptions from the requirement to hold a marketing authorisation. Other activities involved in the supply of medicines on a particular patient basis need to be carried out under the appropriate authorisations.

13.3.10.1 Manufacturer's licences

Section 8(2) of the Medicines Act 1968 requires those involved in the manufacture or assembly of a medicinal product to hold a manufacturer's licence. In fact, Schedule 1 to 1994 Regulations requires the manufacturer/assembler in the United Kingdom of an unlicensed product for particular patient supply to hold a particular type of manufacturer's licence (a manufacturer's 'special' licence). It should also be noted that Section 23 of the act prohibits the manufacture of a medicinal product unless that product has a marketing authorisation, or is exempt from the marketing authorisation requirement.

13.3.10.2 Wholesale dealer's licences

Section 8(3) of the act requires those involved in the wholesale dealing of a medicinal product to hold a wholesale dealer's licence. If the product is imported from another Member State, a wholesale dealer's licence will be required. If it is imported from a country outside the European Union, a wholesale dealer's (importation) licence will be required. Schedule 1 to the 1994 Regulations confirms that these provisions apply equally to particular patient supply.

13.3.11   Clinical trials

The widest use of unlicensed medicinal products is in the course of clinical trials. It is important to distinguish between clinical trial use and particular patient use, as very different rules govern these different types of use.

The rules governing clinical trials in the United Kingdom are now set out in the Medicines for Human Use (Clinical Trials) Regulations 2004,[13] which implement Directive 2001/20/EC on good clinical practice in the conduct of clinical trials.

Clinical trials require advance approval from an ethics committee and from the Medicines and Healthcare Products Regulatory Agency. They have different manufacturing and labelling requirements.

Clinical trials are sometimes continued for an open extension period. This is permissible, provided there are genuine scientific reasons for continuing the study (rather than commercial reasons, such as attempting to create demand for the product) and that the appropriate regulatory clearance has been obtained. If the company does not wish to do this, it would be open to the doctor to request further supplies of the product, but the company must not invite him to do this. Any further supply to the doctor would then need to comply with the provisions regarding particular patient supply, unless the doctor has decided to carry out his own clinical trial.

The distinction between supply for use by particular patients and supply for use in a clinical trial is therefore important, particularly since the rules in the latter case are stricter, and companies must be certain about the basis upon which supply of unlicensed products is made. Various factors are relevant in determining the basis of supply, such as the purpose of the administration (particular patient supply is concerned with treatment; clinical trials are concerning with testing the effects of treatment), the number of patients being treated and the degree of organisation and coordination between physicians treating patients.

13.4   Product Liability Issues

Paragraph 1 of the schedule states that the supply of the unlicensed product must be for use by a doctor's or dentist's individual patients on his direct personal responsibility. Doctors should be aware of the product liability implications of using such products.

The Leaflet MAL 30, issued by the Medicines and Healthcare Products Regulatory Agency to give guidance on the provisions of the legislation affecting doctors and dentists, states that:

> It should be remembered that a practitioner prescribing an unlicensed medicine does so entirely on his own responsibility, carrying the total burden for the patient's welfare and, in the event of an adverse reaction, may be called upon to justify his actions. Under these circumstances it may be advisable for the practitioner to check his position with his medical defence union before prescribing such unlicensed products.

In theory, the practitioner, as a professional person, is able to assess the risks and potential benefits to his patient, and to decide that the balance lies in favour of the use of a particular unauthorised product. A company receiving a request from that practitioner will therefore assume that the doctor will exercise reasonable care and skill in using the product in a way that avoids causing injury to his patients. However, the principle that supply is the doctor's sole responsibility does not provide companies with total protection against liability where a patient is injured by treatment with an unlicensed product.

Companies should therefore respond with great care to requests for unlicensed products from practitioners, bearing in mind that there is no legal obligation to comply with such requests. If they do not act with caution, those companies risk becoming involved in a negligence claim, or in a product liability action under the Consumer Protection Act 1987 for supplying a defective product (one which does not provide the safety which persons are entitled to expect, taking account of all the circumstances, including the information supplied).

Where a company suspects that the product is to be used in a way that is not safe for patients, its duty to those patients may involve warning the doctor that it considers the proposed use to be hazardous and, if necessary, refusing or terminating supply. While there is no general obligation to provide product information with unlicensed medicines (and, as noted above, the use of promotional material is prohibited), from a product liability standpoint, the provision of basic safety information about the product is a sensible precaution.

At the operational level, manufacturers must apply proper care and rigorous quality control during production, to ensure that they supply unlicensed medicinal products of the highest quality. They must also have in place proper systems for dealing with requests for particular patient supply and for keeping all the necessary records.

Companies are advised to have in place a standard operating policy for dealing with requests for particular patient supply, even though this can never act as a guarantee against a patient making a claim at a later stage. As part of this, it is useful to have a standard physician consent form, highlighting the unlicensed status of the product and reminding the requesting physician that he has a personal responsibility for his use of the product.

In Guidance Note 14, the Medicines and Healthcare Products Regulatory Agency states that hospital trusts, health authorities and independent hospitals should have clear policies on the use of unlicensed medicines, explaining liability considerations and requiring all those involved in the supply chain to ensure that the unlicensed status of a product is communicated and fully understood.

Doctors are, of course, under an obligation to inform their patients adequately about proposed treatments, but a company may be concerned that a patient may not know that he is being treated with an unlicensed medicine. One option would

be for the company to provide a form for patients to sign, recording their consent to treatment with the unauthorised product. As a matter of English law, such a consent form could not exclude the manufacturer's liability for personal injury for negligence or under the Consumer Protection Act 1987.[14] Nevertheless, it might be helpful in qualifying the patient's expectations of safety from the product.

13.5 Conclusion

There are compelling pragmatic reasons for allowing the supply of unauthorised medicines for particular patient use. Doctors are able to select the treatment that they consider most appropriate for each patient, even though that treatment may not have a marketing authorisation. Companies are permitted to respond to requests for such products, provided that they, and the doctors, comply fully with the provisions of the Medicines for Human Use (Marketing Authorisations etc.) Regulations 1994. Where the product in question can cause serious adverse reactions or requires very careful monitoring, the company must ensure that it takes particular care, in order to avoid liability in negligence or under the strict liability provisions of the Consumer Protection Act 1987. Any failure to comply with the 1994 Regulations would be regarded unfavourably in any such litigation.

References

1. These will come into force on 20 November 2005.
2. The Medicines (Exemption from Licences) (Special and Transitional Cases) Order 1971 (SI 1971/1450).
3. The Medicines (Exemption from Licences) (Special Cases and Miscellaneous Provisions) Order 1972 (SI 1972/1200).
4. The Medicines (Exemption from Licences) (Importation) Order 1984 (SI 1984/673).
5. The Medicines for Human Use (Marketing Authorisations Etc.) Regulations 1994 (SI 1994/3144).
6. Medicines (Administration of Radioactive Substances) Regulations 1978 (SI 1978/1006).
7. The Medicines (Advertising) Regulations 1994 (SI 1994/1932).

8. Guidance Note 14: The supply of unlicensed relevant medicinal products for individual patients.

9. The Medicines (Standard Provisions for Licences and Certificates) Amendment Regulations 1999 (SI 1999/4).

10. The Medicines (Standard Provisions for Licences and Certificates) Regulations 1971 (SI 1971/972).

11. The Misuse of Drugs Act 1971; the Misuse of Drugs Regulations 2001 (SI 2001/3998).

12. The Medicines (Labelling) Regulations (SI 1976/1726).

13. The Medicines for Human Use (Clinical Trials) Regulations 2004 (SI 2004/1031).

14. Unfair Contract Terms Act 1977, section 2; Consumer Protection Act 1987, section 7.

CHAPTER 14

14 Legal and ethical issues relating to medicinal products

Christine H Bendall and Christopher JS Hodges

Other chapters in this book deal with the evolution of the legal controls over medicinal products and the structure of the European Union regulatory systems set up to authorise business activities and dealings in these products, and to enforce the rules and restrictions the law places upon them. This chapter aims to select some specific legal and ethical issues that arise in relation to product development, authorisation and sale and supply both within the United Kingdom and within the context of the European systems.

14.1 The Chronology of Production, Development and Marketing

The laws and ethical codes that apply to the various stages of pharmaceutical product development are aimed at controlling and placing limits upon defined activities, thereby maximising the protection of the public. In practice, these objectives are supported not only by powers granted to competent regulatory authorities to enforce compliance with medicines laws through compulsory action, but also by the application of relevant principles of the general criminal and civil law.

14.1.1 Development

In the course of product development, testing in both animals and humans is subject to varying degrees of legal control, supplemented by a significant quantity of ethical or 'good practice' guidelines.

14.1.1.1 Animal testing

The legal controls on animal testing were introduced at the European level by a Directive in 1986.[1] The central objectives cited in the formulation of the controls were: to avoid disparities in the controls applied across Member States that might affect the functioning of the common market, and also to limit to a minimum the number of animals used in product development whose use was necessary to meet testing requirements, and to ensure, as far as possible, the best care and treatment of the animals during the conduct of the research and in the method of their disposal.

'Whereas such harmonisation should ensure that the number of animals used for experimental or other scientific purposes is reduced to a minimum, that such animals are adequately cared for, that no pain, suffering, distress or lasting harm are inflicted unnecessarily and to ensure that where unavoidable, they should be kept to a minimum. Whereas, in particular, unnecessary duplication of experiments should be avoided'.

In summary, Directive 86/609/EEC requires the premises in which animal research is undertaken and persons conducting such research, to be subject to local registration and inspection and imposes limitations upon the breeding and supply of experimental animals. There are specific provisions regarding the care of experimental animals, including, for example, minimum caging and temperature requirements. As a Directive, 86/609/EEC required implementation in each Member State to take effect at national level (cf. Regulations which are immediately effective at national level without the need for national legislative or administrative action). Therefore, the systems for applying the requirements of the Directive do vary from country to country; the function of the Directive being to achieve a harmonisation of the principles, aims and objectives to be achieved at local level. Accordingly, enforcement, monitoring and inspection are all matters of local control and design.

In the United Kingdom, by the time of the adoption of the Directive, the authorities had already introduced legislation for the control of animal experimentation in the form of the Animal and Scientific Procedures Act 1986. Its content and coverage was already relatively comprehensive of the requirements set out under the Directive, and so relatively little needed to be done to bring the UK law in line with the European provisions.

The conduct and control of animal experimentation are matters that give rise to strong public feeling. During 1996/1997, extensive UK media coverage of the conditions in testing facilities put the issue of experimentation and effective controls in the public eye. For the product developer using external facilities to generate the preclinical data necessary to make an application for a marketing authorisation, the cost and time of the developmental process is too high for risks to be taken with the acceptability of data for regulatory purposes, whether generated in animal or human experiments. Delays are always costly. Under the European rules[2] (Directives 75/318, 65/65, 92/25, 75/319, 92/28 are now consolidated into Directive 2001/83) specifying the content of a market authorisation application, compliance with testing rules is essential because the preclinical data that are submitted must have been generated from studies complying with 86/609 EEC and with *Good Laboratory Practice*.[3] Under the latter, compliance with the animal testing directive is mandatory. Any evidence to suggest that the data have not been properly generated will allow a competent regulatory authority to discount them in the evaluation of the application.

It is now a well-known theme in European pharmaceuticals legislation that the use of animals should be minimised as far as possible:

'The Commission and Member States should encourage research into the development and validation of alternative technologies which could provide the same level of information . . . . . .' (86/609/EEC Article 23).

The climate of public opinion is strongly supportive and there are several initiatives looking at the potential for conducting tests *in vitro*, where an animal model may previously have been used, but may not be essential to generate useful data. The law tends to follow developments in public moral/ethical thinking and it is not surprising, therefore, that the same theme arises in different sectors of the European law. In the cosmetic sector, for example, the use of animals for further substance testing is now prohibited. In the pharmaceutical sector, however, a complete ban, at least for the foreseeable future, would be highly unlikely where there is no other means of generating the required data. However, the inadequacy of most animal models for predicting human response is a recurrent issue and inescapable fact. Accordingly, many of the provisions concerning the generation of preclinical data, and particularly those set out in the Annex to Directive 2001/83/EEC [as amended (the Annex specifies the requirements for the content of an application for a marketing authorisation in the EU)], leave considerable discretion to the developer to design and justify studies appropriate to the product concerned. In many cases, it is possible for the applicant to justify objectively the omission of certain studies, or the conduct of studies in only one, rather than two, species. The conduct of tests simply for the sake of following a 'traditional', or general, approach without evaluating what the product and the objective justify is wasteful and may not be either scientifically, morally or legally justified.

14.1.1.2   Testing in human beings

The conduct of clinical research in humans raises numerous legal and ethical issues of significant importance. After a lengthy process of gestation, the European Commission has now officially adopted a Directive on clinical research.[6] At the time of writing this chapter the Directive has been implemented in most Member States. Interpretation and enforcement, will remain a local matter. The extent to which the Directive has had a truly harmonising impact upon clinical trial regulation across the European Union is debateable. Variation in the implementation of EU Directives is common and will complicate the conduct of multicentre, multinational research projects, with the associated impact on costs and time.

Arguably there has been greater progress in the development of international ethical practice guidelines.

The development of good research practice guidelines (which were *not* legally binding) began following the Nuremberg Trials, with the Nuremberg Code being published in 1949.[7] The basic principles contained in the Code were designed to protect the well-being (physical and mental), personal rights and integrity of research subjects, asserting the individual's fundamental right to choose whether to become involved in the research. The later Declaration of Helsinki (amended on several occasions, most recently in 2000) followed in 1964,[8] and established international principles for appropriate research practice. The Declaration also distinguished between research that had the potential for therapeutic effect in the volunteers recruited and research conducted for the greater good, that is, the expansion of knowledge without the expectation of direct benefit to the human volunteers. Significantly, in 1975 the Declaration was amended to include the requirement for research projects to be subject to independent ethical review.

From this and other guidelines have developed current principles of good clinical practice ('GCP') centred on ethical review by committee, with a favourable opinion being at least a moral precondition of the commencement of any human research project. In 1989, the CPMP (the Committee for Proprietary Medicinal Products) adopted GCP guidelines (based on a previous 1987 version) for the European Union. Although they were not in themselves legally enforceable, the pharmaceutical industry saw compliance with the guidelines as a means of ensuring that they met the requirements of what was then part four of the Annex to Directive 75/318/EEC nonconsolidated within Directive 2001/83/EEC to submit clinical trial data that had been obtained in compliance with 'GCP'. In some Member States (e.g. The Netherlands), the guidelines were actually incorporated into local legislation. The EU-wide guidelines have since given way to an international guideline (in use since 17/1/97) developed within the International Conference of Harmonisation (ICH), to which European Union, United States of America and Japanese regulators and industries subscribe.[9] It is specifically mentioned in the Clinical Trials Directive, although it is not specifically adopted as the GCP standard by the Directive. The Commission has recently introduced further GCP legislation.

Directive 2001/20/EEC was designed to address the functioning, structure and funding of ethics committees across Europe. In the United Kingdom, prior to 1st May 2004 as a matter of law, it was not a universal requirement that all research (whether concluded for the purposes of obtaining a marketing authorisation by or on behalf of a pharmaceutical company, or by doctors/academics) should be subject to prior ethical review. In fact, there was relatively little law concerning ethical review, or the way in which research itself is conducted. UK law focused instead upon regulating the activities of production of clinical research supplies, labelling and distribution and upon the sponsor (or responsible doctor) having obtained a form of clearance from the competent authorities, usually in the form of either a clinical trial exemption certificate ('CTX') or a doctor's and dentist's exemption certificate ('DDX'). Neither of these authorisations was conditional upon ethical review, and there was only one mention of the review process in the CTX provisions,[10] where the refusal (and presumably withdrawal) of ethical approval had to be notified by the holder to the authorities (although the consequences of this notification are not spelt out). This situation changed with the implementation of the Directive by the Medicines for Human Use (Clinical Trial) Regulations 2004. There are now extensive provisions relating to the requirement for and obtaining of an ethics committee opinion and regarding the establishment and registration of ethics committees.

As mentioned, pharmaceutical company-sponsored research conducted in the United Kingdom (and other Member States) for purposes of regulatory submission has always been affected by the requirement formerly in the Directive 75/318, EEC that the data derived from studies in humans, which are submitted as part of an authorisation application, must have been generated in a study conducted according to standards of 'GCP'. Although the Directive itself does not specify the version of GCP to be followed – and there are several around the world – the ICH guidelines are currently the obvious yardstick in Europe against which to judge the adequacy of the conditions and manner in which research is conducted (especially as the new Directive also cross-refers). Indeed, in the absence of further EU legislation on GCP, the United Kingdom decided to make reference to the ICH guidelines in its implementing legislation. This reference to ICH was to be modified when the GCP Directive completed its legislative process. The sanction provided by the law is that the competent authorities may discount any data not generated in accordance with good practice standards during their evaluation of a product. (This would clearly include studies that had not been ethically reviewed.) In the case of a pivotal study, this could be crucial to the success of the application, and therefore constitutes a strong incentive to comply with the practice standards set out in the guidelines. GCP is also relevant in the context of any claims for personal injury. In the assessment of whether negligence has occurred, compliance with accepted practice guidelines is relevant to judging whether a sponsor (or investigator) has acted reasonably or in a manner that falls below accepted current standards of conduct. As stated, law and ethics coincide in their aim to protect the interests of volunteers recruited for clinical research purposes. The issues of consent, confidentiality and access to compensation for personal injury tend to be uppermost in the minds of lawyers and ethicists.

14.1.1.3 Consent

In both legal and ethical terms, the consent of an individual to his/her participation in research is fundamental. There are few exceptions to this 'golden rule'. The Directive (Articles 3–5) and the UK implementing legislation lay down a specific requirement for the consent of the trial subject or his/her 'legal representative' to participation in any 'clinical trial' (as defined) widely by the legislation. In the United Kingdom, failure to adhere to the principles on GCP, which include the requirements for consent, is a criminal offence. Failure to obtain consent could also give rise to civil claims for damages, for example, on the basis of assault and battery, or trespass to the person. Failure adequately to inform a participant about a study may undermine the consent given and constitute negligence, for which, again, a claim for damages in respect of any personal injury suffered as a consequence may lie. In these cases, the individual would have to show that the receipt of more complete information would have resulted in their withholding consent, thereby avoiding exposure to the risk of the hazard that in fact materialised.

For consent to be legally valid, a volunteer (or legal representative) must be competent to assess the proposed research and to make a considered decision. They must be properly informed, (the term 'informed consent' is often used although, strictly speaking, tautologous, it is not possible to have consent that is legally recognised, which is uninformed in the legal sense) that is, they must have been given 'sufficient' accurate information to appreciate the nature of the study, what would be involved in participation, and what hazards and level of risk attach to the project in question. The decision must be made voluntarily without the exertion of any pressure, or influence from other persons. There must be no incentive offered that would encourage an individual to agree to what, in other circumstances, he/she would refuse. Reliable 'evidence' that a consent process has been properly followed and consent properly obtained, is valuable for legal and ethical reasons. The Directive defines informed consent as a 'decision which must be written' [Article 2(j)] and makes consent in writing the norm, except in 'exceptional cases as provided for in national legislation' [Article 3.2(d)].

There are, of course, some cases where the consent of the trial subject cannot be obtained. This may be because the individual is not competent to make a decision, either because of some mental illness or intellectual deficit, or because of injury resulting in unconsciousness. The legislation addresses the position of both incompetent minors (under-16s in the United Kingdom) and incompetent adults, setting specific conditions that must be met and the requirements for obtaining the consent of a legal representative. In the United Kingdom, the concept of a legal representative who may consent on behalf of an incompetent adult is a new one and applies only in the field of research and not, as yet, in relation to cases of treatment and therapy.

The rules in the United Kingdom for consent on behalf of minors to participation in research are now different from those that apply to consent to treatment. The law in relation to research classifies minors as under 16 years and requires the consent of a person with parental responsibility or other legal representative, although the 'explicit wish' of a minor should be considered by an investigator, there are no 'Gillick competent' minors capable of consenting in their own right in the legislation.[11] [In the Gillick case (concerning the prescribing of contraceptives to teenage girls) the UK courts accepted that minors might be fully capable of consenting in their own right to treatment procedures, provided that in the view of the doctor concerned, they had grasped the nature of the treatment and its potential benefits and risks and were sufficiently mature intellectually and emotionally to make a judgement.]

14.1.1.4 Confidentiality

It is a clear ethical principle that the privacy of the individual should be respected and maintained. The law too, both in common law (i.e. judge-made law) and through certain statutory provisions (specifically Member States' implementation of the 1995 Directive on the protection of personal data 95/46/EEC)

recognises a right to confidentiality in personal data. In the United Kingdom, there have been practice rules[15] within the NHS (National Health Services) for several years and more recently, legislation has been enacted (to address issues concerning health data stored in special registries and databases) concerning the treatment and confidentiality of medical records. All electronically recorded data must be stored and handled by persons/institutions registered under the Data Protection Act of 1998. The 'processing' (widely interpreted) of such data must be done in compliance with the principles of good practice that the Act lays down. The Clinical Trials Directive makes specific the need to adhere to the rules of personal data protection in the clinical trial context [Article 3.2(c)].

At common law, a right to confidentiality can arise either because of: (1) the nature of the information, (2) the circumstances in and conditions upon which it is imparted, or (3) the status of the person to whom the information is given, for example, a doctor. The concern is with data that identify an individual, or from which an unnamed person could be identified. The common law upholds the right to confidentiality by providing that disclosure of confidential information, without the consent of the person concerned, is a breach of that right and may be subject to civil penalty (e.g. damages or even an injunction to prevent disclosure, i.e. breach). In cases where the maintenance of confidentiality in certain data is a contractual obligation, such as in employment contracts, a breach of confidence may lead to disciplinary action and/or loss of employment. Professional codes of conduct may also give rise to other sanctions (e.g. General Medical Council proceedings).

There are a few circumstances in which confidentiality will not be deemed to have been breached so as to give rise to legal sanctions. These include situations where disclosure is warranted as a matter of public interest, and also where disclosure is ordered within court proceedings, etc.

In the context of research in individuals, all personal data should be safely and securely stored and handled. Confidentiality should also be assured by ensuring that no publication of study results includes any identifying, personal information with regard to study subjects. Participants should be well aware, from the outset, of the extent of disclosure that will be necessary with regard to their 'sensitive' personal data, to whom it will be disclosed and for what purpose, and should agree to this when they sign a consent form after being given full information about the project. Where the subject agrees to disclosure to identified persons, disclosure will not constitute a breach of confidence. For this reason, specification of the scope of disclosure, the purpose, and the types of people who may need to have sight of trial data, is extremely important. With express consent, there is no issue with regard to breach of an individual's confidence. However, in some cases data obtained may subsequently have value in the context of a different piece of research. The issue then is whether the consent obtained was sufficiently broad to cover use for the further purposes. This will be a matter of the wording used previously (and, possibly, what might be implied), but consent is referable only to the matters disclosed (whether specifically or generally) to the individual. In most research, where individuals are recruited to a study, issues of confidentiality should not create practical, ethical or legal problems. However, in pure records-based research, where gathering large numbers of individual consents is not practical and in the absence of specific enabling provisions in legislation, there remain issues surrounding the protection of confidentiality. Anonymisation of data is a possible solution.

14.1.2 Compensation – liability issues

Ethical evaluation of a study automatically involves consideration being given to the provision made for the payment of compensation (if any), and the basis upon which it may be payable to a subject injured by participation in proposed research. The Directive makes it a prerequisite of conducting a trial that 'provision' for insurance or indemnity has been

---

Box 14.1 Criteria for negligence

$D + L + F + C = N$

Duty of Care	Owed to the claimant
+**L**ack of reasonable Care	Evidenced by a failure to conduct a project according to accepted standards applicable at the time breach of regulatory requirements, failure to take account of or apply (industry) guidelines
+**F**oreseeable Injury	Of the type likely to occur, for example, side-effect of the drug
+**C**ausation	The act(s) or omission(s) constituting the alleged lack of reasonable care must have caused/contributed to the injury
=**N**egligence	

---

made [Article 3.2(f)]. The basis of legal liability for personal injury generally falls under two headings: (1) negligence and (2) so-called 'strict liability'.[16] Each of these causes of action requires certain elements to be proved (i.e. all of them) (Box 14.1) before the legal claim can be established and damages obtained. This can be a difficult process for a claimant, particularly in terms of proving causation, that is that it was participation in the research that, on the balance of probability, caused the alleged injury.

In the United Kingdom and a number of other Member States there are industry guidelines or professional/ethical codes under which making specific compensation provision for research-related injuries is addressed (for example ABPI in the United Kingdom).[17] In other Member States there have been specific legal provisions in place with regard to the compensation of research subjects[18] for some time and also with regard to the means of ensuring that adequate funds are available to meet such claims, such as by insurance.[19] In practice, in the United Kingdom there has never been a case of a claim for personal injury arising in the context of research that has reached trial conclusion. Where potential claims arise in industry-sponsored research (which is relatively uncommon), experience indicates that they tend to be dealt with under the ABPI (1991 Compensation, or 1988 Healthy Volunteers Research) Guidelines resulting in, where appropriate, settlements at financial levels that would have been ordered by the court had the matter gone to trial.

Most UK ethics committees will look for confirmation of the intention to apply the ABPI guidelines in the case of company-sponsored studies, even from non-member companies. Where the research is 'non-therapeutic', ABPI guidance provides for a contractual promise to be made to the volunteer to pay for injury sustained by reason of participation in the study (whether due to the experimental drugs used or to procedures required by the study protocol), irrespective of whether anyone conducting or responsible for the project was at fault. In 'therapeutic research', no such contractual relationship or obligation is required, and there are some limitations to the circumstances in which voluntary payment will be made.

In the absence of any 'no fault' scheme, the participant who suffers injury and believes it to be trial related must rely only on his/her ability to claim compensation through the courts – often a difficult and lengthy process. Most ethical guidelines require a study participant to be told in advance, what provision has been or will be made – if any. However, in practice some ethics committees are unhappy that there are different approaches applicable to compensation in research, depending upon the identity of the sponsor/initiator.

14.2 Contractual Arrangements in Clinical Research

14.2.1 The legal background

The arrangements made for the conduct of clinical research will usually give rise to a number of legal contracts. For example, there will be a contract between a sponsor and any appointed clinical research organisation (CRO); between the

---

Box 14.2 Criteria for strict liability

$D + D + C = SL$

Defect
  Widely defined

  – product design defect
  – manufacturing error
  – deficiency in 'presentation'
  (for example poor/ incomplete information)

  so that the product is less safe than persons generally would be entitled to expect

+ **D**amage
  To persons (or property) flowing from the defect

+ **C**ausation
  see Box 14.1: there must be a link between the defect and the alleged injury

= **S**trict **L**iability

---

sponsor or CRO and the investigator and/or the institution in which the investigator works.

It would be unusual for there to be a contract between a patient participant and the sponsor or investigator, although this may arise where the participant is a private patient of the investigator. However, in the United Kingdom, in non-therapeutic research that is conducted in accordance with ABPI guidelines, there would normally be a written contract between the sponsor and the participant in which the obligations on both sides are recorded, including the undertaking by the sponsor to provide compensation to a research subject in the event of trial-related injury, irrespective of fault.

Under English law, it is not necessary that a contract should be in writing for it to be legally enforceable (unless the sale of land is involved). Therefore, an oral agreement, perhaps even by telephone, between a sponsor, CRO or investigator may be perfectly valid and enforceable, although, in practice it may be very difficult to prove what the terms of an agreement concluded in this way had been. Individual recollection in such circumstances will generally differ.

However, there are certain legal tests that must be satisfied before any agreement may be deemed to be legally enforceable. The requirements are:

1. *It must be an agreement.* The normal approach to determining whether an agreement has been reached is to identify whether an 'offer' has been made by one party and accepted, on its terms, by another. The test is objective. Communications that are merely preliminary, such as requesting or giving information, or constituting merely an 'invitation to treat' (i.e. encouragement given to another to make an offer), do not constitute an offer.[20] The acceptance must be a final and unqualified expression of agreement to the terms of the offer.[21] Acceptance may be by conduct,[22] but must be communicated to the offerer. A rejection terminates an offer. A counter-offer is also a rejection of the initial offer.

2. *There must a certainty of terms.* The terms of the agreement must be clear and enable the parties to ascertain and perform their obligations.

3. *There must be 'consideration'.* As a rule, a promise is not binding in English law unless it is either made under seal or supported by some form of 'consideration'. In simple terms, both parties must each be bound to contribute 'something of value'. This is usually money, goods or services,[23] and it is normally not difficult to identify the consideration flowing between the parties to commercial transactions. In the context of clinical research, a sponsor will, among other promises, provide information, pay fees and disbursements and provide product, and the investigator will give professional services.

4. *There must be an intention to create legal relations.* The parties must intend their agreement to be legally binding. This is not usually an issue in commercial transactions.

Although it can simplify matters, particularly if a query or dispute arises, if the legal contract is contained in a single document, this is not essential. An agreement may be contained in more than one document. Quite often, for example, a research agreement will cross-refer to a protocol and SOPs that are to be treated as incorporated into its terms. The important matter is that the

relevant documentation is adequately identified and accessible.

In order to provide minimum standards, certain terms are implied by law into any contract for the supply of goods or services[24] unless they are expressly excluded. The actual terms of the agreement may 'exceed' the minimum standards implied. For example, it would be implied by statute that services supplied in the course of a business must be carried out with reasonable care and skill and within a reasonable time. These terms may be substituted by more specific terms of agreement between the parties or by a course of dealing.

One further basic point, which is an important principle in contract terms, is that in general (although there have recently been some changes in the law) the law applies a doctrine of 'privity'. That is, a contract only binds the parties to it, and only the parties (or their appointed representatives or legal substitutes) may enforce or sue upon the agreement. This means that a contract between sponsor and CRO does not bind the investigator or any other person.

14.2.1.1 Standard contract terms

In contracts relating to clinical research – in effect between a sponsor, CRO or investigator/institution – much of the detailed provisions concerning precisely how the research will be conducted will be contained in the trial protocol. If there is no other document that constitutes the legal contract, the terms set out in the protocol will generally be taken to form or will be implied into the oral agreement to conduct the study. However, proper practice is to have a specific agreement, contained in a separate document, which includes a term that the study will be carried out in accordance with the protocol, identified by its title, date and individual reference number (as it may be amended from time to time, by written agreement between the parties).

There is no prescribed format for clinical research contracts. Although there is an agreed template in use in the United Kingdom agreed between industry and the NHS applicable to research sponsored by companies conducted within the NHS. In some situations, it may be inappropriate to use standard-form documents. A standard form must always be adapted to fit the particular study. However, the following are a non-exhaustive checklist of points that might be considered for inclusion in a contract:

14.2.1.2 Study details

1. The protocol should be incorporated by reference into the contract.
2. The protocol must not be deviated from, except (1) as agreed in writing between the parties and approved by the ethics committee, (2) or where, in the opinion of the investigator, it is necessary to do so immediately in order to protect the health and safety of a research subject.
3. A 'key person' clause should be considered. This might specify that identified individuals, or a certain number of staff with specified minimum qualifications, will work on the study, perhaps exclusively.
4. The contract should address whether the CRO or investigator is allowed to subcontract any of their obligations and, if so, which of them.

14.2.1.3 Compliance

1. A specified party must hold or obtain (and maintain) all necessary authorisations, for example, under the UK Medicines for Human Use (Clinical Trial) Regulations 2004, and subordinate/related legislation, the Data Protection Act 1998 and the Animals (Scientific Procedures) Act 1986.
2. All legal and regulatory requirements (including on labelling) must be complied with.
3. Compliance with the ICH *Good Clinical Practice Guidelines* (incorporates the Declaration of Helsinki) or equivalent should be required.
4. The investigator must obtain ethical approval from relevant ethics committees before beginning the study and refer all amendments.
5. The study must be carried out to the highest professional standards.
6. Identified SOPs must be observed.
7. All clinical data generated must be recorded properly and promptly. The data and case report

forms will be complete and accurate; amendments to be made only according to agreed procedure. Appropriate secure storage must be provided for all study records.
8. Provision for monitoring and audit of study site and ongoing cooperation and liaison between sponsor, monitor and CRO/ investigator must be made.

14.2.1.4 Timing

1. Start date, duration/end date should be identified. The terms should identify at what point the study will be considered concluded, for example, upon delivery or finalised agreed trial report.
2. The number of subjects to be recruited by specified dates should be addressed (it is difficult to be too specific in this regard however).
3. The options if the recruitment rate is not on target.
4. Provision for making status reports, providing interim analysis reports and submitting the final report by specified dates should be made.

14.2.1.5 Data

1. Save for the purposes of the study and as required by law, the data must be kept confidential.
2. Retention of title by specified parties (in particular the sponsor) in identified documents and materials should be spelled out.
3. Protection of the intellectual property rights of the sponsor must be covered.
4. The investigator's right to publish the anonymised results, subject to affording the sponsor reasonable notice and other conditions (e.g. method of analysis to be used) must be addressed.
5. Arrangements for maintaining safety and security of data, documents and trial supplies should be identified. An archiving provision should be included consistent with GCP; the investigator will maintain all records relating to the study, including case report forms, for as long as is practicable.
6. Rights of access to, removal or delivery of the data, documents, samples and materials must be specified.

7. Responsibility and procedure for notification of Adverse Drug Reactions (ADRs) or other unexpected or unusual occurrences in compliance with the legislation needs to be described.

14.2.1.6 Payment
The contract should specify:

1. The amounts and timing (advance, stage or interim and final) of payments and the payment of reasonable expenses/disbursements.
2. Whether separate accounts are to be established, for example, for payments due to investigators, passing through a Case Report Forms (CRO).
3. Provision for alteration of budget in the event of amendment of the protocol, and/or extent of services to be provided, and early termination.

14.2.1.7 Materials

1. Supply of the investigator brochure, updates, product and documentation by the sponsor. (CRO may produce study documents such as CRFs must be comprehensively set out.)

14.2.1.8 Product liability
In relation to liability issues, the contract should cover:

1. Indemnity to be provided by the sponsor for any liability costs and expenses of the investigator arising out of personal injury claims, subject to conditions (see below).
2. Indemnity by the CRO or investigator in favour of the sponsor in respect of negligence, malpractice or breach of contract by the CRO or investigator.
3. Observance of applicable local guidelines, for example, ABPI in the UK.
4. Financial provision for handling of claims (e.g. insurance arrangements).

14.2.1.9 Termination
Appropriate provision for termination, especially early termination, is essential:

1. On specified grounds; sensible to provide for termination by the sponsor on notice without reason, but subject to the obligation to pay for work done at that point.
2. The rights of termination, if any, consequent upon a breach of contract by either party should be described.
3. Termination upon the insolvency, administration or liquidation of either party, or long-term suspension of the agreement due to 'force majeure' (i.e. circumstances beyond the control of either party) should be addressed.

14.2.1.10 General
A number of 'boiler-plate' clauses are also needed including:

1. The law of the country that is to govern the agreement.
2. Submission to the jurisdiction of the courts of a particular country in relation to any disputes. Possibly a clause specifying that disputes will be resolved by arbitration.
3. Notice – methods of effecting notice and contact points.
4. Signature of the contract by authorised signatories.

14.2.2 Indemnities

It would be normal practice for a company-sponsor to indemnify an investigator in relation to any claim for compensation for personal injury that may be made against the investigator by a research subject in the event of trial-related injury or death, except for claims resulting from the malpractice or negligence of the investigator or his staff.[25] In the early 1990s in the UK, the ABPI, the Department of Health and some health authorities agreed upon a standard form indemnity for clinical studies in relation to research carried out by, or involving, NHS or NHS trust employees, equipment or facilities.

This standard form provides that if a claim should be made, the sponsor will indemnify and hold the relevant health authority/trust/institution and its employees and agents harmless against all such claims (1) brought by, or on behalf of, research subjects taking part in a study, and (2) arising out of, or relating to, the administration of the product(s) under investigation, or any clinical intervention or procedure provided for or required by the protocol, to which the subject would not have been exposed, *but for* his/her participation in the study. Among other things it is conditional upon compliance with the protocol, there having been no negligence or other default on the part of the investigator, staff, institution, etc., and upon the sponsor being promptly informed of claims (actual and potential) and having the right to conduct them.

14.3 Postauthorisation – controls and protection of investment

14.3.1 Regulatory controls

After a product has been authorised, the regulatory system operates to keep the quality, safety and efficacy of that product under review and to control the way in which it is manufactured, marketed and distributed. The pharmaceutical legislation in Europe has recently been consolidated and, pursuant to Commission consultation and review, amended. The majority of the amendments are due to come into effect in November 2005. What follows, reflects the state of legislation as at close of 2004.

Manufacturers of medicinal products (this includes those who undertake full or partial manufacture of the product, and those who package or 'assemble' the product) must have manufacturing authorisations and are subject to regular plant and system inspections where they are judged against appropriate standards, in particular good manufacturing practice (GMP) rules under European Directive 2003/94/EEC. Any subcontracting undertaken by a manufacturer of a manufacturing process (or any part of it) must be subject to a detailed technical agreement between the parties, setting out the specification for the work subject to contract and the responsibilities, as they are divided between the parties, so as to ensure that all aspects of the process are properly conducted in compliance with the legal and regulatory requirements.

Those operating at wholesale level must similarly hold an appropriate authorisation[27] and

are also subject to inspection to ensure that they are operating in accordance with legal requirements, including good distribution practice ('GDP') rules established under Directive 2001/83/EEC (Article 76–85). Specified paperwork and records must be kept (in particular to facilitate tracing of product and batch recall) and proper systems and operating procedures adhered to.

For the marketing authorisation ('MA') holder, there are numerous obligations and conditions attaching to the authorisation and, as with all authorisations held under pharmaceutical legislation, failure to comply will give rise to the imposition of regulatory sanctions. Enforcement measures are pursued at local level.

Increasingly there is a tendency in European pharmaceutical legislation to assign compliance duties to an identified service or a particular individual operating on behalf of, or within the MA holder's organisation. For example, a manufacturer must have 'permanently and continuously at his disposal' a 'qualified person' whose personal responsibility it is to test product and certify it as performing to the authorised specification before it is placed on the EU market. In some Member States, where breach of certain regulatory requirements is subject to criminal sanction, this approach has an obvious 'advantage' in terms of enforcement and in encouraging compliance. For example, MA holders must have a person who will take responsibility for the system for conducting pharmacovigilance and safety monitoring of the MA holder's products in the market. This involves collecting and reviewing data, making reports to the competent authorities, and generating corporate decisions about how best to respond to signals arising as a result of safety monitoring (e.g. whether to make labelling changes to include new or stronger warnings, contraindications, precautions, etc.) or whether a problem warrants the restriction of the product in the marketplace (e.g. sales to hospitals and specialist clinics only) or the total or partial removal of the product from the distribution chain.[28]

MA holders must also establish 'within' their organisation an information and scientific service to serve the needs and requirements of the

competent authorities and healthcare professionals using, prescribing and supplying product.[29]
Although the legal text does not require the naming of a specific individual, none the less the
identification of the service and its location and
capabilities is becoming part of the information
requirements of the competent authorities in considering the suitability of an application for an
MA, and of the applicant as a potential MA
holder. (See Notice to Applicants Part IIA, of
the Rules Governing Medicinal Products in the
European Union.) The trend in pharmaceutical
legislation (designed after all to try to achieve
levels of harmonisation across Member States
in the interests of promoting free movement of
pharmaceutical goods) is to streamline the production and sale of product and to ensure that the
responsible party is accessible to the authorities
and readily identifiable within the Community.

14.3.1.1 Safety

Since the introduction in 1995 of new procedures for the authorisation of products in the
European Union, the handling of product safety
crises has essentially become a European Community matter, handled at community level.
Under 'New Systems', serious concerns with
regard to product safety where the product is
on the market of more than one Member State,
will be considered at European level: centralised
product issues are automatically a matter for the
European Medicines Evaluation Agency (EMEA)
and therefore the CPMP (including its working
parties) and, in respect of products that may have
been authorised nationally (including through
mutual recognition), the legislation (Regulation
2309/93 and Directive 2001/83/EEC) provides
for references to the CPMP for the resolution of
European concerns and the implementation of an
EU-wide solution.

14.3.1.2 The relationship between local and European laws

All national legislation must be consistent and
read in line with European legislation. National
legislation that is at odds with European law
cannot generally be relied upon locally. EC law

now covers almost all aspects of pharmaceutical development, manufacture and supply.
However, there is still variation in the approach of
Member States to the determination of whether a
product is a 'medicinal product' falling within the
European pharmaceutical legislation, or should
be classified as some other product type, such as
a food or cosmetic, despite the existence of the
definition of 'medicinal product' in Article 1.2 of
Directive 2001/83/EEC. Within the Community,
it remains possible to see the same products
accorded different categorisations and therefore,
supplied subject to different constraints, in different Member States.

14.3.1.3 Advertising, labelling and legal status

There are specific sets of European controls,
implemented by national laws, concerning
product advertising, labelling and leafleting, and
their legal status for purposes of supply (see
Directive 2001/83/EEC Titles VIII, V and VI,
respectively).

14.3.1.4 Advertising

Directive 92/28/EEC first introduced European
controls on the advertising of medicinal products
for human use. Particular concerns involved the
moderation of advertising directed at members of
the public and the setting of high standards with
regard to advertising and promotion directed at
'healthcare professionals' (a term that is broadly
interpreted in the United Kingdom to include,
e.g., administrators with purchasing responsibility in hospitals and clinics). The Directive also
sought to limit the supply of free samples by
companies, and to ensure that companies had
the resources to provide objective information
to those healthcare professionals who required
it. It also required Member States to set up systems through which to monitor and enforce the
advertising controls.

The important first principle with regard to
advertising and promotion is that it cannot
be undertaken in respect of any unauthorised
product. Not only does this include products
in respect of which there is no authorisation to

market at all, but it also means that there can be no advertising of products for unauthorised indications: for those purposes, products are treated as being without a registration.

Further, the term 'advertising' is very broadly defined (see Article 86.1 2001/83/EEC) and the intent behind an activity – that is, whether it is 'designed to promote the prescription, supply, sale or consumption of medicinal products' – is material in assessing an activity or printed material. Certain items are specifically excluded from the scope of the Directive: labelling and package leaflets; correspondence and material of a non-promotional nature needed to answer a specific question about a product; factual and informative announcements; reference material relating to pack changes; adverse reaction warnings, etc.; and statements concerning health and disease that are not referable (even indirectly) to individual medicinal products.

There can be no advertising to the public of products available on prescription only or that are intended and designed for use only with the intervention of a medical practitioner. There are also restrictions on the indications that may be included in advertising destined for the general public. (For e.g., references to tuberculosis, STDs, cancer and diabetes, among others, are prohibited.) There can be no supply of samples to the public for promotional purposes. The Directive also produces a very significant list of 'don'ts' with regard to the content of advertising material.

Some of the more controversial provisions are contained in the sections of the Directive relating to advertising to health professionals, and in particular the extent to which pharmaceutical companies may support and sponsor pharmaceutical conferences and offer hospitality, gifts, etc. in the promotional context. The fundamental limitations that the EC legislation introduces include the following.

1. All advertising to health professionals must include certain 'essential information compatible with the summary of product characteristics or SPC'.
2. Medical sales representatives must be given adequate training and must have SPCs available

for the products they promote at all visits to medical practitioners. They are also under an obligation to pass on information they receive with regard to the use of the product, and in particular suspected adverse reactions, to their employers.
3. No gifts, 'pecuniary advantages' or benefits in kind may be supplied to healthcare professionals 'unless they are inexpensive and relevant to the practice of medicine or pharmacy'.
4. Hospitality available at sales promotions must always be 'reasonable' in level and secondary to the main purposes of the meeting. It may be offered only to healthcare professionals.
5. No healthcare professionals may solicit or accept inducements prohibited by the Directive.
6. Hospitality may be offered at events for professional and scientific purposes provided it is reasonable in level and subordinate to the scientific objective of the meeting. Again, it cannot be extended to persons other than healthcare professionals.
7. There are limits on the number of free samples for prescription-only products that may be left with practitioners each year, and in any event, these must be supplied in response to a written request from the recipient.

The current trend in the United Kingdom is for regulators to seek to take a restrictive line in the enforcement of advertising controls. In the United Kingdom, it has long been the case that the Association of British Pharmaceutical Industry (for 'ethicals' manufacturers) and the Proprietary Association of Great Britain (for the over-the-counter products manufacturers) have each participated in a voluntary 'system' of advertising review, monitoring and control. In the case of the ABPI, which has its own detailed Code of Advertising Practice, a quasi-judicial process was introduced for reviewing and dealing with complaints against member companies with regard to advertising practices. In more recent years, this has given rise to the Prescription Medicines Code of Practice Authority (now independent of the ABPI), to whom complaints are directed, whether from industry, practitioners or other individuals. The PAGB is organised to pre-vet advertising and promotional material with a view to averting breaches of advertising rules in the United Kingdom. Advertising regulations to implement EC law were introduced into the United Kingdom in 1994.

14.3.1.5 Labelling

The leaflets and labels Directive, 92/27/EEC, now part of Directive 2001/83/EEC, was introduced as part of a large package of legislative measures in 1992. It established a requirement for patient information leaflets to be placed in all product packaging, and specified the content and the order of the content for such leaflets. The introduction of the requirement produced an ongoing debate about the language used and the scope of information supplied to patients. The function of a leaflet is potentially two-fold: to help a patient to recognise the fact and to cope with the consequences in the event of side effects or problems arising, but also to allow them to decide whether to take or continue to take a product in the light of information provided. The Directive also introduced specific requirements for the labelling of external, 'immediate' and container packaging for all pharmaceutical products, with the particular concern that the patient should be able to identify the responsible source of the product within the European Community.

However, the provisions with regard to labelling do allow for differences to arise between labels for products destined for different Member States. The variation in material is intended to be located in one place on a product label, which has come to be known as the 'blue box'. Within the blue box, Member States are allowed to require information about the price of the product, reimbursement conditions, legal status and other information that goes to product 'identification and authenticity'. This permissive aspect of the Directive is notable, as it means that even in relation to products that have been authorised through the centralised procedure, where the authorisation is in all other respects identical, it is rarely possible to produce one label that (when translated) is acceptable and appropriate for every Member State in which the product will

be marketed. It also tends to make less attractive the multilanguage label, where the combination of two or more languages and the different information required in the blue box, make design and printing overly complicated, expensive and/or impractical.

So far as the United Kingdom is concerned, the leaflet and labelling requirements are incorporated into UK law through Statutory Instrument 1994 No 3144, otherwise known as the Medicines for Human Use (Marketing Authorisations, etc.) Regulations of 1994. Under Regulation 4, *'every application for the grant renewal or variation of the UK marketing authorisation for a relevant medicinal product shall be made in accordance with the relevant Community provisions ... and the applicant shall comply with so much of the relevant Community provisions as include obligations on applicants as are applicable to the application or the consideration of it'*. Under Regulation 7 *'every holder of a UK marketing authorisation for a relevant medicinal product shall comply with all obligations which relate to him by virtue of the relevant Community provisions including in particular obligations relating to providing or updating information to making changes to applying to vary the authorisation to pharmacovigilance and to labels and package leaflets'*. This represents a fairly common approach in the United Kingdom to the implementation of European legislation, which is either to cross-refer to the relevant European provisions, as here, or to 'import' the text of the European provisions directly and without alteration into the relevant implementing local statutory instrument. From a legal point of view, this approach can give rise to some difficulties in the event of complaints or disputes, as the drafting of European legislation is undertaken on a rather different basis from that in the United Kingdom, where a very literal approach is taken to the interpretation of precise wording. By contrast, European provisions are written more loosely and are intended to be read in line with the stated rationale of the legislation (i.e. the recitals in the Directive or Regulation), rather than by strict reference to the wording used. It is a fact of life that the implementation of European legislation can result in rather different provisions across Member States, each of which interprets the legislation according to its own understanding.

From a liability point of view, MA holders need to bear in mind that the way they present a product (not just its standard of manufacture or inherent design), both to the professionals and to patients, whether through direct advertising to patients of OTC products or through the label and patient information leaflet, is an area upon which focus will be placed in the event of a claim for personal injury that appears to have been caused or contributed to, by shortcomings in product presentation. Such shortcomings can amount to a 'defect' in the product and/or to a manifestation of negligence, and could be sufficient to justify a claim for damages.

14.3.1.6   Status

In the UK Directive 92/26/EEC (now part of Directive 2001/83/EEC) made a relatively minor impact on the matter of assigning legal status to products for supply purposes across the Member States. It laid down the criteria to be applied to determining whether a product should be on prescription only (or subject to restricted limited supply) or available without prescription. It otherwise continued to allow Member States to preserve multi-tier categorisation of product, such as applies in the United Kingdom, where a product may be prescription only pharmacy only or on 'general sale'.

14.3.1.7   Litigation

In recent years, the healthcare industries have seen a very high level (relatively speaking) of personal injury suits (often multiparty), with claims based both on negligence and under the Consumer Protection Act 1987 (which implemented the Product Liability Directive of 1985). However, the cases tend to be complex scientifically, with causation being a particular issue, both as to the general and to the specific arguments, that is, can the product in question cause the injuries alleged and, if so, did the product cause the injuries in the specific case? The changes made in the United Kingdom to the process of litigation pursuant to the Woolf Report, the

increasingly controlled availability of legal aid and conditional fees will all have an impact upon the incidence of claims in years to come. However, in ensuring regulatory compliance, in determining corporate policy and practice, and in all aspects of manufacturing and sales, companies seek to limit the public's exposure and hence their exposure to the risks of avoidable personal injury.

14.3.2   Protecting investment

14.3.2.1   Intellectual property

There are other aspects to the maintenance of a product in the market. The ability to protect and recoup investment is vital if new products and the development of existing products are to be sustained. Intellectual property rights provide various methods of protecting products and can be an important and a valuable asset in providing legitimate barriers against domestic and foreign competition.

The principal method of protecting 'novel' products and processes is by patents. A patent confers an absolute monopoly on the holder, in the territory for which it is granted, but in order for the patent to be valid, everything covered by the patent claim must be a new invention. In Europe, patents generally last for 20 years from the date of application, whereas in the United States the period is 17 years from the date of grant.

The adoption and registration (where possible) of trademarks is another important commercial decision. Any words or symbols, and in some cases colour codings (e.g. the SK & F speckled capsules), that identify the goods of one manufacturer or trader and that are distinctive of those goods may be protected. A trademark may be registered in respect of goods or of services, but will generally be protectable only if it is used, or is to be used, in the course of trade by the owner. Even an unregistered trademark can confer a level of protection upon its holder, who may be able to bring a 'passing-off' action against a competitor using the mark in order to benefit from the reputation built up by its owner.

Copyright applies automatically to literary and artistic works, including industrial designs, plans and drawings. In the pharmaceutical industry, copyright is likely to be of relatively minor importance compared to the levels of protection afforded by patents or registered trademarks. It may, however, be relevant to the packaging used for pharmaceutical products, both as to the layout (artistic copyright) and to the text itself. The right exists to prohibit the unauthorised copying of the whole or a substantial part of a protected copyright work.

Finally, registered designs should be mentioned, although they are of little relevance to pharmaceutical products themselves. Nevertheless, it may be possible to obtain a degree of protection for some goods by registering the designs for the packaging in which they are sold, or the shapes of the products themselves.

It should be borne in mind that European law applies a doctrine of 'exhaustion of rights' in relation to the use of intellectual property rights. In effect, once the right has been used by its owner, for example to put a patented product on the market in a Member State, the owner may not assert that right to prevent the product moving round the Community thereafter. This principle limits the circumstances in which these rights trade in the EU for example in relation to parallel imports.

14.3.2.2   Patents in the United Kingdom

In order to be patentable a product or process must:

- Be new
- Involve an inventive step
- Be capable of industrial application and
- Not be otherwise excluded.

To be new, the invention must never have been disclosed publicly in any way, anywhere, before the date on which an application for a patent is filed. This may be checked in advance by searching trade and technical journals and patent specifications or by filing a patent application with relatively broad claims and leaving it to the Patent Office to make its search through such 'prior art'.

To have an inventive step the invention, when compared with what is already known, that is,

the 'state of the art', must not be obvious to someone with good knowledge and experience of the subject – generally referred to in the trade as the person 'skilled in the art'. Further, it must be capable of being 'industrially applied', and must therefore be either an apparatus or device, a product or substance, or an industrial process or method of operation.

Various things are excluded from patentability, for example, a mathematical method, a scientific theory or a mere discovery. New animal or plant varieties are also excluded from being patentable at present in the United Kingdom and the rest of Europe (though not in the United States), although this is an area in which policy and law are developing under the challenge of new technologies. Also excluded are methods of treatment of humans and animals (e.g. by surgery or therapy) and diagnostic methods, these being deemed to be not 'capable of industrial application'. Nevertheless, a patent may be obtained for the use of a substance/composition in any such method, if this use is otherwise novel and inventive. Microbiological processes and products of microbiological processes are patentable, as may be novel genes and other DNA molecules.

14.3.2.3   Application for a patent

Applications can either be made separately in every country where protection is sought – a process that is both costly and time consuming – or under one of the international conventions that exist. The one most relevant to UK applicants is the European Patent Convention (EPC). Under this, an application is made to the European Patent Office in Munich, designating the signatory states in which a patent is required. This replaces the procedures in the National Patent Offices and results, upon acceptance of the application, in separate national patents in each of the designated states. All European Community Member States are parties. It should be noted that there is no single patent available for all the European Community countries: a so-called 'Community Patent' is envisaged for the future, but is still some way off.

Another convention is the Patent Co-operation Treaty, to which the United Kingdom is a party along with members in both North and South America, Africa, Asia and the Pacific, as well as most of the EPC countries and other European countries. This facilitates, making many national applications by filing in the single Patent Office. Thereafter, the individual national procedures operate independently, leading again to separate national patents.

Generally speaking, every patent application must include sufficient disclosure of the invention for it to be capable of being put into practice by the person 'skilled in the art' after its expiry. The price of temporary monopoly is the disclosure of the invention for later general use. There is invariably a considerable delay between the date of filing an application and the eventual patent grant, during which the relevant examining officers make searches and report any relevant prior documents they may find to the applicant. He may then amend his specification to take these into account to avoid claiming what is known or obvious, and make a further examination of the specification as amended to ensure it meets the requirements of novelty and inventive step.

As already mentioned, a patent gives the patentee a monopoly protection during its life, but it is up to the patentee to enforce his rights by detecting whether someone is infringing the patent, and then initiating legal action if the matter cannot be settled.

14.3.2.4   Trademarks in the United Kingdom

A trademark is a means of identifying the origin of goods or services. It is a symbol, whether in words or a device, or a combination of the two, that a person uses in the course of trade so that his goods may be readily distinguished by the purchasing public from similar goods of other traders. To achieve this, the trademark must be distinctive in itself. Broadly, the more descriptive a trademark is in relation to the goods to which it is applied, the less distinctive it is likely to be. The more a mark is likely to fall into common use by persons trading in goods of a similar description, the less likely it is to be distinctive. Therefore, trademarks that are increasingly used as generic descriptions of classes of goods generally lose their special qualities and protection as trademarks.

Registration of a trademark confers a statutory monopoly over the use of that trade mark in relation to the class of goods for which it is registered (e.g. pharmaceuticals), and the registered owner has the right to sue in the courts for infringement of that mark by a person seeking to apply it, or something confusingly similar to it, to his own goods/services. Because registration confers this statutory monopoly, it is clear that it would not be right to allow the registration of trademarks that are identical, or that can be confused with words or symbols, which other traders in the same class of goods should be free to use in the ordinary course of business.

Goods and services are divided for registration purposes into classes, in respect of which a mark may be registered. Pharmaceuticals fall within Class 5, but the scope of many of the classes (of which there are 42) is very wide. Class 5, in fact, covers pharmaceuticals, veterinary and sanitary substances, infant and invalid foods, plasters, material for bandaging, material for filling teeth and dental wax, disinfectants and preparations for killing weeds and destroying vermin.

A separate application has to be made to cover the goods in each class. Across the European Union, each mark must be separately registered for the appropriate class or classes of goods in each individual country, either according to the applicable procedure or through the recent 'Community trade mark' registration system.

In many cases it will not be possible to obtain a registration of the same trade mark in all countries, for various reasons, such as the existence of conflicting marks already held by others in those countries, or owing to unfortunate associations arising in particular languages. This variation in registration opportunities means that the same product may be marketed in different parts of the European Community under different trade marks, for example Septrin and Eusaprim.

14.3.2.5 Supplementary patent certificate

Patent protection under general law usually lasts for up to around 20 years. This creates a difficulty in relation to medicinal products, as it can take some 12 years for the products to undergo research, development, the extensive clinical trials that are required in order to obtain a marketing authorisation and the authorisation process itself. These steps are also extremely expensive. The amount of time that remains during which the patent holder can exploit his patent and recoup his massive investment can be severely curtailed in relation to medicinal products. For this reason, the European Community has provided a form of additional patent-related protection for medicinal products authorised within the European Community, by means of a Supplementary Protection Certificate.[30] A patent holder may apply for a certificate that takes effect at the end of the term of the basic patent, for a period equal to the period that elapsed between the date on which the application for the basic patent was lodged and the date of the first authorisation to place a product derived from the patent on the market in the Community, reduced by a period of 5 years. The maximum duration of the certificate is 5 years. The certificate applies to all medicinal products derived from the basic patent, but the additional time that can be obtained under the SPC is calculated in relation to the *first* product derived from the patent, authorised in the EU.

Example	Product A
Patent application	1990
Patent granted	2000
First MA in the EU	2004

SPC: 2004–1990 – 14 years less 5 years
Leaves SPC of 9 years, rounded down to the maximum 5 years, to run from 2010.

14.3.2.6 Market exclusivity

Irrespective of patent law, the MA holder may be afforded a period of marketing exclusivity under the European regulatory provisions, that is, a period of freedom from competition and competitors, who do not themselves propose to generate and submit their own full data set in order to obtain an MA. A company that applies for an MA will be required to produce the results of pharmacological and toxicological tests and the results of clinical trials at the cost of considerable time and expense, unless:

1. The holder of the original MA consents to the authorities referring to his data in order to evaluate the second application; or
2. Detailed references in published scientific literature are sufficient to demonstrate that the constituents of the product have a 'well-established medicinal use', with recognised efficacy and an acceptable level of safety; or
3. The 'second' product is 'essentially similar' to a product that has been authorised within the Community for not less than either 6 or 10 years (as determined by the Member State; always 10 years for high-technology products).[31]

The general effect of the latter provision is to afford the holder of the 'first' marketing authorisation a period of marketing exclusivity for 6 or 10 years, irrespective of the patent position,[32] during which time the second applicant cannot make an MA application and enter the market unless he produces the full data required under Directive 2001/83/EEC.

These provisions have been consistently controversial and ambiguous, and as a result have been much litigated upon. They were designed to acknowledge and reward the innovator who goes to the time and cost of researching a product and producing a full data package, but their interpretation varied across the Community and the scope of the 'protection' has been constantly the subject of, arguably limiting, ECJ decisions. Changes to these provisions are a specific and significant part of the revised pharmaceutical legislation due to come into effect at the end of 2005 (see Directive 2004/27/EEC and Regulation 726/2004/EEC).

14.3.2.7 Exemptions from authorisation requirements

As a matter of law, there is very little in the European pharmaceutical legislation dealing with licensing exemptions. Directive 2001/83/EEC Article 5 merely states that: *'The Member State may in accordance with legislation in force and to fulfil special needs exclude from the provisions of this Directive medicinal products supplied in response to a bona fide unsolicited order formulated in accordance with the specifications of an authorised healthcare professional and for use by his individual patients on his direct personal responsibility.'* Therefore, all licensing exemptions with regard to marketing authorisations are determined at local level. In the United Kingdom, they are to be found in Schedule 1 to Statutory Instrument 3144 of 1994 that 'rewrote' large parts of the Medicines Act 1968 in order to bring UK legislation in line with European rules. European law does not address exemptions from holding manufacturing or wholesale distribution authorisations and, where these are necessary to enable supplies to be made to fulfil 'special needs', they are dealt with as a matter of local provision.

As a matter of law, activities that fall within the exemptions and comply with all the criteria and conditions upon which the exemptions operate will be lawful, but as a matter of policy, there are certain circles of thought which believe that to utilise available exemption provisions for large-scale supply is not within the 'spirit' of the exemptions. There is certainly a strong argument that exemption provisions are to allow manufacture and supply in response to needs that are 'special' in that they cannot be met through the use of products already authorised and available on the market.

In the United Kingdom, manufacturers who provide special products must have an authorisation allowing 'special manufacture'. A wholesale distributor will not be in breach of wholesale distribution rules and conditions if he handles a 'special' product, provided that there is no departure from the terms of the rules. The exclusions facilitate 'compassionate use' programmes where product is not authorised, either because it is still at the experimental stage or because it has been withdrawn from the market (for commercial or for safety reasons); or the product may simply never have been intended for full-scale

marketing, as it meets the needs of a very small population only or may not be amenable to large-scale manufacture.

From a liability point of view, although the legislation and comments made by the licensing authority in the United Kingdom (in a Medicines Act leaflet, MAL8, dealing with the doctors' and dentists' exemption) highlight the responsibility of the practitioner choosing an unlicensed option in order to treat his patient, clearly the manufacturer and supplier must also be concerned with the quality of the product, seeking to avoid manufacturing defects and concerned with the accuracy of any labelling, including instructions for use, warnings, etc. that may be supplied with the product.

Although the legislation assumes that a doctor requiring a 'special' has made a clear decision and has evaluated the product and its use in the patient(s) concerned, it seems clear from a liability standpoint that if a company has information relevant to the safe and effective use of a special product, it should supply that scientific/factual information to the practitioner. Moreover, it is not acceptable for a company to make a supply despite reservations it may have about the intended use of the product. In circumstances such as these, both the regulatory and the product liability considerations would demand careful reconsideration of a decision to supply product, and may dictate a refusal.

Notes and References

1. Animal Testing Directive 86/609/EEC.
2. Directive 2001/83/EEC Annex (as amended).
3. 'GLP': Directive 87/18/EEC.
4. Directive 2001/20/EEC.
5. Nuremberg Code – Trials of war criminals before Nuremberg Military Tribunals under Control Council Law No 10 Vol 2 (Washington DC: US Government Printing Office 1949).
6. Declaration of Helsinki (amended 1975, 1983, 1989, 1996 and 2000). World Medicinal Association Inc. Ferney-Voltaire, France.
7. ICH guideline: adopted in the EU by the CPMP 135/95/EEC.

8. CTX SI 1981 No 164, now replaced by SI 1995 No 2808; The Medicines (Exemption From Licences) (Clinical Trials) Order.

9. *Gillick -v- West Norfolk and Wisbech* AHA (HL) [1986] AC 112.

10. The Protection and Use of Patient Information HSG 96 (18); See also Caldicott Report, December 1997 and Protecting and using patient information – A manual for Caldicott Guidelines 1999 (as amended), HSC 1998/089.

11. Product Liability Directive 85/374/EEC and Consumer Protection Act 1987 (UK). NB. In some EU countries, claims under the Directive and its implementing legislation can not be made in relation to investigational medicinal products.

12. Guidelines for Compensation in Clinical Trials (1991) (ABPI); The Use of Healthy Volunteers in Research (ABPI 1988) as amended.

13. e.g. in Ireland.

14. Spanish Law No. 25 of 1990 and subordinate Decrees.

15. *Harvey v Facey* (1893) AC 552.

16. *Peter Lind & Co Ltd v Mersey Docks and Harbour Board* [1972] 2 Lloyds Rep 234.

17. *Harvey v Johnson* (1848) 6 CB 305.

18. *Currie v Misa* (1875) LR 10 EX 153.

19. Supply of Goods and Services Act 1982.

20. ICH guidelines: Clause 5.8.

21. See Directive 2001/83/EEC Title VII.

22. See both Regulation 2309/93 Articles 19 *et seq* and Directive 2001/83/EEC Articles 101 *et seq.*

23. See Directive 2001/83/EEC Article 98.

24. Regulation 1768/92.

25. Regulation 2309/93.

26. Although it was open to Member States to decide not to allow an exclusivity period to run beyond patent expiry.

CHAPTER 15

15 The safety of medical products

A Peter Fletcher and Susan Shaw

15.1 Introduction

In this, the fifth edition of this textbook, the title of the present chapter has been changed to 'The Safety of Medical Products' in order to include devices which are now included in the remit of the Medicines and Healthcare Products Regulatory Agency (MHRA). It has also been decided to revise the chapter so as to reflect more closely the current needs of the pharmaceutical physician whose experience may have been entirely in the field of clinical medicine.

The pharmaceutical industry presents many new challenges to such a person which include the interface with pharmacy and pharmacology, toxicological research, human volunteer studies, clinical trials and post-marketing surveillance to name just a few. Product safety is a factor which impacts on all of those endeavours and the pharmaceutical physician will be expected to work and provide advice within that framework. It will be clear to anyone that evidence of lack of safety in a medical product is not good news for the company concerned and that some level of protective action will often be required which in extreme circumstances may involve product withdrawal. It is, therefore, essential that the pharmaceutical physician should be absolutely clear what constitutes lack of safety in relation to the intended use of the product.

Unfortunately, the public perception of such concepts as safety, risk, hazard, tolerance, toxicity, etc. are notoriously inconsistent in that the same person may consider a drug unacceptably hazardous if it is associated with serious adverse reactions that are slightly more frequent than 1 in 10 000 exposures and yet they will go hang gliding at weekends without a qualm. On the other hand, patients with troublesome joint pain may be willing to take high doses of non-steroidal anti-inflammatory drugs (NSAIDs) even though their pain poses minimal risk to life whereas the drug may rarely cause a fatal outcome from gastrointestinal (GI) haemorrhage.

Nevertheless, pharmaceutical physicians will have to take in their stride these irritating whims when they are faced with a new publication describing 20 cases of cardiac dysrrhythmia apparently triggered by their drug. Dealing with such a problem will require careful judgement based upon a comprehensive review of all the available evidence. Experience tells us that almost always jumping to conclusions is unwise, whether that is a declaration of the product's 'complete' safety or instant withdrawal from the market.

What is 'safe' may be quite different from the points of view of the patient, the doctor in charge of the case, the regulatory authority or the pharmaceutical company. Responsibility for ensuring acceptable safety lies mainly with the the pharmaceutical company and/or the licence holder who may or may not be the same. However, to a not inconsiderable extent, that burden is shared by the regulatory authority which determines the granting of marketing authorisation and the terms under which the product may be used. The doctor trusts the drug development capabilities of the company and the judgement of the licensing authority when he prescribes the product within the terms of the licence. The patient trusts the doctor to prescribe the product appropriately. Sometimes the effect on the patient is an adverse reaction which is out of proportion to any amelioration or cure of the condition being treated. The cause and consequences of such an event may lead to much arduous work for the pharmaceutical physician.

At one end of the spectrum, the event may be a simple dosage problem which could be an error on the part of the prescriber or an unanticipated hypersensitivity for that particular patient. At the other end of the spectrum, is an uncommon, serious adverse reaction not revealed in pre-marketing clinical trials. Somewhere between those two extremes are more or less serious adverse events which are not entirely unexpected but appear to be more common than is accepted for comparable products in the same therapeutic category. This may be a real increase in frequency or may be due to patient selection bias. The later has arisen with new products which claim a lower incidence of certain adverse reactions which encourages doctors to prescribe them preferentially for patients who have suffered such reactions with older products.

15.2   The Concept of Safety

All activities in life are associated with some level of risk, although in most circumstances the potential dangers are so small that we are unaware of their existence.[1] For example, when, on a sunny day, we take a stroll along a sandy beach listening to the distant cries of seagulls and the gentle sound of waves lapping on the shore the awareness of danger (risk) is far from our minds, and yet a boulder may fall from the cliff above us and have serious consequences. There is no such thing as absolute safety, and we live in a world where we continually make judgements on the level of risk we are willing to accept.

This inconsistency also applies to our perception of risk associated with medicinal products, even though most are remarkably safe. This is not the impression given by reports in the popular press and in television programmes which purport to provide the public with a factual view of medicine but which in fact emphasise the most sensational aspects and spread alarm. A useful review of safety and risk may be found in *The BMA Guide to Living with Risk*,[2] which brings into perspective the dangers encountered in everyday life.

The Office of Health Economics has also published a review entitled *What are My Chances Doctor?*[3] which takes into account not only treatment by drugs but also the hazards of surgery. People perceive risk in many different ways that would seem to the objective scientist alarmingly irrational. The distinction between risk and hazard has been nicely illustrated by Ferner[4] (Figure 15.1), who has defined risk as 'the probability that a particular adverse outcome occurs during a given quantum of exposure to a hazard'.

The risks of dying in any particular year (Table 15.1) from a variety of causes gives some idea of the relative risks of a variety of life events, but in the case of drugs it is not only death that is a concern: it is the possibility of survival with long-term or permanent disability. The mortality risks from a number of diseases (Table 15.2) make useful comparisons when considering the relative risks of taking medication. Similar tabulations of the risks associated with life events (Table 15.3) in the United States shows the estimated effects of certain common activities when continued for defined periods of time.

In a somewhat arcane context, Chapman and Morrison,[5] in the scientific journal *Nature*, have provided a list of comparative risks of death in the United States (Table 15.4) from a number of causes. The purpose of their paper was to assess the hazard of an asteroid or comet impact on the earth. Such an event does not immediately come to mind when considering the safety of medicines, but according to their estimates the chances of being killed by an asteroid/comet impact are about the same as dying in an air accident, which

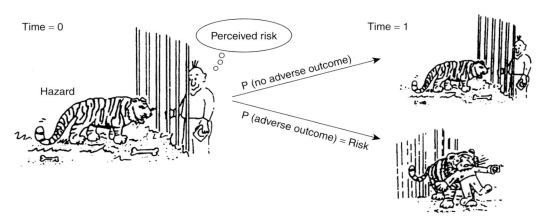

Fig. 15.1 Hazard and risk. The tiger behind bars is the *hazard*, as it could lead to harm. The *risk* is the probability that an adverse outcome will occur in unit time, or for some other specified denominator, such as 'per caged tiger'. The *perceived risk* is the man's intuitive estimate of the risk. He may *express* it ('more dangerous than crossing the road') or *reveal* it, by avoiding the tiger's cage, even if he risks falling into the penguins' pool.

is about 1 in 20 000. This is, of course, a somewhat misleading figure because it refers to an extremely rare event that carries the probability of killing many thousands of people at one time; however, it is interesting that the risk of death from chloramphenicol is about the same.

15.2.1 The quantification of risk

A previous Chief Medical Officer in the United Kingdom has expressed concern that the public's perception of risk with respect to adverse drug reactions (ADRs) is not consistent with other kinds of risk to which people are exposed on a day-to-day basis. In a paper entitled 'Risk Language and Dialects', published in the *British Medical Journal*, Calman and Royston[6] proposed a logarithmic scale for risk probabilities that may be relevant in the United Kingdom. This is probably a good way of presenting numerical information that covers a very wide range of values, even though the concept may be rather too mathematical for the general public. We live in an age in which people are constantly reminded of the many hazards they may encounter, and the media waste no time in sensationalising all manner of disasters. The fact that there is no such thing as zero risk is curiously difficult to transmit, in spite of the fact that virtually every action we

take involves some kind of hazard. Calman and Royston[6] advocate the idea of 'negligible risk' even though it begs the question of what is negligible in any particular situation. Griffin[7] has commented on the Calman paper and questioned whether or not risk assessment is an achievable goal. If serious concern exists with respect to fatal or life-threatening adverse reactions occurring at a rate of 1 in 50 000 to 1 in 100 000, then there are very few drugs with prescription volumes sufficiently large for such reactions to be detected even under the most favourable circumstances. Moreover, it is not simply the perception of level of risk that is difficult to convey realistically to patients, but also the severity of an adverse reaction. These problems are compounded by the fact that everyday life frequently involves appreciably greater risks than those posed by treatment with drugs. People do not stop driving cars, riding motorcycles, taking skiing holidays or smoking even when they know the risks they are taking.

If the risk of death from a road traffic accident is taken as some sort of 'gold standard' then we have to assume that most people are willing to accept a 1 in 10 000 chance of death in a single year, or 1 in 300 over a lifetime without great concern. So how does this picture match up with people's view of medicines?

Table 15.1 Risk of dying in 1989 in England and Wales by cause

Cause	In 1989	Due to a given cause
Any cause	1 in 88	1 in 1
Disease of the circulatory system	1 in 190	1 in 2.2
Neoplasm	1 in 350	1 in 4
Accident and violence	1 in 3000	1 in 33
Motor traffic accidents	1 in 10 000	1 in 130
Poisoning by drugs	1 in 30 000	1 in 330
Toxic effect of carbonmonoxide	1 in 40 000	1 in 450
Fire and flames	1 in 90 000	1 in 1000
Poisoning by antidepressants	1 in 160 000	1 in 1899
Homicide	1 in 180 000	1 in 2000
Toxic effect of ethanol	1 in 420 000	1 in 4800
Railway accidents	1 in 700 000	1 in 8000
Poisoning by salicylates	1 in 800 000	1 in 9500
Assault by poison	1 in 4 200 000	1 in 48 000
Any cause	2 in 88	2 in 1

Source: Based on 1989 Mortality Statistics for England and Wales. DH2 No 16, Office of Population Censuses and Surveys.

Table 15.2 Selected mortality risk levels, England and Wales 1984

Cause	Number of deaths in 1984	Probability of mortality
All causes	566 881	1.0×10^{-2}
Cancers	140 101	2.8×10^{-3}
Coronary heart disease	157 506	3.2×10^{-3}
Strokes	14 211	2.9×10^{-4}
Diabetes	6 369	1.3×10^{-4}
Asthma	1 764	3.5×10^{-5}
Cirrhosis	2 280	4.5×10^{-5}
Ulcers (stomach and duodenum)	4 483	9.0×10^{-5}
Pregnancy	52	1.4×10^{-6}
Measles	10	2.0×10^{-8}
Whooping cough	1	4.0×10^{-8}

15.2.2 The balance of benefit and risk in modern society

The fact that the public, the media, patients and probably the medical profession itself, have a distorted view of the risks involved in taking medicines does not in any way diminish the need for continuing research into the safety of drugs. The fact that the major drugs advisory body in the United Kingdom is called the Committee on Safety of Medicines is not without significance. The Medicines Act (1968) charges the committee with the assessment of the quality, safety and efficacy of drugs before they are granted a product licence.

It is clear that continuing awareness of ADRs, as a major problem in the treatment of most diseases, by doctors, patients, pharmaceutical companies and national regulatory authorities has had little effect in improving safety evaluation over the past 20–30 years. During the period covered by the last two editions of this chapter drug withdrawals, exemplified by the hypoglycaemic agent, troglitazone and the cholesterol lowering agent, cerivastatin, have continued to the dismay of patients, doctors and the pharmaceutical industry. At the time

If products intended for use in clinical conditions that are not life threatening in the relatively short term, then experience suggests that regulatory authorities start to be concerned at a potentially drug related death rate of about 1 in 10 000 exposures. Non-steroidal anti-inflammatories, minor tranquillisers, or products for the relief of common acute GI disorders would come into this category; so, in such cases, patients' expectations of safety are approximately the same as in circumstances that are acceptable in everyday life. It has to be questioned whether or not this is a realistic expectation and, in particular, whether methods are available for detecting, measuring and assessing risks at that level.

Table 15.3 Risks estimated to increase chance of death in any year by one part in a million (United States)

Activity	Cause of death
Smoking 1.4 cigarettes	Cancer, heart disease
Drinking 0.5 L of wine	Cirrhosis of liver
Spending 1 h in a coal mine	Black lung disease
Spending 3 h in a coal mine	Accident
Living 2 days in Boston or New York	Air pollution
Travelling 6 min by canoe	Accident
Travelling 10 miles by bicycle	Accident
Travelling 150 miles by car	Accident
Flying 1000 miles by jet	Accident
Flying 6000 miles by jet	Cancer caused by cosmic radiation
Living 2 months in average stone or brick building	Cancer caused by natural radioactivity
One chest X-ray in a good hospital	Cancer caused by radiation
Living 2 months with a cigarette smoker	Cancer, heart disease
Eating 40 tablespoons of peanut butter	Cancer caused by aflatoxin B
Drinking 30 cans of diet soda	Cancer caused by saccharin
Living 150 years within 20 miles of a nuclear plant	Cancer caused by radiation

Table 15.4 Chances of dying from selected cause as lifetime risk (USA)

Causes of death	Chances
Motor vehicle accident	1 in 100
Murder	1 in 300
Fire	1 in 800
Firearms accident	1 in 2500
Asteroid/comet impact (lower limit)	*1 in 3000*
Electrocution	1 in 5000
Asteroid/comet impact	*1 in 20 000*
Passenger aircraft crash	1 in 20 000
Flood	1 in 30 000
Tornado	1 in 60 000
Venomous bite or sting	1 in 100 000
Asteroid/comet impact (upper limit)	*1 in 250 000*
Fireworks accident	1 in 1 million
Food poisoning by botulism	1 in 3 million
Drinking water with EPA limit of TCE*	1 in 10 million

* EPA, Environmental Protection Agency; TCE, trichloroethylene.

of the present edition the COX 2 inhibitor rofecoxib (Vioxx) has been withdrawn as a consequence of cardiovascular adverse reactions. It is disheartening that all the efforts made to develop new methods of safety evaluation should have failed yet again. It has to be questioned whether this failure is a consequence of not using the most appropriate methods available, or whether the detection of such adverse reactions is inherently unattainable. It seems obvious that pre-marketing clinical trials, which seldom study more than a few thousand patients, are incapable of evaluating safety for any but the most common adverse reactions of short latency, and that spontaneous reporting, which is so inefficient that a 10–15% reporting rate would be considered quite exceptional, is not an appropriate method for new drugs.

From the pharmaceutical industry's point of view, the evaluation of safety for a new product begins from the time that it is first tested in living material. It is for this reason that the great majority of potential new drugs are abandoned before they go beyond animal toxicology. At the first sign of unacceptable toxicity it is highly likely that all research will be stopped, and other related compounds investigated in the hope that they will be less toxic. This is undoubtedly a wasteful process, and it is certain that drugs which would ultimately prove to be safe and effective are abandoned unnecessarily. An excessive concern with safety is certainly part of the problem, but the lack of predictive precision of animal tests[8] and the inability to identify groups of patients that may be at high risk ensure that a very cautious attitude prevails.

The great majority of ADRs are dose related and may be readily understood as excessive responses to the expected pharmacological and physiological effects of the substance. A very small number of reactions do not fall into this category and, although they are rare, create considerable alarm because they are sometimes serious and always unexpected.

Potential new drugs that show acceptable toxicity in animals are usually first tested in healthy human volunteers before being investigated in patients. Chapters 3–6 deal with these aspects of new drug development, and it is the purpose of this chapter to consider how safety should be evaluated at the time of the product licence application and in the post-marketing phase.

15.3 General Considerations

By the time that an application for a product licence is ready, a certain amount of evidence on the safety of the drug will be available. In a review of product licence applications to the Committee on Safety of Medicines (CSMs), Rawlins and Jefferys[9] presented data on the number of patients who were available for the assessment of safety and efficacy (Table 15.5). When it is considered that many of the patients included would have been in short-term clinical trials (up to 28 days), and that other trials would have been conducted on formulations and doses that were different from those recommended in the product licence application, then the relevant numbers are substantially reduced.

In addition, some patients could well have been studied for conditions other than those finally selected, thereby reducing the numbers still further.

If data are available on 1000 patients, then on the assumption that there were no confounding factors, an adverse effect with an incidence of about 1 in 300 might be detected. If there were confounding factors, such as a significant background level of the adverse drug event (ADE), not associated with the drug, then the level of detection could fall to 1 in 100 or even less. Most ADEs that have caused problems occur less frequently than 1 in 1000 patients, and may be as rare as 1 in 10 000 or 50 000, so the evidence available in the product licence application is wholly inadequate for such an assessment. The need for the continuing evaluation of safety is, therefore, a matter of considerable importance, and has been the subject of numerous publications.[10–24]

Many of the major new products reaching the market in the last few years will have had total databases of 5000 or more patients, but when the subtractions are made for formulation, dose and indications that are no longer relevant, then, perhaps, no more than 2500–3500 remain. This is still far short of the number required to make an assessment of safety that would be appropriate for its expected performance when it reaches the market.

There are many uncertainties in the information available on ADEs, as estimated from premarketing clinical trials, and even the 'incidence' figures quoted are frequently guesses rather than

Table 15.5 Median numbers (range) of volunteers and patients exposed to new active substances during premarketing studies[9]

	Healthy volunteers	Efficacy studies	Safety database
All applications	60 (0–819)	861 (41–4906)	1171 (43–15 962)
Successful applications	92 (0–819)	1126 (122–4906)	1480 (129–9400)
Unsuccessful applications	64 (0–431)	785 (41–4786)	1052 (43–15 962)

precise quantitative estimates. Indeed, many words – 'incidence', 'prevalence', 'frequency' and so on – that have specific definitions are used indiscriminately without considering their precise meaning. They are used to suggest some sort of magnitude of risk by which the acceptability of the drug may be judged. There is no harm in this so long as the lack of precision is understood. A major problem is that the chances of suffering an ADE from a particular drug depend on a number of factors that may be specific to that drug or that class of drug, and not to others. Such factors might be duration of administration, route of administration, need for dose titration, and a whole range of precautions in special groups of patients.

15.4 Methods of Post-marketing Safety Evaluation

Many methods have been used for the evaluation of safety in the Post-marketing period, but these can be reduced to five basically different approaches to the problem:

- Clinical trials
- Spontaneous reporting
- Computerised databases
- Prescription event monitoring (PEM)
- *Ad hoc* methods.

Each group of methods will be considered in some detail in order to identify their strengths and weaknesses, and to determine those circumstances in which their use is most appropriate. There has in the past been a hope that some new method – a 'holy grail' – might be discovered that would fulfill all the requirements for post-marketing safety evaluation but, not surprisingly, this has not been realised, and it is now accepted that each situation has different needs and the most appropriate method or methods have to be determined according to the circumstances.

A continuing problem is the lack of attention that has been paid to the capabilities of each method. Too often the temptation to accept the currently fashionable method has taken precedence over a well-considered appraisal of what is available, resulting in a study that fails to measure up to the requirements. Each of the methods has serious defects; numbers of patients and costs are negative factors for cohort studies; completeness of data and validation are problems for computerised systems; and lack of a clear hypothesis or poorly defined diagnostic criteria are incompatible with high-quality case–control studies. Clinical trials pose even greater problems with respect to patient numbers, cost and the logistics of conducting large-scale controlled studies on a multicentre basis. To a great extent this lack of discrimination is a consequence of the predominant influence of clinical trial methodology on clinical research. For example, it has proved difficult to persuade clinical trial lists that purely observational studies do not have 'dropouts': they merely have patients who discontinue or change their medication. The patients are still being observed and are therefore still in the study. There are no 'protocol violations' in observational studies because there are no exclusive or inclusive criteria, and it is just medical practice in the real world that is being recorded. Another factor that is often overlooked is time. This is a vital matter in the pre-marketing phases of new drug development, when the time taken to achieve marketing authorisation is paramount. However, it is also frequently forgotten that the safety of a new product and supporting its position on the market should not be the subject of undue delay.

A recent Editorial in the *BMJ* by Ioannidis *et al.*[25] has questioned the widely held view that the only scientifically acceptable studies are randomised controlled clinical trials, and that observational studies are unreliable and unreproducible. They cite two papers[26,27] reviewing more than 20 studies which show that the correlation between observational and randomised controlled studies was remarkably close, and that the reproducibility of observational studies was good.

In the following sections the case of an orally administered drug intended for long-term use in a commonly occurring condition will be taken as the classic example. Drugs administered by different routes, for acute conditions, for life-threatening diseases or in other special circumstances will require modifications not only in study design but also in analysis and interpretation. The way in which post-marketing safety will be monitored in the new 'biotech' products and gene therapy has yet to be determined, but will certainly involve the development of new methods. It has already been suggested (Rawlins, MD. Personal communication, 1993) that patients receiving gene therapy will have to be monitored for the rest of their lives. It might also be thought necessary to monitor any children they may have in the same way.

15.5 Clinical Trials

The vast subject of clinical trials in new drug development is the subject of Chapter 6 and will be dealt with here only with respect to their use after marketing for the further evaluation of safety.

Clinical trials are specifically designed as experiments to test the many and various aspects of a new drug's characteristics, in particular the determination of appropriate diagnostic indications and the correct dose and dosage regimen. There are clear-cut patient inclusion and exclusion criteria, there may be stringent requirements to confirm the diagnosis, and there will be specific limitations on dosage and duration of treatment. In most clinical trials, a control or comparator group will be included, and patients will be randomly allocated to either the treatment or the control group. These requirements, therefore, create an entirely artificial set of circumstances which are quite unlike the situation that exists in the real world of clinical practice. Such trials are essential in drug development, when efficacy and dosage determination are dominant factors. They are of much less value in the evaluation of safety.

As has already been stated, major new drugs intended for long-term use in common conditions may have been tested in several thousand patients by the time marketing permission is granted. This may seem to be a substantial number but, as has already been pointed out, many of the patients will have been in relatively short-term trials and many will have been in studies conducted on different doses, different dosage regimens and for different indications from those finally agreed upon for marketing. Many other patients may also have been studied in countries in which the standards of clinical research are below an acceptable level. A survey of 118 product licence applications considered by the Committee on Safety of Medicines[9] found that the median number of patients included in the safety database was 1480 (range 129–9400) which, when corrected for studies involving inappropriate formulations, doses and indications and short durations of treatment, would only be able to detect adverse reactions occurring more frequently than 1 in 1000 at the very best. In the great majority of cases the detection capability would be as low as 1 in 2–300, which by any standards is totally inadequate. The reader is referred to some examples of large-scale clinical trials used mainly for the evaluation of safety, but also for better defining drug use.[28–32]

It will be seen that the use of controlled clinical trials to evaluate safety in new drugs is very limited, both from the point of view of the relatively small number of patients that can be studied and because they are, of necessity, conducted in an artificial, experimental setting. The commoner conditions may be detected in this way, but ill-defined and less common adverse events will usually be missed, and will not be discovered until the drug has been used by large numbers of patients in the real world of everyday clinical practice. It is not just that increasing the size and range of controlled clinical trials is impractical for reasons of cost and the time involved in their completion, but because they are essentially experimental in nature they can never provide information on the way in which a drug will be used in the real world. It is well known that even in the best of circumstances drugs are used in ways that are not recommended in the official literature. Dosage levels and dosage regimens, diagnostic indications and durations of treatment, to mention just a few examples, are frequently extended beyond what is permitted in the licence. It is in just these, unapproved, circumstances, which are excluded from clinical trials, that adverse drug-related events are most likely to occur.

The great majority of new drugs will therefore come to the market with only a superficial evaluation of safety. As a consequence, it is now universally agreed that the assessment of safety must be continued into the post-marketing phase, and probably for the entire life of the drug. This is a major challenge for the pharmaceutical industry, all those involved in clinical research and the regulatory authorities. A serious legal problem arises from the fact that drug law in most countries, and in particular the Medicines Act (1968) in the United Kingdom, has little power after a product licence has been granted. It is true that there are requirements for companies to submit any new information that may become available in the post-marketing period if it has relevance to the quality, safety or efficacy of the product, but there are no formal powers to demand specific studies for the evaluation of safety. If a product should become the subject of serious adverse event reports or other evidence that its safety is in doubt, then the licensing authority may request further information on which to base regulatory action if it should be appropriate. It has long been hoped that formal studies continued into the post-marketing period might counteract the ever-present demand for bigger and longer clinical trials, but unfortunately this has never been put into effect. A combination of the legal limitations of the regulatory authorities and a lack of will on the part of the pharmaceutical industry has effectively blocked any progress in this direction.

The granting of a product licence in the United Kingdom, or its equivalent in other countries, is a dividing line that places firm constraints on what studies can and cannot be done in the pre- and post-marketing periods. Because it would be medically and ethically unacceptable to permit doctors (investigators) to use an unapproved drug in unrestricted circumstances, it is essentially impossible to conduct clinical trials

that would mimic real-world use rather than a controlled experimental situation. The result is obvious. The real world is inaccessible in the pre-marketing period. Conversely, once in the post-marketing phase, it is difficult or impossible to constrain drug use to the situations that were defined in clinical trials.

It is no exaggeration to say that nearly 30 years have passed since the Medicines Division, as it was then called, began a campaign to encourage the pharmaceutical industry to continue pre-marketing safety evaluation into the post-marketing phase, which on the one hand, would provide the licensing authority with greater assurance of safety and on the other would safeguard the licence holder from the possible disaster of unexpected adverse reactions. This incentive to self-regulation has never been more than moderately successful and it may well be that this will not be achieved until the post-marketing period is included in the legally recognised period of new drug development. When post-marketing safety evaluation becomes an integral part of the R&D process, a more uniform approach may be achieved.

It is now necessary to consider the various methods that are available for studying drugs in the context of actual clinical practice with the assessment of safety as a primary objective.

15.6 Spontaneous Event Reporting

Spontaneous adverse event reporting may be defined as any system of safety data collection which, in the United Kingdom, relies upon certain healthcare professionals physicians, dentists, other healthcare workers and sometimes patients[33] to report adverse clinical events which, they suspect, may be causally related to the administration of a drug or drugs. The present yellow card scheme invites such reports from doctors, dentists, pharmacists, coroners radiographers, optometrists and nurses. Discussions are in progress to include patient reporting, and pilot studies will be evaluated to determine their effectiveness. It is these systems which are sponsored by the governments of virtually all developed countries and, increasingly, by developing countries as well. For the physician in the pharmaceutical industry it is this method of safety evaluation that will most frequently be encountered and, in spite of its numerous defects and limitations, will take up much working time.

It is one of those illogical quirks of new drug development that a method which is almost universally agreed to be seriously inadequate is, nevertheless, a major consideration in the organisation and running of the pharmaceutical company medical department. For this reason alone it is necessary to look into spontaneous reporting systems in some detail. Misunderstanding and confusion start at the very beginning. Is the clinical condition that is the subject of a report an event or a reaction? At the very least, in the eyes of the reporter it is potentially an adverse reaction, as there was the suspicion of a causal relationship with a drug or drugs. For the personnel of a regulatory agency, who receive thousands of such reports each year, the perception may be totally different, knowing that the reporting doctor usually has little evidence to support an attribution of causality. This is no fault of the doctor, as the well known common ADRs are of little interest and the uncommon ones are so infrequent that any individual doctor may only observe a handful in his/her entire career. The reporting doctor thus has no frame of reference by which to assess possible causality and has to fall back on clinical judgement, which is largely subjective.

The entire basis of medicine is, quite properly, moving from the 'art of medicine' to the 'science of medicine', and the reporting of clinical events observed while a patient is receiving a drug should reflect this change of attitude. At the time of observation, apart possibly from a temporal relationship between the administration of a drug and the event, there may be no other evidence on which to base an attribution of causality. In these circumstances, it would be correct to term the observation an 'event' and not a 'reaction', the latter term being strictly reserved for the situation in which a causal relationship has been reasonably established. The vast majority of spontaneous reports, apart from those

recording well-established ADRs, are, therefore, with respect to clinical events, not reactions. The next stage of the process may be aimed at collecting further data which could provide evidence of causality, particularly when the event is either serious or unexpected or both.

At the present time, several countries have well-organised and experienced spontaneous reporting systems which contribute the bulk of ADE reports. In particular the United States, the United Kingdom, France and the Scandinavian countries have records going back several decades, and can claim to have in their possession data of reasonable quality. The section on p. 438 considers the various methods of causality assessment that are available and the data that are required for their application.

In Europe, the term 'pharmacovigilance' is now used to cover the continuing evaluation of safety into the post-marketing period, and is intended to include all methods of data collection. In practice this has not happened, and 'pharmacovigilance' is almost always used synonymously with spontaneous reporting, which further adds to the existing confusion over definitions and terminology. A mythology now surrounds spontaneous reporting that is disproportionate to its true value and which allows conclusions to be drawn and decisions to be made which, in any other science, would be rejected as unjustifiable speculation. This is not to say that spontaneous reporting is valueless: it has its proper place in safety evaluation but must be used appropriately and its capabilities and limitations recognised. The recently published EU document 'Notice to Marketing Authorisation Holders – Pharmacovigilance Guidelines No PhVWP/108/99' is now the principal source of information and instruction on the reporting of suspected ADRs in the European Union. This document is considered further on p. 441 *et seq.*

In the United Kingdom, the present 'yellow card' system had its origins in 1965, when Witts,[23] who was then a member of the Committee on Safety of Drugs (the precursor to the CSM), published a method for the collection of suspected adverse reactions to drugs.

Table 15.6 Spontaneously reported adverse reactions in WHO database from EU countries

Country	1985	1986	1987	1988	1989	Mean
Belgium	54	52	53	47	36	48
Denmark	213	379	372	346	160	294
France	5	44	95	108	53	61
German Fed. Rep.	38	41	48	23	1	30
Ireland	293	336	227	147	74	215
Italy	17	21	21	17	3	16
The Netherlands	69	68	65	24	6	46
Spain	30	42	58	57	28	43
United Kingdom	217	273	301	314	254	272

The thalidomide tragedy[34–38] was a powerful stimulus for the setting up of an effective system of adverse event monitoring. An excellent early publication which set out many of the basic principles and definitions of terms and procedures is that of Finney.[39]

Since then there have been many publications and reviews of the UK yellow card system and spontaneous reporting systems internationally.[40–49] A summary of the capabilities and limitations of the method is given in Table 15.6. Although these have been discussed in the greatest detail over the past three decades, the obligations that exist for pharmaceutical companies in the reporting of adverse events to the regulatory authorities at both national and international levels make it essential to review them in this chapter.

The European Pharmacovigilance Research Group (EPRG) sponsored by the EU Biomed Programme, which has now been discontinued, examined methods of ADE reporting that would be appropriate for multinational studies within the European Union. As part of the programme an attitudinal survey was carried out in Denmark, France, Ireland, Italy, The Netherlands, Portugal, Spain, Sweden and the United Kingdom to investigate the reporting characteristics of healthcare professionals in those countries. EPRG recognised that underreporting is a universal problem for spontaneous reporting systems, and sought to identify the factors that discouraged reporting. The survey was conducted by sending self-administered questionnaires to approximately 1% of medical practitioners in each country. There was a large variation in response from country to country, as might have been expected, although inhibitory factors seemed to be more similar. Lack of availability of report forms was a common problem, as was the lack of address and telephone number of the reporting agency. Inadequate information on how to report and shortage of time in which to report were also general complaints. Issues that did not discourage reporting included concern about patient confidentiality, fear of legal liability or appearing foolish, reluctance to admit that harm had been caused to a patient, or ambition to collect and publish a personal series of cases.

Another disincentive to reporting is uncertainty in the mind of the doctor or other health professional in judging the seriousness or severity of a suspected adverse reaction. Serious reactions are those that are fatal, life threatening, disabling, incapacitating or which result in prolonged hospitalisation and/or are medically significant. On the other hand, severe reactions may be those that are not life threatneing or disabling but in individual patients are extreme.

15.6.1 Underreporting

It has always been known that only a very small proportion of adverse events were ever the subject of spontaneous reports. There are various reasons for this, the most common probably being a lack of enthusiasm on the part of the doctor, although more serious disincentives may be a fear of criticism, a fear of displaying ignorance or a genuine and entirely understandable failure to recognise a potential ADR when it occurs. Various estimates, usually based on the known number of reporting doctors taken as a proportion of the total, suggest that reporting levels are seldom, if ever, higher than 10% and are almost always much lower.[50] The Nordic countries have claimed levels of 15%, which may be possible in countries with small populations, socialised medicine, legally enforceable requirements and constant motivation by the authorities.

Estimates based upon data from large-scale observational cohort studies[51,52] which involved data collection by event monitoring and spontaneous reporting suggest that the level is more often in the region of 5%, and is frequently below 2%. These are estimates taken across the full range of ADE reports, which include a high proportion of irrelevant observations relating to trivial, symptomatic conditions that are dubiously related to the administration of drugs. There has always been an optimistic hope that the more serious, pathologically distinct conditions may be more frequently recorded and reported as potential ADRs. The papers referred to above do not support that view, but seem to show that many relatively serious conditions, such as photodermatitis, hyper- and hypothyroidism, Cushing's syndrome and extrapyramidal symptoms are only rarely reported, even though they have all been identified as occasionally being causally related to particular drugs. It seems possible that high-profile, well-publicised serious ADRs, such as aplastic anaemia or acute hepatic failure, which have come to be regarded as drug-associated conditions, may be much less affected by underreporting.

Another contributory factor in underreporting is the background incidence of the condition in the overall patient population. The chances of identifying a clinical condition that occurs in the population only extremely rarely as a drug-related event is clearly much greater than if it occurred commonly. The case of thalidomide is the classic example, phocomelia being exceptionally rare as a background condition, which permitted the detection of an increased incidence at an early stage. Had the defect been one of a variety of minor abnormalities which are relatively common, then the detection of the thalidomide problem might have taken much longer. In order to detect ADRs that may be confused with commonly occurring conditions it is essential to use a monitoring method that can provide data containing precise denominator values, so that incidence may be calculated. It is also necessary to know the background incidence with which to compare the ADR data. These requirements are seldom met, and usually the situation remains inconclusive.

An example of this involved the combination product Debendox (Bendectin in the United States), which was indicated for the relief of vomiting in pregnancy. In the formulation that was marketed in the United Kingdom Debendox contained dicyclomine hydrochloride, doxylamine sulphate and pyridoxine, but in formulations used in some other countries the dicyclomine hydrochloride was left out. In 1983, the company withdrew the product from the market because of increasing media pressure and the risks of litigation arising from unfounded suspicions that it was associated with birth defects. No specific defect was referred to, although it was implied that there was a general increase in minor midline and skeletal abnormalities. These occur sporadically, with a total incidence that is estimated to be about 1% of live births. Numerous large-scale studies were conducted,[53–59] which failed to demonstrate any association with Debendox. From the regulatory point of view the drug was no longer under suspicion, but for the company it was off the market. In the period leading up to its withdrawal from the market, regulatory action had reduced the pregnancy indications to severe hyperemesis gravidarum, which is a relatively uncommon condition and is itself associated with an increase in birth defects. In this situation there was, quite literally, no way in which a possible association between Debendox and birth defects could ever be proved. Even if every use of the product were to be monitored the numbers would have been insufficient to reach a statistically significant conclusion. It cannot be stressed too strongly that there are occasions when the size of the total patient population relevant to the problem is too small to provide any answers.

Another serious deficiency with spontaneous reporting is the possibility of bias in the data. The problem is particularly difficult because, often, it is not possible to detect the existence of bias until the lengthy process of collecting additional data has been completed. Increases or decreases in reporting levels may result from numerous external and largely uncontrollable factors. At the 'macro'-level it is known that reporting levels differ greatly from country to country as a consequence of social, medical, religious and other national influences.[43] At the 'micro'-level, publications in the medical literature, media pressure, regulatory agency activities and a host of other ill-defined factors may enhance or inhibit reporting. To add to the difficulties, these biases are capricious in their effects, sometimes causing a flood of reports relating to a particular drug or clinical condition and on other occasions apparently demotivating doctors in reporting.

Other factors causing bias are related to the particular drug or class of drugs, and to the particular clinical condition or organ system involved. As an example, in the United Kingdom the class of NSAIDs has always been heavily over-represented in the yellow card figures, possibly as a consequence of a high level of regulatory activity and media pressure. Many of these biases are shown in the spontaneous reports held on the WHO Collaborative Centre database in Uppsala, Sweden, particularly when comparisons are made between country, drug and clinical condition[24,60] (Edwards, IR. Personal communication) (Tables 15.6–15.9). Potential dangers are involved in combining spontaneous reporting data when it derives from different sources, at different times, for different drugs and relating to different clinical conditions. The current developments in the European Union (EU), with the establishment of a central agency and an increasingly integrated approach to drug registration and post-marketing safety evaluation, will have

to proceed with caution if erroneous decisions are to be avoided. A similar trend towards the extrapolation of data derived from one source to problems occurring in another area is happening in the United States and Canada, where the large multipurpose databases are being used in this way.

15.6.2 The need for denominators

Underreporting and bias are both serious problems, but the greatest deficiency of spontaneous reporting is its lack of denominator values. This means that, without recourse to information derived from other sources, spontaneous reporting can only provide absolute numbers. It may be true that there are rare circumstances when absolute numbers are all that is required to make a regulatory decision. This might happen when a drug with no exceptional benefits in a non-life-threatening condition is shown to have a causal relationship to a serious and potentially fatal condition. In such circumstances, three or four well-documented reports may be sufficient to withdraw the product from the market. In all other circumstances, it is necessary to use one or more denominator values in order to calculate an incidence for the suspected ADR.

The choice of a suitable denominator may not be simple, as the aetiology and pathology of the adverse effect have to be taken into account and these may not be known with any certainty. For example, a particular adverse event may only occur after the drug has been taken for an extended period, and is related to the total amount of drug administered. It could be that only a small minority of patients are in that category, and for whom the risk is high. For the great majority, who only take the drug short term, the risk may be negligible. Similarly, the adverse effect may only occur in a subgroup of patients who, coincidentally, have another pathological condition which predisposes to the ADE. In this case, the incidence in those at risk depends on the selection of an appropriate denominator.

The absolute numbers of spontaneous reports relating to any particular clinical event are dependent on a number of fairly obvious factors.

Table 15.7 Adverse reaction reports in WHO database from EU countries. Distribution of reports per therapeutic drug group as percentage of total number of reports

Country	ATC groups			CNS
	Cardiovascular	**Anti-infective**	**Musculoskeletal**	
Belgium	22.2	13.9	11.8	17.8
Denmark	17.4	17.1	10.1	13.7
France	18.2	4.2	9.5	19.2
German Fed. Rep.	9.6	22.5	11.1	10.8
Ireland	17.7	15.7	10.1	15.1
Italy	9.5	16.6	14.4	15.3
The Netherlands	20.7	12.6	8.8	14.1
Spain	16	20.8	9	15.2
United Kingdom	19.9	15	17.5	13

Table 15.8 Adverse reaction reports in WHO database from EU countries. Distribution of reports per body system organ class as percentage of total number of reports

Country	Body system organ class			
	Skin	**CNS**	**Gastrointestine**	**Liver**
Belgium	19.2	11	10.8	4.5
Denmark	30.3	7.7	8.9	4.3
France	17.6	9.1	8	8.4
German Fed. Rep.	12.4	10.1	15	2.5
Ireland	13.9	13.1	15.4	1.6
Italy	17.7	8	18.2	1.9
The Netherlands	17.5	10.6	9.3	5.4
Spain	18.6	11.9	17.2	1.7
United Kingdom	20.7	11.1	12.9	2.4

The extent to which a drug is used is clearly important, but may be complicated by the pathological mechanism of the adverse reaction. The significance of prescription volume is different for reactions associated with the initiation of treatment from reactions that do not become apparent until the drug has been taken for an extended period.

The extent to which a drug is used is at least partly dependent on the success of the pharmaceutical company's promotional programme, but also on the total number of patients with the relevant clinical indications, which in turn is dependent on the population of the country concerned. For some rare ADEs, small countries such as Belgium or Denmark, which have fewer than 15 million inhabitants, may never have enough patients to make detection possible. In these cases the serious problems involved in using data from other countries arise, and great care must be exercised before conclusions are drawn.

The problem is further complicated by the fact that drug use is spread unevenly over the patient

Table 15.9 Adverse reactions in WHO database from EU countries

Country	Skin reactions		Total	R/T (%)	S/T (%)
	Rash	SJS			
Belgium	257	4	642	40	0.6
Denmark	2 086	0	3 241	64.4	0
France	2 290	69	4 778	47.9	1.4
German Fed. Rep.	1 872	22	4 348	43.1	0.5
Ireland	549	9	956	57.4	0.9
Italy	578	8	1 207	47.9	0.7
The Netherlands	468	4	969	48.3	0.4
Spain	1 445	20	2 757	52.4	0.7
United Kingdom	12 645	203	24 382	51.9	0.8

population, with age and sex having a strong influence on prescribing patterns.[61] For example, if age is split into decades, then in general there is a predominance of first prescriptions in the first three decades and a predominance of repeat prescriptions in the sixth, seventh and eighth decades. The proportion of people who are patients also differs from decade to decade, and this may be an important factor to take into account. On the day of our birth virtually 100% of us are patients, and the same is true on the day of our death, but between these two extremes there is a varying proportion of people who are patients to people who ate not patients. It is possible to imagine a number of scenarios in which this might be of decisive importance in assessing the importance of an adverse reaction. For example, over the total patient population, and taking into account total drug use, a serious ADR may appear to be at an acceptable level. However, further investigation might show that 90% of drug use was in patients in the first five decades of life, whereas 90% of the ADRs were in patients in the seventh, eighth and ninth decades. This would almost certainly arouse great concern and require major changes in the package insert or data sheet.

These denominators may be regarded as scaling factors by which the clinical, regulatory, ethical or social importance of an ADR may be measured, but they are still inadequate if truly balanced decisions are to be taken. Within these constraints there are the ever-present problems of underreporting and bias that have already been discussed. Unfortunately, these two defects of the system are not evenly spread across disease, drugs or patients, making it impossible to apply any simple, generally applicable correction factor. In recently published appraisals of spontaneous reporting,[51,52] it was shown that, within the limitations of the studies reviewed, there were wide variations in underreporting, depending on the clinical event reported. The range probably extends from about 15% at best (85% underreporting) to less than 1% (99% underreporting) at worst. The problem of bias is even more difficult to quantify, and apart from the certain knowledge that it exists there is little objective evidence on its extent.

Overall reporting levels in differing circumstances are an essential requirement if comparisons are to be made between countries, or even comparisons between drugs in a particular class. In the first case it is clear that different correction factors would have to be applied if data from a country with an overall reporting rate of 10% were to be compared with those from a country with a rate of only 5%. The second case would be exemplified by a drug such as triazolam, which has been the subject of high-profile media and regulatory attention, compared with a similar drug such as temazepam, which has not been so closely scrutinised.

The selection of a relevant denominator or denominators is thus a matter for careful consideration. The following factors should be taken into account and, wherever possible, quantified so that appropriate corrections may be made:

- total population of country
- total patient population for the indicated clinical condition(s)
- total prescriptions over a defined period of time
- number of first prescriptions over a defined period of time
- overall reporting rates for country, clinical condition, drug, etc.

The above factors should be subdivided by sex and age (in decades or other appropriate bands).

15.6.3 Special circumstances

There are a number of situations in which spontaneous reporting is essentially inappropriate for the detection of ADEs.

Occasionally, the appearance of an ADE is delayed for an extended period after the initiation of treatment with the drug in question. These ADEs of long latency have been reviewed by Fletcher and Griffin,[62] and in none of the examples cited had they been detected by spontaneous reports. Attention was most often first drawn to the possible drug association by individual case reports in the medical literature. Indeed, it may be that this is the route by which knowledge of potential new ADRs is most commonly gained, whether they are of long latency or immediate. Up to a few years ago no other method had been available for the detection of delayed ADEs, but now, with the development of computerised systems for recording patient information in the doctor's surgery, it is possible to conduct retrospective surveys of drug use over relatively long periods. Many of the important drug disasters of the past three decades, such as thalidomide (drug taken during pregnancy causing phocomelia in the new born), stilboestrol (drug taken during pregnancy causing carcinoma of the vagina in daughters)[63] and practolol (causing the oculomucocutaneous syndrome many months after administration),[64–66] have been of this type of ADR.

Carcinogenicity is always a concern with drugs that are administered chronically, and as the lag period before the development of a detectable tumour and first administration may be as long as 20 years this is a particularly severe problem. It seems unlikely that conventional prospective drug monitoring could ever be a practical method in these circumstances. The problem would more likely be seen as an unexplained rise in the incidence of a particular neoplasm. Surveys conducted by the National Cancer Institute[67,68] in the United States and by others[69] have investigated the possible carcinogenicity of an extensive list of drugs. The effective use of aggressive chemotherapy in conditions such as Hodgkin's disease is now known to be associated with an increase in second primary malignancies.[69]

Another situation in which spontaneous reporting is unlikely to be of help is when the ADE closely resembles another common disease and the prescribing doctor is unable to distinguish between them. In order to recognise such an ADE it is necessary to know the background incidence of the condition, and also to be in a position to see an otherwise unexplained increase in its incidence. Needless to say, these conditions are seldom met, and it is only after long experience with the drug that an increase in ADEs may be detected. Large-scale cohort studies involving 10 000 or more patients are probably the most powerful way of discovering and quantifying such ADEs, provided they occur more frequently than about 1 in 1000 patients taking the drug. This is the situation for many of the better-known examples, such as cough with ACE inhibitors, tremor with beta-agonists and debility with beta blockers, so there is a real place for the cohort study in post-marketing safety evaluation. The wealth of other clinical data provided by cohort studies is an additional benefit in the continuing evaluation of the drug.

The advent of computerised databases that link the prescribed drug to diagnosis and record patient histories over extended periods provides another method by which the incidence of the more common ADEs may be estimated.

Related to the ADE that mimics another condition is the ADE that is a deterioration or alteration of the disease being treated. In this case, it is necessary to know the natural history of the disease when treated by established therapies, and to be in a position to observe an alteration in that process. Once again, these conditions are not often met and so detection may be long delayed.

A failure to detect these classes of ADE may have serious consequences, as the ADE itself may be disabling or even life threatening, but even when it is relatively trivial it may be a reason for the patient's discontinuing effective treatment, which in turn may cause a deterioration in their condition. An example would be the patient who discontinues the treatment of his asthma with a beta-agonist because of tremor and then goes into status asthmaticus, with fatal consequences.

The UK MHRA has recently drawn special attention to several areas of interest and have highlighted adverse reactions in children and the elderly. Children pose a particular problem because they are seldom studied in clinical trials that form the basis of marketing authorisation submissions. The consequence of this is that children are prescribed medicines which are not licensed for that age group and little experience of possible adverse effects is available. The elderly are also under-represented in pre-marketing clinical trials and are also subject to diminished metabolic activity in respect of numerous commonly used drugs.

The preoccupation of many regulatory agencies with rare and serious ADRs as detected by spontaneous reporting systems may provide partial protection against the political and media excesses of the classic drug disaster, but are of little help in detecting the kind of drug-related conditions that endanger patients by limiting effective therapy and preventing optimal drug treatment. It should be remembered that the health of nations is unaffected by rare and exotic ADRs, which may be fascinating for the collector but are of little value in the better treatment of patients. On the other hand, the health of nations *is* affected by the common, but sometimes less serious, drug-related clinical conditions

that place constraints on the most effective treatment.

15.6.4 Can spontaneous reporting be improved?

Much time and discussion has gone into this question over the past several years.[70-74] The cynics would say that more is already being expected of spontaneous reporting than it can ever deliver, and that it has probably reached its limits. The more optimistic – or possibly the more naive – would say that improvements are possible and that we should set about achieving them.

Broadly speaking, there are two areas where improvement might be possible. First, there is the input side[75] of the ADE report that is provided by the prescribing physician, and second, there is the output – the analysis and evaluation of the report.

Anyone who has examined a few hundred spontaneous reports will know that there is great variability in both the quantity and the quality of their content. The reports range from the totally useless to excellent records of important clinical observations. In between, the great majority reflect the real dilemma faced by the reporting physician. Is the observation worth reporting or is it just an irrelevance? Is this going to cause trouble for me? for the company? for the authorities? for the patient? How is it possible to judge potential causality?

The answers are elusive, and although virtually all regulatory agencies limit their requirements to events that meet the accepted definition of 'serious', in the real world this definition is inadequate. For example, is abdominal pain serious? According to the definitions, if it is disabling, life threatening, causing hospitalisation, etc. it is, but not otherwise. If it did not come into any of the defined categories the doctor would not be required or expected to report the event even though it might herald the perforation of a peptic ulcer. There are, similarly, many other symptomatic drug-related events that, although not serious by definition, are nevertheless important indicators of potentially serious conditions. Improving the quality of the input, however desirable, is not a simple matter, as it inevitably relies to a considerable extent on the clinical judgement of the reporting doctor. Improving the education of physicians may help, but there would seem to be a limit to what is possible.

Assuming that the quality of the input is maximal then improving the output will be dependent upon the analysis and evaluation of the data. Because the spontaneous report alone will seldom, if ever, contain sufficient information to determine causality satisfactorily, it is usually necessary to seek additional data which may be available from hospital records, laboratory investigations or post-mortem reports. It is highly desirable that comparable methods and formats of reporting should be used as widely as possible, particularly if international comparisons are to be made. A major benefit of formalised systems of causality assessment, which will be considered in greater detail later in this chapter, is the element of standardisation that is brought to the process of interpretation.

15.6.5   Cohort studies

The basic essentials of a cohort study are a group of patients of defined size, a system of data collection over a defined period, and a system for handling, analysing and presenting the findings. The methods available range from paper-based manual systems to fully computerised technology for all stages of the process. Phase IV clinical trials are a special kind of cohort study which have been dealt with separately, leaving this section to cover purely observational, non-interventional studies. The main objective of observational studies is to monitor drug use in the actual circumstances of everyday clinical practice. Study design should make all possible provision for data collection to proceed without influencing the normal course of treatment. Observational methods will, of course, record inappropriate as well as appropriate drug use, in contrast to clinical trials which involve

patient selection and defined dosages and durations of treatment. Observational cohort studies are therefore also capable of monitoring for those ADEs that are predominantly associated with misuse of the product. By definition, such ADEs are inaccessible to clinical trials. It is for this reason that, in the case of a potential drug disaster, there is little to be gained by simply conducting more, longer and larger clinical trials, which can only measure the effects in an artificial, experimental situation. In fact, it should be emphasised that patient exclusions or drug use limitations should never be included in observational study plans unless there are exceptional circumstances. Provision of the package insert or summary of product characteristics (SPC) is an adequate way of bringing the attention of the doctor to the correct use of the product. In principle, limitations beyond those in the manufacturer's approved literature should always be excluded unless there are compelling safety requirements to be observed. If such compelling requirements do exist then their inclusion in the data sheet should be considered.

A critical review[76] of observational cohort studies conducted by, or on behalf of, pharmaceutical companies in the United Kingdom drew attention to a number of deficiencies in study design which, in certain cases, limited the value of the study. The authors, from the Medicines Control Agency and the Committee on Safety of Medicines, were motivated by the wish to improve the standard of post-marketing cohort studies, but they failed to distinguish between the good and the bad studies that were included in their review, and in doing so created the impression that the observational cohort study as a method was of little value in the assessment of safety. It is unfortunate that none of the good studies (there were at least three that met the highest standards) was cited in greater detail to emphasise that it is not the method which is at fault but the adequacy of the performance. As a consequence of these failings the paper has had a powerful inhibiting effect on companies' enthusiasm for all kinds of post-marketing safety studies. There is little doubt that, quite unintentionally, a great deal of damage has been done, and that some long time may elapse before a more balanced view is regained.

One aim of this paper, which has been achieved, was to stimulate the revision of the existing PMS Guidelines which, it was hoped, would improve the overall standard of cohort studies. The new guidelines, which are entitled 'Guidelines for Company Sponsored Safety Assessment of Marketed Medicines (SAMM)', have had a mixed reception from the industry and their effect on the conduct of relevant studies has yet to be assessed. Ten years on from the MCA/CSM paper[76] there is little interest in observational cohort studies. Whether this has been due to an inhibitory effect of the paper or to a real disenchantment with the method is difficult to assess, but the result has been the virtual loss of a valuable way of assessing post-marketing safety. A recent overview by Linden[77] has drawn attention to the importance of observational studies for research into the actual treatment of patients in every day clinical practice, in contrast to the highly restricted circumstances of randomised controlled clinical trials. In the same journal, Schafer[78] also points out the shortcomings of pre-marketing clinical trials and advocated the use of large-scale observational studies conducted in routine medical practice.

The strengths of observational cohort studies are the depth and quality of data that may be collected. Even though these studies are unstructured in the sense that there are no limiting criteria in respect of patient, drug or dosage, they are defined in size and duration and data collection methods, whether on paper forms or on computer screens, and they can draw the attention of the participating doctor to particular pieces of information that are highly desirable. Should data be deficient or inconsistent then it is a relatively simple matter to go back to the doctor for clarification.

Of considerable importance is the possibility of collecting data on other clinical conditions the patient may have and other drugs that may also be prescribed. It must be emphasised that the elderly are the largest users of drug therapy, they frequently suffer from more than one pathology and they are consequently often being treated with a multiplicity of drugs. It is in these circumstances that ADEs are most likely to occur, and so data covering concomitant disease and medication are an essential part of safety evaluation.

The weaknesses of cohort studies are limits on the numbers of patients that may be included, organisational difficulties, the handling of vast quantities of complex data, and the often quoted but less well-quantified high costs. It is a strange thing that although when companies are faced with the need to conduct a large post-marketing study the first question often concerns cost, remarkably little information is available for each of the different methods.

There are undoubtedly fairly severe problems of a practical nature in conducting cohort studies on numbers of patients in excess of 10–15 000. It is certainly true that larger studies have been done, but usually on drug classes or disease areas where adequate numbers of patients are more readily available. In the case of a drug newly introduced to the market, it is a major challenge to enlist a cohort of 10 000 patients within 2 years of launch unless it is one of the few 'blockbuster' products that will be used in hundreds of thousands of patients. These, and the problems of organisation and data handling, are practical matters rather than scientific ones, and the benefits of plentiful high-quality data have to be balanced against the methodological limits that exist. For the identification and quantification of both expected and unexpected ADEs that occur at a frequency of more than 1 in 3000 patients, and to have the capability of assessing the possible influences of concomitant disease and concomitant medication, the prospective observational cohort study is the best method available.[79,80]

The SAMM Guidelines have been supplemented by a useful review entitled 'International Guidelines on Post-authorisation Research and Surveillance' by Herbold.[81]

15.7 Computerised Databases

In the United Kingdom approximately 80% of general practices are computerised, about half of which use their computers for maintaining patient records as well as for practice management, and there is little doubt that these numbers will continue to increase in the years ahead. The existence of detailed patient records extending over prolonged periods is a new resource for a broad range of clinical and related healthcare research. Perhaps their greatest value lies in the area of retrospective observational studies, where information on actual clinical practice is required. As these databases are the records of patient healthcare at the time of general practitioner (GP)/patient contact, the normal course of treatment is uninfluenced by the conduct of the study itself. Indeed, it is probably true to say that for the long-term evaluation of drug safety, which is one of the more important research applications of these new systems, there is no other method that could provide years of continuous data together with a wealth of information on morbidity and co-medication. The databases may also be used for prospective studies by identifying patients currently receiving healthcare and following their clinical courses at defined future time points.

Because of their recent development, the full range of their research potential has not, as yet, been exploited or even explored. The evaluation of drug safety has already been mentioned, and it is a small step for studies that investigate the consequences of non-serious but troublesome side effects on the continuity of drug treatment and drug switching.[82,83] The importance of factors that adversely affect drug compliance and which therefore have both therapeutic and economic consequences has been sadly neglected, to the detriment of both patients and healthcare providers. Applications to research in the fields of epidemiology, the natural history of disease, case–control studies and pharmacoeconomics, to mention just a few, have yet to be developed.

The fact that the great majority of the data needed for a retrospective study are already present in the database demands an entirely new conceptual approach. The situation can be compared to that of a sculptor faced by a massive block of stone from which he plans to carve a much smaller but absolutely precise statue. The sculptor has to cut away all the unwanted stone

so as to leave just those parts that are required for the statue. A large computerised database contains the elements of the study, and all that has to be done is to strip away the unnecessary data. To do this, the required data must be selected by carefully defining those elements as accurately as possible. This may sound simple, but in practice it is frequently extremely difficult to achieve. A single data element, such as an age in years, a diagnosis or a particular drug, presents no problem, but millions of data elements related in extremely complex chronological ways are a completely different matter. To obtain the maximum value from these new systems, it is desirable to utilise their full potential. This means drawing upon the complete range of demographic, diagnostic and therapeutic data, and their chronological relationships. Any study that fails to incorporate all the data elements in the database which are relevant to the investigation runs the risk of reaching incomplete or erroneous conclusions.

In the randomised, controlled clinical trial the structure of the study is determined by the preparation of a detailed protocol, which is designed to ensure that all essential data elements will be provided. In the case of studies conducted with computerised patient databases the study has to be designed within the limitations of the data already in the database. These existing data may be supplemented by seeking extra information from the doctor, as has been done in several studies conducted by Jick and co-workers,[84–87] but this adds to the cost and the time taken to complete the study. The fact that patient demographics, diagnosis, drug(s) prescribed, dosage, duration of treatment, laboratory investigations and many other factors have already been determined and are in the past, which demands a major new conceptual approach.

In the United States, there are several computerised healthcare systems, sometimes referred to as multipurpose databases, which have been used for post-marketing surveillance purposes. The best-known include Group Health Cooperative of Puget Sound, Kaiser-Permanente, Medicaid, Rhode Island and the Saskatchewan database in Canada.[88–103]

Some confusion exists because these databases may be used in two essentially different ways. Most commonly, they have been used to investigate in greater detail previously identified clinical conditions that are suspected of being drug related. A recent example would be the suspicions raised by several reports in the medical literature that the use of human insulin was associated with an excess of hypoglycaemic episodes in the absence of prodromal signs or symptoms, compared with the use of animal insulins. In this case, databases could be searched retrospectively to find all insulin-dependent diabetics being treated in a defined period, and then to determine how many were on each of the two kinds of insulin and the number of hypoglycaemic episodes suffered by each group. Similar database searches could be made starting, for example, from the identification of all patients being prescribed short-acting benzodiazepines and then determining all adverse clinical events associated with their administration. The identification of patients with particular characteristics for cost–control studies, which will be considered in the next section, may be facilitated by computerised database searching.

The second way in which the databases may be used is to identify all patients on a particular drug or with a particular clinical condition and then to follow them up over a defined period to determine what clinical events subsequently occur. For all practical purposes this method is a cohort study conducted through a computerised database, using screens and electronic data transmission rather than paper.

The advantages and disadvantages of computerised systems may be summarised as follows.

15.7.1 Advantages

1. In the right circumstances, very large patient groups may be identified and studied, retrospectively, over extended periods.
2. Retrospective database searching has no influence on the treatment of the patient and is thus free from any inducements to change treatment for the purposes of the study.
3. Data collection and management may be quicker, more efficient and more sophisticated than by other methods.
4. The database is continually being added to and is thus an increasing resource for research.
5. Comparator data may be readily available.
6. It is possible to conduct case–control studies by identifying the relevant groups of patients from the database.

15.7.2 Disadvantages

In the case of retrospective studies, the data items that have been entered into the database are, essentially, the data that are available. If data items are missing, then for all practical purposes they are not available for the study. It is possible to go back to the physician in the hope that other records or memory may be of help, but after months or years this could be a costly and unprofitable procedure.

1. In the absence of intensive training programmes, with their considerable cost implications, the quality of data is highly variable from doctor to doctor.
2. Within any computerised system the physicians involved are a fixed group with its own idiosyncrasies and limitations in number.
3. Any particular system may contain certain fixed biases. In some of the US systems, patients may be predominantly of particular age groups, of particular social classes or in other ways atypical of the total population.
4. The multiplicity of hardware and software that is available creates incompatibilities between systems, which in turn makes the combination or comparison of data difficult or impossible.

Since the first edition of this book, developments have continued in this area, particularly with respect to computerised databases as a source of detailed and reliable data for use in the pharmacoeconomic assessment of new drugs. The creation of specialised databases, such as HIV Insight, which contains the detailed clinical records of about 2500 patients who are either

HIV seropositive or have the disease AIDS, has been very successful and plans are being made to develop other specialised databases in diabetes, oncology, Alzheimer's, osteoporosis and other similar chronic diseases.

15.8 Case–Control Studies

These studies are of greatest value when a potential ADR has already been identified, that is, they are hypothesis testing rather than hypothesis generating. The case–control method has been used in a wide range of circumstances where risks to health have been identified. The classic examples are the relationship between smoking and bronchial carcinoma, and the association of the oral contraceptive (OC) with thromboembolic disorders. Case–control studies have also been used when no potential ADE has been identified, but these can be little more than 'fishing trips' conducted in the hope that something of interest may be caught.

The foundations of the method were laid by Cornfield, Dorn, Mantel and Haenszel[104–108] in the 1950s, and it was rapidly adopted by epidemiologists as a major new technique. An interesting historical account of case–control studies has been given by Lilienfeld and Lilienfeld,[109] who trace the method back to Louis and his study of tuberculosis in 1844.[110] Later developments have been reviewed by Cole,[111] who provides a useful assessment of the strengths and weaknesses of such studies. Emphasis is placed upon the need for precise case definition and the futility of attempting to get meaningful results in studies on broad diagnostic descriptions, such as depression or bone cancer. Further methodological problems have been addressed by Feinstein,[112] and the particularly serious problem of bias was reviewed by Sackett.[113]

There is little doubt, on the one hand, that case–control studies have a valuable place in pharmacoepidemiology, and therefore in the evaluation of drug safety. There is also little doubt that without minute attention to detail and, possibly, a little luck, the method may be unreliable or even completely misleading. A list of 56 topics was reviewed by Mayes et al.[114] because the case–control studies on them had provided conflicting results. A total of 265 studies were considered, of which 137 were supportive of the hypothesis and 128 were not. On this basis it would be unwise to draw conclusions from a single case–control study, it being prudent to wait until further studies confirm or refute the original findings.

The basic principle of the method is simple. A cohort of patients with the disease in question is identified, and then a cohort of patients without the disease (usually two to three times as many) is matched with respect to a number of critical characteristics and used as the control group. Differences between the two groups with respect to exposure to the suspected causative agent are then measured. A major advantage is that uncommon or rare conditions are accessible to study, which is not the case for cohort studies or for computerised systems, where the total number of patients available is less than the several millions that might be needed.

In practice, the method is considerably more difficult than the simplicity of the design suggests. The series of studies conducted on the possible relationship of the Rauwolfia derivatives to various cancers is testimony to the conflicting findings that may result. Indeed, the 11 case–control studies[115–126] on reserpine and other Rauwolfia alkaloids reviewed by Labarthe,[127] and the additional study by Friedman,[128] could well be regarded as the classic example of the uncertainties inherent in this method of safety evaluation. The first three studies to be published strongly suggested a causal association between reserpine and breast cancer, although each of them urged caution in their interpretation. In spite of this plea for a carefully considered approach there was a flurry of regulatory activity by both the Food and Drug Administration (FDA) in the United States and the CSM in the United Kingdom. Both agencies considered the possibility of removing the products from the market, but decided to await further studies before coming to a final conclusion. Later studies did not confirm the original findings, no regulatory action was taken, and it was concluded that a causal relationship between reserpine and breast cancer was unlikely.

It is not the purpose of this chapter to analyse in detail the shortcomings of the original studies which resulted in weeks of work for the FDA and CSM, but there are one or two important lessons to be learnt. The importance of case definition referred to earlier was clearly not heeded in these studies. The condition studied was 'breast cancer', which is almost certainly too broad as a diagnostic classification.

Depending upon the pathology textbook of your choice, somewhere between 15 and 20 different kinds of malignant tumours of the breast are recognised, all of which would fall within the description 'breast cancer'. There is an enormous variation in the characteristics of these tumours with respect to originating tissue, histological type, malignancy, hormone dependence and tendency to metastasise. It is highly unlikely that any single agent could be the cause of such a wide variety of neoplasms. The most common malignant breast tumour is the scirrhous adenocarcinoma, which is usually very slow growing. It is known to have low growth fractions, with cell production exceeding cell loss by only about 10%, with the consequence that many years may pass from the time of tumorigenesis to the point at which the tumour becomes detectable. In the Boston Collaborative study six out of the 11 cancer cases had first been exposed to reserpine 5 years or less before the diagnosis. From these facts alone the role of reserpine as a carcinogen would seem to be very unlikely, and fully justified the cautious approach taken by FDA and CSM.

In the assessment of causality, Bradford Hill[129] cited biological plausibility as a major factor to take into consideration. If existing knowledge of physiological or pathological mechanisms is difficult to reconcile with the findings of a study, then much thought should be given to any attribution of causality.

Even in situations in which the diagnosis is straightforward, difficulties may arise if an assessment of severity or the presence of associated disease is required. However, it is in the selection of control cases that major difficulties

occur. There is the assumption, in the methodology, that all the relevant criteria for matching cases to controls are known, which in some cases is certainly not true. The hope is that cases and controls will be the same for all essential characteristics except the presence or absence of the disease. The finding that the test group exhibited excess exposure to the suspected toxin would then be interpreted as a positive result and the existence of a causal relationship inferred.

Case–control studies are powerful tools for the further investigation of suspected rare and uncommon ADEs, provided the factors discussed above are carefully controlled. The literature contains numerous examples of the method that should be evaluated critically.[130,131]

15.9   Prescription Event Monitoring

This form of adverse event monitoring was pioneered and developed by the Drug Safety Research Unit (DSRU) in Southampton. The aim is to monitor all new products that are expected to be widely used in general practice, with studies starting as soon as possible after the drug is first launched in the United Kingdom. PEM can be used to generate safety signals about new medicines that participating doctors may not have suspected to have been caused by the drug.

All patients who are prescribed the drug are identified from prescriptions submitted to the Prescription Pricing Authority (PPA). Copies of the prescriptions are sent to the DSRU to provide exposure data on patient and prescribing doctor. After a certain interval, typically 12 months, each GP is contacted and asked to complete a simple questionnaire (the 'green form') describing any 'event' that might have been recorded since the first prescription to the individual patient.

An 'event' is defined as a diagnosis, sign or symptom, accident, operation, change of treatment or any other incident that the doctor had considered important enough to enter into the patient's notes. For example, a fall would be considered an event, but not necessarily an ADR. The GP is not required to decide whether events are drug related or not.

The green forms are returned, scanned and the data entered on to computer. Important medical events, serious possible ADRs, all deaths from uncertain causes, pregnancies and events of interest are followed up. The response rate from green forms is very high (55.75%) compared to spontaneous reporting (yellow cards). The incidence densities (IDs) are then calculated for all the events occurring during treatment with the drug during a specified time period (t). The figures are expressed as ID per 1000 patient–months of treatment:

$$ID_t = \frac{\text{Number of reports of an event during treatment for period } t}{\text{Number of patient–months of treatment for period } t} \times 1000$$

Event rates are compared between the first month of treatment and the second to sixth months, and also during and after drug exposure. 'Reasons for stopping' are identified and medically qualified staff assess the causal relationship between the drug in question and selected events, using the following categories: probable, possible, unlikely or not assessable. The incidence of a particular event in patients who have not been exposed to the drug is examined (easier in those illnesses which are rarer), and event rates are compared between drugs of the same class and with similar indications. Safety signals, if present, can then be generated.

The system has several qualities that are very desirable in observational studies which include access to a large and widely distributed patient population and applicability to most new and generally used medicines. Reporting can be commenced as soon as the product reaches the market and observation may be extended over relatively long time periods. Disadvantages are the probability that there is considerable bias due to self-selection or exclusion by the doctor, impracticality of providing comprehensive clinical information on many chronically ill patients, recent low response rates, concerns in respect of confidentiality and increasing time constraints on GPs. Two recent studies[132,133] have also

suggested that response rates may be affected by the extent of prescribing for non-approved indications which would be perceived as increasing liability for the prescriber. An example of this is the widespread use of non-steroidal anti-inflammatory agents as general analgesics even when particular products are not licensed for those indications.

Examples of recent work carried out by the DSRU includes the examination of mortality rates and cardiac arrhythmias between sertindole and two other atypical antipsychotics, olanzapine and risperidone.[134] Tolterodine, an agent often used for urinary frequency and bladder instability, is the latest drug to be examined by the DSRU.[135]

15.10 Some Examples

It would be useful for pharmaceutical physicians to have some examples of medical products that have been the subject of serious adverse reactions requiring regulatory action. In the following subsections a number of products have been selected that illustrate different drug safety problems. Major attention has been paid to psychotropic agents because they are widely used and have been the subject of regulatory evaluation and action over the past several years which has resulted in restrictions to use and in some cases withdrawal from the market.

15.10.1 Psychotropic agents

Before the late 1980s there were very limited options in terms of pharmaceuticals for the psychiatric patient. With the advent of fluoxetine (Prozac), which was first launched in Belgium in 1986, the whole area of neuroscience became of much greater interest, especially given the fact that it was an area which had been relatively neglected up until that point. Options for treatment are now much more varied and offer the psychiatrist and patient far more choice. This has come at a price though; several drugs have had to be taken off the market while some remain available but with restricted use. In this section antidepressants and antipsychotics will be examined.

15.10.1.1 Clozapine

Clozapine is considered to be the gold standard of treatment of schizophrenia with patients usually moving onto it after treatment failure with two other antipsychotics. Yet the history of it is quite chequered. When it was first introduced onto the European market in 1975 it was used freely with no restrictions on use. Following the death of eight patients in Finland from agranulocytosis, a very rare (<1%) but often fatal condition occuring normally within the first few months of use, it was voluntarily taken off the market.

Thirty years later it is widely used throughout the United Kingdom and is growing in popularity. Indeed, the National Institute for Clinical Excellence (NICE) guidance on schizophrenia now encourages its use and mental health NHS trusts will soon be assessed on whether it is being prescribed enough. Further trials were carried out showing that up to 60% of patients who had been unresponsive to other antipsychotic treatment, did respond to long-term clozapine therapy. In 1990, clozapine gained a product licence and was relaunched with concurrent weekly monitoring of the white cell count for the first 16 weeks followed by fortnightly monitoring for the first year. Stringent measures were introduced such that hospital pharmacies were not permitted to dispense the drug until they had received notification of a 'green' result from the CPMS (clozapine patient monitoring service). An amber result (white count lowered) requires a repeat result which must be green, before dispensing can take place and a red result means that the patient has to stop the drug immediately. With such monitoring the incidence of agranulocytosis is 0.38%.

The successful relaunch of clozapine illustrates how life-threatening side effects can be managed as long as (1) they are detected quickly enough both in clinical practice and in pre-registration clinical trials and (2) stringent enough measures are put in place to prevent dispensing of drugs if necessary. It is interesting to note that clozapine now prevents more deaths from suicide in patients with schizophrenia than it does in causing death from agranulocytosis.

15.10.1.2 Cardiac dysrhythmias associated with antipsychotics

Sertindole, an atypical antipsychotic was introduced into the UK market in 1996 and initially it appeared that the drug would be useful, despite recommendations for ECG monitoring before and during sertindole therapy. QTc prolongation (rate corrected QT interval) was known to effect approximately 2% of patients in clinical trials. The drug was voluntarily suspended in 1998[134] following reports of sudden unexpected deaths and is now only available on a named-patient basis for those patients already stabilised on it, for whom other antipsychotics are inappropriate. Although 2% might seem a relatively insignificant figure for a side effect, given the fact that the consequences of a prolongation of the QT interval can be fatal, the pharmaceutical physician needs to be mindful of the type of side effect and potential seriousness of it. A side effect of perhaps 10% of patients experiencing headache would not, potentially lead to the withdrawal of a drug, unlike a 2% risk of QTc prolongation or 1% risk of agranulocytosis.

Reilly et al.[136] in their seminal review of antipsychotics and QTc-interval prolongation further highlighted the potential risks of such drugs. They noted that thioridazine and droperidol were at higher risk of causing such abnormalities. Thioridazine had been used for many years both with psychiatric patients and the elderly as a means of sedation. It is likely that many elderly patients may have died as a result of the drug because 'old age' was thought to be the cause. It is now available as a second-line treatment, under specialist supervision only. Droperidol is a long-established antipsychotic of high potency which was used in the maintenance of schizophrenia and for acutely agitated patients. Droperidol was withdrawn for use in the United Kingdom in 2002. Ziprasidone,[137] another atypical antipsychotic which can cause QT interval prolongation, although available in the United States, has never received approval in the European Union.

15.10.1.3 Antipsychotics and stroke

Risperidone and olanzapine have been widely used in patients with dementia exhibiting behavioural problems. Following the withdrawal of thioridazine from the market, old age psychiatrists and GPs were increasingly atypical antipsychotics, in particular risperidone as it was the only atypical which had been examined in randomised clinical trials (RCTs) with the elderly. In 2004, the CSM[138] advised that both risperidone and olanzapine caused an increased three-fold risk of cerebrovascular events in elderly patients with dementia compared with placebo. Consequently, the CSM advised that these drugs should be used with caution in patients with risk factors for cerebrovascular disease and in fact many thousands of patients have now been taken off the atypical antipsychotics.

15.10.1.4 Antipsychotics and diabetes/hyperlipidaemia

Atypical antipsychotics[139,140] have also been linked with the development of Type II diabetes and hyperlipidaemia in patients with schizophrenia. In several studies, olanzapine[141-143] has been more strongly linked than risperidone and there is a caution for use in patients with diabetes. Many psychiatrists now carry out a baseline glucose before initiating patients on it. The development of diabetes and hyperlipidaemia is of great concern, as patients with schizophrenia often neglect their physical health, smoke heavily and are at greater risk of developing diabetes than the normal population, even before they start to take antipsychotics. It is a problem that has emerged over several years and thus illustrates the importance of yellow card reporting and the pharmaceutical physician paying close attention to case reports and the company database. Side effects that can seem relatively minor in clinical trials can take on a much greater significance, once a drug has been on the market for several years and had huge patient exposure, and thus increasing numbers of cases.

15.10.1.5 Selective serotonin reuptake inhibitors and major depressive disorder in children and adolescents

In 2003, the CSM[138] advised that paroxetine and venlafaxine should not be used in children under the age of 18 to treat depression, following advise that the risks of self-harming behaviours outweighed the benefits of treatment. An expert working party was then set up to examine the safety and efficacy of the other selective serotonin reuptake inhibitors (SSRIs). All the clinical trial data available for citalopram, escitalopram, sertraline, fluvoxamine and fluoxetine was examined. Only fluoxetine was shown to have a favourable risk/benefit ratio in children and adolescents and is now the only SSRI recommended for use in this age group. In the other SSRIs, clinical trial data did not demonstrate efficacy in this age group and were associated with serious side effects such as suicidal thoughts and an increased rate of self-harm. Given that approximately 20 000 children under the age of 18 were estimated to be taking SSRIs other than fluoxetine at the time of this advice, clearly this had huge implications for treatment and confidence in the use of these drugs. The CSM have now set up a further working party to examine the efficacy and safety of SSRIs in adults, which has published its report in 2004.

Thus, the psychiatric drugs which showed so much hope when they were initially launched, and indeed for some years afterwards, are now increasingly being linked with serious and potentially fatal side effects. Clinical trials either do not detect these problems or detect it in such small figures that problems do not emerge until widespread use. This is the reason that extremely large Phase IV trials which are naturalistic are so vital in order to be able to detect these types of side effects. Phase IV trials are, of course, costly but necessary, if useful drugs can be made available to patients in a safe manner. Clozapine is one such drug that illustrates so well how a potentially lethal drug can still be prescribed with confidence by the clinician. The pharmaceutical physician must be alert to these potential problems and be creative in advising how they can be managed.

For instance, if patients taking olanzapine are obliged to be warned of these serious side effects before taking the drug and health advice is given initially, the weight gain usually seen in the first few months may be prevented and hence the onset of Type II diabetes, which is of course associated with obesity. As ever, the risks and benefits of drugs must be weighed up and not ignored, even if it leaves the treating clinician with few options.

15.10.2 Third generation OCs

The two OCs containing gestodene and desogestrel as progestogens were licensed for marketing in the early 1980s, the first being Marvelon in 1982, largely upon the claims that they had improved safety characteristics when compared with those previously available due to a lower oestrogen content. They soon became known as third generation products following on from the earlier ones that had become known as the second generation. It is of interest that in the mid- and late 1970s a commonly held view in the UK regulatory authority was that the evolution of OCs had probably reached its final stage. Levels of safety and efficacy were widely accepted and the regulatory requirements had become so demanding that it was difficult to see how a new product could be developed as an economically viable replacement for the numerous well-tried and clinically acceptable products on the market. To a greater or lesser extent the same view prevailed in the United States and other developed countries. In particular, the second generation products had demonstrated safety levels that would be difficult to improve upon in principle and even more difficult to determine objectively. It is possible that the companies concerned were encouraged by the chequered regulatory history of existing OCs and the financial prize that awaited a product that was demonstrably an advance on the second generation products.

However, soon after licensing, an increased incidence of venous thromboembolism (VTE) was suspected. By 1990–1 there were three main sources of information that could have been regarded as possibly generating hypotheses.

All third generation Combined Oral Contraceptives (COC) had been subject to UK and EU spontaneous reporting systems which are accepted as the primary systems of pharmacovigilance. The shortcomings of spontaneous reporting are well known, as has been discussed earlier in this chapter, but are nevertheless regarded as a major source of ADR reports by all licensing authorities. Sales figures had been used as denominators for all these ADR reports and no excess of VTEs was found.

In June 1987, Brill *et al.*[144] started a study which recruited a total of 96 000 patients in Germany. The study was completed by June 1989 and was published in 1990. Numerous criticisms have been raised which doubt its reliability but the findings did not provide evidence of a high level of VTEs. There were expressions of concern from Germany, mainly from the media, and although this raised questions regarding safety no demands or recommendations were made by the regulatory authority.

In spite of the widespread doubts concerning the validity of these data sources which, apparently, inhibited immediate regulatory action, stronger warnings were included in official literature by the mid-1990s which suggested that the third generation products carried an excess risk of VTEs of about 1.7. Following these warnings, several groups of patients started a legal action in the United Kingdom under the Consumer Protection Act (CPA) claiming that the two OCs concerned were defective within the meaning of the Act. The Judge closed the case prematurely on the grounds that the claimants had no possibility of proving an excess risk that was two or greater, which had been agreed as the level required for establishing the products as defective.

15.10.3 Vaccines

A trivalent vaccine containing the live attenuated viruses for measles, mumps and rubella was first introduced in the United States in the early 1970s by Merck and Co Inc. Since that time, other triple vaccines have been developed using various different viral strains and many countries have licensed them either as the sole vaccine available or alongside the monovalent vaccines. In 1988, three triple vaccines were licensed in the United Kingdom and although the original intention seems to have been to retain the single measles vaccine it was soon withdrawn leaving parents with no alternative choice for the protection of their children from that disease.

In the following years, it gradually emerged that a number of parents suspected that the triple vaccines, now referred to by the single name – MMR, might be associated with the development of autism, a poorly defined condition now better known as autistic spectrum disorder (ASD). These initial reports presented the typical picture of a new and unexpected adverse effect. It so happened that the rise in MMR associated reports paralleled fairly closely an apparent general increase in the diagnosis of ASDs particularly in the United Kingdom and the United States. This, almost certainly, boosted the reporting rate even though there was no objective evidence to support causality. Nevertheless, the number of reports, which extended into the hundreds, raised the question for the pharmaceutical physician and the regulator – how many reports do there have to be before they cannot all be explained by chance?

At the same time Wakefield and co-workers[145–148] described an inflammatory bowel condition apparently related to young children with an ASD. As a tentative suggestion the possibility that this might also be related to MMR vaccination was raised which resulted in cries of dismay, mostly from the UK Department of Health but also from certain sections of the medical profession. There is certainly good evidence that these disorders are chronologically related to the time of MMR vaccination and, in addition, measles virus, sometimes claimed to be of vaccine origin, has been found in bowel tissue but a convincing causal relationship has been widely discounted.

At the time of writing this chapter the problem remains unresolved which has created considerable anxiety for many parents. Vigorous denial of causality by health authorities has inhibited the revision of official literature which, for many other medicinal products, would have been required even in the absence of proof of causality. The withdrawal of single component measles vaccine has accentuated the difficulties in that parents in the United Kingdom now have no alternative to the triple vaccine.

15.10.4 Rofecoxib (Vioxx)

The cyclooxygenase 2 (COX 2) inhibitors were first licensed for sale at the end of the 1990s as more effective and better tolerated NSAIDs which, it was hoped, would provide improved therapy for patients with rheumatoid and osteoarthritis. One of the first of those was rofecoxib which quickly achieved dominance in the market and seemed to have lived up to its expectations over its first 2 years. Other similar agents, which included valdecoxib, celecoxib and meloxicam, were granted product licences and became competitor products. As might be expected, the major comparative clinical trials which were conducted in support of the products concentrated almost exclusively on GI adverse effects which are generally accepted as being limiting factors in the use of earlier NSAIDs. Two of the studies concerned (CLASS and VIGOR[149,150]) demonstrated clear GI advantages but only VIGOR noted a lower incidence of myocardial infarction in the comparator group although the authors stated that the overall mortality from cardiovascular causes was not increased.

In September 2001, however, a news item in the *British Medical Journal*[151] reported that further analyses confirmed the increase in rates of myocardial infarction and questioned whether this was an adverse reaction affecting the whole class of COX 2 drugs. The debate continued for the next 3 years with the main emphasis remaining on GI toxicity. A PEM study[152] that included more than 15 000 patients made no mention of cardiovascular adverse events. However, a second paper[153] compared rofecoxib and meloxicam with respect to thromboembolic events which showed that both, to a variable extent were associated with cardiovascular, cerebrovascular and peripheral venous pathology. A meta-analysis published recently in *The Lancet*[154] suggests that Merck, the licence holder for Vioxx, was aware of cardiovascular problems as early as 2000 and there is the implication that the US FDA failed to act on the basis of this information. Indeed, there are growing doubts concerning the independence and impartiality of drug regulatory authorities in general. The Vioxx saga culminated in the withdrawal of the product from the market by Merck in September 2004 with disastrous results for the company.

15.10.4.1 Overall conclusions

The above examples have been selected to illustrate the complexity of managing suspected and actual adverse reactions to medical products. The pharmaceutical physician should take careful note of two vital factors. First, the initial recognition that a product may be related to a series of AE reports could be a slow process extending over months or even years and second that proof of causality is usually difficult and frequently impossible. This does not mean that regulatory action is not required or that a legal case may not follow. However, what is certain is that a potentially developing situation must not be neglected and every effort should be made to investigate the problem as scientifically as possible. The case of MMR illustrates very well the regrettable fact that epidemiologically based studies may not be capable of recruiting a sufficient number of patients to provide statistically significant conclusions. This is a particularly serious problem for vaccines that are commonly administered to a major proportion of the relevant population which results in comparator groups that are too small to permit meaningful results.

It has long-been recognised that individual patient susceptibility may be a major factor in the causality of adverse reactions. Recent advances in human genetics hold out the promise of identifying individuals or families that may be at greater risk than others but the application of these opportunities to improved prescribing has been extremely disappointing. It is clear from simple observational studies that ADRs occur in only relatively small subsets of the patient population leaving the majority unaffected. The unfortunate subset remains undetected until after the event.

There has never been any incentive for the pharmaceutical industry to pursue research along these lines even though, as in the case of Vioxx, the end results of neglecting adverse effects may be very costly. The aim of the industry has usually been to extend the market size irrespective of potential risk and attempts to implement effective post-marketing surveillance has received little enthusiasm. It is to be hoped that company medical departments and pharmaceutical physicians will continue to support the need for a broad range of safety evaluation studies to be conducted on new medicinal products.

15.11 Causality Assessment

Lack of safety in medicinal products arises from the recurrence of undesired adverse effects associated with their use. The first requirement for the assurance of safety is the ability to detect such adverse effects. This has been dealt with in an earlier section of this chapter. Once detected, it is highly desirable that a significantly convincing causal relationship between the use of the product and the adverse effect should be established.

In previous editions of this textbook a number of methods of determining causality have been described and an attempt made to evaluate their relative reliability and validity. It has to be understood that such statistically based methods have, over several dacades, been in competition with common observation and 'inspired guesswork' for the assessment of adverse effects in respect of the need for regulatory action. This is not just a matter of idiosyncratic personal preference but is frequently imposed by the clinical and numerical evidence available.

The most familiar story of a new and unexpected adverse effect starts in a dense fog of uncertainty. The pharmaceutical company may have received a few reports from doctors or other healthcare workers, there may be a letter in the medical press describing six or so cases of a suspected adverse effect or the regulatory authority may tentatively draw attention to a possible problem. The pharmaceutical physician may, quite reasonably, assess the small number of reports and conclude that they are slightly worrying but, probably, chance associations. Time passes and similar reports accumulate and the level of concern rises. This increasing concern may well be more apparent in the medical departments than those responsible for sales, and the pharmaceutical physician should not be inhibited from further investigations. A point is reached as the numbers increase, 20, . . . , 30, . . . , 40, . . . , 50 at which chance becomes a receding explanation. The physician may question him/herself, 'can I realistically believe that all these reports are spurious, that not a single one is a true bill?' This has little to do with objective clinical science but it has a real impact on further action. If the answer is 'no' then numbers, in themselves, have assumed the status of evidence.

This turning point in the decision process anticipates the continuing accumulation of case reports which may provide the quantity of data required by objective statistical methods. In the case of medical products which are in widespread use for common, well-understood clinical conditions this may be readily available but for products not having these attributes the data demanded for scientifically supported causality may be unobtainable.

The aims of causality assessment are manifold. Adverse events need to be classified, a decision needs to be made whether a drug has caused this event, regulatory requirements need to be satisfied, signal recognition can be aided, and finally, at the end of this process, a label change may be necessary.

Attributing causality is a major problem with spontaneous reports of suspected drug-related events. Clinical event reports arising from cohort studies or from computerised databases may also raise similar problems, particularly when they are in isolation or in such small numbers that a conventional statistical approach is not appropriate. If ADRs occur a long time after the original use of the drug, or there are delayed consequences of long-term use (e.g. tardive dyskinesia with the use of typical antipsychotics), then detection becomes difficult. In addition, clinical trials often do not include special populations, such as pregnant women, the elderly, children or patients with severe hepatic or renal disease, who may be at special risk of an ADR.

In the time that has elapsed since the previous edition of this book, it has been the authors' impression that enthusiasm for formal methods of causality assessment has decreased to the extent that few, if any, pharmaceutical companies still use them. Nevertheless, brief comments on methods that have been developed over the years are needed to complete the picture.

In a typical situation, two or three individual case reports may be published in the medical literature, to be followed by another half dozen spontaneous reports (yellow cards) to the regulatory agency that draw attention to a possible ADR to a particular product. The scientific value of such reports ranges from situations in which a causal relationship is a near certainty, to those in which any attribution of causality would seem to be a forlorn hope. The former would include reports on patients with a single disease, who are administered a single drug for the first time, with a clearly described adverse clinical event occurring within hours of administration and resolving on withdrawal of the drug. Even if the event occurs many years later, as in the cases of clear-cell adenocarcinoma in young women exposed to stilboestrol, it can be detected if the rate of this illness in this population would otherwise be negligible. Needless to say, this is seldom the case. At the other end of the scale is the patient with multiple pathologies, on 10 or more drugs, who develops a vague symptomatic adverse event 10 days after the introduction of a new medication, with partial resolution after its withdrawal. Often the reporting physician has no idea whether the drug in question has caused the effect or not. Even beyond such confused and nebulous accounts are reports of so little clinical or scientific value that they can only be described as frivolous and have to be disregarded as useless.

In between these two extremes lie the great majority of spontaneous reports for which the attribution of causality is at best doubtful, and always difficult. It is not surprising, therefore, that considerable work has been done to devise mathematical methods to give numerical values to the varying degrees of certainty or uncertainty.

These methods are applicable to individual cases either singly, or for relatively small groups of selected cases where there are high-quality data and few confounding factors. It may be questioned whether assigning numerical values, in which a degree of precision is implicit, to data which are, to a substantial extent, subjective in nature can produce better results than the clinical judgement of experts. Whatever the answer to this question may be, there is no doubt that the application of a formalised system of assessment to ADE evaluation may produce a level of consistency that would not be possible by clinical judgement alone.

Meta-analysis is a method often used to determine the effectiveness of a drug but to date it has rarely been used to assess safety. One case illustrates how this technique can help. Six studies examining the use of intravenous lidocaine for acute myocardial infarction did not, on an individual basis, give strong enough evidence to support the hypothesis that this technique could cause excess mortality. The meta-analysis, however, was able to demonstrate this.[133]

A useful review of causality assessment methods has been produced by Stephens,[169,176] one of which he has developed for use by Glaxo Group Research. Because most of the methods are relatively time consuming and rely on high-quality clean data, they are not readily applicable to situations in which hundreds or even thousands of reports have to be assessed. It is possibly true to say that most pharmaceutical companies still rely heavily upon clinical judgement, with occasional use of one or other of the described methods of causality assessment. In many cases, the continuing accumulation of similar ADE reports becomes the most convincing evidence that some unexpected reaction is occurring. This may be scientifically unsatisfactory, but is a reminder of the uncertainties that are an inseparable part of clinical medicine.

Edwards and Aronson[155] have suggested a way of coding whether an adverse event is an ADR. This depends on factors such as the time relation between the use of the drug and the occurrence of the reaction being assessed; pattern recognition; dechallenge and rechallenge of the drug in question and laboratory investigations.

Another system has been devised by Benichou and Danan[156] which assigns numerical values to factors of importance in the assessment of causality (Table 15.10).

In recent years, a method of causality assessment based on Bayes' theorem has been developed by a number of workers in the United States.[157–161] Its application to the evaluation

Table 15.10 Method for causality assessment of ADRs

Criteria	Score
1. Time to onset of the reaction	
Highly suggestive	+3[a]
Suggestive	+2
Compatible	+1
Inconclusive	0[a]
If incompatible, then case 'unrelated'	
If information not available, then case 'insufficiently documented'	
2. Course of the reaction	
Highly suggestive	+3
Suggestive	+2
Compatible	+1
Against the role of the drug	−2
Inconclusive or not available	0
3. Risk factor(s) for drug reaction	
Yes	+1[b]
No	0
4. Concomitant drug(s)	
Time to onset incompatible	0
Time to onset compatible but unknown reaction	−1
Time to onset compatible and known reaction	−2
Role proved in this case	−3
None or information not available	0
5. Non-drug-related causes	
Ruled out	−2
Possible or not investigated	−1
Probable	−3
6. Previous information on the drug	
Reaction unknown	0
Reaction published but unlabelled	+1
Reaction labelled in the product's characteristics	+2

continued

Table 15.10 Continued

Criteria	Score
7. Response to re-administration	
Positive	+3
Compatible	+1
Negative	−2
Not available or not interpretable	0
Plasma concentration of the drug known as toxic	+3
Validated laboratory test with high specificity, sensitivity and predictive values	
Positive	−3
Negative	+3
Not interpretable or not available	0

[a] Qualifying terms in italics are not to be used for assessing acute drug-induced liver injuries.
[b] One additional point for each validated risk factor.

of ADEs is shown in Table 15.11 and a practical method (from Hutchinson) is shown in Table 15.12 and Figure 15.2. This is probably the most sophisticated system developed so far, and it has been applied to a number of actual drug problems. An integrated approach to ADE assessment which permits the prediction of incidence extends the method beyond individual case evaluation.

In 1968, an international collaboration to identify rare adverse events not detected in clinical trials was set up under the auspices of the World Health Organisation (WHO) in Uppsala, Sweden. The Uppsala Monitoring Centre maintains an international database with data collected from 58 official member countries (those with a formally recognised national ADR monitoring centre) and six associate member countries (those with strong pharmacovigilance capacity but no formally recognised ADR monitoring centre).[162] Reports are published two or three times a year giving updated information on ADRs and the work of the centre. These are available online at: http://www.who-umc.org. A new signalling process using Bayesian logic applied to data mining, within a confidence propagation neural network, has been developed, with initial work suggesting that this approach has a high predictive value that can identify early signals of ADRs.[163]

15.12 The Legal Framework and its Implications for Future International Developments

In the pre-marketing phase of new drug development national regulatory authorities encourage and evaluate a broad range of experimental methods that come within the definition of clinical trials.

In the evaluation of safety in the post-marketing phase, regulatory agencies are greatly more restricted in their enthusiasm for data derived from some of the methods available than from others. Indeed, the EC national agencies separately and the CPMP collectively have developed a legislative framework that is predominantly concerned with spontaneous adverse event monitoring and which is, for all practical purposes, silent on the matter of safety data collected by other methods.

The starting point was set out in Directive 65/65/EEC which states:

The competent authorities of the Member States shall suspend or revoke an authorisation to place a proprietary medicinal product on the market where that product proves to be harmful in the normal conditions of use, or where its therapeutic efficacy is lacking when it is established that therapeutic results cannot be obtained with the proprietary product.

This is a very general statement, giving no guidance on what might be seen as harmful or what would constitute lack of efficacy.

In 1989, in Article 33 of Directive 89/341/EEC, the situation was dealt with in more detail.

1. Each Member State shall take all the appropriate measures to ensure that decisions authorizing marketing, refusing or revoking a marketing authorization, prohibit supply, or withdrawing a product from the market together with the reason on which such decisions are based, are brought to the attention of the Committee forthwith.

Table 15.11 Hand-held Bayesian ADR assessment

Instructions

Case parameters

Read the case and write down those elements in the following categories that best describe the generic type of case and which most facilitate assessment of the prior. This may mean picking descriptions that fit with other cases reported in the literature or on which you have other sources of information.

Clinical background. Usually includes patient's age, sex, underlying illness. It should include anything else that changes the likelihood for different causes of the event, but which will not be used later in the case findings.

Adverse event type. Usually a general description of the event that would allow you to look it up in a reference source, e.g. acute renal failure, diarrhoea. Does not usually include all details of the event.

Time to onset. The interval between starting the suspected drug and the occurrence or detection of the adverse event.

Evolution of the event and drug withdrawal. What was there about the course of the event and its response (or non-response) to drug withdrawal that helped differentiate between the causes?

Rechallenge. As for behaviour of the event on restarting the suspected drug.

Other. List other items that you feel have diagnostic value.

Scoring

For each category of assessment consider the list of possible causes. Identify the one least likely to lead to the particular finding being considered (in the case of the prior, the finding is the adverse event type). Give this cause a score of 1 in that category. Identify the next lowest cause likely to lead to the findings and assign it a number between 1 and infinity that represents by how many times more likely it is to lead to the finding that the least likely cause. Proceed in this way for each cause using the cause that received a score of 1 in that category as the comparator in each case.

Time horizon. An arbitrary time chosen to be longer than the actual time of occurrence and longer than expected timings for the drug cause being considered. Using these guidelines, choose the time that most facilitates the assessment.

Possible causes. List the suspected drug, other drugs that you consider potential causes, and other possible causes (such as the patient's underlying disease). The list should include all the causes you consider possible. Note that if you consider a drug interaction a possible cause, this should appear as a separate item on the cause list.

Case findings

Read the case and write down those elements in the following categories that you feel help distinguish between the potential causes you are considering. This does not mean the whole case report, and will generally be a very brief list of information that you feel has diagnostic values.

Specific background. Those elements of the patient's background that were not included in the general but that make one or more of the causes more (or less) likely.

For the next category of assessment pick a new 'least likely cause' and assign it a score of 1. Proceed as for the previous category. Continue in this way until all categories of assessment in which there is relevant information have been completed.

To obtain the final score, multiply the scores under each cause to obtain a product fot that cause. Add the products to obtain a total. Divide each product by the total to obtain the probability that the particular cause led to the ADR. Note that the categories in which there is no information do not receive a score and are ignored in the final scoring. Note also that if you encounter a finding whose likelihood for occurrences is 0 for one of the causes on the list, you should simply remove that cause from further consideration and assign a 1 to the next most unlikely cause for that finding. The scores for the other causes that were obtained before 'ruling out' finding was assessed remain valid and can be used unaltered to obtain the products used in the final score.

Table 15.12 Hand-held Bayesian ADR assessment: data and scoring sheet

Case (DSD) number

Case parameters (used for assessing prior)	Case findings (for other assessment categories)
General background	Time to onset
	Specific background
Adverse event type	Evolution of event
Time horizon	Drug withdrawal
Possible causes	Rechallenge
	Other
	1.
	2.
	3.
	Possible causes

Assessment category	Drug	Other (1)	Other (2)	Other (3)
Prior				
Time to onset				
Specific background				
Evolution of event				
Drug withdrawal				
Rechallenge				
Other				
1.				
2.				
3.				Total
	+	+	+	=

Products.

Products ÷ total

2. The person responsible for the marketing of a medicinal product shall be obliged to notify the Member States concerned forthwith of any action taken by him to suspend the marketing of a product or to withdraw a product from the market, together with the reason for such action if the latter concerns the efficacy of the medicinal product or the protection of the public health. Member States shall ensure that this information is brought to the attention of the Committee.

3. Member States shall ensure that appropriate information about action taken pursuant to paragraphs 1 and 2 which may affect the protection of public health in third countries is forthwith brought to the attention of the World Health Organisation, with a copy to the Committee.

4. The Commission shall publish annually a list of the medicinal products which are prohibited in the Community.

The term 'pharmacovigilance' has now been adopted by all Member States for the activities involved in the study and evaluation of drug safety. Although pharmacovigilance covers a broad range of data collection methods, it is the spontaneous reporting systems sponsored by all European governments to which the term usually refers.

Since the previous edition, numerous lengthy documents have become available which address

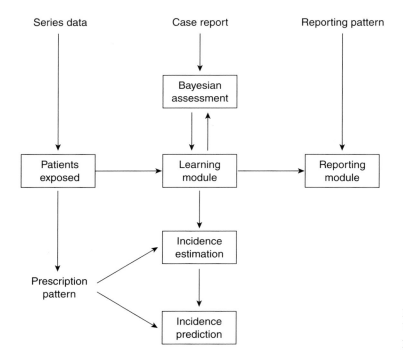

Series data   Case report   Reporting pattern

Fig. 15.2 An integrated Bayesian system for predicting ACR incidence.

the ADR reporting requirements in greater detail and in a more comprehensible way. It is not the purpose of this chapter to review each of these individually, but the reader is recommended to become familiar with those listed below.

1. Directive 75/319/EEC (Amended) on the approximation of provisions laid down by law, regulation or administrative action relating to medicinal products.
2. Regulation (EEC) No 2309/93. Council Regulation (EEC) No 2309/9 of 22 July 1993 laying down Community procedures for the authorisation and supervision of medicinal products for human and veterinary use and establishing a European Agency for the Evaluation of Medicinal Products.
3. Regulation (EC) No 540/95. Commission Regulation (EC) No 540/95 of 10 March 1995 laying down the arrangements for reporting suspected unexpected adverse reactions which are not serious, whether arising in the Community or in a third country, to medicinal products for human

or veterinary use authorised in accordance with the provisions of Council Regulation (EEC) No 2309/93.
4. Conduct of Pharmacovigilance for Centrally Authorised Products: EMEA April 1997.
5. Conduct of Pharmacovigilance for Medicinal Products: authorised through the mutual recognition procedure EMEA June 1997.
6. ICH Topic E1A Population Exposure: the extent of population exposure to assess clinical safety.
7. ICH Topic E2A Clinical Safety Data Management: definitions and standards for expedited reporting.
8. ICH E2B(M) Clinical Safety Data Management: data elements for transmission of individual case safety reports.
9. ICH Topic E2C Clinical Safety Data Management: periodic safety update reports for marketed drugs.
10. CPMP Note for Guidance on Electronic Exchange of Pharmacovigilance Information for Human and Veterinary Medicinal Products in the European Union August 1999.

11. CPMP Joint Pharmacovigilance Plan for the Implementation of the ICH E2B M1 and M2 Requirements Related to the Electronic Transmission of Individual Case Safety Reports in the Community.

Since the last edition of this book was published, a plethora of new updating information has become available on the internet. The sheer volume of this is such that it is beyond the reach of this chapter. Attempts to create a standard set of procedures and requirements in the new and enlarged European Union have certainly made progress although the pharmaceutical physician will have to consult the most recent regulations and guidelines if errors are to be avoided. Even such basic concepts as a suspected 'serious' adverse reaction may vary between countries.

The following is a generally accepted listing of serious events:

- Fatal
- Life threatening
- Results in persistent or significant disability/incapacity
- Results in or prolongs hospitalisation.

This also includes congenital abnormalities/birth defects and serious adverse clinical consequences with use outside the terms of the Summary of Product Characteristics (SPC) including overdoses or abuse.

The generally expected reporting requirements for serious adverse reactions (expedited reporting) are as follows:

All such reports should be reported immediately and in no case later than 15 calendar days from receipt. The clock for expedited reporting starts as soon as one or more of the following has received the minimum information required for the submisssion of an adverse reaction report:

1. Any personnel of the marketing authorisation holder – including sales representatives.
2. The qualified person responsible for pharmacovigilance or persons working for or with this person.

3. Where the marketing authorisation holder has entered into relationships with a second company for the marketing of, or research on, the suspected product, the clock starts as soon as any personnel of the marketing authorisation holder receives the minimum information; however, wherever possible, the time frame for regulatory submission should be no longer than 15 from the receipt by the second company. Explicit procedures and detailed agreements should exist between the marketing authorisation holder and the second company to facilitate the achievement of this objective.
4. In the case of relevant worldwide scientific literature, the clock starts with awareness of the publication by any personnel of the marketing authorisation holder; the marketing authorisation holder is expected to maintain awareness of possible publications by accessing a widely used systematic literature review and reference database, such as Medline, Excerpta Medica or Embase, no less frequently than once a week, or by making formal contractual arrangements with a second party to perform this task; marketing authorisation holders are also expected to ensure that relevant publications in each Member State are appropriately reviewed.

Some comments are required in respect of the document entitled 'Notice to Marketing Authorisation Holders – Pharmacovigilance Guidelines' and identified as MCA EuroDirect Publication No PhVWP/108/99. This guideline was issued from the European Medicines Evaluation Agency (EMEA) in January 1999 and probably has more practical importance for the reader of this book. It has to be said that it is not without a number of shortcomings that make it less clear than it should be. Nevertheless, it does outline the actual procedures involved in ADR reporting and the responsibilities of all those concerned. Like many other publications from the various European authorities it is likely to be the subject of revisions and amendments as time goes by, so vigilance is advised.

As in other areas in which self-regulation has been relied upon, the response has been disappointing. Even though all major companies would agree that the safety evaluation of new drugs should be continued into the post-marketing phase, remarkably little enthusiasm has been apparent when the time actually comes. The solution to the problem probably lies in the integration of post-marketing studies into the overall drug development procedure in such a way that new drug applications would only be considered if a detailed and realistic post-marketing plan were to be included.

Back in the mid-1970s the Association of the British Pharmaceutical Industry (ABPI) was very concerned by the increasing demands being made with respect to the numbers of patients in clinical trials and the duration of treatment. They entered into discussion with the CSM to see if there were ways in which the demands for the better assessment of safety could be met without enlarging clinical trials to the point where new drug development would be stifled. It was recognised nearly 20 years ago that there were limitations on what clinical trials could achieve, and that at the time of marketing the new product emerged from a very carefully controlled environment to the largely uncontrolled world of everyday clinical practice. It was at this time that the Medicines Division in the United Kingdom was becoming very active in creating the yellow card system, experimenting with monitored release, post-marketing surveillance and pre-scription event monitoring, and there were hopes that one or more of these systems would provide a solution to the problem.[164] It has to be said that those hopes have never been realised, and we are no further ahead than we were then except that clinical trial demands have continued to increase, albeit probably more slowly than had been feared.

The hope had been that stopping escalating demands for bigger clinical trials could be off-set by continuing large-scale studies into the post-marketing period. This could not be done, because the CSM had only limited powers after the granting of a product licence and so could not require post-marketing studies.

A similar pattern seems to have occurred in other countries of the European Union, and it is now difficult to believe that progress could

be made in this direction without fairly substantial changes in existing legislation. The insubstantial legal framework provides no incentives for companies to set up realistic post-marketing programmes. They will therefore continue to put their faith in spontaneous reporting systems and to receive unpleasant surprises when unexpected adverse events arise. The concentration of regulatory authority efforts on spontaneous reporting, which is essentially the only method envisaged in the present legal structure, focuses attention upon uncommon, bizarre and usually serious conditions and neglects commoner problems which, although they may be less serious, are nevertheless limiting factors in drug treatment.

This policy may well be shortsighted, but competition is such that pharmaceutical companies would prefer to accept the risk and save the money. It is this attitude that is a major contributor to the poor image of the industry in the eyes of the public and the media. Unfortunately, in this and many other fields, self-regulation has not worked, so we probably have to look to strengthening legal framework and setting down requirements if improvements are to be made.

15.13 Other Considerations and Conclusions

There is no doubt that the continuing evaluation of the safety of medicines into the post-marketing period is an expanding and still developing area of research. Matters relating to safety spread over into efficacy, which together imply risks and benefits which, in the present international climate of healthcare provision, have consequences for outcomes and costs. A whole new field of research – pharmacoeconomics – is in the process of development and it is to be anticipated that many of the methods used for safety evaluation will be modified and applied in this area.

Then there are questions of ethics, patient confidentiality, informed consent and ethics committee approval to be addressed, as well as the whole new range of legislation already referred to. At present, purely observational studies, which have no influence on the normal course of the patient's treatment, require neither informed consent nor ethics committee approval. Whether this will continue to be the case in the new Europe and internationally remains to be seen. There are certainly concerns for the privacy and protection of the patient as an individual, but there are also the broader questions of the delivery of efficient and effective healthcare to large populations, which depends on the continuation of high-quality clinical research.

Phase IV clinical trials and prospective observational cohort studies have been criticised as no more than promotional devices used by aggressive pharmaceutical companies. The fact that misuse has sometimes happened should not be allowed to obscure the greatly more important needs of safety evaluation and the further development of new and improved therapies. A set of guidelines[165] has been published in the United Kingdom which are specifically intended to provide the high standards of study design and methodology necessary for observational cohort studies. It is to be hoped that similar procedures will be adopted internationally.

In addition to the methods reviewed in this chapter there has been the development of a procedure known as 'meta-analysis',[164–166] which seeks to combine as many clinical studies as possible in a formal and structured way, so that patient numbers may be increased to a level at which conclusions may be drawn that would not be possible from single studies. Needless to say, there are strongly held views both for and against meta-analysis, but at present it would probably be true to say that the jury is still out.

Another area of research is growing within the established fields of biochemistry, metabolism, immunology and genetics which is aimed at the elucidation of mechanisms[167] involved in ADRs. The importance of this development is hard to overemphasise when it is considered that the risk for patients not susceptible to a particular ADR is probably zero, whereas for the susceptible patient it approaches certainty. The detection of susceptible patients through knowledge of genetic or metabolic characteristics would be a major advance in knowledge.

Since the last edition of this book, the internet has become a valuable source of information on ADRs and pharmacovigilance. The various directives, regulations and guidelines referred to in this chapter are now readily available from this source, and the reader will be able to obtain the full versions of all such documents. A paper by Cobert and Silvey[168] contains much useful information and many internet addresses.

A hope for the future would be to limit the massive burden of pre-marketing testing of new drugs, which threatens the continuation of research in the pharmaceutical industry, and to establish methods of investigation in the post-marketing phase that would provide the necessary safeguards. It should be remembered that the cost of a patient in a controlled clinical trial may be 10–20 times greater than that of the same patient in an observational study. There is certainly a difference in the type and quantity of data available, but as a means of evaluating safety in the real-life situation the observational cohort study is the method of choice.

A recent Editorial in the *BMJ* entitled 'Using Drugs Safely'[169] has reported that the Audit Commission found that nearly 1100 people had died in England and Wales in the previous 12 months as a result of medication errors or adverse reactions and that this was a five-fold increase in just 10 years. The Editorial emphasises the need for improvements in medical education in order to foster good prescribing and an awareness of ADRs. It is a sobering observation in the revision of this chapter that so little progress has been made since the first edition.

References

1. Royal Society Study Group. *Risk Assessment.* London: Royal Society, 1983.
2. British Medical Association. *The BMA Guide to Living with Risk.* London: Penguin Books, 1987.
3. O'Brien B. *'What are My Chances Doctor?' A Review of Clinical Risks.* London: Office of Health Economics, 1986.
4. Ferner RE. Hazards, risks and reality. *Br J Clin Pharmacol* 1992;**33**:125–8.

5. Chapman CR, Morrison D. Impacts on the Earth by asteroids and comets: assessing the hazard. *Nature* 1994;**367**:33–40.

6. Calman KC, Royston HD. Risk language and dialects. *BMJ* 1997;**315**:939–42.

7. Griffin JP. Realistic risk assessment – an unachievable goal. *Scr Mag* 1997;March:22–4.

8. Fletcher AP. Drug safety tests and subsequent clinical experience. *J Roy Soc Med* 1978;**71**:693–6.

9. Rawlins MD, Jefferys DB. Study of United Kingdom product licence applications containing new active substances. *BMJ* 1991;**302**:223–5.

10. Inman WHW. Lets get our act together. In: Dukes MNG, ed. *Side Effects of Drugs Essay*. Amsterdam: Elsevier, 1990:115–35.

11. Lawson DH. Postmarketing surveillance of drugs. *Proc Roy Coll Phys Edinb* 1990;**20**:129–42.

12. Mann RD. CSM monitoring today. *Pharm Med* 1988;**3**:275–89.

13. Rawlins MD. Spontaneous reporting of adverse drug reactions I: the data. *Br J Clin Pharmacol* 1988;**26**:1–5.

14. Rawlins MD. Spontaneous reporting of adverse drug reactions II: uses. *Br J Clin Pharmacol* 1988;**26**:7–11.

15. Rawson NSB, Pearce GL, Inman WHW. Prescription event monitoring: methodology and recent progress. *J Clin Epidemiol* 1990;**43**:509–22.

16. Tilson HH. *Postmarketing Surveillance. The Way Forward*. Centre for Medicines Research, MTP press.

17. Venning GR. Identification of adverse reactions to new drugs. I: what have been the important adverse reactions since thalidomide? *BMJ* 1983;**286**:199–202.

18. Venning GR. Identification of adverse reactions to new drugs. II: how were 18 important adverse reactions discovered and with what delay? *BMJ* 1983;**286**:365–8.

19. Venning GR. Identification of adverse reactions to new drugs. III: alerting processes and early warning systems. *BMJ* 1983;**286**:458–60.

20. Venning GR. Identification of adverse reactions to new drugs. IV: verification of suspected adverse reactions. *BMJ* 1983;**286**:544–7.

21. Venulet J. Possible strategies for early recognition of potential drug safety problems. *Adv Drug React Ac Pois Rev* 1988;**1**:39–47.

22. Winstanley PA, Irvin LE, Smith JC, *et al.* Adverse drug reactions: a hospital pharmacy-based reporting scheme. *Br J Clin Pharmacol* 1989;**28**:113–16.

23. Witts LJ. Adverse reactions to drugs. *BMJ* 1965;**2**:1081.

24. WHO Anniversary Symposium Proceedings. *Adverse drug reactions: a global perspective on signal generation and analysis.* Uppsala, 1988.

25. Ionnidis JPA, Haidich A-B, Lau J. Any casualties in the clash of randomised and observational evidence? *BMJ* 2001;**322**:879–80.

26. Benson K, Hartz AJ. A comparison of observational studies and randomized, controlled trials. *N Engl J Med* 2000;**342**:1878–86.

27. Concato J, Shah N, Horwitz RI. Randomized, controlled trials, observational studies and the hierarchy of research designs. *N Engl J Med* 2000;**342**:1887–92.

28. Daneshmend TK, Hawkey CJ, Langman MJS, *et al.* Omeprazole versus placebo for acute upper gastrointestinal bleeding: randomised double blind controlled trial. *BMJ* 1992;**304**:143–7.

29. Ferguson J, Addo HA, McGill PE, *et al.* A study of benoxaprofen induced photosensitivity. *Br J Dermatol* 1982;**107**:429.

30. GREAT Group. Feasibility, safety, and efficacy of domiciliary thrombolysis by general practitioners: Grampian region early anistreplase trial. *BMJ* 1992;**305**:548–53.

31. ISIS-3. ISIS-3: a randomised comparison of streptokinase vs tissue plasminogen activator vs anistreplase and of aspirin plus heparin vs aspirin alone among 41 299 cases of suspected acute myocardial infarction. *Lancet* 1992;**339**:753–70.

32. Jacobson SJ, Jones K, Johnson K, *et al.* Prospective multicentre study of pregnancy outcome after lithium exposure during the first trimester. *Lancet* 1992;**339**:530–3.

33. Campbell JPM, Howie JGR. Involving the patient in reporting adverse drug reactions. *J Roy Coll Gen Pract* 1988;**38**:370–1.

34. McBride WG. Thalidomide and congenital abnormalities. *BMJ* 1962;**5320**:1681.

35. Lenz W. Thalidomide and congenital abnormalities. *Lancet* 1962;**1**:45.

36. Lenz W. Malformations caused by drugs in pregnancy. *Am J Dis Child* 1966;**112**:99–106.

37. Lenz W, Knapp K. Die thalidomidembryopathie. *Dtsch Med Wochenschr* 1962;**87**:1232.

38. Burley DM. Thalidomide and congenital abnormalities. *Lancet* 1962;**1**:271.

39. Finney DJ. The design and logic of a monitor of drug use. *J Chronic Dis* 1965;**18**:77–98.

40. Edlavitch SA. Adverse drug event reporting. *Arch Int Med* 1988;**148**:1499–503.

41. Faich GA. National adverse drug reaction reporting. *Arch Int Med* 1991;**151**:1645–7.

42. Faich GA. Special report – adverse drug reaction monitoring. *N Engl J Med* 1986;**314**:1589–92.

43. Griffin JP. Survey of adverse drug reaction reporting schemes in fifteen countries. *Br J Clin Pharmacol* 1985;**22**:83S–100S.

44. Griffin JP, Weber JCP. Voluntary systems of adverse reaction reporting. Part I. *Adv Drug React Ac Pois Rev* 1985;**4**:213–30.

45. Griffin JP, Weber JCP. Voluntary systems of adverse reaction reporting. Part II. *Adv Drug React Ac Pois Rev* 1986;**5**:23–55.

46. Griffin JP, Weber JCP. Voluntary systems of adverse reaction reporting. Part III. *Adv Drug React Ac Pois Rev* 1989;**8**:203–15.

47. Lawson DH. The yellow card: mark II. *BMJ* 1990;**301**:1234.

48. Sachs RM, Bortnichak EA. An evaluation of spontaneous adverse drug reactions monitoring systems. *Am J Med* 1986;**81**:49–55.

49. Walker SR, Lumley CE. The attitudes of general practitioners to monitoring and reporting adverse drug reactions. *Pharm Med* 1986;**1**:195–203.

50. Lumley CE, Walker SR, Hall GC, *et al*. The underreporting of adverse drug reactions seen in general practice. *Pharm Med* 1986;**1**:205–12.

51. Fletcher AP. Spontaneous adverse drug reaction reporting vs event monitoring: a comparison. *J Roy Soc Med* 1991;**84**:341–4.

52. Fletcher AP. An appraisal of spontaneous adverse event monitoring. *Adv Drug React Toxicol Rev* 1992;**11**:213–27.

53. Smithells RW, Sheppard S. Teratogenicity testing in humans; a method demonstrating safety of Bendectin. *Teratology* 1978;**17**:31–6.

54. Harron DWG, Griffiths K, Shanks RC. Debendox and congenital malformations in Northern Ireland. *BMJ* 1980;**281**:1379–80.

55. Jick H, Holmes LB, Hunter JR, *et al*. First trimester drug use and congenital disorders. *JAMA* 1981;**246**:343–6.

56. Mitchell AA, Rosenberg L, Shapiro S, *et al*. Birth defects related to Bendectin use in pregnancy. *JAMA* 1981;**245**:2311–14.

57. Cordero JF, Oakley GP, Greenberg F, *et al*. Is Bendectin a teratogen? *JAWM* 1981;**245**:2307–10.

58. Correy JF, Newman NM. Debendox and limb reduction deformities. *Med J Aust* 1981;**1**:417–18.

59. Clarke M, Clayton DG. Safety of Debendox. *Lancet* 1981;**1**:659–60.

60. Edwards IR, Lindquist M. The WHO database II. *Drug Inf J* 1992;**26**:481–6.

61. Mann RD, Rawlins MD, Fletcher P, *et al*. Age and the spontaneous reporting of adverse reactions in the UK. *Pharmacoepidemiol Drug Safety* 1992;**1**:19–23.

62. Fletcher AP, Griffin JP. International monitoring for adverse reactions of long latency. *Adv Drug React Ac Pois Rev* 1991;**10**:189–210.

63. Herbst AL, Ulfelder H, Poskanzer DC. Adenocarcinoma of vagina: association of maternal stilboestrol therapy with tumour appearance in young women. *N Engl J Med* 1971;**284**:878–81.

64. Wright P. Skin reactions to practolol. *BMJ* 1974;**2**:560.

65. Wright P. Untoward effects associated with practolol administration: oculomucocutaneous syndrome. *BMJ* 1975;**1**:595–8.

66. Wright P. Ocular reactions to beta-blocking drugs. *BMJ* 1975;**4**:577.

67. Friedman GD, Ury HK. Screening for possible drug carcinogenicity: second report of findings. *J Natl Cancer Inst* 1983;**71**:1165.

68. Williams RR, Feinleit M, Connor RJ, *et al*. Case–control study of anti-hypertensive and diuretic use by women with malignant and benign breast lesions detected in a mammography screening program. *J Natl Cancer Inst* 1978;**61**: 325–7.

69. Swerdlow AJ, Douglas AJ, Vaughan Hudson G, *et al*. Risk of second primary cancers after Hodgkin's disease by type of treatment: analysis of 2846 patients in the British National Lymphoma Investigation. *BMJ* 1992;**304**:1137–43.

70. McEwen J. Improving adverse drug reaction reporting. *Med Toxicol* 1987;**2**:398–404.

71. CIOMS Working Group. *International Reporting of Adverse Drug Reactions*. Geneva: CIOMS, 1990: 45–7.

72. CIOMS. Standardisation of definitions and criteria of causality assessment of adverse drug reactions – drug-induced cytopenia. *Int J Clin Pharmacol Ther Toxicol* 1991;**29**:75–81.

73. CIOMS. Basic requirements for the use of terms for reporting adverse drug reactions. *Pharmacoepidemiol Drug Safety* 1992;**1**:39–45.

74. CIOMS. *Working Group II Final Report*. Geneva: Council for International Organisations of Medical Sciences, 1992.

75. Edwards IR, Lindquist M, Wiholm B-E, *et al*. Quality criteria for early signals of possible adverse drug reactions. *Lancet* 1990;**336**:156–8.

76. Waller PC, Wood SM, Langman MJS, *et al.* Review of company postmarketing surveillance studies. *BMJ* 1992;**304**:1470–2.

77. Linden M. Phase IV research and drug utilisation observation studies. *Pharmacopsychiatry* 1997;**30** (Suppl):1–3.

78. Schafer H. Post-approval drug research: objectives and methods. *Pharmacopsychiatry* 1997;**30** (Suppl):4–8.

79. Fletcher AP. Profile of a large scale cohort study. *Drugs* 1990;**40** (Suppl 5):43–7.

80. Hill PL, Bridgman KM. A multicentre postmarketing surveillance study to evaluate the safety of bisoprolol in the treatment of hypertension and ischaemic heart disease. *Br J Clin Res* 1992;**3**:85–98.

81. Herbold M. International guidelines on post-authorisation research and surveillance. *Pharmacopsychiatry* 1997;**30** (Suppl):62–4.

82. Hall GC, Luscombe DK, Walker SR. Postmarketing surveillance using a computerised general practice database. *Pharm Med* 1988;**2**:345–51.

83. Johnson N, Mant D, Jones L, *et al.* Use of computerised general practice data for population surveillance: comparative study of influenza data. *BMJ* 1991;**302**:763–5.

84. Jick H. Use of automated databases to study drug effects after marketing. *Pharmacotherapy* 1985;**5**:278–9.

85. Jick H, Madsen S, Nudelman PM, *et al.* Postmarketing follow-up at Group Health Cooperative of Puget Sound. *Pharmacotherapy* 1984;**4**:99.

86. Jick H, Walker AM, Watkins RN, *et al.* Oral contraceptives and breast cancer. *Am J Epidemiol* 1980;**112**:577.

87. Jick H, Dinan BJ, Hunter JR, *et al.* Tricyclic antidepressants and convulsions. *J Clin Psychopharmacol* 1983;**3**:182.

88. Faich GA, Fishbein HA, Ellis SE. The epidemiology of diabetic acidosis: a population based study. *Am J Epidemiol* 1983;**117**:551.

89. Friedman GD, Collen MF, Harris LE, *et al.* Experience in monitoring drug reactions in outpatients: the Kaiser-Permanente Drug Monitoring System. *JAMA* 1971;**217**:2498.

90. Guess HA, West R, Strand LM, *et al.* Fatal upper gastrointestinal hemorrhage or perforation among users and nonusers of nonsteroidal anti-inflammatory drugs in Saskatchewan, Canada 1983. *J Clin Epidemiol* 1988;**41**:35.

91. Morse ML, LeRoy AA, Strom BL. COMPASS: a population-based post-marketing drug surveillance system. In: Inman WHW, ed.

92. Ray WA, Griffin MR. The use of Medicaid data for pharmacoepidemiology. *Am J Epidemiol* 1989;**129**:837.

93. Saskatchewan Health: International symposium on drug database uses, Regina, Canada, 7–8 Nov 1984. Proceedings. Regina: Saskatchewan Health, 1985.

94. Schnell BR. A review of the use of prescription drugs in Saskatchewan. *Can Pharm J* 1981;**7**:267.

95. Shapiro S. The role of automated record linkage in the post-marketing surveillance of drug safety: a critique. *Clin Pharmacol Ther* 1989;**46**:371–86.

96. Skoll SL, August RJ, Johnson GE. Drug prescribing for the elderly in Saskatchewan during 1976. *CMAJ* 1979;**121**:1974.

97. Stergachis A. Record linkage studies for postmarketing surveillance: data quality and validity considerations. *Drug Intell Clin Pharm* 1988;**22**:157.

98. Strand LM. Drug epidemiology resources and studies: the Saskatchewan database. *Drug Info J* 1985;**19**:253.

99. Strom BL, Carson JL, Halpern AC, *et al.* Using a claims database to investigate drug-induced Stevens–Johnson syndrome. *Stat Med* 1991;**10**:565–76.

100. Strom BL, Carson JL, Morse ML, *et al.* The Computerised On-line Medicaid Pharmaceutical Analysis and Surveillance System: a new resource for post-marketing drug surveillance. *Clin Pharmacol Ther* 1985;**38**:359.

101. Strom BL, Carson JL, Morse ML, *et al.* Hypersensitivity reactions associated with zompirac sodium and other nonsteroidal anti-inflammatory drugs. *Arthritis Rheum* 1987;**30**:1142.

102. Carson JL, Strom BL, Morse ML, *et al.* The relative gastrointestinal toxicity of the nonsteroidal anti-inflammatory drugs. *Arch Int Med* 1987;**147**: 1054.

103. Tilson H. Getting down to bases: record linkage in Saskatchewan. *Can J Public Health* 1985;**76**:222.

104. Cornfield J. A method of estimating comparative rates from clinical data. Application to cancer of the lung, breast and cervix. *J Natl Cancer Inst* 1951;**11**:1269–75.

105. Dorn HF. Some applications of biometry in the collection and evaluation of medical data. *J Chronic Dis* 1955;**1**:638–69.

106. Dorn HF. Some problems arising in prospective and retrospective studies of the etiology of disease. *N Engl J Med* 1959;**261**:571–9.

Monitoring for Drug Safety. Philadelphia: JB Lippincott, 1986.

107. Mantel N, Haenszel W. Statistical aspects of data from retrospective studies of disease. *J Natl Cancer Inst* 1959;**22**:719–48.

108. Cornfield J, Haenszel W. Some aspects of retrospective studies. *J Chronic Dis* 1960;**11**:523–34.

109. Lilienfeld AM, Lilienfeld DE. A century of case–control studies: progress? *J Chronic Dis* 1979;**32**:5–13.

110. Louis PCA. *Researches on Phthisis. Anatomical, Pathological and Therapeutical.* (Trans. by WH Wolshe). London: Sydenham Society, 1844.

111. Cole P. The evolving case–control study. *J Chronic Dis* 1979;**32**:15–27.

112. Feinstein AR. Methodologic problems and standards in case–control research. *J Chronic Dis* 1979;**32**:35–41.

113. Sackett DL. Bias in analytic research. *J Chronic Dis* 1979;**32**:51–63.

114. Mayes LC, Horwitz RI, Feinstein AR. A collection of 56 topics with contradictory results in case–control research. *Inf J Epidemiol* 1988;**17**:680–5.

115. Armstrong B, Stevens N, Doll R. Retrospective study of the association between use of Rauwolfia derivatives and breast cancer in English women. *Lancet* 1974;**2**:672–5.

116. Boston Collaborative Drug Surveillance Program. Reserpine and breast cancer. *Lancet* 1974;**2**:669–71.

117. Friedman GD. Rauwolfia and breast cancer: no relation found in long-term users aged fifty and over. *J Chronic Dis* 1983;**36**:367.

118. Heinonen OP, Shapiro S, Tuominen L, *et al.* Reserpine use in relation to breast cancer. *Lancet* 1974;**2**:675–7.

119. Laska EM, Siegl C, Meisner M, *et al.* Matched pairs study of reserpine use and breast cancer. *Lancet* 1975;**2**:296–300.

120. Lilienfeld AM, Chang L, Thomas DB, *et al.* Rauwolfia derivatives and breast cancer. *Johns Hopkins Med Bull* 1975;**139**:41–50.

121. Armstrong B, Skegg D, White G, *et al.* Rauwolfia derivatives and breast cancer in hypertensive women. *Lancet* 1976;**2**:8–12.

122. Aromaa A, Hakama M, Hakulinen T, *et al.* Breast cancer and use of Rauwolfia and other antihypertensive agents in hypertensive patients: a nationwide case–control study in Finland. *Int J Cancer* 1976;**18**:727–38.

123. Kewitz H, Jesdinsky HJ, Shroter PM, *et al.* Reserpine and breast cancer in West Germany. *Eur J Clin Pharmacol* 1977;**11**:79–83.

124. Mack IM, Henderson BE, Gerkins VR, *et al.* Reserpine and breast cancer in a retirement community. *N Engl J Med* 1975;**292**:1360–71.

125. Christopher LJ, Crooks J, Davidson JF, *et al.* A multicentre study of Rauwolfia derivatives and breast cancer. *Eur J Clin Pharmacol* 1977;**11**:409–17.

126. O'Fallon WM, Labarthe DR, Kinland LT. Rauwolfia derivatives and breast cancer. *Lancet* 1975;**2**:292–6.

127. Labarthe DR. Methodologic variation in case–control studies of reserpine and breast cancer. *J Chronic Dis* 1979;**32**:95–104.

128. Friedman GD. Rauwolfia and breast cancer: no relation found in long-term users aged fifty and over. *J Chronic Dis* 1983;**36**:367.

129. Hill AB. The environment and disease: association or causation. *Proc Roy Soc Med* 1965;**58**:295–300.

130. Jick H, Vessey MP. Case–control studies in the evaluation of drug-induced illness. *Am J Epidemiol* 1978;**107**:1–7.

131. Nienhuis H, Goldacre M, Seagroatt V, *et al.* Incidence of disease after vasectomy: a record linkage retrospective cohort study. *BMJ* 1992;**304**:743–6.

132. Layton D, Heely E, Hughes K, *et al.* Comparison of the incidence rates of selected gastrointestinal events reported for patients prescribed rofecoxib and meloxicam in general practice in England using prescription-event monitoring data. *Rheumatology* 2003;**42**:622–31.

133. Layton D, Riley J, Wilton LV, *et al.* Safety profile of rofecoxib as used in general practice in England: results of a prescription-event monitoring study. *Br J Clin Pharmacol* 2003;**55**:166–74.

134. Wilton LV, Heeley El, Pickering RM, *et al.* Comparative study of mortality rates and cardiac dysrhythmias in post-marketing surveillance studies of sertindole and two other atypical antipsychotic drugs, risperidone and olanzapine. *J Psychopharmacol* 2001;**15**:120–6.

135. Layton D, Pearce G, Shakir S. Safety profile of tolterodine as used in general practice in England: results of prescription event monitoring 2001. *Drug Safety* 2001;**24**:703–13.

136. Reilly JG, Ayis SA, Ferrier IN, *et al.* QTc-interval abnormalities and psychotropic drug therapy in psychiatric patirents. *Lancet* 2000;**355**:1048–52.

137. Taylor D. Ziprasidone in the management of schizophrenia: the QT interval issue in context. *CNS Drugs* 2003;**17**:423–30.

138. Committee on Safety of Medicines: www.mca.gov.uk/aboutagency/regframework/csm/csmframe.htm

139. Gianfresco FD, Grogg AL, Mahmoud RA, *et al.* Differential effects of risperidone, olanzapine, clozapine, and conventional antipsychotics on type 2 diabetes: findings from a large health plan database. *J Clin Psychiatry* 2002;**63**:920–30.

140. Sernyak MJ, Leslie DL, Alarcon RD, *et al.* Association of diabetes mellitus with atypical neuroleptics in the treatment of schizophrenia. *Am J Psychiatry* 2002;**159**:561–6.

141. Koro CE, Fedder DO, L'Italien GJ, *et al.* Assessment of independent effect olanzapine and risperidone on risk of diabetes among patients with schizophrenia: population based nested case–control study. *BMJ* 2003;**326**:283.

142. Meyer JM. A retrospective comparison of weight, lipid and glucose changes between risperidone- and olanzapine-treated inpatients: metabolic outcomes after 1 year. *J Clin Psychiatry* 2002;**63**:425–33.

143. Koro CE, Fedder DO, L'Italien GJ, *et al.* An assessment of the independent effects of olanzapine and risperidone exposure on the risk of hyperlipidemia in schizophrenic patients. *Arch Gen Psychiatry* 2002;**59**:1021–6.

144. Brill K, Norpoth T, Schnitker JA, *et al.* Clinical experience with a modern low-dose oral contraceptive in almost 100 000 cases. *Contraception* 1990;**43**:101–10.

145. Wakefield AJ, Murch SH, Anthony A, *et al.* Ileal-lymphoid-nodular hyperplasia, non-specific colitis and pervasive developmental disorder in children. *Lancet* 1998;**351**:637–41.

146. Furlano RI, Anthony A, Day R, *et al.* Colonic CD8 and $\chi\delta$ T-cell infiltration with epithelial damage in children with autism. *J Pediatr* 2001;**138**: 366–372.

147. Wakefield AJ, Anthony A, Murch SH, *et al.* Enterocolitis in children with developmental disorders. *Am J Gastroenterol* 2000;**95**:2285–95.

148. Torrente F, Ashwood P, Day R, *et al.* Small intestinal enteropathy with epithelial IgG and complement deposition in children with regressive autism. *Mol Psychiatry* 2002;**7**:375–82.

149. Silverstein FE, Faich G, Goldstein, *et al.* Gastrointestinal toxicity with celecoxib vs nonsteroidal anti-inflammatory drugs for osteoarthritis and rheumatoid arthritis: the CLASS study: a randomised controlled trial. *JAMA* 2000;**284**:1247–55.

150. Bombardier C, Laine L, Reicin A, *et al.* Comparison of upper gastrointestinal toxicity of rofecoxib and naproxen in patients with rheumatoid arthritis. VIGOR study group. *N Engl J Med* 2000;**343**:1520–8.

151. Gottlieb S. COX2 inhibitors may increase risk of heart attack. *BMJ.* 2001; **323**:471.

152. Layton D, Riley J, Wilton LV, *et al.* Safety profile of rofecoxib as used in general practice in England: results of a prescription event monitoring study. *Br J Clin Pharmacol* 2003;**55**:166–74.

153. Layton D, Heeley E, Hughes K, *et al.* Comparison of the incidence rates of thromboembolic events reported for patients prescribed rofecoxib and meloxicam in practice in England using prescription event monitoring. *Rheumatology* 2003;**42**:1342–53.

154. Juni P, Nartey L, Reichenbach S, *et al.* Risk of cardiovascular events and rofecoxib: cumulative meta-analysis. *Lancet* 2004;**364**:2021.

155. Edwards RI, Aronson JK. Adverse drug reactions: definitions, diagnosis and management. *Lancet* 2000;**356**:1255–9.

156. Benichou C, Danan G. Causality assessment in the European pharmaceutical industry: presentation of preliminary results of a new method. *Drug Inf J* 1992;**26**:589–92.

157. Hutchinson TA. Computerised bayesian ADR assessment. *Drug Inf J* 1991;**25**:235–41.

158. Lane DA, Hutchinson TA, Jones JK, *et al. A Bayesian Approach to Causality Assessment.* University of Minnesota School of Statistics Tech Reps No 472 (no date available).

159. Lane DA, Kramer MS, Hutchinson TA, *et al.* The causality assessment of adverse drug reactions using a Bayesian approach. *Pharm Med* 1987;**2**:265–83.

160. Naranjo CA, Busto U, Sellers EM, *et al.* A method for estimating the probability of adverse drug reactions. *Clin Pharmacol Ther* 1981;**30**:239–45.

161. Naranjo CA, Lanctot KL. Microcomputer-assisted Bayesian differential diagnosis of severe adverse reactions to new drugs: a 4-year experience. *Drug Inf J* 1991;**25**:243–50.

162. Olsson S. The role of the WHO programme on international drug monitoring in coordinating worldwide drug safety efforts. *Drug Safety* 1998;**19**:1–10.

163. Lindquist M, Stahl M, Bate A, *et al.* A retrospective evaluation of data mining approach to aid finding new adverse drug reaction signals in the WHO international database. *Drug Safety* 2000;**23**:533–42.

164. Grahame-Smith DG. Report of the adverse reactions working party to the Committee on Safety of Medicines. London: Department of Health and Social Security, 1983.

165. Joint Committee of ABPI, BMA, CSM, and RCGP. Guidelines on postmarketing surveillance. *BMJ* 1988;**296**:399–400.

166. Eysenck HJ. Meta-analysis, sense or non-sense? *Pharm Med* 1992;**6**:113–19.

167. Rawlins MD, Thompson JW. Mechanisms of adverse drug reactions. In: Davies DM, ed. *Textbook of Adverse Drug Reactions*. Oxford: Oxford University Press, 1985:18–38.

168. Cobert B, Silvey J. The Internet and drug safety. What are the implications for pharmacovigilance? *Drug Safety* 1999;**20**:95–107.

169. Maxwell S, Walley T, Ferner RE. Using drugs safely. *BMJ* 2002;**324**:930–1.

PART III
Regulatory aspects

CHAPTER 16

16 History of drug regulation in the United Kingdom

John P Griffin and Rashmi R Shah

16.1 Introduction

Our concepts on how medicines should be tested and regulated have evolved very gradually over time, perhaps dating back to 120 BC. This chapter is a brief account of some of the major events that have guided drug regulation to what it is today in the United Kingdom.[1]

Mithridates VI, 120 BC, King of Pontus, concocted a compound preparation called 'Mithridatium' that was held as a panacea for almost every illness until the 1780s. Having investigated the powers of a number of single ingredients, which he found to be antidotes to various venoms and poisons individually, he evaluated them experimentally. The required 'clinical trials' were conducted on condemned criminals! Once an ingredient was found to be effective, Mithridates proceeded to incorporate it into his compound preparation, which included 41 individual components when fully formulated. Another formulation of Mithridatium, known as 'Galene', which included 55 components, was also available from the days of Andromachus (*c.* AD 50). 'Galene' means 'tranquility' and also became known as a 'theriac'. The concoction took some 40 days to prepare, after which the process of maturation began. Galen considered 12 years as the proper period to keep it before use. The quality of Mithridatium

and Galene was important since, as late as 1540, failure of their efficacy was attributed to the use of poor quality of their ingredients.

Mithridatium and Galene had also found their way into England, where, after the founding of the Royal College of Physicians in 1518, their manufacture was made subject to supervision under the Apothecary Wares, Drugs and Stuffs Act of 1540. This Act was one of the earliest British statutes on the control of drugs and it empowered the physicians to appoint four inspectors of 'Apothecary Wares, Drugs and Stuffs'.

Standards for the manufacture of Mithridatium and Galene were laid down in *The London Pharmacopoeia* in 1618 (see Figure 16.1). The manufacture of these theriacs took place in public with much pomp and ceremony (Figure 16.2). It was commonly thought by those in authority that if Mithridatium did not produce the desired cure, this was due to incorrect preparation (perhaps with adulterated or poor quality materials) or to incorrect storage after use. However, Galen records that Marcus Aurelius consumed the preparation within 2 months of its being compounded without ill effect.

In 1665, during the Great Plague of London, Charles II turned to the Royal College of Physicians for advice. This advice recommended, among other measures, that the victims of the plague who developed buboes were to be treated

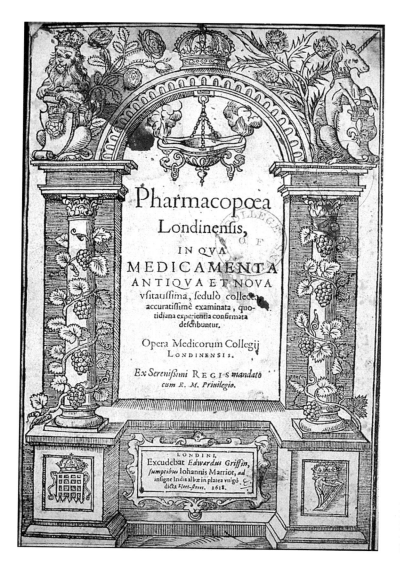

Fig. 16.1 Frontpiece of *The London Pharmacopoeia*, 1618. (Reproduced with kind permission from The Hunterian Libraries, The Royal College of Physicians, London.)

with a plaster of either Mithridatium or Galene applied hot, thrice daily.

Many physicians in the early eighteenth century had doubts as to whether Mithridatium was the universal panacea of all illness as claimed. The ultimate mortal attack on the remedy came from Dr William Heberden (1710–1801) (see Figure 16.3), better known clinically for his description of the 'Heberden's nodes' in osteoarthritis. Consequently, the 1746 edition of *The London Pharmacopoeia* was the last in

which references to Mithridatium appear. With its disappearance, the long-used complex remedy attributable to an experimental toxicologist from the first century BC came to an end. Perhaps in the final analysis, the contribution of Mithridatium to modern medicine was that concerns about quality stimulated the earliest concepts of medicines regulation.

Concerns on the safety of medicines began to emerge when the laws on vaccination against smallpox were tightened in 1853 and later

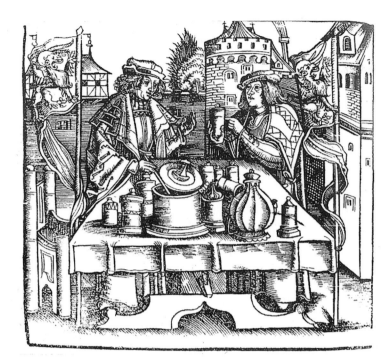

Fig. 16.2 Manufacture of Mithridatium.

in 1871[2] when a House of Commons Select Committee, set up to investigate the efficacy of the compulsory system, was concerned by a report by Dr Jonathan Hutchinson who gave an account of the transmission of syphilis in two patients by arm-to-arm inoculation.

Following the discovery and clinical use of chloroform in 1847, The Royal Medical and Chirurgical Society (later to become The Royal Society of Medicine) had already set up in 1864 a committee to enquire 'into the uses and the physiological, therapeutical and toxicological effects of chloroform'. There had been 109 fatalities following administration of chloroform. A critical relationship had been demonstrated between the dose and effect of this anaesthetic. The committee commented on the need for animal experiments to compare chloroform with ether and also on the relative cardiac safety of ether.

At the British Medical Association (BMA) meeting in Manchester in 1877, Spencer Wells strongly advocated urgent investigations into

how anaesthesia, effective as it was, might be rendered safe for the future. The BMA too set up its own working party in 1877, to investigate sudden deaths following chloroform anaesthesia and had suggested setting up an independent body to assess its safety. This BMA working party published its report in 1880 but this had little impact on generating public or political concern to set up a regulatory authority. The safety of chloroform was to resurface as late as 1978 (see later).

The stimulus to drug regulation ultimately came following the publications of two BMA papers entitled 'Secret Remedies' in 1909 and 'More Secret Remedies' in 1912. These prompted a Parliamentary Select Committee on Patent Medicines to be set up. This Select Committee reported in 1914, but the outbreak of war resulted in the shelving of all proposed legislation.

Following the discovery of arsphenamine (Salvarsan) in Germany in 1907, it was imported into the United Kingdom until the beginning of World War I, when the Board of Trade issued licences to certain British manufacturers

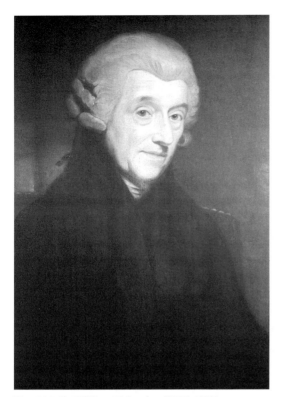

Fig. 16.3 Dr William Heberden (1710–1801). (Reproduced with kind permission from The Hunterian Libraries, The Royal College of Physicians, London.)

to produce it. Each batch had to be submitted to the Medical Research Council (MRC) for approval before marketing.

The forerunner to monitoring of adverse reactions can be traced to a recommendation in 1922 by the MRC Salvarsan Committee. This Committee, set up to investigate epidemics of jaundice and hepatic necrosis following the use of Salvarsan, encouraged reporting 'to the Ministry of Health of details concerning such accidents, for it is only in the light of such information that investigation and measures with regard to their prevention can be successfully undertaken'.

Following concerns on impurities and standardisation, the Therapeutic Substances Act was passed in 1925 with the aim of regulating the manufacture of biological substances, providing the standards to which they must conform and

regulating their labelling. This Act recognised the significance of the manufacturing process and factory inspection and in-process controls played a large part in supervision by the Ministry of Health. This Therapeutic Substances Act was later consolidated and strengthened in 1956 when Part II was added, which dealt with control of sale and supply. Records of sale had to be kept and the container had to identify both the manufacturer and the batch. The first schedule to the 1956 Act included the substances commonly known as vaccines, sera, toxins, antitoxins and antigens.

The Venereal Disease Act of 1917 and The Cancer Act of 1939 had already prevented public advertisement and promotion of drugs for these conditions to protect sufferers from inadequate or unsuitable treatment and fraudulent claims (of efficacy).

Clearly, by the 1950s, fragments of legislation controlling the quality, sale and promotion of drugs had existed in the United Kingdom for many years but these had in general been disease orientated and had little relevance to the therapeutic revolution that was taking place at the time. There seemed to be no major concerns in Europe with the way the drugs were manufactured, placed on the market, and, in a broad sense, controlled.

In France, 102 people had died and 100 more were affected by paraplegia in 1957 as a result of the administration of Stalinon capsules for the treatment of boils. The Stalinon episode had resulted from a formulation error – Stalinon capsules for marketing contained 15 mg diiodoethyltin and 100 mg isolinoleic acid esters. Clinical trials were carried out with capsules containing only 3 mg of diiodoethyltin (one-fifth of the marketed dose)! Subsequent studies in animals and in humans confirmed the neurotoxicity of diiodoethyltin, which was characterised by intramyelinic vacuolation and astrocyte swelling with no evidence of neuronal degeneration. This tragedy, however, was a foretaste of an even much greater disaster – that due to thalidomide.

The thalidomide disaster in 1961 was to blow apart the complacency on regulation of drugs. The confidence in the therapeutic revolution promised by the pharmaceutical industry was shattered and there followed considerable public outcry.

16.2 The Thalidomide Disaster and its Immediate Aftermath

Thalidomide[3] was a sedative and a hypnotic that first went on sale in 1956 in West Germany. Between 1958 and 1960, it was introduced in 46 countries under 51 different trade names. It was first introduced in the UK market in April 1958 under the name Distaval. It enjoyed good sales because of its prompt action, lack of hangover and addiction observed with barbiturates, and apparent safety.

Following anecdotal reports of benefit in the treatment of vomiting in early pregnancy, it was heavily promoted for this purpose. This use in early pregnancy was soon followed by an epidemic of a previously unknown congenital malformation of the limbs, termed 'phocomelia' due to its resemblance to the flippers of a seal, and other associated internal malformations. The first cases were reported from Germany beginning in 1959 but the malformation also began to make an appearance in other countries where the drug was on sale. Curiously, among the West European countries the drug was not marketed in France, which was spared the tragedy. The Stalinon disaster had resulted in new regulatory requirements being published in February 1959 by the French Health Authority. The manufacturers had to have recourse to an officially appointed expert committee for the preparation of registration file. This registration file had to provide evidence of the therapeutic interest of the product and of its safety under normal conditions of use as well as of the manufacturing process associated with adequate testing to guarantee the quality of the product on an industrial scale.

Of considerable concern, was the scale of the disaster resulting from its protracted marketing, the manufacturer continuing to deny all evidence of a causal relationship between these congenital abnormalities and the drug. Worldwide, there were an estimated 10 000 babies with phocomelia and other allied deformities, including more than 500 in England. The frequency of the malformations in Germany followed the absolute sales of the drug with a time lag of a little less than 1 year. The drug was withdrawn from the market in Germany in November 1961, in the United Kingdom in December 1961 and, over the next 10 months thereafter, from most countries of the world. After the withdrawal of the drug from the market, 8 to 9 months later the wave of the unique malformations disappeared as suddenly as it had appeared and with the same time lag that it had followed the introduction of the drug. The drug was soon confirmed as a potent teratogen in a number of animal studies.

Governments throughout the Western world were now galvanised into introducing effective drug regulation. Even in the United States, despite the strength of the prevailing legislation on safety, news reports on the role of Dr Frances Kelsey, a medical officer at the Food and Drug Administration (FDA), in keeping the drug off the US market, aroused much public support for even stronger drug regulation.

For their part, the UK Government set up in August 1962 the Joint Subcommittee of the English and Scottish Standing Medical Advisory Committees, under the Chairmanship of The Lord Cohen of Birkenhead, with the following terms of reference:

To advise the Minister of Health and the Secretary of State for Scotland on what measures are needed:

1. To secure adequate pharmacological and safety testing and clinical trials of new drugs before their release for general use.
2. To secure early detection of adverse effects arising after their release for general use.
3. To keep doctors informed of the experiences of such drugs in clinical practice.

16.3 Voluntary Controls in the United Kingdom (1963–71)

In its interim advice delivered on 2 November 1962, the Joint Subcommittee of the English and

Scottish Standing Medical Advisory Committees, set up in the aftermath of the thalidomide disaster, made three main recommendations that:

1. The responsibility for the experimental laboratory testing of new drugs before they are used in clinical trials should remain with the individual pharmaceutical manufacturer.
2. It was neither desirable nor practical that at this stage of their evaluation the responsibility for testing drugs should be transferred to a central authority.
3. There should be an expert body to review the evidence and offer advice on the toxicity of new drugs, whether manufactured in Great Britain or abroad, before they were used in clinical trials.

Following further consideration and consultations, the Joint Subcommittee proposed to formulate detailed advice on the composition and terms of this expert advisory body. On 6 November 1962, the Minister of Health announced that the Government had accepted the first two recommendations and would await the advice on the third.

In the period intervening between its interim advice and its final report, the Joint Subcommittee received memoranda from, and met representatives of, the Association of the British Pharmaceutical Industry (ABPI), the BMA, the Pharmaceutical Society of Great Britain and the College of General Practitioners.

Despite reservations expressed by a number of these bodies, the Joint Subcommittee took the view that public opinion was unlikely to be content with anything short of Ministerial responsibility for verifying that adequate precautions had been taken to secure the safety of drugs, the more so because of the number and nature of new drugs.

The Joint Subcommittee issued its Final Report on 'Safety of Drugs'[4] in March 1963, which states in paragraph 10:

'We think that a Committee on Safety of Drugs should be established with subcommittees to advise it on each of the three aspects, namely:
(i) toxicity
(ii) clinical trials and therapeutic efficacy and
(iii) adverse reactions'.

16.3.1　Committee on Safety of Drugs (CSD)

The three Health Ministers of the United Kingdom, in consultation with the medical and pharmaceutical professions and the ABPI, set up the Committee on Safety of Drugs (CSD) in June 1963. The three Health Ministers were the Secretary of State for Scotland, the Minister of Health and the Minister of Health and Social Services, Northern Ireland.

The Committee had the following terms of reference:

1. To invite from the manufacturer or other person developing or proposing to market a drug in the United Kingdom, any reports they may think fit on the toxicity tests carried out on it; to consider whether any further tests should be made and whether the drug should be submitted to clinical trials; and to convey their advice to those who submitted reports.
2. To obtain reports of clinical trials of drugs submitted thereto.
3. Taking into account the safety and efficacy of each drug, and the purposes for which it is to be used, to consider whether it may be released for marketing, with or without precautions or restrictions on its use; and to convey their advice to those who submitted reports.
4. To give to manufacturers and others concerned any general advice they may think fit.
5. To assemble and assess reports about adverse effects of drugs in use and prepare information thereon that may be brought to the notice of doctors and other concerned.
6. To advise the appointing Ministers on any of the above matters.

The Committee consisted of a panel of independent experts from various fields of pharmacy, medicine and pathology among others, with Sir Derrick Dunlop as its first Chairman. In tribute to his personal charm, considerable skills and foresight, it soon became popularly known as the 'Dunlop Committee'.

The Committee had no legal powers but worked with the voluntary agreement of the ABPI and the Proprietary Association of Great Britain (PAGB). These associations promised that none of their members would put on clinical trial or release for marketing a new drug against the advice of the Committee and whose advice they would always seek. In an attempt to make sure that the manufacturers adhered to this, the Health Ministers undertook, in a circular sent to all dentists and doctors in the United Kingdom, to inform the prescribers of any cases of drugs being marketed or put to clinical trials without the Committee's approval.

A number of subcommittees were also established to assist the main Committee. These were the Subcommittee on Toxicity and the Subcommittee on Clinical Trials and Therapeutic Efficacy. Against the background of the thalidomide tragedy, an important subcommittee established was the Subcommittee on Adverse Reactions. The memberships of the main

Committee and its three Subcommittees when first established in 1963 are shown in Table 16.1.

The Committee spent the first 6 months of its existence (the latter half of 1963) in completing its preparatory work. By 1 January 1964, the Committee was in a position to invite submissions (this is what they were called, and not 'applications') on drugs intended for clinical trials or about to be released for the market.

In 1967, the Subcommittee on Toxicity and the Subcommittee on Clinical Trials and Therapeutic Efficacy were merged since the interests of the two were shown by experience to overlap considerably. The new subcommittee, the Subcommittee on Toxicity, Clinical Trials and Therapeutic Efficacy, was chaired by Professor AC Frazer with Professor EF Scowen (later Sir Eric Scowen) as the Deputy Chairman.

Table 16.1 Membership of the Committee on Safety of Drugs and its Subcommittees (1963)

Committee on Safety of Drugs	Subcommittee on Adverse Reactions	Subcommittee on Toxicity	Subcommittee on Clinical Trials and Therapeutic Efficacy
(All committee papers to be printed on white paper)	*(All subcommittee papers to be printed on yellow paper)*	*(All subcommittee papers to be printed on green paper)*	*(All subcommittee papers to be printed on pink paper)*
Sir Derrick Dunlop *(Chairman)*	Professor LJ Witts *(Chairman)*	Professor AC Frazer *(Chairman)*	Professor RB Hunter *(Chairman)*
Professor AC Frazer *(Deputy Chairman)*	Professor OL Wade *(Deputy Chairman)*	Professor EF Scowen *(Deputy Chairman)*	Professor GM Wilson *(Deputy Chairman)*
Professor LJ Witts	Dr EV Kuenssberg	Dr F Hartley	Dr W Linford-Rees
Professor EF Scowen	Professor DJ Finney	Dr LG Goodwin	Sir Austin Bradford Hill
Professor GM Wilson	Dr KR Carper	Professor GJ Cunningham	Professor TNA Jeffcoate
Professor OL Wade	Professor WW Mushin	Dr PN Magee	Professor DR Laurence
Professor WW Mushin		Mr TC Denston	
Dr EY Kuenssberg			
Dr F Hartley			
Mr TC Denston			
Sir Austin Bradford Hill			
Professor RB Hunter			

16.3.2   CSD Secretariat

The CSD was serviced by a professional secretariat of pharmacists and medical officers who undertook the assessment of the submissions and presented these to the Committee and its various subcommittees. The secretariat initially included three doctors and two pharmacists. In 1965, the number of professional staff had been increased to six doctors and three pharmacists. Among the six doctors was Dr Denis Cahal, who headed the secretariat. Others were Drs J Broadbent, M Hollyhock, WH Inman, D Mansel-Jones and C Ruttle. The secretriat, known as the Medicines Division, was created as a branch of the Department of Health. The close collaboration between Dr Cahal and Sir Derrick Dunlop was pivotal in guiding the Medicines Act through Parliament in 1968 and setting the foundation of a system that became a model to the rest of the world for fairness and efficiency.

The Medicines Division was originally based at Queen Anne's Mansions, Queen Anne's Gate, London SW1, where the Committee and the Subcommittees also held their meetings. The secretariat was moved on 1 April 1971 to a new accommodation at Finsbury Square House, 33/37a Finsbury Square, London EC2A 1PP. Still later in March 1980, it moved to its current imposing location, overlooking the River Thames, at Market Towers, 1 Nine Elms Lane, Vauxhall, London SW8 5NQ.

Each manufacturer was given a four-digit company number for identification and this number was to be used for all their product-related documents – a system that prevails even today. For example, Geigy (UK) Ltd was 0001, Glaxo Group Ltd was 0004, John Wyeth & Brother Ltd was 0011, Astra-Hewlett Ltd was 0017, Parke Davis & Co. was 0018, AB Kabi was 0022, ER Squibb & Sons Ltd was 0034, Abbott Laboratories Ltd was 0037 and for those who are given to reminisce and remember it, Beecham Research Laboratories was 0038. The order of the allocation of these numbers was determined by the order in which the submissions were received by the new regulatory body from the companies. Thus, Geigy (UK) Ltd was the first company ever to make a submission to the CSD. A second set of four-digit numbers followed the company number (i.e. 0000/0000) and related to the individual products licensed for sale to that company, again in a numerical order in which the submissions for marketing authorisations were received.

16.3.3   The legacy of the Committee on Safety of Drugs

Even in these embryonic days, the Committee was to establish many important principles that still dominate drug regulation today.

The Committee had required as a minimum, teratogenicity testing in two species, one of which should preferably be a non-rodent, for one generation only. They also recognised the limitations of teratogenicity tests in animals but emphasised that only in the most exceptional circumstances would they release any drug for clinical trial in women of child-bearing age until the appropriate tests on animals had been carried out satisfactorily.

The Committee also required a wider interpretation of the term 'new drugs' to include *new formulations of existing drugs, drugs to be presented for a new purpose, and existing substances not previously used as drugs, covering virtually all new products introduced*'. The Committee had clearly appreciated that new formulations ought to be subject to scrutiny since reformulation did occasionally introduce additional hazards.

Perhaps, one of the most important years in drug regulation in the United Kingdom was 1965. That year, the manufacturers began to challenge the right of the Committee to require under its terms of reference evidence of efficacy of a drug. The Committee took the view that for serious diseases failure of efficacy constituted an unacceptable risk, while for trivial diseases where efficacy may be irrelevant, even a trivial safety hazard is not acceptable – the concept of modern day 'risk/benefit'. The Committee also emphasised that it was not concerned with efficacy and its clearance of a drug for the market did not necessarily imply its approval of the drug as a valuable remedy. The Committee also noted *'Medicines are not sacrosanct however, simply because they have been in use for a long time'*.

During the year there were a number of reports in the press of deaths associated with phenacetin. The Committee emphasised that the hazard was associated with the abuse of the drug (excessive doses taken over a long term) and reiterated that, consequently, no special action was necessary. Furthermore, because a drug (including phenacetin) could be marketed under different proprietary names, it could confuse a doctor. Therefore, the Committee decided that they would not consider an application by a manufacturer to market a new substance unless the applicant gave an assurance that an approved name had been obtained or applied for.

When considering new drug submissions, the Committee also paid attention to the claims and indications that the promoter intended to include on the label of a drug or in its promotional literature. Another significant step taken by the Committee related to labelling of the prescribed medicines by pharmacists. The practice of labelling the container as 'The Tablets' was no longer considered acceptable (unless the prescribing doctor specified otherwise). After canvassing the opinions of many professional bodies, including all Royal Colleges, the BMA and the Pharmaceutical Society of Great Britain had agreed by 1971 to the proposal of marking of prescriptions 'Nomen Proprium'.

The period 1966–7 was one of consolidation. The Committee had received considerable support for and re-emphasised all their previous recommendations. Between 1964 and 1967 the Committee received representatives from the World Health Organisation (WHO) and many European and Far and Middle Eastern countries, as well as from Canada and the United States, to study its methods.

In 1966, the Committee made observations on a hazard that increasingly plagues many drugs even today – the problems of drug–drug interactions. The Committee noted

It is now well known that the administration of one drug may considerably modify the actions of another being given at the same time. Both the toxicity and the metabolism of each drug

may be affected by the other. This applies to combinations of drugs in one preparation as well as to those separately administered. However, it is still too readily assumed by some manufacturers that no additional hazard is incurred by combining two or more drugs in one preparation.

The first drug–drug interaction alert issued by the Committee in 1966 concerned the risks from interactions between preparations containing adrenaline or noradrenaline and monoamine oxidase (MAO) inhibitors used for the treatment of depression.

In its final report, in 1969–70, the Committee expressed safety concerns arising from the names of products that differ, for example, only by a suffixed letter, and expressed a desire to see the naming of products put on a more rational basis.

It is interesting that for entirely new chemical entities, submissions in these early days of drug regulation were *'often voluminous: a submission containing over 1000 pages of reports, drafts and tables was not unusual'*. Rejection of drugs outright was a comparatively minor part of the Committee's operations; by far the more important actions involved persuading manufacturers to make changes in their intentions (formulation, indication, etc.).

In 1965, a great majority of submissions had concerned reformulation of established drugs. The number of submissions for reformulated preparations of established drugs was even higher in 1966, a matter that concerned the Committee in respect of *'the extent to which the drug houses have tended to flood the market with so many similar preparations'*. As a result, Mr CA Johnson (a pharmacist) and Dr DFJ Mason (a toxicologist) were then appointed to the Subcommittee on Toxicity. The work of the Committee during their tenure from January 1964 to 31 August 1971 in terms of submissions received and determined is shown in Table 16.2.

From time to time, the Committee received submissions related to vaccines or immunological products. When considering these, the Committee felt the need to seek advice of experts in that special field. Therefore, in November 1969 it was decided to set up a Vaccine Advisory Group. This initiative ultimately culminated in the establishment of the Subcommittee on

Table 16.2 Submissions to the Committee on Safety of Drugs (1964–1971)

	1964	1965	1966	1967	1968	1969	1970	1971
Clinical trial submissions	66	168	203	202	239	218	178	122
	(11.0%)	(19.2%)	(22.4%)	(26.4%)	(30.2%)	(25.7%)	(24.9%)	(22.0%)
Marketing submissions	534	706	705	563	552	630	536	432
Total (inc.NCEs)	600	874	908	765	791	848	714	554
	(55)	(69)	(66)	(56)	(56)	(66)	(69)	(??)
Approved	386	807	771	698	669	694	499	411
Rejected	15	19	24	36	36	33	53	38
	(2.5%)	(1.8%)	(2.4%)	(4.1%)	(4.1%)	(3.5%)	(6.3%)	(5.0%)
Withdrawn by applicant	32	119	86	70	83	86	79	66
	(5.3%)	(11.4%)	(8.6%)	(7.9%)	(9.5%)	(9.2%)	(9.4%)	(8.7%)
Further information	99	49	39	43	34	47	68	74
requested	(16.5%)	(4.7%)	(3.9%)	(4.8%)	(3.9%)	(5.0%)	(8.1%)	(9.7%)
Pending further	68	47	84	41	53	75	137	170
consideration								
Total	600	1041	1004	888	875	935	836	759

NCEs: New chemical entities.

Biological Substances, and the Biological Standards Act received the Royal Assent in February 1975. This Act provided for the establishment of a National Biological Standards Board to manage the activities carried out at the National Institute for Biological Standards and Control. The Institute undertook the control of testing of biological substances used for therapeutic, prophylactic and diagnostic purposes (e.g. vaccines, sera, antibiotics) to discharge their obligations under the Therapeutic Substances Act 1956 and the Medicines Act 1968.

In 1969, it came to the attention of the Committee that unidentified tablets of a drug purporting to be nitrazepam were being distributed in the United Kingdom. The Ministers issued a press statement warning those concerned not to use any other but the branded product that the Committee had cleared. Likewise, in early 1970 it came to public notice that one manufacturer was proposing to market L-dopa, a drug which at the time was still under clinical trial for the treatment of Parkinsonism, without first making a submission to the Committee. The Department of Health responded by issuing a statement advising strongly against the use of this drug from any source that had not been approved by the Committee. By the end of 1969, the Committee was able to 'fast track' the only two submissions for approval of clinical trials with L-dopa for its use in Parkinsonism. These manufacturers were encouraged by the Committee to submit the data early and it was possible to release some L-dopa preparations for marketing during the earlier part of 1970.

The membership of the Committee on Safety of Drugs and its subcommittees changed further following the resignation of Sir Derrick Dunlop in May 1969, as a result of his appointment as the first Chairman of the Medicines Commission (MC), established under the Medicines Act 1968. Professor AC Frazer was appointed to succeed Sir Derrick but unfortunately he died shortly thereafter. During 1969, therefore, Professor EF Scowen succeeded Professor Frazer as the Chairman of the Committee. In June 1970, the membership of the Committee was revised to correspond with that of the then newly established (under section 4 of the Medicines Act 1968) Committee on Safety of Medicines (CSM). The full

Table 16.3 Membership of Committee on Safety of Drugs and its Subcommittees (December 1970)

Committee on Safety of Drugs	Subcommittee on Adverse Reactions	Subcommittee on Toxicity, Clinical Trial and Therapeutic Efficacy
Professor EF Scowen (*Chairman*)	Professor WRS Doll (*Chairman*)	Professor GM Wilson (*Chairman*)
Professor WI Cranston	CW Barrett	Professor CT Dollery
Professor T Crawford	Professor WI Cranston	Sir Austin Bradford Hill
Professor CT Dollery	Professor J Crooks	Professor PJ Huntingford
Sir Austin Bradford Hill	Dr DM Davies	Professor DR Laurence
Dr DC Garratt	Professor DJ Finney	Professor PN Magee
Professor PJ Huntingford[a]	DR MJ Linnett	Dr DFJ Mason
Dr EV Kuenssberg	Professor GR Lowe	Professor DVW Parke
Professor DR Laurence	Professor WW Mushin	Professor W Linford-Rees
Professor PN Magee	Professor DA Price Evans	
Professor WW Mushin	Dr DW Vere	
Professor DVW Parke	Professor RD Weir	
Professor W Linford-Rees		
Professor JB Stenlake		
Professor GM Wilson		
Professor JS Scott[a]		

Notes: [a] Appointed to a new post abroad. Therefore Professor PJ Huntingford resigned and he was replaced by Professor JS Scott in September 1971.

membership of the Committee on Safety of Drugs as on 31 December 1970 is shown in Table 16.3.

16.3.4 Voluntary adverse reactions reporting system: the 'yellow card scheme'

The CSD had also started studies of adverse reactions to drugs (ADRs) by the beginning of 1964. Sir Derrick Dunlop wrote to all the doctors (4 May 1964) and dentists (15 June 1964), inviting them *'to report to us promptly details of any untoward condition in a patient which might be the result of drug treatment'*. They were assured that *'all the reports or replies that the Committee receive from them will be treated with complete professional confidence by the Committee and their staff. The Health Ministers have given an undertaking that the information supplied will never be used for disciplinary purposes or for enquiries about prescribing costs'*.

This spontaneous adverse reaction reporting system was the brainchild of Professor Leslie Witts and was, and still is, based upon the submission of ADR reports by doctors and dentists by means of reply-paid yellow cards, and hence it is popularly known as the 'Yellow Card Scheme'.

In the first year, up to 100 yellow card reports were received each week. In the case of *'serious suspected adverse reactions that might call for action it is necessary, therefore, to have more information about the reported incident and a number of doctors have been appointed throughout the country who will help the Committee on a part-time basis by following up reports'*. At the end of 1965, there were 35 such part-time doctors helping with the follow-up of serious reports. During the first 5 years, the number of reports received averaged about 60 per week, but the problem of determining number of prescriptions was soon recognised. The Committee needed to relate the number of reports with exposure. It concluded, 'it is possible to determine the ratio of adverse reactions only by asking a number of doctors who have prescribed a drug about their experience of it with special reference to the adverse reactions which, from reports, appear to be associated with its use'.

The Committee, as early as 1964, seemed to have anticipated Prescription Event Monitoring as well as the need for compiling large databases. It thought of a scheme that 'involves taking a sample of prescriptions written by doctors for the drugs being investigated. In the United Kingdom the assembly of National Health Service prescriptions for pricing purposes offers a unique opportunity for this sort of analysis that is not available anywhere else in the world and the pricing bureaux have kindly offered their help.' Regarding large databases, it went on 'prescription scripts are not at present filed in a way which allows easy identification of particular drugs but with the cooperation of the pricing bureaux, the Committee are developing a satisfactory procedure'.

Since new drugs are often at first used in hospitals and 'it is at this stage that serious adverse reactions are likely to be noticed', a pilot scheme was set up with a number of hospitals for recording prescriptions and the Committee devised a 'list of specially monitored drugs' which at 'any time will contain all the new substances introduced during the previous 2 years and a number of older drugs that still need special observation'. This clearly was the forerunner to the present 'Black Triangle' Scheme that operates today to identify drugs requiring intensive monitoring for at least 2 years.

When a safety problem was suspected, the promotion of information on safety of drugs was an important remit of the Committee and this they discharged by issuing a series of leaflets to all the doctors and dentists in the United Kingdom. The first alert leaflet in this series entitled 'Adverse Reactions Series' was issued by the Committee on Safety of Drugs in February 1964. It dealt with reports of liver damage and blood pressure changes following the use of MAO inhibitor drugs. Nine such alert leaflets were issued over the next 5 years to December 1969. The contents of these alerts are summarised in an earlier account.[3]

In 1967, computer facilities were installed for handling the yellow card reports and, after consultation, a method of confidential feedback to the profession was designed. A doctor reporting an ADR was automatically sent a summary of all the reports received by the Committee on the drug and on similar drugs. Where possible, an estimate of the extent to which the drug was prescribed was also given.

By 1965, the value of the Yellow Card Scheme was clearly established and two other countries had introduced a similar scheme. By the beginning of 1967, the Committee was also cooperating in the WHO's Pilot Study on the Monitoring of ADRs at an international level. By the end of 1968, a total of 10 countries were participating in this Pilot Study. This study matured into the international WHO ADR Monitoring Centre based in Uppsala (Sweden), with a membership that now stands at 67 countries with six others enjoying associate status.

The Yellow Card Scheme was soon beginning to pay dividends. In early 1966, the Yellow Card Scheme had identified methyldopa as a cause of haemolytic anaemia and an appropriate advice was issued. Another success was the detection of a faulty batch of a particular product, which the manufacturer immediately withdrew, underlining the value of an efficient procedure for tracing a batch. During June 1967, the Committee distributed a leaflet on the use of aerosols in asthma. This was prompted by the death rate amongst asthmatic patients aged 5 to 34 years that had risen some 300% above the level in 1959–60 when such preparations were introduced. By September 1968, the rate had dropped to only 50% above that seen in 1959–60 despite sales having dropped only 20%.

Among the first three 'old' drugs to be withdrawn from the market during the tenure of the CSD were benziodarone, a vasodilator launched in 1962 and withdrawn in 1964 due to reports of jaundice, pronethalol, a β-blocker introduced in 1963 and withdrawn in 1965 due to animal carcinogenicity and phenoxypropazine, an antidepressant introduced in 1961 and withdrawn in 1966 due to its hepatotoxicity.

The first major new drug to be approved and withdrawn from the market by the CSD was ibufenac, the first of the non-steroidal anti-inflammatory drugs (NSAID) to be marketed. Ibufenac was a precursor of ibuprofen and its use in the United Kingdom was associated with serious and frequent hepatotoxicity. Two other drug withdrawals (also approved during their tenure by CSD) were chlormadinone and fenclozic acid.

During 1969–70, the nephropathic hazards of phenacetin again attracted much attention and the Committee made a seminal observation that has profoundly influenced our regulatory philosophy even today: '*It is the safety of drugs in normal usage that is the Committee's concern, and because all drugs have their hazards when abused, particularly by over-dosage, the Committee has not considered that it should take special action in connection with phenacetin*'.

The 'demise' of the CSD was marked by a reception at Lancaster House in December 1971. It was attended by the Secretary of State together with the Health Ministers of Scotland, Wales and Northern Ireland as well as by the current and previous members of CSD, its first Chairman, Sir Derrick Dunlop, the Presidents of the Royal Colleges and representatives of the medical and pharmaceutical professions and pharmaceutical industry.

The CSD had already set the pattern for effective drug controls in the future.

16.4   The Medicines Act 1968

The Joint Subcommittee of the English and Scottish Standing Medical Advisory Committee, chaired by The Lord Cohen of Birkenhead, had included as its members seven distinguished clinicians and pharmacists of the day.[4] They were:

- Professor S Alstead, CBE, MD, FRCP, FRFPS
- AB Davies, BSc, MD, ChB, MRCS, LRCP
- Professor Sir Charles Dodds, MVO, MD, DSc, FRCP, FRS
- JB Grosset, MPS, DBA
- Sir Hugh Linstead, OBE, LLD, FPS, MP

- Professor EJ Wayne, MD, FRCP, FRFPS
- Professor GM Wilson, MD, FRCP

The Joint Subcommittee had concluded that testing was the responsibility of the manufacturers and they appeared to favour a voluntary scheme of control.

Para 25: Sanctions under a Voluntary Scheme While a voluntary scheme could have no formal legal sanctions, we think that the following measures might help, nevertheless, to ensure that new drugs were subject to adequate toxicity testing and clinical trials. . .

However, the two eminent pharmacists, John Grosset and Hugh Linstead, appended to the report a lengthy note of dissent that was forceful and stated with uncompromising clarity:

Voluntary or Statutory Control of Toxicity Testing and Clinical Trials?

Our main disagreement with our colleagues lies in the answer to this question. They favour a voluntary system until time can be found for legislation. We believe that any voluntary system must have so many loopholes that it can offer no real additional safeguards to the public. In consequence, we consider that there is no satisfactory alternative to early legislation.[4]

In their note, they also commented extensively on the deficiencies of a voluntary system. Grosset and Linstead concluded their note with a plea '*to set on foot, with or without further enquiry, the preparation of a comprehensive statute dealing with drugs and medicines that will bring the whole field, including the supervision of toxicity testing and clinical trials, under the responsibility of the Health Ministers advised by a central body of experts*'.

Full voluntary cooperation was clearly not as assured as might have been anticipated. During 1965, the CSD itself seemed to articulate in its Annual Report a carefully concealed aspiration for the introduction of statutory controls on drug regulation. After a period of review and consultation, a White Paper 'Forthcoming Legislation on the Safety, Quality and Description of Drugs and Medicines' was published in September 1967 and the Medicines Act based on these proposals received the Royal Assent on 25 October 1968. The CSD *'welcomes the statutory provisions that provide a firm basis for the continued evaluation of drug safety in the future'*.

The Medicines Act 1968 is a comprehensive set of measures replacing most of the previous legislation on the control of medicines for human use and for veterinary use in the United Kingdom. It is a consolidation into a single Act of the most desirable features of all previous rules, regulations and Acts in the United Kingdom and also includes controls on promotion and sale of drugs. The Act has 136 sections divided into eight Parts (Parts I to VIII) and has a further eight schedules appended to it. Among the important sections for licensing and monitoring purposes are:

• Sections 18–24 regarding applications for, and grant and renewal of, licences with section 19 requiring evidence for safety, efficacy and quality when determining an application.
• Sections 28–30 in respect of suspension, revocation and variation of licences.
• Sections 31–39 on clinical trials.
• Sections 51–59 on sale and supply.
• Sections 85–88 on labelling and leaflets.
• Sections 92–97 on promotion and advertising.
• Sections 104–128 on enforcement.

Under section 118 of the Act, all data submitted by a company in support of an application to conduct clinical trials or market a medicinal product are confidential; indeed even the existence of such an application is confidential. Breach of confidentiality attracts penalties and 'any person guilty of an offence under this section shall be liable (1) on summary conviction, to a fine not exceeding £400; (2) on conviction on indictment, to a fine or to imprisonment for a term not exceeding 2 years or to both'.

The Act has been frequently amended as appropriate to ensure that it is in line with the European community legislation. Given the remarkable degree of similarity between the requirements under the Medicines Act 1968 and the legislations prevailing at the time in the United States and the European Economic Community (EEC), the existence of four major legislations, together with their amendments and

consequential secondary legislations, is worth bearing in mind.

One was the Federal Pure Food and Drugs Act (also known as the 'Wiley Act') that was introduced in the United States in 1906. This law was enacted in response to revelations of worthless, impure and dangerous patent medicines that were claimed to cure almost anything. Another was the Federal Food, Drug and Cosmetic Act 1938 that had been passed following the Elixir Sulfanilamide disaster in the United States during 1937 in which 107 people (mostly children) had died from renal failure associated with its therapeutic use. As the drug was called 'elixir', implying that the preparation contained alcohol, the FDA could only make seizure of the product for misbranding. In reaction to this calamity, the US Congress passed the 1938 Act, which, for the first time, required proof of safety before release of a new drug. However, no proof of efficacy was required. Following the thalidomide tragedy in Western Europe, a subsequent New Drug Amendment (the Kefauver–Harris Amendment) was introduced in 1962 that required the FDA to monitor all stages of drug development. As a result of the Kefauver–Harris Amendment, even investigational drugs then required comprehensive animal testing before extensive human trials could be started. Proof of efficacy and safety was mandatory and the time constraints for disposition of new drugs, previously deemed approved by default if the FDA had failed to consider the new drug application by 60 days, were removed.

The EEC had already in place the Council Directive 65/65/EEC on the approximation of provisions laid down by law, regulation or administrative action relating to medicinal products. Many of the requirements under Council Directive 65/65/EEC had already formed part of the Medicines Act. When Directives 75/318/EEC and 75/319/EEC were adopted by the Council of Ministers on 20 May 1975, they only supplemented and amended the original Directive 65/65/EEC. Therefore, when the United Kingdom joined the EEC in 1973, the provisions of these two new Directives did not substantially affect the licensing system that operated in the United

Kingdom under the Medicines Act, although certain relatively minor amendments were necessary.

The first provisions laid down in the Medicines Act regarding licensing of medicinal products and other aspects of control came into effect on 1 September 1971 – the 'duly appointed day'. The Act was administered by the Health and Agriculture Ministers of the United Kingdom acting together as the Licensing Authority or in some cases acting separately as the health ministers or the agriculture ministers in respect of human and veterinary medicines respectively. The Act allows for Orders and Regulations to be made implementing its provisions and 98 Statutory Instruments had been made by the end of 1977. The first four were made in 1970 (SI 1970/746, 1257, 1304 and 1256), establishing respectively the Medicines Commission, Committee on Safety of Medicines, Veterinary Products Committee and the British Pharmacopoeia Commission. A full list of these is contained in the Annual Reports for 1976 and 1977 of the Medicines Commission and the section 4 Committees.

16.4.1 The Licensing Authority

Under section 6 of the Medicines Act 1968, the Licensing Authority (LA) is the authority responsible for the grant, renewal, variation, suspension and revocation of licences and certificates. In 1971, the LA was constituted of a body of Ministers consisting of the Secretary of State for Social Services, the Secretary of State for Scotland, the Secretary of State for Wales, the Minister of Health and Social Services for Northern Ireland, the Minister of Agriculture, Fisheries and Food and the Minister of Agriculture in Northern Ireland.

16.4.2 Medicines Division (DHSS)

The day-to-day administration of the Act for human medicines was delegated to the Medicines Division of the Department of Health and Social Security (DHSS) and was managed jointly by an Under Secretary and the professional head of the division. The professional head of the

Medicines Division held the rank of senior principal medical officer.

Over the period, the successive professional heads of the Medicines Division have been Dr DA Cahal (1964–70), Dr D Mansel-Jones (1970–4), Dr EL Harris (1974–7), Dr JP Griffin (1977–84) and Dr G Jones (1984–9). In 1989, when the Medicines Division was reorganised into the Medicines Control Agency (MCA) (see section 16.7), Dr KH Jones was appointed the first Director of the new Agency.

Before the United Kingdom joined the European Union, the Medicines Division had developed close links with other authorities both within and outside the European Union. Notable among these were the 'Tripartite Meetings' held biannually with the US FDA and the Canadian Health Protection Branch. These meetings, lasting a few days, discussed all areas of drug regulation generally and problems with specific drugs. Having first started in 1971, these meetings continued, while the EU system was evolving during the UK membership, until 1991 (apart from a very brief lull during the mid-1980s). By 1991, the International Conference on Harmonisation (ICH) initiative (see later) had fully matured into the first ICH meeting, to be held in Brussels in November 1991.

16.5 Statutory Controls in the United Kingdom (1971 and thereafter)

16.5.1 Medicines Commission

The Medicines Commission, provided for in section 2 of the Act, was established by the Ministers to give them advice generally relating to the execution of the Act (SI 1970/746), with Sir Derrick Dunlop as its first Chairman.

The scope of the functions of the Commission is very wide, but as defined in 1975 may be summarised as follows:

1. to advise the LA on matters relating to the execution of the Medicines Act.
2. to recommend to the Ministers, the number and functions of committees to be established

under section 4 of the Act and to recommend such persons as they consider well qualified to serve as members of such committees.

3. to advise the LA in cases where it consults the Commission, including cases where the LA arranges for the applicant for the grant of a licence to have an opportunity of appearing before, and being heard by, the Commission.

Sir Derrick Dunlop's tenure of office ended on 31 December 1971. The Medicines Commission has since then been successively chaired by Lord Rosenheim (from January 1972 to 2 December 1972, when he died suddenly), Professor A Wilson (Acting Chairman December 1972 to the middle of 1973), Sir Ronald Bodley Scott (middle of 1973 to December 1975), Professor WJH Butterfield (later Sir John Butterfield and later still Lord Butterfield, January 1976 to December 1981), Professor Rosalinde Hurley (later Dame Rosalinde Hurley, January 1982 to December 1993), Professor DH Lawson (January 1994 to December 2001) and Professor Parveen Kumar (January 2002 to October 2005).

The establishment of the Medicines Commission in May 1969 was followed by the establishment of a number of expert committees with specific advisory functions, appointed by Ministers after considering the recommendations of the Commission as proposed in section 4 of the Medicines Act. These expert committees, whose members are appointed by Ministers on the advice of the Medicines Commission, advise the LA and consist of independent experts such as hospital clinicians, general practitioners, pharmacists and clinical pharmacologists, and not the staff of the DHSS.

The relevant advisory committees with a remit for medicines for human use established under the Medicines Act 1968 were the Committee on Safety of Medicines (CSM), set up in June 1970 (SI 1970/1257) under the Chairmanship of Professor EF Scowen and the British Pharmacopoeia Commission (BPC), also set up in June 1970 (SI 1970/1256) under the Chairmanship of Dr F Hartley (later Sir Frank Hartley). The Veterinary Products Committee (VPC), chaired by Professor CSG Grunsell (with a remit for

medicines for veterinary use and administered through the Ministry of Agriculture Food and Fisheries), was also established in June 1970 (SI 1970/1304). Other important bodies set up were the Joint Subcommittee on the Use of Antibiotics and Related Substances and Standing Joint Subcommittee on the Classification of Proprietary Preparations, both of which reported directly to the Medicines Commission.

The products already on the market on 1 September 1971, the date for implementation of the Medicines Act, were given the Product Licences of Right (PLR) that were subject to a review process at a later date. This proposal for review of PLRs is reminiscent of the FDA contract with the National Academy of Sciences/National Research Council (NAS/NRC) in 1966, to evaluate the effectiveness of some 4000 different drug formulations approved on the basis of safety alone between 1938 and 1962 – the year of the Kefauver–Harris Amendment.

In 1977, the Medicines Commission reached a significant milestone when the work on classification of medicines was completed. New arrangements provided for three categories of medicines according to their safety factor – those available on prescription only (POM), those sufficiently safe to be on general sale to the public through any retail outlet (GSL), and an intermediate category of those that should only be sold at pharmacies (P). Under section 59 of the Medicines Act, all new medicinal products, not previously on the market, are prescription only for the first 5 years. A conscious decision is made for reclassification of each before the 5-year period expires. This requires updating the Prescription Only Medicines (POM) Order or the General Sales List (GSL) Order.

Rule 13(1) of the Poisons Rules (1972) allowed a pharmacist to supply a POM medicine without a prescription when, by reason of some emergency, a doctor was unable to furnish a prescription immediately.

Section 96 of the Medicines Act provided that after the duly appointed day (1 September 1971), no advertisement relating to medicinal products may be sent to a practitioner unless a data sheet had been sent some time in the previous

15 months. Final regulations on long term arrangements for data sheets appeared in 1972.

The issue of chloroform had surfaced again in 1978. In June 1977, a consultation letter was issued by the LA (MLX 90) introducing a proposal to make an Order under section 62 of the Act prohibiting the sale, supply and importation of any medicinal products containing chloroform (with certain exceptions such as its use as a preservative in pharmaceuticals). Many organisations, including the Joint UK Working Party on Chloroform, made representations and the Commission considered the safety of chloroform in the context of its alleged carcinogenicity in animals and safety in humans. It was concluded that chloroform was not mutagenic and hence did not present a carcinogenic risk to humans. It was also concluded that the upper permitted level of chloroform in medicinal products should be that of the saturated aqueous solution, which is 0.5% volume in volume. The exceptions to the prohibition included the use of chloroform as an anaesthetic agent, its use in dental surgery and the right of doctors and dentists to exercise clinical judgement to have prepared for their patients, products containing a higher concentration.

Over the period, the Commission has continued to discharge its functions and has been pivotal not only in implementing the provisions of Medicines Act 1968 but also advising the Ministers on broader policies relating to public health and drug regulation in the United Kingdom. For example, apart from deregulating medicines from prescription control and to GSL, the Commission has deliberated and advised on sale, supply and administration of medicines by health professionals under patient group directions, administration of POMs by ambulance paramedics, review of the process for reclassification (change of legal status) of medicines in the United Kingdom, proposals for supplementary prescribing by chiropodists, physiotherapists, radiographers and optometrists and proposed amendments to the POM (Human Use) Order 1997 and access to yellow card scheme.

Currently, the Commission has some 24 members (the Act requires it to have a minimum of eight) and meets five to six times per year. Members are appointed for 4-year terms. However, the work of the Commission has steadily diminished over recent years because of changes in licensing arrangements (e.g. the growth of EU licensing under the centralised and mutual recognition procedures) and other procedural changes within the Medicines and Healthcare products Regulatory Agency (MHRA) (e.g. reclassification procedures). For example, the Commission heard a total of three appeals in 2002 and none in 2003, compared with an average of four or five per year for the previous 10 years. Given also that there are profound changes in the European regulatory structure, environment and legislation (see Section 16.9 and Chapter 17), the MHRA is about to implement amalgamation of the functions of MC and CSM. This proposal is discussed later under Section 16.8.

16.5.2 Committee on Safety of Medicines (CSM)

The CSM, first chaired by Professor EF Scowen, replaced the previous CSD and first met on 25 June 1970. Its functions may be summarised as follows:

1. Giving advice with respect to safety, quality and efficacy, in relation to human use, of any substance or article (not being an instrument, apparatus or appliance) to which any provision of the Act is applicable.
2. Promoting the collection and investigation of information relating to adverse reactions, for the purpose of enabling such advice to be given.

A number of subcommittees assisted the main Committee. Originally, these were the Subcommittee on Toxicity, Clinical Trials and Therapeutic Efficacy, the Subcommittee on Chemistry, Pharmacy and Standards, the Subcommittee on Adverse Reactions and the Subcommittee on Biologicals.

In order to permit a smooth transition, the two committees (that on Safety of Drugs and that on Safety of Medicines) met simultaneously from June 1970 onwards, the CSD continuing to appraise products for clinical trials and marketing while the CSM had been concerned with preparation for the implementation of the Medicines Act. On 1 September 1971, the 'duly appointed day', the CSM took over the work formerly done by the CSD and the applicants, responsible for submissions still awaiting consideration by the CSD on 1 September 1971, were invited to convert those submissions into applications for Clinical Trial Certificates or for Product Licences. The CSD, however, continued to meet several times after 1 September 1971 to deal with some residual matters arising directly from its own decisions.

Commensurate with the emphasis on drug safety, the terms of reference of the Subcommittee on Adverse Reactions were reviewed in 1971 and revised as follows:

1. To promote and assemble reports about possible adverse effects of medicinal products administered to man
2. To assess the meaning of such reports
3. To recommend to the Committee any special or extended investigations that it considered desirable
4. To keep under review the methods by which adverse reactions are monitored
5. To make recommendations to the Committee based on its assessment of any action that it considers should be taken; and
6. To advise the Committee on communications with the professions relating to the work of the Subcommittee.

The LA was already empowered by the Medicines Act to suspend, revoke or vary licences under section 28 and to control clinical trials in patients under section 36. At the outset in 1971, the Committee recognised the need to adhere to the policy stated by the CSD in respect of considering efficacy but took a much firmer line in 1972, bearing in mind section 19 of the Act. The Committee stated explicitly that, in future, it would require applications to be supported by some evidence of efficacy before advising that a product licence should be granted.

Since its establishment, the CSM has been chaired successively by Professors EF Scowen (June 1970 to March 1976), GM Wilson (April 1976 to December 1976), EF Scowen (January 1977 to June 1980), A Goldberg (later Sir Abraham Goldberg, July 1980 to December 1986), AW Asscher (later Sir William Asscher, January 1987 to December 1992), MD Rawlins (later Sir Michael Rawlins, January 1993 to December 1998), AM Breckenridge (later Sir Alasdair Breckenridge, January 1999 to March 2003) and G Duff (April 2003 to date).

16.5.3 Committee on the Review of Medicines (CRM) and Committee on Dental and Surgical Materials (CDSM)

The proposed review of PLRs was already considered necessary by the United Kingdom but became a requirement when it joined the European Union. It was to correspond to the requirements under Directives 65/65/EEC and 75/318/EEC of the European Community that required that, throughout the Community, proprietary medicinal products granted licences before 22 November 1976 should be reviewed by 20 May 1990. All Member States of the European Community were similarly required to review the quality, safety and efficacy of products on their market.

Therefore, under the Act, the CRM was established in 1975 (SI 1975/1006), under the Chairmanship of Professor EF Scowen with Professor OL Wade as the Deputy Chairman, to review all PLRs.

This Committee first met in October 1975. Initially, the review was organised in approximately 30 therapeutic categories such as analgesics, NSAIDs, psychotropics, etc. The priority was antirheumatics first, followed by analgesics and psychotropics, the priority being determined by the fact that adverse reactions related to these drugs were reported frequently. Therefore, a number of subcommittees, such as the Subcommittee on Anti-Rheumatic Agents, Subcommittee on Analgesics and Subcommittee on Psychotropic Agents, were established. This approach proved slow and it was modified to a review of products of all companies, each company in two 5-yearly cycles. The Herbal

Standards Subcommittee of the CSM also contributed to the review of PLRs.

In 1974, the Health Ministers consulted the UK Medicines Commission on a proposal to set up a committee under section 4 to advise the LA on applications for product licences for dental and other surgical materials.

The CDSM was also established (SI 1975/1473) in 1975 under the Chairmanship of Professor RA Cawson to advise on dental and ophthalmic products and surgical materials. It dealt with PLRs within its area of expertise and held its first meeting in October 1976.

These two main review Committees had their own dedicated professional secretariat with a remit to review the evidence of safety, quality and efficacy of all 39 035 PLRs. Of these some 6000 PLRs related to homeopathic or blood products, vaccines, toxins, sera and radiopharmaceuticals that were excluded from review requirements since these were excluded from Directives EEC/65/65, 75/318 and 75/319 as they stood in 1976. Subsequently, however, the Extension Directive brought even these products within the scope of review.

The number of PLRs that were allowed to lapse by the manufacturers or were revoked or suspended in the United Kingdom between 1971 and 1982 was 22 376, and by 1988 this number had increased to 27 938. By 1982, the number of PLRs that were converted into full product licences was only 598. At the completion of the review in 1990, the number of applications received for full product licences was 6272 and of these just under 5300 were converted into full licences, most after changes had been agreed to the terms of the licences.[5] Of the 6272 applications, only 706 required referral to CRM or CDSM for advice. The CRM was deemed to have completed its work in 1991 and was disestablished on 31 March 1992 (SI 1992/606) while similarly, the CDSM was disestablished on 31 December 1994 (SI 1994/15).

During their existence, the CRM and the CDSM had four chairmen each – Professors EF Scowen (October 1975–December 1978), OL Wade (January 1979–December 1984), W Asscher (January 1985–December 1986) and DH Lawson (January 1987–March 1992) chairing the CRM,

while Professors RA Cawson (October 1976–December 1979), R Hurley (January 1980–December 1981), CL Berry (later Sir Colin Berry, January 1982–December 1992) and D Poswillo (January 1993–December 1994) chaired the CDSM.

16.5.4 Earlier controls on conduct of clinical trials in the United Kingdom

The Medicines Act 1968 included the definitions of a clinical trial and of a medicinal product. Clinical studies involving healthy volunteers did not meet this definition of a clinical trial and, as a result, did not come under the remit of regulatory controls. Such studies were subject to self-regulation by the pharmaceutical industry. Consequently, only the clinical trials in patients had to be covered by a clinical trial certificate (CTC).

The LA did not lay down rigid requirements concerning the data that must be provided before authorisation can be given for a certificate for the clinical trial of a new drug. It did, however, issue guidelines for applicants.

In view of the regulatory delay that was caused by the need to apply for a CTC, a Statutory Order (SI 1974/498) was made during 1974, to provide an exemption from the need to hold a CTC in such cases, subject to certain conditions. This order applied to trials conducted by doctors and dentists on their own responsibility (DDX). The basis of the clinical trial exemption (CTX) scheme, introduced in 1981, to include studies initiated by the pharmaceutical industry, was that together with a detailed clinical trial protocol and summaries of chemical, pharmaceutical, pharmacological, pharmacokinetic, toxicological and human volunteer studies, a clinical trial in patients may proceed without the need for the additional details normally required for a CTC or Product Licence application. This exemption scheme was based on the requirements that:

- A doctor must certify the accuracy of the data
- The applicant undertook to inform the LA of any refusal to permit the trial by an ethical committee; and

- The applicant also undertook to inform the LA of any data or reports concerning the safety of the product.

The LA had 35 days to respond to the notification to proceed with a clinical trial but could in exceptional circumstances require a further 28 days to consider the notification. If the CTX was refused, the applicant could apply for a CTC, in which case complete data had to be filed. If the CTC application was refused the statutory appeal procedures came into play if the applicant company wished to avail itself of this provision.[6] These appeal procedures were identical with those applying to marketing applications. The CTX scheme proved highly successful in encouraging inward investment into research in the United Kingdom. In a sample of 42 companies, an increase in research investment of 10% or more was attributed to the scheme by 23 of them.[7,8] Its implementation was criticised by consumer groups and its effect was carefully monitored every 6 months to ensure that no added risk to patients had been introduced.

This introduction of the CTX scheme is widely cited as an example of the benefits of deregulation. Australian drug regulatory authorities subsequently also introduced a similar scheme.

With a view to harmonising the conduct of clinical trials across the European Union, Directive 2001/20/EEC was finally agreed on 14 December 2000 and was formally adopted in May 2001 with a 3-year transition period for its implementation. The Directive is now fully implemented in the United Kingdom and further information on clinical trials there can be accessed at the MHRA website. Under the provisions of the Directive, all clinical trials now require a Clinical Trial Authorisation (CTA). This is discussed in detail in Chapter 17.

16.5.5 CSM and monitoring adverse reactions

One of the most important aspects of the UK regulatory system is the scheme that provides for the voluntary reporting of adverse reactions to a marketed drug. Since most serious ADRs are rare

events, they are unlikely to be detected in early clinical trials.

In order to stimulate a decreasing rate of reporting, the CSM in 1971 adopted a new version of the yellow card that was simple to complete but provided for more information to be included. The trial proved successful. In addition, to promote reporting of adverse drug reactions from general practitioners, the Subcommittee on Adverse Reactions convened a conference at the Royal College of General Practitioners in September 1973. In order to explore the ways of improving the dissemination of information about ADRs, a conference was also organised at the Royal College of Physicians in October 1975. Sustaining the efforts of the CSD, the CSM continued close cooperation with the WHO and with other regulatory authorities, in particular on matters relating to adverse reactions to medicinal products.

The first two safety letters from CSM to the doctors were sent out in 1973. One in May dealt with a range of issues, including the reports of subacute myelo-optic neuropathy (SMON) in association with clioquinol (some 10 000 cases in Japan but in the United Kingdom none of SMON and only a few cases of reversible neurotoxicity following prolonged exposure) and vaginal adenocarcinoma in daughters of mothers who had taken stilboestrol during pregnancy (80 cases in the United States but none in the United Kingdom). The other dated 3 January 1974 reported on 130 cases (66 fatal) of halothane-induced jaundice, 94 of which were associated with repeated exposures to this anaesthetic.

During 1974, the Committee discussed the introduction of a special mark to identify recently introduced products. This resulted in the introduction in January 1976 of the 'Black Triangle' Scheme to identify drugs requiring intensive monitoring. This involves the Product Name to be followed immediately by an inverted black triangle (▼) as a superscript next to it in all product literature. Products requiring this symbol would include new drugs, established products having significantly new indications or new routes of administration and entirely novel combinations of potent medicinal substances. In 1977, the Committee also produced detailed guidelines for the improved post-marketing surveillance of drugs. Following consultations in 1978, final guidelines were agreed with the ABPI and BMA.

The Yellow Card Scheme, at first restricted to receive reports from doctors, dentists and coroners, has been gradually expanded to receive reports from other sources. From October 1996, the Scheme was extended to include reporting of suspected adverse reactions to unlicensed herbal remedies. In April 1997, the Yellow Card Scheme was further extended to include hospital pharmacists as recognised reporters of suspected ADRs. In addition, there are specially targeted extensions of the Scheme such as adverse reactions to HIV medicines and adverse reactions in children. Over the period, the Scheme has been gradually extended further to receive reports from community pharmacists and in October 2002, from nurses, midwives and health visitors.

On 21 July 2003, the Parliamentary Under Secretary of State for Health (Lords), Lord Warner, announced an Independent Review of the 'Yellow Card Scheme', under the Chairmanship of Dr Jeremy Metters. Dr Metters convened a multidisciplinary Steering Committee and on 6 October 2003, undertook a 3-month public consultation on the potential implications of increasing access to yellow card data. This full report of the Independent Review is available at MHRA website on: http://medicines.mhra.gov.uk/ ourwork / monitorsafe-qualmed / yellowcard/ yellowcardreport.pdf. Among the 24 main recommendations contained in the Report of the Steering Committee on Access to the Yellow Card Scheme was one to enable and encourage patients to directly report suspected ADRs to the MHRA. As a result, on 17 January 2005, a pilot scheme was initiated whereby patients too could report suspected ADR. Thus, for the first time in the United Kingdom, the Scheme was being opened to patients, parents and carers. The CSM/MHRA have set up a special Patient Reporting Working Group.

Direct reporting of adverse drug reactions to national regulatory authorities has been possible in the United States and Germany since the mid-1980s.[9]

In compliance with Data Protection legislation and the General Medical Council guidelines on confidentiality, the Yellow Card was updated in September 2000 to ask for an *identification number* for the patient; for instance, a practice or hospital number. The CSM no longer asked for personal patient identifiers on Yellow Cards; all that is now required is the patient's initials and age instead of their name and date of birth. The inclusion of the identification number enables the patient to be identifiable to the reporter but not to the CSM, thus allowing the reporter to know to whom the report refers for any potential future correspondence.

Apart from these changes necessary to keep pace with the changing times, the system has continued unchanged from when it was first set up, and the number of reports and fatal reactions each year of the Scheme's operation to 2004 is shown in Table 16.4. By then, the CSM had received well over 450 000 reports since 1964. Despite relatively low reporting rates (a common feature of all spontaneous reporting systems worldwide), the UK Yellow Card Scheme has enjoyed a remarkable success and international recognition and has been responsible for uncovering many important drug safety hazards.

Communication with the profession was at first maintained by continuing (until January 1985) the *Adverse Reaction Series* leaflets started by CSD, and later by a regularly published bulletin on 'Current Problems'. The first issue of *Current Problems* in September 1975 led with the adverse oculo-cutaneous effects and sclerosing peritonitis associated with β-adrenergic receptor blocking agents and also included items on loss of consciousness associated with prazosin and on the risks of anti-inflammatory agents and asthma.

Major drugs withdrawn between 1971 and 1982 for safety reasons included polidexide (introduced 1974 and withdrawn 1975), oral formulation of practolol (1970 and 1976), alclofenac (1972 and 1979), tienilic acid (1979 and 1980), clomacron (1977 and 1982) and indoprofen (1982 and 1982).

Table 16.4 Annual number of total and fatal Adverse Reaction Reports to the CSD and CSM

Year	Total ADR reports	Total fatal reports	Fatal reports (% of total)
1964	1 415	86	6.1
1965	3 987	169	4.2
1966	2 386	152	6.4
1967	3 503	198	5.7
1968	3 486	213	6.1
1969	4 306	271	6.3
1970	3 563	196	5.5
1971	2 851	203	7.1
1972	3 638	211	5.8
1973	3 619	224	6.2
1974	4 815	275	5.7
1975	5 052	250	4.9
1976	6 490	236	2.6
1977	11 255	352	3.1
1978	11 873	396	3.3
1979	10 881	286	2.6
1980	10 179	287	2.9
1981	13 032	303	2.3
1982	10 922	340	3.1
1983	12 689	409	3.2
1984	12 163	340	2.8
1985	12 652	348	2.8
1986	15 527	403	2.6
1987	16 431	390	2.4
1988	19 022	410	2.2
1989	19 246	475	2.5
1990	18 084	377	2.1
1991	20 272	541	2.7
1992	20 161	478	2.4
1993	18 078	480	2.7
1994	17 556	412	2.3
1995	17 748	467	2.6
1996	17 109	393	2.3
1997	16 637	455	2.7
1998	18 062	529	2.9
1999	18 505	560	3.0
2000	33 147	610	1.8
2001	21 467	650	3.0
2002	17 622	666	3.8
2003	19 257	737	3.8
2004	20 206	861	4.3

Practolol illustrated well not only the value of a spontaneous reporting system but also the depth to which the Committee would investigate a signal of a serious ADR. Practolol-induced eye damage first came to light as a result of a publication by an ophthalmologist. Prior to this, the Committee had received only one report over a period of nearly 3 years. Subsequent to the publication, more than 200 cases of eye damage were reported retrospectively. In January 1975, a warning leaflet in the *Adverse Reaction Series* was issued and the Committee continued to receive additional reports. Later that year, the manufacturer proposed restrictions in the use of practolol. Ultimately, the oral formulation was withdrawn from the market.

The full might of the statutory control on regulation of drugs and their safety became evident in 1982 with the suspension of benoxaprofen, the first drug to be suspended from the UK market.[10] Benoxaprofen, also an NSAID, was approved in 1980 and marketed by Eli Lilly under the name Opren. It was launched amidst massive publicity and its marketing was 'explosive'. However, reports of serious ADRs and associated fatalities began to appear at an alarming rate. The first reports of deaths associated with benoxaprofen appeared in April and May 1982, when there were reported a total of eight cases of elderly women who developed jaundice while taking benoxaprofen; six of them died. Many other reports soon followed and the incidence of hepatotoxicity was estimated to be 2–4%. Before long, there were 61 fatalities associated with benoxaprofen and the drug was immediately suspended from the market on 3 August 1982.[10]

Experience with benoxaprofen and later with other drugs given to elderly patients was ultimately to result in a clinical guideline, adopted by the European Community's Committee for Proprietary Medicinal Products (CPMP) in September 1993, requiring the 'Investigation of Medicinal Products in Geriatrics' focusing on pharmacokinetics, pharmacodynamics and drug interactions as well as on the influence of renal or hepatic diseases on drug disposition. This also illustrates how guidelines frequently evolve with experience.

At the time the yellow card system celebrated its Silver Jubilee in 1989 at the Royal College of Physicians in London, the number of ADR reports in the CSM register was well in excess of 210 000. In relation to the size of the population, this represented a reporting rate in Britain that was among the highest in the world. The United Kingdom is a major contributor to the reports held by the WHO ADR Monitoring Centre in Uppsala, who have over three million reports in their database.[11] In 1991, the existing computer system was completely replaced by inauguration and introduction of ADROIT (Adverse Drug Reactions On-line Information Tracking), that was developed by the Medicines Control Agency (MCA). This system makes use of state-of-the-art information technology and highly interrelational databases including a medical dictionary designed by the agency staff. All major regulatory authorities now use this dictionary, MedDRA, for the purposes of monitoring and communicating information on adverse drug reactions. Data held on the previous system were transferred to ADROIT, which allowed assessors to set up complex enquiries of the database and respond rapidly to emerging safety issues.

On 4 May 2004, the CSM/MHRA celebrated fortieth anniversary of the Yellow Card Scheme.

16.6 General Safety Measures

The Commission and the CSM also made recommendations on the introduction of many other broad safety measures. These included the Phenacetin Prohibition Order (SI 1974/1082), presentation of medicines in relation to child safety (SI 1975/2000), and declaration of alcohol in medicinal products on their package as active ingredient where this is likely to be pharmacologically active. Other labelling issues culminated in an Order (SI 1976/1726) that set out the standard particulars that must be shown on the containers and packaging of medicinal products. Consultations on other generally applicable warnings on the labels of certain medicines to protect children and to ensure that more general advice and information is provided resulted in SI 1977/996.

In the United States, the FDA had first required patient information leaflets in 1970. Following consultations with the Pharmaceutical Society, the ABPI, BMA, Health Council and other bodies, regulations on leaflets (SI 1977/1055) were introduced to make sure that the public had greater information on the medicines they were prescribed.

Concerns on promotion of drugs were beginning to emerge and regulations were introduced under section 95 of the Act to control advertising to practitioners (SI 1975/298 and 1326). The former dealt with the advertising of products covered by PLRs while the latter dealt with specifying the information that must appear in all advertisement, including succinct statements on contraindications, warnings and adverse effects relevant to the indications. In addition, the generic name and the NHS cost were also required to appear. Further regulations (SI 1978/41) were also introduced on 1 February 1978 in respect of advertising direct to the public. Part of this made it an offence to advertise any product for certain serious diseases.

In 1975, the Medicines Division set up the Advertising Action Group to monitor advertising. The group included doctors, pharmacists, lawyers and administrators. In 1977, agreement was also reached with the ABPI for voluntary control and monitoring of advertisements by the industry and the ABPI instituted a Code of Practice and a Committee to supervise its implementation. Although a number of small companies had been prosecuted by the LA for breaching the regulations on advertising, these cases attracted little attention or interest within the industry at large. However, in 1984, monitoring of advertisements reached its climax with the successful prosecution of a major pharmaceutical company in respect of its advertisement for its drug Surgam (tiaprofenic acid).[12] The outcome of this prosecution has greatly influenced the behaviour of, and within, the industry and strengthened the case for the professional independence and responsibilities of physicians working in the industry.

16.7 Medicines Control Agency

Because of the rising future demands and delays in licensing, the Minister of Health announced on 11 March 1987 that he had commissioned a study of the control of medicines in the United Kingdom. The terms of reference were:

To examine the issues for DHSS arising from continued increase in licence applications and other work under the Medicines Act and to recommend ways of dealing expeditiously with this work, while maintaining adequate standards for the safety, efficacy, and quality of human medicines in the UK.

The study was undertaken by Dr John Evans, a previous Deputy Chief Medical Officer at the DHSS, and Mr Peter Cunliffe, Chairman of the Pharmaceutical Division of ICI. In 1988 the DHSS was split into two Departments, the Department of Health (DoH) and the Department of Social Security (DSS). Following the Cunliffe/Evans report, the Medicines Division of the DoH was reorganised in April 1989 to become the Medicines Control Agency under a Director and Dr Keith Jones was appointed the first Director of the Agency. The Agency was expected to be self-funding from fees commensurate with the services provided. In July 1991, the Agency became an Executive Agency of the DoH under the Government's 'Next Steps' initiative. Dr Jones therefore became the Chief Executive and was thereafter accountable directly to the Secretary of State for Health.

The Agency was the competent national authority responsible for human medicinal products in the United Kingdom and continued to discharge the functions of its predecessor, the Medicines Division, in implementing the Medicines Act and all European legislation. As at January 2001, the total staff had increased to 530 of whom 153 were working in the Licensing Division and 152 in the post-licensing Division. These 305 included 49 medical, 53 pharmaceutical and 85 preclinical or scientific staff.

The Agency continued to thrive and play a key role in Europe and also in all the regulatory and scientific activities of the European Committee for Proprietary Medicinal Products (see Section 16.9) and all its Working Parties. Dr Susan Wood represented the United Kingdom at CPMP and until her death in 1998 was the first Chairperson of its Pharmacovigilance Working Party. Dr PC Waller who succeeded her as the UK representative at CPMP also chaired this important Working Party. Mr AC Cartwright, another officer from the United Kingdom, chaired the Quality Working Party. Over the period, the United Kingdom has remained among the leading regulatory authorities in the European Union in terms of rapporteurship for the applications going through the Centralised Procedure, acting as a Reference Member State for the applications intended to go through the Mutual Recognition Procedure and as a coordinator of scientific advice from the CPMP.

At a European level, the United Kingdom has continued to contribute extensively to the many subsequent EU Directives and Regulations that control drugs in the European Union. All these, once adopted, have been incorporated into UK national legislation. In the UK, for example, Council Directive 92/27/EEC of 31 March 1992 regulated labelling and leaflets while Council Directive 92/28/EEC of 31 March 1992 regulated advertising of medicinal products for human use.

16.8 The Medicines and Healthcare products Regulatory Agency (MHRA)

On the 12 September 2002, the Health Minister, Lord Philip Hunt announced that the MCA and the Medical Devices Agency (MDA) would merge with effect from 1 April 2003. The merged agency would be known as the Medicines and Healthcare products Regulatory Agency (MHRA).

Effective from 1 January 2004, Professor Kent Woods, Professor of Therapeutics at the University of Leicester, was appointed Chief Executive of the MHRA.

Having been established under section 4 of the Medicines Act, 1968, the CSM advises on the safety, efficacy and quality of medicines for human use and to promote the collection and investigation of information relating to ADRs. Applications for national marketing authorisations cannot be refused by the LA on grounds of safety, efficacy or quality unless first referred to the CSM. Similarly, proposals to revoke or suspend a national authorisation on those grounds, or to refuse certain applications to vary a marketing authorisation, must be referred to the CSM. As a matter of practice, all applications for national authorisations for medicines containing new chemical entities are also referred to CSM. It is also the 'appropriate committee' that must be consulted on proposals to make regulations and orders under Part III of the Medicines Act 1968, which relates to the sale and supply of medicines. For example, the CSM is consulted on amendments to the POM (Human Use) Order 1997 when changes are required in relation to matters such as nurse prescribing, and on prohibition orders under Section 62 of the Act. In addition, the views of the CSM are sought by the MHRA on those centralised applications to the European Medicines Agency (EMEA) where the United Kingdom is rapporteur or co-rapporteur, and also on applications received under the mutual recognition procedure where a marketing authorisation is sought in the United Kingdom. The CSM's views are also sought on matters relating to the safety of marketed medicines. To fulfil these roles, the CSM has created three subcommittees: The Chemistry, Pharmacy and Standards Subcommittee (CPS); The Biologicals Subcommittee and The Subcommittee on Pharmacovigilance (SCOP) all of which report to the main Committee. In addition, the CSM creates working parties to deal with specific regulatory issues, usually relating to safety, and where it considers that it requires advice that is not available from within its membership. The CSM currently has 34 members and meets twice monthly, most members attending one meeting per month. Members are appointed for 3-year terms. As stated earlier, the MHRA is planning amalgamation of the functions of MC and CSM.

The MHRA issued a Consultation Letter (MLX No 300) in February 2004 seeking wider views on the proposed amalgamation of CSM and MC.

Following the consultation process, the restructuring of the advisory procedure was in progress at the time of writing this chapter in September 2005. In summary, from Autumn 2005, the new advisory structure will comprise:

- A new Commission on Human Medicines (CHM) that amalgamates the responsibilities of the present Medicines Commission and the Committee on Safety of Medicines, which will advise Ministers direct on matters relating to medicines for human use.
- A number of other committees established by Ministers, which will be able to advise Ministers direct on issues for which they are responsible. These are:
  - The Advisory Board on the Registration of Homeopathic Products (ABRH);
  - A new Herbal Medicines Advisory Committee (HMAC);
  - and The British Pharmacopoeia Commission (BPC).
- A number of Expert Advisory Groups (EAGs) that will advise the Commission, ABRH, HMAC and BPC on certain specific and technical matters.
- A panel of experts (including toxicology and statistics) to provide specialist advice to the above bodies and EAGs if required;
- A panel that brings together the lay (patient and consumer) representatives on the various bodies and EAGs.

Commission on Human Medicines

The new Commision (CHM) would be a newly appointed body, rather than an amalgamation of the current bodies. Its membership would be subject to a full appointments exercise, with a view to appointing the Chairman and members. On 27 July 2005, Professor Gordon Duff, previously the Chairman of the last CSM, was appointed the first Chairman of CHM, for a term of 4 years effective from 30 October 2005.

Functions of the new Commission

The new Commission would take on the functions currently performed by the MC and the

CSM in relation to medicines for human use. In particular it would be responsible for:

1. Advising Ministers and the Agency on policy matters relating to the regulation of medicinal products;
2. Advising on the safety, quality or efficacy of medicinal products (e.g. advising the Agency on those licensing applications that are currently considered by the CSM);
3. Promoting the collection and investigation of information relating to adverse reactions;
4. Advising on the establishment and membership of committees established under section 4 of the Medicines Act 1968. For example, the British Pharmacopoeia Commission (BPC) and Veterinary Products Committee (VPC) would be retained.

Subcommittees and Expert Advisory Groups

To facilitate the fullest participation in the new EU regulatory environment it is proposed that, in addition to the new Commission, provision would be made for the establishment of Expert Advisory Groups (EAGs) in defined therapeutic areas. CHM or relevant Section 4 Committee will make the appointments to the EAGs, Expert Panels and list of Experts. These EAGs would advise them on scientific issues which apply across therapeutic areas, or which relate to relatively self-contained substance-types. It is intended that EAGs would be expert groups set up to advise and make recommendations to the new CHM on specific issues, and they would not themselves have decision-making powers.

There is likely to be a continuing need for some subcommittees of the new Commission, such as those serving the present CSM. Although their current role and remit in relation to the CSM would not change under the new arrangements, it is proposed that these too should become known in the future as EAGs.

How the Commission and EAGs would operate

The CHM and the EAGs will most likely operate under the following arrangements:

1. The CHM would comprise approximately 10-12 core members, appointed by Ministers. Rather than restricting membership within the areas currently specified in the Medicines Act for the MC, the CHM would need members with high level scientific expertise and an ability in critical appraisal, a capacity to contribute beyond individual speciality and, where possible, experience in the NHS clinical practice and the regulatory field.
2. A number of EAGs would be created by the new Commission, with members selected and appointed by them and comprising national experts.
3. Recommendations from EAGs to the new Commission would be in the form of either a paper or a personal presentation by the EAG Chair who would attend as an invited member;
4. The majority of EAGs would exist as standing committees, each with certain members 'on retention'. Permanent members would include the Chair; and one or two permanent experts. MHRA would supply the secretariat and MHRA designated assessors may need to attend. Other experts would be invited for specific topics. Referrals from and between the various committees and groups would be arranged as necessary;
5. It will be an important task of the secretariat both to manage the logistics of EAG membership and to ensure that appropriate issues are referred to EAGs for their timely consideration;
6. The new Commission would meet once monthly;
7. EAGs would meet as required depending on the nature of the advice required by the new Commission. It would be possible for an EAG to 'meet' by tele- or TV-conference rather than by holding an actual meeting. UK representation at a European Therapeutic Advisory groups could, where relevant, be provided from a national EAG.

Initially, there will be EAGs in the following therapeutic areas and disciplines:

- Pharmacovigilance
- Biologicals and vaccines (including clinical issues for vaccines)
- Pharmacy and Standards (including pharmacokinetics)

(The chairs of the above three EAGs will also be full members of the CHM.)

In addition, there are likely to be EAGs for:

- Paediatrics
- Cardiology, diabetes, renal
- Respiratory and allergy
- Oncology and haematology
- Endocrine, obstetrics and gynaecology and bone metabolism
- Gastrointestinal and hepatology
- Anti-infectives and HIV/AIDS
- Neurology and pain management
- Psychiatry and old-age psychiatry
- Rheumatology, immunology
- Patient information
- Dermatology

Other expert advice

For other areas where advice is less frequently required there will be panels of experts who may supplement the EAGs or be called upon by the CHM as experts for the day.

Under the proposed new arrangements, if a marketing authorisation for a product (or a certificate of registration) was refused by the licensing authority, after a hearing before the CHM, the applicant would still be able to appeal to a 'person appointed' as provided for in the legislation. In particular, there would be scope for involving EAGs in clarification meetings to maximise predictability of outcome for companies and to resolve issues without the necessity of involving formal statutory appeals procedures.

In view of the increasing profile and use of herbal medicines, the European union has established a Committee for Herbal Medicinal Products (see chapter 17). The MHRA consulted and has also established a Herbal Medicines Advisory Committee (HMAC). This Committee would advise Ministers directly on areas for which the Committee is responsible. The remit of HMAC would be the registration scheme to be introduced under the Directive 2004/24/EC on Traditional Herbal Medicinal Products and unlicensed herbal medicines. However, CHM will be responsible for advice in relation to marketing authorisations for herbal medicines. Professor Philip Routledge was appointed the first Chairman of HMAC, for a term of 4 years effective from 30 October 2005.

16.9 European dimensions

The United Kingdom joined the European Community in January 1973 but the data requirements for granting marketing authorisations have, since the implementation of the Medicines Act 1968, been in accordance with European Community Directive 65/65/EEC and the subsequent Directive 75/318 as amended, which elaborated on the requirements for preclinical testing, pharmaceutical quality and manufacture. It was vital that during 1973, following the entry of United Kingdom into the Community, the CSM also had the opportunity to consider and comment extensively on the two draft directives (later to become 75/318/EEC and 75/319/EEC). Directive 75/318/EEC introduced the common dossier that harmonised the standards and requirements across the European Union while Directive 75/319/EEC established the CPMP, introduced the Mutual Recognition Procedure and brought in the requirements for expert reports.

The European Union's advisory Committee, the CPMP, was set up in 1975 under Directive 75/319. The first meeting was held on 26 November 1976 and Mr Leon Robert from Luxembourg was appointed its first Chairman. The Professional Head of the then UK Medicines Division, Dr EL Harris, who was also the UK Representative to CPMP, was elected a Deputy Chairman. Dr JP Griffin, initially his alternate but later the UK representative during 1977–84, was appointed Chairman of the CPMP Working Party on Safety. Dr NMG Dukes from the Dutch regulatory authority was appointed Chairman of the Efficacy Working Party at the same time. Dr Dukes was later succeeded by Professor JM Alexandre (from the French regulatory authority) who then proceeded to become the Chairman of the CPMP (1995 to 2000).

The proposed review of PLR in the United Kingdom, already considered necessary, was to correspond to the requirements under European Directives. These Directives required that throughout the Community proprietary medicinal products granted licences before 22 November 1976 should be reviewed by 20 May 1990. Indeed, the United Kingdom was among the first to complete this review on time. This review eliminated from the market all medicinal products that were released for clinical use previously without scrutiny and that were ineffective, unsafe or that had an unacceptable benefit to risk ratio.

Much later, Directive 83/570 required the applicants to produce a draft Summary of Product Characteristics (SPC) as an integral part of the documentation. In September 1995, an order was made (SI 1995/2321) to the effect that, in the United Kingdom, data sheets were no longer required where a product had an approved SPC and also that data sheets no longer had to be sent to all doctors and dentists prior to advertising.

In the United Kingdom, healthy volunteer studies were subject to self-regulation by the pharmaceutical industry and consequently only the clinical trials in patients had to be covered by a CTC. However, as stated earlier, clinical trials in the UK are now regulated under EU Clinical Trials Directive (2001/20/EEC) fully implemented in the UK.

The EU Clinical Trials Directive contains specific provisions regarding the conduct of clinical trials, including multicentre trials, on human subjects. It defines 'clinical trial' as any investigation in human subjects intended to discover or verify the clinical, pharmacological and/or other pharmacodynamic effects of one or more investigational medicinal product(s), and/or to identify any adverse reactions to one or more investigational medicinal product(s) and/or to

study absorption, distribution, metabolism and excretion of one or more investigational medicinal product(s) with the object of ascertaining its (their) safety and/or efficacy and defines 'subject' as an individual who participates in a clinical trial as either a recipient of the investigational medicinal product or a control. Thus, healthy volunteer studies are included.

Further stringent requirements have evolved over time in respect of investigations to be carried out during the clinical development of drugs, the data required before they are approved for marketing, and subsequently the requirements for safety monitoring during the post-marketing period (pharmacovigilance).

The raft of rules, regulations, guidelines and procedures (both the European Union and ICH) governing the human medicinal products in the European Union can be found in the following five volumes published by the European Commission:

Volume 1 Pharmaceutical Legislation
Volume 2 Notice to Applicants
    2A: Procedures for Marketing Authorisation
    2B: Presentation and Content of the Dossier
    2C: Regulatory Guidelines
Volume 3 Guidelines
    3A: Quality and Biotechnology
    3B: Safety, Environment, and Information
    3C: Efficacy
Volume 4 Good Manufacturing Practice
Volume 9 Pharmacovigilance

(Volumes 5–8 relate to veterinary medicinal products)

Many of the Directives originally adopted have been frequently amended over the period. In the interests of clarity and rationality, a whole range of the latest versions of these Directives was codified by assembling them in a single text, that is Directive 2001/83/EC of 6 November 2001. Therefore, the reader should also cross-refer to this Directive, which codifies the following:

1. Council Directive 65/65/EEC of 26 January 1965, on the approximation of provisions laid down by law, regulation or administrative action relating to medicinal products.

2. Council Directive 75/318/EEC of 20 May 1975, on the approximation of the laws of Member States relating to analytical, pharmacotoxicological and clinical standards and protocols in respect of the testing of proprietary medicinal products.

3. Council Directive 75/319/EEC of 20 May 1975 on the approximation of provisions laid down by law, regulation or administrative action relating to proprietary medicinal products.

4. Council Directive 89/342/EEC of 3 May 1989 on immunologicals (vaccines, toxins or serums and allergens).

5. Council Directive 89/343/EEC of 3 May 1989 on radiopharmaceuticals.

6. Council Directive 89/381/EEC of 14 June 1989 on products derived from human blood or human plasma.

7. Council Directive 92/25/EEC of 31 March 1992 on the wholesale distribution.

8. Council Directive 92/26/EEC of 31 March 1992 on classification for the supply.

9. Council Directive 92/27/EEC of 31 March 1992 on labelling and package leaflets.

10. Council Directive 92/28/EEC of 31 March 1992 on advertising.

11. Council Directive 92/73/EEC of 22 September 1992 on homeopathic medicinal products.

Directive 2001/83/EC was subsequently amended by (1) Directive 2002/98/EC of 27 January 2003, setting standards of quality and safety for the collection, testing, processing, storage and distribution of human blood and blood components, (2) Commission Directive 2003/63/EC of 25 June 2003, replacing Annex 1 of Directive 2001/83/EC (detailing scientific and technical requirements) with a new Annex (detailing scientific and technical requirements in CTD terms) and (3) Directive 2004/24/EC of 31 March 2004 as regards traditional herbal medicinal products.

Regarding all activities for the regulation of pharmaceuticals at the European Union level, Article 71 of Regulation EEC/2309/93 required that 'Within 6 years of the entry into force of this Regulation, the Commission shall publish a general report on the experience of the procedures laid down in this Regulation, in Chapter III of Directive 75/319/EEC and in Chapter IV of Directive 81/851/EEC'. The tender for review was awarded to a consortium of Cameron McKenna and Arthur Anderson. The full report from Cameron McKenna, entitled 'Evaluation of the Operation of Community Procedures for the Authorisation of Medicinal Products', is a comprehensive and highly constructive document.

Following extensive discussions among all interested parties, such as the national authorities, the EC and the European Federation of Pharmaceutical Industries and Associations (EFPIA), the EC proposed comprehensive reform of the EU pharmaceutical legislation. The amending legislations are (1) Directive 2004/27/EC of the European Parliament and of the Council of 31 March 2004, amending Directive 2001/83/EC, on the Community code relating to medicinal products for human use and (2) Regulation (EC) No 726/2004 of the European Parliament and of the Council of 31 March 2004, laying down Community procedures for the authorisation and supervision of medicinal products for human and veterinary use and establishing a European Medicines Agency – thus replacing Regulation EEC/2309/93. The adoption this reformed legislation just preceded the enlargement of the European Union on 1 May 2004 when the EU membership was increased from 15 to 25 Member States by the accession of 10 new Member States, namely Cyprus, Czech Republic, Estonia, Hungary, Latvia, Lithuania, Malta, Poland, Slovak Republic and Slovenia. Directive 2004/27/EC must come into force in all Member States by 30 October 2005, although Member States are able to implement early any of the provisions should they wish. Regulation 726/2004 has a transposition date of 20 November 2005, from which date its provisions will apply in all Member States.

Article 5 of Regulation (EC) No 726/2004 created a Committee for Medicinal Products for Human Use (CHMP) that shall be responsible for drawing up the opinion of the Agency on any matter concerning the admissibility of the files submitted in accordance with the centralised procedure, the granting, variation, suspension or revocation of an authorisation to place a medicinal product for human use on the market and pharmacovigilance. The CPMP therefore became the CHMP and consists of one member (with an alternate) appointed by each of the EU Member States, after consultation with the Management Board, for a term of 3 years, which may be renewed, and a chairperson. The Committee also includes one member appointed by each of the EEA-EFTA States, for a term of 3 years, which may be renewed.

The Committee, in order to complement its expertise, has appointed five coopted members chosen on the basis of their specific scientific competence, from among the experts nominated by Members States or the Agency. Coopted members are appointed for the term of the committee, which may be renewed, and do not have alternates. The Chairman of CPMP, Dr Daniel Brasseur was elected the Chairman of CHMP during its inaugural meeting on 1–3 June 2004.

Article 55 of Regulation (EC) No 726/2004 created the European Medicines Agency, comprising of a Management Board, an Executive Director, a Secretariat, the CHMP, the Committee for Medicinal Products for Veterinary Use (CVMP), the Committee on Orphan Medicinal Products (COMP) and the Committee on Herbal Medicinal Products (HMPC). Thus, the former European Medicines Evaluation Agency (EMEA) became the European Medicines Agency. However, for technical reasons, it had to retain the acronym EMEA (the acronym EMA belongs to European Medical Association).

16.10   International Dimensions

In June 1984, the Commission decided that a meeting with the Japanese authorities, attended by Mr F Sauer and the Chairman and Vice-Chairman of the Safety Working Party, Dr JP Griffin and Professor R Bass respectively, and the Chairman of the Efficacy Working Party, Professor JM Alexandre, should take place in Tokyo. The efforts following this initial meeting were ultimately to culminate in the ICH.

The main players at ICH are now the European Commission/EMEA, EFPIA, Japanese Ministry of Health Labour and Welfare (MHLW), Japanese Pharmaceutical Manufacturers Association (JPMA), US FDA and Pharmaceutical Research and Manufacturers of America (PhRMA). The WHO, Canadian Health Protection Branch and the European Free Trade Area (EFTA) countries enjoy an observer status at ICH meetings.

The ICH Steering Committee establishes expert working groups to discuss areas where harmonisation is possible and to produce universally acceptable guidelines. Thus under the auspices of the ICH, a large number of guidelines have been issued in the areas of quality, safety and efficacy, with the objective of achieving harmonisation of requirements for registration between regulatory authorities and thereby reducing the need to duplicate studies. It must be made clear that these documents are guidelines and not requirements.

These guidelines may not be at the cutting edge of science but they represent acceptable compromises based on sound science. As of January 2004, there were at least 13 safety, 17 efficacy (clinical safety is included in these), 19 quality and 8 multidisciplinary guidelines accepted since the first meeting of ICH in Brussels in November 1991. Once adopted by the CPMP and published, the guidelines resulting from the ICH process are locally implemented and applied as EU Community guidelines.

Regarding pharmacovigilance, the corner stone of post-marketing safety of drugs, there are a number of ICH/CPMP guidelines and a Joint Pharmacovigilance Plan (CPMP/PhVWP/2058/ 99 Revision 1) for the Implementation of the ICH guidelines E2B, M1 and M2. Two major advances were the acceptance of MedDRA (ICH topic M1) as a common medical dictionary for regulatory work and the acceptance of Periodic Safety Update Reports for marketed drugs (PSUR) (ICH topic E2C). The ICH pharmacovigilance guidelines adopted by the CPMP include ICH/135/95 [Good Clinical Practice, (E6)], ICH/285/95 [Guidance on Recommendations on Electronic Transmission of Individual Case Safety Reports Message

Specification (M2)], ICH/287/95 [Guidance on Clinical Safety Data Management: Data Elements for Transmission of Individual Case Safety Reports (E2B)], ICH/288/95 [Guidance on Clinical Safety Data Management: Periodic Safety Update Reports for Marketed Drugs (E2C)], and ICH/377/95 [Clinical Safety Data Management: Definitions and Standards for Expedited Reporting (E2A)].

If harmonisation could be achieved, as it has been, across a broad range of areas in quality, safety and efficacy, there seemed no logical reason why a Common Technical Document or dossier could not be prepared that would be acceptable to all drug regulatory authorities. At the ICH meeting in November 2000 in San Diego (USA), an agreement was reached on a Common Technical Document (CTD) that represented a common format for the submission of dossiers to the three regions of the United States, the European Union, and Japan. Effective from July 2003, the format of the EU dossier must conform to the CTD format. CTD is common to all the three major regions of drug regulation (European Union, United States and Japan) and most of the other major non-ICH authorities have also agreed to accept the dossier in this format. Information on the CTD 'Presentation and format of the dossier CTD' can be accessed from the EC website. This document also shows the correspondence of the previous format with the CTD format. It is important to appreciate that the introduction of CTD has not resulted in a change in the qualitative or quantitative nature of data required – only the format in which these data are presented has changed. Even applications for line extensions must be submitted using the new EU-CTD format. However, references can be made to already assessed and authorised 'old' parts of the dossier, but only if no new additional data are submitted in these parts. In such cases, it is not necessary to reformat already assessed and authorised 'old' documentation.

In order to expedite and optimise drug development, clinical trials are now conducted in different parts of the world. Recognising that drug development is a global process and in order that the data from one ethnic group can be confidently extrapolated to another, an ICH guideline (CPMP/ICH/289/95) has been agreed taking into account the genetic and non-genetic influences on drug responses. Application of this and all other national, regional and international guidelines relevant to quality, toxicity testing and demonstrating efficacy in clinical trials has ensured that public safety is not compromised while still ensuring that safe and effective medicines are made available to the UK public without the need for repeating lengthy clinical trials.

16.11 Conclusions

This chapter has provided a brief but hopefully, an interesting account of the events that have been responsible for the evolution of the present drug controls in the United Kingdom. Importantly, it highlights how the broad pattern of drug regulation was already set during the early period that led to the implementation of the Medicines Act in 1971 and how this pattern was consolidated during the three decades thereafter.

Contrary to what is generally believed, the need for an effective control was always recognised, and indeed demanded, and there was a sort of control. However, it was patchy, very limited in its scope, erratic in its implementation and of little relevance to the drugs that were beginning, and were likely in the future, to appear in the market as a result of progress in pharmacology and medicinal chemistry.

Thalidomide generated an outcry and a demand that could no longer be ignored, and spurred the Government into not only consolidating all previous legislation and extending its scope but also creating a formal regulatory structure by which to ensure that the legislation was adequately and fully implemented.

The Medicines Act, together with the associated EU legislation and EU and ICH guidelines, should ensure that the safety of drugs made to the highest quality, the acceptability of their risk/benefit ratio and the promotion of correct information to the prescribers and consumers are the dominant features of the controls that operate today.

References

1. Griffin JP. Venetian treacle and the foundation of medicines regulation. *Br J Clin Pharmacol* 2004;**58**: 317–25.
2. Penn RG. The state control of medicines: the first 3000 years. *Br J Clin Pharmacol* 1979;**8**:293–305.
3. Shah RR. Thalidomide, drug safety and early drug regulation in the UK. *Adverse Drug React Toxicol Rev* 2001;**20**:199–255.
4. Ministry of Health, Scottish Home and Health Departments. *Safety of Drugs*. Final Report of the Joint Sub-Committee of the Standing Medical Advisory Committees. Her Majesty's Stationery Office, London, 1963.
5. Winship K, Hepburn D, Lawson DH. The review of medicines in the United Kingdom. *Br J Clin Pharmacol* 1992;**33**:583–7.
6. Griffin JP, Long JR. New procedures affecting the conduct of clinical trials in the United Kingdom. *Br Med J* 1981;**2**:477–9.
7. Speirs CJ, Griffin JP. A survey of the first year of operation of the new procedure affecting the conduct of clinical trials in the United Kingdom. *Br J Clin Pharmacol* 1983;**15**:649–55.
8. Speirs CJ, Saunders RM, Griffin JP. The United Kingdom Clinical Trial Exemption Scheme – its effects on investment in research. *Pharm Int* 1984; **5**:254–6.
9. Griffin JP. Survey of the spontaneous adverse drug reactions reporting schemes in 15 countries. *Br J Clin Pharmacol* 1986;**22** Suppl **1**:83S–100S.
10. Shah RR. Drug-induced hepatotoxicity: pharmacokinetic perspectives and strategies for risk reduction. *Adverse Drug React Toxicol Rev* 1999;**18**: 181–233.
11. 'WHO Pharmacovigilance: Ensuring the safe use of medicines' WHO Policy Perspectives on Medicines No 9. Geneva, October 2004.
12. Collier J, Herxheimer A. Roussel convicted of misleading promotion. *Lancet* 1987;**i**:113–4.

Other Sources of Information

Committee on Safety of Drugs. Report of the Committee on Safety of Drugs for the year ended December 31, 1964. Her Majesty's Stationery Office, London, 1965.

Committee on Safety of Drugs. Report for the year ended 31 December 1965. Her Majesty's Stationery Office, London, 1966.

Committee on Safety of Drugs. Report for the year ended 31 December 1966. Her Majesty's Stationery Office, London, 1967.

Committee on Safety of Drugs. Report for the year ended 31 December 1967. Her Majesty's Stationery Office, London, 1968.

Committee on Safety of Drugs. Report for the year ended 31 December 1968. Her Majesty's Stationery Office, London, 1969.

Committee on Safety of Drugs. Report for 1969 and 1970. Her Majesty's Stationery Office, London, 1971.

Medicines Commission. First Annual Report to end of 1970. Her Majesty's Stationery Office, London, 1971.

Medicines Commission. Annual Report for 1971. Her Majesty's Stationery Office, London, 1972.

Committee on Safety of Medicines. Report for the year ended 31 December 1971. Her Majesty's Stationery Office, London, 1972.

Committee on Safety of Medicines. Report for the year ended 31 December 1972. Her Majesty's Stationery Office, London, 1973.

The Medicines Commission. Annual Report for 1973 (together with annual reports of standing committees appointed under section 4 of the Medicines Act 1968). Her Majesty's Stationery Office, London, 1974.

The Medicines Commission. Annual Report for 1974 (together with annual reports of standing committees appointed under section 4 of the Medicines Act 1968). Her Majesty's Stationery Office, London, 1975.

The Medicines Commission. Annual Report for 1975 (together with annual reports of standing committees appointed under section 4 of the Medicines Act 1968). Her Majesty's Stationery Office, London, 1976.

The Medicines Commission. Annual Report for 1976 (together with annual reports of standing committees appointed under section 4 of the Medicines Act 1968). Her Majesty's Stationery Office, London, 1977.

The Medicines Commission. Annual Report for 1977 (together with annual reports of standing committees appointed under section 4 of the Medicines Act 1968). Her Majesty's Stationery Office, London, 1978.

The Medicines Commission. Annual Report for 1978 (together with annual reports of standing committees appointed under section 4 of the Medicines Act 1968). Her Majesty's Stationery Office, London, 1979.

CHAPTER 17

17 Regulation of human medicinal products in the European Union

Rashmi R Shah and John P Griffin

17.1 Introduction

The thalidomide disaster, described in Chapter 16, resulted in an epidemic of a previously unknown malformation ('phocomelia'). The scale of the disaster reached such proportions that not only was the drug withdrawn from the market worldwide but there was also a public outcry on the lack of controls on human medicinal products in Europe. The United States was essentially spared the thalidomide tragedy because of the concerns of the Food and Drug Administration (FDA) over the neurotoxicity of thalidomide. This had resulted in the application being stalled in the United States. The US Federal Pure Food and Drugs Act (1906) and the Federal Food, Drug and Cosmetic Act (1938) were already in place but following the thalidomide tragedy in Western Europe, a subsequent New Drug Amendment (the Kefauver-Harris Amendment) in 1962 called for the FDA to monitor all stages of drug development. As a result, even investigational drugs then required comprehensive animal testing before extensive human clinical trials could be started. Under the Kefauver-Harris Amendment, proof of efficacy and safety was mandatory and the time constraints on the FDA for disposition of new drug applications were removed.

The thalidomide disaster was to provide the impetus to the introduction, for the first time in most non-US countries (including those in Western Europe), of regulatory control of drugs to be marketed for clinical use. In the United Kingdom the result was the Medicines Act 1968 and the establishment of the Licensing Authority.

Although the United Kingdom joined the European Community in 1973, the data requirements for granting marketing authorisations under the Medicines Act 1968 had been in accordance with European Community Directive 65/65/EEC and the subsequent Directive 75/318/EEC as amended. It is to be noted that the requirements, and also the general nature of the regulatory controls envisaged under the Medicines Act, 1968, are remarkably similar to those under other legislations prevailing at the time in the United States and the European Economic Community (EEC). In particular, the existence of four major pieces of legislation is worth bearing in mind:

- The US Federal Pure Food and Drugs Act (1906)
- The US Federal Food, Drug and Cosmetic Act (1938)
- US New Drug Amendment (the Kefauver–Harris Amendment) (1962)
- The EU Council Directive 65/65/EEC (1965).

Since the United Kingdom joined the European Community all EU pharmaceutical regulation and legislation is transposed into the UK national pharmaceutical regulation and legislation. The primary aim of the Community legislation is laid down in the preamble to the Council Directive of 26 January 1965 (65/65/EEC), which states that:

The Council of the European Economic Community, having regard to the Treaty establishing the European Economic Community and in particular Article 100 thereof . . .

– Whereas the primary purpose of any rules concerning the production and distribution of medicinal products must be to safeguard public health;

– Whereas, however, this objective must be attained by means which will not hinder the development of the pharmaceutical industry or trade in medicinal products within the Community;

– Whereas trade in medicinal products within the Community is hindered by disparities between certain national provisions, in particular between provisions relating to medicinal products (excluding substances or combinations of substances which are foods, animal feeding stuffs or toilet preparations); and whereas such disparities, directly affect the establishment and functioning of the common market;

– Whereas such hindrances must accordingly be removed; and whereas this entails approximation of the relevant provisions;

– Whereas, however, such approximation can only be achieved progressively; and whereas priority must be given to eliminating the disparities liable to have the greatest effect on the functioning of the common market;

has adopted this Directive.

The breadth of the regulatory definition of a medicinal product defined the scope of the legislation. The legislation defined a medicinal product as any substance or combination of substances presented for treating or preventing disease in human beings or animals or that may be administered in human beings or animals with a view to making a medical diagnosis or to restoring, correcting or modifying physiological functions in human beings or animals. Substance was further defined as any matter that may be of human, animal, vegetable or chemical origin.

The definition of a medicinal product has been changed following the recent review of the EU pharmaceutical legislation (Directive 2004/27/EC). The new definition states that to be a medicine a product must be:

1. Any substance or combination of substances presented as having properties for treating or preventing disease in human beings; or
2. Any substance or combination of substances that may be used in or administered to human beings either with a view to restoring, correcting or modifying physiological functions by exerting a pharmacological, immunological or metabolic action, or to making a medical diagnosis.

A new provision has also been added to remove any uncertainties, which states that:

'In cases of doubt, where, taking into account all its characteristics, a product may fall within the definition of a product covered by other Community legislation the provisions of this Directive shall apply.'

Taken together, these provisions are intended to ensure that where doubt exists over whether a product – those on the 'borderline' between, for example, medicines and medical devices, medicines and cosmetics, medicines and food supplements, etc., – should be regulated under medicines or other sectoral legislation, the stricter medicines regulatory regime should apply.

17.2 Regulatory Controls in the European Union

In the European Union, a medicinal product may only be placed on the market when the competent authority of a Member State for its own territory (national authorisation) has issued a marketing authorisation or when the European Commission (EC) has granted an authorisation for the entire Community (Community authorisation).

Subsequent to Directive 65/65/EEC (1965), Directive 75/318/EEC introduced the requirements relating to analytical, pharmacotoxicological and clinical standards and protocols in respect of the testing of proprietary medicinal products in order to establish their quality, safety and efficacy, while Directive 75/319/EEC established the Committee for Proprietary Medicinal Products ('old' CPMP) and introduced the multistate procedure (known now as the mutual recognition procedure). Directive 87/22/EEC introduced the concertation procedure (known now as the centralised procedure) relating to the placing on the market of high technology medicinal products, particularly those derived from biotechnology.

Since these original requirements, further stringent legislation and requirements have evolved in respect of investigations during the development of a drug, data necessary for its approval, its promotion and monitoring the safety of medicines during the post-marketing period (pharmacovigilance).

In order to enable the reader to appreciate better the development of regulatory controls in the European Union, we have referred to various Directives by their original citations in this chapter. However, these Directives have been frequently amended subsequent to their original adoption. In the interests of clarity and rationality, they were all assembled in a single text, namely Directive 2001/83/EC of 6 November 2001, codifying a whole range of the latest versions of these Directives. Therefore, the reader should also cross-refer to this Directive, which codifies the following:

1. Council Directive 65/65/EEC of 26 January 1965 on the approximation of provisions laid down by law, regulation or administrative action relating to medicinal products.

2. Council Directive 75/318/EEC of 20 May 1975 on the approximation of the laws of Member States relating to analytical, pharmacotoxicological and clinical standards and protocols in respect of the testing of proprietary medicinal products.

3. Council Directive 75/319/EEC of 20 May 1975 on the approximation of provisions laid down by law, regulation or administrative action relating to proprietary medicinal products.

4. Council Directive 89/342/EEC of 3 May 1989 on immunologicals (vaccines, toxins or serums and allergens).

5. Council Directive 89/343/EEC of 3 May 1989 on radiopharmaceuticals.

6. Council Directive 89/381/EEC of 14 June 1989 on products derived from human blood or human plasma.

7. Council Directive 92/25/EEC of 31 March 1992 on the wholesale distribution.

8. Council Directive 92/26/EEC of 31 March 1992 on classification for the supply.

9. Council Directive 92/27/EEC of 31 March 1992 on labelling and package leaflets.

10. Council Directive 92/28/EEC of 31 March 1992 on advertising.

11. Council Directive 92/73/EEC of 22 September 1992 on homeopathic medicinal products.

It may be helpful for the reader to appreciate that the highest legislative instrument in the European Union is a Regulation. It is directly applicable in all Member States and therefore, the consistency of the law throughout the EU territory is safeguarded with no discrepancies and has a full legal certainty. In contrast, the next lower level of legislative instrument is a Directive that is 'not directly applicable' and requires national implementation by transposition into national law. Discrepancies may arise during the process of national implementation. A guideline has no legal force and is not binding.

Directive 2001/83/EC was subsequently amended by (1) Directive 2002/98/EC of 27 January 2003, setting standards of quality and safety for the collection, testing, processing, storage and distribution of human blood and blood components, (2) Commission Directive 2003/63/EC of 25 June 2003, replacing Annex 1 of Directive 2001/83/EC (detailing scientific and technical requirements) with a new Annex (detailing scientific and technical requirements in CTD terms) and (3) Directive 2004/24/EC of 31 March 2004 as regards traditional herbal medicinal products.

As will be discussed later, following a comprehensive review of European pharmaceutical legislation, Directive 2001/83/EC was further amended extensively by Directive 2004/27/EC of the European Parliament and of the Council of 31 March 2004.

17.2.1 Committee for Proprietary Medicinal Products

The CPMP [now replaced by Committee for Medicinal Products for Human use (CHMP) – see Section 17.2.4 below] was the pharmaceutical advisory committee to the EC in respect of human medicinal products. It had an elected chairman and was constituted of two members from each Member State. This 'old' CPMP met for the first time on 26 November 1976. Its last meeting was on 13–14 December 1994. Article 1 of Council

Regulation EEC/2309/93 of 22 July 1993 established formally the European Medicines Evaluation Agency (EMEA) and article 5 re-established the CPMP established by Article 8 of Directive 75/319/EEC. This 'new' CPMP was responsible for formulating the opinion of the Agency on any question concerning the admissibility of the files submitted in accordance with the centralised procedure, the granting, variation, suspension or withdrawal of an authorisation to place a medicinal product for human use on the market arising in accordance with the provisions of this regulation, and pharmacovigilance. The 'new' CPMP met for the first time in January 1995 at which Professor Jean-Michel Alexandre elected as its first Chairman. It was also constituted of two members from each of the 15 Member States. On completion of his two terms in December 2000, Professor Alexandre retired and was succeeded in January 2001 by Dr Daniel Brasseur from Belgium. The last meeting of this 'new' CPMP took place on 20–22 April 2004 and the May 2004 meeting was postponed to 1–3 June 2004. Effective from 1 June 2004, the functions of the CPMP were transferred to CHMP (see below).

The EMEA, based in London since 1995, has the executive functions of a professional (administrative and scientific) Secretariat and works in very close liaison with the national authorities of the Member States. The EMEA includes the Committee for Orphan Medicinal Products (COMP – see below), the Committee for Medicinal Products for Veterinary Use (CVMP), the Committee for Herbal Medicinal Products (HMPC) and the CHMP and their various working parties. These are the Efficacy Working Party, Safety Working Party, Quality Working Party, Pharmacovigilance Working Party, Biotechnology Working Party, Blood and Plasma Products Working Party, Gene Therapy Working Party, Vaccine Working Party, Scientific Advice Working Party, Herbal Remedies Working Party (now a full statutory Committee, see Section 17.2.3) and Paediatric Working Party. Among the emerging technologies, pharmacogenetics is being rapidly integrated in the drug development in order to optimize this process. Therefore, in February 2005, the Ad Hoc Expert group on Pharmacogenetics was

converted into a formal Pharmacogenetics Working Party, in accordance with the implementation of the Title IV of Regulation (EC) No 726/2004 of the European Parliament and of the Council, to provide recommendations to the CHMP on all matters relating directly or indirectly to this discipline. Representatives on these working parties are nominated by the national authorities and represent either Member States or are chosen on the basis of expertise. The working parties are responsible for regularly producing a number of concept papers, points to consider documents and guidelines relevant to their scientific fields. Of late, the documents are no longer classified as 'Points to Consider' documents since their status was unclear. Following initial consultation with CPMP and subsequently with interested organisations, the final drafts are adopted by the CPMP for implementation. In addition, the CPMP also sets up when necessary special ad hoc groups of experts to deal with specific issues or scientific subjects of particular regulatory interest (for e.g. drug-induced QT interval prolongation or pharmacogenetics in drug development).

17.2.2 Committee for Orphan Medicinal Products

Following the success of the US orphan drug legislation passed in 1983, a number of countries introduced similar legislation (Japan in 1993 and Australia in 1998). Orphan diseases are those that are sufficiently rare that there are no commercial incentives to research these diseases and develop effective therapy. In 1999, the European Union also passed legislation relating to this important area of drug development. There are two primary pieces of orphan drug legislation in the European Union. The first is the Regulation (EC) No 141/2000 of the European Parliament and of the Council of 16 December 1999 on orphan medicinal products. This is concerned with the purpose, definitions, criteria for designation, establishing the COMP, procedures, provision of protocol assistance, access to centralised procedure without further justification for community marketing authorisation, market exclusivity and other incentives. The other is the Commission Regulation (EC) No 847/2000 of 27 April 2000 laying down the provisions for implementation of the criteria for designation and definitions of the concepts of 'similar medicinal product' and 'clinical superiority'. The COMP considers and gives opinions on the applications for designation of drugs as orphan drugs.

In order to encourage pharmaceutical companies to invest in orphan drug development, legislation provides for a number of incentives. These include application fee waiver (the extent of reduction varies with the region of the world, and in the European Union it is 50% for all fees since 2002), market exclusivity and protocol assistance. In the European Union, there is 100% reduction in the fee applicable to the provision of any scientific advice. The fund made available by the Community for fee exemptions for orphan medicinal products amounts to € 3 700 000 in 2005.

The period of market exclusivity is 10 years from authorisation of the product. In the context of market exclusivity in the European Union, a Member State must not accept another application for a marketing authorisation or grant a marketing authorisation or accept an application to extend an existing marketing authorisation for the same therapeutic indication in respect of a *similar medicinal product*. However, exclusivity may be lost by the first applicant consenting to a second application from another applicant, if the first is unable to meet demand, if a similar product is found to be *clinically superior*, if the criteria are no longer met or if, at the end of 5 years, a Member State can show that the product is (excessively) profitable.

COMP held its inaugural meeting in April 2000 and until May 2004, was constituted of a member from each Member State, three nominated by the EC to liase with CPMP and three from patient organisations, making a total of 21 representatives. As far as the authors know, it is at present the only advisory committee (associated with drug regulation) in the world with such direct patient representation. Following the accession of the 10 new Member States, the membership

has now increased to 31 members. In addition to these 31 members, the Committee also includes one member appointed by each of the European Economic Area-European Free Trade area (EEA-EFTA) states. The current Chairman is Professor Joseph Torrent-Farnell from Spain who is serving his second term. The COMP has access to the expertise of all the working parties setup by CPMP/CHMP and is highly proactive in promoting the development of orphan drugs and interacting with academia, industry and patient groups.

17.2.3 Committee for Herbal Medicinal Products

Herbal medicines of long tradition are in wide use in a number of Member States of the European Union. A significant number of these medicinal products, despite their long tradition, do not fulfill the requirements of a well-established medicinal use with recognised efficacy and an acceptable level of safety and are not eligible for a marketing authorisation. The long tradition of these medicinal products makes it possible to reduce the need for clinical trials, in so far as the efficacy of the medicinal product is plausible on the basis of long-standing use and experience. Preclinical tests do not seem necessary, where the medicinal product on the basis of the information on its traditional use proves not to be harmful in specified conditions of use. However, even a long tradition does not exclude the possibility that there may be concerns with regard to the product's safety, and therefore the competent authorities should be entitled to ask for all data necessary for assessing the safety. The quality aspect of the medicinal product is independent of its traditional use so that no derogation is made with regard to the necessary physico-chemical, biological and microbiological tests. These products should comply with quality standards in relevant European Pharmacopoeia monographs or those in the pharmacopoeia of a Member State.

A herbal medicinal product is defined as any medicinal product, exclusively containing as active ingredients one or more herbal substances or one or more herbal preparations, or one or more such herbal substances in combination with one or more such herbal preparations.

Herbal substances are defined as all mainly whole, fragmented or cut plants, plant parts, algae, fungi, lichen in an unprocessed, usually dried form, but sometimes fresh. Certain exudates that have not been subjected to a specific treatment are also considered to be herbal substances. Herbal substances are precisely defined by the plant part used and the botanical name according to the binomial system (genus, species, variety and author).

Herbal preparations are defined as preparations obtained by subjecting herbal substances to treatments such as extraction, distillation, expression, fractionation, purification, concentration or fermentation. These include comminuted or powdered herbal substances, tinctures, extracts, essential oils, expressed juices and processed exudates.

To maintain these products on the market, the Member States had enacted differing procedures and provisions. These differences might hinder trade in traditional medicinal products within the Community and lead to discrimination and distortion of competition between manufacturers of these products. They might also have an impact on the protection of public health since the necessary guarantees of quality, safety and efficacy are not always provided at present. Having regard to the particular characteristics of these medicinal products, especially their long tradition, it was therefore desirable to provide a special, simplified registration procedure for certain traditional medicinal products.

Starting as an *Ad Hoc* Working Group on Herbal Medicinal Products in May 1997, there evolved a Herbal Medicinal Products Working Party (HMPWP) which had been operational as regards traditional herbal medicinal products until August 2004. However, Article 16h of Directive 2004/24/EC of 31 March 2004 formally established the Committee for Herbal Medicinal Products (HMPC).

Each Member State appoints, for a 3-year term which may be renewed, one member and one alternate to this Committee. These members and alternates are chosen for their role and experience in the evaluation of herbal medicinal products and represent the competent national authorities.

The Committee may also coopt a maximum of five additional members chosen on the basis of their specific scientific competence. These members are appointed for a term of 3 years, which may be renewed, and do not have alternates. The inaugural meeting of the HMPC took place on 23–24 September 2004 and the current Chairman is Dr Konstantin Keller from Germany.

Article 16a provides for a simplified registration procedure for herbal medicinal products which fulfill all of the following criteria:

1. They have indications exclusively appropriate to traditional herbal medicinal products which, by virtue of their composition and purpose, are intended and designed for use without the supervision of a medical practitioner for diagnostic purposes or for prescription or monitoring of treatment.
2. They are exclusively for administration in accordance with a specified strength and posology.
3. They are an oral, external and/or inhalation preparation.
4. The period of traditional use for the medicinal product in question, or a corresponding product in medicinal use throughout is a period of at least 30 years preceding the date of the application, including at least 15 years use within the community.
5. The data on the traditional use of the medicinal product are sufficient; in particular the product proves not to be harmful in the specified conditions of use and the pharmacological effects or efficacy of the medicinal product are plausible on the basis of long-standing use and experience.

However, this simplified procedure should be used only where no marketing authorisation can be obtained through procedures for typical medicinal products. In order to promote harmonisation, Member States are expected to recognise registrations of traditional herbal medicinal products granted by another Member State based on community herbal monographs or consisting of substances, preparations or combinations thereof contained in a list to be established. The simplified registration should be acceptable only where the herbal medicinal product may rely on a sufficiently long medicinal use in the community. Medicinal use outside the community should be taken into account only if the medicinal product has been used within the community for a certain time. Where there is limited evidence of use within the community, it is necessary to assess carefully the validity and relevance of use outside the community.

The HMPC is expected to establish community herbal monographs for herbal medicinal products. These herbal remedies have their product particulars and literature. Apart from other controls, any advertisement for a medicinal product registered is required to contain the following statement: 'Traditional herbal medicinal product for use in specified indication(s) exclusively based upon long-standing use.'

The Member States are required to take the necessary measures to comply with this Directive by 30 October 2005.

17.2.4 Review 2001 and Committee for Medicinal Products for Human Use

Effective from June 2004, the CHMP replaced the CPMP. The membership of the CPMP/CHMP has been established so that it is a technically expert committee that advises the EC.

Regarding all activities for the regulation of pharmaceuticals at the EU level, Article 71 of Regulation EEC/2309/93 that established the EMEA and the CPMP required that 'Within 6 years of the entry into force of this Regulation, the Commission shall publish a general report on the experience of the procedures laid down in this Regulation, in Chapter III of Directive 75/319/EEC and in Chapter IV of Directive 81/851/EEC'. The tender for review was awarded to a consortium of Cameron McKenna and Arthur Anderson. The full report from Cameron McKenna, dated October 2000 and entitled 'Evaluation of the Operation of Community Procedures for the Authorisation of

Medicinal Products', is a comprehensive and highly constructive document that made a large number of recommendations for reform.

Following extensive discussions among all interested parties, such as the national authorities, the EC and the European Federation of Pharmaceutical Industries and Associations (EFPIA), the EC proposed comprehensive reform of the EU pharmaceutical legislation. The amending legislations are:

1. Directive 2004/27/EC of the European Parliament and of the Council of 31 March 2004, amending Directive 2001/83/EC, on the Community code relating to medicinal products for human use and
2. Regulation (EC) No 726/2004 of the European Parliament and of the Council of 31 March 2004, laying down Community procedures for the authorisation and supervision of medicinal products for human and veterinary use and establishing a European Medicines Agency – thus replacing Regulation EEC/2309/93.

Directive 2004/27/EC must come into force in all Member States by 30 October 2005, although Member States are able to transpose and implement early any of the provisions should they wish. Regulation 726/2004 has an implementation date of May 2004 for part of it and final date of 20 November 2005, from when all provisions will apply in all Member States.

The adoption of these legislative reforms just preceded the enlargement of the European Union on 1 May 2004 when the EU membership was increased to 25 Member States by the accession of 10 new Member States, namely Cyprus, Czech Republic, Estonia, Hungary, Latvia, Lithuania, Malta, Poland, Slovak Republic and Slovenia.

Article 55 of Regulation (EC) No 726/2004 created the European Medicines Agency, comprising of a Management Board, an Executive Director, a Secretariat, the CHMP, the CVMP, the COMP and the HMPC. Thus, the former EMEA became the European Medicines Agency. However, for technical reasons, it had to retain the acronym EMEA (the acronym EMA belongs to European Medical Association). The Agency may give a scientific opinion, in the context of cooperation with the World Health Organisation, for the evaluation of certain medicinal products for human use intended exclusively for markets outside the community.

Article 5 of Regulation (EC) No 726/2004 created the CHMP, which is responsible for drawing up the opinion of the Agency on any matter concerning the admissibility of the files submitted in accordance with the centralised procedure, the granting, variation, suspension or revocation of an authorisation to place a medicinal product for human use on the market and pharmacovigilance. The CPMP therefore became the CHMP and consists of one member and one alternate appointed by each of the EU Member States, after consultation of the Management Board, for a term of 3 years, which may be renewed, and a chairperson. The alternates represent and may vote for the members in their absence and can also act as rapporteurs in their own right. In addition, the CHMP also includes one member and one alternate appointed by each of the EEA-EFTA States, for a term of 3 years, which may be renewed. The members appointed by the EEA-EFTA States may not be elected Chairperson or Vice-Chairperson of the Committee and may not vote but their positions shall be stated separately in the opinion, where relevant, in the minutes of the Committee and in case of divergent opinions appended to the Committee's opinion. Their position is not counted in reaching the Committee's opinion. However, they may act as rapporteurs. Indeed, Norway and Iceland have been represented at the CPMP since January 2000. Although Liechtenstein is entitled to participate, it more frequently than not adopts the decisions made by Swissmedic – the Swiss Agency for Therapeutic Products. As permitted by the Regulation, the Committee, in order to complement its expertise, has appointed five coopted members chosen on the basis of their specific scientific competence, among the experts nominated by Members States or the Agency. Coopted members are appointed for the term of the committee, which may be renewed, and do not have alternates. The Chairman of CPMP, Dr Daniel Brasseur was elected the Chairman of CHMP during its inaugural meeting on 1–3 June 2004. Each national competent authority shall monitor the level and independence of the evaluation carried out and facilitate the activities of nominated members and experts. Members States shall refrain from giving Committee members and experts any instruction that is incompatible with their own individual tasks or with the tasks and responsibilities of the Agency. The quorum required for the adoption of scientific opinions or recommendations by the Committee is reached when two thirds of the total members of the Committee eligible to vote are present. A scientific opinion or recommendation is adopted if supported by an absolute majority of the members of the Committee (i.e. favourable votes by at least half of the total number of Committee members eligible to vote plus one, that is 16).

The CHMP has three levels of expertise available to it. These are (1) individual experts consulted by the rapporteur/co-rapporteur or coordinators within the framework of centralised applications, referral and scientific advice, (2) ad hoc groups such as that on QT interval and (3) scientific advisory groups (SAGs). Three SAGs have already been set up – oncology, anti-infectives and diagnostics. The next series of SAGs will be established for HIV/viral diseases, diabetes and central nervous system diseases. The SAGs could be consulted on centralised applications, scientific advice and protocol assistance, referrals, guidelines or any other scientific issues at the request of CHMP.

The details of the reform and the large number of legislative changes introduced in relation to medicines for human use are beyond the scope of this chapter. However, the key objectives of the review of EU medicines legislation and reform of the regulatory regime can be summarised as follows:

1. To guarantee a high level of health protection for EU citizens, in particular, by making safe, innovative products available to patients as quickly as possible.
2. To guarantee tighter surveillance of the market, in particular by strengthening pharmacovigilance procedures.

3. To complete the internal market for pharmaceuticals while taking globalisation into account.

4. To set up a legal framework that fosters the competitiveness of the European pharmaceutical industry.

5. To take the opportunity to rationalise and, if possible, simplify the regulatory system, thereby improving its consistency, profile and transparency.

6. To take the opportunity to prepare the regulatory system for enlargement of the European Union.

The changes to the legislation are intended to strengthen the protection of public health of EU citizens through the effective regulation of medicines for human use while improving the competitiveness of the EU pharmaceutical industry. The following measures have been adopted to provide the greatest public health benefits:

1. More effective market surveillance of medicinal products on the markets by:

   a. The introduction of a more robust and integrated approach to pharmacovigilance (by sharing safety data between Member States and a common approach to the collection, verification and presentation of information on adverse drug reactions).

   b. Increased frequency of periodic safety update reports (PSUR).

   c. The extension of good manufacturing practice to new areas, such as active pharmaceutical ingredients (APIs).

   d. The introduction of the ability of the competent authorities to carry out unannounced inspections by the competent authority of manufacturers of APIs.

2. Effective provision of appropriate high-quality information to patients by:

   a. Reordering the information to be included in the Summary of Product Characteristics (SPC), a key document for marketing a medicinal product in the European Union.

   b. Introducing requirements for Marketing Authorisation Holders (MAH) to include the name of the medicinal product in Braille on the outer packaging, and make the package leaflet available on request from patients' organisations in formats appropriate for blind and partially sighted people.

   c. The publication of Assessment Reports.

3. Increasing the attractiveness of the EU pharmaceutical market by:

   a. More effective and timely procedures for assessing marketing authorisation applications by refining the mutual recognition procedure to take into account lessons learned since its introduction and the introduction of an alternative decentralised procedure.

   b. Increasing the competitiveness of the EU regulatory regime by harmonising data and market exclusivity periods across the community at 8 and 10 years respectively, with the possibility of an extension to 11 years if certain criteria of innovation are met.

   c. The introduction of legislative definitions of 'generic' and 'reference' medicinal products, which will bring greater clarity and certainty in operating the rules for both the innovative and generics sectors of industry.

   d. The introduction of a provision to allow the development of generic copies of medicinal products and other products without infringing patent protection.

   e. Deregulatory measures, such as changes to the requirement that a marketing authorisation has to be renewed every 5 years, complemented by increasing the frequency of PSURs, which is a less bureaucratic and more safety focused means of ensuring public health protection.

Some of the key features of the Directive 2004/27/EC are summarised below.

Apart from changing the definition of a medicinal product, the definition of 'risks related to use of the medicinal product' has also been changed. The definition now has four components – in addition to the current definition which defines risk to public health in terms of the quality, safety and efficacy of the product, the revised legislation requires an assessment of any undesirable effects on the environment from use of the product.

Under Article 26, the grounds for refusing a marketing authorisation have been amended under the review. The new provision allows a refusal if the risk–benefit balance of the product is not favourable, if the therapeutic efficacy is insufficiently substantiated, or if its qualitative and quantitative composition is not as declared. The application may also be refused if the documents are not submitted in accordance with the requirements set out in the Directive. The MA holder/applicant is responsible for the accuracy of the data and documentation submitted. The unfavourable risk–benefit balance is the additional ground for refusal, although in practice this has previously been applied.

Article 1(28)a of Directive 2004/27/EC defines the risk–benefit balance as an evaluation of the positive therapeutic effects of the product in relation to the risks to patients' or public health. The environmental component of the definition of risks is excluded from the risk–benefit balance. Under the new legislation, the risk–benefit balance is considered as part of Article 23 (which enables the competent authority to continuously assess the risk–benefit balance by requesting relevant data from MAH), and Article 104 (relating to the submission by MAH of PSURs).

The new Regulation allows Member States to supply, on 'compassionate use' grounds to certain groups of patients, unauthorised human medicinal products that are required to use the centralised procedure. This will allow patient access to certain unauthorised products, provided there are adequate public health and safety grounds. In addition, for centrally authorised products, a new provision will be introduced that allows the conditional authorisation of medicinal products in defined circumstances, provided there are justified reasons (such as the products of public health interest). The conditions under which the authorisation is made would be reassessed on an annual basis. The EC has also agreed to establish the circumstances in which small and medium-sized companies may pay reduced fees, defer payment of fees or receive administrative assistance.

Article 126a allows a Member State to authorise on public health grounds the marketing of a product on its territory even if the MAH has not made an application for an authorisation to that competent authority. It requires, nonetheless, that the authorising Member State ensures that the following requirements of the legislation can still be met: titles V (leaflets and labels), VI (classification), VIII (advertising), IX (pharmacovigilance) and XI (supervision and sanctions).

Generic versions of centrally approved reference medicinal products may use the centralised procedure (for definitions of these products, see Section 17.8.3). To harmonise data protection, the revised legislation provides for 10 years' *market* exclusivity following initial authorisation for innovative products authorised under Articles 6 and 8 of the amending Directive. Second applicants for generic product authorisations based on abridged dossiers may submit applications no earlier than 8 years (the *data* exclusivity period) from the date of initial authorisation of the innovative reference product and obtain a marketing authorisation. However, they may not place their products on the market until the 10-year period has elapsed. The 10-year period of market exclusivity for innovative products may be extended to a maximum of 11 years if, during the first 8 years from the date of initial authorisation, the MAH obtains an authorisation for one or more new therapeutic indications which are deemed to bring a significant clinical benefit in comparison with existing therapies. Presumably, significant clinical benefit would be expected to include new indications and/or new categories of patients. It is anticipated that whether a new indication represents a significant clinical benefit and hence whether the product qualifies for an additional year of market exclusivity, will be evaluated as part of the product assessment and will be included in the assessment report. Where these reports are shared with EMEA and other Member States for purposes of centralised, decentralised or mutual recognition procedures for authorisation, there will be an opportunity for the Member States to establish an agreement on the significance, or otherwise of the new indication.

There is a reordering of the information to be included in the SPC. With regard to generic medicines, the final paragraph of Article 11 states that for authorisations under Article 10, those parts of the SPC of the reference product referring to indications or dosage forms that are still covered by patent law at the time when a generic medicine is marketed need not be included. This provision will allow the authorisation of generic products with indications that vary between Member States to take account of usage patents in force on the innovative product in certain Member States. Under the current rules, some Member States would only accept an authorisation of the generic with those indications that did not have a usage patent anywhere in the European Union. The United Kingdom takes the view that while it may be acceptable to omit reference to certain indications and dosage forms it may not be permissible to omit associated warnings or contraindications where those are important for the protection of public health. Therefore the extent of modifications possible for a particular generic product SPC will be judged on a case-by-case basis.

Articles 21(3) and 21(4) oblige the competent authorities to make publicly available without delay the marketing authorisation, SPC, Assessment Report and reasons for the opinion after deletion of commercially confidential information.

The provisions of Article 23(a) require the MAH to inform the competent authority about various activities associated with the availability of the product on the market. Under Article 24 of the revised legislation only a single renewal is required when the product has been authorised for 5 years. A second renewal may take place after a further 5 years if there are justified pharmacovigilance grounds. In addition, any authorisation, which is not followed by placing the product on the market within 3 years (or which is not present on the market for 3 years), shall cease to be valid. Member States may grant exemptions from the 3-year rule, if justified on public health grounds.

Article 102 includes a provision that requires Member States to share information collected through their pharmacovigilance system with other Member States and the EMEA. The central database 'EudraVigilance' has been developed to allow Member States and the EMEA to share information on adverse drug reactions once all Member States have populated it.

The text of Article 104–107 includes a new requirement for the MAH to submit adverse drug reactions data in electronic format except in exceptional circumstances. The text also increases the frequency of PSURs by increasing the frequency of reporting from the fifth year. After authorisation, a MAH will be required to submit PSURs on request by the competent authority, but at least every 6-monthly from date of the authorisation until the product is marketed, then 6-monthly for 2 years after marketing, yearly for the following 2 years then 3-yearly. The increased frequency of PSURs links with the changes to the renewals procedure and will ensure regular examination of safety issues, undertaken in a coordinated manner across the European Union.

Where, as a result of the evaluation of pharmacovigilance data, a Member State considers that a marketing authorisation should be suspended, revoked or varied in accordance with the guidelines referred to in Article 106(1), it shall forthwith inform the Agency, the other Member States and the MAH. Where urgent action to protect public health is necessary, the Member State concerned may suspend the marketing authorisation of a medicinal product, provided that the Agency, the EC and the other Member States are informed no later than the following working day.

In February 2005, the EC issued a draft consultation regulation for laying down the procedure to adopt the maximum amounts and the conditions and methods for collection of financial penalties imposed by the EC under Regulation No (EC) 726/2004. The scope of this Regulation is wide and includes (but not restricted to) pharmacovigilance and market surveillance, in accordance with chapter 3 of Title II, chapter 3 of Title III of Regulation (EC) No 726/2004 and any other provisions adopted pursuant to them and with Article 9(1) of Regulation (EC) 1085/2003.

17.3 Procedures for Clinical Trials

Since the implementation of the EU Directive 2001/20/EEC on clinical trials in the United Kingdom on 1 May 2004, all clinical trials now require a Clinical Trial Authorisation (CTA). Prior to this, a different system of controls operated in the United Kingdom.

17.3.1 Previous control of clinical trials in the United Kingdom

The primary legislation regarding the clinical trials in the United Kingdom was the Medicines Act 1968, which included the definition of a clinical trial and of a medicinal product. Clinical studies involving healthy volunteers did not meet this definition of a clinical trial and, as a result, did not come under the remit of the Medicines Act 1968 or Medicines and Healthcare products Regulatory Agency (previously known as Medicines Control Agency). Such studies were subject to self-regulation by the pharmaceutical industry. However, the legislative basis and the procedures involved in initiating clinical trials in the United Kingdom changed following the introduction of the EU Clinical Trials Directive (see Section 17.3.2) relating to the implementation of good clinical practice in the conduct of clinical trials on medicinal products for human use.

Prior to the introduction of EU Clinical Trials Directive, there were four ways of seeking approval for the commencement of clinical trials in the United Kingdom. These were by means of a Clinical Trial Certificate (CTC), a Clinical Trial Exemption (CTX), a Doctor's and Dentist's Exemption (DDX) or as a Clinical Trial on a Marketed Product (CTMP). Each required provision of a detailed protocol of the proposed trial.

17.3.1.1 Clinical trial certificate
A CTC was granted for a period of 2 years and may be renewed. Variations to the certificate were possible. The applicant for a CTC was required to provide full information on the quality and safety of the product to be used in the trial along with any early evidence of efficacy. This information was provided under the same headings as a marketing authorisation application and, thus, consisted of data on the chemical or biological/biotechnological and pharmaceutical aspects of the drug substance and drug product

(Part II), preclinical data on the pharmacodynamics, pharmacokinetics, safety pharmacology and toxicology of the material (Part III), and any clinical data already generated (Part IV).

The full data package was submitted and assessed by assessors from each of the three disciplines. The Committee on Safety of Medicines and its sub-committees then considered their assessment report. If the decision was positive then a certificate was issued. If the decision was negative, then the applicant had the same appeal rights as those that apply to a marketing authorisation application (see Section 17.8.1).

The disadvantage of the CTC approach was that it could be slow. There were no statutory timelines for the process. As a result, most applicants used the CTX scheme. A CTC was, however, required for any proposed trials involving xenotransplantation.

17.3.1.2 Clinical trial exemption
This was an exemption from the need to hold a CTC and this scheme had been available since 1981. It was introduced in an attempt to avoid delay to medical research and had the advantage of statutory timelines. Summary data, under the same headings as for a CTC, were submitted and were assessed by assessors from each of the three disciplines on behalf of the Licensing Authority. If the Exemption was granted, it was valid for a period of 3 years. If it was refused then the applicant could submit a revised application, taking account of the reasons for refusal, which were always on safety grounds. This process could be repeated as often as was required until an Exemption could be granted. In the event of a refusal, the applicant also had the option of applying for a CTC.

The advantage of the CTX scheme was its speed, since a decision had to be made by the Licensing Authority within 35 days with the possibility of one 28-day extension to this period. The maximum time for determination of a CTX application was therefore 63 days.

17.3.1.3 Doctor's and Dentist's Exemption
This was an exemption, which was available to doctors or dentists who were undertaking clinical

trials initiated by them and not at the request of a pharmaceutical company. Outline information about the trial was required and a decision was made within 21 days. Where the product to be used was unlicensed and was complex, further information might be requested and the 21-day time period might be extended.

17.3.1.4 Clinical trials on marketed products

Where a clinical trial was proposed with a marketed product then the CTMP scheme could be used. This was a streamlined process based on the fact that there were no quality issues with a product that had already been granted a marketing authorisation. The applicant submitted a copy of the trial protocol, provided information on the investigators and, depending on whether or not the applicant was the MAH, information on the procedures for reporting adverse drug reactions. It was only possible to use this procedure for UK marketed products. It did not apply to unauthorised products manufactured specifically for trial or to products, which were licensed only in countries other than the United Kingdom.

17.3.2 Current control of clinical trials in the United Kingdom and throughout the European Union

With a view to harmonising the conduct of clinical trials across the European Union, Directive 2001/20/EEC was finally agreed on 14 December 2000 and was formally adopted in May 2001 with a 3-year transition period for its implementation. The Directive is now fully implemented in the United Kingdom and further information on clinical trials in the UK can be accessed at the MHRA website (see end of this chapter). As stated earlier, all clinical trials now require a CTA.

The EU Clinical Trials Directive contains specific provisions regarding the conduct of clinical trials, including multicentre trials, on human subjects. It sets standards relating to the implementation of good clinical practice and good manufacturing practice, with a view to protecting clinical trial subjects. All clinical trials, including

bioavailability and bioequivalence studies, must be designed, conducted, and reported in accordance with the principles of good clinical practice. It proposes the introduction of procedures in the community that will provide an environment where new medicines can be developed safely and rapidly. The Directive is very detailed and comprehensive in terms of clarifying ethical and scientific standards.

It defines 'clinical trial' as any investigation in human subjects (including healthy volunteer studies that were previously exempt from the UK legislation) intended to discover or verify the clinical, pharmacological and/or other pharmacodynamic effects of one or more investigational medicinal product(s), and/or to identify any adverse reactions to one or more investigational medicinal product(s), and/or to study absorption, distribution, metabolism and excretion of one or more investigational medicinal product(s) with the object of ascertaining its (their) safety and/or efficacy, and defines 'subject' as an individual who participates in a clinical trial as either a recipient of the investigational medicinal product or a control. Thus, healthy volunteer studies are included.

If the competent authority of the Member State notifies the sponsor of grounds for non-acceptance, the sponsor may, on one occasion only, amend the content of the request to take due account of the grounds given. There are specific measures before the commencement and end or early termination of a clinical trial, including a time limit not exceeding 60 days for Member States to consider a valid request. No further extension to this period is permissible except in the case of trials involving medicinal products for gene therapy or somatic cell therapy or medicinal products containing genetically modified organisms for which an extension of a maximum 30 days is permitted. For these products, this 90-day period may be extended by a further 90 days under certain circumstances. In the case of xenogenic cell therapy no time limit to the authorisation period is allowable. It is important to note that 'The Member States may lay down a shorter period than 60 days within their area of responsibility if that is in compliance with current practice', and that 'The competent authority can nevertheless notify the sponsor before the end of this period that it has no grounds for non-acceptance.'

The Directive contains detailed articles on the conduct of a clinical trial, exchange of information between Member States, EMEA, and the EC, the reasons and procedures for suspension of the trial by a Member State, and notification of adverse events, including serious adverse reactions.

The Directive lays down specific obligations for the Member States. As required by the Directive, EC in consultation with the Member States was required to issue guidance in consultation with the Member States before the Directive can be implemented in all Member States by 1 May 2004. In April 2003, the EC issued a detailed guidance on several aspects including (1) the application format and documentation to be submitted in an application for an Ethics Committee opinion on the clinical trial on medicinal products for human use, (2) the European clinical trials database (EUDRACT Database) and (3) European database of suspected unexpected serious adverse reactions in clinical trials. In April 2004, the EC also issued a detailed guidance for the request for authorisation of a clinical trial on a medicinal product for human use to the competent authorities, notification of substantial amendments and declaration of the end of the trial. Recently, the EC adopted Directive 2005/28/EC of 8 April 2005 laying down principles and detailed guidelines for good clinical practice as regards investigational medicinal products for human use, as well as the requirements for authorisation of the manufacturing or importation of such products. Also released for consultation is a guideline (185401/2004) on the requirements for the chemical and pharmaceutical quality documentation concerning investigational medicinal products in clinical trials (ICH).

Most of the procedures and criteria contained in the Directive were already part of the UK clinical trials practice under the Medicines Act, 1968. Nevertheless, the legislative basis and the procedures involved in initiating clinical trials in the United Kingdom changed following the implementation of the EU Directive on clinical trials.

This clinical trial Directive was among the most contentious to be implemented and much has been written on its merits, demerits and effect on pharmaceutical research (for example, see References 1–7).

17.4 Applications for Marketing Authorisations in the European Union

17.4.1 Legislation and guidance notes

As stated earlier, Council Directive 65/65/EEC, referred to earlier, was the first Directive on pharmaceuticals. It had been frequently amended and other Directives had extended the scope of legislation for authorising medicines and introducing new procedures.

Needless to add that the key legislative pieces at present are (1) Directive 2004/27/EC of the European Parliament and of the Council of 31 March 2004, amending Directive 2001/83/EC, on the Community code relating to medicinal products for human use and (2) Regulation (EC) No 726/2004 of the European Parliament and of the Council of 31 March 2004, laying down Community procedures for the authorisation and supervision of medicinal products for human and veterinary use and establishing a European Medicines Agency and replacing Regulation EEC/2309/93.

For human medicinal products, the relevant legislation is presented in Volume 1 of *The Rules Governing Medicinal Products in the European Union*, published by the European Commission. Volume 2 comprises the *Notice to Applicants for Marketing Authorisations for Medicinal Products for Human Use in the European Union*. Procedures for marketing authorisations are described in Volume 2A, the presentation and the content of the dossier are described in Volume 2B, and various regulatory guidelines in Volume 2C. Volume 3 gives guidance notes for medicinal products for human use, Volume 4 relates to good manufacturing practice, and Volume 9 is concerned with pharmacovigilance (both for human and veterinary use). The remaining volumes (5–8) are concerned with veterinary medicinal products.

The reader may be interested to know that it is possible to create one's own CD with the whole pharmaceutical legislation (human and veterinary) and an integrated search engine. The CD is similar to the EudraLex section of the web site, but clearly has the advantage of off-line use. All the documents are in PDF format and without protection.

Guidance notes produced by the CPMP through its working parties or its membership of the International Conference on Harmonisation (ICH) are compiled in Volumes 3A (quality and biotechnology), 3B (pharmacotoxicological) and 3C (clinical) and are now on-line on the EMEA website. These guidelines have been prepared by experts, have undergone input from academia and the industry during consultation, and have been adopted only thereafter. None of these guidelines is legally binding and they are intended to be sufficiently flexible so as not to impede scientific progress in drug development. However, where an applicant chooses not to follow a guideline, the decision must be explained and justified in the dossier.

17.4.2 Format of the dossier

The basic requirements for the contents of the dossier of information accompanying the application for a marketing authorisation are the same whether it is submitted nationally or centrally and were laid out in detail in Directive 715/318/EEC and its subsequent amendments. These requirements were included as Annex 1 of the codified Directive 2001/83/EC.

Subsequently, following agreement on Common Technical Document (CTD) format for the dossier, Commission Directive 2003/63/EC of 25 June 2003, replaced Annex 1 of Directive 2001/83/EC (detailing scientific and technical requirements) with a new Annex (detailing scientific and technical requirements in CTD terms). Provisions are made in the legislation for the omission of data in certain circumstances where information is already available to the regulatory authorities from other sources, for example,

in the case of applications for line extensions to existing products or for generic drugs. Applications that do not include a full dossier of information are referred to as 'abridged applications'. The complex legal basis for the different types of generic or abridged applications for marketing authorisations will not be considered further in this chapter.

17.4.2.1 Previous format of the dossier

Directive 75/318/EEC required that the dossier be presented in four highly structured parts: Parts I, II, III, and IV. Directive 83/570/EEC was the amending Directive, which introduced the requirements for a draft SPC to be produced by the applicant. Volume 2B of *The Rules Governing Medicinal Products in the European Union* gave a detailed breakdown of the structure of a European regulatory dossier. This format was accepted until the end of June 2003 when a new format known as the Common Technical Document (CTD) became mandatory (see later).

An application for a marketing authorisation must be accompanied, among other items, by specified pharmaceutical, preclinical and clinical particulars and documents (the 'dossier'). Three important summary documents in the dossier are the SPC, a Package or Patient Information Leaflet (PIL), and the sales presentation of the product (label). The SPC has a formally prescribed structure (Box 17.1), and forms the basis for *authorised* clinical prescribing of the medicinal product concerned.

Part I was a summary of the information presented in the whole dossier and included the application forms and administrative particulars on fees, various declarations and the type of application as well as particulars of the marketing authorisation (IA), proposed SPC (IB1), proposals for packaging, labels and package or patient information leaflets (IB2), and any SPCs already approved in the Member State(s) for the particular product (IB3). Also included were separate Expert Reports on chemical and pharmaceutical (IC1), pharmacotoxicological (preclinical) (IC2), and clinical documentations (IC3), as required under Directive 75/319/EEC. These Expert Reports were the summaries of the dossier with a critical appraisal of the data presented by an expert on behalf of the applicant. Detailed regulatory guidance, supported by various Directives, is available on the content of each of these documents.

Part II related to the quality of the product and gave details of its chemical, pharmaceutical and biological testing. In cases where the active ingredient was made by a manufacturer other than the applicant or product manufacturer, some of the information required in Part II might be presented in a separate file, the Drug Master File, to maintain the confidential nature of the synthetic process. Part III described the pharmacotoxicological tests conducted with the drug in animals (preclinical tests). Part IV described the clinical documentation. The details of requirements for these four parts are annexed to Directive 2001/83/EC. This Directive is a very important document since it codifies into a single document a number of previous Directives that have been amended frequently.

Regardless of the format in which the dossier is submitted, pharmaceutical data should be provided in respect of qualitative and quantitative particulars of the constituents, description of the method of preparation, control of starting materials, control tests on intermediate products, control tests on the finished product and stability tests. In cases where the active ingredient is made by a manufacturer other than the applicant or the product manufacturer, some of the information may be presented in a separate file, the Drug Master File, to maintain the confidential nature of the synthetic process. Pharmacotoxicological data should include pharmacology, safety pharmacology, pharmacokinetics, single- and repeat-dose toxicological evaluation, reproductive function, fertility, embryofoetal and perinatal toxicity, mutagenic potential and data on carcinogenicity. The clinical data are divided into detailed clinical pharmacology of the medicinal product and the clinical experience. Clinical pharmacology data should provide characterisation of the pharmacodynamics and the pharmacokinetics of the drug. It is not only the primary pharmacology (responsible for the therapeutic effect of the drug) but also its secondary pharmacology (responsible for unwanted effects) that needs to be investigated. Pharmacokinetics requires full characterisation, with all the aspects that embody the term in its broadest sense, together with data on the effects of age, gender, renal or hepatic dysfunction and food.

Genetic factors are assuming greater importance and information should be provided on the effect of genetic factors on the pharmacology of a drug and the ethnic structure of the trial population.

Arising from pharmacokinetic studies there should be a detailed and well-designed programme of drug interaction studies. It is important that the dose schedule is scientifically supported by the pharmacokinetics and pharmacodynamics of the drug. Equally critical are the considerations of the time to steady state and whether the pharmacodynamic effects lag behind changes in plasma concentrations. An ideal dose-ranging studies programme should provide definitive information on the risk/benefit of a range of doses and dosage regimens.

Each study in the clinical dossier, whether clinical pharmacology or clinical experience, should be presented in a structured manner to include a summary, study objectives, detailed study design (including doses selected, duration, planned number of patients, all efficacy variables, assessment time-points and statistical methods), results, conclusion and bibliography if necessary. The safety database (both clinical and laboratory but dealt with separately) should be presented overall and by subpopulation exposed in terms of dose, duration, age, gender and special populations, such as those with hepatic dysfunction or renal impairment. Safety data should also include any post-marketing experience from countries (EU and non-EU) where the product is already approved and on the market. Information should be provided on the intensity and outcomes of these effects. To put these data in their perspective, data should be included on the estimated patient exposure. Every attempt should be made to obtain details of the patients withdrawn from studies, serious adverse events, and those that resulted in deaths. Expert reports required are not a promotion platform for the product but an assessment of the data generated, an explanation of the results and an interpretation. Reports should also make clear whether or not the preclinical studies submitted have been conducted according to good laboratory practice, and whether the clinical studies have been conducted according to good clinical practice

principles and in accord with the Declaration of Helsinki.

17.4.2.2   CTD – *the current standard*

Following agreement at the ICH meeting in November 2000, the format of the EU dossier described above changed to conform to the new format known as the 'Common Technical Document'. This new format (CTD) is common to all the three major regions of drug regulation (European Union, United States and Japan) and most of the other major non-ICH authorities have also agreed to accept the dossier in CTD format. Information on the CTD 'Presentation and format of the dossier CTD' can be accessed from the EC website (see end of this chapter). This document also shows the correspondence of the previous format with the CTD format. It is important to appreciate that introduction of CTD has not resulted in a change in the qualitative or quantitative nature of data required – only the format in which these data are presented has changed. Even applications for line extensions must be submitted using the new EU-CTD format. However, references can be made to already assessed and authorised 'old' parts of the dossier, but only if no new additional data are submitted in these parts. In such cases, it is not necessary to reformat already assessed and authorised 'old' documentation.

CTD consists of four modules, preceded by a Module 1 that is region-specific and includes administrative and prescribing information. Module 2 comprises of CTD summaries and overviews of the quality, non-clinical and clinical data, Module 3 contains data on quality, Module 4 consists of the non-clinical study reports and Module 5 comprises the clinical study reports. There are guidelines on the details to be included in each module and these are summarised in Box 17.2. The non-clinical and clinical overviews and summaries are equivalent to the previous Expert Reports submitted under sections IC2 and IC3 respectively of part I, data.

The objectives behind the CTD are to reduce the time and resources needed to compile applications, to facilitate electronic submissions,

Box 17.2   Summary of the contents of the modules of the CTD
Module 1 EU-specific requirements

1.1 Module 1 Comprehensive table of contents (Module 1–5)
1.2 Application form
1.3 Product literature
  1.3.1 Summary of product characteristics (SPC)
  1.3.2 Labelling
  1.3.3 Package leaflet
  1.3.4 Mock-ups and specimen
  1.3.5 SPCs already approved in the Member States
1.4 Information about experts
1.5 Specific requirements for different types of applications Annex: Environmental risk assessment

Module 2 CTD Summaries

2.1 CTD table of contents (Module 2-5)
2.2 CTD introduction
2.3 Quality overall summary
2.4 Nonclinical overview
2.5 Clinical overview
2.6 Nonclinical written and tabulated summary
  Pharmacology
  Pharmacokinetics
  Toxicology
2.7 Clinical Summary

  Biopharmaceutics and associated analytical methods
  Clinical pharmacology studies
  Clinical efficacy
  Clinical safety
  Synopsis of individual studies

Module 3 Quality

3.1 Module 3 table of contents
3.2 Body of data
3.3 Key literature references

Module 4 Non-clinical Study Reports

4.1 Module 4 table of contents
4.2 Study reports
4.3 Literature references

Module 5 Clinical Study Reports

5.1 Module 5 table of contents
5.2 Tabular listing of all clinical studies
5.3 Clinical study reports
5.4 Literature references

regulatory reviews and communications and to facilitate exchange of information between regulatory authorities. It is not intended to indicate what studies are required – these are essentially the same as before – but to indicate merely an appropriate internationally harmonised format for the presentation of the data that have been generated.

17.5   Integrated Regulatory Assessment

A typical dossier for a new active substance (NAS) included 4–6 volumes of administrative (previously known as Part I), 6–10 volumes of pharmaceutical (Part II), 20–40 volumes of pharmacotoxicological (Part III), and 60–100 volumes of clinical (Part IV) data – each volume being approximately 400 pages. As stated above, it is now mandatory to submit the dossier in the CTD format.

During the assessment process, there is a documented interactive dialogue between each assessor and the applicant to clarify points that are complex or ambiguous or to enable the applicant to provide additional raw data, statistical appendices and detailed protocols to facilitate the assessment process. However, none of the various parts of the dossier is self-standing or independent of others. There are areas within each, which are intricately linked to the others. In preparing a comprehensive and integrated regulatory assessment report, it is important that these areas of common interest are appropriately addressed.

17.5.1   Integration of preclinical and pharmaceutical data

The drug substance and finished product specification of any product allow for the presence of low levels of impurities, depending on daily dose and duration of treatment. The permitted levels are specified. It is important that the safety of these allowable impurities is confirmed. The preclinical dossier requires careful scrutiny to ensure that these impurities were present in the test product administered to animals and in quantities sufficient to provide a confident and reassuring margin of safety.

If this has not been done, then the impurities present in relatively high concentration(s) need to be isolated or synthesised and a limited programme of toxicity studies, probably consisting of acute toxicity and genotoxicity, should be conducted directly with these.

17.5.2 Integration of preclinical and clinical data

The clinical dossier has to be scrutinised to ensure that the effects observed in preclinical general toxicity studies have been looked for in the clinical studies and, if present, the level of the risk established. Typical examples would include the preclinical effect of the drug on drug metabolising enzymes or specific target organs for toxicity. Likewise, it is easier to appreciate the significance of an unexpected finding in the clinical studies if there was a corresponding finding in the animal studies.

Often, unusual preclinical findings may require specific studies in man to exclude their clinical significance. While for others, such as testicular or thyroid tumours in animals, the mechanism of their induction is sufficiently well understood that usually no additional studies are warranted.

Of course, any metabolite-related toxicity can only be relied upon if the metabolic profile of the drug in man and in the animal species concerned was similar. While some drug metabolising isoforms show polymorphism in man, the same may not apply to the animal species used in the preclinical programme. As with impurities, any unusual metabolite, if found at a significant level in man, would have to be tested preclinically in separate studies. This is more likely if the impaired metabolism of a drug in man is likely to activate alternative pathways and generate atypical metabolites. In case of drugs with chiral centre, the enantioselectivity in pharmacokinetics in man and in animals should be similar if the

findings from clinical and preclinical studies are to be correlated.

The most important areas of preclinical and clinical integration are the results of the genotoxicity, oncogenicity and reproductive studies. The findings from the latter studies are central to approving the use of the drug during pregnancy and breast-feeding and in children.

17.5.3 Integration of pharmaceutical and clinical data

Frequently, the formulation used in clinical trials is not the one that is ultimately marketed. The pharmaceutical dossier is scrutinised for these variations and to ensure that studies have been carried out to prove the bioequivalence of the two. The same applies if more than one dose strength or dosage form is to be marketed, for example, tablets for adults and liquid preparations for use in children.

Devices used for delivery of the drug (such as inhalers) are another area requiring an integrated clinical and pharmaceutical assessment for their performance, ease of use, and implications for safety and efficacy.

The content uniformity and the finished product specifications are critical for drugs with a very narrow therapeutic index. In such cases, the specifications may have to be tightened.

17.6 Medicines for Paediatric Use

It is estimated that over 50% of the medicines used in children have never actually been studied formally for use in children in specifically designed studies. The absence of suitably tested and evaluated medicinal products authorised to treat children has been an issue of concern for some time. Since existing EU medicines frequently do not include information on safe and effective use in paediatric populations, their use is largely 'off-label' and may result in significant risks, including lack of efficacy and/or unexpected adverse effects, even death. The approach and various initiatives of the EU regulatory authorities reflect this concern and a desire to remedy this. A number of Member States, including the United Kingdom, have been particularly active in this area. For example, in the United Kingdom, the Committee on Safety of Medicines (CSM) established a Paediatric Medicines Working Group in July 2000. Its terms of reference is to advise the Licensing Authority on the key regulatory issues and appropriate action in relation to unlicensed use of medicines in children.

A note for guidance on clinical investigation of medicinal products in the paediatric population (CPMP/EWP/462/95) was adopted by CPMP and came into operation in September 1997. Following a round table meeting at the EMEA in 1997 organised by the EC, one of the conclusions at that time was that there was a need to strengthen the legislation, in particular by introducing a system of incentives.

An ICH guideline (CPMP/ICH/2711/99) on paediatric medicines was agreed and subsequently adopted as a European guideline in July 2000 to come into operation in January 2001. This superseded the original CPMP/EWP/462/95 guideline of September 1997. Directive 2001/20/EC on Good Clinical Practice (in clinical trials), which was adopted in April 2001, also takes into account some specific concerns of performing clinical trials in children, and in particular lays down criteria for their protection in clinical trials.

It had been suggested that a new set of legislative provisions might be necessary to achieve the objectives outlined. At a meeting in November 2001, the importance of taking a European-wide approach was stressed which took into account single market considerations and development efficiencies. A consultation paper was issued in February 2002. However, even if there was a clear therapeutic need for the product, there was no legal provision for obliging these studies to be performed if the company did not present the product for use in the paediatric population. The paper proposed an obligation for companies to perform paediatric studies as a marketing authorisation requirement, unless the medicine was unlikely to be used for children.

Aware of the unmet medical needs of the paediatric population, the CHMP took the initiative to create an *ad-hoc* Paediatric Expert Group (PEG). Dr Daniel Brasseur, chairman of the CHMP and a paediatrician himself, chairs this group. The group comprises 14 experts representing the main areas of specific expertise (e.g. pharmaceutical formulations, pharmacokinetics, trials methodology and several paediatric specialities such as neonatology, immunology, nephrology, adolescent medicine). In addition, several members ensure active links with other CHMP Working Parties (Safety, Efficacy, Pharmacovigilance, Quality), and the COMP. The PEG has prepared a number of Concept Papers such as:

- Pharmaceutical formulations of choice for children use
- Evaluation of Pharmacokinetics in children
- Pharmacovigilance of medicines used in children (CPMP/PhVWP/4838/02)

In addition, the CPMP adopted in May 2002 a concept paper (CPMP/EWP/968/02) on a proposal to develop a 'CPMP Points to Consider' document on the evaluation of the pharmacokinetics of medicinal products in the paediatric population.

A discussion paper (35132/03) on the implications of renal immaturity in neonates when investigating a medicine for paediatric use has been released for consultation. It is anticipated the PEG will finalise by 2005 the work commenced in 2002/2003 in assessing the paediatric needs in three therapeutic areas – gastroenterology, anti-HIV and pain. A very comprehensive work plan for PEG for 2004–5 attests to the importance of this area of drug development.

Such is the emphasis on the scientific development of medicines for paediatric use that Section 4 of the application for marketing authorisation specifically requires the applicant to state whether or not there is a paediatric development programme. Following the Council Resolution of December 2000, in February 2002 the EC published a consultation paper on 'Better Medicines for Children – proposed regulatory actions in paediatric medicinal products'. This paper represented one of the first proposals of the EC to address the problem (see end of chapter).

The PEG has been transformed into Paediatric Working Party in relation to implementation of Regulation (EC) No 726/2004. On 29 September 2004, the EC released the first proposal for a Regulation on Medicinal Products for Paediatric Use together with an explanatory memorandum, the Extended Impact Assessment and questions and answers document. The proposal has now been presented to the Council of Ministers and the European Parliament and it will go through the co-decision procedure. The earliest that the proposal is likely to become law is late 2006.

17.7   Scientific Advice and Protocol Assistance

In order to optimise drug development, it is often necessary to obtain scientific views ('scientific advice') from the authorities on issues that are not regulatory in nature and that are *not* covered by existing guidelines, or when the applicant is proposing to deviate from these guidelines. Scientific advice also facilitates the evaluation of the dossier, as there are no ambiguities or inconsistencies between Member States. It is particularly important to seek this advice before embarking on Phase III studies. 'Protocol Assistance' is the term used for scientific advice for the development of orphan medicinal products.

Applicants are free to solicit advice from individual Member States and according to various surveys conducted by the European Federation of Pharmaceutical Industries and Associations, they often do. Apart from the FDA, these surveys reveal, the EU Member States most often consulted are Germany, France, Sweden and the United Kingdom. However, it is often important to secure a pan-European advice. Article 51 of Council Regulation EEC/2309/93 requires the EMEA to provide the Member States and the institutions of the Community with the best possible scientific advice on any question relating to the evaluation of the quality, the safety and the efficacy of medicinal products for human or veterinary use: 'To this end, the EMEA shall undertake (subsection j) where necessary, advising companies on the conduct of the various tests and trials necessary to demonstrate the quality, safety and efficacy of medicinal products.'

The CPMP had established a procedure for companies to obtain scientific advice and this was formalised in January 1999 and then greatly improved in January 2003. There were standard operating procedures (SOP) for giving scientific advice and protocol assistance (EMEA/SOP/H/3037) and for organisation of oral explanation meetings for scientific advice and protocol assistance (EMEA/SOP/H/3042). The procedure was highly structured to strengthen and to widen the CPMP input and to guarantee the availability of proper expertise.

The Scientific Advice Review Group (SciARG) of the CPMP was the body in charge as of 1999, and this became Scientific Advice Working Group (SAWG) in 2003 – it brought forward to the CPMP an integrated view of all the Member States. Its membership consisted of some CPMP members, two members from the COMP, experts nominated by coordinators for each request, and representatives of different working parties. The SAWG met on the Monday before the CPMP meeting.

Article 56(3) of the new Regulation (EC) 726/2004 provides that 'The Executive Director, in close consultation with the CHMP and the CVMP, shall set up the administrative structures and procedures allowing the development of advice for undertakings, as referred to in Article 57(1)(n), particularly regarding the development of new therapies. Each committee shall establish a standing working party with the sole remit of providing scientific advice to undertakings.'

In view of the ever increasing number of requests, the SAWG has now been restructured and renamed the Scientific Advice Working Party (SAWP) which meets for 2, or sometimes even 3 days about 2 weeks before the CHMP meetings. SAWP is a multidisciplinary expert group and includes 21 members. These are a Chairperson, a Vice-Chairperson and 19 members including three members from the COMP. The chairpersons of Efficacy Working Party and Safety Working

Party are invited members. The mandate states that the SAWP includes at least the following expertise:

- Preclinical safety: at least two representatives
- Pharmacokinetics: at least one representative
- Methodology and Statistics: at least two representatives. Experience in small population methodology and pharmacoepidemiology
- Therapeutic fields for which there are frequent requests and/or defined in the annex of the new Regulation.

A pre-submission meeting with the EMEA Secretariat is encouraged and is free. It is especially advisable if it is the applicant's first experience in seeking scientific advice, and should usually be scheduled about 1 to 2 months before submitting a request. This meeting is valuable for guidance on the scientific advice procedure and for help with the structure/content of the request. There is an EMEA Scientific Advice Guidance Document available to the applicants. The applicant should inform the EMEA Secretariat of the intention to submit an application about 2 weeks before the submission of request and then, once the appropriate fees have been paid, the procedure can start.

At the SAWP meeting, two coordinators are appointed, to whom the applicant should submit the full documentation. These two coordinators have a deadline of 20 days by when they should circulate to all the members their individual first reports on draft CHMP advice. These are discussed at the next meeting of SAWP (Day 30) and, if there is no disagreement, a Joint Report is adopted and the final scientific advice letter is prepared for adoption by the CHMP (Day 40). Typically, however, there is often a lack of consensus between the two coordinators or other members of SAWP and there is a need for further discussion. Therefore, the applicant is invited for an oral explanation and a Joint Report is prepared which is discussed at the following meeting (Day 60). This may result in a final scientific advice letter being prepared (Day 60) for adoption by CHMP on day 70. Exceptionally, a decision is made on whether to constitute an expert meeting (and if necessary, when to do so) or request

a discussion meeting with the applicant. Subsequently, the events follow a highly structured course and by day 100 of the procedure, a final scientific advice is prepared for approval by CHMP.

Protocol assistance for orphan drugs is essential in view of the unique challenges associated with the development of these products (small sample sizes, widely distributed patient population, study designs, use of comparators versus placebo, the choice of endpoints and making sure that all criteria for designation are likely to be addressed, especially demonstrating significant benefit over authorised products). The pharmaceutical activity resulting from the EU orphan drug legislation is reflected in the number of products designated by COMP and the number of protocol assistances delivered by the SAWP. The CHMP has emphasised repeatedly that scientific advice is not a pre-submission evaluation of the data available but is intended to provide clarification on issues of science. The plans for adequate development of the drug remain a company responsibility and the scientific advice is *not* binding on either side, especially if there have been significant scientific advances of relevance to the advice in the interim.

More recently, effective from 1 January 2005, there is an initiative for a Pilot Scheme for Parallel Scientific Advice Meetings between SAWP and FDA. The goal of this pilot is to provide a mechanism for EMEA and FDA assessors and sponsors to exchange their views on scientific issues during the development phase of new medicinal products (i.e. new human drugs and biologics). This pilot will last 1 year, and will commence with the first meeting being held no sooner than January 2005. At the end of 1 year, EMEA and FDA will assess the experience and value, if any, and determine a future course. These parallel scientific advice meetings usually occur at the request of the sponsor, but, in special circumstances, may also be initiated by either EMEA or FDA in cooperation with the sponsor. Prime candidates for parallel scientific advice under this pilot should be important (e.g. products for orphan indications or paediatric populations) or breakthrough medicinal products, especially if the product is being developed for indications for which development guidelines do not exist or, if guidelines do exist, those from the EMEA and from the FDA differ significantly. Most parallel scientific advice meetings conducted under this pilot should be a single occurrence focused on a specific development issue raised. Each agency will provide their independent advice to the sponsor on the questions posed during the parallel scientific advice, according to their usual procedures. The advice of each agency may still differ after the joint discussion.

Details of guidance for companies requesting scientific advice and protocol assistance can be accessed on the EMEA website (see end of chapter).

17.8 Procedures for Marketing Authorisation Applications

The MAH must be established within the EEA, which consists of the EU plus Norway, Iceland and Liechtenstein.

The applications for national authorisations are submitted to the national competent authority which, in the United Kingdom, is the Licensing Authority (LA), whose functions are discharged by the Medicines and Healthcare products Regulatory Agency (MHRA, previously Medicines Control Agency, MCA) of the Department of Health. The LA/MHRA are advised by the CSM, a multidisciplinary scientific body consisting of clinical, preclinical and pharmaceutical members well known for their expertise in their respective fields. Lay members are also included.

Marketing authorisations in the European community can be obtained at present by two main procedures – mutual recognition of a national authorisation from one Member State or a community-wide authorisation through a procedure known as the centralised procedure. In November 2005, a new procedure, known as the decentralised procedure, will be introduced under the new legislation.

Applications through mutual recognition or decentralised procedure are submitted to national authorities. The applications for community

authorisations are submitted to the EMEA, based in Canary Wharf, London. The European Commission is advised by the CHMP of the EMEA, a scientific body that consists of one member representing each Member State of the European Union and in addition, five members coopted for their expertise. These members are chosen by reason of their role and experience in the evaluation of medicinal products and they represent their competent authorities and may be accompanied by their experts. In addition to providing objective scientific opinions, these members ensure that there is appropriate coordination between the tasks of EMEA and the work of the competent national authorities, including the consultative bodies. As discussed later, while NASs or innovatory medicinal products *may* use this 'centralised' procedure, there are certain classes of medicinal products that *must* use the centralised procedure.

17.8.1 UK national authorisations

The following advisory system prevailed until October 2005 when a new advisory structure was put in place (see Section 16.8 in Chapter 16).

When an application is received by MHRA, it is validated to ensure that it is submitted in the correct format, with all requirements for contents and procedure satisfied, and that an appropriate fee has been paid.

The data are then assessed and an integrated assessment report prepared for discussion at the CSM. It is possible to appoint special member(s) for the day in case of drugs that require unique expertise at the Committee. Following in-depth discussion, the Committee communicates its *provisional* advice to the applicant. This may be a refusal to grant a marketing authorisation and the reasons for this rejection, grant of a marketing authorisation, or, as is more often the case, grant of a marketing authorisation subject to any number of amendments to the SPC and other conditions for data to be provided. If the advice of the CSM is other than in the terms of the application, this is conveyed to the applicant in a Notice under Para. 6(1) of Schedule 2 to the Medicines for Human Use (MA, etc.)

Regulations 1994 (previously Section 21(1) of the Medicines Act).

In the event of a refusal or a conditional grant, the applicant either accepts the provisional advice or exercises a right of appeal. This appeal is supported by additional data or clarification of concerns from data already available. Most or all of the CSM concerns/conditions may (or may not) be resolved at the appeal and the CSM has no further role after delivering their *final* advice to the LA. If the final advice is to reject the application, this is conveyed to the applicant in a Notice under Para. 7(4) of Schedule 2 to the Medicines for Human Use (MA, etc.) Regulations 1994 (previously Section 21(3) of the Medicines Act).

If the applicant is still unhappy with refusal or revised conditions, the only option available is an appeal to the Medicines Commission. The Medicines Commission will consider only the outstanding issue(s) and their decision is final. If the applicant is still not content with the outcome, the only course open to the applicant is to seek a judicial review in the High Court. The High Court is concerned primarily with ensuring that the due legal processes were adhered to and is not concerned with the science behind the rejection.

The procedures described above for UK marketing authorisations will of course change in their details when a new advisory structure is implemented. The MHRA has issued a consultation letter on its proposal to change to advisory structure (see Chapter 16).

Apart from some differences in detail, similar procedures operate for national authorisation in almost all EU Member States.

When an applicant has obtained one national authorisation (within an European Union country), any ongoing assessment of that product in other EU Member States is suspended and the first authorisation granted is entered for mutual recognition by all or selected (depending on the choice of the applicant) Member States.

17.8.2 Mutual recognition procedure

Information on the mutual recognition procedure can be accessed from the EC website (see end of chapter). The procedure has a time frame of 90 days following the validation of an application and entry of a marketing authorisation for mutual recognition. At the completion of the procedure, the applicant should anticipate receiving a number of essentially identical marketing authorisations' the only differences being in the authorisation number, product name or pack size.

This procedure applies when a medicinal product has been granted a marketing authorisation by one of the Member States or when the same medicinal product is being examined by more than one Member States. Where a Member State notes that another application for the same medicinal product is being examined in another Member State, the Member State concerned shall decline to assess the application and shall advise the applicant that Articles 27 to 39 apply.

Once a medicinal product has been granted a marketing authorisation by one of the Member States, the marketing authorisation is entered into this procedure for mutual recognition by other Member States. During this procedure, the original competent authority and the applicant act jointly. The applicant submits an identical application (with the dossier updated if necessary) to each Member State from whom the applicant seeks a marketing authorisation. The original competent authority (called the Reference Member State, RMS) transmits the assessment report (updated if necessary), together with the SPC approved by it, to each Member State (called the Concerned Member States, CMS). The role of RMS is to act as the scientific assessor of the dossier, regulatory advisor to the applicant, a moderator in facilitating discussions between the applicant and the CMSs, to arrange, chair and administer the face-to-face meeting ('Breakout Session') between the applicant and the CMSs and to close the procedure appropriately.

From then on, each CMS treats the application almost as a national application with the important differences that, first, they deal with the RMS (rather than the applicant) in respect of any concerns, queries or need for clarification, and secondly, the procedure is driven by predetermined immutable deadlines.

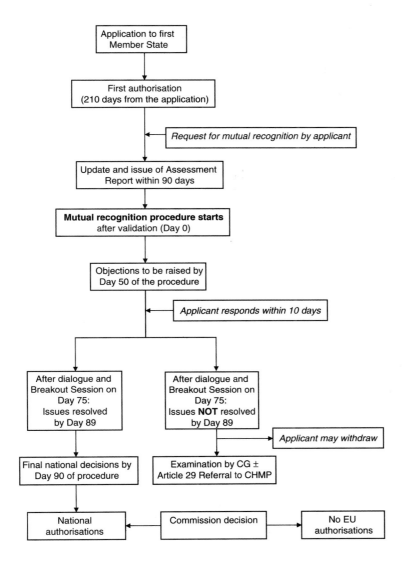

Fig. 17.1 Mutual recognition procedure.

The mutual recognition procedure is shown in Figure 17.1.

By day 50, all CMSs are required to have communicated their concerns to the RMS. By day 60, the applicant, with the help of the RMS, responds to all CMSs, addressing their concerns and enclosing an RMS-approved revised SPC. At day 75, outstanding issues of major concerns are discussed in a face-to-face meeting, known as the 'Breakout Session', between the RMS, CMSs and the applicant. The SPC is still revised further if necessary with the agreement of the RMS. By day 85 (but more frequently day 89) any CMS that still has major public health concerns declares its position and reasons for concerns. The procedure is closed on day 90 with a final revision to the SPC. The applicant may withdraw the applications from those CMSs (on average one or two), which still have major public health concerns. If the applicant refuses to withdraw the application from a CMS that has major public health concerns, the CMS has no choice but to refer the application for arbitration. The applicant too is free to refer the application to arbitration (known as a referral) if it considers any major objection to be unreasonable. The arbitration procedure has its own timetable.

In contrast to the earlier process described above, the new legislation requires that the arbitration by CHMP is preceded by an examination of any question relating to marketing authorisation by a Coordination Group (CG) set up in accordance with the procedures laid down. If a Member State cannot approve the assessment report, the SPC, the labelling and the package leaflet on the grounds of potential serious risk to public health, it is required to give a detailed exposition of the reasons for its position to the RMS, to the other CMSs and to the applicant. The points of disagreement are forthwith referred to the Coordination Group. The EMEA provides the secretariat of this Coordination Group. This Group will be composed of one representative per Member State appointed for a period of 3 years, renewable. Members of the Coordination Group may arrange to be accompanied by experts.

Within the Coordination Group, all Member States are expected to use their best endeavours to reach agreement on the action to be taken. They shall allow the applicant the opportunity to make his point of view known orally or in writing. If, within 60 days of the communication of the points of disagreement, the Member States reach an agreement, the RMS shall record the agreement, close the procedure and inform the applicant accordingly. Each Member State in which an application has been submitted shall adopt a decision in conformity with the approved assessment report, the SPC and the labelling and package leaflet as approved and grant a marketing authorisation within 30 days after acknowledgement of the agreement.

If the Member States fail to reach an agreement in the Coordination Group within the 60-day period, the Agency shall be immediately informed, with a view to proceeding with the arbitration by CHMP (Article 29 referral, of Directive 2001/83/EC). The Agency shall be provided with a detailed statement of the matters on which the Member States have been unable to reach agreement and the reasons for their disagreement. A copy shall be forwarded to the applicant. As soon as the applicant is informed that the matter has been referred to the Agency, he shall forthwith forward to the Agency a copy of relevant information and documents referred to in the first subparagraph of Article 28(1). Member States that have approved the assessment report, the draft SPC and the labelling and package leaflet of the RMS may, at the request of the applicant, authorise the medicinal product without waiting for the outcome of the referral procedure laid down in Article 32. In that event, the authorisation granted shall be without prejudice to the outcome of that procedure.

Some of the finer details of the procedure under the new legislation are yet to be confirmed.

Following the reform of the legislation, the EC issued on 22 February 2005, a draft guideline on the definition of a potential serious risk to public health. As proposed in the draft consultation guideline, serious risk to public health could arise from inadequate scientific justification for the claims for efficacy, evaluation of the preclinical toxicity/safety pharmacology and clinical safety data that do not provide adequate support for the conclusion that all potential safety issues for the target population have been appropriately and adequately addressed in the proposed labelling, the absolute level of risk from the product is considered unacceptable or the proposed production and quality control methods cannot guarantee that a major deficiency in the quality of the product will not occur, that might have a negative impact on the safety or efficacy of the product. Serious risk to public health can also arise from an adverse overall risk-benefit balance in target population or from unsatisfactory product information. According to the draft guideline, examples of efficacy and safety issues that *would not* be considered as grounds for a serious risk to public health are:

- Efficacy:
  a. The absence of an active comparator study versus a specific medicinal product
  b. The absence of clinical trials in non-target populations: the elderly

c. The absence of evidence demonstrating added therapeutic value of the new medicine in comparison to existing medicines

d. The length of the treatment varies according to national medical practices in the various Member States.

- Safety:

  a. The targeted population is too narrow, and should include patients who are allergic or intolerant to medicinal products approved for the same indications

  b. A Member State requires a special interaction study with a medicinal product that is not usually prescribed or used together with the new medicinal product

It must be stressed that at the time of writing this chapter, these proposals were at a draft stage and yet to be agreed by all Member States.

It is easy to see why an SPC coming out of this procedure is usually a highly effective document in terms of the therapeutic claims allowed, a dose schedule that is carefully scrutinised, and detailed safety information and/or monitoring requirements. In rare instances, the SPC comes out too restricted or unbalanced because of the differences in medical practices and cultures among the Member States.

Once a product goes through the mutual recognition procedure, all its post-approval activities are undertaken by the original RMS and go through the same procedure.

17.8.3 Community authorisations

Information on the centralised procedure can be accessed from the EC website (see end of chapter). The EMEA is required to ensure that the opinion of CHMP is given within 210 days after the receipt of a valid application. When an application is submitted for a marketing authorisation in respect of medicinal products for human use which are of major interest from the point of view of public health and in particular from the viewpoint of therapeutic innovation, the applicant may request an accelerated assessment procedure. If the applicant duly substantiates the request and if the CHMP accepts

the request, the time limit shall be reduced to 150 days. A successful application under the centralised procedure delivers a single marketing authorisation (a single document from the EC) for a medicinal product valid throughout the Community under a single trade name and a common SPC. Some of the finer details of the procedure under the new legislation are yet to be confirmed.

Conceptually, this procedure for Community authorisations (also known as the centralised procedure) resembles a hybrid of the national procedure and the mutual recognition procedure, with the differences that first, the application is submitted to EMEA; second, the dossier supporting the application undergoes a detailed assessment by the CHMP before approval in any Member State of the EU; third, the applicant is provided with an opportunity to clarify any issues raised by any of the EU Member States; fourth, the procedure naturally has an extended time frame but still with predetermined deadlines; and finally, the applicant ends up with an approval or a refusal to market the product in all or any Member States of the EU. The centralised procedure is shown in Figure 17.2.

Through the EEA agreement, three European Free Trade Area (EFTA) states – Iceland, Liechtenstein and Norway – have adopted a complete Community *acquis* on medicinal products, and are consequently parties to the centralised procedure. The only exemption from this is that legally binding acts from the Community, for example EC decisions, do not directly confer rights and obligations in these countries but first have to be transposed into legally binding Acts in these states.

The types of product that fell within the scope of Council Regulation (EEC) No. 2309/93 as amended, were set out in the Annex to that Regulation. For medicinal products falling within the scope of Part A of the Annex, applicants were obliged to use the centralised procedure and send their application to the EMEA. For those falling within the scope of Part B of the Annex, applicants may, at their discretion, also use the centralised procedure. Unlike the previous concertation procedure (Council Directive

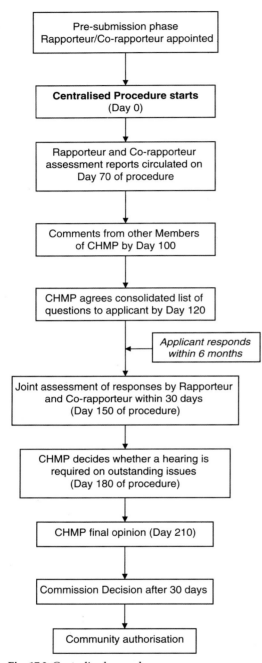

Pre-submission phase Rapporteur/Co-rapporteur appointed

↓

Centralised Procedure starts (Day 0)

↓

Rapporteur and Co-rapporteur assessment reports circulated on Day 70 of procedure

↓

Comments from other Members of CHMP by Day 100

↓

CHMP agrees consolidated list of questions to applicant by Day 120

← *Applicant responds
within 6 months*

Joint assessment of responses by Rapporteur and Co-rapporteur within 30 days (Day 150 of procedure)

↓

CHMP decides whether a hearing is required on outstanding issues (Day 180 of procedure)

↓

CHMP final opinion (Day 210)

↓

Commission Decision after 30 days

↓

Community authorisation

Fig. 17.2 Centralised procedure.

87/22/EEC), there is no provision for an application for a Part A medicinal product intended to be marketed in only one Member State to be exempted from the scope of the centralised procedure.

Box 17.3 shows the *original* scope of products covered by Parts A and B of this Annex. The scope of the medicinal products that must go through the centralised route has been gradually extended by Regulation (EC) No 726/2004. Apart from the products originally covered by Part A (shown in Box 17.3), the scope of medicinal products (under the new legislation) which must go through the centralised route was extended to new active substances used to treat HIV/AIDS, cancer, neurodegenerative diseases and diabetes. It also now includes orphan medicinal products. In addition, human medicinal products used to treat auto-immune diseases and other immune dysfunctions and viral diseases will be added after 4 years, at which time a review may also take place. Even generic versions of centrally approved products may also use the centralised procedure. To this end, Article 10(2)a of Directive 2004/27/EC defines a reference medicinal product and Article 10(2)b goes on to define a generic medicinal product as 'a medicinal product which has the same qualitative and quantitative composition in active substances and the same pharmaceutical form as the reference medicinal product, and whose bioequivalence with the reference medicinal product has been demonstrated by appropriate bioavailability studies'. The different salts, esters, ethers, isomers, mixtures of isomers, complexes or derivatives of an active substance shall be considered to be the same active substance, unless they differ significantly in properties with regard to safety and/or efficacy. In theory, therefore, a copy of a biological/biotechnology reference medicinal product may be regarded as a 'biogeneric' product but for obvious reasons, different criteria will apply when it comes to defining these. The scope of Part B products will be extended to include any new active substance that was not authorised in the Community before and also products concerned with interest of patients at Community level. In certain cases, companies may wish to obtain more than one marketing authorisation for the same medicinal product, through either simultaneous

Box 17.3   Products *originally* covered by Part A and Part B (see text for details)

Part A   Medicinal products derived from bio-technology

Any medicinal product developed by means of one of the following biotechnological processes:

- Recombinant DNA technology
- Controlled expression of genes coding for biologically active proteins in prokaryotes and eukaryotes, including transformed mammalian cells
- Hybridoma and monoclonal antibody methods

Any medicinal product in the composition of which there is a proteinaceous constituent obtained by means of recombinant DNA technology irrespective of whether or not the constituent is an active substance of the medicinal product. This also applies where a recombinant DNA technology step is introduced into the manufacture of a proteinaceous product after the granting of a marketing authorisation.

Part B   Innovative medicinal products

- New active substance (this is also defined further)
- Medicinal products developed by other biotechnological processes which, in the opinion of the EMEA, constitute a significant innovation
- Medicinal products administered by means of new delivery systems which, in the opinion of the EMEA, constitute a significant innovation
- Medicinal products presented for an entirely new indication which, in the opinion of the EMEA, are of significant therapeutic interest
- Medicinal products based on radio-isotopes which, in the opinion of the EMEA, are of significant therapeutic interest
- New medicinal products derived from human blood or human plasma
- Medicinal products, the manufacture of which employs processes which, in the opinion of the EMEA, demonstrate a significant technical advance such as two-dimensional electrophoresis under micro-gravity
- Medicinal products intended for administration to human beings, containing a new active substance which, on the date of entry into force of the Regulation, was not authorised by any Member State for use in a medicinal product intended for human use

or subsequent applications. A specific procedure has been agreed for this between the EMEA and the EC. Under this procedure, companies should inform both the EMEA and the EC Services, at the latest 4 months prior to submission of their intentions, in particular providing the EC with an explanation of the underlying motives for the multiple applications and their intentions regarding exploitation of any authorisations granted.

At the time of receipt of the letter of intent, the proposed invented (trade) name will be checked. However, review of the trade name more than 6 months in advance of the submission date is also acceptable, although such an early checking will only serve to detect objections that exist at that time and not later. This check is performed by the EMEA in liaison with the national competent authorities, in order to determine whether the name would raise any identifiable public health concern, for resolution 1 month thereafter.

For applications to be processed via the centralised procedure, the CHMP appoints one of its members to act as rapporteur for the coordination of the evaluation of an application for a marketing authorisation. The CHMP may, and usually does, also appoint a second member to act as co-rapporteur. For line extensions, the CHMP will decide on the need for appointment of a co-rapporteur on a case-by-case basis. All members have an equal opportunity to act as the rapporteur or co-rapporteur, and therefore the CHMP members are invited to express their preference regarding rapporteurships in writing in advance of the meeting at which rapporteurs are appointed. Rapporteurs are usually appointed at every other meeting to facilitate the decision making process as regards (co)-rapporteurships.

Appointments of rapporteur and co-rapporteur were made on the basis of two criteria: first, the preferences expressed by the applicant, and second, the preferences of CHMP members based on their expertise. The CHMP will no longer take into account preferences expressed by applicants in selecting rapporteurs. A member of staff of the Pre-authorisation Evaluation of Medicines for Human Use Unit of the EMEA is officially appointed as EMEA project manager, and the applicant is notified of the project manager's identity. The project manager remains responsible for providing procedural guidance during the pre-submission phase, coordinating the validation of the application submitted, monitoring compliance with the time frame, preparing the CHMP assessment report and coordinating all the activities (between the applicant, EMEA, CHMP and the rapporteurs) with regard to the progression and final determination of the application.

On receipt of a valid application via the EMEA, the rapporteur and the co-rapporteur both prepare their separate detailed assessment reports, which are circulated to the EMEA and all other Member States by day 70 from the start of the procedure. The new Regulation requires that the duration of the analysis of the scientific data in the file concerning the application for marketing authorisation must be at least 80 days, except in cases where the rapporteur and co-rapporteur declare that they have completed their assessment before that time.

By day 100, rapporteur, co-rapporteur, CHMP members and EMEA receive comments from all other members of the CHMP. A consolidated draft list of questions is prepared by the rapporteur and circulated to the members by day 115. A final consolidated list of questions is agreed by the CHMP on day 120 and communicated to the applicant, and the clock of the procedure is stopped (usually up to 6 months maximum). This consolidated list includes any major public health concerns, points for clarification and changes to the SPC, raised by all Committee members.

The applicant, after seeking clarification from the rapporteur if necessary, responds to these issues (the maximum time allowed for responding is usually no longer than 6 months) and the clock is restarted. These clarification meetings between the applicant and the rapporteurs are crucial. During the procedures in 2004, 61% of the applicants had requested such meetings and the vast majority found these very useful in terms of formulating their responses. The rapporteur and co-rapporteur prepare a joint

assessment (of responses) report that is circulated by day 150 to all members of the CHMP. The deadline for comments from CHMP members to be sent to rapporteur and co-rapporteur, EMEA, and other CHMP members is day 170. Any issue(s) still outstanding are discussed on day 180 of the procedure at the CHMP and a decision may be made on whether to issue a positive CHMP opinion. If there still are any outstanding issues, these are communicated to the applicant and may be addressed at a hearing before the CHMP. If oral explanation is needed, the clock is stopped (usually for no longer than 1 month) to allow the applicant to prepare the oral explanation. Day 181 is the start of the clock when the oral explanation takes place. Days 181–210 of the procedure involves preparation of the final draft of English SPC, labelling and package leaflet sent by applicant to the rapporteur and co-rapporteur, EMEA and other CHMP members. The deadline for adopting an opinion is day 210 of the procedure. A positive opinion requires an absolute majority (at least 16 positive votes of the potential 30) in support; otherwise a negative opinion is issued. If positive, the CHMP opinion is communicated to the EC for their decision. Should the CHMP want to record any follow-up measures they will be included in the Assessment Report and referenced in a letter of undertaking signed by the applicant, which will be annexed to it. Once the medicinal product is authorised and in all cases *before* the medicinal product is placed on the market, specimens of the final outer and immediate packaging and the package leaflet must be submitted to the EMEA within a timeframe agreed between the EMEA and the MAH.

A negative opinion may be the subject of an appeal (now called re-examination), a procedure that has its own time frame. The EMEA immediately informs the applicant when the opinion of the CHMP is that the application does not satisfy the criteria for authorisation set out in the Regulation. The following documents are annexed and/or appended to the opinion: first, the CHMP assessment report stating the reasons for its negative conclusions, and second, when appropriate, the divergent positions of committee members, with their grounds. The applicant may notify the EMEA/CHMP of their intention to appeal within 15 days of receipt of the opinion (after which, if the applicant does not appeal, they are deemed to have agreed with the opinion and it becomes the final opinion). The grounds for appeal must be forwarded to the EMEA within the next 45 days, that is 60 days from receipt of the negative opinion. If the applicant wishes to appear before the CHMP for an oral explanation, this request should also be sent at this stage. The CHMP may decide to appoint a new rapporteur and co-rapporteur to coordinate the appeal procedure, accompanied, if necessary, by additional experts. Within 60 days from the receipt of the grounds for appeal, the CHMP will consider whether its opinion should be revised. If considered necessary, an oral explanation can be held within this 60-day time frame.

Once the CHMP issues a final opinion (positive or negative), it is forwarded (with the required annexes) within 15 days of its adoption, to the EC, the Member States, Norway and Iceland and to the applicant, stating the reasons for its conclusion. On receipt of the CHMP opinion, the EC has now 15 days in which to issue the decision. It is important to appreciate that the CHMP only provides a scientific opinion on quality, safety and efficacy; it is the EC that issues a decision that is binding upon all Member States. A European Public Assessment Report (EPAR) for each of the products approved through the centralised procedure can be obtained via the EMEA website (see end of chapter). Under the new legislation, if an applicant withdraws an application for a marketing authorisation submitted to the Agency before an opinion has been given on the application, the applicant shall communicate its reasons for doing so to the Agency. The Agency shall make this information publicly accessible and shall publish the assessment report, if available, after deletion of all information of a commercially confidential nature.

Once a product goes through the centralised procedure, all its post-approval activities are undertaken by the same rapporteur and go through this procedure.

17.8.4 Decentralised procedure

This is a new procedure introduced under Directive 2004/27/EC. In contrast to the mutual recognition procedure, the decentralised procedure applies to products for which the centralised procedure is not mandatory and which are not authorised in any EU Member State. It facilitates the parallel submission to both RMS and CMSs, involvement of the CMS during the national evaluation phase, and parallel granting of national marketing authorisations after the positive finalisation of the European step of the procedure. Some of the finer details of this new procedure established under the new legislation are yet to be confirmed.

Where an applicant wishes to market a product in more than one Member State, an identical dossier will be sent to all relevant Member States. If an authorisation has not been previously granted, one Member State will be appointed by the applicant to act as RMS who will prepare a draft assessment report with a draft SPC and a draft of the labelling and package leaflet. The CMSs will have the opportunity to review and approve the documents. Therefore, conceptually, the decentralised procedure resembles the centralised procedure without the involvement of CHMP, representing consultation between the Member States before even the first marketing authorisation is granted.

The Member State appointed as RMS will have 120 days in which to prepare the draft documents. During this step, the clock may be stopped for a period of up to 3 months (which could be extended) for the applicant to prepare responses to any issues that may have merged. This will be followed by a 90-day European step during which to reach an agreement. If an agreement is reached, this will be followed by a national step in each Member State for the grant of the marketing authorisation.

As with the mutual recognition procedure, if no agreement can be reached during the 90-day European step, the matter is referred to the Coordination Group for resolution and if still unresolved, the CHMP will arbitrate and deliver an opinion. Consequently, the grounds for refusal are the same irrespective of whether the CMS evaluates an Assessment Report, SPC, package leaflet and labelling from the RMS in a mutual recognition procedure, or a draft Assessment Report, SPC, package leaflet and labelling from the RMS in a decentralised procedure.

17.9 Applications for Orphan Designation

The definition of what constitutes a 'rare' disease varies in different regions of the world. The prevalence figure accepted in the European Union is no more than five individuals per 10 000 of the EU population. In the United States, it is defined as a disease that affects less than 200 000 of the population. This size of population is approximately equal to a prevalence of 7.5 individuals per 10 000 of the United States population. Similarly, the prevalence figures accepted in Japan and Australia are no more than 4.2 and 1.1 individuals respectively per 10 000 of their corresponding populations.

The sponsor proposing to develop a drug for an orphan indication is required to submit an application for the designation of a drug as orphan for a defined clinical entity. To meet the criteria for a successful orphan designation, the applicant should establish:

- that the prevalence of the condition in the European Union is ≤ 5 in 10 000 or that the product is unlikely to generate sufficient return on investment;
- the life-threatening or debilitating nature of the condition;
- that no satisfactory methods exist for the treatment of the condition or if there is a product already authorised in the European Union, the medicinal product will be of significant benefit.

All claims should be substantiated by data or references.

The applicants are generally advised to have a pre-submission meeting with the EMEA Secretariat. On receipt of a valid application, COMP appoints an EMEA coordinator and a COMP member as a coordinator (Day 0). These two prepare a joint report for discussion at the following

meeting (Day 30). If COMP is satisfied that the criteria are met, a positive opinion is issued. More often, there are issues that require clarification and a list of issues to be addressed or questions is sent to the applicant. The responses are assessed by the coordinators and discussed at the next meeting (Day 60). If there are still any outstanding issues, these can be dealt with during an oral hearing on day 90 when an opinion is issued. In case of a negative opinion, the applicant has full appeal rights.

Following its consideration of an application, COMP adopts an opinion, which is transmitted to the EC, which is responsible for issuing a binding decision on the orphan designation status of the drug for the indication concerned. This is similar to the EC decisions on CHMP opinions in respect of a centralised application for a marketing authorisation or a variation.

Products designated as orphan products have automatic access to the centralised procedure but an applicant may opt to take the mutual recognition route until November 2005. In this event, no withdrawals are permissible in order to obtain market exclusivity, as are possible with the conventional drug application going through this route. The option to use the mutual recognition procedure will be abolished after November 2005. Applications for marketing authorisation of orphan medicinal products are evaluated with the same scientific rigour as the normal drugs.

Details about orphan drug legislation, its application and associated procedures and guidance notes are available at the EMEA website (see end of chapter).

17.10 Sale and Supply of Human Medicines

Regarding the sale and supply, the natural tendency of medicinal products approved in the United Kingdom was a pharmacy sale under the supervision of a pharmacist, unless restrictions were relaxed or tightened. Legislation had already existed in the United States (Durham–Humphrey Amendment of 1951) that defined the kinds of drugs that could not be safely used without medical supervision and restricted their sale to prescription by a licensed practitioner, and in 1958 the FDA published the first list of Substances Generally Recognised as Safe (GRAS). The list contains nearly 200 substances. With a similar objective in mind, the Medicines Commission recommended the appointments of a 'Committee on Prescription Only Medicines and Related Matters' and a 'General Sales Lists Committee'.

In the United Kingdom, a significant milestone was reached in 1977, when the work on classification of medicines was completed and the new arrangements provided for three categories according to their safety factor – those available on prescription only (POM), those sufficiently safe to be on general sale to the public through any retail outlet (General Sales List, GSL) and an intermediate category of those which, while not requiring a prescription, should only be sold at pharmacies (P). Under section 59 of the Medicines Act, all new medicinal products containing an NAS (new active substance) and not previously on market are prescription only for the first 5 years. A conscious decision is made for reclassification of each before the 5-year period expires. This requires updating the POM Order or the GSL Order.

Restriction of medicinal products to the POM list had been recommended where they contain substances that present a toxicity hazard, are dependence-producing or present a community hazard. In special circumstances and subject to special provisions, a pharmacist is allowed to supply a POM medicine without a prescription when, by reason of some emergency, a doctor was unable to furnish a prescription immediately. This emergency exemption was originally designed to enable diabetic patients to obtain an emergency supply of insulin which, at that time, was a POM. The GSL list included products that were pre-packed and could 'with reasonable safety' be sold or supplied by retail at shops other than registered pharmacies. These were the products where the hazard to health, the risk of misuse, or the need to take special precautions in handling was small and where wider sale would be a convenience to the purchaser – the concept of 'with reasonable safety'. Inclusion in the General Sales List in no way implied that the product had any therapeutic value. Nor does it imply that no harm could ever come from its use.

17.10.1 Harmonisation across the European Union

The classification for supply of medicinal products for human use to the public varied appreciably from one Member State to another, whereas medicinal products sold without prescription in certain Member States could be obtained only on medical prescription in others. Council Directive 92/26/EEC 'Concerning the classification for the supply of medicinal products for human use' was adopted as an initial step towards harmonising the basic principles applicable to the classification for the supply of medicinal products in the Community or in the Member States concerned. The relevant articles in Directive 2001/83/EC are 70–75.

Article 1 of Council Directive 92/26/EEC provides two classifications for the supply of medicinal products for human use in the community:

- Medicinal products subject to medical prescription
- Medicinal products not subject to medical prescription.

Article 3 provides the criteria for classifying a medicinal product as subject to medical prescription. These are products that are likely to present a danger either directly or indirectly, even when used correctly, if utilised without medical supervision; or are frequently and to a very wide extent used incorrectly, and as a result are likely to present a direct or indirect danger to human health; or contain substances or preparations thereof, the activity and/or adverse reactions of which require further investigation; or are normally prescribed by a doctor to be administered parenterally. Thus a medicinal product that meets any of these criteria is subject to a medical prescription and a medicinal product that does not meet these criteria is not subject to a medical prescription.

The Directive provides discretion and options to Member States for subcategories for medicinal products that are available on medical prescription only but is silent on the subcategorising of non-prescription products.

Under the Directive, the competent authorities are required to draw up a list of the medicinal products subject, on their territory, to medical prescription, specifying, if necessary, the category of classification. They should update this list annually. The Directive also requires that on the occasion of the 5-yearly renewal of the marketing authorisation or when new facts are brought to their notice, the competent authorities should examine and, as appropriate, amend the classification of a medicinal product. Each year, Member States have to communicate to the EC and to the other Member States the changes that have been made to the list referred to above.

With regard to reclassification, the new legislation requires that where a change of classification of a medicinal product has been authorised on the basis of significant pre-clinical tests or clinical trials, the competent authority shall not refer to the results of those tests or trials when examining an application by another applicant or another MAH for a change of classification of the same substance for 1 year after the initial change was authorised.

There is also an EU guideline (dated 29 September 1998 and in operation since January 1999) on changing the classification for the supply of a medicinal product for human use. Article 3 predetermines the POM products. Therefore, the criteria in Article 3 have been used as a basis for this guideline. This guideline does not address the different restrictions that may be available for medicinal products not subject to a medical prescription, such as available in pharmacies only following initial medical diagnosis, or available on general sale, as the case may be.

Part 2 of this guideline describes the data required for changing the classification. The documentation required concerning safety and efficacy in support of an application for a change in the classification for the supply will depend on the nature of the active substance and the extent of any changes to the marketing authorisation. In order to facilitate the evaluation of safety in relation to benefit it should be presented in a logical and concise manner.

17.10.2 Expert report or the clinical overview

In all cases, an Expert Report (or its CTD equivalent, the Clinical Overview), which is a critical analysis of the proposed availability of the product without a medical prescription with the dose and indications as stated in the application, must be provided. The expert is expected to take a clear position, defend the proposal in light of current scientific knowledge, and demonstrate why none of the criteria that determine classification for supply subject to a medical prescription applies to the product.

17.10.3 Safety

Safety data are vital in supporting any application for a change in the classification. Such data will cover the following aspects.

1. A summary should be given of, or references to, animal studies or studies on humans that show low general toxicity and no relevant reproductive toxicity, genotoxic or carcinogenic properties relevant to the experience/exposure of the product.

2. Experience in terms of patient exposure to the substance needs to be considerable and should be outlined. Normally, active substances that are suitable for supply without a medical prescription will have been in widespread use for 5 years, in medicinal products subject to a medical prescription. However, provided enough data is available, this does not exclude the possibility of an authority accepting a shorter time. Adverse drug reactions to the pharmaceutical form and dose proposed for supply not subject to a medical prescription should in normal conditions be minor and should cease on discontinuing therapy.

3. Information should be provided on adverse reactions, including experience of use without medical supervision, for example in another Member State or in a third country.

4. Risks of drug interactions should be detailed.

5. Consequences concerning misuse, for example use for longer periods than recommended, as well as accidental or intended overdose and the use of higher doses, should be discussed.

6. Consequences of the use of the product by a patient who has incorrectly assessed his or her condition or symptoms should be considered.

7. The application should consider the consequences of incorrect or delayed diagnosis of a patient's condition or symptoms due to self-medication with the product.

17.10.4 Efficacy

Evidence of the product's efficacy is not normally considered in the application for changing the classification for supply, unless this application also includes changes to the indications or posology. If other parts of the dossier are changed, for example indication, posology or strength, then supporting data should be provided. A suitable time period for treatment of the suggested indication(s) should be justified and given, together with a proposed pack size.

17.10.5 Product information

For a medicinal product classified for supply without a medical prescription, the proposed product label and leaflet are important elements of the application and will be closely examined for comprehensive information and effectiveness in protecting patients from any safety hazards.

17.11 Communications

Communication with healthcare professionals and the general public is essential to promoting safe and effective use of medicines. Legislation is in place in the European Union to ensure not only that these avenues of communications are not abused but also to impose appropriate penalties when the legislative code is breached.

17.11.1 Package leaflet

The package or patient information leaflets and labels were regulated by Council Directive 92/27/EEC of 31 March 1992 on the labelling of medicinal products for human use and on package leaflets. Article 6 of Directive 92/27/EEC requires the inclusion within the packaging of all medicinal products of a leaflet for the information of users. This is obligatory unless all the information required by Article 7 is directly conveyed on the outer packaging or on the immediate packaging. Article 7 specifies that the package leaflet shall be drawn up in accordance with the SPC and that it shall include the information in an order which is specified in the Directive. The requirements are now codified as articles 54–69 of Directive 2001/83/EC as amended by Directive 2004/27/EC. An acceptable package information leaflet is expected to contain the details shown in Box 17.4.

Article 8 requires that the package leaflet must be written in clear and understandable terms for the patient and be clearly legible in the official language or languages of the Member State where the medicinal product is placed on the market. This provision does not prevent the package leaflet being printed in several languages, provided that the same information is given in all the languages used. In order to address this issue of readability, the European Union has issued a detailed guideline, dated 29 September 1998, on the readability of the label and package leaflet of a medicinal product for human use and this came into operation in January 1999. This guideline makes recommendations on the print size and type as well as print colour. Regarding the syntax, it recommends that as far as possible, overlong sentences (i.e. more than 20 words) should be avoided.

Moreover, it is recommended that lines of a length exceeding 70 characters are not used. Different fonts, upper and lower case letters, length of words, number of clauses per sentence, and length of sentences can all influence readability. A group of bullet points should be introduced with a colon and a single full stop should be placed at the end of the group. A list of bullet

Box 17.4 Contents of a patient information leaflet

- Identification of the medicinal product
    - the name of the medicinal product, followed by the common name
    - the pharmaceutical form and/or the strength
    - full statement of the active ingredients and excipients expressed qualitatively and a statement of the active ingredients expressed quantitatively, using their common names, in the case of each presentation of the product
    - the pharmaceutical form and the contents by weight, by volume or by number of doses of the product, in the case of each presentation of the product
    - the pharmacotherapeutic group, or type of activity in terms easily comprehensible for the patient
- The name and address of the holder of the authorisation
- The name and address of the holder of the manufacturer
- The therapeutic indications
- A list of information which is necessary before taking the medicinal product
    - contraindications
    - appropriate precautions for use
    - forms of interaction with other medicinal products and other forms of interaction which may affect the action of the medicinal product
    - special warnings, taking into account the particular condition of certain categories of users (e.g. children, pregnant or breastfeeding women, the elderly, persons with specific pathological conditions)
- Mention, if appropriate, of potential effects on the mental alertness
    - ability to drive vehicles or to operate machinery
- Details of excipients
    - knowledge of which is important for the safe and effective use of the medicinal product and included in the guidelines published
- The necessary and usual instructions for proper use, in particular
    - the dosage
    - the method and, if necessary, route of administration
    - the frequency of administration, specifying if necessary the appropriate time at which

Box 17.4 Contd

the medicinal product may or must be administered
- depending on the nature of the product, the duration of treatment where it should be limited

- The action to be taken in the case of an overdose
- The course of action to take when one or more doses have not been taken
- Indication, if necessary, of the risk of withdrawal effects
- A description of the undesirable effects
    - which can occur under normal use and, if necessary, the action to be taken in such a case; patients should be expressly invited to communicate any undesirable effect which is not mentioned in the leaflet to their doctor or to their pharmacist
- A reference to the expiry date indicated on the label, with
    - a warning against using the product after this date
    - where appropriate, special storage precautions
    - if necessary, a warning against certain visible signs of deterioration
- The date on which the package leaflet was last revised

points should begin with the uncommon and specific case and end with the common or general case, unless this is inappropriate for the product. A minimum number of words should be used in the bullet points and never more than one sentence. There should be no more than nine items where the bullet points are simple and no more than five when they are complex. Abbreviations should be avoided.

Under Directive 2004/27/EC, there are various changes to the information to be included on the product label and certain provisions relating to the product's package leaflet. There is also a new requirement for the name of the medicinal product to be expressed in Braille format on the label. For products containing up to three active substances, the legislation specifies that the international non-proprietary name (INN) must also appear on the labelling. The MAH must also ensure that the package leaflet is made available on request from patients' organisations in formats appropriate for the blind and partially sighted. Articles 59(3) and 61(1) require user testing of patient information leaflets.

17.11.2 Promotion and advertising

Advertising was regulated by Council Directive 92/28/EEC of 31 March 1992 on the advertising of medicinal products for human use. The requirements are now codified as articles 86-100 of Directive 2001/83/EC as amended by Directive 2004/27/EC.

For the purposes of these Directives, advertising of medicinal products includes any form of door-to-door information, canvassing activity or inducement designed to promote the prescription, supply, sale or consumption of medicinal products. The legislation regulates in particular the advertising of medicinal products to the general public and to persons qualified to prescribe or supply them, visits by medical sales representatives to persons qualified to prescribe medicinal products, the supply of samples, the provision of inducements to prescribe or supply medicinal products by the gift, offer or promise of any benefit or bonus, whether in money or in kind, except when their intrinsic value is minimal, sponsorship of promotional meetings attended by persons qualified to prescribe or supply medicinal products, sponsorship of scientific congresses attended by persons qualified to prescribe or supply medicinal products, and in particular payment of their travelling and accommodation expenses in connection therewith.

There are special provisions for advertising to the general public as well as to the health professions.

Member States have an obligation to prohibit any advertising of a medicinal product in respect of which a marketing authorisation has not been granted in accordance with Community law. Member States must prohibit the advertising to the general public of medicinal products for therapeutic indications specified in the Directive. When permissible, all advertising to the general public of a medicinal product has to be set out in a prescribed manner.

All parts of the advertising of a medicinal product must comply with the particulars listed in the SPC. The advertising of a medicinal product should encourage only the rational use of the medicinal product, by presenting it objectively and without exaggerating its properties, and not so as to be misleading.

In respect of advertising to health professionals, there are detailed requirements in respect of provision of information, free samples and gifts and hospitality as well as the training and duties of medical sales representatives.

Member States have an obligation to monitor advertising and are required to ensure that there are adequate and effective methods to monitor the advertising of medicinal products. Such methods, which may be based on a system of prior vetting, must in any event include legal provisions under which persons or organisations regarded under national law as having a legitimate interest in prohibiting any advertisement inconsistent with the Directive may take legal action against such an advertisement, or bring such an advertisement before an administrative authority competent either to decide on complaints or to initiate appropriate legal proceedings.

Under the legal provisions, Member States must confer upon the courts or administrative authorities powers enabling them, in cases where they deem such measures to be necessary, taking into account all the interests involved and in particular the public interest, to order the cessation of, or to institute appropriate legal proceedings for an order for the cessation of, misleading advertising, or if misleading advertising has not yet been published but publication is imminent, to order the prohibition of, or to institute appropriate legal proceedings for an order for the prohibition of, such publication, even without proof of actual loss or damage or of intention or negligence on the part of the advertiser. Member States must also make provisions for the statutory measures that confer various powers upon the courts or administrative authorities.

The Directive, however, does not exclude the voluntary control of advertising of medicinal products by self-regulatory bodies and recourse to such bodies, if proceedings before such bodies are possible in addition to the judicial or administrative proceedings referred to above.

17.12 Pharmacovigilance

Every Member State has local legislation and obligations for maintaining effective pharmacovigilance and there are criminal, civil, and/or regulatory penalties for non-compliance by MAH.

The harmonisation of pharmacovigilance within the European Union is also gaining momentum. Not surprisingly, there were significant variations between Member States (and also from other major regulatory regions such as the United States and Japan) in terms of reporting requirements generally. Neither were there any consistent requirements for periodic reporting of clinical trials or post-authorisation safety studies. Despite most Member States using Regulation EEC/2309/93 as the basis for expedited reporting, there were a number of variations between Member States in terms of reports requiring expedited reporting.

However, rapid progress is being made to eliminate inconsistencies and to harmonise procedures generally. There is an active Pharmacovigilance Working Party (PhVWP) that meets every month, with the Chairman reporting to the plenary meeting of the CHMP. This Working Party not only discusses an approach for ongoing safety issues but also interacts with industry with regard to guidelines as necessary. Regular video-conferences and exchange of urgent information are held with the FDA in the margins of each meeting of the Working Party.

The legislative framework for pharmacovigilance across the European Union is already provided in a number of regulations, directives and guidelines. These consist of Council Regulation EEC/2309/93, Commission Regulation 540/95, Council Directive 75/319/EEC as amended and Commission Directive 2000/38/EC. Various legislations have been codified as Articles 101–108 of Directive 2001/83/EC as amended by Directive 2004/27/EC. Volume 9 of

the Notice to Applicants is a compilation of all the guidelines on pharmacovigilance.

PhVWP has already adopted a number of guidelines. Of particular interest are the following two.

17.12.1 Notice to MAHs: pharmacovigilance guidelines (CPMP/PhVWP/108/99)

This guideline lays down the roles and responsibilities of the MAH and of the national competent authorities in respect of the products authorised through the national procedures (including the mutual recognition procedure). Also defined are the roles and responsibilities of the Reference Member States (for mutual recognition products) and of the rapporteur and EMEA for centrally approved products. The role and responsibilities of the MAH include having a named, qualified person responsible for pharmacovigilance at the EU level, and there may be a need for an additional named person at the national level when this is required.

The duties of the qualified person include:

1. The establishment and maintenance (*recently changed to 'manage'*) of a system for collection, evaluation and collation of all suspected adverse reaction information so that it may be accessed at a single point in the Community;
2. Preparation of reports referred to in Council Directive 75/319/EEC for competent authorities and for centrally authorised products, for competent authorities and EMEA, reports referred to in Council Regulation EEC/2309/93;
3. Reporting to the Member State concerned within 15 days of receipt of information on all suspected serious adverse reactions within the Community;
4. Preparation of Periodic Safety Update Reports (PSURs) as required by the legislation.
5. Answering fully and promptly any request from competent authorities for the provision of additional information necessary for the evaluation of the benefits and risks afforded by a medicinal product.

There are provisions for pharmacovigilance inspections with each Member State having a responsibility for this activity. However, there is currently no EU guideline and Member States have different rules and practices with regard to pharmacovigilance inspections.

17.12.2 Note for guidance on procedure for competent authorities on the undertaking of pharmacovigilance activities (CPMP/PhVWP/175/95 Rev. 1)

This guideline lays down the requirements and procedures for national competent authorities regarding the collection, evaluation and management of pharmacovigilance data on medicinal products, however authorised in the community.

17.12.3 Other guidelines adopted by ICH/CPMP/PhVWP are listed below

1. Clinical Safety Data Management: Definitions and Standards for Expedited Reporting (E2A) (ICH/377/95).
2. Note for Guidance on the Rapid Alert System (RAS) and Non-Urgent Information System (NUIS) in Human Pharmacovigilance (CPMP/PhVWP/005/96, *Revision 1*).
3. Two major advances were the acceptance of MedDRA (ICH topic M1) as a common medical dictionary for regulatory work and the acceptance of PSURs (ICH topic E2C, ICH/288/95) for drugs marketed in the European Union.
4. Joint Pharmacovigilance Plan for the Implementation of the ICH E2B, M1 and M2: Requirements related to the Electronic Transmission of Individual Case Safety Reports in the Community (ICH M2) (ICH/285/95 or CPMP/PhVWP/2058/99)
5. Note for Guidance on Electronic Exchange of Pharmacovigilance Information for Human and Veterinary Medicinal Products in the European Union (CPMP/PhVWP/2056/99)
6. Position Paper on Compliance with Pharmacovigilance Regulatory Obligations (CPMP/PhVWP/1618/01) (Adopted November 2001).

7. Note for Guidance on Regulatory Electronic Transmission of Individual Case Safety Reports (ICSRs) in Pharmacovigilance (EMEA/H/31387/01) (EudraVigilance TIG adopted March 2002)
8. Note for Guidance on the Electronic Data Interchange (EDI) of Individual Case Safety Reports (ICSRS) and Medicinal Product Reports (MPRS) in Pharmacovigilance during the Pre- and Post-Authorisation Phase in the EEA (EMEA/115735/2004) (EudraVigilance TIG adopted September 2004)

The need for a more structured monitoring of the post-marketing safety of products approved by centralised and mutual recognition routes, and for a very interactive relationship with other regions and principles for providing the WHO with pharmacovigilance information, has been set out in the following papers:

1. Conduct of Pharmacovigilance for Centrally Authorised Products (CPMP/183/97). Volume 9 of the Pharmacovigilance (EudraLex) provides a summary of the role and the responsibilities of all partners involved in the conduct of pharmacovigilance for centrally authorised products. These include the Member States, Rapporteurs/ Co-Rapporteurs, EMEA Secretariat, Pharmacovigilance Working Party, the CHMP and the Commission. There is also in place a Crisis Management Plan regarding centrally authorised products for human use.
2. Conduct of Pharmacovigilance for Medicinal Products Authorised through the Mutual Recognition Procedure (Rev. 1)
3. Principles of Providing the World Health Organisation with Pharmacovigilance Information (CPMP/PhVWP/053/98).

As stated earlier, a Concept Paper on Pharmacovigilance of medicines used in children (CPMP/PhVWP/4838/02) has also been adopted.

The following draft guideline was released for consultation in June 2004: Note for Guidance on the Exposure to Medicinal Products during Pregnancy: Need for Post-Authorisation Data (EMEA/CHMP/1889/04).

More recent activities to proactively improve pharmacovigilance include discussions on Risk Management at ICH. A tripartite, harmonised guideline is considered necessary to define how principles of risk management can be more effectively applied and consistently integrated into decisions, both by regulators and industry, regarding the quality of pharmaceuticals across the product lifecycle, including GMP compliance. This guideline will include a framework of risk management for pharmaceutical quality, which will contribute to more consistent, science-based, decision-making and support the establishment and revision of quality related practices, guidelines, requirements and standards.

At ICH6 meeting in November 2004, final agreement was reached on the guideline 'Pharmacovigilance Planning' (Topic E2E) which sets out a format for documenting the safety profile of new medicines and a pharmacovigilance plan.

17.12.4   Periodic Safety Update Reports (PSUR)

Once a medicinal product is authorised in the European Union, even if it is not marketed, the MAH is required to submit a PSUR. These PSURs were previously required to be prepared at 6-monthly intervals for the first 2 years following the medicinal product's authorisation in the European Union, annually for 2 years, at the first renewal, and then 5-yearly at renewal thereafter. However, as shown later, Regulation 726/2004 has increased the frequency of PSURs.

For medicinal products authorised under the centralised procedure PSURs should be submitted to the competent authorities of all Member States and to the Agency in accordance with Council Regulation (EEC) No 2309/93 Articles 21 and 22, Commission Regulation (EC) 540/95 Articles 2 and 3 and other current legislations. In the PSUR, MAH are expected to provide succinct summary information together with a critical evaluation of the benefit to risk balance of the product in the light of new or changing post-authorisation information. This evaluation should ascertain whether further investigations need to be carried out and whether changes should be made to the marketing authorisation, the SPC, PIL or product advertising.

Where a product is authorised to more than one MAH, the submission of joint PSURs is acceptable provided that the products remain identical and provided that the PSURs are submitted independently by, or on behalf of, the respective MAH for its product. The data lock point should be based on the birth date used for the first authorised product.

When data received from a partner company(ies) might contribute meaningfully to the safety analysis and influence any proposed or effected changes in the product information of the reporting MAH, these data should be included, with source indicated, and discussed in the PSUR, even if it is known that they are included in the PSUR of another MAH.

Unless other requirements have been laid down as a condition for the granting of the marketing authorisation by the Community, a PSUR should be submitted, to the Agency and Member States, immediately upon request or at least every six months after authorisation until the placing of the product on the market. PSURs shall also be submitted immediately upon request or at least every six months during the first two years following the initial placing of the product on the Community market and once a year for the following two years. Thereafter, the reports shall be submitted at three-yearly intervals, or immediately upon request. Multiples of 6-monthly PSURs, are acceptable, provided that the MAH submits a PSUR bridging summary report.

The EC has also awarded a contract for an 'Assessment of the European Community system of pharmacovigilance' to a joint bid from 'Fraunhofer Institute Systems and Innovation Research' and 'Coordination Centre for Clinical Studies at the University of Tubingen' (KKSUKT). A report is expected by the end of 2005.

17.13   Referrals to and Arbitration by CHMP

The European Union has a highly structured legislative framework for resolution of referrals to its scientific advisory committees – for new applications as well as for products already authorised. Community pharmaceutical legislation has created a binding community arbitration mechanism, which may be invoked on the basis of the following articles:

1. Article 29 of Directive 2001/83/EC as amended ('Mutual Recognition referral')
2. Article 30 of Directive 2001/83/EC as amended ('Divergent decision referral')
3. Article 31 of Directive 2001/83/EC as amended ('Community interest referral')
4. Articles 35, 36 and 37 of Directive 2001/83/EC as amended ('Follow-up referrals' with regard to variations)

The elements of the referral procedure are laid down in 32, 33 and 34 of Directive 2001/83/EC as amended. These procedural elements are similar for all types of Community referrals. They give clear practical guidance on what needs to be done in the referral procedure.

For mutual recognition applications, Article 29 of Directive 2001/83/EC provides that where a Member State considers that there are grounds for supposing that the marketing authorisation of the medicinal product concerned may present a risk to public health, it shall forthwith inform the applicant, the RMS, other CMSs, and the EMEA. The Member State must state its reasons in detail and indicate what action may be necessary to correct any defect in the application.

Article 30 provides for a situation where several applications have been made for a particular medicinal product, and Member States have adopted divergent decisions concerning the authorisation of the medicinal product or its suspension or withdrawal. A Member State, or the EC, or the MAH, may refer the matter to the CHMP for application of the procedure laid down in Article 32. The Member State concerned, the MAH or the EC must clearly identify the question which is referred to the CHMP for consideration and, where appropriate, must inform the holder.

Under Article 31, the Member States or the EC or the applicant or holder of the marketing authorisation may, in specific cases where the interests of the Community are involved, refer the matter to the CHMP for the application of the procedure laid down in Article 32 before reaching a decision on a request for a marketing authorisation or on the suspension or withdrawal of an authorisation, or on any other variation to the terms of a marketing authorisation that appears necessary, in particular to take account of the information collected in accordance with Title IX of the Directive 2001/83/EC. The Member State concerned or the EC must clearly identify the question which is referred to the CHMP for consideration and must inform the MAH.

Article 32 describes the timelines and the procedures to be followed following a referral. When reference is made to the procedure described in this Article, the CHMP has to consider the matter concerned and issue a reasoned opinion within 90 days of the date on which the matter was referred to it. However, in cases submitted to the CHMP in accordance with Articles 30 and 31, this period may be extended by 90 days. In case of urgency, on a proposal from its Chairman, the CHMP may agree to a shorter deadline.

17.14 Summary of Product Characteristics

For all practical purposes, the most important document is the SPC. Its terms are carefully scrutinised by the competent authority in light of the dossier accompanying the application. The approved SPC sets out the agreed position of the medicinal product as distilled during the course of the assessment process. It is the definitive statement between the competent authority and the MAH and it is the common basis of communication between the competent authorities of all Member States. As such, the content cannot be changed except with the approval of the originating competent authority. The agreed SPC forms the basis for subsequent marketing of the medicinal product and includes all information which may/should be made available to health professionals and the patients.

Involving as it does the scrutiny of pharmaceutical, preclinical and clinical assessors from each of the Member States, the Euro-SPC of a NAS is a highly effective document, doing full justice to the efficacy of the product and delineating precise indications and dose schedules for its clinical use while providing all information aimed at or necessary for safeguarding the public.

The MAH needs the approval of the competent authority should it wish to vary the terms of the SPC. Such variations require supporting data.

There are, of course, special provisions when a Member State can suspend or revoke an authorisation where the product proves to be harmful in the normal conditions of use or where its therapeutic efficacy is found to be lacking or where its qualitative and quantitative composition is not as declared. An authorisation may also be suspended or revoked where the particulars in the dossier are incorrect or have not been amended or when the controls on the finished product have not been carried out.

17.15   Regulatory Activities under National Authorities

Essentially, four major activities still remain entirely within the remit of national competent authorities.

17.15.1   Manufacturers licences

Manufacturers Licences were issued by the UK LA from the inception of the Medicines Act to cover all manufacturing operations including those previously embraced by the Therapeutic Substances Act (TSA). The Medicines Inspectorate laid down standards in its *Guide to Good Manufacturing Practice* (GMP), otherwise known as 'The Orange Guide'. The most recent edition was issued in 1997. Although the issue of Manufacturers Licences remains a national regulatory function, it is governed by the standards set in Commission Directive 91/356/EEC, which can be summarised as follows.

The Directive lays down the principles and guidelines of manufacturing practice to be followed in the production of medicines, and requirements to ensure that manufacturers and Member States adhere to its provisions. Manufacturers must ensure that production occurs in accordance with GMP, and the manufacturing

authorisation. Imports from non-EU countries must have been produced to standards at least equivalent to those in the European Union, and the importer must ensure this. All manufacturing processes should be consistent with information provided in the marketing authorisation application, as accepted by the authorities. Methods have to be updated in the light of scientific advances, and modifications must be submitted for approval.

In 2003, the provisions of Commission Directive 91/356/EEC had to be extended to accommodate the Directive on clinical trials when the EC issued a Directive 2003/94/EC of 8 October 2003 laying down the principles and guidelines of GMP in respect of medicinal products for human use and investigational medicinal products for human use. This Directive replaces Commission Directive 91/356/EEC and lays down the principles and guidelines of GMP in respect of medicinal products for human use whose manufacture requires the authorisation referred to in Article 40 of Directive 2001/83/EC and in respect of investigational medicinal products for human use whose manufacture requires the authorisation referred to in Article 13 of Directive 2001/20/EC. This new Directive on GMP deals with issues relating to inspections, compliance with marketing authorisation, conformity with GMP, quality assurance system, personnel, premises and equipment, documentation, production, quality control, work contracted out, complaints, product recall and emergency unblinding, self-inspection and labelling.

Good manufacturing standards in the United Kingdom are enforced by the Medicines Inspectorate of the Medicines and Healthcare products Regulatory Agency (see Box 17.5). The United Kingdom has been involved in the Pharmaceutical Inspection Convention (PIC) since its inception and through the Orange Guide set standards which are now reflected in the EU Directives. Articles 111–121 of Directive 2001/83/EC define the obligations of the Member States in respect of supervision and sanctions.

Fees are charged for inspections. Usually, there is mutual recognition of inspections undertaken by countries which are members of the PIC.

Box 17.5 Principles and guidelines for GMP

- Quality management: Implementation of quality assurance system
- Personnel: Appropriately qualified with specified duties, responsibilities and management structures
- Premises and equipment: Appropriate to intended operations

Documentation

- Production: According to pre-established operating procedures with appropriate in-process controls, regularly validated
- Quality control: Independent department, or external laboratory, responsible for all aspects of quality control. Samples, from each batch must be retained for 1 year, unless not, practicable
- Work contracted out: Subject to contract, and under the same conditions, without subcontracting
- Complaints and product recall: Record keeping and arrangements for notification of competent authority
- Self inspection: By the manufacturer of his own processes with appropriate record keeping

---

Membership of the PIC is wider than that of the European Union.

17.15.2 Wholesale dealers licences

This activity, established under the Medicines Act, still remains wholly within the remit of national authorities but in accordance with Council Directive 92/25/EEC of 31 March 1992 on the wholesale distribution of medicinal products for human use (now Articles 76–85 of Directive 2001/83/EC).

In accordance with Article 10 of Council Directive 92/25/EEC, a guideline has been prepared on Good Distribution Practice of medicinal products for human use (94/C63/03). There are strict controls and requirements placed on the wholesalers in respect of premises, installations and equipment for appropriate conservation and distribution of medicines, and for record keeping. All these activities must comply with Council Directive 92/25/EEC and Good Distribution Practice guideline. The guideline does not cover commercial relationships between parties involved in distribution of medicinal products nor questions of safety at work.

17.15.3 Routes of sale and supply

As stated earlier, the Medicines Act 1968 assumes that in the United Kingdom all medicinal products will be sold through a pharmacy unless it is decided by the LA that supply of the product should be limited to being dispensed only on a registered medical practitioner's prescription. Such products appear on the POM list and their packaging is marked POM. Similarly, products available through outlets other than pharmacies and designated as GSL products, are listed in the General Sales List and their packaging is marked GSL.

Additional restrictions on supply are imposed by the Misuse of Drugs Act 1971 and the Misuse of Drugs Regulations. Substances that have a potential for abuse are scheduled under three categories, Class A, B and C.

Class A includes: alfentanil, cocaine, dextromoramide, diamorphine (heroin), dipipanone, lysergide (LSD), methadone, morphine, opium, pethidine, phencyclidine, and class B substances when prepared for injection.

Class B includes: oral amphetamines, barbiturates, codeine, ethylmorphine, glutethimide, pentazocine, phenmetrazine and pholcodine.

Class C includes: certain drugs related to the amphetamines such as benzphetamine and chlorphentermine, buprenorphine, diethylpropion, mazindol, meprobamate, pemoline, pipradrol, cannabis, cannabis resin and most benzodiazepines.

Cannabis and cannabis resin were reclassified from Class B to Class C in January 2004. On 18th

March 2005 the Home Secretary, Charles Clarke, asked the Chairman of the Advisory Council on the Misuse of Drugs (ACMD) to consider returning cannabis and cannabis resin to Class B listing. This request was made as a result of 'emerging evidence' of a link between cannabis consumption and deteriorating mental health. The Misuse of Drugs Regulations 1985 define the classes of person who are authorised to supply and possess controlled drugs while acting in their professional capacities and lay down the conditions under which these activities may be carried out. In the Regulations, drugs are divided into five schedules each specifying the requirements governing such activities as import, export, production, supply, possession, prescribing and record keeping which apply to them.

Schedule 1 includes drugs such as cannabis and lysergide that are not used medicinally. Possession and supply are prohibited except in accordance with Home Office authority.

Schedule 2 includes drugs such as diamorphine (heroin), morphine, pethidine, quinalbarbitone, glutethimide, amphetamine and cocaine and which are subject to the full controlled drug requirements relating to prescriptions, safe custody (except for quinalbarbitone), the need to keep registers, etc. (unless exempted in Schedule 5).

Schedule 3 includes the barbiturates (except quinalbarbitone, now in Schedule 2), buprenorphine, diethylproprion, mazindol, meprobamate, pentazocine, phentermine and temazepam. They are subject to the special prescription requirements (except for phenobarbitone and temazepam) but not to the safe custody requirements (except for buprenorphine, diethylpropion and temazepam) nor to the need to keep registers (although there are requirements for the retention of invoices for 2 years).

Schedule 4 includes 33 benzodiazepines (temazepam is now in Schedule 3) and pemoline which are subject to minimal control. In particular, controlled drug prescription requirements do not apply and they are not subject to safe custody.

Schedule 5 includes those preparations which, because of their strength, are exempt from virtually all controlled drug requirements other than retention of invoices for 2 years.

The European Monitoring Centre for Drugs and Drug Addiction (EMCDDA) is one of the European Union's decentralised agencies. Established in 1993 and based in Lisbon, it is the central source of comprehensive information on drugs and drug addiction in Europe. However, there is no 'harmonised' comprehensive legislation to control drugs of abuse under an EU Directive.

17.15.4   Pricing policy

The provisions of the new Regulation (EC) 726/2004 do not affect the powers of Member States' authorities as regards setting the prices of medicinal products or their inclusion in the scope of the national health system or social security schemes on the basis of health, economic and social conditions. In particular, Member States shall be free to choose from the particulars shown in the marketing authorisation those therapeutic indications and pack sizes which will be covered by their social security bodies.

Each Member State of the European Union operates its own policy regarding the pricing of pharmaceutical products. In the United Kingdom, the primary tool is the Pharmaceutical Price Regulation Scheme (PPRS), which is better described as a profit-regulating scheme. This is dealt with in detail in Chapter 26.

The EC has in the past tried to achieve a harmonisation of prices but this could not be achieved and produced the Transparency Directive (89/105/EEC). The contents of this Directive can be summarised by its various Articles as follows:

Article 1   If the authorities fix prices of the medicinal products, they must comply with the rules of this Directive

Article 2.1   Time limit to comply with rules is 90 days

Article 2.2   Reasons must be given by authorities if the price is other than that sought by the person putting the product on the market

Article 3   Deals with procedures where price increases are sought

Article 4 Imposed price freezes

Article 5 Deals with profit regulation schemes

Article 6 Deals with Limited Lists (Positive lists)

Article 7 Deals with Limited Lists (Negative lists)

Article 8 Classification of products by therapeutic class for inclusion or exclusion

Article 9 Report on the operation of the Directive to be made within 2 years of its adoption

Article 10 A Committee to be set up

Article 11 Demand that all Member States conform.

Essentially, the Directive allowed Member States to operate whatever scheme they chose provided they operated to 'objective and verifiable criteria'.

Undoubtedly, in the future steps may be taken to encompass even these activities, which are at present within the remit of each national authority.

Acknowledgement

The authors are most grateful to Dr Agnes Saint Raymond, Head of Sector Scientific Advice and Orphan Drugs and Acting Head of Sector Safety & Efficacy, European Medicines Agency, London for her valuable and constructive comments during the preparation of this chapter. Any errors, however, are entirely the responsibility of the authors.

References

1. Boyce M, Warrington S. Analysis of 312 studies of investigational medicinal products in healthy subjects to assess the impact of European Union Clinical Trial Directive. *Int J Pharm Med* 2002;**16**:179–184.

2. Kurz R, Crawley FP. The Clinical Trial Directive's ethical impact on research into disease that cause incapacity and diseases of children: perspectives from non-commercially funded research in hospitals. *Int J Pharm Med* 2003;**17**:7–9.

3. Rouesse J. Opinion of the French National Academy of Medicine on the legislative framework for the application of the European Directive on biomedical research in humans [Article in French]. *Bull Acad Natl Med* 2003;**187**:1001–15.

4. Tiner R. The European Clinical Trails Directive: will it promote clinical research in Europe? *Int J Pharm Med* 2004;**18**: 3.

5. Daniels M. Impact of Clinical Trials Directive on the research-based pharmaceutical industry. *Int J Pharm Med* 2004;**18**:5–8.

6. Baeyens AJ. Impact of the European Clinical Trials Directive on academic clinical research. *Med Law* 2004;**23**:103–110.

7. Calder N, Boyce M, Posner J, *et al*. Clinical pharmacology studies in UK Phase 1 units: an AHPPI survey 1999–2000. *Br J Clin Pharmacol* 2004;**57**:76–9.

Consolidated List of Useful Website Addresses

Directive 2001/83/EC: http://pharmacos.eudra. org/F2/eudralex/vol-1/DIR_2001_83/DIR_2001_83_EN.pdf

Review 2001: http://pharmacos.eudra.org/F2/pharmacos/docs/Doc2000/nov/reportmk.pdf

Report from the Commission on the EMEA/CPMP Experience from 1995–2000: http://pharmacos.eudra.org/F2/review/doc/reviewrapport/rap_fv.pdf

Directive 2004/27/EC: http://pharmacos.eudra.org/F2/review/doc/final_publ/Dir_2004_27_20040430_EN.pdf

Regulation (EC) No 726/2004: http://pharmacos.eudra.org/F2/review/doc/final_publ/Reg_2004_726_20040430_EN.pdf

Orphan drug Regulation (EC) No 141/2000: http://pharmacos.eudra.org/F2/orphanmp/doc/141_2000/141_2000_en.pdf

Orphan drug Regulation (EC) No 847/2000: http://pharmacos.eudra.org/F2/eudralex/vol-1/REG_2000_847/REG_2000_847_EN.pdf

Commission Communication Regulation (EC) n° 141/2000 on orphan medicinal products: http://pharmacos.eudra.org/F2/orphanmp/doc/com_0703/com_orphan_en.pdf

Other information with regard to orphan medicines: http://pharmacos.eudra.org/F2/orphanmp/index.htm.

Clinical Trial Directive 2001/20/EEC: http://pharmacos.eudra.org/F2/eudralex/vol-1/DIR_2001_20/DIR_2001_20_EN.pdf

Clinical Trials in the United Kingdom: http://
medicines.mhra.gov.uk/ourwork/licensingmeds/
types/clintrialdir.htm

The rules of procedure for CHMP: http://www.emea.
eu.int/pdfs/human/regaffair/11148104en.pdf

The rules of procedure for COMP: http://www.
emea.eu.int/pdfs/human/comp/821200en.pdf

The rules of procedure of SAWP: http://www.emea.
eu.int/pdfs/human/sciadvice/6968604en.pdf

Eudralex volumes on EU pharmaceutical legislation and procedures: http://pharmacos.eudra.org/
F2/eudralex/index.htm

Mutual recognition procedure: http://pharmacos.
eudra.org/F2/pharmacos/docs.htm

Centralised procedure: http://pharmacos.eudra. org/
F2/pharmacos/docs.htm.

Information on the Common Technical Document
'Presentation and format of the dossier CTD':
http://pharmacos.eudra.org/F2/eudralex/vol-2/
B/ctd2003july.pdf.

Details about orphan drug legislation, its application, and associated procedures and guidance notes:
http://www.emea.eu.int/sitemap.htm.

Details of guidance for companies requesting scientific
advice and protocol assistance: http://www.emea.
eu.int/pdfs/human/sciadvice/426001 en.pdf

Information regarding each of the products approved
through the centralised procedure (European Public
Assessment Report – EPAR): http://www.emea.eu.
int/htms/human/epar/epar.htm

Report from Round Table meeting on drugs for paediatric use: http://www.emea.eu.int/pdfs/human/
regaffair/2716498en.pdf

Commission consultation paper on 'Better Medicines for Children – proposed regulatory actions in
paediatric medicinal products': http://pharmacos.
eudra.org/F2/pharmacos/docs/Doc2002/feb/
cd_pediatrics_en.pdf

Regulation on Medicinal Products for Paediatric Use
together with an explanatory memorandum, the
Extended Impact Assessment and questions and
answers document: http://pharmacos.eudra.org/
F2/Paediatrics/index.htm

Work plan for Paediatric Expert group (PEG) for 2004–
2005: http://www.emea.eu.int/pdfs/human/peg/
2289603en.pdf

CHAPTER 18

18 European regulation of medical devices

Christopher JS Hodges

18.1 Introduction

The regulatory system for medical devices is quite different from that for pharmaceuticals. It does not involve the assessment of a product by a medicines agency or the grant of a marketing authorisation. Instead, the onus of ensuring and declaring that a product conforms to the legal essential requirements is placed on the manufacturer, but in many instances this is subject to approval by an independent technical organisation (known as a *notified body*).

A manufacturer must apply an appropriate *conformity assessment* procedure to their device in order to ensure that it complies with the essential requirements, after which they must certify this fact by completing a *declaration of conformity*. There is usually a choice of conformity assessment procedures open to a manufacturer, depending on a risk-based classification of the class into which the device falls. The two main approaches to conformity assessment are based either on an approved total quality management system audited to ISO 9000 series standard, as customised for medical devices with EN 46 000 series standard, or individual product assessment.

The essential requirements relate to the safety in use of the device, including labelling requirements, but are principally expressed in terms of scientific and technical performance characteristics. Efficacy, as such, is not a criterion. Confirmation of conformity must include evaluation of clinical data for many devices, generated from either a compilation of scientific literature or the results of clinical investigations on the product, for which prior ethical and regulatory approval is required. Conformity of a device with the essential requirements is denoted by affixing a *CE marking* to the device. CE marking, which must be marked on the device, acts in effect as the passport that authorises the device to be placed on the market and to circulate freely within the European Economic Area (EEA).

The legal obligation is that a product must comply with the relevant essential requirements, but where the manufacturer chooses to apply a national standard that adopts a European harmonised standard (EN series) to an aspect of the product, conformity will be *prima facie* presumed in respect of the aspects of the essential requirements covered by that standard. Other national or international standards do not have this regulatory benefit. Compliance with the essential requirements at the time of placing the device on the market, or declaration of this fact, should mean that the device is safe but it may later transpire that this is not the case. Manufacturers therefore have some post-marketing vigilance requirements. If a marketed device is unsafe, the competent authority of a Member State has power under a safeguard clause in each Directive to take regulatory action to effect the withdrawal of the product from the market in its jurisdiction: the matter is then referred to the Commission and all Member States who then coordinate their actions.

European pharmaceutical regulation has been in existence since the mid-1960s and over three decades has successively extended from control of the requirements for placing a product on the market and the data necessary to justify this, coupled with control on manufacture, to virtually all aspects of dealing with a medicine, including wholesale dealing, advertising and clinical research. In contrast, systematic regulation of medical devices is more recent and dates from the 1990s. It essentially covers the requirements for placing a product on the market, coupled with aspects of manufacture, labelling and clinical investigation, but does not cover aspects, such as distribution or advertising. The central difference is that many activities with pharmaceuticals require prior competent authority approval, which is not the case with devices.

Before the medical-devices Directives came into being, most medical devices were unregulated in most European states. In some states some were regulated (illogically, but this was the only available mechanism) as if they were medicines. Examples of products formerly regulated as medicines in the United Kingdom include: contact lens products; intrauterine contraceptives; certain medicated dressings, surgical ligatures and sutures; absorbent or protective materials and dental filling substances.

18.2   Law on Specific Devices

The EEA law on the marketing of medical devices is governed by three principal Directives each of which adopt the Community's scheme for product regulation known as the 'new approach'.[1] The new approach applies to many product sectors, such as machinery, personal protective equipment, low voltage equipment and electromagnetic compatibility (EMC) requirements but not to pharmaceuticals or cosmetics. There are three device Directives.

1. Directive 90/385/EEC on active implantable medical devices ('AIMDs') came into force on 1 January 1993 and is mandatory from 1 January 1995. This covers all powered implants or partial implants that are left in the human body, such as a heart pacemaker.

2. Directive 93/42/EEC on medical devices (MDs) came into force on 1 January 1995 and became mandatory on 14 June 1998. This covers a wide range of devices ranging from first aid bandages, tongue depressors and blood collection bags to hip prostheses and active (powered) devices.
3. Directive 98/79/EC on *in vitro* diagnostics ('IVDs') came into force on 7 June 2000 and is mandatory from 7 December 2003. This covers products such as pregnancy tests, blood glucose monitoring and tests for transmissible diseases.

A transitional period is provided under each of these Directives so that during the period from the coming into force of the Directive until it is mandatory, manufacturers may choose whether to apply the Directive to their device or the national rules that were in force immediately prior to the date on which the Directive came into force. From the date a Directive becomes mandatory, a device that is covered by national law implementing that Directive must comply with it.

Under Community law, a Directive is binding on each Member State, which is obliged under the EC Treaty to implement the Directive into its national law. A Member State has the discretion to choose the manner in which the Directive may be implemented so long as the effect of the Directive is achieved under its national legal order. Most Member States transpose Directives into their national law by enacting domestic legislation that follows the text of the Directives closely, if not *verbatim*. However, differences between implementing laws can arise, particularly in relation to enforcement and sanctions for non-compliance, which are aspects only governed by Directives in broad terms so are in any event matters for the national authorities. It is the national law that is directly binding on people, companies and operations within a particular state, not the Directive. However, since the Directive ultimately governs the national law, people often colloquially refer to the Directive rather than the national law and this approach will be adopted in this chapter. Nevertheless, in any given situation, one must always check the relevant national law and consider, first, what its provisions are, second, to what extent they differ from the Directive and third, whether any difference constitutes a breach of Community law by the Member State and what consequences might follow, such that the national provision might be unenforceable.

The UK legislation is the Medical Devices Regulations 2002/618.

The basic structure, concepts and terminology of the three Directives on AIMDs, MDs and IVDs are identical; the differences that exist among them arise out of the different nature of these products. The following discussion will therefore focus on the medical devices directive (MDD), since this is the central Directive and covers most products. Short sections follow on AIMDs and IVDs. Detailed analysis of the relevant provisions would fill a large book: what is intended here is to highlight the important aspects which should be considered.

The basic purpose of the MDDs, as with all product Directives based on Article 95 (formerly 100a) of the EC Treaty, is to ensure that devices placed on the EEA market ensure *a high level for the protection of safety and health* of patients, users and others, when properly maintained and used in accordance with their intended purpose.[2] The reference to a 'high level' of protection should be noted: the standard of safety and protection required by the legislation is significant. Strictly speaking, this high level only applies where a device is properly maintained and used in accordance with its intended purpose. In practice, however, danger arising where a device has not been properly maintained or as a result of misuse would be highly likely to lead to action by the authorities.

Despite the emphasis of the legislation on safety, an equally important basic purpose of the legislation relates to the EEA's commerce and the economy. All Directives have as a basic purpose the creation of a European internal market without internal barriers to trade and with a single harmonised set of laws governing the placing of a product on the market and its free movement within the market.[3]

The intention behind the legislative scheme is that a product should essentially be regulated under a single product-specific regime as a medicinal product,[4] AIMD, MD, IVD, cosmetic,[5] blood or blood product,[6] or personal protective equipment.[7] However, certain other Directives might apply to particular medical devices, including:

1. Directive 89/336/EEC on electromagnetic compatibility (the EMC Directive): EMC requirements are included within the essential requirements of the MDDs so the EMC Directive only applies to MDs before the relevant MDD is applicable.
2. Directive 2001/95/EC on general product safety (GPS): this applies to all consumer products, some of its obligations apply to MDs used by consumers.

18.3 Resolution of Uncertainties

Since this legislation is extensive, complex, frequently written in generalised terms and seeks to create an entirely new regulatory system for products that were formerly largely unregulated, difficulties of interpretation or application are bound to arise. Since the Directives constitute a legal system, ultimate authority for interpretation rests with the courts, fundamentally with the Court of Justice of the European Communities in Luxembourg, to which questions of interpretation of Community law may be referred by national courts. A mechanism exists, however, under the MDDs by which measures and interpretations may be formally adopted: in the case of the MDD this is the Article 7 Committee, which is a committee of representatives of Member States chaired by the Commission. Under the Article 7 procedure, the Commission may submit to the Committee a draft of measures to be taken, on which the Committee delivers its opinion based on a weighted majority of representatives. The Commission will adopt the measures envisaged if they are in accordance with the opinion of the Committee. If there is divergence, the Commission then permits a proposal to the Council of Members, which acts by a qualified majority of votes.

Less formal, non-binding procedures also exist. There are frequent meetings between representatives of the Commission, Member States and notified bodies. The Commission is also assisted by a Working Group of Experts. A sequence of guidance notes have been issued by the Commission (MEDDEV series), by certain competent authorities (such as the UK Medical Devices Agency's Bulletins) arising out of the meeting of notified bodies, by trade associations and others.

18.4 Competent Authorities and Notified Bodies

Each Member State has designated a competent authority, which is the governmental authority responsible for implementing the Directive in that Member State. In the case of the United Kingdom, the competent authority is the Medicines and Healthcare Products Regulatory Agency (MHRA). The principal function of a competent authority in practice is to ensure the safety and health of patients and users of MDs.

A competent authority is not involved in the assessment or authorisation for placing an MD on the market. As stated above, the legal responsibility in each case rests with the individual manufacturer. However, in many cases the manufacturer is required to obtain independent certification from a third-party testing house, called a notified body. Such testing houses are private, commercial enterprises who may apply for, and be approved for, the purposes of the legislation by the competent authority in their Member State and are then notified within the Community by their approval being published in the Official Journal. Notified bodies may be approved for all devices or only for specific classes of devices. Criteria which they must satisfy in order to be approved are set out in an Annex to the relevant Directive (Annex XI for the MDD). In effect, therefore, notified bodies, although private entities, perform certain delegated regulatory functions. A manufacturer who is required by law to utilise the services of a notified body may choose any notified body within the Community who has the appropriate certification, irrespective of where either of them is located. The relationship between manufacturer and notified body is based

on contract even though certain actions of the notified body have regulatory authority.

18.5 What is an MD

An MD is defined as any instrument, apparatus, appliance, material or other article, whether used alone or in combination, including the software necessary for its proper application intended by the manufacturer to be used for human beings, for the purpose of:

1. Diagnosis, prevention, monitoring, treatment or alleviation of disease.
2. Diagnosis, monitoring, treatment, alleviation or compensation for an injury or handicap.
3. Investigation, replacement or modification of the anatomy or of a physiological process.
4. Control of conception.

and which does not achieve its principal intended action in or on the human body by pharmacological, immunological or metabolic means, but which may be assisted in its function by such means.[8]

An accessory is also considered to be an MD. An accessory is defined as: an article which while not being a device is intended specifically by its manufacturer to be used together with a device to enable it to be used in accordance with the use of the device intended by the manufacturer of the device.[9]

18.5.1 The drug and device borderline

Difficult borderline questions arise in relation to a significant number of products, particularly whether they are to be classified as medicinal products or as MDs. As a general rule, a relevant product is regulated either under the MDDs or by the medicinal products Directives (MPDs). Normally, the procedures of both Directives do not apply cumulatively. The Commission has issued guidelines on this drug–device borderline issue[10] and also on what constitutes MDs, AIMDs and accessories. In order to decide which regime applies, the relevant criteria are:

1. The intended purpose of the product, taking into account the way the product is presented

(this is likely to establish if either the MDD or MPD apply, rather than distinguish between the two regimes).

2. The method by which the principal intended action is achieved. This is crucial in the definition of a medical device. Typically, the MD function is fulfilled by physical means (including mechanical action, physical barrier, replacement of, or support to, organs or body functions). The action of a medicinal product is achieved by pharmacological or immunological means or by metabolism.

The principal intended action of a product may be deduced from:

- the manufacturer's labelling and claims
- scientific data regarding mechanism of action.

Although the manufacturer's claims are important, it is not possible to place the product in one or other category in contradiction with current scientific data. Manufacturers may be required to justify scientifically their rationale for classification of borderline products.

Medical devices may be assisted in their function by pharmacological, immunological or metabolic means, but as soon as these means are not any more ancillary with respect to the principal purpose of a product, the product becomes a medicinal product. The claims made for a product, in accordance with its method of action may, in this context, represent an important factor for its classification as MD or medicinal product. Examples of MDs incorporating a medicinal substance with ancillary action include catheters coated with heparin or an antibiotic, bone cements containing antibiotic and blood bags containing anticoagulant.[11]

18.5.2 Drug–device combinations

The MDD specifies the following approaches[12]:

1. A device that is intended to administer a medicinal product (e.g. an unfilled syringe) is a medical device. The medicinal product itself remains regulated as a medicine.

2. If the device and the medicinal product form a single integral product which is intended exclusively for use in the given combination and which is not reusable (e.g. a pre-filled syringe), that single product is regulated as a medicine. An application for a marketing authorisation must be made under Directive 2001/83/EC. However, the safety and performance of the device features of the integral product are assessed in accordance with the essential requirements of Annex I of the MDD.

3. Where a device incorporates, as an integral part, a substance which, if used separately, may be considered to be a medicinal product and which is liable to act upon the body with action ancillary to that of the device (e.g. a heparin-coated catheter), the product is classed as a medical device. However, the medicinal product is to be assessed in accordance with the requirements of Directive 75/318/EEC (replaced by 2001/83/EC and updated by 2003/63/EC). A notified body undertaking conformity assessment on a medical device which incorporates a medicinal substance having ancillary action has a responsibility to consult a national medicines agency about the medicinal substance, to verify its safety, quality and usefulness by analogy with the appropriate methods specified in Directive 75/318/EEC.

18.6 Classification of Devices

The purpose of classification of devices is simply so as to provide options for conformity assessment methods. Under the MDD, medical devices are categorised into four classes, generally according to the degree of risk that they represent. In summary, Class I covers those that do not enter or interact with the body, Classes IIa and IIb are invasive or implantable devices or those that do interact with the body, Class III is for devices that affect the functions of vital organs. Implantables with an energy source are covered by the AIMDD. The detailed classification rules are lengthy and are set out in Annex IX of Directive 93/42/EEC. A sequence of rules must be worked-through: charts and software are available to assist this.

The classification system uses three basic criteria, in various combinations: duration of contact with the body, degree of invasiveness and the anatomy affected by the use of the device.

Duration is based on continuous use (i.e. uninterrupted actual use) and categorised as transient (<60 min), short term (±30 days) and long term (>30 days). Invasive devices penetrate wholly or partly inside the body by way of an orifice or via the surface of the body. A body orifice is a natural opening in the body and includes the external surface of the eyeball and any permanent artificial opening, such as a stoma. Surgically invasive devices penetrate via the surface to the inside of the body by surgical intervention. Implantable devices are surgically invasive devices intended to be totally introduced to the body, to replace an epithelial surface or the surface of the eye and intended to remain in place after the procedure, and also includes those partially introduced surgically invasive devices remaining in place for at least 30 days. The central circulatory system is defined by the following vessels: arteriae pulmonales, aorta ascendens, arteriae coronarieae, arteria carotis communis, arteria carotis externa, arteria carotis interna, arteriae cerebrales, truncus brachicephalicus, venae cordis, venae pulmonales, vena cava superior, vena cava inferior. The central nervous system consists of the brain, meninges and spinal cord. Active medical devices depend on a power source, such as electricity, for its operation, but not sources of power generated by the human body or gravity.

Non-invasive devices are covered by rules 1–4 and include the following classes.

1. Class I, for example, ostomy pouches, wheelchairs, eye glasses, incontinence pads, cups and spoons for administering medicines, wound dressings, such as cotton wool and wound strips.
2. Class IIa, for example, transfusion equipment, storage and transport of donor organs, polymer film dressings, hydrogel dressings.
3. Class IIb, for example, haemodialysers, dressings for chronic extensive ulcerated wounds.

Invasive devices are covered by rules 5–8 and include the following classes.

1. Class I, for example, dressings for nose bleeds, hand-held dentistry mirrors, enema devices, reusable surgical instruments
2. Class IIa, for example, contact lenses, urinary catheters, tracheal tubes connected to a ventilator,

needles used for suturing, infusion cannulae, dental bridges and crowns
3. Class IIb, for example, urethral stents, insulin pens, devices supplying ionising radiation, prosthetic joint replacements, intraocular lenses, maxillofacial implants
4. Class III, for example, prosthetic heart valves, rechargeable non-active drug delivery systems, absorbable sutures, spinal stents, neurological catheters, temporary pacemaker leads.

Active devices, while covered under the above rules, are largely covered by rules 9–12 and include the following classes.

1. Class I, for example, examination lights, surgical microscopes, wheelchairs, thermography devices, recording, processing or viewing of diagnostic images
2. Class IIa, for example, suction equipment, feeding pumps, anaesthesia machines, ventilators, hearing aids
3. Class IIb, for example, lung ventilators, incubators for babies, surgical lasers, X-ray sources.

Special rules 13–18 govern several hazardous characteristics that may be found in certain devices and require a certain level of control and conformity assessment. Rule 13 deals with devices incorporating a medicinal substance whose action is ancillary to that of the device – Class III, for example, antibiotic bone cements, condoms with spermicides, heparin-coated catheters.

Rule 14 deals with devices used for contraception or the prevention of transmission of sexually transmitted diseases – Class IIb, for example, condoms, contraceptive diaphragms and if they are implantable or long-term invasive; Class III, for example, intrauterine devices.

Rule 15 deals with devices for specific disinfecting, cleaning and rinsing and includes contact lens disinfecting, cleaning, rinsing and hydrating – Class IIb, for example, contact lens solutions, comfort solutions, and devices specifically intended for disinfecting medical devices; Class IIa, for example, disinfectants for use with endoscopes.

Rule 16 classifies non-active devices specifically intended for recording X-ray diagnostic images as Class IIa, for example, X-ray films.

Rule 17 classifies all devices utilising animal tissues or derivatives rendered non-viable and coming into contact with breached skin as Class III, for example, biological heart valves, porcine xenograft dressings, catgut sutures, collagen implants and dressings.

Rule 18 puts blood bags into Class IIb.

If several rules apply to a device, the strictest rule resulting in the higher classification applies.

It must be reiterated that classification is based on the manufacturer's intended use and thus the listing of devices into classes must be taken as guidance only. No classification system can be perfect and thus the aim is to capture the majority of products while recognising that there will always be products that are borderline either between classes or with other product types, such as drugs and cosmetics, and also new innovative products that do not fit the criteria laid down.

18.7 Conformity Assessment Procedures and CE Marking

Depending on the class of the device, a manufacturer may be able to choose between a number of alternative conformity assessment procedures in the assessment of whether a medical device conforms to the essential requirements. Although the rules should be considered in detail in each case,[13] the basic options might be summarised as follows:

1. For all products in Classes IIa, IIb and III, and AIMDs, *a full quality assurance* system, audited periodically by a notified body (Annex II of the MDD), which includes examination and certification by the notified body of the design dossier of each product covered. The manufacturer must keep documentation on the quality system and the design dossier of each product plus other documentation. The quality system obligations include post-marketing and vigilance aspects. Compliance with Annex II may be achieved (this is not mandatory but is invariably adopted voluntarily) by compliance with the EN 29 000 and 46 000 series standards, which apply the ISO 9000 series.

2. For products in Classes IIa, IIb and III, and AIMDs, examination and certification by a notified body of a specimen product (type examination: Annex III of the MDD) coupled with a varying degree (partially restricted by product class) of product or production quality assurance (MDD Annexes IV, V and VI), which ensures that the manufacturing process produces products that conform to the certified type and might involve a quality system for manufacture and final inspection (Annex V), or a quality system for final inspection and testing (Annex VI).

3. For products in Class I, the manufacturer must have specified technical documentation on the design of the product showing that it conforms to the essential requirements: manufacturing aspects are not covered and a notified body is not involved unless there is a measuring function and/or the product is sterilised. (Annex VII: EC declaration of conformity.)

In all cases, the specified documentation must be kept for 5 years after the last product has been manufactured. The Annex VII procedure is also available for Class IIa devices if coupled with the Annex IV or V or VI procedure.

18.7.1 Registration

The manufacturer of a Class I device or of a custom-made device, or a person who markets a system or procedure pack, must inform the competent authority of the manufacturer's registered place of business and the description of the devices concerned.[14] Such manufacturers who are located outside the EEA must designate persons established within the Community who are responsible for such registration.

18.7.2 Harmonised standards

Manufacturers may voluntarily decide to apply any standard to their product or business. Devices that are in conformity with a national standard adopted pursuant to a harmonised EC standard published in the *Official Journal of the*

European Communities are presumed by Member States to comply with those aspects of the essential requirements that are covered by the standard. Harmonised standards are those adopted by the EC standards bodies pursuant to a mandate issued by the Commission, in this case the European Committee for Standardisation (CEN) and the European Committee for Electrotechnical Standardisation (CENELEC). A large number of standards are contemplated but may take time to be written and adopted. Standards may be horizontal (covering aspects common to all or a number of product types) or vertical (dealing only with a specific aspect or specific product type). Important harmonised standards exist on the following:

- EN 29 000 and EN 46 000 series quality systems for medical devices
- EN 1041 information and labelling for medical devices
- EN 980 graphical symbols
- EN 30 993 series biological evaluation of medical devices
- EN 14 155 clinical investigation of devices
- EN 60 601 series medical electrical equipment
- EN 14 971 risk analysis
- EN 1174 sterilisation.

18.7.3 Custom-made devices

A new device that is specifically made in accordance with a duly qualified medical practitioner's written prescription and which gives, under the practitioner's responsibility, specific design characteristics, and is intended for the sole use of a particular patient is permitted to be marketed without CE marking under provisions referring to custom-made devices.[15] The prescription may be made by any person authorised by virtue of their professional qualifications to do so. Mass produced devices that need to be adapted to meet the specific requirements of the medical practitioner or any other professional user are not considered to be custom-made devices.

The manufacturer must undertake to keep available for the competent authorities documentation on the design, manufacture and performance of the product so as to allow assessment of conformity with the essential requirements. He must also draw up a statement containing the following information:

1. Data allowing identification of the device in question.
2. A statement that the device is intended for exclusive use by a particular patient, together with the name of the patient.
3. The name of the medical practitioner or other authorised person who made out the prescription and, where applicable, the name of the clinic concerned.
4. The particular features of the device as specified in the relevant medical prescription.
5. A statement that the device in question conforms to the essential requirements set out in Annex I of the Directive and, where applicable, indicating which essential requirements have not been fully met, together with the grounds. The manufacturer must inform the competent authorities of his registered place of business and the description of the devices concerned.

18.7.4 Systems and procedure packs

A number of items are sometimes assembled and marketed together as a particular system or to be used with a particular medical procedure. The individual items might or might not already bear CE marking. Where all the devices bear CE marking and are put together within the intended purposes specified by their manufacturers, a person or manufacturer who puts them together must draw up a declaration stating the following:

1. They have verified the mutual compatibility of the devices in accordance with the manufacturers' instructions and have carried out their operations in accordance with these instructions.
2. They have packaged the system or procedure pack and supplied relevant information to users incorporating relevant instructions from the original manufacturers.
3. The whole activity is subjected to appropriate methods of internal control and inspection.

The system or procedure pack must not bear additional CE marking and must be accompanied by the original manufacturers' information. The declaration must be kept for 5 years.

Where the above conditions are not met, as in cases where the system or procedure pack incorporates devices that do not bear CE marking or where the chosen combination of devices is not compatible in view of their original intended use, the system or procedure pack must be treated as a device in its own right and the appropriate conformity assessment procedure must be followed.

18.7.5 Essential requirements

The essential requirements contained in Annex I of each new approach Directive specify the aspects of safety and performance that must be satisfied at the time at which a relevant product is placed on the market. Essential requirements are stated as principles or as generalised aspects and exclude detailed technical requirements. The scheme of the Community's new approach is that detailed technical aspects are not required as legal obligations but, if they are generally accepted, may be applied voluntarily by manufacturers through being included in official standards.[16] The essential requirements are intended to be comprehensive and all must be satisfied save for those requirements that do not apply to a particular product as a matter of common sense.

The essential requirements in the MDD fall under two headings: general requirements and requirements regarding design and construction. The general requirements include the following provisions:

1. The devices must be designed and manufactured in such a way that when used under the conditions and for the purposes intended, they will not compromise the clinical condition or the safety of patients, or the safety and health of users or, where applicable, other persons, provided that any risks that may be associated with their use constitute acceptable risks when weighed against the benefits to the patient and are compatible with a high level of protection of health and safety.

2. The solutions adopted by the manufacturer for the design and construction of the devices must conform to safety principles, taking account of the generally acknowledged state of the art. In selecting the most appropriate solutions, the manufacturer must apply the following principles in the following order:

a. eliminate or reduce risks as far as possible (inherently safe design and construction);

b. where appropriate, take adequate protection measures including alarms if necessary, in relation to risks that cannot be eliminated;

c. inform users of the residual risks due to any shortcomings of the protection measures adopted.

3. The devices must achieve the performances intended by the manufacturer and be designed, manufactured and packaged in such a way that they are suitable for one or more of the functions as specified by the manufacturer.

4. The characteristics and performances referred to in sections 1, 2 and 3 above must not be adversely affected to such a degree that the clinical conditions and safety of the patients and, where applicable, of other persons are compromised during the lifetime of the device as indicated by the manufacturer, when the device is subjected to the stresses that can occur during normal conditions of use.

5. The devices must be designed, manufactured and packed in such a way that their characteristics and performances during their intended use will not be adversely affected during transport and storage, taking account of the instructions and information provided by the manufacturer.

6. Any undesirable adverse effect must constitute an acceptable risk when weighed against the performances intended.

Section 2 above implies that a manufacturer must carry out a risk analysis. A harmonised standard is available on this topic, EN 14 971, which amplifies the methodology for risk analysis, elimination or reduction required by section 2.

The essential requirements regarding design and construction are too extensive to be summarised here. They cover the following headings:

- Clinical, physical and biological properties
- Infection and microbial contamination
- Construction and environmental properties
- Devices with a measuring function
- Protection against radiation
- Requirements for medical devices connected to, or equipped with, an energy source
- Information supplied by the manufacturer (this is discussed further below).

18.7.6   Information supplied by the manufacturer

The general principle is that each device must be accompanied by the information needed to use it safely and to identify the manufacturer, taking account of the training and knowledge of the potential users. This information comprises the details on the label and the data in the instructions for use. A series of 13 particular requirements are specified for inclusion in the label and the same 13 requirements plus a further 15 categories of information must be included in the instructions for use.

As far as practicable and appropriate, the information needed to use the device safely must be set out on the device itself and/or on the packaging for each unit or, where appropriate, on the sales packaging. If individual packaging of each unit is not practicable, the information must be set out in the leaflet supplied with one or more devices. Instructions for use must be included in the packaging for every device. By way of exception, no such instructions for use are needed for devices in Class I or IIa if they can be used safely without any such instructions.

Where appropriate, this information should take the form of symbols. Any symbol or identification colour used must conform to the harmonised standards. In areas for which no standards exist, the symbols and colours must be described in the documentation supplied with the device.

It will be noted that in the above three paragraphs, which are quoted verbatim from Annex I, certain flexibility is permitted through use of the words 'where appropriate': this is a feature of many of the other essential requirements. The manufacturer is permitted some discretion over compliance with the essential requirements, based on an application of common sense to the circumstances of his particular product.

18.7.6.1   Who is a manufacturer?

A manufacturer is defined as the natural or legal person with responsibility for the design, manufacture, packaging and labelling of a device before it is placed on the EU market under that manufacturer's own name, regardless of whether these operations are carried out by that manufacturer or on their behalf by a third party. The Directives also apply to those who assemble, package, process, fully refurbish or label a product and in certain other situations.

The intention is that the person (more normally, the company) who assumes the legal responsibility of 'manufacturer' need not be the person who assembles the product. One or more of the activities of design, manufacture, packaging or labelling may be subcontracted by the legal manufacturer. The name or tradename and address of the legal manufacturer must appear on the label and instructions for use.[17] In addition, for devices imported into the Community, the label, or the outer packaging, or instructions for use, must contain the name and address of either the authorised representative of the manufacturer established within the Community, or of the importer established in the Community (this is in effect for devices whose importation is not authorised by the manufacturer), or for the person who has the responsibility to register with the competent authorities in the case of Class I or custom-made devices.

18.7.6.2   Manufacturers outside the EEA

A non-EEA manufacturer may place a Class I or custom-made medical device or a system or procedure pack on the EU market under their own name provided it has undergone a relevant conformity assessment procedure and bears CE marking, and the competent authorities in the relevant Member State have been informed of either

1. The manufacturer's registered place of business in that Member State, if they have one, and the description of the device, or
2. The registered place of business in that Member State of a person designated by the manufacturer as responsible for marketing the device in the European Union, and the category of the device.[18]

In relation to devices in Classes II, IIa and IIb, a manufacturer must certify conformity personally under the Annex II procedure, but an authorised representative established in the European Union may do this in place of the manufacturer under the Annex III and IV procedures.

The functions of an authorised representative are not precisely defined in the Directives except for the IVDD, but such a person is explicitly designated by the manufacturer, and acts and may be addressed by authorities and bodies in the Community instead of the manufacturer with regard to the latter's obligations.[19] It would be good practice for the manufacturer to have a written contract recording their relationship.

18.7.7 'Placing on the market' and 'putting into service'

The Directives provide that devices may be placed on the market and put into service only if they comply with the requirements laid down in the Directive when duly supplied and properly installed, maintained and used in accordance with their intended purpose.[20] Devices, other than devices that are custom-made or intended for clinical investigations, that are considered to meet the essential requirements set out in Annex I of the relevant Directive must bear the CE marking of conformity when they are placed on the market.[21]

The CE marking of conformity, as specified in MDD Annex XII, must appear in a visible, legible and indelible form on the device or its

sterile pack, where practicable and appropriate, and on the instructions for use. Where applicable, the CE marking must also appear on the sales packaging. It must be accompanied by the identification number of the notified body responsible for implementation of the relevant conformity assessment procedure. It is prohibited to affix marks or inscriptions that are likely to mislead third parties with regard to the meaning or the graphics of the CE marking. Any other mark may be affixed to the device, to the packaging or to the instruction leaflet accompanying the device provided that the visibility and legibility of the CE marking is not thereby reduced.

The concepts of 'placing on the market' and 'putting into service' are standard in Community 'new approach' Directives. For the purposes of the MDD, they are defined as follows:

1. *Placing on the market* means the stage of first making available in return for payment or free of charge a device other than a device intended for clinical investigation, with a view to distribution and/or use on the Community market, regardless of whether it is new or fully refurbished.
2. *Putting into service* means the stage at which a device has been made available to the final user as being ready for use on the Community market for the first time for its intended purpose.[22]

The European Commission has issued guidance on these concepts in the context of all 'new approach Directives'.[23] In essence, a device is placed on the market when it is first put into the stream of distribution or commerce by its manufacturer. A device which is fully refurbished is treated as if it were a new device and must be subject afresh to the requirements of the Directive. Difficulties arise over the definition of what constitutes refurbishment (simple servicing is clearly not included) and aspects, such as upgrading.

18.8 Clinical Investigation

Confirmation of conformity with the essential requirements must be based on clinical data in the case of:

• (as a general rule) implantable and long-term invasive devices falling within Classes IIa and IIb, and all Class III devices under the MDD.[24]

• all active implantable devices under the AIMDD.[25]

The adequacy of such clinical data must be based on either:

• a compilation of the relevant scientific literature and, 'if appropriate', a written report containing a critical evaluation, or

• the results of all clinical investigations made.

Thus, *evaluation* of the clinical safety and performance is required for all devices, whereas a clinical *investigation* of each device may or may not be necessary (the term 'clinical trial' is not used in relation to devices). The Directives give some latitude over the circumstances in which a clinical investigation of a non-CE marked device is required. Guidance issued by the MHRA[26] states that an investigation would be required where:

1. There is the introduction of a completely new concept of device into clinical practice where components, features and/or methods of action, are previously unknown.

2. An existing device is modified in such a way that it contains a novel feature, particularly if such a feature has an important physiological effect; or where the modification might significantly affect the clinical performance and/or safety of the device.

3. A device incorporates materials previously untested in humans, coming into contact with the human body or where existing materials are applied to a new location in the human body, in which case compatibility and biological safety will need to be considered.

4. A device, either CE marked or non-CE marked, is proposed for a new purpose or function.

Clinical investigation will also be required where a CE marked device is to be used for a new purpose.

The regime of the Directives is that if clinical evaluation is required, it must be subject to ethical approval in accordance with the principles of the Declaration of Helsinki.[27] The Directives specify[28] that the purpose of a clinical investigation is to:

1. Verify that, under normal conditions of use, the performance of the devices conform to (those intended by the manufacturer, viz. the device should be designed and manufactured in such a way that it is suitable for the functions specified by the manufacturer).

2. Determine any undesirable side effects, under normal conditions of use, and assess whether they are acceptable risks with regard to the intended performance of the device.

The Directives also specify the methodology to be adopted in clinical investigations. Adverse incidents occurring in the investigation must be reported to the competent authority. A general requirement in the MDD is:

Clinical investigations must be performed on the basis of an appropriate plan of investigation reflecting the latest scientific and technical knowledge and defined in such a way as to confirm or refute the manufacturer's claims for the device; these investigations must include an adequate number of observations to guarantee the scientific validity of the conclusions.[29]

The primary consideration of a clinical investigation of a device is assessment verification of the manufacturer's claims for the technical performance of the device. Safety considerations are, nevertheless, relevant in that the clinical investigation should determine and assess any undesirable adverse effects, but the main thrust of the clinical evaluation, and in particular of the conformity assessment by a notified body or the manufacturer to permit marketing, is on technical performance rather than a complete evaluation of safety. It is an essential requirement for marketed devices that '[A]ny undesirable side-effect must constitute an acceptable risk when weighed against the performances intended'.[30]

Both the AIMDD[31] and the MDD[32] specify that a manufacturer must submit a statement [in the specified form (MDD Annex VIII) containing information as detailed as design drawings, manufacturing methods, descriptions and explanations and the results of calculations and technical tests] to the competent authority of the Member State in which the investigation is to be conducted. For Class II devices and implantable and long term devices in Classes IIa and IIb the investigation may commence either after 60 days unless the authority has objected, or earlier if the authority so authorises, provided a favourable ethics committee opinion is available. For devices other than those just specified, the Member State may authorise immediate commencement after receipt of notification, provided a favourable ethics committee opinion has been issued. A device which is intended for clinical investigation must not bear CE marking.

Compliance with the requirements relating to clinical investigations (AIMDD Annex VII; MDD Annex X) is assisted by adoption of standard EN 540 on 'Clinical Investigation of Medical Devices for Human Subjects', which is very similar to pharmaceutical GCP.

Clinical investigation is not required for IVDs.

18.8.1 *In vitro* diagnostics

An IVD medical device is defined as any medical device which is a reagent, reagent product, calibrator, control material, kit, instrument, apparatus, equipment or system, whether used alone or in combination, intended by the manufacturer to be used *in vitro* for the examination of specimens, including blood and tissue donations derived from the human body, solely or principally for the purpose of providing information (1) concerning a physiological or pathological state or congenital abnormality; (2) to determine the safety and compatibility with potential recipients; or (3) to monitor therapeutic measures. For the purpose of this Directive, a specimen receptacle, whether evacuated or not, specifically intended by its manufacturer to contain a specimen for the purposes of an IVD examination, is considered to be a device. Products for general laboratory use are not devices unless such products, in view of their characteristics, are specifically intended by their manufacturer to be used for IVD examination.[33]

The IVD Directive follows the same general 'new approach' scheme as the other MDDs with the following major differences. IVDs are divided

into two classes: Annex II devices and everything else. Annex II devices are themselves divided into List A (high risk) and List B which include the following (each case also including calibrators and control materials):

1. List A
   a. Reagents and reagent products for determining the following blood groups: ABO system, Rhesus (C, c, D, E, e) anti-Kell.
   b. Reagents and reagent products for the detection, confirmation and quantification in human specimens of markers of HIV infection (HIV 1 and 2), HTLV I and II, and Hepatitis B, C and D.
2. List B
   a. Reagents and reagent products for determining the following blood groups: anti-Duffy and anti-Kidd.
   b. Reagents and reagent products for determining irregular antierythrocytic antibodies.
   c. Reagents and reagent products for the detection and quantification in human samples of the following congential infections: rubella, toxoplasmosis.
   d. Reagents and reagent products for diagnosing the following hereditary disease: phenylketonuria.
   e. Reagents and reagent products for determining the following human infections: cytomegalovirus, chlamydia.
   f. Reagents and reagent products for determining the following HLA tissue groups: DR, A, B.
   g. Reagents and reagent products for determining the following turmoral marker: PSA.
   h. Reagents and reagent products, including software, designed specifically for evaluating the risk of trisomy 21.
   i. The following device for self-diagnosis: device for the measurement of blood sugar.

One of the following two conformity assessment procedures may be followed for devices covered by Annex II:

1. The EC Declaration of Conformity procedure (full quality assurance: Annex IV), or
2. the EC type examination procedure (Annex V) coupled with either the EC verification procedure

(Annex VI) or the EC Declaration of Conformity (production quality assurance: Annex VII).

All devices other than those covered by Annex II are subject to the EC Declaration of Conformity procedure (Annex III), which does not involve the intervention of a notified body, but which includes supplementary requirements for devices for self-testing, which does involve a notified body (Annex III).

Common technical specifications (CTS) are to be adopted by the Article 7.2 Committee (a working group of scientific experts appointed by the Member States) which will apply to devices in Annex II List A and, when required, devices in Annex II List B. There is some uncertainty about the circumstances in which the requirement might apply to List B devices. CTS establish appropriate performance evaluation and re-evaluation criteria, batch release criteria, reference methods, and reference materials. If, for duly justified reasons, manufacturers do not comply with the CTS, they must adopt other solutions which are at least equivalent to these specifications. CTS are intended mainly for the evaluation of the safety of the blood supply and organ donations.

Manufacturers shall notify competent authorities:

1. For reagents, reagent products, reference and control materials, of information concerning common technological characteristics and/or analytes, as well as any important and subsequent modification, including suspension of marketing authorisation.
2. For other IVDs' appropriate indications.
3. For devices in Annex II and devices for self-testing, all data allowing identification and the analytical parameters and, where applicable, for diagnostic products in Annex I.3, results of evaluation of performance in accordance with Annex VIII and certificates of notified bodies.

Clinical evaluation is not appropriate for IVDs but a procedure is specified for performance evaluation studies in clinical laboratories or in other appropriate environments outside the manufacturer's premises (Annex VIII). Manufacturers who place devices on the market under their own name must notify the competent authorities of the Member State in which they have their registered place of business of the address of that registered place of business, the categories of devices as defined in terms of common characteristics of technology and/or analytes, and of any significant change thereto.

18.9   Adverse Event Reporting: Vigilance

All adverse events with medical devices of which the manufacturer becomes aware must be recorded. The detailed legal requirements in relation to recording and reporting are, curiously, more onerous in relation to MDs than AIMDs. However, the Commission's guidance is that they should be treated the same in practice. In general, a manufacturer of general medical devices should report, and a Member State record and evaluate,

1. Any malfunction or deterioration in the characteristics and performance of a device, or inadequacy in the labelling, which might lead to, or have led to, the death of a patient or user or to a serious deterioration in their state of health.
2. Any technical or medical reason in relation to the characteristics or performance of a device for the reasons referred to above, leading to systematic recall of devices of the same type by the manufacturer.

Guidance is issued by the European Commission on medical device vigilance[34] which includes an explanation of the difficult concept of when a deterioration in state of health should be considered serious:

• Life-threatening illness or injury.
• Permanent impairment of a body function or permanent damage to a body structure.
• A condition necessitating medical or surgical intervention to prevent permanent impairment of a body function or permanent damage to a body structure.

Regulatory data is (to be) stored on a European Database on medical devices accessible only to competent authorities. This will include data on registration, certificates issued or withdrawn and vigilance.[35]

18.10 General Product Safety Directive

Directive 2001/95/EEC imposes GPS obligations on producers and distributors (as defined) of products 'intended for consumers or likely to be used by consumers'.

The obligations on producers are that they must:

1. Place only safe products on the market.
2. Provide consumers with the relevant information to enable them to assess the risks inherent in the product throughout the normal or reasonable foreseeable period of its use, where such risks are not immediately obvious without adequate warnings, and to take precautions against those risks.
3. Adopt measures commensurate with the characteristics of the products which they supply, to enable them to be informed of risks which these products might present.
4. Take appropriate action to avoid these risks including, if necessary, withdrawing the product in question from the market or recalling it.
5. Batch-mark products.
6. Immediately notify the competent authorities in each Member State in which the product is in circulation if a product placed on the market no longer complies with the definition of a safe product.
7. Inform the competent authorities of actions taken, or intended, to prevent risks.
8. Collaborate with the authorities on action taken to avoid risks.

Other obligations apply to distributors of consumer products. The GPS obligations apply in the absence of other specific rules of Community law governing the safety of such products. It is clear that the obligations under the medical device Directives cover most, if not all, producers' obligations which arise under the GPS Directive as set out above. Manufacturers are

obliged, for example, under MDD Annex II, to undertake their notified body that they will institute and keep up to date a systematic procedure to review experience gained from devices in the post-production phase and to implement appropriate means to apply any necessary corrective action. This undertaking includes an obligation to notify the authorities of reportable adverse events. Whatever the strict legal position on whether GPS obligations do or do not apply to medical device manufacturers, their general principles should be followed as a matter of prudence and for product liability reasons.

18.10.1 Recall

A manufacturer may have a number of post-marketing obligations arising under either the medical devices legislation and/or the GPS legislation, and under product liability or negligence law. The precise legal provisions constitute a somewhat incomplete matrix, although the UK Medical Devices Agency has issued guidance on the subject of recall (defined to include the return, modification, exchange, destruction or retrofit of a device) which covers in general terms the circumstances in which a recall might be appropriate and how it should best be implemented.[36]

18.10.2 Enforcement and sanctions

The medical device Directives authorise Member States to take enforcement action against medical devices which prove to be unsafe. The specific powers, offences, sanctions and penalties are subject to the discretion of Member States. Accordingly, these matters are provided for under national legislation and practice. It must be remembered that relevant national provisions may be found not only within national legislation implementing the relevant medical device Directive but also in other provisions such as general consumer protection, trade descriptions or criminal legislation. Where a Member State invokes the 'safeguard clause' under a medical device Directive, removing a product from the market on grounds of safety, a mechanism must be followed under which the Commission and other Member States are notified, the position discussed, and a unified approach taken by the authorities.

Enforcement provisions are generally of two types: first, powers to investigate and take action against a product and, second, offences that may be committed by individuals for breach of which they may be prosecuted by the authorities and subject to criminal sanctions. In the United Kingdom, for example, the first category of provisions arise under the product-specific regulations and Part II of the Consumer Protection Act 1987. The offences are as specified in the product-specific regulations. There is a considerable variation between Member States in the number and wording of criminal offences which may be committed and in the penalties which might be imposed.

Different national agencies have different practices on what action they may take when faced with dangerous products. The UK Medical Devices Agency, for example, operates a practice of issuing a sequence of three advisory notices to UK health services, for which the criteria for the various safety warning categories are as follows.[37]

- Hazard notices are issued:
  a. In cases of actual death or serious injury, or where death or serious injury would have occurred but for the fortuitous circumstances or the timely intervention of healthcare personnel (or a carer).
  b. Where the medical device is clearly implicated.
  c. Where immediate action is necessary to prevent recurrence.
- Device alerts are issued:
  a. In cases where there is the potential for death or serious injury, or there may be implications arising from the long-term use of the medical device.
  b. Where the medical device is likely to be implicated.
  c. Where the recipient is expected to take immediate action on the advice.

- Safety notices are used to recommend or inform:
  a. Where action by the recipient will improve safety.
  b. Where it is necessary to repeat warnings on long-standing problems.
  c. To support or follow-up manufacturers' field modifications.

References

1. Council resolution of 7 May 1985 on a new approach to technical harmonisation and standards, OJ 1985 No. C 136/1, 4.6.85.
2. Directive 93/42/EEC, recitals 2, 3 and 5 and Article 2.
3. For example, Directive 93/42/EEC, recital 1.
4. Directive 65/65/EEC as amended and related Directives.
5. Directive 76/768/EEC as amended.
6. A Directive or Directives will be forthcoming on these products.
7. Directive 89/686/EEC as amended.
8. Directive 93/42/EEC, Article 1.2(a); Directive 90/385/EEC, Article 1.2(a).
9. Directive 93/42/EEC, Article 1.2(b).
10. *Guidelines*, European Commission, MEDDEV 2.1/3 rev. July 2001.
11. Draft Commission Guidelines, MEDDEV 14/93 rev. 2.
12. Directive 93/42/EEC, Recital 6 and Article 1.3 and 1.4.
13. Directive 93/42/EEC, Article 11.
14. Directive 93/42/EEC, Article 14.
15. Directive 93/42/EEC, Articles 1.2(d), 12.6 and Annex VIII.
16. Council Resolution of 21 December 1989 on a global approach to conformity assessment, OJ 1989 No. C10/1, 16.1.90.
17. Directive 93/42/EEC, Annex I, paragraph 13.1.
18. Directive 93/42/EEC, Article 14.
19. Directive 98/79/EC, Article 1.2(g).
20. For example, Directive 93/42/EEC, Article 2.
21. For example, Directive 93/42/EEC, Articles 17 and 3.
22. Directive 93/42/EEC, Article 1.2(h) and (i) as amended by Article 21 of Directive 98/79/EC.
23. *Guide to the Implementation of Directives Based on the New Approach and the Global Approach*, European Commission, 2000.

24. Directive 93/42/EEC, Annex X and Article 15.

25. Directive 93/42/EEC, Article 9, Annex 2 paragraph 4.1 and Annex 3 paragraph 3.

26. *Guidance Notes for Manufacturers or Clinical Investigations to be carried out in the UK*, Medical Devices Agency, September 1996.

27. Directive 93/42/EEC, Annex 7, paragraph 2.2 and Directive 93/42/EEC, Annex X, paragraph 2.2.

28. Directive 93/42/EEC, Annex 7 and Directive 93/42/EEC, Annex X.

29. Directive 93/42/EEC, Annex X, Requirement 2.3.1.

30. Directive 93/42/EEC, Annex I, Requirement 6.

31. Directive 93/42/EEC, Article 10.

32. Directive 93/42/EEC, Article 15.

33. Directive 98/79/EC, Article 1.2(b).

34. *The Medical Devices Vigilance System: European Commission Guidelines*, Medical Devices Agency, undated.

35. Directive 93/42/EEC, Article 14a.

36. Medical Devices Agency, *Guidance on the Recall of Medical Devices*, 2000.

37. Medical Devices Agency, *Safety Notices*, 2001.

CHAPTER 19

19 Technical requirements for registration of pharmaceuticals for human use: the ICH process

D W G Harron

19.1 Introduction

The International Conference on Harmonisation of Technical Requirements for Registration of Pharmaceuticals for Human Use (ICH) is a unique project that brings together the regulatory authorities of Europe, Japan and the United States and experts from the pharmaceutical industry in the three regions to discuss scientific and technical aspects of product registration. The purpose is to make recommendations, on ways to achieve greater harmonisation in the interpretation and application of technical guidelines and requirements for product registration. This is in order to reduce or obviate the need to duplicate the testing carried out during the research and development of new medicines. The objective of such harmonisation is a more economical use of human, animal and material resources, and the elimination of unnecessary delay in the global development and availability of new medicines while maintaining safeguards on quality, safety and efficacy, and regulatory obligations to protect public health.

19.2 ICH Organisation

19.2.1 Members

Harmonisation, under ICH, involves the European Union, Japan and the United States of America, with the assistance initially of observers from WHO, EFTA (European Free Trade Association) and Canada. The six co-sponsors of the Conference are:

- European Commission – European Union (EU);
- European Federation of Pharmaceutical Industries' Association (EFPIA);
- Ministry of Health and Welfare, Japan (MHW);
- Japan Pharmaceutical Manufacturers Association (JPMA);
- US Food and Drug Administration (FDA);
- Pharmaceutical Research and Manufacturers of America (PhRMA).

In addition, the International Federation of Pharmaceutical Manufacturers Associations (IFPMA) participates as an 'umbrella' organisation for the pharmaceutical industry, and provides the ICH secretariat.

19.2.2 The Steering Committee

The ICH Steering Committee (SC) oversees the preparations for ICH conferences, and the harmonisation initiatives that are undertaken under the ICH Process. The Committee normally meets two or three times a year.

19.2.3 Expert Working Groups (EWGs)

The SC is advised, on technical issues concerned with harmonisation topics, by the EWGs.

These are joint regulatory/industry Working Groups for which experts are nominated from the six co-sponsors of the conference. The Working Groups deal with individual harmonisation topics under general headings; 'Safety' (pre-clinical toxicity and related tests), 'Quality' (pharmaceutical development and specifications), 'Efficacy' (clinical testing programmes and safety monitoring) and 'Multidisciplinary' (cross-cutting topics including regulatory communications and timing of toxicity studies in relation to clinical studies).

In October 1994, the ICH SC announced a 'new direction' in the harmonistaion work coming within the review of ICH. In response to developments in communications technology and the need to avoid divergence in the three regions, which could affect the efficiency of the regulatory process, it was agreed that two aspects on *Regulatory Communications* should be included in the ICH programme; these are the development of an international *Medical Terminology* and agreement on *Electronic Standards for the Transfer of Information and Data.*

19.3 The ICH Process

On the basis of experience to date, the SC has outlined a step-wise *ICH Process* (Figure 19.1) for monitoring the progress of the harmonisation work and identifying the action that is needed in order to reach a defined end point.

19.3.1 ICH meetings and conferences

It was agreed, from the start, that the focus for discussions of tripartite harmonisation should be an international conference or series of conferences. The Steering Committee recognised the importance of ensuring that the process of harmonisation is carried out in an open and transparent manner and that ICH discussions and recommendations are presented in open forums.[1–4]

1. *The First International Conference on Harmonisation* (ICH 1) Brussels, November 1991, hosted by the European Commission and EFPIA.

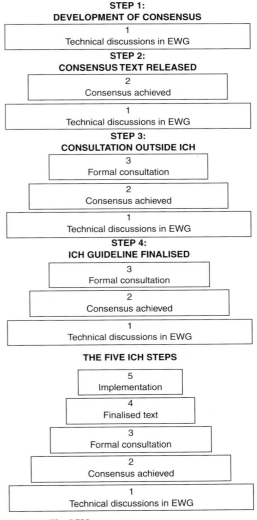

Fig. 19.1 The ICH process.

2. *The Second International Conference on Harmonisation* (ICH 2) Orlando, FL, 27–29 October 1993.

3. *The Third International Conference on Harmonisation* (ICH 3) Yokohama, Japan, 29 November to 1 December 1995.

4. *The Fourth International Conference on Harmonisation* (ICH 4) Brussels, 16–18 July 1997.

5. *The Fifth International Conference on Harmonisation* (ICH 5) San Diego, USA, 9–11 November 2000.

6. *The Sixth International conference on Harmonisation* (ICH 6) Osaka 12–15 November 2003.

19.3.2 Status of ICH harmonisation initiatives

It was generally assumed that following the ICH 4 meeting in 1997 that International Harmonisation had reached an interim conclusion and that the future would focus on developing a Common Technical Document (CTD), to improve efficiency in documenting new medicines for regulatory purposes. However, the ICH process has continued not only for developing the CTD but also ICH 5 and ICH 6 conferences have been convened; the total number of finalised tripartite guidelines has now reached 59[5–11] (20 quality, 13 safety, 17 efficacy, 7 multidisciplinary, 2 eCTD), for examples see Tables 19.1–19.5. For full details www.ich.org.

19.3.3 Common technical document

The adoption of the CTD was a major event that required a global level conference (ICH 5),

---

Table 19.1 ICH: guidelines (quality examples)

Topic	Guidelines	Step
Stability		
ICH Q1A(R2)	Stability testing of new drugs and products (revised guideline)	Step 5 (2003)
ICH Q1B	Photostability testing of new drug substances and products	Step 5 (1996)
ICH Q1C	Stability testing for new dosage forms	Step 5 (1996)
ICH Q1D	Bracketing and matrixing designs for stability testing of drug substances and drug products	Step 5 (2002)
ICH Q1E	Evaluation of stability data	Step 5 (2003)
ICH Q1F	Stability data package for registration in climatic zones III and IV	Step 5 (2003)

Table 19.2 ICH: guidelines (safety examples)

Topic	Guidelines	Step
Safety		
ICH S1A	Guideline on the need for carcinogenicity studies of pharmaceuticals	Step 5 (1995)
ICH S1B	Testing for carcinogenicity of pharmaceuticals	Step 5 (1997)
ICH S1C	Dose selection for carcinogenicity studies of pharmaceuticals	Step 5 (1994)
ICH S1C(R)	Addendum to SIC: addition of a limit dose and related notes	Step 5 (1997)
Genotoxicity Studies		
ICH S2A	Genotoxicity: guidance on specific aspects of regulatory tests for pharmaceuticals	Step 5 (1997)
ICH S2B	Genotoxicity: a standard battery for genotoxicity testing for pharmaceuticals	Step 5 (1997)

Table 19.3 ICH: guidelines (efficacy examples)

Topic	Guidelines	Step
Good Clinical Practice		
ICH E6	Good clinical practice consolidated guideline	Step 5 (1996)
Clinical Trials		
ICH E7	Studies in support of special populations geriatrics	Step 5 (1993)
ICH E8	General considerations for clinical trials	Step 5 (1997)
ICH E9	Statistical principles for clinical trials	Step 5 (1998)
ICH E10	Choice of control group in clinical trials	Step 5 (2000)
ICH E11	Clinical investigation of medicinal products in the pediatric population	Step 5 (2000)
Guidelines for Clinical Evaluation by Therapeutic Category		
ICH E12A	Principles for clinical evaluation of new antihypertensive drugs (ICH principle document)	Step 5 (2000)
ICH E14	Clinical evaluation of QT/QTc interval prolongation and proarrhythmic potential for non-antiarrhythmic drugs	Step 2 (2003)

Table 19.4 ICH: guidelines multidisciplinary

Multidisciplinary topics		
ICH M1	Medical terminology (MedDRA)	
ICH M2	Electronic standards for transmission of regulatory information (ESTRI)	
ICH M3	Timing of pre-clinical studies in relation to clinical trials	
ICH M4	Organisation including the granularity documents that provides guidance on document location and paginations (The common technical document) (Revised annex: granularity document, November 2003)	Step 5
	CTD: Q&As (updated November 2003)	Step 5 (2003)
ICH M4Q	Quality: the section of the application covering chemical and pharmaceutical data including data for biological/biotechnological products (re-edited)	Step 5 (2002)
	CTD quality; Q&As	Step 5 (2003)

both to present the final document and consider implementation issues.

The arguments in favour of a CTD have been forcefully presented. Having harmonised the technical requirements for the demonstration of quality, safety and efficacy of a new medicinal product under the first phase of the ICH process, it seemed reasonable that the three regions should now agree on the way in which this information should be presented for the purpose of obtaining authorisation to place the medicinal product on the therapeutic market.

Table 19.5 ICH: guidelines multidisciplinary/eCTD

ICH M4S	The non-clinical section of the application (re-edited)	Step 5 (2002)
	CTD safety: Q&As (updated November 2003)	Step 5 (2003)
ICH M4E	The clinical section of the application (re-edited)	Step 5 (2002)
	CTD efficacy: Q&As (updated November 2003)	Step 5 (2003)
eCTD	The electronic CTD	Step 5 (2002)
	eCTD: Q&As (updated November 2003)	Step 5 (2003)
ICH M5	Data elements and standards for drug dictionaries	Step 1 (2003)

This would obviously save unnecessary duplication and reworking and would decrease the time and resources required for submission of the regulatory documents, ultimately benefiting patients in the three regions and in the rest of the world.

The industrialists performed a feasibility study in Europe and the United States to determine some of the resource requirements for producing a CTD. They evaluated the time and resources required to convert a New Drug Application (NDA) to a EU application and vice versa. For eight international companies, it took an average of 3 to 4 months to convert one submission to the other; obviously a costly operation in terms of time and resources. But, the report showed the feasibility of developing the CTD and this was presented to regulators in advance of an ICH Steering Group Meeting. The feasibility report revealed slight differences between the three regions in the proposed format of technical dossiers. Agreed harmonisation of format was considered to be relatively easy to achieve, but harmonising content was considered to be harder as differences were greatest between the three regions with regard to the details required in reports submitted to the regulatory authorities.

Thus the CTD is feasible, but it is a formidable challenge. ICH has already demonstrated its ability to deliver and enforce consensus decisions, based upon good science and mutual trust. There is therefore an opportunity to develop in common a more logical, a more efficient, a more user-friendly way of compiling the technical requirements for registration purposes, taking into account the most recent advances of regulatory science and the extraordinary potentials of new information technologies. The ICH SC agreed to a two-year schedule to produce a document. It was also considered, and this is an important development, that the CTD would apply to generics and OTC products and that their manufacturers should also be involved in discussions as to content. Up to this point, generic manufacturers and OTC producers had been largely ignored by ICH.

19.4   ICH 5 Meeting Report

19.4.1   CTD

Prior to the Conference, during which the ICH Expert Working Group and Steering Committee met, the ultimate objective of ICH 5 was achieved.[5] The Common Technical Document (CTD) was agreed (see Table 19.6 for finalised CTD), setting out a harmonised format (see below) for regulatory submissions.

Module 1: Administrative information and prescribing information. This contains documents specific to each region including (e.g. application forms or the proposed label for use in the region); the content and format of this module will be specified by the relevant regulatory authorities.

Module 2: Summaries. In addition to a table of contents and a one-page introduction, this module contains the quality overall summary,

Table 19.6 Organisation of the Common Technical Document (CTD) for the registration of pharmaceuticals for human use

Module 1: Administrative information and prescribing information
Table of contents
Documents specific to each region (e.g. application forms, prescribing information)

Module 2: Common technical document summaries
Overall common technical document table of contents
Introduction
Quality overall summary
Non-clinical overview
Clinical overview
Non-clinical summary
  Pharmacology
    Written summary
    Tabulated summary
  Pharmacokinetics
    Written summary
    Tabulated summary
  Toxicology
    Written summary
    Tabulated summary
Clinical summary
  Summary of biopharmaceutics and associated analytical methods
  Summary of clinical pharmacology studies
  Summary of clinical efficacy
  Summary of clinical safety
  Synopses of individual studies

Module 3: Quality
Table of contents
Body of Data
Key literature references

Module 4: Non-clinical study reports
Table of contents
Study reports
Literature references

Module 5: Clinical study reports
Table of contents of clinical study reports and related information
Tabular listing of all clinical studies
Clinical study reports
Literature references

the non-clinical overview, and the clinical overview; these are followed by the non-clinical written summaries, the non-clinical tabulated summaries, and the clinical summary; [separate documents (M4Q, M4S and M4E) give guidance on the format and content of the summaries].

Module 3: Quality. This covers information on manufacture, specifications, quality control and stability that must be presented in the structured format described in guideline M4Q.

Module 4: Non-clinical study reports. This covers reports on animal and *in vitro* tests that must be presented in the order described in guideline M4S.

Module 5: Clinical study reports. This covers human study reports and related information presented in the order described in guideline M4F.

19.4.2 Implementation of the CTD

All three of the ICH regulatory parties: the European Commission, FDA and MHW, made firm commitments to implement the CTD, when their representatives spoke in a panel on *What the CTD will mean to Regulators* in the closing plenary.

By common agreement, at the ICH SC meeting, all three parties would accept applications in the CTD format from 1 July 2001. This would be on a so-called 'voluntary' basis, as the time required before implementation could become mandatory and vary according to the formal steps needed in the three regions. It was apparent that a question in the minds of many in the audience was whether the new format would really replace current requirements. At several points in the CTD, there is provision for authorities to ask for additional information according to 'regional requirements'.

Background

Each region has its own requirements for the organisation of the technical reports in the submission and for the preparation of the summaries and tables. In Japan, the applicants must prepare the GAIYO, (summary) which organises and presents a summary of the technical information. In Europe, Expert Reports and tabulated summaries are required, and written summaries are recommended. The U.S. FDA has guidance regarding the format and content of the New Drug Application. To avoid the need to generate and compile different registration dossiers, this guideline describes a format for the Common Technical Document that will be acceptable in all three regions.

> Organisation of the Common Technical
> Document (M4)

Harmonisation of the requirements for summaries (Module 2) has been the most challenging task for the CTD Working Groups. A background note in the CTD text (see box above) identifies the current requirements that will be changed by

CTD, but there was concern, for example, that the FDA would still retain an additional 'regional' requirement for the Integrated Safety Summary (ISS) and Integrated Efficacy Summary (IES).

Dr Janet Woodcock, Director of the FDA, Centre for Drug Evaluation and Research (CDER) confirmed that implementation of the CTD would require changes in the Code of Federal Regulations (CFR) and hoped that it would be possible to 'rewrite a more flexible and less specific CFR'. She cautioned, however, that this would take time and that the full consultations required under FDA's Good Guidance Practices must be followed. In response to questions about the ISS, she indicated that this was still regarded as a 'crucial document' in assessment of safety but that FDA recognised the need to address the subject further in order to achieve the goal of a single clinical summary.

Ms Emer Cooke, Principal Administrator in the pharmaceuticals and cosmetics unit of the European Commission Enterprise Directorate-General, presented a timetable under which the CTD could be fully implemented in the European Union by July 2002.

- revision of *Notice to Applicants*, Vol IIB, first quarter of 2001;
- acceptance of applications in the new format, July 2001;
- proposal for revision to Directive 75/318/EEC (technical directive), mid- to end-2001;
- date for CTD to become mandatory, provisionally July 2002.

Dr Yoshinobu Hirayama, Director, Evaluation Division 1, of the MHW Pharmaceuticals and Medical Devices Evaluation Centre confirmed that 'the current GAIYO (Expert Report) will be replaced by CTD Module II documents'. He cautioned, however, that although the CTD provides a common content and format, there will be cases where differences would necessarily occur in dossiers for the three regions (e.g. there may be different dosage recommendations and different quality requirements). He sympathised its the impact on industry who would feel 'the burden of transition more than regulators' and indicated that the transition time before the CTD became mandatory might depend on how much preparatory work needs to be done by industry. Progress on the electronic version of the CTD was discussed. It was anticipated that the (e-CTD) specification would reach draft consensus (or Step 2 of the ICH process) in May 2001 and be finalised (Step 4) by the end of 2001.

The SC for ICH 5 issued a statement on the future of ICH that emphasises the intentions of ICH to focus its activities on: implementing and maintaining existing guidelines, preventing disharmony, encouraging scientific dialogue and harmonisation in new areas (e.g. new technologies or therapies), and undertaking efforts towards global cooperation with non-ICH regions and countries. At its May 2001 meeting, the SC discussed practical aspects, including the possibility of harmonisation efforts in the area of the post-marketing activities.

19.5   The CTD Post-ICH 5

19.5.1   Organisation of the CTD

The common format of the CTD[6,13] has been changed slightly compared to the Step 2 version agreed in July 2000 (e.g. the 'Overall Summary' is now called 'Overview'). The new version of the Organisation is shown in Table 19.6.

19.5.2   Benefits for authorities and applicants

A common format is of value to both applicants and reviewers as the order of documents is logical, more user-friendly, shortens review time, saves resources and facilitates the exchange of information and discussions. Janet Woodcock, Director of FDA's CDER, speaking at ICH 5, expects more 'reviewable' applications, more complete, well-organised submissions, a format that is more predictable, and as a consequence, more consistent reviews.

19.5.3   Hurdles for harmonisation of the content of Module 3

19.5.3.1   Quality

Unfortunately, up to now it was not possible to harmonise the content of the quality dossier in addition to the format also. One of the major reasons for this is the fact that there are some areas where there has never been an ICH guideline developed (e.g. for synthesis of drug substances, manufacturing of drug products, process validation and packaging material). These points were also highlighted by Cone (2004). That means that national guidelines apply. Also, it seems to be of high priority for FDA to develop new national guidelines and regulations incorporating ICH guidelines where they exist. In consequence, applicants may be able to submit common dossiers but should not expect identical query letters or common decision issued by the various regulatory agencies concerned.

The other reasons for disharmony of the content, is the fact that the three major pharmacopoeias are different in terms of monographs and methods required, with the consequence that industry is forced to duplicate testing and generate different specifications, analytical testing, validation of methods, stability testing and summaries. In order to harmonise General Methods of Analysis and Excipient Monographs, the Pharmeuropa (*Ph. Eur*), the *Japanese Pharmacopoeia* (JP) and the *United States Pharmacopeia* (USP) formed a Pharmacopoeial Discussion Group (PDG) in 1989. At the time of ICH 5, only four of 11 general chapters defined as essential in Q6A have reached stage 6 of the PDG procedure, six are still in stage 4, and one in stage 3. Only one Excipient Monograph out of 50 reached stage 6, 31 are in Stage 5 and nine in Stage 4 (Table 19.7) only three general monographs moved forward between ICH 5 and ICH 6.[12] These were bacterial endotoxins, residue on ignition and sterility.

In addition to these regulatory issues there are some homemade limitations to common quality documentation (e.g. normally, pharmaceutical companies prefer to market tablets in polyethylene bottles in the United States, in contrast to blister packs for the European market and different trade names, colours or pack sizes are also unavoidable in certain cases). The consequence of these differences is the fact that a common Module 3 (Quality) and therefore a common Quality Summary in Module 2 cannot be compiled.

Table 19.7 The pharmacopoeial discussion group process

PDG stage no.	Status
Stage 1	Selection of subjects to be harmonised and nomination of a coordinating pharmacopoeia for each subject
Stage 2	Investigation on the existing specifications, on the grade of products marketed and on the potential analytical methods Preparation of a first draft text ('Stage 3 draft')
Stage 3	Publication of the draft text in the forum of each pharmacopoeia: *Pharmeuropa (Ph Eur), Japanese Pharmacopoeial Forum (JP)* and *Pharmacopoeial Forum (USP)* Comments received and consolidated Preparation of a second draft text ('Stage 3 draft')
Stage 4	Publication of the Stage 4 draft Comments received and consolidated Preparation of a revised version ('Stage 5A draft')
Stage 5A	Stage 5A draft reviewed and commented on Revised provisional harmonised document prepared and reviewed until consensus is reached by all three pharmacopoeias ('Stage 5B draft')
Stage 5B	Consensus document is signed off by the three pharmacopoeias
Stage 6	Adoption of the signed-off document by the organisation responsible for each pahrmacopoeia Publication of the adopted document by the three pharmacopoeias in supplements or new editions
Stage 7	Implementation of published document in each region

19.5.3.2 Safety

Safety CTD is causing the fewest problems.[13]

19.5.3.3 Efficacy

The efficacy CTD discussions are dominated by the debate on the need for, and positioning of, ISS and ISE that are required for FDA applications.[13,14]

19.5.4 Other problems facing regulatory agencies and the pharmaceutical industry

In addition and in parallel to the legal changes to be made, several internal aspects have to be faced by the regulatory agencies concerned, for example:

• the impact of the new format on the current review process has to be checked;

• current good review practices need to be adapted;

• new templates and technical guidelines are to be set up;

• internal training of reviewers and document staff will be required; and

• a feed-back mechanism for applicants based on experience in the voluntary phase will have to be created.

Internationally-operating pharmaceutical companies as well as CROs are busy these days with similar activities in order to gain first-hand experience with the new format, and to take part in the voluntary phase by filing applications simultaneously as soon as possible.

Sooner rather than later, CTD-formatted dossiers should also be made acceptable for other types of products (e.g. generics, line extensions, herbals, radiopharmaceuticals and blood products). Also applications for clinical trials [e.g. CTX in the United Kingdom, Investigational new Drug Application (IND) in the United States], as well as applications for variations, and Drug Master Files could be formatted according to the CTD guideline. However, before this becomes a reality, national regulations and guidelines need to be adapted accordingly.

19.5.5 Impact on non-ICH countries

In addition to the ICH regions United States, European Union and Japan that agreed to accept a CTD-formatted dossier as of July 2001, other authorities in non-ICH countries announced they will also accept this, in particular the ICH observers, Canada and Switzerland.

The Swiss authorities made the CTD format mandatory as of 1 July 2002 for new chemical entities (NCEs), as of 1 January 2003 for generics, and as of 1 July 2003 for OTC products and herbals. The same applies to the other EFTA countries (i.e. Iceland, Norway and Liechtenstein).

Mike Ward, representing the Canadian authorities' point of view in San Diego, supports a simultaneous filing of applications, and therefore expects an early acceptance of CTD formatted dossiers. He also mentioned, however, some challenges linked to the implementation of the CTD in Canada (e.g. defining and adopting requirements, systems and procedure for CTD-based NDS which is a complex task; also, the electronic submissions that need to be adjusted to the CTD format). An implementation master plan has been drafted and just needs to be completed. The Canadian authorities seem to be committed to ICH and the CTD. Health Canada will continue with their templates used since 1996 for the comprehensive summaries and evaluation reports, adapted to the CTD guideline accordingly.

South Africa, Australia, New Zealand and countries in Latin America, the Middle East and South East Asia are expected to adopt the CTD guideline, or at least will hopefully not insist in any particular national format. That means, in consequence, that applicants would just need to compile one common dossier in a modular approach following the CTD format, and would be able to submit this to the authorities concerned in all their target countries at the same time.

19.5.6 Developments: Brussels, February 2002

The ICH process is continuous and the SC met in Brussels on February 2002 reporting on the CTD, eCTD, and MedDRA (Medical Dictionary for Regulatory Activity) terminology, the setting up of the Global Cooperation Group, and the status of the technical guidelines. This information can be obtained from the website: www.ifpma.org. As has been stated the success of the ICH process and full implementation of the CTD is fraught with difficulties, not only from current regional reporting differences but also from the impact of local factors such as disease prevalence, ethnicity and local medical practice. The integration of these disparate views will be encouraged with the eCTD, which will provide a medium to transfer data through the world instantaneously. These changes will require companies to develop their own technical and human resources to meet the 'e' demand.

With the adoption of the ICH CTD from July 2002 and mandatory use in the European Union and Japan from July 2003 (and its use strongly encouraged by the USFDA), 'aids' to finding our way round the CTD are beginning to appear. One of these is produced by Quintiles Regulatory Affairs Europe as a teaching aid and is reproduced in the *Regulatory Affairs Journal*.[8]

19.5.7 Developments: Washington, September 2002

- Electronic version of Common Technical Document (eCTD) has been adopted and would move forward for adoption in the three ICH regions.
- Paper version of CTD upgraded/clarification on Quoting References in the Scientific Literature.
- ICH has published a list of frequently asked questions (FAQs) on its website.

• ICH guidelines on pharmacovigilance have been further developed.

• Open workshop on gene therapy convened and recommended amongst other topics; the need to review the safety issue relating to germ-line integration following administration of either viral or non-viral based vectors.

• The SC agreed to establish an EWG to develop harmonised Guidelines on bioequivalence of biotech products (Q5).

• Implementation Working Group (IWG) set up to develop recommendations and clarifications for the E5 Guideline on ethnic factors in acceptability of foreign clinical data.

• Other guidelines being further developed include
  • residual solvents [Q3C(M)];
  • impurities in new drug products (Q3B);
  • safety pharmacology studies for assessing the potential for delayed ventricular repolarisation (QT interval prolongation) by human pharmaceuticals (S7B).

• MedDRA Version 5.1 released.

19.6   ICH6: November 2003 Osaka

The issues discussed at this Conference included[10]

1. *Harmonisation with countries outside the ICH remit.* This enlargement process was mediated through an expanded ICH Global Cooperation Group (GCG). The new members include representatives from
   a. Asia-Pacific Economic group (APEC)
   b. Association of Southeast Asian Nations (ASEAN)
   c. Southern African Development Community (SADC)
   d. Pan American Health Organisation (PAHO) WHO and the Pan American Network for Drug Regulatory Harmonisation (PANDRH) were also included.

2. *MedDRA.* The global standard medical terminology for regulatory activities (MedDRA) continued to evolve. Version 6.1 was released in September 2003, Version 7.0 and 7.1 are issued in March 2004 and September 2004 respectively.

A Spanish Version 6.1 was issued in December 2003.

3. *Gene therapy.* This is a relatively new ICH initiative (September 2002); whose current issues include:
   a. the safety and design of lentiviral vectors;
   b. the characterisation and use of adenoviral reference material and other reference materials;
   c. detection of replication competent adenovirus (RCA) and adenovirus by infectivity PCR;
   d. cytoplasmic gene therapy using Sendai virus vectors;
   e. current requirements on inadvertent germline integration;
   f. insertional mutagenesis/oncogenesis.

4. *Common Technical Document (CTD).* The meeting discussed the implementation of both the paper and electronic versions of the CTD with particular relevance to biotech products and new chemical entities.

5. *Assessment of innovative therapies.* Discussions focused on the new ICH initiative regarding risk-based approach to drug product quality and GMP. Talks also focused on new technologies to enhance drug development, challenges in the area of biotechnology and pharmacogenetics and targeted medicines.

6. *Quality.* Guidelines discussed included:
   a. comparability of biotechnological and biological products subject to changes in their manufacturing processes (ICHQ5E);
   b. bracketing and matrixing designs for stability testing of new drug substances and drug products (ICHQ1D);
   c. evaluation of stability data (ICHQ1E);
   d. stability data package for registration in climatic zones III and IV (ICHQ1F);
   e. impurities in new drug substances [ICHQ3A(R)];
   f. impurities in new drug products [ICHQ3B(R)];
   g. impurities – residual solvents (maintenance) [ICHQ3C(M)];
   h. specifications for new drug substances and products – chemical substances (ICHQ6A and ICHQ4).

7. *Safety and efficacy.* It was announced that concerted discussions would continue on the following:

    a. clinical evaluation of QT/QTc interval prolongation and proarrhythmic potential for non-antiarrhythmic drugs (ICH E14);

    b. safety pharmacology studies for assessing the potential for delayed ventricular repolarisation (QT interval prolongation) by human pharmaceuticals (ICHS7B);

    c. ethnic factors in the acceptability of foreign clinical data (ICH E5).

8. *Pharmacovigilance.* The implementation issues concerning the standard of electronic reporting – data elements for the transmission of individual base safety reports [ICH E2B(M)] were adopted as was post-approval safety data management – definitions and standards for expedited reporting (ICH E2D). Pharmacovigilance planning (ICH E2E) reached Step 2 in November 2003. Also discussed were: Addendum to E2C – perodic safety update reports for marketed drugs (ICH E2 Cadd), ICHE2D and ICH E2E.

9. *Future work (as of January 2004).* Areas for future scientific dialogue included:

    a. new technologies to enhance drug discovery;

    b. specific areas regarding biological medicines derived from new biotechnology processes;

    c. pharmacogenetic/pharmacogenomic techniques to target medicines. These are in addition to three existing new initiatives:

        • risk management (Adopted ICH Q9)

        • data elements and standards for drug dictionaries (ICH M5)[13]

        • immunotoxicology studies (ICH 5B).

19.7 Developments: Washington, June 2004

At meetings of the SC and EWGs, discussions focused on:

1. how to streamline and optimize working practices and improve the management of the ICH process;

2. the ICH global cooperation group with significant progress on pharmaceutical development (Q8) and GMP risk management (Q9) and a new proposal on GMP quality systems;

3. the PDG, developed a position paper on interchangeability and identified three chapters for harmonisation;

4. QT/QTc (E14 topic);

5. Q&A documents that had reached Step 4: E2BM, CTD General, CTD efficacy and eCTD.

19.8 Developments: Yokohama November 2004

The ICH SC and EWGs from regulatory agencies and industry from the ICH regions of Europe, the US and Japan, plus observers from Health Canada and the generic industry, agreed on the text of a new ICH guideline — *Q8 Pharmaceutical Development*. The guideline describes the suggested contents for the P2 pharmaceutical development section of a regulatory submission in the ICH M4 Common Technical Document (CTD) format.[15]

The most important points of the guideline are as follows:

- There is no escalation of current requirement;
- It defines the baseline for any new submission according to the CTD;
- It defines optional opportunities for:
  - Regulatory flexibility;
  - Continuous improvement; and
  - Real time release;
- It opens the door for submitting quality by design data;
- It provides for optional update of P2 for adding knowledge for postapproval change;
- It defines what is a critical parameter; and
- If defines 'design space' and what is and is not a change.

The document is open for public consultation on www.ich.org/MediaServer/jser?@ ID=1707&@ MODE=GLB.

Also at this meeting which included, as well as he above, WHO, EFTA and the self-medication industries, work continued on the text of a guideline on Quality Risk Management for the pharmaceutical industry (Draft 4 was produced and will be finalised in April 2005)[16] Other topics discussed included Pharmacopoeial Convergence.[17]

19.9   Conclusion to date

The whole ICH process is continually changing – the concept is universally accepted but it is a dynamic process that has to be modified to suit new technologies and the aspirations of all the participants.

References

1. Cone M, D'Arcy PF and Harron DWG. ICH international conference on harmonisation of technical requirements for registration of pharmaceuticals for human use. *Int Pharm J* 1996;**10**: 104–6.
2. D'Arcy PF. ICH 3: a report and background. *Adverse Drug React Toxicol Rev* 1996;**15**:125–7.
3. D'Arcy PF. ICH 4: a report and background. *Adverse Drug React Toxicol Rev* 1997;**16**:199–206.
4. D'Arcy PF and Harron DWG. Proceedings of the Fourth International Conference on Harmonisation, Brussels 1997. Published at The Queen's University of Belfast. 1998:1–1158.
5. Cone M. Meeting Report: Fifth International Conference on Harmonisation. *The Regulatory Affairs Journal-Pharma* 2000;**11**: 954–5.
6. Zahn M. The Common Technical Document (CTD) Post-ICH 5. *The Regulatory Affairs Journal-Pharma* 2001;**12**:113–7.
7. Nick C. The CTD and beyond: surviving the impact. *The Regulatory Affairs Journal-Pharma* 2002;**13**:373–4.
8. Winzenrieth A. CTD roadmap. *The Regulatory Affairs Journal-Pharma* 2002;**13**:463–8.
9. Cone M. ICH Update. *The Regulatory Affairs Journal-Pharma* 2002;**13**:814–6.
10. Anon. Worldwide update: ICH6. *The Regulatory Affairs Journal-Pharma* 2004;**15**:30–2.
11. Anon. Worldwide update: ICH Guidelines. *The Regulatory Affairs Journal-Pharma* 2004;**15**:63–8.
12. Potter C. Pharmacopoeial Harmonization Revisited. *The Regulatory Affairs Journal-Pharma* 2004;**15**: 97–9.
13. Cone M. Reflections on the International Conference on Harmonisation. *The Regulatory Affairs Journal-Pharma* 2004;**15**:87–92.
14. De Crémiers. ICH6 – CTD Efficacy. *The Regulatory Affairs Journal-Pharma* 2004;**15**:174.
15. Erni F. Consensus on New ICH Pharmaceutical Development Guidelines. *The Regulatory Affairs Journal–Pharma* 2005;**16**:89–90.
16. Cough P. and Roenninger S. New Guideline on Quality Risk Management for the Pharmaceutical Industry takes shape. *The Regulatory Affairs Journal–Pharma* 2005;**16**:91–93.
17. Potter C and Zhan M. Pharmacopoeial Convergence 2005;**16**:94–96.

CHAPTER 20

20 The regulation of drug products by the United States Food and Drug Administration

Peter Barton Hutt

20.1 Introduction

The regulation of drug products by the Food and Drug Administration (FDA) in the United States is extraordinarily detailed and complex, and has enormous public costs as well as public benefits.[1] This chapter provides only a broad overview of this subject. Entire books,[2] and thousands of articles, have been devoted both to a comprehensive review of the area and to specific aspects. Anyone who wishes to understand it in greater detail must consult the governing statutes, regulations and guidance, as well as the experience of experts who have spent their entire careers working in the field. This chapter therefore presents a bare outline, permitting a glimpse into this extremely important and fascinating area but not a definitive analysis of any of its myriad aspects.

20.2 Regulatory Framework

20.2.1 Federal regulatory requirements

In the United States, regulatory policies are established by statutes enacted by Congress and signed by the President. These laws govern all regulatory requirements imposed by FDA upon drug products. No additional or different requirements can be imposed by any administrative official, but the statutory requirements are continually subject to reinterpretation and thus expansion as they are implemented by administrative action.

Laws are usually written by Congress in relatively general terms. They are intended to be implemented and enforced by administrative officials, in this instance located in FDA. Under the Federal Food, Drug and Cosmetic Act (FD&C Act) of 1938,[3] FDA is empowered to promulgate regulations implementing the statute, in accordance with the procedural requirements established by the Administrative Procedure Act.[4] These procedural requirements require that most regulations initially be published as proposals in the Federal Register, accompanied by a lengthy preamble explaining the purpose and meaning of the proposed regulations.[5] Time is then given for public comment. After the public comment has been received, FDA reviews the comment, makes a final decision on the regulations and promulgates the final regulations, together with a preamble explaining the decision with respect to each comment received and the reasons for the final version of the regulation. The regulations are then codified in the Code of Federal Regulations, without the explanatory preambles.

Following the promulgation of a federal regulation, any interested person may challenge the legality of the regulation in the courts.[6] The primary grounds for any such legal challenge are that the regulation exceeds the FDA statutory authority or that it is arbitrary or capricious.

Any person who challenges an FDA regulation in this way has a heavy burden to demonstrate that the regulation is illegal, and in most instances the FDA regulations are upheld by the courts.

Even though the FDA regulations are more detailed than the governing statute, they are, nonetheless, still often worded in general terms, and thus it becomes important to have more specific and detailed documents to guide daily decision-making in the agency. Such detailed policy comes in many forms, including the preambles to the regulations, written guidance, letters, speeches and a host of other documents, as well as unwritten tradition and practice. It is this area that largely governs daily FDA action. Because the vast bulk of FDA policy is not set forth either in the statute or in the regulations, it is uniquely a field where experience and judgement play a very large role.

20.2.2   State regulatory requirements

Decades ago, the individual states played an important part in the regulation of pharmaceutical products. As pharmaceutical science has become more complex and as the FDA regulation of the pharmaceutical industry has become more intense and pervasive, however, the states have shifted their traditional regulatory responsibilities to concentrate more heavily on food products and other items that are more appropriate for local control. Thus, state regulation of drug products is a relatively insignificant aspect of drug regulation in the United States today.

The individual states have retained their statutes governing both non-prescription and prescription drugs, however, and on occasion will exercise their authority to regulate in these areas. In recent years, this regulation has largely been limited to non-prescription drugs. For example, California has guidelines for slack fill in the packaging of non-prescription drugs.[7] On some occasions, states have also switched a non-prescription drug to prescription status in order to address a local abuse problem – usually only for a short duration. State regulation of drugs is not considered further in this chapter.

20.2.3   Product liability

The one aspect of state 'regulation' of pharmaceutical products that has increased is that of product liability. Drawing upon common law precedent extending back to medieval English origins, an individual harmed by a pharmaceutical product may bring a civil tort action under state law against the manufacturer or distributor of the drug for damages sustained. This can be a potent form of regulation. If a pharmaceutical product causes widespread damage to patients, the resulting tort liability could endanger the future of the manufacturer. One example is the Dalkon Shield, the damage actions from which resulted in the bankruptcy of AH Robbins. Further discussion of the field of product liability is beyond the scope of this chapter.

20.3   FDA History

The US Patent Office began its interest in agricultural matters in the 1830s. Eventually, an Agricultural Division was established in the Patent Office, and a chemical laboratory was funded in that division.[8]

When Congress created the United States Department of Agriculture (USDA) by statute in 1862,[9] the Agricultural Division of the Patent Office, and its chemical laboratory, were transferred to form the nucleus of the new department. A Chemical Division was immediately formed within USDA. This became the Division of Chemistry in 1890,[10] the Bureau of Chemistry in 1901,[11] the Food, Drug and Insecticide Administration in 1927[12] and the FDA in 1930.[13]

The FDA remained a part of USDA until it was transferred to the new Federal Security Agency in 1940.[14] When the Department of Health, Education and Welfare (HEW) was established in 1953, as a successor to the Federal Security Agency, FDA became a part of HEW.[15] HEW was renamed the Department of Health and Human Services (HHS) in 1979.[16]

Throughout this period, FDA (and its predecessor agencies) were created by administrative action, not by Congress. The governing statutes were all officially delegated for implementation and enforcement to the Secretary of Agriculture/HEW/HHS, not to the Commissioner of Food and Drugs. It was not until the Food and Drug Administration Act of 1988[17] that Congress officially established FDA as a government agency. To this day, however, the governing statutes delegate responsibility for implementation and enforcement to the Secretary of HHS.

Throughout this history, the Commissioner of Food and Drugs and his predecessors have also occupied a position that was created solely by administrative action, not by Congress. The Food and Drug Administration Act of 1988 also officially created the position of the Commissioner of Food and Drugs, and required that the Commissioner be appointed by the President and with the advice and consent of the Senate.

The Secretary of HHS is a Cabinet position, appointed by the President with the advice and consent of the Senate. The Commissioner of Food and Drugs reports to the Secretary of HHS.

Within FDA, there is an Office of the Commissioner and five product-oriented centres (for food, drugs, biologics, medical devices and veterinary medicine) located in the Washington DC area.[18] The Center for Drug Evaluation and Research and the Center for Biologics Evaluation and Research are responsible for regulation of drug products. Outside Washington DC, FDA has an extensive field force located in regions and districts throughout the United States, where FDA employees inspect drug establishments and conduct enforcement activities. The FDA field force is also responsible for the inspection of foreign drug establishments located throughout the world.

20.4 Historical Overview of Drug Regulation Statutes

Government concern about the adulteration and misbranding of pharmaceutical products extends back to ancient times.[19] Pliny the Elder, for example, in the first century AD, criticised 'the fashionable druggists' shops which spoil everything with fraudulent adulterations'.[20] As a result, various forms of government control to prevent the adulteration and misbranding of

food and drugs can be found in virtually every recorded civilisation. These regulatory controls were brought to the American colonies by early settlers, were enacted into state law following the American Revolution, and eventually were adopted by Congress as nationwide requirements in a series of federal statutes.

During most of the nineteenth century regulation of food and drug products was thought to be a matter of state and local concern, not appropriate for federal legislation, under the US Constitution. During this period, most federal laws governing food and drugs, therefore, related to foreign commerce rather than to domestic commerce. It is only since 1900 that regulation of food and drugs in the United States has been concluded to be a matter of national concern that justifies the enactment of federal statutes. The following paragraphs present a brief chronology of the major federal regulatory statutes governing non-prescription and prescription drug products in the United States.

20.4.1 The Vaccine Act of 1813

Following Edward Jenner's discovery of a smallpox vaccine in 1798, and the demonstration by Benjamin Waterhouse in the United States in 1800 that the vaccine was effective, fraudulent versions of the vaccine were marketed throughout the country. A Baltimore physician, John Smith, initially convinced the Maryland legislature to enact a statute designed to ensure the availability of an effective smallpox vaccine supply, and then persuaded Congress to enact the Vaccine Act of 1813[21] for the same purpose. This statute authorised the President to appoint a federal agent to 'preserve the genuine vaccine matter and to furnish the same to any citizen' who requested it.

The President promptly appointed Dr Smith as the first and, as it turned out, only federal vaccine agent. Following an outbreak of smallpox in North Carolina in 1821 that was thought to be caused by a contaminated lot of vaccine supplied by Dr Smith under the 1813 statute, the matter was investigated by two committees of the House of Representatives. The second committee concluded that regulation of smallpox vaccine should be undertaken by state and local officials rather than by the federal government, and as a result the 1813 Act was repealed in 1822.[22] As will be discussed below, 80 years later another drug tragedy led to the enactment of a new statute in 1902 under which vaccines are currently regulated by FDA.

20.4.2 The Import Drug Act of 1848

A congressional investigation in 1848 discovered that a wide variety of drugs imported into the United States for use by American troops in Mexico were adulterated. Congress therefore enacted a statute dealing solely with imported drugs. The 1848 Act[23] required that all imported drugs be labelled with the name of the manufacturer and the place of preparation, and be examined and appraised by the US Customs Service for 'quality, purity and fitness for medical purposes'. The Customs Service was directed to deny entry, into the United States, of any drug determined to be so adulterated or deteriorated as to be 'improper, unsafe or dangerous to be used for medical purposes'. This law remained in effect until it was replaced by another statute in 1922.[24]

20.4.3 The Biologics Act of 1902

As the result of a series of problems with biological drugs during the late 1890s, culminating in the death of several children in St Louis from a tetanus-infected diphtheria antitoxin, Congress enacted the Biologics Act of 1902.[25] This statute is the first known regulatory law in any country that required pre-market approval. It required approval of both a product licence application (PLA) and an establishment licence application (ELA) before any biological product could be marketed in interstate commerce. Although it was recodified in 1944[26] and 1997,[27] it has remained in effect without significant change since 1902. It was initially implemented by the Public Health Service, but was transferred to FDA in 1972.[28] Today it is implemented partly by the Center for Biologics Evaluation and Research (CBER) within FDA, which is located in buildings

on the campus of the National Institutes of Health, where it had been located prior to the 1972 transfer to FDA, and partly by the Center for Drug Evaluation and Research (CDER).

20.4.4 The Federal Food and Drugs Act of 1906

The first legislation to establish comprehensive nationwide regulation of all food and drugs was introduced in Congress in 1879. Largely because regulation of food and drugs was at that time thought to be a matter for state and local control, Congress debated this legislation for 27 years, ultimately enacting the Federal Food and Drugs Act in 1906.[29] This law broadly prohibited any adulteration or misbranding of drugs marketed in interstate commerce. Although it was quite short, and very broad and general in nature, it was extremely progressive for its time and included sufficient authority to permit FDA to take strong enforcement action against the unsafe, ineffective and mislabelled products that flooded the US market in the late 1800s. Unlike the Biologics Act of 1902, however, it contained no provisions requiring pre-market testing or approval for new drug products. An attempt by FDA to obtain this type of authority in 1912 was unsuccessful. Thus, Congress initially provided pre-market approval authority for biological drugs but not for other drugs.

20.4.5 The Federal Food, Drug and Cosmetic Act of 1938[30]

Shortly after President Franklin D Roosevelt took office in 1933, the Commissioner of Food and Drugs persuaded the new administration to propose a legislation to modernise the Federal Food and Drugs Act of 1906. The legislation was introduced in 1933, and ultimately enacted as the Federal Food, Drug and Cosmetic Act of 1938 (the FD&C Act), and debated by Congress for 5 years. Initially, it was intended primarily to add cosmetics and medical devices to the 1906 Act and to require additional affirmative labelling for food and drug products. In September 1937, however, more than 100 people died of diethylene glycol poisoning following use of Elixir Sulfanilamide, which used this chemical as the solvent without any form of safety testing. As a result, Congress added a pre-market notification requirement for new drugs to the pending legislation and enacted the new law in June 1938. Under this statute, a 'new drug' was defined as a drug that was not generally recognised as safe for its intended use. Before a new drug could be marketed, it was required to be tested on humans in accordance with investigational new drug (IND) regulations promulgated by FDA. When sufficient data were obtained under the IND to demonstrate the safety of the drug, the manufacturer was required to submit a new drug application (NDA) for the drug to FDA. If FDA did not disapprove the NDA within 60 days after filing, the NDA became effective and the drug could be marketed. The FD&C Act has been amended more than 100 times since 1938, and is now a very lengthy, detailed and complex law. The more important amendments relating to drugs are summarised below.

20.4.6   The Insulin and Antibiotics Amendments

Following enactment of the FD&C Act in 1938, insulin, penicillin and other antibiotic drugs were developed and marketed. Because of the unique production processes for these new pharmaceutical products, Congress enacted special provisions in the law requiring both that FDA approve each of them as safe and that FDA have the authority to require that each batch be certified by FDA as conforming to standards established for them by the agency. Thus, insulin and antibiotics were regulated by FDA under provisions that were similar to, but nonetheless different from, those established both for biologics and for chemical drugs.[31]

20.4.7   The Durham–Humphrey Amendments of 1951

The FD&C Act made no distinction between non-prescription and prescription drugs. A company could label a drug either way, depending upon marketing strategy. In 1939, however, FDA promulgated regulations declaring that any drug for which adequate directions for lay use could not be prepared must be sold only on prescription, thereby for the first time creating a mandatory prescription class of drugs. In order to make certain that the same drug, at the same dosage and for the same indication, could not be marketed both as a non-prescription and a prescription drug, in 1951 Congress codified the FDA regulations into law by enacting the Durham–Humphrey Amendments.

20.4.8   The Drug Amendments of 1962

Although thalidomide was marketed throughout Europe, the NDA for this drug was not marketed in the United States. When it was learned in mid-1962 that thalidomide was a potent human teratogen, Congress immediately enacted the Drug Amendments of 1962 to strengthen the new drug regulatory system to make certain that FDA had adequate statutory authority to ensure that no such drug could be marketed in the future.[33] The 1962 Amendments made a number of important changes. First, and most important, the amended law requires FDA explicitly to approve an NDA, rather than simply allowing the NDA to become effective through FDA inaction. Thus, the new drug provisions of the law were converted in 1962 from pre-market notification to pre-market approval, making them parallel with the Biologics Act of 1902. Second, a new drug was required to be shown to be effective as well as safe. Third, FDA was given additional authority to require compliance with current good manufacturing practices (GMP), to control the advertising of prescription drugs, to register drug establishments and to implement other regulatory requirements. Finally, FDA was required to review all NDAs that had become effective during 1938–62, to determine whether these drugs were effective as well as safe.

20.4.9   The Controlled Substances Act of 1970

Beginning in the early 1900s, Congress enacted a series of laws to control narcotic drugs and other drugs subject to abuse. All of these laws were repealed in 1970 and replaced by the Controlled Substances Act.[34] Responsibility for enforcement rests with the Drug Enforcement Administration (DEA) of the Department of Justice. FDA may approve an NDA for any controlled substance that has a legitimate medical use, but DEA may impose upon any new drug that is also a controlled substance additional regulatory requirements to prevent abuse and misuse by classifying it into one of four categories: schedules II (most restrictive)–V (least restrictive).

20.4.10 The Poison Prevention Packaging Act of 1970

In response to concern about household poisoning of children with hazardous household products, Congress enacted the Poison Prevention Packaging Act[35] to require the use of special child-resistant packaging. In accordance with regulations established by the Consumer Product Safety Commission, this type of packaging is now common for virtually all prescription drugs and for most non-prescription drugs.[36]

20.4.11 The Drug Listing Act of 1972

The Drug Amendments of 1962 included a requirement that every owner of a US drug establishment register that establishment with FDA. Congress enacted the Drug Listing Act of 1972[37] to add the requirement that every person who registers an establishment shall include a list of all drugs manufactured at that establishment.

20.4.12 The Orphan Drug Act of 1983

An orphan drug is one that is intended for use in rare diseases and thus for which there is not a sufficient market to justify the investment needed to demonstrate safety and effectiveness in order to obtain approval of an NDA. For more than 20 years FDA had permitted orphan drugs to be distributed through a permanent IND, with little or no thought that it would ever progress to an approved NDA. In 1983, Congress enacted the Orphan Drug Act[38] to provide

economic incentives for the industry to make the investment necessary to develop this category of drugs. When that proved insufficient, the Act was amended in 1984 to expand its coverage substantially, by providing that any drug with a use that has a target patient population of fewer than 200 000 people is automatically classified as an orphan drug.[39] Although the Orphan Drug Act does not provide for any different regulatory requirements from those applied to non-orphan drugs, the tax incentives and, in particular, a 7-years period of market exclusivity during which no competing NDA may be approved by FDA, combined with the extraordinary expansion in 1984 of the number of drugs covered by this statute, has had a major impact on drug development in the United States.

20.4.13 The Drug Price Competition and Patent Term Restoration Act of 1984

Under the new drug provisions as initially enacted in 1938 and as amended in 1962, all information in an IND and NDA was regarded as confidential proprietary business information that could not be revealed by FDA to the public or any competitor, and could not be used as the basis for any subsequent approval of a generic version of the pioneer new drug. Even after the patent for a pioneer new drug expired, competitors were unable to obtain an approved NDA for a generic version without duplicating all the animal and human testing needed to demonstrate safety and effectiveness. Congress, therefore, enacted the Drug Price Competition and Patent Term Restoration Act of 1984,[40] which authorised FDA to approve an abbreviated NDA for a generic version of a pioneer new drug after the patent and the statutory period of market exclusivity for the pioneer drug had expired. The result has been a substantial increase in the number of generic drugs available in the United States.

At the same time, Congress recognised that the effective patent term of pioneer drugs was dramatically reduced because of the time required for drug development by the FDA IND/NDA requirements prior to marketing. On average, the effective patent life for a pioneer drug was less than half the 17-years period then specified by Congress under the patent law, as of the time of NDA approval. For some drugs, no patent could be obtained. As part of the 1984 legislation, Congress therefore directed the Patent Office to extend the patent for a pioneer drug for up to 5 years in order to compensate for the lost patent life resulting from FDA regulatory review requirements. Congress also specified a minimum period of 3 or 5 years of market exclusivity during which no generic version could be approved by FDA even if there was no patent protection.

20.4.14 The Drug Export Amendments Act of 1986

Under the FD&C Act as enacted in 1938, adulterated and misbranded drugs may lawfully be exported but an unapproved new drug could not. This was a drafting error, but it was nonetheless enforced by FDA. Congress therefore enacted the Drug Export Amendments Act of 1986,[41] which authorised the limited export of unapproved new human drugs and biological products after FDA had approved an export application. An export application could be approved only if

- There was an active IND
- Approval of an NDA was actively being pursued in the United States
- The product was for export to one or more of 21 listed countries with sophisticated regulatory systems
- The product was currently approved and marketed in the receiving country
- FDA had not disapproved the product
- The product was manufactured in conformity with GMP and was not adulterated
- The product's labelling listed the countries to which FDA permitted it to be exported
- FDA had not determined that domestic manufacture of the drug for export was contrary to the public health and safety of the United States
- The product was properly labelled for export.

Not surprisingly, these restrictions were so tight that most US companies preferred to move their manufacturing facilities overseas, and thus to source the drug from abroad, rather than to make it in the United States and attempt to obtain FDA approval for an export application. As a result, in 1996 the 1986 Amendments were repealed and replaced with substantially more flexible provisions.[42]

20.4.15 The Prescription Drug Marketing Act of 1987

Congressional investigations in the mid-1980s demonstrated that pharmaceutical products were being exported from the United States and later imported back into the country without adequate assurance that they had not become adulterated or misbranded while abroad. Congress responded by enacting the Prescription Drug Marketing Act[43] of 1987, which makes the importation of US drugs by anyone other than the manufacturer illegal. It also prohibits the sale of drug samples and the resale of drug products initially sold to healthcare institutions. Distribution of drug samples by pharmaceutical manufacturers is permitted only in response to a written request, for which a receipt is obtained. The provisions requiring state licensure of wholesale distributors of prescription drugs were subsequently clarified in the Prescription Drug Amendments of 1992.[44]

20.4.16 The Generic Drug Enforcement Act of 1992

Following enactment of the Drug Price Competition and Patent Term Restoration Act of 1984, FDA embarked upon a major campaign to expedite approval of abbreviated NDAs for generic versions of important pioneer drugs for which the patents had expired. Because of the enormous economic profit that could be made by the generic drug company that marketed the first generic version of an important pioneer drug, a number of generic drug manufacturers submitted fraudulent data to FDA as part of abbreviated NDAs, and even paid illegal bribes to FDA officials in an attempt to obtain preferential handling of their applications. When this scandal came to light, in addition to the criminal prosecution of the individuals and companies involved, Congress enacted the Generic Drug Enforcement Act of 1992[45] to increase the penalties for such illegal behaviour. These new penalties include mandatory and permissive debarment of corporations and individuals, suspension and withdrawal of approval of abbreviated NDAs and civil money penalties. Although the 1992 Act applies primarily to generic drugs, it also provides mandatory and permissive debarment for individuals who engage in wrongdoing with respect to any drug, whether generic or pioneer. All of the provisions of the Act apply to both non-prescription and prescription drugs.

20.4.17 The Prescription Drug User Fee Act of 1992[46]

Following enactment of the Drug Amendments of 1962, the time needed to develop the data and information to demonstrate the safety and effectiveness of a new drug, and to obtain FDA approval of an NDA, escalated. As a result, a 'drug lag' developed between the pharmaceutical products available in the rest of the world and those available in the United States. FDA on many occasions pointed out that the time needed for FDA review of an IND or an NDA was at least in part a function of the resources available to the agency. Although both FDA and the pharmaceutical industry initially opposed the imposition on the industry of 'user fees' that would generate additional revenue to permit FDA to hire additional people to review INDs and NDAs, both abruptly reversed their earlier positions and agreed to enactment of the Prescription Drug User Fee Act of 1992.[46] Under this statute, FDA was authorised to collect user fees for 5 years based on annual fees levied for each pioneer prescription drug and each pioneer prescription drug establishment, as well as a one-time fee for each NDA for a pioneer new drug. The fees do not apply to generic or pioneer drugs after they become subject to generic competition. All of the revenue from these user fees is required to be in addition to the existing FDA budget and must be used solely for the IND/NDA review

system. User fees were extended for another 5 years under the Food and Drug Modernization Act of 1997,[47] and for another 5 years under the Prescription Drug User Fee Amendment of 2002.[48]

20.4.18 The FDA Export Reform and Enhancement Act of 1996[49]

Following the November 1994 elections, in which the Republican Party won control of both the House of Representatives and the Senate for the first time in 40 years, Congress began to consider statutory reform of FDA in earnest. When the reform legislation became stalled in 1996, the provisions dealing with the export requirements of the FD&C Act were separated out and enacted. The 1996 Act repealed the Drug Export Amendments Act of 1986[50] and adopted a much more liberal and expansive approach. A drug that is not approved in the United States may now be exported to any country in the world if it complies with the laws of that country and has valid marketing authorisation by the appropriate authority in any country included in a new list of 25 countries with sophisticated regulatory systems. A drug that is not approved in the United States may be exported for investigational use in any listed country. FDA approval of the export of a drug that is not approved in the United States is required only if it is exported for investigational use in a non-listed country. Although the 1996 Act is a major improvement over the 1986 Act, the export provisions of the FD&C Act continue to be the most stringent in the world, and thus many US companies continue to manufacture products abroad in order to avoid its cumbersome requirements.

20.4.19 The Food and Drug Administration Modernization Act of 1997

One year after the drug export provisions of the FD&C Act were reformed, Congress enacted the remainder of the reform legislation that it had been considering. The Food and Drug Administration Modernization Act of 1997[51] is a lengthy, comprehensive and complex statute. Although the impact of this statute has been modest at best, it is the first statute since the FD&C Act was enacted in 1938 that has attempted significant reform. The following brief summary of the major provisions in the 1997 Act is sufficient to convey the broad scope of this legislation.

• Reauthorises prescription drug user fees for another 5 years.
• Establishes for a period of 5 years an additional 6 months of market exclusivity for paediatric studies of new drugs.
• Establishes a fast-track system for the study and approval of new drugs that address unmet medical needs related to serious or life-threatening conditions.
• Establishes a data bank in NIH to provide information on research relating to new drugs for serious or life-threatening diseases, for use by the general public.
• Establishes new criteria for permitting healthcare economic information relating to new drugs in labelling and advertising.
• Clarifies the requirements for NDA approval to say that data from one adequate and well-controlled study, together with confirmatory evidence, may, in the discretion of FDA, constitute substantial evidence of effectiveness of a new drug.
• Requires FDA to consult with NIH and representatives of the pharmaceutical industry to review and develop guidance on the inclusion of women and minorities in clinical trials.
• Adds a provision that is intended to reduce the number of post-market manufacturing changes requiring FDA approval and otherwise to make it easier to implement manufacturing changes for approved new drugs.
• Reduces the amount of information required to be submitted to FDA as part of an IND application.
• Clarifies the power of FDA to prevent or halt a clinical investigation of a new drug through use of a clinical hold.
• Requires FDA to issue guidance describing when abbreviated reports may be submitted in lieu of full reports for clinical and non-clinical studies required to be included in an NDA.

• Requires FDA to issue guidance for NDA reviewers relating to promptness in conducting the review, technical excellence, lack of bias and conflict of interest, and knowledge of regulatory and scientific standards.
• Requires FDA to meet with a sponsor upon reasonable written request for the purpose of reaching agreement on the design of pivotal trials, and provides that, after testing begins, the agreement cannot be changed unilaterally by FDA unless the director of the reviewing division issues a written decision that the change must be made because of a safety or effectiveness issue identified after the testing has begun.
• Provides that a decision by the reviewing division is binding on the FDA field and compliance personnel unless the reviewing division agrees to change its decision.
• States that no action of the reviewing division may be delayed based on a delay in action by field personnel.
• Provides for the use of scientific advisory committees to provide expert advice and recommendations to FDA regarding clinical investigation and approval of new drugs.
• Requires FDA to promulgate separate regulations governing the approval of radiopharmaceuticals.
• Amends the Public Health Service Act to eliminate the requirement of separate product and establishment licences and directs FDA to harmonise the review and approval requirements for biological products and new drugs to the extent possible.
• Provides that a drug manufactured in a pilot or other small-scale facility can be used to establish safety and effectiveness and to obtain marketing approval prior to scale-up unless FDA determines that a full-scale facility is necessary to ensure safety or effectiveness.
• Eliminates the separate regulatory requirements for insulin and antibiotics, and makes these drugs subject to the IND and NDA requirements.
• For prescription drugs replaces the old label statement 'Caution: Federal Law prohibits dispensing without a prescription' with a new 'Rx Only' designation.

- Deletes the obsolete statutory provisions relating to labelling of 17 listed 'habit-forming' drugs.
- Establishes an entire new programme to control pharmacy compounding.
- Reauthorises a clinical pharmacology programme in FDA.
- Establishes new requirements for Phase IV studies that the manufacturer has agreed to conduct as a condition for NDA approval.
- Requires notice to FDA from the sole manufacturer of a life-supporting product 6 months before the manufacturer discontinues production.
- Establishes national uniformity in the regulation of non-prescription drugs.
- Requires the label of a non-prescription drug to bear the quantity or the proportion of each active ingredient.
- Requires the label of a non-prescription drug to bear the name of each inactive ingredient, listed in alphabetical order.
- Authorises manufacturers of new drugs to disseminate information on unapproved (off-label) uses of approved products under very limited conditions.
- Authorises expanded access to drugs that are still undergoing investigation for serious diseases and conditions.
- Attempts to reduce the disincentives to the submission of supplemental NDAs by reducing the cost and increasing the efficiency of handling them within FDA.
- Establishes dispute resolution mechanisms for the resolution of scientific controversies relating to new drugs.
- Requires FDA to promulgate a regulation regarding the development, issuance and use of guidance documents, and requires FDA to ensure that employees do not deviate from guidance without appropriate justification and supervisory concurrence.
- Establishes a statutory mission statement for FDA, which includes both the promotion of public health by taking appropriate action on the marketing of regulated products in a timely manner and the protection of public health by ensuring that regulated products are safe, effective and properly labelled.

- Requires FDA to publish a plan to bring the agency into compliance with each of the obligations established under the FD&C Act, and to review and revise the plan biennially.
- Requires FDA to publish an annual report in the Federal Register on its performance under the agency plan.
- Requires FDA to establish an information system regarding all submissions to the agency requesting agency action.
- Requires FDA to provide training and education programmes for employees relating to their regulatory responsibilities.
- Requires FDA to support the office of the US Trade Representative to reduce the burden of regulation and harmonise international regulatory requirements consistent with the purposes of the FD&C Act.
- Requires FDA support of efforts to move towards the acceptance of mutual recognition agreements between the European Union and the United States.
- Requires FDA to participate in meetings with foreign governments to discuss and reach agreement on methods and approaches to harmonise regulatory requirements.
- Provides that an environmental impact statement prepared in accordance with the FDA regulations shall be considered to meet the requirements of the National Environmental Policy Act, notwithstanding any other provision of law.
- Requires FDA to implement programmes and policies that will foster collaboration between FDA, NIH and other science-based federal agencies in order to enhance the scientific and technical expertise available to FDA in discharging its duties with respect to regulating drugs.
- Authorises FDA to enter into contracts with any organisation or individual with relevant expertise to review and evaluate any application or submission for the approval or classification of an article, for the purpose of making recommendations to the agency on the matter.
- Provides that a person who submits an application or other submission under the FD&C Act may ask FDA for a determination respecting the proper regulatory classification of the product

and the organisation within FDA that will regulate the product.

- Requires registration of foreign drug establishments.
- Establishes a rebuttable presumption of interstate commerce for drugs.
- Provides that any report or information relating to the safety of a drug that is submitted to FDA shall not be construed to reflect necessarily a conclusion that the report constitutes an admission that the product caused or contributed to an adverse experience.
- Repeals the former provision in the FD&C Act that prohibited any representation in labelling or advertising that FDA had approved an application for a new drug.

Only some of these provisions have been implemented by FDA, and the full impact of most of them remains to be determined.

20.4.20   The Medicine Equity and Drug Safety Act of 2000

The Prescription Drug Marketing Act of 1987 prohibited the reimportation into the United States of any prescription drug that had been exported. In response to public concern about the high cost of prescription drugs in the United States, Congress passed the Medicine Equity and Drug Safety Act of 2000[52] to authorise the reimportation of prescription drugs if the Secretary of HHS certified to Congress that its implementation would impose no risk to the public health and safety and that it would result in a significant reduction of the cost of covered products to the American consumer. The Secretary of HHS under both the Clinton and the Bush administrations determined that these certifications could not be made and this law has therefore never been implemented.

20.4.21   The Best Pharmaceuticals for Children Act

The paediatric drug testing provisions in the Food and Drug Administration Modernization Act of 1997 had an automatic 5-years sunset limitation. In January 2002, Congress enacted the Best Pharmaceuticals for Children Act[53] reauthorising these provisions, with changes, for another 5 years. The 2002 Act, like the 1997 provisions, relies upon incentives for voluntary industry testing of drugs used for children.

20.4.22   The Public Health Security and Bioterrorism Preparedness and Response Act of 2002

Congress passed the Public Health Security and Bioterrorism Preparedness and Response Act of 2002[54] as part of the Homeland Security Act, in response to the terrorism attacks of 11 September, 2001. The new law contains several provisions that are designed to strengthen the public health system generally and the availability of drugs, biological products and medical devices for countering bioterrorism, in particular.

20.4.23   The Pediatric Research Equity Act of 2003

Following enactment of the Best Pharmaceuticals for Children Act in 2002, a court ruled that the FDA regulation requiring mandatory paediatric testing of new drugs is not authorised under the FD&C Act and is thus illegal.[55] Congress responded by enacting the Pediatric Research Equity Act of 2003,[56] providing specific authorisation for FDA to require mandatory paediatric testing for new drugs.

20.5   Other Pharmaceutical Products

In addition to biological and chemical drugs, two other categories of pharmaceutical products deserve brief mention: animal drugs and human medical devices. Both are beyond the scope of the present chapter.

20.5.1   Animal drugs

Under the Federal Food and Drugs Act of 1906 and the FD&C Act of 1938 animal feed and drugs were regulated under the same provisions as human food and drugs. A separate statute, the Animal Virus, Serum and Toxin Act of 1913,[57] was enacted by Congress to authorise USDA to regulate biological drugs intended for use in animals, and USDA retains jurisdiction over that statute to this day. To simplify FDA regulation of animal feed and drugs, Congress enacted the Animal Drug Amendments of 1968.[58] Following the approach of the 1984 statute authorising FDA approval of generic versions of human new drugs, Congress also enacted the Generic Animal Drug and Patent Term Restoration Act of 1988,[59] the Animal Drug User Fee Act of 2003,[60] and the Minor Use and Minor Species Animal Health Act of 2004.[61]

20.5.2   Medical devices

Medical devices were first made subject to FDA regulation under the FD&C Act of 1938. At that time, the statute included no requirement for pre-market testing or approval. Congress enacted the Medical Device Amendments of 1976[62] to require pre-market notification for all medical devices, and pre-market approval for some old and new devices for which there is no adequate assurance of safety and effectiveness. The 1976 Amendments established a broad new array of statutory requirements and enforcement provisions. This new regulatory approach was supplemented by the Safe Medical Devices Act of 1990[63] and further refined by the Medical Device Amendments of 1992,[64] the Food and Drug Administration Modernization Act of 1997,[65] and the Medical Devise User Fee and Modernization Act of 2002.[66]

20.6   Two Classes of Drug Products

There are two classes of drugs under the FD&C Act in the United States: non-prescription and prescription. Neither the Federal Food and Drugs Act of 1906 nor the FD&C Act of 1938 distinguished between non-prescription and prescription drugs or established a class of mandatory prescription drugs. Shortly after the FD&C Act

was enacted in 1938, however, FDA promulgated regulations establishing criteria for a class of drugs that could only lawfully be sold by prescription.[67] Those regulations were later codified into law by Congress in the Durham–Humphrey Amendments of 1951.[68] Under this statute, prescription status is mandatory for drugs that are not safe for use except under a practitioner's supervision, and drugs limited to prescription sale under an NDA. The statutory criteria for determining prescription status are toxicity, other potential for harmful effect, and the method of use and collateral measures necessary to use the drug. In all instances today, the prescription or non-prescription status of a new drug is determined by the NDA.

A drug may be switched from prescription to non-prescription status.[69] Prior to 1970 this was most often accomplished by FDA promulgation of a regulation. During 1970–90, a switch from prescription to non-prescription was most frequently accomplished as part of the FDA OTC Drug Review, discussed in detail below. Now that the OTC Drug Review is substantially complete, and with the availability of market exclusivity under the Drug Price Competition and Patent Term Restoration Act of 1984, a switch from prescription to non-prescription status is accomplished primarily through a supplemental NDA.

Non-prescription drugs may be sold at any kind of retail store in the United States, ranging from a pharmacy to a grocery store to a gasoline filling station. There are no criteria or limitations on their method of distribution and sale. Pharmacy groups have contended that FDA should establish a 'third class' of drugs that would be available only through a pharmacy, and have used those prescription drugs that are in the process of being switched to non-prescription status as one example of the need for such a new class. FDA has declined to establish such a third class, on both policy and legal grounds.[70] First, FDA has stated that any drug switched by the agency from prescription to non-prescription status is sufficiently safe for sale in any retail establishment, and that a requirement limiting sale to a pharmacy would provide an unjustified monopoly to pharmacists. Second,

FDA has stated that the FD&C Act provides no authority for FDA to restrict distribution of a non-prescription drug to pharmacies.

20.7 Regulation of Non-prescription Drugs

20.7.1 Adulteration and misbranding

Since 1906, the adulteration or misbranding of a non-prescription drug has been illegal in the United States.[71] Both 'adulteration' and 'misbranding' are terms of art, defined in the FD&C Act. Adulteration includes such acts as the failure to comply with good manufacturing practices; the use of a container that may render the contents injurious to health; the use of an illegal colour additive; failure to comply with *United States Pharmacopeia* requirements; failure to meet labelled strength or purity and related prohibited acts. Misbranding includes

- such labelling violations as any false or misleading labelling
- the failure to contain mandatory information relating to the name and address of the manufacturer and the net quantity of contents
- the failure to bear adequate directions for use and warnings against unsafe use
- the failure to meet packaging and labelling requirements established by the *United States Pharmacopeia*
- the failure to use packaging and labelling to reduce product deterioration
- danger to health when used as recommended in the labelling
- the failure to obtain batch certification for an antibiotic for which such certification is required
- the failure to comply with a large number of other statutory requirements, including drug establishment registration and product listing, and poison prevention and tamper-resistant packaging.

The adulteration and misbranding provisions of the statute itself are continually expanded by FDA regulations that impose additional requirements either for all non-prescription drugs or for specific categories. Accordingly, current requirements can be determined only by consulting FDA regulations and other policy statements, as well as the statute itself.

20.7.2 The IND/NDA system

Since 1938, non-prescription drugs have been subject to the new drug provisions of the Act as well as the adulteration and misbranding provisions. As a practical matter, however, the new drug provisions cover only those non-prescription drugs that have been switched from prescription status through a supplemental NDA. Almost all new chemical entity drugs are initially restricted by FDA to prescription status. Only a handful of new chemical entity drugs that require an NDA – perhaps one per decade – are marketed initially with non-prescription status. For those non-prescription drugs that do go through the IND/NDA system, the requirements are no different than for a prescription drug. These requirements are discussed in detail below.

20.7.3 The OTC drug review

During the period beginning with enactment of the new drug provisions in the FD&C Act in 1938 and ending with enactment of the Drug Amendments of 1962, there were approximately 420 NDAs for non-prescription drugs. Many of these NDAs were for long-established ingredients for which no NDA was actually required, but it was so simple to obtain an effective NDA during that time that many were submitted simply to obtain a perceived marketing advantage. As part of the Drug Amendments of 1962, FDA was required to review these 420 NDAs and to determine whether the drugs were effective as well as safe. Rather than limit its inquiry to these 420 specific non-prescription drug products, FDA decided instead to broaden the scope of its review to all active ingredients used in all non-prescription drugs on the market at that time. The agency also decided to review the safety and labelling as well as the effectiveness of the active ingredients in these products.

In 1972, FDA announced the beginning of its massive OTC Drug Review – the largest and most extensive review of the safety, effectiveness and labelling of non-prescription drugs ever undertaken.[72] FDA established panels of experts to review individual categories of non-prescription drugs and to prepare reports on their conclusions and recommendations. Those reports were published as proposed monographs establishing the conditions for safe, effective and properly labelled non-prescription drugs within each category. Following public comment, FDA published a tentative final monograph. Following additional public comment and a public hearing before the Commissioner, FDA established the final monograph. The documents that comprise these public proceedings represent an extremely important record of the status of non-prescription drug active ingredients and finished products in the United States.

By the early 1980s, all of the FDA panels had completed their deliberations and issued their reports. Because the industry largely followed the conclusions and recommendations of these reports, most of the impact of the OTC Drug Review had already been reflected in the marketplace. Nonetheless, a number of monographs remain to be completed and it will be some years before the OTC Drug Review is fully finished.

An OTC drug monograph establishes those conditions under which a non-prescription drug is generally recognised as safe and effective and properly labelled, and thus may be lawfully marketed in the United States without the need for an NDA or any other type of FDA approval. Any person may market a non-prescription drug in the United States today in compliance with one of these monographs (or, where no final monograph has been issued, in accordance with a tentative final monograph). One of the major purposes behind the OTC Drug Review was to establish, by regulations, the criteria under which an NDA is not required. Where a product is marketed with any deviation from an OTC drug monograph, however, some form of NDA is required in order to justify that deviation before marketing will be permitted.[73] In short, complete compliance with

an OTC drug monograph guarantees immediate marketing without any form of pre-market approval. Of course, all non-prescription drugs must comply with the general adulteration and misbranding provisions of the law, including GMP, establishment registration and drug listing.

20.7.4 Tamper-resistant packaging

In September 1982, it was discovered that several people living in Chicago had died from cyanide poisoning after taking Extra-Strength Tylenol capsules. FDA promptly promulgated regulations requiring tamper-resistant packaging for most non-prescription drug products.[74] Congress followed by enacting the Federal Anti-Tampering Act of 1983,[75] which makes it a crime to tamper with a consumer product with reckless disregard for the risk of persons or with intent to cause injury to a business. A number of individuals have in fact been prosecuted for illegal tampering under this statute.

20.7.5 Non-prescription drug labelling

Based on an extensive rule-making, FDA promulgated regulations in March 1999 establishing completely new labelling requirements for all non-prescription drug products.[76] The new regulations require the use of a 'drug facts' box using a standardised format and type size. The new labelling requirements are being phased in, in coordination with the development of final monographs for non-prescription drugs. Industry has petitioned FDA for modification of some of the new requirements, and changes may be adopted through revision of the new labelling regulations, revisions of individual monographs, or the issuance of guidance.

20.7.6 Non-prescription drug advertising

In 1914, Congress enacted a statute to prohibit unfair methods of competition and created the Federal Trade Commission to implement this new law.[77] The FTC and the courts interpreted unfair methods of competition to include false or misleading labelling and advertising of non-prescription drugs and other consumer products. In 1933, when the legislation that became the FD&C Act was first introduced, it proposed to transfer the jurisdiction over food and drug advertising from the FTC to FDA. Not surprisingly, the FTC objected. Congress ultimately resolved this controversy in 1938, by enacting both the Wheeler–Lea Amendments to the FTC Act[78] and the FD&C Act. Congress gave the FTC jurisdiction over advertising and FDA jurisdiction over labelling. Because the FTC was also given jurisdiction over all unfair or deceptive acts or practices, however, it has jurisdiction over labelling as well as advertising. And because the courts have agreed with FDA that the agency may refer to advertising to determine the proper regulatory classification and requirements for a product under the FD&C Act, FDA to some extent indirectly regulates advertising. To clarify the situation, in September 1971 the FTC and FDA entered into a Memorandum of Understanding.[79] Under this agreement, the FTC has primary jurisdiction over advertising and FDA has primary jurisdiction over labelling of non-prescription drugs and other FDA-regulated products.

20.7.7 Industry self-regulation

The Consumer Healthcare Products Association (CHPA), the US trade association representing the non-prescription drug industry, has established a number of voluntary codes and guidelines to supplement FDA regulation of non-prescription drugs. Among these are recommended package sizes for non-prescription drug categories, label 'flags' to bring the attention of consumers to significant product changes, bulk mail sampling of non-prescription drugs, expiry dating of non-prescription drugs, product identification of solid dosage non-prescription drugs and label readability for non-prescription drugs. Although these are not legal requirements, they are widely followed in the non-prescription drug industry.

20.8 Regulation of prescription drugs

It is particularly difficult to summarise FDA regulation of prescription drugs. The statutory provisions are long and complex, the regulations consume hundreds of pages in the Code of Federal Regulations, the preambles cover thousands of pages in the Federal Register and the guidelines and policy directives are numerous and diverse. The discussion will therefore begin with a historical overview of the development of FDA regulation of prescription drugs. This is followed by a brief analysis of how the current system works.

This section is limited to drugs regulated under the FD&C Act. Biological drugs are considered in the next section.

20.8.1 Historical overview[80]

As enacted in 1938, the FD&C Act defined a 'new drug' as any drug that was not generally recognised as safe.[81] Section 505 of the 1938 Act provided that an NDA must be submitted for every new drug, and authorised FDA to permit an NDA to become effective or to disapprove it, but not affirmatively to approve an NDA. If FDA took no action within 60 days after the filing of an NDA, the NDA automatically became effective and the drug could lawfully be marketed.

During the first few years after 1938 the pharmaceutical industry submitted thousands of NDAs. Because FDA was unprepared to deal with this large number, it advised drug manufacturers that NDAs were not required for 'old drugs' that were generally recognised as safe (GRAS), and in fact refused to accept NDAs for these drugs. This substantially reduced the numbers of NDAs that were submitted to, and accepted by, FDA. For example, more than 4000 NDAs had been submitted by 1941 but by 1962 NDAs for only 9457 individual drug products had become effective. Most prescription drugs were marketed on the conclusion of FDA or the manufacturer that they were GRAS, and hence old drugs that did not require an NDA.

Following enactment of the Drug Amendments of 1962, FDA immediately encountered two problems. First, the pharmaceutical industry submitted a substantially increased number of INDs and NDAs, which again overwhelmed the resources of FDA to deal with them. Second, the 1962 Amendments required FDA to review all of the NDAs that had become effective between 1938 and 1962 on the basis of a demonstration of safety, and to determine whether these drugs were also effective. Because of the overwhelming number of current INDs and NDAs for new products, FDA had no resources to devote to this requirement. Accordingly, in June 1966 FDA contracted with the National Academy of Sciences (NAS) to conduct the review of 1938–62 NDAs.

The NAS review was conducted by panels of experts in specific drug categories. Drugs were rated in one or other of the following six categories: (1) effective, (2) probably effective, (3) possibly effective, (4) ineffective, (5) effective but other drugs are preferable or (6) ineffective as a fixed combination. Because roughly half of the drugs were no longer marketed, the NAS ultimately reviewed approximately 4000 different drug formulations. Brief reports, many consisting only of a single sentence, were transmitted to FDA by the NAS in 1967–8. FDA then undertook to implement these reports in the form of notices published in the Federal Register as part of what the agency called the Drug Efficacy Study Implementation (DESI) programme.

In order to implement the NAS reports, FDA found that it must first address a number of important policy issues. First, FDA was required to determine whether the NAS findings would apply only to the pioneer drug for which the NDA was submitted or would also apply to all subsequently marketed generic versions of the drug. FDA determined that the latter approach was required, which led to extensive litigation. The FDA policy on this matter was ultimately upheld by the Supreme Court in June 1973.[82]

Second, FDA had to confront the fact that prior to the 1962 Amendments it had issued hundreds of 'old drug' opinion letters for generic versions of pioneer new drugs. It, therefore, issued a statement of policy in May 1968 revoking all of those opinions.[83]

Third, FDA was confronted with potentially thousands of requests for formal trial-type administrative hearings before it could remove from the market pre-1962 new drugs that were found to be less than effective. The requirement of formal administrative hearings would have effectively precluded implementation of the 1962 Amendments. FDA resolved this by publishing in the Federal Register regulations defining the new statutory requirement of adequate and well-controlled clinical investigations,[84] and issuing summary judgement notices withdrawing approval of new drugs that failed to submit clinical studies which seemingly met the requirements of the new regulations. The regulations defining adequate and well-controlled clinical investigations were upheld in the courts, and the summary judgement procedure was also upheld.[85] Thus, the number of drugs for which formal administrative hearings were required was substantially reduced.

Fourth, FDA established a new procedure for regulating generic versions of pre-1962 pioneer drugs that were found under the DESI programme to be safe and effective. FDA established the 'abbreviated' NDA, which required the submission of information to FDA on bioequivalence and manufacturing controls only, and not on basic safety and effectiveness.[86] Any manufacturer who wished to market a generic version of a pre-1962 pioneer drug found to be safe and effective under the NAS review could obtain FDA approval through an abbreviated NDA.

In 1972, 10 years after the 1962 Amendments were enacted, three lower court rulings threatened to destroy the FDA approach to these matters. The agency successfully took all three cases, as well as a fourth in which FDA had prevailed, to the US Supreme Court, and in June 1973 the Supreme Court sustained FDA on all of the legal issues involved.[87] From then on, the basic approach to FDA implementation of the 1962 Amendments was established and strengthened.

The FDA pace of implementation of the 1962 Amendments was, however, necessarily slow. The American Public Health Association therefore brought a lawsuit to require FDA to complete its DESI programme for pre-1962 new drugs, and the federal district court entered an order requiring completion within 4 years.[88] Although FDA to this day has still not completed this programme, the court order did impose a greater sense of urgency and led FDA to devote greater resources to the matter.

Throughout this time, FDA was groping for a consistent approach to the handling of generic drugs. Initially, it revoked all 'old drug' opinion letters. Later, it proposed a procedure for determining old drug status for products.[89] Following that, it concluded that an abbreviated NDA should be submitted for all generic versions of pre-1962 new drugs.[90] In 1975, it again reversed itself and decided to develop old drug monographs, similar to the non-prescription drug monographs, for which an NDA would not be required.[91] Still later, it abandoned that approach and again stated that an abbreviated NDA would be required for all generic versions of pre-1962 new drugs.[92] That position was challenged in the courts, but was upheld by the Supreme Court.[93]

An attempt was made during 1977–80 to resolve all of these issues through a comprehensive revision of the new drug provisions of the FD&C Act. The legislation passed the Senate in 1979[94] but did not reach the floor of the House and, because the legislation was so detailed and complex, it was never again seriously considered.

By 1980, a new problem had emerged. FDA had administratively created the concept of an abbreviated NDA to handle generic versions of pre-1962 pioneer new drugs, but there was no similar mechanism for the approval of generic versions of post-1962 new drugs. As time went by, more and more post-1962 pioneer new drugs lost patent protection, but retained an equivalent protection under the FD&C Act because FDA had no authority to approve any form of an abbreviated NDA for generic versions of these drugs. FDA therefore began to search for a solution to this problem. In 1978, FDA announced it would approve a 'paper' NDA for a generic copy of a post-1962 pioneer new drug based on the published scientific data for the drug. This policy was upheld in the courts,[95] but it had relatively little impact because there were insufficient published animal and human data to approve generic versions of most post-1962 new drugs. Thus, relatively few paper NDAs were approved by FDA.

Another drug tragedy in early 1984 focused FDA on yet another aspect of regulating prescription new drugs. An intravenous vitamin E product marketed without an NDA produced serious adverse reactions that required a nationwide recall.[96] FDA concluded that there were approximately 5000 prescription drugs marketed without an approved NDA of any kind. Some 1800 would eventually be subject to the requirement for an abbreviated NDA when the DESI programme was fully implemented, but another 2400 were never subject to the NAS review because they were on the market prior to the FD&C Act of 1938, or were otherwise grandfathered. FDA was forced to concede that these products could remain on the market until the agency could find the resources to review them and consider appropriate regulation.[97] Indeed, new versions of these products can still be marketed as long as they are identical to the previously marketed versions. FDA did promulgate a regulation requiring adverse drug reaction reports for all prescription drugs marketed without an approved NDA, in order to track any potential public health problem.[98]

In the past three decades, FDA has proceeded slowly but surely with the DESI programme implementing the NAS review of pre-1962 new drugs. Where drugs have been found ineffective, most have been taken off the market using the summary judgement procedure. A few manufacturers have succeeded in requiring an administrative hearing, but none has prevailed before an administrative law judge, the Commissioner or the courts.

In a surprisingly large number of instances, manufacturers decided to market new drugs without any NDA, and outside the 1984 FDA policy that permits such products if they are identical to old products that never had an NDA, solely on the basis that they were old drugs because they were generally recognised as safe and effective (GRAS and GRAE) and therefore did not require an approved NDA. FDA brought enforcement actions against dozens of these products, and because the agency prevailed in every case, this approach is rarely tried today.

As indicated above, the status of generic versions of both pre-1962 and post-1962 new drugs was settled by Congress in the Drug Price Competition and Patent Term Restoration Act of 1984.[99] That statute will be discussed in greater detail below.

Accordingly, the large conceptual issues that confronted FDA following enactment of the Drug Amendments of 1962 have now been resolved, and most (but not all) of the large categories of DESI prescription drug products on the market have been brought under regulatory control. The major category of products that remains without any form of NDA approval are the pre-1962 new drugs that were never the subject of an NDA and for which FDA has not yet conducted some form of regulatory review. It is estimated that the number of these unapproved drug products has grown from about 2400 in the 1980s to about 12 000 today.

20.8.2   Regulatory categories of prescription drugs

There are two primary categories of prescription drugs: those not currently subject to any form of NDA approval, and those subject to some form of NDA approval.

20.8.2.1   No NDA

Those not subject to any form of NDA approval consist largely of products for which an NDA has never been required or obtained, and which thus were not subject to the NAS review of 1938–62 new drugs. This is a limited category.

In its 1984 policy statement,[100] FDA stated that until some form of regulatory control was instituted, new versions of these drugs could be marketed only if the new version was in all significant respects identical to the old version. The life of one of these products is, of course, uncertain. FDA could at any time decide to regulate any or all of these products in a more comprehensive way. FDA announced a new draft Compliance Policy Guide in October 2003 that confirmed

and strengthened the 1984 FDA policy.[101] The precise status of any of these drugs can be determined only by a detailed review of all of the facts available for the specific product involved.

20.8.2.2   Three forms of NDA

The vast bulk of prescription drugs on the market today are subject to the requirement for some form of an approved NDA. Following enactment of the Drug Price Competition and Patent Term Restoration Act of 1984, there are now three clearly established types of NDA: a full NDA, a paper NDA [now called a Section 505(b)(2) NDA, after the provision in the FD&C Act that created it], and an abbreviated NDA. Each of these is discussed in the sections that follow.

20.8.2.2.1   The full NDA

For any new chemical entity drug, whether or not it has been first marketed abroad, and whether or not it is chemically related to some other approved new drug, FDA requires compliance with the full IND/NDA process.

The IND.   Before submitting an NDA to FDA, the sponsor of a drug must conduct, or arrange to be conducted, various types of non-clinical (*in vitro* and animal) tests and clinical (human) studies designed to demonstrate that the drug is safe and effective for its intended use.[102]

For non-human studies no IND is required. Companies may perform *in vitro* testing, for example, to obtain chemical information necessary to set exact specifications for the active ingredient or to obtain stability data. The company may also conduct animal toxicology tests to establish an adequate margin of human safety. Animal toxicology testing must be conducted in accordance with the FDA good laboratory practice (GLP) regulations,[103] but no IND or any other type of notice to FDA is required for any type of non-human studies. FDA also has both formal and informal guidelines to govern animal toxicity testing.

After adequate preclinical testing has been completed, an IND must be submitted to FDA to justify clinical investigation in humans. The content and format of an IND are set out in detail in the FDA regulations, and therefore need not be repeated here. The IND must contain all relevant information about the safety and effectiveness of the new drug, the protocols intended to be used in the investigations, the chemistry, manufacturing and control information, pharmacology and toxicology information, previous human experience and other pertinent information. In all respects, the FDA IND regulations must be followed in detail.

After submission, FDA has 30 days within which to evaluate the IND. By the end of 30 days, one of several things will have occurred. First, FDA may approve the IND, in which case testing can begin. Second, FDA may place the IND on formal clinical hold, in which case testing cannot begin.[104] Third, FDA may say nothing, or may raise questions, or may offer suggestions, or may say virtually anything in response to the IND. The sponsor must then determine whether to proceed in light of these developments, or to delay testing until the matter is clarified. Many sponsors conclude that the only reasonable thing to do is to delay testing until all issues are fully resolved, but others proceed in the face of open questions.

Once the initial 30-day period has expired, the IND may be amended and updated periodically. For example, additional protocols may be added. There is no 30-day delay for any subsequent amendment. Once again, however, sponsors must determine whether to delay testing until FDA is consulted and any issues are fully resolved.

An essential element of the IND is approval of the investigation by an institutional review board (IRB), either constituted by the institution in which the drug will be tested or established as a for-profit private IRB.[105] The IRB is charged with reviewing the ethical and moral dimensions of the study as well as the scientific merit. IRB approval does not guarantee FDA approval, nor does FDA approval guarantee IRB approval. They are separate and independent requirements, and both must be fulfilled before testing may begin under an IND.

Adherence to the IND by the sponsor is essential: deviations from any aspect of it are not permitted. Before there can be any change in

any aspect of the IND – including the specifications of the drug, the nature of the manufacturing process, the protocol for the investigation and the identity of the investigators, to name just a few – the IND must be amended.

No investigational new drug may be promoted or otherwise commercialised. No charge may be made for an investigational new drug without the prior approval of FDA.

The FDA IND regulations contain requirements for various types of records and reports, which must be adhered to without exception.[106] Immediate reports to FDA are required for any serious and unexpected adverse experience associated with the drug. Annual reports are required for every IND. Records must be kept to document all aspects of the IND.

Clinical testing under an IND is usually regarded as proceeding through three phases. Phase I includes the initial introduction of an investigational new drug into humans under closely monitored conditions, usually in a teaching hospital. This phase involves a relatively small number of subjects and is intended to obtain basic information on the pharmacology of the drug. Phase II includes controlled clinical studies conducted to evaluate the effectiveness and optimum dosage of the drug, and to determine common side effects and other risks. It involves a greater number of subjects, but is not a large-scale trial. Phase III involves expanded controlled and uncontrolled trials to gather additional information about safety and effectiveness that is needed to evaluate the overall benefit–risk relationship, and may involve up to several thousand subjects. In recent years, these three phases have tended to overlap substantially, and approval has been obtained on the basis of Phase II or Phase II/III studies for a number of important drugs.

Three types of unusual IND situations deserve special mention. First, the regulations contain a provision governing emergency use of an investigational new drug. Where FDA will permit such use by telephone or other rapid communication means.[107] In these situations, the IND must subsequently be amended to reflect the new situation. Second, FDA will approve specific treatment protocols for compassionate use of an investigational new drug. Where the drug is intended to treat a serious or immediately life-threatening disease, there is no satisfactory alternative; the drug is under clinical investigation pursuant to an IND, and marketing approval is actively being pursued with due diligence.[108] After a treatment IND has been approved, the sponsor may provide the drug to any patient who meets the criteria in the treatment IND, and may charge in order to recoup the cost of the drug. Third, FDA will approve 'parallel track' protocols for AIDS where there is no therapeutic alternative and individuals cannot participate in the controlled clinical trials, in order to assure widespread use of the most promising drugs at the earliest possible stage.[109] As a practical matter, it is difficult, if not impossible, to distinguish between a parallel track IND and a treatment IND.

Compassionate use of investigational new drugs has been permitted by FDA since the 1950s in order to assure that individual patients who have no other alternative are not denied any promising treatment. The more recent terminology of 'treatment IND' and 'parallel track' is therefore simply a continuation of this longstanding policy, with no significant substantive change. In addition to these new forms of compassionate-use INDs, the pharmaceutical industry continues to use the traditional form of compassionate-use protocol as well.

The results of clinical trials conducted under an IND have traditionally been regarded as confidential business information that FDA was prohibited from releasing to the public under the Freedom of Information Act and that the publication of which was determined solely by the drug sponsor. The Food and Drug Administration Modernization Act of 1997 established a clinical trial data bank for drugs for serious or life-threatening disease and required the inclusion of information on all effectiveness trials for these drugs. As a result of widespread concern about the lack of public availability of information about all clinical trials and their results, individual companies and the Pharmaceutical Research and Manufacturers of America have announced programmes to make this information public; the editors of important scientific and medical journals have determined that they will not publish studies unless this information is made public.[110] The National Institutes of Health has also announced that such information from NIH trials will be made public.

The NDA. After the sponsor has completed all non-clinical and clinical testing necessary to demonstrate the safety and effectiveness of the drug, the test results must be compiled in an NDA for submission to FDA.[111] As with the IND, the content and format of the NDA are set forth in the FDA regulations and must be followed in detail. The NDA must begin with a summary, to be followed by technical sections relating to (1) chemistry, manufacturing and controls, (2) non-clinical pharmacology and toxicology, (3) human pharmacokinetics and bioavailability, (4) microbiology, (5) clinical data and (6) statistics. Proposed labelling must also be included. The typical NDA comprises tens of thousands or even hundreds of thousands of pages.

The statute requires that a new drug should be shown to be both safe and effective. Because no drug has ever been shown to be completely safe or effective, in all cases this has been interpreted to mean that the benefits of the drug outweigh its risks under the labelled conditions of use for a significant identified patient population. The statute is very broadly worded with respect to the required proof for safety and effectiveness, and FDA has exercised substantial discretion in applying these requirements. New drugs have been approved on the basis of only one study, on the basis of Phase II studies that have never progressed to Phase III, on the basis of foreign studies alone and with results that could not be regarded as definitive from a scientific standpoint.

In most instances, FDA requires more than one adequate and well-controlled clinical trial. In the FDA Modernization Act of 1997, however, Congress clarified the law by providing that FDA may base the approval of an NDA on data from one adequate and well-controlled clinical investigation and confirmatory evidence.[112]

The FDA has in practice implemented this provision only when the single adequate and well-controlled clinical investigation has statistical significance that is an order of magnitude greater than is normally required, that is, 0.005 or greater than 0.05.

Under the FD&C Act, FDA has always been required to evaluate the NDA and approve or disapprove it within 180 days. Until 1992, this almost never occurred. The average time for approval of an NDA was between 2 and 3 years. This time remained largely unchanged for the years between 1962 and 1994, in spite of repeated promises and attempts by FDA to speed up the process. FDA was able to avoid the 180-day statutory time deadline in several ways. First, the agency started the clock when it accepted the NDA for filing, not when it was submitted. Second, FDA stopped the clock, and restarted it, whenever new submissions were made. Third, FDA requested an extension of time from the applicant, who had no choice but to agree. Fourth, FDA simply ignored the 180-day deadline, and there was nothing that the applicant could do about it anyway.

For many years it was proposed that user fees should be assessed on NDAs and that the proceeds should be used to hire sufficient FDA personnel to process applications more expeditiously. In 1992, the regulated industry and FDA finally agreed on this approach and Congress enacted the Prescription Drug User Fee Act (PDUFA) of 1992.[113] PDUFA was initially authorised for 5 years, and was reauthorised for another 5 years under the FDA Modernization Act of 1997[114] and another 5 years under the Prescription Drug User Fee Amendments of 2002.[115] The legislation provides for 3 types of user fee: drug applications, drug products and drug establishments. These fees have allowed the FDA to more than double the number of personnel reviewing NDAs. As a result, the time for NDA approval was initially halved. In 1999 and 2000, however, this trend has reversed and the time for approval has begun to increase significantly. Reflecting this increase in approval time, FDA has begun to issue 'approvable' letters within the user-fee time guidelines, and then

to take a substantial additional period to negotiate remaining issues (often including labelling) before a final approval letter is sent.

In response to criticism that the agency was not moving quickly enough to approve new drugs for AIDS and other serious or life-threatening illnesses, in 1992 the FDA established regulations to establish an accelerated approval process.[116] This is commonly referred to as the subpart H process, after the designation in the FDA regulations. The regulations describe two subpart H procedures. Under the first, FDA is authorised to approve a new drug based on a surrogate endpoint that has not yet been validated but that is 'reasonably likely . . . to predict clinical benefit', if the sponsor agrees to conduct and submit data from post-marketing studies. Under the second procedure, FDA may grant accelerated approval to beneficial but highly toxic drugs if the sponsor agrees to post-approval distribution restrictions. Under the regulations, both of these procedures are voluntary. FDA has no legal authority to impose either procedure on an NDA sponsor.

Subsequent to the establishment of subpart H, Congress enacted separate 'fast-track' procedures for new drugs to treat a serious or life-threatening condition that had the potential to address unmet medical needs under the FDA Modernization Act of 1997.[117] FDA is required to respond to requests for designation of new drugs as fast-track products within 60 days, and must expedite the development and review of a fast-track NDA. Approval may be based on a determination that the product has an effect on a clinical endpoint or on a surrogate endpoint. If it is based on a surrogate endpoint, post-approval studies can be required to confirm the effect on the clinical endpoint. The NDA sponsor must submit copies of all promotional materials prior to NDA approval and subsequently. Approval of a fast-track product may be withdrawn using expedited procedures. FDA has issued a guidance, but no regulations, to implement this provision.

Following market withdrawal of several new drugs because of toxicity that had not been uncovered in the non-clinical or IND studies, in 1998 FDA established a Task Force on Risk

Management to evaluate the FDA system for managing the risks of FDA-approved medical products. The task force concluded that the rates of drug withdrawals and adverse events remain low, but recommended a new risk management approach in order to better identify and control these risks as early as possible in the NDA process.[118] Implementation of this report has had a substantial impact on the IND/NDA process. FDA reviewers are requiring more patients in clinical trials, longer follow-up and more trials. A number of NDAs that had been expected to obtain FDA approval were disapproved and will require additional evidence of safety and effectiveness. As already noted, the time for NDA approval has increased significantly following the release of the report. The release in late 1999 of the widely publicised Institute of Medicine report on the number of deaths caused by medication errors undoubtedly contributed to the new FDA wave of conservatism.[119] Patients have complained that their interests are not being considered, as drugs have been withdrawn or withheld because of concern about toxicity to a few individuals, and the benefits to large numbers of patients are not being taken into account. It is uncertain whether the recent widespread publicity about the potential risk from Cox-2 inhibitor drugs, and the withdrawal of Vioxx from the market, will propel FDA or Congress into another wave of conservatism.

The FDA divides NDAs into two categories for the purpose of review: priority drugs and all other drugs. For priority drugs, FDA sets a target of NDA review within 6 months. For all other drugs, the target is 10 months. These targets are subject to periodic adjustment when the Prescription Drug User Fee Act is renegotiated every 5 years, but it is unlikely that they will be substantially reduced.

During the NDA evaluation there are no guidelines or rules that require open communication between FDA and the applicant. It is impossible to generalise about the relationship between drug applicants and FDA reviewers. The CDER review divisions have quite varied reputations for openness, promptness and cordiality. Thus, discussion between an FDA review division and the applicant varies all the way from virtually no communication to constant discussion. Relations range from friendliness to near hostility. The NDA review process is, in short, entirely an *ad hoc* and informal process of negotiation that may go very well or very poorly, and over which the applicant has virtually no control. Attempts to obtain resolution of disputes through the FDA ombudsman or by appealing issues to higher officials are almost never successful, and often worsen relations with the NDA reviewers. Pharmaceutical companies uniformly fear retaliation unless they cooperate fully with every request from the NDA reviewers.

For every NDA, some clinical study is almost certain to remain in progress at the time when the NDA is submitted. Safety update reports are therefore required to be submitted to FDA by the applicant while the NDA is pending, and particularly following receipt of an approvable letter.[120] Detailed systems and procedures are required to ensure that the data in the NDA and the safety updates are accurate and complete, and failure to meet these requirements is regarded by FDA as a serious deficiency.

It is customary for FDA to submit one or more letters of disapproval as part of the NDA review process. These frequently lead to the submission of new information, a revision of labelling and further negotiation. In a relatively small number of cases, FDA will issue a definitive disapproval letter determining that there is no additional information on the basis of which the drug could be approved. There are then various administrative and judicial appeals that the applicant can make. In no instance since 1938, however, has any applicant successfully challenged FDA denial of approval of an NDA.[121] For this reason, it is generally understood that there is no practical way to challenge whatever FDA requires during the NDA process, and that the only realistic alternative is to negotiate the best possible approach with FDA in a cooperative spirit.

Confidentiality of information. Under the Freedom of Information Act, all information in government files is subject to public disclosure unless it falls within a specified exemption.[122] Both the FD&C Act[123] and the Federal Trade Secrets Act[124] prohibit the public disclosure of confidential commercial information and trade secrets. FDA has promulgated detailed regulations governing the status of general categories of data and information in its files,[125] and particularly data and information submitted as part of an IND or NDA.[126] In general, no data or information submitted to FDA as part of an IND or NDA will be made public prior to FDA approval or disapproval of the NDA. Even the existence of an IND or NDA will be kept confidential by FDA if it has not been disclosed by the sponsor. Upon approval, FDA issues a summary of the basis for the agency approval of the product, which describes the safety and effectiveness data on which the agency relied.[127] Whether FDA will also release the reports and data relating to the testing for safety and effectiveness will depend upon whether the company can convince the agency that these data retain value as 'confidential commercial information'.[128] In general, FDA will release the full data and information on safety and effectiveness after a drug becomes subject to generic competition, but not before. Agency regulations spell out FDA's confidentiality policies in great detail, but there still are often disputes about their application to any particular set of facts.

Advisory committees. There is no statutory requirement that FDA review the approval of an NDA with an advisory committee before final action is taken. Since the 1970s, however, this has been the customary practice, particularly with important new drugs. This prompted Congress to enact a specific provision dealing with the establishment of drug advisory committees under the FDA Modernization Act of 1997.[129]

The review of an NDA by an advisory committee is an extremely important step in the approval process. It represents the best opportunity that the applicant has to address the agency and the public about the evidence of safety and effectiveness and the importance of the drug to public health. In the vast majority of cases, FDA accepts the recommendation of the advisory committee for approval, further testing or outright disapproval. Where the advisory committee recommends approval and FDA disagrees, however, the agency will almost always take a long time to implement the advisory committee recommendations, or may even add additional testing requirements before approval is eventually obtained. The importance of advisory committee review is widely recognised in the pharmaceutical industry, and it is common for a company to engage in extensive preparation for the company presentation and to seek supportive statements from independent outside experts and patients as well.

Post-approval requirements. Following approval of an NDA, FDA requires the submission of three different types of reports by the owner of the NDA.[130] First, serious and unexpected adverse drug experiences must be immediately reported to FDA regardless of whether or not the company believes they are causally related to the drug. Second, all adverse drug experiences, as well as other safety and effectiveness information, must be reported periodically to FDA, at intervals specified in the FDA regulations. Third, information relating to all other aspects of the drug must be reported immediately to FDA if they represent a potential problem, but otherwise may be included in an annual report. Foreign as well as domestic adverse experiences and other information must be included in these reports.

Changes in the NDA after approval. Any significant change from the detailed terms and conditions specified in the approved NDA must be the subject of a supplemental NDA and cannot be put into effect until the supplemental NDA has been approved by FDA.[131] The only changes in an approved NDA that may be made without approval of a supplemental NDA are set forth in the FDA regulations, and those exceptions must be reflected in the annual report submitted to FDA. Where FDA finds that changes have been made from an approved NDA, beyond those permitted without a supplemental NDA, very stringent regulatory action can be taken, including recall of the product and the inability to manufacture any more product until the unapproved changes are eliminated or approved. Accordingly, it is essential that all aspects of an approved NDA be followed in detail unless a clear exception is created in the FDA regulations. In close cases, FDA should be consulted.

Summary suspension of approval. The statute provides that the Secretary of HHS may summarily suspend approval of an NDA upon a finding that the drug represents an imminent hazard to the public health.[132] This authority is delegated to the Secretary of HHS alone, and cannot be exercised by FDA or anyone else. It has been used only once, and its use was upheld in the courts.[133]

Antibiotic drugs. New antibiotic drugs are subject to the same IND and NDA requirements contained in the FDA regulations as other new drugs. Although the FD&C Act initially provided that FDA could require batch certification for antibiotics, in 1982 FDA exempted all classes of antibiotic drugs from this requirement because of the high level of manufacturer compliance with antibiotic standards. Because the FDA Modernization Act of 1997 repealed the old antibiotic provisions of the FD&C Act,[134] antibiotics today are regulated in basically the same way as all other new drugs.

User fees. Under the Prescription Drug User Fee Act of 1992, as extended 5 more years by the FDA Modernization Act of 1997 and another 5 years by the Prescription Drug User Fee Amendments of 2002, FDA has authority to collect user fees for pioneering drugs until such time as generic competition is approved.[135] The fees include (1) a one-time NDA fee, (2) an annual product fee and (3) an annual establishment fee. The precise amount of each fee escalates each year and is subject to modification according to detailed provisions in the statute. The funds obtained from these fees must be in addition to the existing congressionally appropriated resources for the IND/NDA system as adjusted for cost-of-living increases, and must be used solely for the IND/NDA process. In return for receiving user fees, FDA has committed to specific goals for improving the drug review process, by reducing the backlog of applications, meeting specified time deadlines, and making improvements in the process. The extent to which these commitments can be kept will become apparent only in the coming years.

20.8.2.2.2   The paper NDA

When Congress enacted the Drug Price Competition and Patent Term Restoration Act of 1984, it included a provision based on the concept of a paper NDA but which in fact expanded that concept significantly. The former paper NDA is therefore now called a Section 505(b)(2) NDA, after the statutory provision that creates it.[136] It applies to those situations where a pioneer drug is no longer protected by patents or market exclusivity but where an applicant is unable to submit an abbreviated NDA because the modified drug differs in some substantial way from the pioneer drug. A Section 505(b)(2) NDA relies upon the pioneer NDA for all information except the data needed to support the element of substantial difference. Thus, the Section 505(b)(2) NDA need not include any data relating to the basic safety and effectiveness of the drug, except insofar as the difference between the pioneer drug and the applicant's modification of that drug bears upon safety or effectiveness.

As will be discussed below, minor differences between a pioneer drug and a generic version of that drug may be approved by FDA as appropriate for an abbreviated NDA pursuant to a 'suitability petition'. Where those differences become substantial, however, FDA will deny the suitability petition and will require the approval of a more complete NDA. In these circumstances, the Section 505(b)(2) paper NDA will be sufficient, and a full NDA will not be required. Thus, the Section 505(b)(2) NDA is midway between a full NDA and an abbreviated NDA. The same regulations and requirements apply to a Section 505(b)(2) paper NDA under the 1984 Act as it applies to a full NDA. FDA interprets Section 505(b)(2) to authorise the agency to rely on confidential commercial information in a pioneer NDA in order to approve a generic competitor's version of the drug. The regulated industry takes the position that this would be illegal under the FD&C Act. This disagreement must ultimately be resolved in the courts.

20.8.2.2.3   The abbreviated NDA

All of the regulations and requirements for an abbreviated NDA developed by FDA in the late 1960s as part of the implementation of the Drug Amendments of 1962, and all of the proposed changes that FDA considered to adapt those requirements to post-1962 new drugs, were eliminated when Congress enacted the Drug Price Competition and Patent Term Restoration Act of 1984. The 1984 Act established detailed requirements that supersede everything that went before.[137]

Under the 1984 Act, an abbreviated NDA may be approved by FDA for a generic version of a pioneer new drug after (1) all relevant product and use patents have expired for the pioneer drug and (2) all relevant periods of market exclusivity for the pioneer drug have also expired. The statute contains detailed and complex rules for determining precisely how this system works. No attempt will be made here to discuss the specific provisions, but they are extremely important in determining the commercial value of a pioneer new drug because they govern when the drug will become subject to generic competition. Of particular importance, Congress expanded the length of protection granted under the 1984 Act in the FDA Modernization Act of 1997, as extended by the Best Pharmaceutical for Children Act in 2002, by providing an extra 6 months of market exclusivity at the end of the extended patent term (or market exclusivity term, if the patent has already expired) when the sponsor conducts paediatric testing requested and approved by FDA.[138]

There are basically two types of situation where an abbreviated NDA may be submitted. The first situation is where the generic version is the same as the pioneer version in all material respects. Where this is true, the applicant for the generic product simply submits the abbreviated NDA and FDA may approve it without further consideration about the basic safety and effectiveness of the drug. The second circumstance is where the generic version is different from the pioneer drug in any significant respect (e.g. a different active ingredient, route of administration, dosage form or strength). In these circumstances, the generic applicant must first submit to FDA a 'suitability petition' demonstrating that the difference between the drugs is not sufficient to preclude an abbreviated NDA, and that additional studies to show safety and effectiveness are not needed. If FDA grants the suitability petition, an abbreviated NDA may be submitted. If the suitability petition is denied, the applicant must submit either a Section 505(b)(2) paper NDA or a full NDA. In all other respects, the regulations and requirements for an abbreviated NDA are the same as those for a full NDA.

20.8.3   The Applications Integrity (Fraud) Policy

As a result of the generic drug scandal described above, where generic drug manufacturers submitted fraudulent data and bribed FDA officials, the FDA adopted a 'fraud policy' in September 1991, which was later called the Applications Integrity Policy, to cover situations where FDA concluded that an applicant who had engaged in a wrongful act would need to take corrective action to establish the reliability of data submitted to FDA in support of pending applications and to support the integrity of products already on the market.[139] Under this policy, FDA issues a formal letter invoking the policy and requiring the applicant to cooperate fully with the FDA investigation. The applicant is required to identify all individuals associated with the wrongful act and to ensure that they are removed from any substantive authority on matters under FDA jurisdiction. A credible internal review must be conducted to identify all instances of wrongful acts, to supplement FDA's own investigation. The internal review should involve an outside consultant or team qualified by training and experience to conduct such a review. Finally, the applicant must commit in writing to developing and implementing a corrective action operating plan. Although this fraud policy was developed in response to the generic drug scandal, it also applies to pioneer drug companies and to data in full NDAs.

20.8.4 Labelling and advertising

The labelling for a new drug must be included as part of the NDA and must be explicitly approved by FDA. No significant change may be made in the labelling without prior FDA approval through a supplemental NDA. Because this rule is so clear and so stringent, the pharmaceutical industry seldom takes chances with deviations in product labelling that could result in FDA enforcement action.

The Drug Amendments of 1962 gave FDA the authority to regulate advertising for prescription drugs, as well as labelling.[140] However, the FD&C Act was not amended to give FDA pre-market approval over advertising, similar to its pre-market approval over labelling. Accordingly, FDA must rely upon general policing of prescription drug advertising to determine whether it is false or misleading.

In accordance with its statutory authority, FDA has promulgated regulations that illustrate ways in which prescription drug advertising may be false, lacking in fair balance, or otherwise misleading.[141] As the pharmaceutical industry has expanded its promotional activities, FDA has also issued a variety of policy statements on various types of advertising practice that do not fall within the existing regulations. These policy statements deal with such issues as press conferences, medical seminars, journal supplements, TV and radio talk shows and a wide variety of other means of communication.[142] It is essential that anyone engaging in prescription drug marketing be fully familiar with the latest FDA policy in these areas.

A recent innovation has been direct-to-consumer (DTC) prescription drug promotion in the broadcast media. Because FDA regulations require a summary of the entire approved package insert to appear with any prescription drug advertisement, it was extremely difficult to use radio or television advertising for this purpose. Most consumer advertising for prescription drugs was therefore limited to the print media. Beginning in July 1997, however, FDA has issued guidance that allows the package insert requirement to be satisfied with more flexible ways to provide the same information to consumers.[143] This has resulted in an explosion of DTC prescription drug advertising on television. FDA reviews these advertisements very carefully, and thus caution must be used in preparing them. It is sound practice to review proposed advertising of this type with FDA prior to its use. Because of criticism that DTC prescription drug advertising may contribute to unwarranted use of prescription drugs and to higher drug prices, FDA is conducting a thorough review of the current requirements for this category of advertising. It is likely that the agency will require greater emphasis on the potential risk of prescription drugs in future DTC prescription drug advertising.

20.8.5 Good manufacturing practices

One of the most important parts of an NDA is the description of the chemistry, manufacturing and controls (CMC).[144] FDA has traditionally placed substantial reliance upon this part of the NDA in ensuring the safety and effectiveness of the drug. One study conducted a decade ago found that more questions were raised by FDA reviewers about this section of the NDA than about the safety and effectiveness of the drug itself.

Beginning in 1991, moreover, FDA announced a new enforcement technique designed to assure adequate GMP compliance before an NDA is approved.[145] Prior to FDA approval of the NDA, the FDA field force now conducts a pre-approval inspection (PAI) of the establishment where the new drug is to be manufactured. If the manufacturing facility deviates in any way from either the description in the NDA or the general requirements for GMP in the FDA regulations,[146] the NDA will be held hostage and will not be approved until full compliance is achieved. Pursuant to this policy, the approval of numerous NDAs has been substantially delayed. Compliance with GMP is therefore essential to any NDA approval. Because of widespread concern about this practice, Congress included in the

FDA Modernization Act of 1997 a specific provision stating that an NDA approval may not be delayed because of unavailability of information from, or action by, the FDA field personnel unless the reviewing division determines that a delay is necessary to assure the marketing of a safe and effective drug.[147] In spite of this provision, FDA continues to hold drugs hostage as a result of a PAI without a finding that this is necessary to ensure the marketing of a safe and effective drug.

After approval of an NDA, FDA periodically inspects a drug establishment for two purposes. First, FDA determines whether any unapproved changes have been made in the manufacturing process from those set forth in the approved NDA. If any such changes are made beyond those permitted without a supplemental NDA, FDA may well bring stringent enforcement action. Second, FDA routinely inspects all establishments to determine compliance with GMP. Although FDA has not changed its GMP regulations, the interpretation and application of those regulations by FDA inspectors are thought by the pharmaceutical industry to have been substantially tightened and made more strict in the past few years.

Where FDA determines any deviation from GMP, the inspector leaves a form, FDA-483, specifying the manufacturing deficiencies. It is essential in these circumstances that the company immediately make all corrections and respond to FDA in writing about them. It can be expected that FDA will reinspect the establishment and look both for what has been done to correct the prior deficiencies and for any new deficiencies that can be found. The pharmaceutical industry believes that FDA often lists insignificant matters, that establishments which have passed without observed deficiencies in the past suddenly will be the subject of major deficiencies because of a change of inspectors or of interpretation, and that the requirements vary widely from individual inspector to individual inspector and from FDA district to FDA district. The industry has found, however, that its complaints fall on deaf ears, and thus that it must comply with whatever is required by the individual inspector or face the threat of serious regulatory action.

Realising that the agency had not reviewed its drug GMP regulations and requirements since 1979, FDA announced in 2002 an initiative to conduct a thorough evaluation of all aspects of its implementation of drug GMP requirements. In 2004, FDA issued a final report announcing a number of reforms relating to drug GMP.[148] Of primary importance, drug GMP decisions will, in the future, be based upon scientific principles of risk analysis and risk management. FDA also established a technical dispute resolution process for GMP disputes between FDA inspectors and the regulated industry.

20.8.6 Pharmacy compounding

Prior to 1997, there was no provision in the FD&C Act that explicitly authorised pharmacy compounding. FDA policy recognised the practice of pharmacy compounding, but the agency brought action against compounding pharmacists when they began to advertise specific drugs or to stockpile substantial quantities of drugs.[149]

Under the FDA Modernization Act of 1997, Congress for the first time addressed the requirements and limitations of pharmacy compounding. To take advantage of the authority to compound, a pharmacy would have been precluded from advertising that specific compounded drugs were available from that pharmacy. In 2002, the Supreme Court held that this restriction was unconstitutional, in violation of the right of free speech under the First Amendment to the US Constitution.[150] Because a lower court had ruled that the advertising restriction could not be separated from the other pharmacy compounding provisions, the result is that none of these provisions remains effective. Accordingly, pharmacy compounding is now back to where it was before the 1997 Act. FDA has reiterated its views regarding when pharmacy compounding becomes illegal manufacture.[151]

20.8.7 Distribution controls

On one occasion, FDA sought to limit the distribution of a new drug to hospital-based pharmacies and to prohibit it through community pharmacies. Upon challenge by the pharmacy profession, the courts ruled that this was an illegal restriction that was not authorised by the FD&C Act.[152] Since then, FDA has approved the labelling for new drugs under which the sponsor has voluntarily included restrictions on distribution, including under subpart H,[153] but the agency has not itself imposed distribution controls on any new drug.

20.8.8 Import and export

20.8.8.1 Import

In general, a prescription drug may lawfully be imported into the United States only in full compliance with all the laws and regulations applicable to domestic drugs. There is, however, one exception. Since 1977, FDA has stated that the agency will not detain unapproved new drugs imported for personal use.[154] This became important when patients suffering from AIDS began to import drugs not available in the United States. Subsequently, AIDS organisations established buying clubs to import drugs for all of their members. FDA has not sought to prohibit this activity except where it is done for commercial profit or involves unsafe or fraudulent products for which the agency has issued an import alert (such as RU-486). Where FDA has considered cracking down on such imports, public pressure has forced the agency to back off from enforcement action.

The United States is the only country in the world that does not fix the prices for prescription drugs. Patented prescription drug costs in the United States are therefore higher than in any other country, and the cost of generic drugs in the United States are lower than in any other country. Because of the large price differential between the United States and other countries for patented prescription drugs, internet pharmacies and other organisations have begun to ship prescription drugs illegally into the United States, without an approved NDA or in violation of the prohibition against reimportation under the Prescription Drug Marketing Act of 1987. FDA has

vigorously opposed these illegal imports as well as any legislation designed to change the current statutory requirements for imported new drugs. Under both the Clinton and the Bush administrations, the Secretary of HHS has declined to certify that importation of unapproved drugs from abroad could be undertaken safely and would result in significant cost savings to the American consumer. Accordingly, the provisions of the Medicine Equity and Drug Safety Act of 2000 that would have provided for prescription drug imports have never gone into effect.

20.8.8.2 Export

The FD&C Act of 1938, and even the Drug Export Amendments Act of 1986, placed such stringent limitations on the export of unapproved drugs from the United States that they raised enormous commercial potential for foreign countries. Many US pharmaceutical companies reasonably anticipated that their drugs would receive approval for use outside the United States before they were approved by FDA, and could not take the risk that they would be able to obtain and maintain FDA approval of an export application. Under these circumstances, they had no option other than to build their manufacturing facilities abroad rather than in the United States. For that reason, foreign countries competed in attempting to attract these pharmaceutical factories.

The FDA Export Reform and Enhancement Act of 1996 eliminated many, but far from all, of the restrictions on FDA export of unapproved new drugs. For example, although unapproved new drugs may be exported to any of the 25 listed countries for investigational use, these drugs may not be shipped to any other country for the same purpose without FDA approval – which can take a year or more. No other country in the world controls exports in the same way as the United States, and thus a pharmaceutical establishment may be located anywhere other than the United States without fear of unreasonable limitations on international trade. Accordingly, it is essential for any US or foreign company to be able to source its drugs abroad, rather than in the United States, if it is to be assured of the ability to investigate and market its new drugs throughout the world.

20.8.9   Orphan drugs

Under the Orphan Drug Act of 1983[155] and its numerous amendments, an orphan drug is eligible for two types of benefit. The first, which is often of minor significance, consists of tax credits. The second type, which has proved to be of enormous importance, is the market exclusivity provided by the prohibition against any form of FDA approval of the same drug for another company for 7 years. The company that obtains FDA approval of an NDA for an orphan drug is thus assured of greater protection under the Orphan Drug Act than under any other statute, including the patent laws.

As enacted in 1983, the Orphan Drug Act had relatively little impact because the scope of the term 'orphan drug' was considered by FDA to be relatively narrow. When Congress amended the law in 1984[156] to define an orphan drug as any drug, or any single indication for a drug, for a condition afflicting fewer than 200 000 patients in the United States, however, the impact of the law changed dramatically. Some orphan drugs are now blockbusters on which entire companies can be founded. Although Congress has considered legislation to cut back some of the provisions of the Orphan Drug Act, one such bill was vetoed by the President[157] and no other has since come close to enactment. Even if the benefits available from the Orphan Drug Act are changed, they are likely to remain important to drug companies for the foreseeable future.

20.8.10   Physician prescribing

The FD&C Act has been interpreted by FDA as applying only to the labelling, advertising and marketing of a new drug, not to the practice of medicine as reflected in the physician's prescription of the drug for a particular patient. In a policy first published in 1972[158] and reiterated many times,[159] the FDA has stated that the physician may, within the practice of medicine, lawfully prescribe an approved drug for

an unapproved use. Because the Drug Price Competition and Patent Term Restoration Act of 1984 provides no significant market protection for companies that obtain FDA approval of new uses for previously approved new drugs, companies rarely submit supplemental NDAs to request FDA approval of an unapproved use for an approved drug. As unapproved uses expand, the prescription drug package insert approved by FDA has become substantially outdated. In many areas, the unapproved uses of a new drug overwhelm the approved uses. Although the FDA has deplored this fact, it has thus far done nothing to find an adequate resolution.

Although the FDA has stated since 1938 that the agency has no authority to require an NDA sponsor to conduct testing for uses that the sponsor has not included in the proposed labelling, FDA nonetheless promulgated regulations in late 1998 to require paediatric testing of new drugs in most situations in order to reduce unapproved use of new drugs in infants and children.[160] The FDA regulation on paediatric testing was determined to be illegal by a court in 2002, but was restored by Congress in the Pediatric Research Equity Act of 2003. In the FDA Modernization Act of 1997 as extended for another 5 years by the Best Pharmaceutical for Children Act in 2002, Congress included not only 6 months of marketing exclusivity for paediatric testing,[161] but also a provision to allow dissemination of information on unapproved uses of approved new drugs under specific limited conditions.[162]

While the 1997 Act was being considered by Congress, the FDA policy prohibiting dissemination of information on unapproved uses of approved new drugs was being challenged in the courts. The US District Court held that the FDA policy violated the First Amendment to the US Constitution, even taking into consideration the new statutory provision added by the 1997 Act, and issued an injunction that permitted a drug manufacturer to disseminate to physicians and other medical professionals information on unapproved uses of approved new drugs from a peer-reviewed professional journal or a reference textbook, or to suggest content or speakers to an independent programme adviser for a continuing medical education (CME) programme. The injunction permitted FDA to require the drug manufacturer to disclose the company's interest in the drug and the fact that the use of the drug had not been approved by FDA.[163] FDA then changed its legal position and argued on appeal that its policy merely constituted a 'safe harbour', and that a violation would not necessarily bring an enforcement proceeding. As a result, the US Court of Appeals reversed the District Court's decision on procedural grounds, without in any way disagreeing with it.[164] The District Court then revoked its injunction, although indicating that it had not changed its opinion on the matter.[165] The FDA subsequently published a notice stating its continued intent to enforce its policy,[166] and the Washington Legal Foundation has returned to court on the matter. It is extremely unlikely that FDA will enforce its unapproved use policy under the circumstances permitted by the now-dissolved District Court injunction, regardless of the outcome of this case, and FDA officials have so stated. Thus, the First Amendment right of free speech in the United States makes it even more difficult for FDA to attempt to force NDA sponsors to submit supplemental NDAs for unapproved uses, absent unequivocal statutory authority to require that drugs be tested for these uses, and that applications be submitted for including them in approved labelling. To the extent that a drug loses its patent status, of course, the problem of requiring the generic and the pioneer sponsors to conduct such testing is substantial.

20.8.11   Patient freedom of choice

Beginning with enactment of the Drug Amendments of 1962, organised patient groups have argued strenuously that they should have the freedom to purchase whatever drugs they may wish to use, regardless of their FDA status, particularly where individuals are suffering from life-threatening diseases. Cancer patients argued for the use of Krebiozen and Laetrile, but FDA sought to prohibit those drugs by every means

available, and the courts ultimately supported the agency.[167]

With the dramatic rise in AIDS, however, a larger, more vocal and more politically active interest group challenged the authority of FDA to deny experimental and unapproved drugs to any patient who wishes to use them. This time, the activists had a greater impact.[168] FDA has declined to take enforcement action in many instances where it would have done so in the past. The agency has also expedited the approval of AIDS drugs on the basis of scientific information that would not have been accepted as sufficient for any other disease area. Thus, FDA has bent its rules for putative AIDS treatments but has refused to expand its flexibility to include other disease areas as well. The result is an inconsistent series of decisions approving drugs for one disease on the basis of preliminary information and withholding approval of more extensively tested drugs for other diseases.

20.8.12   The costs and benefits of the IND/NDA system

There have been hundreds of investigations and reports on the IND/NDA system.[169] Numerous analyses have been done of the costs and benefits, and hundreds of recommendations have been made about ways to improve the system. Feelings run deep on these subjects, and the philosophical and emotional element often dwarfs the factual and analytical element.

A 1991 study demonstrated that the average NDA requires an investment of about $231 million.[170] In the last year of NDA approval, the average carrying cost (cost of capital) alone was $31 million. Today, these figures have escalated to an estimated $1.7 billion.[171] Critics argue that this is largely the result of unrealistic regulatory requirements that cause higher drug prices, that the delay in drugs reaching the market substantially harms the public health and that the high cost of drug development discourages drug R&D and directly hinders the development of life-saving drugs for the future. Supporters of the system point to drug tragedies of the past, argue that any relaxation of regulatory controls will dramatically increase drug risks and reduce drug effectiveness, and state that the only sound way to protect the public health is to continue and indeed to strengthen the present system. Supporters of biotechnology charge that the present system is destroying the opportunity presented by this new technology, and critics of biotechnology applaud that result.

20.9 Biological Drugs

For a full century, biological drugs have been regulated under the Biologics Act of 1902, in accordance with statutory requirements that have not significantly changed.[172] When FDA was delegated the responsibility for regulating biologics in 1972, however, the agency promulgated regulations adding a number of the drug regulatory provisions under the FD&C Act to those already available under the Biologics Act. Current regulation of biologics therefore incorporates requirements from both statutes.

20.9.1 The biologics licence application

Prior to 1996, FDA required the submission and approval of both an ELA and a PLA. This bifurcated submission and approval process was widely criticised as inefficient. Following the November 1994 elections and the realisation that FDA would be a major target for legislative reform, the agency revised its regulations to eliminate the requirement for a separate ELA and to substitute a single biologics licence application (BLA) for four categories of well-characterised biological products.[173] In the FDA Modernization Act of 1997, however, Congress eliminated the ELA and PLA for all biological products and substituted the single BLA.[174] Congress also ordered FDA to take measures to minimise differences in the review and approval of biological products under Section 351 of the Public Health Service Act and new drugs under Section 505(b)(1) of the FD&C Act. FDA promptly amended the regulations governing biologics licences to implement this requirement.[175]

Before a company may manufacture any biological product, a BLA must be submitted to, and approved by, FDA, for the product involved. Under Section 351 of the Public Health Service Act as it is now revised, the product approval system for a biological drug is the same as for a new drug. Non-clinical studies may be conducted without FDA knowledge or approval. Clinical investigation in humans must be preceded by the submission of an IND, and all the IND regulations discussed above for chemical drugs apply equally to a biological drug. It is only the BLA that has a different name and a somewhat different focus.

A basic premise of the regulation of biological drugs is that, because they come from natural sources, they cannot adequately be characterised by chemical specifications and must instead be regulated very rigidly by rigorous adherence to detailed manufacturing procedures. For this reason, approval of a BLA depends upon the specific establishment specified and approved in that BLA. If the owner of an approved BLA wishes to manufacture all or part of the biological drug in a new establishment, it has long been standard policy under the Biologics Act to require not just that the new product be shown to be the same as the old, but also that new clinical studies independently demonstrate the safety and effectiveness of the new product as manufactured in the new establishment. This goes beyond the requirements that FDA has applied to new drugs.

This FDA policy has important ramifications for the generic drug industry. When Congress enacted the Drug Price Competition and Patent Term Restoration Act of 1984, it included only new drugs and it excluded biological drugs. Nonetheless, a small number of biological products were handled under NDAs rather than BLAs, the most prominent of which is human growth hormone. Generic drug manufacturers have in fact submitted abbreviated NDAs or Section 505(b)(2) NDAs for human growth hormone. Thus, FDA must decide whether generic versions of this biological product may be approved without the requirement of the same type of clinical testing that was required for the pioneer product. For all other biological products that have been licensed through BLAs under the Biologics Act of 1902, however, the advent of generic versions must await a revision of the statute by Congress.

With the advent of biotechnology, the work in the CBER has changed dramatically. For decades, the only biological products regulated under the Biologics Act of 1902 were vaccines, blood, allergenic extracts and other related products that did not pose the difficult problems of balancing benefits against risks that were daily faced by the CDER. As a result, CBER was able to review and approve ELAs and PLAs rapidly, in a fraction of the time that it took CDER to do the same job. Now, the two are indistinguishable. The time required for review and approval of a BLA became even longer than that for an NDA. The backlog at CBER rose dramatically. Critics suggested that review and approval of new pharmaceutical products by CBER was slower and more difficult than by CDER. FDA therefore announced in 2002 that the handling of most biological drugs would be transferred from CBER to CDER, but that regulation of traditional biological products, such as vaccines and blood, will remain in CBER. Approximately one-third of the CBER resources were transferred to CDER as part of this re-organisation.

20.9.2 The Biologics Review

When implementation of the Biologics Act was transferred to FDA in 1972, a process was just being formulated by the Division of Biologics Standards in NIH to review the safety, effectiveness and labelling of the biological products that had been licensed during the past 70 years under the 1902 Act. FDA promptly established written procedures and undertook the Biologics Review.[176] The Biologics Review was patterned after the OTC Drug Review and is similarly not yet completed.

20.10 Enforcement

The FDA has available to it a wide variety of formal and informal enforcement authorities under the FD&C Act. They apply equally to all products regulated by FDA. For generic drugs, FDA also can rely upon the provisions of the Generic Drug Enforcement Act of 1992. The following sections summarise some of the more important enforcement provisions used by FDA to regulate all pharmaceutical products.

20.10.1 Formal enforcement authority

20.10.1.1 Factory inspection
For purposes of enforcing the law, FDA inspectors may at any time inspect any non-prescription or prescription drug.[177] For both, FDA inspectors may see all records and documents except those that relate to financial data, sales data other than shipment data, pricing data, personnel data and research data.[178] An FDA inspector may spend whatever amount of time is necessary to complete such an inspection – even weeks or months. Where significant enforcement issues have been found, FDA inspectors have been known to spend more than a year at a single establishment.

20.10.1.2 Seizure
The FDA has statutory authority to request the Department of Justice to 'seize' any illegal product.[179] If FDA asserts that the drug is dangerous to health or the labelling is fraudulent or misleading in a material respect, the statute authorises multiple seizures throughout the country. Prior to 1997, FDA was required to prove the requisite shipment in interstate commerce in order to establish the agency's jurisdiction. Under the FDA Modernization Act of 1997, Congress established a rebuttable presumption of interstate commerce for purposes of FDA enforcement jurisdiction, thereby making all FDA enforcement action substantially simpler.[180]

20.10.1.3 Injunction
The FDA also has statutory authority to request the Department of Justice to seek a court injunction against continued violations of the law by a prescription drug manufacturer or distributor.[181] FDA has had mixed results in attempting to obtain injunctions from the courts, who realise that an injunction can shut down a company entirely or subject it to arbitrary demands by

FDA. FDA has therefore sought to obtain the equivalent in the form of stipulated agreements with companies that are filed in court as consent decrees and thus are fully enforceable as a requirement of law.

20.10.1.4   Criminal penalties

All violations of the FD&C Act are automatically criminal violations of law.[182] On two occasions the US Supreme Court has held that any person standing in a responsible relationship to a violation of the FD&C Act is criminally liable, regardless of the lack of knowledge or intent.[183] The nature of the offence is the failure of an individual to take action to prevent a violation and to ensure compliance with the law.

This is an extremely harsh statute. As a practical matter, FDA exercises its prosecutorial discretion only to bring cases for continuing violations of law, violations of an obvious and flagrant nature, and intentionally false or fraudulent violations. Although there have been attempts to change the criminal liability standard under the FD&C Act by legislation, none has so far been successful.

20.10.1.5   Section 305 hearing

The FD&C Act provides that, before any violation is reported by FDA for institution of a criminal proceeding, the person against whom the proceeding is contemplated shall be given appropriate notice and an opportunity to present views.[184] In accordance with this provision, it is the custom of FDA to provide an informal hearing to individuals, to show cause why they should not be prosecuted. When a grand jury is convened, however, FDA usually does not provide this type of hearing. Where such a hearing is given, it is obviously important for the individual to demonstrate a good faith attempt to comply with the law and an intent to correct and prevent any deficiencies in the future.

20.10.1.6   Other criminal statutes

The US Code contains a number of criminal provisions related to enforcement of the FD&C Act. These laws prohibit any criminal conspiracy,[185]

false reports to the government,[186] mail fraud,[187] bribery,[188] perjury[189] and other similar illegal activity. FDA has in fact used these provisions on a number of occasions to bring criminal prosecution against individuals and companies who have violated the FD&C Act.

20.10.1.7   Civil money penalties

The Prescription Drug Marketing Act of 1987 includes civil penalties for violation of the drug sample provisions of the FD&C Act.[190] The law provides that a manufacturer or distributor who violates these provisions is subject to a civil penalty of not more than $50 000 for each of the first two violations resulting in a conviction in any 10-year period, and for not more than $1 million for each violation resulting in a conviction after the second conviction in any 10-year period. These penalties may be imposed only by a Federal District Court. FDA has no administrative authority to impose any civil penalties under these provisions.

20.10.1.8   Restitution

One court has interpreted the FD&C Act as not authorising FDA to require restitution by a manufacturer to purchasers of a product that has been found to violate the FD&C Act,[191] but a more recent court decision has upheld restitution.[192] The Medical Device Amendments of 1976 explicitly provide such authority for medical devices.[193]

20.10.2   Informal enforcement authority

20.10.2.1   Recall

For decades, FDA has worked with product manufacturers to request, and to help carry out, the recall of illegal products from the market. Courts have disagreed on whether the FD&C Act authorises an injunction that includes a requirement for product recall.[194] As a practical matter, however, the precise legal authority of FDA on this matter is irrelevant. Manufacturers routinely cooperate with FDA on the recall of any dangerous product. FDA has established detailed administrative policy governing recall procedures.[195]

20.10.2.2 Warning letters

The FD&C Act authorises FDA to decline to institute formal enforcement proceedings for minor violations whenever FDA believes that the public interest will be adequately served by a suitable written notice or warning. In accordance with this provision, in the early 1970s FDA began to issue a 'regulatory letter' in lieu of bringing formal court enforcement action. This permitted more rapid, less costly and more efficient enforcement of the law. In the early 1990s regulatory letters were renamed 'warning letters', and lost their impact because they were no longer approved by FDA top management and the Chief Counsel. Nonetheless, any warning letter must be given immediate attention in order to avoid more serious formal enforcement action in the courts.

20.10.2.3 Publicity

The FDA has explicit statutory authority to issue information to the public.[196] The courts have upheld the right of FDA to publicise illegal activity and to issue publicity about products and practices that it concludes to be harmful to the public health.[197] This is regarded by many as the most potent enforcement tool available to FDA. Instead of using the formal enforcement authority established in the FD&C Act, for example, FDA issued strong negative publicity about the dangers of phenylpropanolamine and ephedra and destroyed the market for both of these products overnight.

20.10.3 Enforcement statistics

In the first few decades of the 1900s FDA brought hundreds of seizure and criminal actions to enforce the FD&C Act. Beginning in the 1970s, the formal court enforcement actions have been replaced in two ways. First, FDA has promulgated hundreds of regulations that establish the precise requirements of the law, thus reducing the need for many court enforcement actions. Second, formal court enforcement actions have been replaced by informal administrative enforcement actions such as recalls

and warning letters. FDA statistics demonstrate that the increase in administrative enforcement actions has been greater than the decrease in formal court enforcement actions, and thus that overall FDA enforcement activity has continued to increase.

20.11   Conclusion

This brief survey of the FDA regulation of pharmaceutical products demonstrates the breadth and depth of FDA activity in this field. Although there are repeated calls for reform of the IND/NDA system, it appears unlikely that any substantial change will occur in the near future. It is therefore important that any person who enters the prescription drug industry in the United States be fully informed about the requirements, understand the regulatory risks involved, and comply adequately with all of the FDA requirements.

References

1. An earlier version of this chapter was published in Burley DM, *et al. Pharmaceutical Medicine, 2nd edn.* 1993, ch. 9.
2. For example, Hutt PB and Merrill RA. *Food and Drug Law: Cases and Materials, 2nd edn.* 1991.
3. 52 Stat. 1040 (1938), 21 U.S.C. 301, *et seq.* FDA's internet website contains a large amount of information about the agency, the statutes it implements, its regulations and guidances, and other pertinent documents: www.fda.gov.
4. 5 U.S.C. 551 *et seq.*
5. 21 C.F.R. 10.40.
6. 21 C.F.R. 10.45.
7. Section 12606 of the California Business and Professions Code.
8. Hutt PB. A historical introduction. *Food Drug Cosmetic Law J* 1990;**45**:17; The transformation of United States Food and Drug Law. *J Association Food Drug Officials* 1996;**60**:1.
9. 12 Stat. 387 (1862).
10. 26 Stat. 282, 283 (1890).
11. 31 Stat. 922, 930 (1901).
12. 44 Stat. 976, 1002 (1927).
13. 46 Stat. 392, 422 (1930).

14. 54 Stat. 1234, 1237 (1940).

15. 67 Stat. 631, 632 (1953).

16. 93 Stat. 668, 695 (1979).

17. 102 Stat. 3048, 3120 (1988).

18. 21 C.F.R. 5.200.

19. Hutt PB and Hutt PB II. A history of government regulation of adulteration and misbranding of food. *Food Drug Cosmetic Law J* 1984;**39**:2.

20. Pliny, *Natural History* 207 (H Rackham ed. 1949).

21. 2 Stat. 806 (1813).

22. 3 Stat. 677 (1822).

23. 9 Stat. 237 (1848).

24. 42 Stat. 858, 989 (1922).

25. 32 Stat. 728 (1902).

26. 58 Stat. 682, 702 (1944).

27. 111 Stat. 2296, 2323 (1997), 42 U.S.C. 262.

28. 37 Fed. Reg. 12865 (29 June 1972).

29. 34 Stat. 768 (1906).

30. Note 3 supra.

31. 55 Stat. 851 (1941); 59 Stat. 463 (1945); 61 Stat. 11 (1947); 63 Stat. 409 (1949).

32. 65 Stat. 648 (1951).

33. 76 Stat. 780 (1962).

34. 84 Stat. 1236, 1242 (1970), 21 U.S.C. 801.

35. 84 Stat. 1670 (1970).

36. 16 C.F.R. part 1700.

37. 86 Stat. 559 (1972).

38. 96 Stat. 2049 (1983).

39. 98 Stat. 2815, 2817 (1984), section 526 (a)(2) of the FD&C Act, 21 U.S.C. 360bb(a)(2).

40. 98 Stat. 1585 (1984).

41. 100 Stat. 3743 (1986).

42. 110 Stat. 1321, 1321–313 (1996), as amended, 110 Stat. 1569, 1594 (1996), section 802 of the FD&C Act, 21 U.S.C. 382.

43. 102 Stat. 95 (1988).

44. 106 Stat. 941 (1992).

45. 106 Stat. 149 (1992).

46. 106 Stat. 4491 (1992); Kuhlik BN Industry funding of improvements in the FDA's new drug approval process: the Prescription Drug User Fee Act of 1992. *Food Drug Law J* 1992;47:483.

47. 111 Stat. 2296, 2298 (1997).

48. 116 Stat. 594, 687 (2002).

49. Note 42 supra; Hutt PB and Kuhlik BN *Export Expertise: Understanding Export Law for Drugs, Devices and Biologics.* 1998.

50. Note 41 supra.

51. 111 Stat. 2296 (1997).

52. 114 Stat. 1549A-35 (2000).

53. 115 Stat. 1408 (2002).

54. 116 Stat. 594 (2002).

55. Association of American Physicians and Surgeons, Inc., v. FDA, 226 F. Supp. 2d 204 (D.D.C. 2002).

56. 117 Stat. 1936 (2003).

57. 37 Stat. 822 (1913), 21 U.S.C. 151.

58. 82 Stat. 342 (1968), section 512 of the FD&C Act, 21 U.S.C. 360b.

59. 102 Stat. 3971 (1988).

60. 117 Stat. 1361 (2003).

61. 118 Stat. 891 (2004).

62. 90 Stat. 540 (1976); Hutt PB. A history of government regulation of adulteration and misbranding of medical devices. *Food Drug Cosmetic Law J* 1989;**44**:99.

63. 104 Stat. 4511 (1990); Flannery EJ. The Safe Medical Devices Act of 1990: an overview. *Food Drug Cosmetic Law J* 1991;**46**:129.

64. 106 Stat. 238 (1992).

65. Title III of 111 Stat. 2296, 2332 (1997).

66. 116 Stat. 1588 (2002).

67. Hutt PB. A legal framework for future decisions on transferring drugs from prescription to nonprescription status. *Food Drug Cosmetic Law J* 1982;**37**:427.

68. Note 32 supra.

69. Note 67 supra.

70. For example, 39 Fed. Reg. 19880, 19881 (4 June 1974).

71. Sections 7 and 8 of the 1906 Act, 34 Stat. 768, 769–71 (1906); sections and 502 of the FD&C Act, 21 U.S.C. 351 and 352.

72. 37 Fed. Reg. 85 (5 January 1972); 37 Fed. Reg. 9464 (11 May 1972); 21 C.F.R. part 330.

73. 21 C.F.R. 330.11.

74. 47 Fed. Reg. 50442 (5 November 1982); 21 C.F.R. 211.132.

75. 97 Stat. 831 (1983), 18 U.S.C. 1365.

76. 62 Fed. Reg. 9024 (27 February 1997); 64 Fed. Reg. 131254 (17 March 1999); 21 C.F.R. 201.66.

77. 38 Stat. 717 (1914).

78. 52 Stat. 111 (1938), 15 U.S.C. 41 *et seq.*

79. 36 Fed. Reg. 18539 (16 September 1971).

80. Note 2 supra at 477–487.

81. 52 Stat. 1040–1042 (1938).

82. *USV Pharmaceutical Corp.* v. *Weinberger*, 412 U.S. 655 (1973).

83. 33 Fed. Reg. 7758 (28 May 1968), 21 C.F.R. 310.100.

84. 34 Fed. Reg. 14596 (19 September 1969); 35 Fed. Reg. 3073 (17 February 1970); 35 Fed. Reg. 7250 (8 May 1970); 21 C.F.R. 314.126.

85. *Upjohn* v. *Finch*, 422 F. 2d 944 (6th Cir. 1970); *Pharmaceutical Manufacturers Ass'n v. Richardson*, 318 F. Supp. 301 (D. Del. 1970).

86. 34 Fed. Reg. 2673 (27 February 1969); 35 Fed. Reg. 6574 (24 April 1970).

87. *USV Pharmaceutical Corp.* v. *Weinberger*, 412 U.S. 655 (1973); *Weinberger* v. *Bentex Pharmaceuticals, Inc.*, 412 U.S. 645 (1973); *Ciba Corp.* v. *Weinberger*, 412 U.S. 640 (1973); *Weinberger* v. *Hynson, Westcott & Dunning, Inc.*, 412 U.S. 609 (1973).

88. *American Public Health Ass'n* v. *Veneman*, 349 F. Supp. 1311 (D.D.C. 1972).

89. 33 Fed. Reg. 7762 (28 May 1968).

90. Note 86 supra.

91. 40 Fed. Reg. 26142 (20 June 1975).

92. 41 Fed. Reg. 41770 (23 September 1976); FDA Compliance Policy Guide 440.100.

93. *United States* v. *Generix Drug Corp.*, 460 U.S. 453 (1983).

94. S. Rep. No. 96–321, 95th Cong. 1st Sess. (1979); 125 Cong. Rec. 2244–75 (26 September 1979).

95. *Burroughs Wellcome Co.* v. *Schweiker*, 649 F. 2d 221 (4th Cir. 1981); *Upjohn Manufacturing Co.* v. *Schweiker*, 681 F. 2d 480 (6th Cir. 1982).

96. 'Deficiencies in FDA's Regulation of the Marketing of Unapproved New Drugs: The Case of E-Ferol', H.R. Rep. No. 98–1168, 98th Cong., 2d Sess. (1984).

97. 49 Fed. Reg. 38190 (27 September 1984); FDA Compliance Policy Guide 440.100.

98. 50 Fed. Reg. 11478 (21 March 1985); 51 Fed. Reg. 24476 (3 July 1986); 21 C.F.R. 310.305.

99. Note 40 supra.

100. Note 97 supra.

101. 68 Fed. Reg. 60703 (23 October 2003).

102. 21 C.F.R. part 312.

103. 21 C.F.R. part 58.

104. Section 505(i)(3) of the FD&C Act, 21 U.S.C. 355(i)(3).

105. 21 C.F.R. parts 50 and 56.

106. 21 C.F.R. 312.32 and 312.33.

107. 21 C.F.R. 312.36.

108. 21 C.F.R. 312.34 and 312.35.

109. 55 Fed. Reg. 20856 (21 May 1990).

110. Clinical trial registration, *J American Medical Association* 2004;**292**:1363.

111. 21 C.F.R. part 314.

112. Section 505(d) of the FD&C Act, 21 U.S.C. 355(d).

113. Note 46 supra.

114. Note 51 supra.

115. Note 48 supra.

116. 57 Fed. Reg. 13234 (15 April 1992); 57 Fed. Reg. 58942 (11 December 1992); 21 C.F.R. part 314, subpart H.

117. Section 506 of the FD&C Act, 21 U.S.C. 356.

118. FDA, *Managing the Risks from Medical Product Use: Creating a Risk Management Framework*. Washington, DC: FDA, 1999.

119. Institute of Medicine, *To Err is Human: Building a Safer Health System*. 1999.

120. 21 C.F.R. 314.50(d)(5)(vi)(b).

121. For example, *Ubiotica* Corp. v. *FDA*, 427 F.2d 376 (6th Cir. 1970); *Edison Pharmaceutical Co., Inc.* v. *FDA*, 600 F.2d 831 (D.C. Cir. 1979).

122. 80 Stat. 250 (1966), 5 U.S.C. 552.

123. Section 301(j) of the FD&C Act, 21 U.S.C. 331(j).

124. 18 U.S.C. 1905.

125. 37 Fed. Reg. 9128 (5 May 1972); 39 Fed. Reg. 44602 (24 December 1974); 21 C.F.R. part 20.

126. 21 C.F.R. 312.130 and 314.430.

127. 21 C.F.R. 314.430(e)(2)(i).

128. 21 C.F.R. 314.430(f); 130 Cong. Rec. 24977–8 (12 September 1984).

129. Section 505(n) of the FD&C Act, 21 U.S.C. 355(n); 21 C.F.R. 14.160.

130. Section 505(k) of the FD&C Act, 21 U.S.C. 355(k); 21 C.F.R. 314.80 and 314.81.

131. 21 C.F.R. 314.70.

132. Section 505(e) of the FD&C Act, 21 U.S.C. 355(e); 21 C.F.R. 2.5.

133. *Forsham* v. *Califano*, 442 F. Supp. 203 (D.D.C. 1977).

134. 111 Stat. 2296, 2325 (1997).

135. Section 735 of the FD&C Act, 21 U.S.C. 379g.

136. Section 505(b)(2) of the FD&C Act, 21 U.S.C. 355(b)(2); 21 C.F.R. 314.50.

137. Section 505(j) of the FD&C Act, 21 U.S.C. 355(j); Flannery EJ and Hutt PB. Balancing competition and patent protection in the drug industry. *Food Drug Cosmetic Law J* 1985;**40**:269.

138. Section 505A of the FD&C Act, 21 U.S.C. 355a.

139. 55 Fed. Reg. 52323 (21 December 1990); 56 Fed. Reg. 46191 (10 September 1991); FDA Compliance Policy Guide 120.100.

140. Section 502(n)(2) of the FD&C Act, 21 U.S.C. 352(n).

141. 21 C.F.R. part 202.

142. 62 Fed. Reg. 14912 (28 March 1997).

143. FDA, *Guidance for Industry: Consumer-Directed Broadcast Advertisements*. Washington, DC: FDA, Draft July 1997, Final August 1999.

144. Section 505(b)(1)(D) of the FD&C Act, 21 U.S.C. 355 (b)(1)(D); 21 C.F.R. 314.50(d)(1).

145. 58 Fed. Reg. 47340 (28 January 1991); 56 Fed. Reg. 3180 (8 September 1993).

146. 21 C.F.R. parts 210 and 211.

147. Section 505(b)(4)(F) of the FD&C Act, 21 U.S.C. 355(b)(4)(F).

148. FDA, *Pharmaceutical CGMPs for the 21st Century – A Risk-Based Approach.* Washington, DC: FDA, 2004.
149. E.g., *Cedars North Towers Pharmacy, Inc.* v. *United States*, 1978–80 FDLI Judicial Record 668 (S.D. Fla. 1978).
150. *Thompson* v. *Western States Medical Center*, 535 U.S. 357 (2002).
151. FDA, *Compliance Policy Guide* Section 460.200 (May 2002).
152. *American Pharmaceutical Ass'n* v. *Weinberger*, 377 F. Supp. 824 (D.D.C. 1974), affirmed per curiam, 530 F.2d 1054 (D.C. Cir. 1976).
153. Note 116 supra.
154. Note 2 supra at 563–565.
155. Note 38 supra.
156. Note 39 supra.
157. 26 Weekly Compilation of Presidential Documents 1796 (9 October 1990).
158. 37 Fed. Reg. 16503 (15 August 1972).
159. For example, 21 C.F.R. 312.2(d).
160. 62 Fed. Reg. 43900 (15 August 1997); 63 Fed. Reg. 66632 (2 December 1998); 21 C.F.R. 314.55.
161. Note 138 supra.
162. Section 551 of the FD&C Act, 21 U.S.C. 360aaa.
163. *Washington Legal Foundation* v. *Friedman*, 13 F. Supp 2d 51 (D.D.C. 1998), 36 F. Supp. 2d 16 (D.D.C. 1999), and 56 F. Supp. 2d 81 (D.D.C. 1999).
164. *Washington Legal Foundation* v. *Henney*, 202 F. 3d 331 (D.C. Cir. 2000).
165. *Washington Legal Foundation* v. *Henney*, 128 F. Supp 2d 11 (D.D.C. 2000).
166. 65 Fed. Reg. 14286 (16 March 2000).
167. *United States* v. *Rutherford*, 442 U.S. 544 (1979); *Rutherford* v. *United States*, 806 F. 2d 1455 (10th Cir. 1986).
168. Note 2 supra at 552–566.
169. Hutt PB. Investigation and reports respecting FDA regulation of new drugs: parts I and II. *Clin Pharmacol Therapeut* 1983;**33**:537,674.
170. DiMasi JA, *et al.* Cost of innovation in the pharmaceutical industry. *J Health Economics* 1991;**10**:107.
171. Gilbert J., *et al.* Rebuilding big pharma's business model. *In Vivo* 2003;**21**.

172. Notes 25, 26 and 27 supra.
173. 61 Fed. Reg. 2733 (29 January 1996); 61 Fed. Reg. 24227 (14 May 1996).
174. Section 123 of the FDA Modernization Act of 1997, 111 Stat. 2296, 2323 (1997), Section 351(a) of the Public Health Service Act, 42 U.S.C. 262(a).
175. 63 Fed. Reg. 40858 (31 July 1998); 64 Fed. Reg. 56441 (20 October 1999); 21 C.F.R. 601.2.
176. 37 Fed. Reg. 16679 (18 August 1972); 38 Fed. Reg. 4319 (13 February 1973); 21 C.F.R. 601.25.
177. Section 704 of the FD&C Act, 21 U.S.C. 374.
178. The non-prescription drug industry traded records inspection for national uniformity under the FDA Modernization Act of 1997, 111 Stat. 2296, 2374, 2375 (1997).
179. Section 304 of the FD&C Act, 21 U.S.C. 334.
180. Section 709 of the FD&C Act, 21 U.S.C. 379a.
181. Section 302 of the FD&C Act, 21 U.S.C. 332.
182. Section 303(a) of the FD&C Act, 21 U.S.C. 333(a).
183. *United States* v. *Dotterweich*, 320 U.S. 277 (1943); *United States* v. *Park*, 421 U.S. 658 (1975).
184. Section 305 of the FD&C Act, 21 U.S.C. 335.
185. 18 U.S.C. 371.
186. 18 U.S.C. 1001.
187. 18 U.S.C. 1341.
188. 21 U.S.C. 209.
189. 21 U.S.C. 1623.
190. Section 303(b) of the FD&C Act, 21 U.S.C. 333(b).
191. *United States* v. *Parkinson*, 240 F. 2d 918 (9th Cir. 1956).
192. *United States* v. *Universal Management Systems, Inc.*, 191 F. 3d 750 (6th Cir. 1999).
193. Section 518 of the FD&C Act, 21 U.S.C. 360h.
194. For example, *United States* v. *Superpharm Corp.*, 530 F. Supp. 408 (E.D.N.Y. 1981); *United States* v. *Barr Laboratories, Inc.*, 812 F. Supp. 458 (D.N.J. 1993).
195. 21 C.F. R. 7.40.
196. Section 705 of the FD&C Act, 21 U.S.C. 375.
197. *Horsey Cancer Clinic* v. *Folson*, 155 F. Supp. 376 (D.D.C. 1957); *Ajay Nutrition Foods, Inc.* v. *FDA*, 378 F. Supp. 210 (D.N.J. 1974), affirmed, 513 F. 2d 625 (3rd Cir. 1975).

21 The US FDA in the drug development, evaluation and approval process

Richard N Spivey, Judith K Jones,
William Wardell and William Vodra

21.1 Introduction

21.1.1 Background

The Food and Drug Administration (FDA) is one of the largest and most complex agencies dealing with drug development, evaluation and approval. Separate centres handle drugs and therapeutic biologics, vaccines and blood products, devices and food. At the same time, personnel within the agency are accessible and a wealth of information is readily available to help guide novice and experienced pharmaceutical personnel alike through the process. The FDA has a website (http//:www.fda.gov) that gives ready access to food and drug law, official guidelines and unofficial guidance documents for drugs, biologics, devices and foods. Also, one can find FDA press releases and 'talk papers' on a variety of topics of current interest as well as information concerning the FDA Advisory Committees. Chapter 21 of the Code of Federal Regulations (21 CFR) contains the official regulations for the FDA. A printed version is available through the US Superintendent of Documents. The Public Health Service Act governs biologics. Regulation of biologics and drug development has recently been largely harmonised and regulation of drugs and therapeutic biologics has been consolidated within the Center for Drug Evaluation and Review (CDER).

The FDA, like all drug regulatory agencies worldwide, is in the midst of rapid change in response to the pressures of consumers and healthcare professionals for more rapid approval of life-saving drugs and from the push for international harmonisation of review and approval procedures. At the same time, the frequent occurrence of safety problems, some of which reach political proportions, acts as a restraining force on too-rapid change. The FDA Modernization Act (FDAMA) of 1997 represents congressional response to some of these pressures. FDAMA is the most extensive legislative changes made to the Food, Drug and Cosmetic Act (FD&C Act) since the landmark 1962 Kefauver–Harris amendments, which added the explicit requirement that drugs demonstrate efficacy in addition to being safe. For the most part, however, FDAMA merely codified current FDA practice rather than making substantial reforms. Specific references will be made to the FDAMA changes in this chapter, but it is important always to check the implementing regulations.

Of late, there has been increasing pressure on FDA from a new front. Access to medication from ex-US sources (parallel importing) is being demanded by consumers, and FDA is being asked to ensure a safe, high-quality supply chain. How this issue is resolved could have significant implications on FDA resources, especially for field inspection staff. In addition, there have surfaced many topics that consume FDA resources, ranging from risk management programs for newly marketed products to identifying drug development impediments and offering advice to the industry on ways to expedite development (the 'Critical Path' Initiative of 2004), as well as very recent renewed concerns on how the FDA assures the safety of drugs. Many of these topics will result in additional draft guidances and formal guidelines; some topics will be addressed in greater detail elsewhere in this chapter, while others are included in a subsequent chapter on development-related issues in the United States.

21.1.2 Phases of drug development

As described in more detail in Section 21.2, initiation of clinical testing must be preceded by submission of an Investigational New Drug Application (IND) to the FDA for review, prior to introduction in humans, that may proceed if a review of the pre-clinical data provides no basis for the agency to place a clinical hold on the testing. Clinical drug development leading to product approval is often described in three phases. In the US regulations Phase 1 is described as the initial introduction into humans. Studies conducted in this phase of development are intended to determine the tolerance (dose range), metabolism and pharmacologic actions of the drug in humans and to characterise the adverse experiences associated with increasing doses. Studies in Phase 1 are usually closely monitored and may be conducted in patients as well as normal subjects, depending on the nature of the drug as well as the type of information being sought. Drug interaction studies are also likely to be conducted.

In Phase 2 the studies are conducted to prove the therapeutic concept and evaluate efficacy and assure that measures of efficacy are adequate. Importantly, dose–response studies are conducted to determine the therapeutically useful dose range and to establish doses to be used in full-scale clinical trials. These studies are closely monitored and well controlled in a small to moderate numbers of patients with the condition of interest. Study results may also give some idea of common dose-related adverse events following short-term therapy.

Phase 3 studies are usually large and placebo-controlled in design. They provide expanded information concerning the efficacy and safety of the drug in the intended patient population. For the FDA, these studies have traditionally been to provide information on benefit versus risk, as well as prescribing information for physicians. Historically, two adequate and well-controlled studies (usually Phase 3) were required for drug approval, often including the use of placebo. In addition, for chronic-use drugs, longer-term experience is required, that is, beyond 6–12 months of treatment. International Conference on Harmonization (ICH) guidelines now describe recommended durations and numbers for chronic testing. For oncology and AIDS drugs, Phase 2 studies have been accepted in support of approval, and in some cases only a single adequate and well controlled study was considered sufficient. To clarify the requirement for the number of studies, FDAMA specifically stated that a single 'adequate and well-controlled' study is sufficient provided that 'confirmatory evidence' is obtained before or after the trial. The acceptability of a single trial should be discussed with FDA.

It is important to note that the phases described above are not mutually exclusive and are not necessarily performed in strict linear order. These definitions have become increasingly blurred with the accelerated development plans seen with drugs for the treatment of serious and life-threatening disorders. It is becoming more important to ask of each study, what will be learned and what the study contributes to proof of either efficacy or safety, or ultimately to the product label. The evidence required for approval increases inexorably year by year. For example, increasing emphasis has been placed on exploring drug use in special populations, such as, the elderly, the young and patients with hepatic or renal impairment, and to characterise possible major drug–drug interactions. The most recent major addition has been studies to address cardiovascular safety (e.g. QTc prolongation) that may alone add a cost of one-to several million dollars to each development program.

21.1.3 FDA meetings: general considerations

The FDA is open to communication. Meetings can be by teleconference, videoconference or face-to-face. The FDA procedure refers to a 'center [FDA] component', which in most cases will be the FDA division responsible for the IND and eventually for the new drug application (NDA) [or in the case of biologics, the biologics licence application (BLA)]. The request must be in writing, usually preceded by a telephone call to the Consumer Safety Officer (CSO) / project manager responsible for the drug to discuss the need for the meeting and to make preliminary arrangements. The written request for the meeting should include a statement on the purpose of the meeting, a list of specific objectives that the sponsor has for the meeting, a proposed agenda, a list of sponsor attendees, a request for FDA attendees and the timing of submission of a background document for the meeting.[1]

The director of the FDA component, usually the Division Director, will determine whether the meeting is appropriate. Normally the background document must be sent to the FDA at least 4 weeks prior to the meeting. Once the Division Director has agreed to a meeting, the reviewing division has 14 days to set a date with the sponsor (the earliest date when FDA participants can be available) within 30–75 days, depending on the type of meeting.

The FDA is usually quite accommodating about meetings, but meetings should not be requested frivolously or prematurely. In preparing for an FDA meeting the sponsor should prepare and submit an agenda and background document to the FDA reviewing division. This should not be too lengthy and large documents should be submitted as appendices to the background document. The sponsor should submit specific questions for FDA to address. Any presentation should conform to the written material submitted and should be succinct and focused. It is rare to obtain more than 1 h and time must be allotted for dialogue. Rehearsal is important to avoid unclear presentations and to clearly focus on key questions and meeting objectives. The agency often decides to dispense with the formal presentation and go straight to the sponsor's questions and discussion. When the FDA requests that presentations be omitted, the sponsor should follow the agency's lead and listen and respond to the comments. If, during the discussion, there are areas that require clarification, there may be parts of the planned presentation that can be used. The timing of the meeting may have some importance in terms of confidentiality; for example, there are regulations concerning the confidentiality of an existing IND that may not apply to a meeting held before an IND has been submitted.

It is very important for the sponsor and the FDA to keep complete and accurate minutes of official meetings, and in some cases these are done at the meeting with both parties agreeing to the wording. Often, FDA provides draft responses to questions posed by the sponsor prior to or at the time of the actual meeting. This greatly facilitates communication of issues and possible pathways to address data requirements. The FDA procedure for meetings outlines distribution within the agency. The minutes of the meeting should be exchanged between agency and sponsor to minimise misunderstandings. These minutes provide a record of agreements reached and they may be very important as development proceeds and at the time of NDA submission. Sponsors may request assessment of specific protocols to determine if they are adequate to meet scientific and regulatory requirements. These protocols include: (1) animal carcinogenicity protocols, (2) final product stability protocols and (3) clinical protocols for Phase 3 trials. These assessments, if agreed to by sponsor and FDA, are reduced to writing.[2]

21.2 The Investigational New Drug Application

21.2.1 General considerations

An IND is required before clinical testing of a new drug can begin in the United States. The information requirements for the IND are found in chapter 21, part 312 of the Code of Federal Regulations (21 CFR 312). The purpose of the IND is to provide a scientific rationale for studying the drug in humans and sufficient information from preclinical studies to warrant the risk of exposure in humans. Although the information to be submitted is specified in the regulations, there is flexibility as to the amount and type of information needed, based on the design of the first trials to be performed under the IND. For example, if all that is needed initially is to test the bioavailability of a drug in man, the requirements for data may be less than for a more extensive Phase 1 programme. Although there are exceptions, FDA generally wants a separate IND for each dosage form and research target (e.g. heart failure and asthma). Cross-referencing to information contained in an existing IND is permitted and reduces the need for duplicate paperwork.

The FDA has clarified the minimum requirements for an IND submission in three areas: chemistry, toxicology reports (draft) and size (2–3 volumes, each 3″ thick) in an attempt to relax current practices somewhat, to the level required for a UK CTX.[3] However, full reports are to be provided within a short time after the initial drafts. (Conversely, however, information needed to conduct human studies in the European Union has increased, recently, with the implementation of the Clinical Trial Directive.)

An individual (rather than an industrial sponsor) may also submit an IND for the purpose of conducting clinical investigations. Such an individual is referred to as an investigator-sponsor. If the investigator plans to study a drug already subject to an IND held by an industrial or other sponsor, he or she can request that the sponsor allow them to cross-reference the existing IND. A letter from the IND sponsor allowing cross-referencing by the investigator-sponsor is usually all that is needed. These situations usually occur when an investigator wishes to pursue a research target not of interest to the industrial sponsor. The request for cross-referencing may be denied if the planned investigation is felt not to be consonant with the development of the drug. An investigator-sponsor may, however, proceed if he supplies

information independent of the industrial sponsor to support the investigator-sponsor application and thus meet FDA data requirements. This is usually beyond the individual capabilities of the investigator-sponsor, especially for drugs not yet approved for any indication.

The question of the benefits and risks of investigator-sponsored INDs is often raised by small pharmaceutical companies, who are attracted to the independence, and often the lower initial cost, that this entails. Investigators are responsible for all the administrative support of their own INDs and maintain responsibility for meeting all IND reporting and performance obligations. Usually the initial costs are indeed less to the small company, as the investigator is often willing to handle the IND requirement because he or she may have independent funding for the conduct of the study. The risk to the company is the lack of control over the study (and the drug) that this independence entails. The investigator may not perform the study to the standards needed, or may fail to report safety data in an appropriate and timely manner. Any of these failures could raise issues for the development of the drug and could have an adverse impact on the drug, the programme and the company.

Similar issues of control and development priorities are raised when studies are conducted under the auspices of any organisation not contractually bound to the company. Examples include National Institutes of Health (NIH) entities such as the National Cancer Institute (NCI) or any of the cancer cooperative study groups, or the AIDS Cooperative Trials Group (ACTG). The company is at the mercy of the priorities, sense of urgency, objectives, standard operating procedures (SOPs), auditing standards, case report forms, coding dictionaries and databases of these groups when the latter are the sponsors independent of the company. At the same time, these groups may well be the most cost-efficient and expeditious way of developing a new drug, and they may control access to specialised resources (e.g. specialised clinical laboratories). These factors (in addition to ownership issues) must be carefully weighed before a decision is taken to rely on any outside sponsorship for drug development.

21.2.2   IND submission and review

An IND is submitted to the appropriate reviewing division within CDER (see 21 CFR 312.23 for IND content and format). If there is uncertainty as to the appropriate reviewing divisions, one should check with the division considered most likely and obtain guidance. For both drugs and biologics, one may also consult the office of the Deputy Director. Once an IND is submitted the reviewing division will acknowledge receipt, and the date of receipt becomes the official date for review purposes. Once an IND is submitted, the FDA reviewing division has 30 days from the official submission date in the acknowledgment letter in which to evaluate the information contained in the IND and to decide whether the information supports going forward with the initial human study protocol. There is no official 'approval' of an IND; rather, it is 'allowed'. If FDA raises no 'hold' issues during the 30-day evaluation period the sponsor is free to proceed. However, it is generally good practice to contact the agency prior to study initiation to confirm that there are no concerns related to starting the planned study.

The FDA may respond to the IND with questions and concerns in writing. These may be requests for clarification or issues that need to be addressed during the drug development process. If the FDA feels that the planned study poses a significant safety risk to human subjects they may inform the sponsor that the study cannot proceed. This act is referred to as placing a 'clinical hold' on the IND. A clinical hold may be complete or partial. In the latter case, the FDA may place a hold on certain aspects of the planned development while permitting the sponsor to proceed with other aspects. For example, the planned study may be a dose-escalation trial and the FDA may only permit a single dose level based on the information provided in the IND. FDAMA has codified FDA obligations to a sponsor whose IND is placed on clinical hold (Section 117). The FDA is obliged to explain its concern and make clear

to the sponsor what is needed to respond. Guidance documents adopted before the legislative changes require the reviewing division to communicate its concerns by telephone and with a written communication within five working days. The sponsor then responds and the FDA must reply within 30 days as to the adequacy of the response. If the hold is not lifted, formal appeal to the office level may be needed to resolve differences of opinion.

21.2.3   IND meetings (see 21 CFR 312.47)

21.2.3.1   Early IND meetings

One of the decisions that a sponsor should make regarding the time immediately before or after filing an IND is whether to request a meeting with the FDA to discuss the submission. The FDA has become more receptive in recent years to offering early advice and counsel. As a result, meetings during early development are much more common than they were a decade ago. Reasons for requesting a meeting in the early phases of an IND are varied. The sponsor may have concerns regarding some element of the IND – for example, they may wish to have as a first study relatively long exposure, and there may be problems with the adequacy of the animal toxicological data to support the exposure planned. The sponsor may wish to introduce the FDA to what they feel is a very interesting and promising development project. Another reason for requesting a meeting might be to determine whether the early development programme is adequate to achieve the stated objectives. If the latter is the primary purpose of the meeting, it is highly recommended that the sponsor present a plan to the FDA for comment and discussion, rather than asking the agency how to proceed. This latter approach can lead to less productive dialogue and perhaps a less than focused or less commercially feasible development programme.

21.2.3.2   End of Phase 2 meeting

For most drugs, one of the most important meetings with the FDA in the new drug development process is the end of Phase 2 meeting. This was initially directed at drugs of specific interest because of either medical need or possible toxicity. This meeting is now standard at the FDA for development planning. Its purpose is to present to FDA the results of studies conducted during Phase 1 and Phase 2 to gain the agency's concurrence that it is safe and reasonable to proceed into Phase 3. More importantly, assuming there is concurrence to proceed, the meeting serves to review plans for Phase 3 development. Under FDAMA, written agreements on the adequacy of design of the key efficacy trials can be obtained (Section 119). Because Phase 3 can be very expensive for the sponsor and critical to the ultimate approval of the drug, it is critical to obtain FDA commitment at this juncture.

The timing of the end of Phase 2 meeting is important. The meeting should be scheduled when sufficient information from earlier phases of development is available, yet early enough to permit planning and preparation for Phase 3. The information available must be in a condition to permit adequate summary and analysis. The background package of information presented to the FDA is critical to achieving the objectives of the meeting. At this stage, one should have ready a 'target package insert' with clearly stated desired claims and careful annotation showing the existing or planned studies that are intended to support these claims. This is pivotal for obtaining detailed advice and opinion from the agency. A clinical development plan has little meaning unless related to the precise language of a package insert 'Indications' section. Also, if any specific safety statements are desired or anticipated these should be highlighted and the data supporting them referenced in the background material. This meeting needs intense preparation. In order to achieve the objectives in the limited time available, any presentations must be concise and focused. If the FDA has reviewed the background material the agency may wish to omit the sponsor's presentations, but the sponsor must still be prepared.

21.2.3.3   IND amendments

The IND evolves with the development programme. It is amended with each new protocol and with each meaningful change in an existing protocol. It is particularly important to remember to amend a protocol when there is a change in design or in the scope of the study. The sponsor may begin a new study or implement a change in protocol when the protocol or protocol amendment has been submitted to the FDA for review and approval obtained from the institutional review board (IRB) responsible for the study.

There are also information amendments submitted to the IND that incorporate new information concerning the drug under study. Examples include new toxicology data or new information concerning chemistry, manufacturing or controls of the drug. These amendments are essential to support new clinical protocols or amendments. There are proposals currently being discussed to determine the feasibility and desirability of submitting the original IND and subsequent amendments electronically. If this is done well, the body of information can be more accessible to the FDA reviewers and lead to a more comprehensive knowledge base in anticipation of a future NDA submission. This concept has been referred to as a 'cumulative' IND.

The IND safety report is another important type of IND amendment. Any serious, unexpected adverse experience associated with the use of the drug occurring in clinical trials *or in animal studies* must be submitted to the FDA; the regulations define 'serious' and 'unexpected' (21 CFR 312.32). 'Associated with' is somewhat more subjectively defined as an event for 'which there is a reasonable possibility that the event might have been caused by the drug'. The sponsor must report to the FDA and notify all participating investigators in writing within 15 calendar days following the initial receipt of the report. It does not matter whether or not the source of the event was a study conducted under the IND for it to be reportable. If the safety report concerns a fatal or life-threatening event of the type described, the FDA is to be notified by telephone within five calendar days. This is to be followed by the written report within 15 calendar days. It is critical that the regulations concerning IND safety reports be reviewed in detail as there are several nuances of interpretation, and strict compliance is essential.

21.2.3.4 IND annual reports

Within 60 days of the anniversary date on which the IND went into effect, the sponsor must submit an annual report. Regulations (21 CFR 312.33) outlines the requirements for this report. It should include a brief summary of the status of each study completed or in progress. If a study is complete, a brief description of the findings should be presented, and if in progress any interim results available should be summarised. A summary of all IND safety reports submitted during the year must be included, along with tabulations of the most frequent and serious adverse experiences observed. Listings of all patients who died or who discontinued from the study because of adverse events (regardless of causality) must also be included. All preclinical studies completed or in progress during the year should be listed and any new findings summarised. New manufacturing information should also be presented. There is flexibility in the format of the report but it is important to submit it in a timely manner. Extensions may be granted upon request to the agency.

21.2.3.5 IND issues for drugs that treat serious or life-threatening conditions

FDAMA widened and codified 'fast-track' procedures that had previously been addressed in part by 21 CFR 312 Subpart E, for drugs intended to treat 'life-threatening and severely debilitating illnesses'. The act refers to drugs 'intended for the treatment of a serious or life-threatening condition and it demonstrates the potential to address unmet medical needs for such a condition' (Section 112). Sponsors apply for 'fast-track' status and, if this is granted, receive expedited review of the application based on clinical or surrogate measures 'reasonably likely to predict clinical benefit'. The Act also codifies the process of a 'rolling review', whereby an incomplete application can be reviewed, while results from ongoing studies are added as the review progresses. Both the Act and existing Subpart E regulations place several conditions and limitations on drugs approved under 'fast track'. These include commitments to carry out definitive studies post approval, pre-clearance of promotional material by the FDA and a procedure for accelerated withdrawal of the drug from the market in cases where clinical benefit is not confirmed. Because development is accelerated under this procedure, sponsor and agency interactions are more frequent and intense than for other applications. For example, the enhanced interactions allow for an end of Phase 1 meeting, where guidance might be offered that would allow an adequate and well controlled Phase 2 study or studies to be used as the basis of approval.

Another set of regulations, 21 CFR 312.34, governs the availability of a treatment IND or protocol. A treatment IND protocol allows a drug to be made available to patients not otherwise eligible to participate in clinical studies that are part of the drug development programme. A treatment protocol may be filed when the drug provides a possible treatment for a serious or life-threatening disorder where no alternative therapy is available. A treatment protocol may be filed during Phase 3, or when all clinical studies have been completed. When the drug is clearly valuable, a treatment IND can be filed as early as Phase 2. The regulations spell out the information that must be provided when submitting a treatment protocol. The FDA must determine that there is sufficient information to suggest that the drug may offer the prospect of efficacy and that the risks for use are acceptable. The sponsor must also give assurances that they are continuing the development of a drug with due diligence. The sponsor should be aware that there is a risk that making the drug available under a treatment protocol may reduce the ability of the sponsor to recruit patients into the controlled trials, thereby delaying ultimate approval of the NDA.

21.3 The new drug application (NDA or BLA)

21.3.1 General considerations

The NDA is an organised presentation of all the information collected during the drug development process assembled into a format allowing

FDA review. The regulations governing the NDA are found in 21 CFR 314. In addition, the FDA has issued detailed guidelines on the content and format of the NDA, which can be accessed on the FDA website. It is important to note, however, that the reviewing division may have specific format or organisational needs for the data to ensure speedy review (see pre-NDA meeting). Commonly, case report forms and data tabulations have been submitted in electronic portable document file (PDF) format, greatly reducing the volume of paper that needs to be submitted to FDA. It is now possible – and soon to be mandatory – that NDAs be submitted entirely in electronic form. Several guidelines have been issued that outline the requirements for such submissions, including the need for electronic signatures.

Recently, FDA has promulgated specific proposed guidances on the structure and activities for pre-marketing risk assessment, and final guidances are forthcoming.[4] This guidance is in the context of an overall initiative by FDA to promote 'Risk Management' planning as part of the NDA process. (There are two additional companion guidances on Risk Minimization Action Plans (RiskMAPs) and pharmacovigilance that relate more to post-marketing activities). The expectation implicit in these proposed guidances and other actions by FDA is that each NDA may need to consider whether a RiskMAP is needed for a particular risk. It is also implied that if this is the case, the NDA should include descriptions of this plan and how it will be evaluated, which may include pre-market testing of the RiskMAP as part of the NDA clinical trials. This testing may include evaluation of communications or other interventions to be used in the post-marketing period.

The NDA is a 'layered' document. There are summary documents, individual study reports and actual data tabulations. It differs in two main ways from the dossier submitted in the European Union: (1) in the amount of raw data contained in the NDA submission, and (2) in the presence of expert reports in the European dossier, compared with well defined integrated summaries in the NDA. This resulted from historical, cultural and structural differences between United States and European regulatory bodies. In general, Europeans have relied more heavily on outside experts to review applications. The ICH Conferences have made considerable progress in harmonising the content of many sections of the US NDA and the EU dossier. ICH has now agreed on the common technical document (CTD) that will, as the name implies, be a common approach to dossiers in the three participating regions of the world, the United States, the European Union and Japan. In addition, work has begun on elaborating the requirements for the electronic version, the eCTD.

21.3.2 The pre-NDA meeting

As preparations for the submission of an NDA begin, there needs to be a pre-NDA meeting with the FDA reviewing division. This meeting focuses on format, not content, and is important to eliminate delays that can occur when an NDA does not meet the specific needs of the assigned reviewers at the FDA (21 CFR 312.47). The sponsor should provide to the FDA an idea of the types and volume of information to be submitted, as well as the plan for data summary, presentation and analysis. The FDA should provide to the sponsor any specific requests for the display and analysis of data. Electronic formats and requests have become more routine, and a good understanding of what is planned and needed can help improve efficiency and minimise later difficulties.

21.3.3 NDA submission

The sponsor submits the NDA along with an appropriate application fee (currently in the range of $600 000), and the FDA reviews the application for completeness, that is to determine whether all parts of the NDA are present, in particular the information critical for their review. If the NDA is complete enough for review it is 'filed' (accepted) by the FDA. The agency has 60 days in which to perform this 'completeness' review. The completeness review is important under user fee legislation, as the review clock starts with FDA's receipt of an NDA for review. If the FDA finds that some critical information is missing, the agency will notify the sponsor that the NDA is not filed (i.e. not complete). In that case the agency must state the nature of the deficiency, so the sponsor can resubmit with the needed information. The sponsor forfeits half of the application fee if the NDA is not accepted for filing. For drugs reviewed under fast-track procedures, an incomplete NDA can be filed for review and additional data submitted during the review process (the 'rolling review' referred to earlier).

The official filing date is 60 days after receipt of the submission, if no significant deficiencies in the application have been found. FDA then has 180 days in which to review the content of the application for its acceptability for approval. This time frame was almost never met in the past, and until recently was usually much longer. The Prescription Drug User Fee Act of 1992 (PDUFA) set specific performance targets for the agency, listed below. Performance has improved considerably since the passage of this Act. There is a 'sunset' clause in PDUFA that requires re-approval every 5 years. It was last renewed in 2002, and is due for renewal by Congress again in 2007.

21.3.4   NDA classification

PDUFA provides for the classification of NDA submissions as being subject to either standard or priority review. Priority applications are targeted for, and tracked to, an action at 6 months. The standard applications are targeted for action at 10 months. The sponsor may request the priority review status to be applied. This request is usually contained in the cover letter, along with the rationale for the request. Although there are general guidelines that address the basis for ascribing priority review status, decisions are not always clear-cut and arguments provided by the sponsor may help guide the agency. Nevertheless, FDA considers for priority review classification, a drug product that would be a significant improvement compared to marketed products, demonstrated by: (1) evidence

of increased effectiveness in treatment, prevention or diagnosis of disease; (2) elimination or substantial reduction of a treatment-limiting drug reaction; (3) documented enhancement of patient compliance; or (4) evidence of safety and effectiveness in a new subpopulation.[5]

21.3.5   Monitoring the review of the NDA

Once the NDA has been filed, the sponsor must monitor the progress of the NDA review in order to detect problems or concerns at the earliest possible moment. This monitoring or tracking must be carried out with great sensitivity. If contacts are too frequent or poorly timed they can quickly become an annoyance, which can hamper further communications. The project manager or consumer safety officer is the usual point of contact. If there is difficulty with a particular review, then the reviewer should be contacted (with consideration, obviously, for the reviewer's time).

One must consider the reviewer's style and preferred method of communication. Some reviewers prefer requests to go through the project Manager or CSO. One reviewer might be very responsive to e-mail, whereas another might prefer a telephone call. The contacts during an NDA review can be numerous – the exact number will vary with the application and the reviewing division. The purpose of contacts should not only be to track or monitor, but whenever possible to assist the reviewer in resolving quickly minor issues that can sometimes cause the reviewer to slow or even halt a review.

All substantial requests, whether received informally or through official notification, must be addressed as promptly and completely as possible. An attempt to gloss over an issue usually leads to further delay. Issues raised by the reviewer represent significant concerns and should be treated as such. The amount and type of any new information needed to answer a request must be carefully considered. Under user fee guidelines, the FDA likes to keep the review moving without the need to review large amounts of new data which, if too large, may cause FDA to 'reset the clock', that is, extend the review timeframe. The effect of such a submission on the review should be discussed with the agency and balanced against the need for the information.

21.3.6 FDA actions

Until quite recently the actions of the FDA concerning an NDA were expressed in either, an approvable letter or a non-approval letter. In the case of a non-approval letter, the deficiencies were noted and were felt by the agency to require substantial action by the sponsor since a positive action by the agency in the present review cycle was not possible. Where the issues could be solved promptly by the sponsor, a non-approval letter was not necessarily a bad result because it officially clarified the remaining issues.

An approvable letter usually stated some minor area of concern that needed to be resolved prior to final approval. The letter usually stated that if these concerns were resolved approval would be granted.

In contrast, an approval letter meant that the submitted information justified approval. The only action usually requested for this type of letter was the submission of final printed labelling and advertising. In some cases, an approval letter could spell out other conditions for approval, such as post-approval studies, or restrictions on distribution or promotion. These conditions were generally discussed with the sponsor and agreed to prior to receipt of the letter.

Efforts are underway to replace the non-approval and approvable letters with a letter that lists all the deficiencies the sponsor will need to correct to obtain approval. If deficiencies are substantial the letter will read more like the old non-approval letter; if the deficiencies are minor, the letter would read more like an approvable letter. To date, the use of such letters has been random at best, and it is still most common to receive one of the three 'action' letters noted above.

The sponsor will usually be made aware of the deficiencies prior to the action letter, and this allows a more rapid response. If post-approval studies are to be performed as a condition of approval, the agency now has clear authority to require the sponsor to report on those studies under Section 130 of FDAMA. Under the previous law, FDA's authority in this regard was never clear, and post-approval studies had been conducted under a 'gentleman's agreement' without a firm legal basis.

21.3.7 Post-approval reporting

Following the approval of an NDA, the sponsor has ongoing reporting responsibilities. The most important of these is the monitoring of clinical safety once the drug is on the market, to ensure that the product's benefits outweigh any risks identified when it is introduced to larger, more diverse populations. Clinical safety regulations for drugs are found at 21 CFR 314.80, and for biologics at 21 CFR 600.80 and basically require that all reports of safety concerns received by the sponsor are captured and reported to FDA. These regulations describe specific and rigidly enforced requirements, as to the timing of submissions of individual spontaneous reports of suspected adverse events, determined by the type of report (e.g. serious and unlabelled events are reported in 15 calendar days, whereas most other events are submitted in periodic reports). The information required is described on a standard form, the 3500A, which closely corresponds to the international Council for International Organizations of Medical Sciences (CIOMS) form for event reporting that is accepted in most countries.

In the past decade, there has been increased emphasis on drug safety, and more public visibility of safety problems. The volume of reports now exceeds 250 000 spontaneous reports per year, and adverse events are highlighted in the medical press and also in the general media. The FDA has released extensive proposed new regulations for post-approval reporting that in part move to harmonise requirements with ICH recommendations for periodic safety update reports (PSURs) in use in many other countries, use of standardised terminology (MedDRA) and standards for electronic reporting of adverse events. These proposed regulations also include broader definitions for reporting serious events as well as actual and potential medication errors. In parallel, the FDA has focused more intently on this area in both NDA reviews and in the post-marketing period. This has been prompted by the need to withdraw a number of products, such as cisapride, phenylpropanolamine, terfenadine, troglitazone, cerivastatin and rofecoxib. Also, there is increased scrutiny of products associated with particular adverse events, such as cardiac arrhythmias (*torsades de pointes*) and hepatic necrosis, because many of the safety problems have involved these events. In the case of many of these drugs, initial attempts to improve the safe use of the products through additions to the product label (e.g. bolded warnings, black boxes) were found not to be heeded by either prescribers or pharmacies dispensing the products.

The agency generally concluded that label changes are insufficient for preventing significant risks. The result has been an emphasis on the concept of risk management of a product. This concept evolved, after open hearings and feedback, into RiskMAPs and is described in Draft FDA Guidance released in May 2004.[6] The Risk Management Draft Guidance identifies the need to (1) identify potential risks in the indication population, (2) determine which tools (information as in labels, active interventions such as patient consent or restricted distribution) can be best applied to prevent them and (3) develop methods to determine whether the interventions are effective or need to be further optimised. Several risk management efforts are already in place (e.g. thalidomide, alosetron, isotretinoin) and are regularly being evaluated by FDA as the guidances are starting to be implemented on a broader scale. Although only draft versions of the guidance have been released, there is a general trend for sponsors to develop at least some general plans for RiskMAPs as part of the NDA.

In addition to the required reporting of spontaneously reported and literature adverse events, there is a requirement for an NDA annual report that contains other information relevant to the NDA. Again, the requirements are detailed in the CFR. Annual reports must contain a brief summary of new information that might bear on the safety, efficacy or labelling of the drug. This summary should also include any actions taken or planned as a result of the new information. The report also contains product distribution data, current labelling with any changes highlighted, as well as new information from preclinical and clinical studies. Updates are also needed for any ongoing studies.

Sponsors are required to submit copies of promotional materials, for example, journal advertisements, detail pieces such as file cards, etc. to FDA at the time of initial dissemination. This means that the sponsor is to submit them to FDA simultaneously with the use of that piece or program. It is also possible for companies to engage FDA in review of proposed programs or advertisements, in order to gain feedback on acceptability. This is particularly important for broadcast advertisements aimed at consumers, such as those viewed on television. If promotional materials are deemed to be violative by FDA, for example, if they are false and misleading, a sponsor must withdraw the advertisements and in some cases undertake new campaigns to correct the objectionable statements.

The NDA is a living document for as long as a drug is marketed. It is also a 'contract' that cannot be modified without notice to (and in most cases approval by) FDA of changes in its terms through the submission of a 'supplement' to the NDA. For example, supplements must be approved for labelling modifications such as new indications, patient populations, dosing instructions or cautionary advice. Similarly, most changes in the chemistry, manufacturing and controls provisions must be approved in advance of implementation, although some can be implemented at the time of notification to FDA (and subject to FDA disapproval) and other, minor changes need only be reported in the annual report to the NDA.

The maintenance of an NDA is nearly as important as the approval, because any neglect in this activity can place the product in jeopardy.

21.4 Conclusions

The roles of the Pharmaceutical Industry and the FDA, and the relationships between them, have evolved considerably since the 1962 effectiveness amendments to the FD&C Act, and today the two parties are engaged in a close, complex, generally supportive – if sometimes fractious – relationship. There is no doubt that the achievements of these two parties, both individually and together, have been spectacular – even historic – as their effectiveness and safety standards have been embraced by the whole world. Indeed, these standards are now recognised as a landmark in post-enlightenment science, as well as a forerunner of the current philosophy of evidence-based medicine.

Now, however, there are growing worries in a new direction; that the drug-development effort has become bogged down in exaggerated regulatory process and compliance activities. The resulting fear is that drug development is slowing down, failing more often and could eventually grind to a halt because of the increasing weight of regulatory demands.

In the next chapter we consider these concerns, and other aspects of the future of the drug development and approval process.

Acknowledgement

The authors wish to acknowledge the contributions of their friend and colleague Dr Louis Lasagna to the field of Clinical Pharmacology and to its wider applications in Regulation, Drug Development, and Pharmaceutical Medicine. Dr Lasagna contributed to the previous edition of this chapter; he died in August 2003 as the present edition was being planned.

References

1. Guidance for Industry: Formal Meetings with Sponsors and Applicants for PDUFA Products (February 2000).
2. Guidance for Industry: Special Protocol Assessment (May 2002).
3. Guidance for Industry: Content and Format of Investigational New Drug Applications (INDs) for Phase 1 Studies of New Drugs, including Well-Characterised, Therapeutic, Biotechnology-derived Products (November 1995).
4. Draft Guidance for Industry Pre-marketing Risk Assessment (May 2004).
5. Manual of Policies and Procedures (MAPP 6020.3) Review Management Priority Review Policy.
6. Draft Guidance for Industry: Development and Use of Risk Minimization Action Plans (May 2004).

CHAPTER 22

22 Past evolution and future prospects of the Pharma Industry and its regulation in the USA

*William Wardell, William Vodra,
Judith K Jones and Richard N Spivey*

22.1 Introduction

In the previous chapter (Chapter 21), we described how the pharma industry and the FDA work together today, respectively, to develop and approve new drugs, and to ensure their safe use in the marketplace. In this chapter, we consider the future course and prospects for regulation and drug development.

Now is an opportune time to make these observations. Both the pharma industry and the agency are under special stresses, which are having negative effects on the discovery and testing of new drugs and on their availability to physicians and patients. To start, we review the enormous changes since the Drug Amendments were enacted in 1962, in order to understand what may (or should) happen in the future.

The United States began regulating drugs in 1906, focusing mainly on the adulteration and misbranding of patent medicines and the control of narcotics. In 1938, Congress adopted a comprehensive overhaul, the Federal Food, Drug and Cosmetic Act. But every year or two since then, the national legislature has found new issues and problems warranting additions to the 1938 Act. The most recent actions occurred in 2003 (the Bioterrorism Act) and 2004 (as part of the addition of prescription drug coverage to the Medicare program).

For purposes of drug research, development and marketing, the Drug Amendments of 1962 (also called the Kefauver-Harris Act) constituted the most significant single piece of legislation. Congress mandated that drugs be proven effective for their intended uses through 'adequate and well-controlled' clinical investigations. This deceptively simple requirement profoundly changed the pharma industry, the FDA and America's – indeed, the whole world's – standards and expectations for therapeutic agents. The Drug Amendments also directed the FDA to become involved in the clinical research process, required companies to adhere to current good manufacturing practices in making pharmaceuticals, allowed FDA greater access to corporate records, and transferred regulatory control over the advertising of prescription drugs from the Federal Trade Commission.

Since 1962, the FDA and the Industry have achieved improvements in the effectiveness and safety of prescription drugs that are unparalleled in the history of medicine. Indeed, the methods of thinking about, analysing and implementing the steps needed to prove the effectiveness and safety of therapeutic drugs, and to guide their proper use in medicine and the marketplace, have led the field of evidence-based medicine and created its most extensive and well-defined example. The influence of drug regulation has extended to the use of all therapeutic or diagnostic interventions – including diet, exercise, watchful waiting, surgical procedures and medical devices – and has set new standards that are still percolating through all branches of medicine and the related sciences. It is probably no exaggeration to say that these conceptual and operational advances in ensuring effectiveness and safety are among the most significant made in the field of therapeutic interventions since the Enlightenment.

In this chapter we first consider, sector by sector, the main components of this achievement, and also the corresponding problems that have arisen. We also discuss two other public policy changes since 1962 that have had enormous impacts on the pharma industry: the introduction of generic competition for pharmaceuticals, and health care cost containment efforts. Lastly we suggest how to overcome the problems and keep the field improving in the future.

22.2 The Evolution of the FDA and the Pharma Industry from 1962 to 2005

22.2.1 Evolution of the FDA's approach to drug effectiveness

22.2.1.1 The 1962 Act and the DESI project

Before 1962, the FDA was legally empowered to evaluate evidence on safety of a proposed new pharmaceutical, but not evidence on effectiveness. In practice, however, the agency did consider efficacy, at least in the case of drugs with major side effects. It reasoned that the decision to approve a drug for marketing had necessarily to involve both safety and efficacy, because the amount of risk allowed had to take into account each drug's efficacy. Nevertheless, this approach was the exception, not the rule, and the agency rarely acknowledged any formal evaluation of effectiveness. By 1962, at least 13 000 New Drug Applications (NDAs), covering approximately 4000 unique formulations of active ingredients and over 16 000 distinct therapeutic claims, became effective under the 1938 statute.

The 1962 legislation changed this situation in several respects. First, it required affirmative agency approval of the NDA. Under the old law, if the FDA failed to object in the first 60 days after an NDA was submitted, the drug could enter the market. Thus, Congress delayed the marketing until FDA had acted. Second, it insisted that a drug be effective for its declared use. Third, the legislation required that effectiveness be proved by adequate and well-controlled investigations, including clinical investigations. Finally, Congress directed the FDA to reassess all drugs that had entered the market under the prior law, to ensure their effectiveness.

This last provision had, in many respects, the most significant impact on the agency and the pharma industry over the next 15 years. Initially, the agency contracted with the National Academy of Sciences – National Research Council (NAS-NRC) to conduct a review of the marketed products. The NAS-NRC in turn hired teams of physicians, pharmacologists and clinical researchers to perform the actual reviews. At the end of 1968, NAS-NRC reported back that, for almost 15% of the claims, the products did not work; for another 24%, the claims were supported, but there were superior products treating these conditions; and for another 42%, the evidence supporting efficacy was equivocal. In short, less than 20% of the efficacy claims were found to be supported without qualification. Moreover, the NAS-NRC found a large number of products ineffective as fixed combinations in that there was no substantial reason to believe that each ingredient added to the effectiveness of the combination.

The NAS-NRC report set the FDA and the pharma industry on a collision course. The agency was under orders from Congress to remove the ineffective products. The industry faced the choice of giving up products (and revenues) or investing in new research for old products. The Drug Effectiveness Study Implementation (DESI) program resulted in protracted litigation and painful disputes between drug companies and the FDA over prescription drugs. In the process, both parties learned a lot more about the nuances and complexities of 'adequate and well-controlled' clinical investigations in many diverse and previously inadequately studied diseases. The agency promulgated the first regulations defining the elements of such investigations and then, after much litigation, applied them to deny formal hearings to NDA holders in order to complete the DESI effort. Companies, physicians and regulators grappled with how to design and interpret clinical trials in virtually all areas of pharmacotherapy. By the time DESI was over (1984), and partly in response to it, the science of drug development had taken an enormous leap forward. Moreover, academia, industry and the FDA had largely replaced disputes over the drug effectiveness requirement with a common understanding and acceptance of the methods and value of adequate and well-controlled studies. In sum, there had been a complete paradigm shift.

The intensity and focus of the DESI program influenced the process of evaluating new NDAs. After 1962, the agency had greatly increased the number of physicians, pharmacologists, toxicologists, statisticians and pharmacists to carry out both DESI and the review of pending NDAs. Many of these technical experts started their careers with a skepticism about the merits of manufacturers' claims for drugs (vindicated by the DESI findings) and with an intense course in the meaning of 'adequate and well-controlled' studies needed to carry out the DESI project. The subsequent adverse effects on products in the pipeline gave rise to the Drug Lag and Patient Access debates, which will be discussed shortly.

Another collateral effect of the DESI project was the development of the 'abbreviated NDA', by which a generic version of the innovator product could satisfy the statutory preconditions for entering the market, without repeating the preclinical and clinical studies of the innovator. This administrative creation, designed to assure that generics were both pharmaceutically equivalent and bioequivalent to the pioneer product, was endorsed by Congress in 1984. As will be seen, this development had a staggering impact on the business model of the pharma industry.

22.2.1.2 FDA organisation and attitudes toward industry

Implementation of the 1962 amendments, and subsequent challenges, led to a series of organisational changes within the agency. In the 1960s, FDA was organised along disciplinary lines (e.g. Bureaus of Medicine, Science and Compliance). In 1970, it was reorganised along product lines (e.g. Bureau of Drugs, Bureau of Foods). Within the new Bureau of Drugs, the old separation between 'new' drugs (NDA evaluation) and 'marketed' drugs (evaluation of supplements and safety information) were eliminated, by creation of the Office of New Drugs. In 1972, a departmental reorganisation resulted in the transfer of the Division of Biologic Standards from the National Institutes of Health to the FDA, which renamed it the Bureau of Biologics. For a brief period in the 1980s, the Bureau of Drugs was consolidated with that for Biologics into the National Center for Drugs and Biologics. The marriage failed, and by the late 1980s the agency created the Centre for Drug Evaluation and Research (CDER) and the Centre for Biologics Evaluation and Research (CBER). In 2002, jurisdiction for many therapeutic biologicals was reassigned from CBER to CDER.

Throughout this period, the agency has undergone a series of reorientations regarding its relationship with the regulated industry. In the 1960s and early 1970s, the attitude was frankly adversarial. The drug industry was characterised as unscrupulous seekers of profits. In a book called *Pills, Profits, and Politics*, Philip Lee (Assistant Secretary for Health in the Lyndon Johnson Administration) and Milton Silverman attacked the pharma industry. Even in the early-to-mid 1970s, Senators Ted Kennedy (Democrat – MA), Gaylord Nelson (Democrat – WI) and Congressman LH Fountain (Democrat – NC) conducted hearings that regularly sought to expose problems with drug safety and alleged misconduct by the pharma industry or the FDA (or often both). While ignoring the obvious slowdown in new drug approvals, these well-publicised congressional investigations attempted to embarrass the FDA for failing to regulate the industry adequately. Among the outcomes of these investigations were greater agency attention both to post-approval adverse event monitoring and to rigorous enforcement of rules to assure the integrity of research data.

By the mid-1970s, however, attitudes within the agency were changing. While some still viewed their role as finding industry errors, a new professional ethic emerged in which the FDA was to judge objectively the evidence presented. By the mid-1980s, the orientation shifted further, in light of the AIDS crisis. The picture changed to one where new drug approval was no longer deemed to be a zero-sum game in which benefit for some was possible only at the expense of harm to others. Drug development was understood to be a process wherein approval could be speeded by efficient and timely review of relevant animal and human data so that every sector could benefit – the sick obviously, but also the medical profession, the FDA and the industry. In the 1990s, the terminology became one of 'stakeholders' in which the agency viewed itself as a neutral party mediating between divergent interests and serving all constituent groups, including industry. This 'customer' focus itself became a target of criticism by those who felt the FDA could not serve both industry and the public at the same time.

22.2.1.3 Investigational New Drug

Prior to 1962, the agency had played no role until the NDA was submitted. After learning, however, that pregnant women were given thalidomide (to prevent morning sickness) without being told what the drug was or that it was experimental, Congress demanded federal oversight and informed consent from all research subjects. The result was the Investigational New Drug (IND) application, and a new series of FDA regulations governing informed consent, protections of the rights and safety of human subjects and good clinical research practices (GCPs).

In response to demands to accelerate the drug review process, however, the FDA perceived opportunities to use the IND process to improve the chances that the subsequent NDA would answer the essential regulatory questions, or eliminate them by answering these questions

before the NDA was submitted. Gradually, the chemistry, manufacturing and controls segments of the IND application moved from merely being adequate to assure the safety and consistency of the investigational product, to being complete and acceptable for NDA purposes. Clinical reviewers provided more guidance on study design, to avoid fundamental flaws that would render the final results scientifically invalid. Pharmacologists and toxicologists urged completion of all preclinical studies early in the IND process, so that issues could be flagged in advance of the NDA filing. Overall, the IND became burdened with regulatory requests that were unnecessary for subject protection but might shorten NDA review times and increase the chances for ultimate drug approval.

22.2.1.4 The drug lag debate and its consequences

By the early 1970s, many observers were questioning the impact and value of FDA review of NDAs for effectiveness. In particular, cardiologists could point to the fact that in a period of almost five full years, the FDA had not approved a single new molecular entity (NME) in their field. The pharma industry was keenly aware of the decline in approvals of NMEs via the NDA process, despite the fact that many new products were available in Europe. William Wardell identified a 'drug lag', showing that the United States had fallen behind other pharmaceutically-advanced countries (as represented, e.g. by the United Kingdom) in terms of the number of new drugs approved and the overall capabilities of the therapeutic armamentarium available. Work on the Drug Lag and the wider issues of pharmaceutical policy in government and industry led in 1974 to the founding of the Centre for the Study of Drug Development (CSDD) by Louis Lasagna and William Wardell at the University of Rochester Medical Center. The CSDD moved to Tufts University in the 1980s.

A few personal touches emerged to underline the drug lag issue, such as the FDA Commissioner's taking propranolol for hypertension at a time when it was not approved by the FDA for that purpose. Meanwhile, the more cautious parties cited the dangers of the perceived rapid and less stringent approvals in Europe and the example of practolol, a beta-blocker that was found to cause a severe 'mucocutaneous syndrome' with sclerosis of eyes and internal organs that was severely debilitating and sometimes fatal. Its prodrome, 'itchy eyes', had been noted and discounted in the clinical trials.

Although the charges of drug lag were greeted with hostility from Congress, the FDA and the anti-drug lobby, they were welcomed by the drug industry. In the end, the proponents had tremendous influence over the future of drug regulation in the United States.

Interestingly, the debate went beyond the regulated parties. Economists and libertarians commenced a campaign to let the marketplace determine which drugs were effective. Advocates of laetrile (a purported cancer cure), fought in court for an exception to the effectiveness requirements for drugs intended for persons with terminal illnesses that could not be treated by any approved or recognised methods.

No one was officially declared the winner in the drug lag debate. The FDA, fearing for the survival of the effectiveness requirement, refused to admit that a lag existed, but pledged to eliminate it anyway. At the same time, the agency presented to Congress a legislative proposal that put the efficacy standard on the table, for ratification or repeal. Leaders in both Houses made clear that repeal was out of the question. At about the same time, the Supreme Court rejected the arguments of the laetrile proponents, observing that the effectiveness requirement also protected patients with incurable diseases from quackery. Industry, moving past DESI and getting more and faster approvals of important new products, lost interest in attacking the efficacy provision and focused its attention on two new objectives. First, it sought restoration of patent life for time lost in the development and review process; this law was enacted in 1984. Second, it agreed to fund the FDA directly to provide more resources to shorten review times. The Prescription Drug User Fee Act (PDUFA) was enacted in 1992, and renewed in 1997 and again in 2002. Under PDUFA, each manufacturer of innovator

prescription drugs pays an annual assessment fee based on the number of establishments it operates. In addition, for each original NDA or supplement that requires review of clinical data, the applicant pays a fee. The revenues are earmarked for drug review activities and may not be used by the agency to offset the funding it receives for these activities from the federal treasury.

By the mid-1990s, after two decades of attention, the drug lag had been eliminated; indeed, the pendulum had swung clearly in favour of the FDA. Whether due to the PDUFA resources, to the advent of more bureaucracy overseas (e.g. the formation of the European Union's central drug approval authority) or to criticism of delays at the agency, today the United States is often the first country to approve new drugs.

22.2.1.5 The patient access debate and its consequences

While the drug lag debate was waning, a new challenge emerged to the FDA standards for drug effectiveness. This time, it was patient advocates who led the charge.

Orphan diseases are those that affect such a small number of patients that the market cannot sustain the cost of research to find treatments. For some time, the agency, the industry and patient support groups had recognised the problem; indeed, the FDA worked with various drug firms to find 'homes' for potentially valuable orphan products. Nevertheless, the economics worked against those with rare diseases.

In 1979 Dr Louis Lasagna wrote a seminal article, 'Who will adopt the therapeutic orphans?' that helped Abby Meyers, the founder of NORD (the National Organisation for Rare Disorders), to obtain enough Congressional attention to start the move towards supportive legislation. Beginning in 1983, Congress responded to this situation by enacting (and in 1985 and 1986 strengthening) the Orphan Drug Act. This legislation allowed sponsors to seek FDA designation of pipeline products as 'orphan drugs' for specific indications. Once designated, the sponsors could seek funding grants and could receive tax credits for research costs. Most significantly, if a sponsor was the first to get a particular product approved for an orphan indication, no other company could obtain FDA approval of an identical product for the same use for 7 years. This exclusivity incentive proved powerful and as a result many new drugs have reached the market.

In the mid-1980s, the AIDS crisis exploded. Activists behaved in ways no patient advocacy group had ever done, including picketing the agency's offices. Initially, they demanded immediate access to any drug that might help the disease, and they objected to placebo-controlled trials as unethical. Libertarians and political conservatives (including in the White House) voices were also heard, calling for a broader suspension of the effectiveness standard. In its first response, the agency rushed through the approval of the first diagnostics for HIV and the first therapies for AIDS and related opportunistic infections. It also adopted regulations (just before the 1988 Presidential elections) to expedite the development, evaluation and marketing of new treatments for life-threatening diseases. These so-called Subpart E rules allowed for early consultations between sponsors and the agency on study requirements, treatment protocols, active FDA monitoring of ongoing studies, Phase 4 studies to delineate additional information after approval and a risk-benefit analysis that explicitly recognised the severity of the disease and the absence of alternative therapies as factors to be considered.

The political pressures to expand early access for patients did not abate. Other policy changes occurred, such as the encouragement of community-based simple studies, and the initiation of fast track review procedures (giving priority for important new drugs over those offering smaller contributions to patient health). In 1992, the agency adopted another set of regulations to provide for the accelerated approval of new drugs for life-threatening illnesses. These rules, called Subpart H, were similar to the Subpart E policies (that remained in place), but now authorised the FDA to approve drugs based on surrogate endpoints rather than mortality effects, to restrict the distribution of drugs so approved

to special settings, to preclearance of advertising copy and to expeditions withdrawal of approval if Phase 4 trials failed to demonstrate a clinical benefit.

It is important to note that the majority of AIDS activists, after initially opposing controlled investigations, came around to recognise that improvements in HIV therapy could only be identified through such studies.

In 1997, Congress stepped in once again to tinker with the Federal Food, Drug and Cosmetic Act. With regard to drug effectiveness, it directed the agency to develop guidelines on those situations in which a single adequate and well-controlled study would be adequate for approval of a new drug or a new indication for an approved product. The FDA issued the guidance the following year. To some observers, it offered little meaningful change from past practice.

Thus, by the end of the 20th century, the effectiveness requirement, requiring proof through more than one adequate and well-controlled clinical investigation, remained the standard to which most new drugs were held. Important therapeutic breakthroughs, however, could reach patients earlier or faster through one or more administrative mechanisms created by the agency. As a result of the resources provided by PDUFA, the FDA has become the largest and best-staffed drug regulatory agency in the world, setting standards that influence all other countries.

Criticisms of slowness, rigidity and authoritarianism are still heard from industry, but with less frequency. One can debate whether the decline is due to improvements within the agency, or to the fact that industry now contains a large number of employees whose careers depend largely on satisfying FDA's demands or to the reluctance of industry to express concerns publicly. The FDA has become a significant 'sponsor' or 'patron' of many diverse elements within the Industry; its laws provide economic benefits to the industry (such as limiting parallel imports and generic competition); it has the power to cripple or destroy individual companies. Thus for many reasons, regulatory decisions may be less vigorously challenged or resisted by industry today than 40 years ago, at the height of DESI.

In 2003, then-Commissioner Mark McClellan, who is both a physician and an economist, recognised the high and increasing cost of drug development and proposed, as part of a strategic plan, that the agency should consider ways to reduce it. The following year, the agency announced its 'Critical Path' initiative, to identify (and, one hopes, ultimately to solve) problems in drug development science that increase costs and add time to the process. A mutual commitment on the part of industry and FDA to boosting efficiency and output represents a critical opportunity for drug developers.

22.2.2 Evolution of FDA's approach to drug safety

The concept of drug safety in 1938, focused on premarket testing and on post-approval adulteration. Adverse events emerging after a drug entered the marketplace were not really considered part of FDA's responsibility. When chloramphenicol was discovered (in the early 1950s) to cause aplastic anemia, the alarm was sounded to the American Medical Association (AMA). The AMA joined with hospital and pharmacy organisations to create a registry for reporting these cases, and later, adverse events associated with other drugs, thus forming the origins of what would ultimately be FDA's adverse reaction system. The registry was transferred to the FDA in 1969.

Later, the Agency developed specific regulations for mandatory reporting of adverse events by holders of NDAs, but not by health care professionals who, instead, were encouraged to report voluntarily. Also, uniquely in the world, the agency accepted reports directly from consumers; and though attempts are made to get medical verification of such reports, this is one feature that has created skepticism over the value of the FDA adverse events data. This structure remains in place today. Voluntary reporting for all drugs tends to spike in the wake of publicity about safety issues requiring withdrawal of a product [e.g. phenformin (1977), benoxaprofen

and ticrynafen (1982), nomefensine (1987) and fenfluramine (1997)].

These episodes also led to regulatory focus on recurring areas of drug toxicity, such as hepatic or renal injury and blood dyscrasias. With the advent of sudden cardiac death due to *torsades de pointes* associated with the antihistamine terfenadine and the gastrointestinal drug cisapride, drug safety entered a newer era. First, it was found that both drug problems were usually associated with drug interactions, specifically at the 3A4 cytochrome p450 metabolising site. Thus, requirements for pre-market testing for these and analogous interactions that might increase toxicity gradually became routine parts of the NDA requirements. Second, for these drugs and several others introduced in the 1990s, the discovery of preventable risks was rapidly followed by labelling changes and 'Dear Healthcare Professional' letters, as had been the agency's routine practice for decades. But now, however, careful studies demonstrated that these warnings had little or no impact on physician's prescribing behaviour; the life-threatening risks due to drug interactions were still occurring. The FDA concluded that label changes had little or no impact. Third, an analysis of drug surveillance studies estimated that adverse events associated with drugs accounted for approximately 100 000 deaths per year, placing this event in the major public health problem arena.

In 1999, the FDA unveiled a new initiative on identifying and preventing risks from medical products, and in May 2004, the agency produced several specific proposed guidances on risk management, covering pre-marketing risk assessment, risk management programs and pharmacovigilance programs, as well as a proposal for regulations that represent the most comprehensive overhaul of the adverse event reporting regulations ever undertaken. In essence, the proposed guidances greatly extend the focus on drug safety from Phase I clinical studies right through the commercial life of a product. The FDA now expects detailed collection and analyses of clinical safety data in the NDA, plus comprehensive pharmacovigilance programs that encompass not only passive spontaneous report surveillance but also proactive programs. The rigor of this examination is most recently reflected in extensive guidelines for the NDA safety review in February 2005. For drugs identified as posing significant risks, FDA will require plans in the NDA, called Risk Management Action Plans, or RiskMAPs, for specific interventions to minimise these risks and/or evaluating the effectiveness of the interventions; if the interventions do not work, additional steps may be necessary.

FDA has also formed a Drug Safety and Risk Management Advisory Committee during this time, provided specific training for the members and has subsequently placed selected members on Advisory Committee Panels to consider various risks or to review existing risk management programs.

As this goes to press, still more dramatic developments have emerged in the drug safety arena. In August 2004, the agency determined that at least some selective serotonin reuptake inhibitors (SSRIs) for depression may increase the risk of suicide in some patients, particularly children. The following month, the manufacturer of rofecoxib, a COX-2 inhibitor nonsteroidal anti-inflammatory drug (NSAID) for arthritis, suspended marketing worldwide because of cardiovascular risks. In both cases, the risks were identified (and only identifiable) through randomised controlled clinical trials, which traditionally have focused only on drug effectiveness. Some experts began suggesting the expanded use of such trials to assess safety. Meanwhile, Congressional hearings unearthed scientific dissent within the agency and called for more effective safety monitoring. In February 2005, the agency announced a new Safety Oversight Board, comprising of experts from the FDA, other government agencies and academia, to provide oversight to the drug safety assessment process.

The FDA's approach to drug safety is thus in great flux. The final guidelines on risk management and the new regulations on adverse event reporting are expected soon. How the Agency will incorporate the learning from the SSRI and COX-2 experiences, and will use the new Safety Oversight Board, remains to be seen.

Nevertheless, there is a growing concern that the FDA is becoming more risk-averse, resulting in more requirements for pre-approval safety testing, more delays in drug approvals and more restrictions on post-approval use of drugs.

22.2.3 The changing economics of the pharma industry

The business model for the pharmaceutical industry has also undergone important changes, especially in the last 20 years. Moreover, the pace of change seems to accelerate, challenging the managers who must guide their companies forward. While many factors are at play, some that are unique to the pharmaceutical industry merit special recognition.

22.2.3.1 The advent of generic drug competition

Generic drugs have always been available in the US market. When the DESI program was underway, the agency estimated that there were between 5 and 13 products without NDAs that were identical, similar or related to each of the 13 000 products that held NDAs under the 1938 Act. These products might contain the same active ingredient in the same amount and dosage form; often, though, they claimed some unique characteristic: a different salt or ester, a different amount, a different dosage form or an extra-added ingredient. As part of the DESI project, the FDA sought to introduce uniformity and control over these products. First, the Agency said that a copy had to be identical, unless the proponent got FDA permission to vary from the innovator. Second, the manufacturer had to obtain an 'abbreviated' NDA (or ANDA) showing that the product was identical and could be made consistently. In essence, it was an application that contained all of the chemistry, manufacturing and controls of a full NDA, but omitted any preclinical or clinical data. A number of generic firms opposed even these requirements, and significant litigation followed.

While the ANDA process was evolving, a new problem arose. Physicians were reporting that congestive heart failure patients who had been titrated carefully to a specific dose of digoxin went out of control upon getting prescriptions refilled. Investigation revealed that digoxin, a pre-1938 drug never subject to an NDA, varied from manufacturer-to-manufacturer, and from lot-to-lot: not in quantity of actual drug per tablet, but in the amount of drug released from the tablet into the body. The consequences could be life-threatening. The agency responded with an order that each manufacturer submit an ANDA that included bioavailability studies showing the rate and extent of absorption into the body. Thus was born the idea of bioequivalence: that competing products must not only be pharmaceutically identical but also show no significant difference in the rate or extent of absorption in controlled bioavailability studies.

The ANDA process and bioequivalence permitted the agency for the first time to declare individual generic products to be therapeutically equivalent to approved brand name versions. The FDA began making such declarations in 1975 or 1976; by 1979, the agency began to publish them in the Orange Book. This step was critically important. Before this point, generics did not pose a great competitive threat, because state pharmacy laws did not permit the substitution of a generic for the innovator drug that had been prescribed. The premise of these laws was that pharmacists were not in a position to assure the equivalency of generic products. But once the FDA gave its imprimatur, the rationale for non-substitution disappeared. In 1979 the Federal Trade Commission unveiled a model state drug product selection law, which guided state legislatures on how to amend pharmacy laws to permit druggists to substitute equivalent generics for innovators, without the permission of the prescribing physician.

Even this step did not have a profound effect, because the ANDA mechanism was only available to generic copies of drugs first approved before 1962. But in 1984, as part of the compromise to obtain restoration of patent life that was being lost during the drug development and review process, the pharma industry agreed to extension of the ANDA requirement to copies

of an approved product, once the patent for the product had expired or was declared invalid. The impact of this change was first felt in the late 1980s, when important innovations went off patent. Whereas, prior to the ANDA process, an innovation could rely on retaining over 80% of its market share for years after generic entry, now companies found themselves losing 90% of the market in 3–6 months.

The effect was staggering to the pharma business model. Henceforth, the only period during which a research-based drug sponsor could plan to profit from the sales of a new product was the time window from approval and launch to the date of patent expiration. Could things get worse? Within the 1984 law were seeds of further troubles for the Pharma Industry. One provision rewarded a generic manufacturer who challenged an innovator patent; if the patent were invalid or not infringed, the challenger would be rewarded with 6 months of exclusive marketing of the generic. During this window, not only would the innovator lose its market share, but the generic could charge a premium price and make substantial profits. Moreover, experience began to reveal that, after three or four generics entered the market, their prices fell to pure competitive or commodity levels, with very low profit margins. The generic firm, to survive and prosper, would have to become aggressive in finding innovator patents to 'break'. By the end of the 1990s, it was increasingly common for generics to contest patents rather than wait for this expiration.

This foreshortening of the commercial life of a pharmaceutical would necessarily affect the projected return on investment for a pipeline product. The incentives were skewed in favour of 'blockbuster' developments that would command both high prices and high demand despite the high prices.

22.2.3.2   The accelerating rate of innovator competition

The marketplace is indeed crowded, especially in the more traditional therapeutic areas. Further, the time lag between when the first member of a class enters the market and a 'me-too' follow-on product is approved is lessening. As a result, the ability of a company to maintain high prices before the entry of generic competition is also compromised.

22.2.3.3 The emerging demand for cost-effectiveness

Health care costs in the United States have become a major issue for government (that subsidises health care for the poor, disabled and elderly), business (that subsidises health care for employees), labour unions (that are increasingly fighting to preserve benefits and jobs, rather than to increase wages) and politicians (who recognise that a huge proportion of the population has no health insurance). Historically, drug costs were a trivial part of the health care budget. Indeed, in 1964, when Congress enacted the original Medicare program, prescription drugs were not covered. The political perception was that the products were inexpensive and not necessarily effective.

Beginning in the 1990s, prescription drug expenditures accelerated as a percentage of total health care costs. This shift should be viewed as a positive development, reflecting the discovery and introduction of agents to address a population whose life expectancy has been extended, thanks to other medical advances. Unfortunately, but realistically, there are limits to the proportion of the economy that can be allocated to health. As a result, third party payers are searching for ways to reduce the total cost. At the same time, for the reasons just discussed, manufacturers introduced 'value-based' pricing for new pharmaceuticals. The first drug to cost more than $10 000 per year for a single patient was AZT, the first AIDS drug. After initial complaints, the high price was accepted, and now products are launched at an annual per person costs that are much higher. Thus it is no surprise that the payers have focused on prescription drugs as a way to control costs.

'Newer' does not automatically mean 'better', and today payers are insisting that innovations be more cost-effective than competitor products, in particular low-price generic competitors. It was once possible to launch profitably an eighth or twelfth beta-blocker or NSAID. But now, so-called 'me-too' products must at least offer some cost–benefit advantage over the innovator. The prizes go to the first-in-class product (because it will have the greatest volume of use to support safety) and to the best-in-class (because it would have been shown to be superior in some way to the others). The rest fight over the crumbs left by those who do not respond to the first- or best-in-class products.

Furthermore, some therapeutic areas are inelastic. For example, in the case of migraine, this market shows no sign of growth, despite the fact that there are now at least seven triptans available for patients, including four distinct dosage forms. New entrants employ large sales forces to launch new products, but often results are meager, until continued investment proves prohibitive to do even that. Meanwhile, managed care organisations decide that only one or two representatives of the class will be reimbursable, thus placing additional pressure on marketing organisations.

The economic implications should be clear. Today's drug development decisions must be made with a careful regard to the drug's place in the queue of likely competitors, and to the sponsor's ability to demonstrate therapeutic advantages. In the case of some drugs, such as proton pump inhibitors, the very mechanism of action limits the potential for significant improvements by later generations. In other areas, such as the calcium channel blockers, diltiazem and verapamil, the chemistry may not permit a second generation molecule.

22.2.3.4 The declining productivity of research and development

The productivity of research and development efforts within the pharma industry has declined significantly in the past decade. While large numbers of INDs are submitted each year, only a small proportion in the pipeline emerges as NDA submissions or approvals. NDA submissions have fallen by half, from a high of 50 in 1995, to 23 and 24 in 2002 and 2003, respectively. Approvals have fallen from a high of 53 in 1996, to 17 and 19 in 2002 and 2003, respectively (although the 2004 result is considerably higher). No clear reasons exist for this decline, especially in the face of record high levels of R&D investment. Speculation has offered suggestions such as: the 'easy' targets have already been exploited; profit potential for products cannot meet ever-increasing financial targets; and safety concerns require inordinately clean safety profiles.

Research technology has advanced particularly rapidly over the past two decades, and techniques such as robotics, high throughput screening and computer-aided design and simulations have been instituted in discovery and early-development labs. Companies have established genomics departments to exploit the much-touted future benefits of pharmacogenomics. Given the declining level of NME NDA submissions, it appears that to date there has not been a high degree of payoff. With respect to genomics, arguments are made that it takes 10 years to exploit such a fundamental technology, or that the industry has failed to adjust its business model to 'personalised' medicine. Overall, however, the decline may be a symptom of a serious, long-term problem, which may necessitate more selective research investments in the future.

22.2.3.5   The increasing costs of drug development

The costs of bringing a new drug to the market keep rising exponentially. This fact compounds the problems of persistently long development time (now averaging 12 years) and a remarkably high failure rate (75%) in the clinical research phase. The latest estimate from the Tufts Center for the Study of Drug Development puts large pharma's average out-of-pocket cost, including failures, of developing a new chemical entity to the point of NDA approval, at $403 million ($121 million preclinical plus $282 million clinical). When the cost of the capital, expended over the 12-year average time of product development, is included, this figure

rises to $802 million ($336 million preclinical plus $466 million clinical). Development speed and failure rates have a large effect on the cost of development: if development time could be cut in half, the $802 million would drop to $568 million. If the failure rate were reduced from 75% to 67%, total costs would be lowered by $217 million.

Some of the more potent causes of these increasing costs include the following:

1. Chronic and complex indications demand longer, larger and more complex studies.
2. Comparative trials, needed to compete in the marketplace, may require larger populations and longer durations to have sufficient power to determine equivalency or superiority.
3. Special preapproval studies are now expected, or required, to explore safety and effectiveness in special subpopulations. These groups include the elderly, children (which has 4 subsets: neonates and infants; toddlers; prepubescent and post-puberty adolescents), women of child-bearing potential, persons with renal or hepatic impairment and persons using foreseeable concomitant medications (looking for dangers such as QTc interval prolongation, a signal for possible *torsades de pointes*).
4. More trials, with greater numbers of subjects, necessitate utilisation of outside consultants and contract research organisations to manage sites, collect and verify data, assure protocol compliance plus adherence to GCP regulations. The number of outside companies who draw their livelihood from the growing size and complexity of the drug development process is itself an ominous portent.
5. Competition for a limited pool of patients has led to recruitment and retention problems and to the need for direct payments to subjects for their participation.
6. Increased use of information technology, such as remote electronic data entry and electronic diaries, creates the further need for additional data integrity controls and audit trails, plus the support of this whole industry infrastructure.
7. More rigorous demands for the format of regulatory submissions. The FDA initiatives to eliminate unnecessary paperwork through electronic

filings can lead to unnecessary technology and expense which, although perhaps leading to economy and efficiency in the long run, is far from that today. The agency's recent 'refusal to file' Neurocrine's NDA – because the reviewer could not use the hyperlinked version that supposedly satisfied the FDA's own specifications – is a case in point.

While any large R&D organisation presents management challenges to overcome inefficiencies, every Pharma R&D organisation has a special dimension: the number of tasks and people that are required to interact with the world's regulatory agencies. This requirement permeates far beyond the staff of the regulatory department itself. It extends to many other departments in which even an 'expression of interest' by the FDA or another agency guarantees the jobs and careers of a large fraction of the department's employees, even if they have no direct participation in the drug development process or in the necessary development activities of the pipeline.

A representative example today is pharmacogenomics. Most would agree that there will in the future be potential contributions from pharmacogenomics to drug discovery, development and approval. But in the meantime, one of the stated justifications today for a pharmacogenomic department to be established in a pharma company is that 'the FDA is very interested in the potential of this technology'. In this way, the discipline is granted a place in the development pathway that may be independent of its actual current value to the process. Numerous other departments and functions in a pharma company enjoy similar privileges under the protection of real or putative FDA requirements or interest.

The compounding effect of so many added burdens from all directions – standards, size, quality and speed – has itself produced new dimensions of complexity and costs not readily apparent to those outside – or even inside – the system. There is a real danger that the system will collapse of its own weight; growth at this pace cannot continue forever.

22.2.4 The economic effects on the Pharma Industry

22.2.4.1 Consolidation of the industry
The steeply rising costs of R&D, combined with a foreshortened period of generic-free competition, has driven pharma into maintaining large sales forces and an efficient supply chain. Its business model has further evolved to focus on blockbuster drugs, ones that today must generate at least $1 billion per year in order to make a profitable return on R&D investments before generics or 'me-too' products enter the market. The declining productivity of R&D has forced the industry to cast a wider net to discover compounds and take them through the initial phases of development, but despite this, the lack of sufficient blockbuster products has forced the consolidation of the industry, in order to support the sales and manufacturing operations and ongoing R&D. Unprecedented consolidation has taken place over the last 10–15 years because of these economic pressures.

While these mergers may yield efficiencies in marketing and production, it is doubtful whether the same efficiencies would hold in drug development. The search for blockbuster drugs has compelled research organisations to be more market-driven than science-driven. One result of consolidation has been the creation of mega-R&D organisations, some of which have 15–20 000 staff or more, with multiple research sites on several continents, creating the further challenge of managing these resources, and the need to hire yet more staff to administer these gigantic bureaucracies. Paradoxically, there is no evidence that consolidation has improved innovation, or that huge R&D organisations have useful economies of scale or efficiencies in discovery or development. It would not be surprising to hear that the consolidation has actually achieved the opposite of its intent in R&D, and that discovery and innovation have declined as a result.

22.2.4.2 The rise of the Biotechnology Industry
A new drug discovery industry has emerged in parallel with the consolidation of the pharma

industry. Beginning in the 1970s, boosted by the Bayh-Dole Act of 1980 (encouraging out-licensing of university-based discoveries made with NIH funds), and funded by venture capital, start-up biotechnology, or 'biotech' companies, proliferated. The term 'biotech' originally applied to the tools offered by recombinant DNA and monoclonal antibody technologies, but now embraces startup and small companies in general, using small molecule design and discovery, genomics and proteomics, bioinformatics, therapeutic vaccines, novel drug delivery systems, combinations of a medical device with a drug or biologic, nanotechnology and other cutting edge biomedical research ideas and tools. Unfortunately, the great potential of these new technologies has not yet been fully realised. A staggering number of products and the start-up companies that spawned them have failed. Other great promises, such as interferon, endorphins and gene therapy have proved so far to have limited clinical applications or unsuspected toxicity. The translation of new technologies to the hospital, pharmacy and bedside is taking longer, and costing more, than was expected in the enthusiasm of the 1990s. Part of the reason is the enthusiastic hype that seems necessary to get new companies and industries started.

Nevertheless, biotechnology has made a very substantial contribution to the pharmaceutical pipeline and the therapeutic armamentarium, with approximately 6–8 NME products reaching the market each year. The largest biotech companies (e.g. Amgen) are now indistinguishable, in the business sense, from traditional pharma companies. The vibrant biotech small-company sector, particularly at the discovery and early-development level, is supplying candidates for licensing or acquisition by pharma companies to supplement their internal research operations. The relationship is mutually beneficial. Pharma cannot afford to finance the scale of drug discovery operations needed to maintain a pipeline; companies funded by venture capital and stock offerings assume much of the risk of early failures; and both parties share the rewards of success. As a result, every major pharma company scouts for new opportunities,

and the most promising candidates become the subjects of intensive bidding competitions.

The rate of biotech discoveries reaching the market needs to increase rapidly if the overall pharmaceutical pipeline is to grow. At the very least, however, the advent of the biotech Industry has greatly changed the face of pharmaceuticals worldwide, and may yet become – as has been touted for decades – the creative force that saves the pharma industry.

22.2.4.3 Outsourcing

The steady rise of outsourcing since the 1960s has greatly expanded the operating capacity and expertise base of the pharma industry. It began with the clinical contract research organisations (CROs) that handled the logistics of clinical trials and with animal testing laboratories compliant with FDA's good laboratory practice regulations. Subsequently, the field expanded to include firms in the areas of formulation development, stability programs, pharmacokinetic studies, biostatistics, data management, clinical site management, auditing for compliance with GCP requirements and preparation of regulatory submissions. Even the duties of institutional review boards (IRBs) are undertaken for multicentre trials by free-standing, for-profit companies.

These diverse businesses have contributed to the rising standards of performance – and, unfortunately the costs – of drug development. Competition in individual areas has forced a 'race to the top' in terms of quality, speed and compliance. Pharma clients cannot risk obtaining data that will not be acceptable to the FDA. Thus, even more so than pharma companies themselves, the outsourcing industry shows a militant enthusiasm for complying with regulatory standards; rather than contesting the wisdom of an agency guidance or interpretation, contractors will embrace it to the letter and pass on the increased cost to the client companies. In addition to the general problem of high costs, this has a particularly dampening effect on the activities of the small, innovative startups from whom so much is expected: increasingly, they cannot afford to pay for a clinical program that they desperately need to proceed with the CRO help.

The future of outsourcing is clearly strong, but it also reveals a growing need for cheaper ways of satisfying the law's requirements for evidence of effeciveness and safety. One recent way that is growing steeply is to move activities out of the United States and other high-cost countries. Both pharma and CROs have invested in operations in Eastern Europe, India and China. One CRO, for example, recently relocated its entire ECG monitoring services to India and promises one-hour 24/7 turnaround, in the same way that American hospitals have contracted for reading of X-rays in that country. Other specific functions such as data management, analysis and information technology can also be performed elsewhere. The United States has thus forced a trend that could end its comfortable near-monopoly in pharmaceutical discovery and development.

22.2.4.4 Front-loading the drug development process

The potentially formidable power of the sciences of drug discovery and early development creates a plausible hope that candidate drugs can be screened earlier in the development process for potential problems, thereby reducing the failure rate at later stages. While this argument is logically appealing, the results to date have been disappointing. Moreover, the opportunity itself creates a new dilemma. By investing more in the numerous technologies available at the early stage of a drug's development, such a strategy 'frontloads' each compound's early development costs. Thus, if the compound still ultimately fails, the cost of failure is even higher than it was before the front-loading strategy. So far, that strategy has not worked well enough to reverse the pitifully low success rate of compounds that enter development. FDA's 'critical path' initiative is a welcome new attempt to address the development-failure problem, but the fact that it depends on further front-loading the activities and costs of the development pathway cannot be overlooked.

The example of pharmacogenomics illustrates this dilemma, although one could equally well cite other new scientific techniques, such as extensive computer modelling and simulation, in this context. In the mid-1990s, in anticipation of the sequencing of the human genome, many new startup pharmacogenomic companies were established, offering the vision of 'individualised therapeutics' or 'personalised medicine', based on the companies' claimed abilities to determine each patient's genomic variations (including single nucleotide polymorphism, SNPs) that they presumed must underlie inter-individual differences in the patients' responses to drugs. It was asserted that this would enable the widespread prediction of responders and non-responders to drug therapy, as well as those at the risk of adverse reactions; and that the result would be smaller, more powerful effectiveness trials, a cleaner safety profile and the salvage of drugs that fail in development ('drug rehab').

With the exception of a few examples (e.g. Herceptin), the basic premise has not yet been widely demonstrated, though this area of tumor markers may well be the most promising in the long run. The prospects for more general applicability and cost-effective utility are still unclear at present. Many pharmacogenomic companies went public with stock offerings in the late 1990s boom, only to disappear in the crash of 2000. Nevertheless, the idea that much pharmacogenomics should be performed in the early development stage of drugs has been endorsed by the FDA, and as a result, taken up enthusiastically by pharma; and is resulting in a very large amount of extra work being added to the early development of essentially all new drugs. For example, a new, more formal agency initiative for early pharmacogenomic work in early development has just been announced. It is still not clear whether these initiatives will turn out to be the salvation of the drug industry, or yet another example of the unproven burdening of the front-end of the drug development process.

In general, the front-loading of the development process by further use of any of the numerous modern available technologies would be attractive if one could be sure unequivocally that it would work. But to date, it has not produced enough successful results to conclude that it is a superior strategy, and the success of clinical programs remains abysmal. The traditional approach of taking a new compound into human studies as early as possible, so that human data can be obtained at an early stage has not yet been improved upon, despite the enormous frontloading of development across the whole industry.

22.2.5 Changing public attitudes toward the pharma industry

In recent years, the drug industry has come under increasing criticism on a wide variety of fronts. The cumulative impact makes the industry look bad. Opinion polls place drug manufacturers among the least respected industries, near tobacco. Politicians score populist points by attacking drug companies. Prosecutors jump on the bandwagon, investigating and bringing actions for alleged violations of the Federal Food, Drug and Cosmetic Act, the laws against fraud, abuse and kickbacks in the Medicare/Medicaid systems, prohibitions of deceptive and unfair advertising, securities statutes and false claims against the government. And in the product liability arena, plaintiffs lawyers are able to secure enormous amounts of punitive damages from juries who are angry with the pharma industry.

The number of books published in the United States in just the past year attacking the pharma industry is sobering. A catalog of the public concerns and objections (real or imaginary) illustrates the complexity of the public relations challenge facing drug firms:

High prices for prescription drugs. Americans are now convinced that they are paying more for drugs than residents in Canada and elsewhere. Moreover, those not covered by health insurance purportedly have to choose between food and their medicines.

Excessive total costs for prescription drugs. Insurers and other third party payers see drugs as the fastest-rising component in total health care spending. For them, it is not merely the question of price per pill, but the aggregate utilisation of drugs. With the advent of 'life-style' drugs and later generation medicines that may offer no convincing advantages over those that are available as generics, there are real concerns about the diversion of limited resources to unnecessary products and the soaring costs for employee benefits that must be built into cost of goods sold.

Dubious practices in promoting prescription drugs. Americans have long had a love–hate relationship with advertising, but the apparent excesses and misconduct linked to prescription drug marketing, call it uniquely into question. Gifts, luxury trips and consulting contracts for physicians smack of bribes. The ratio of sales representatives to prescribing physicians is stunning. The introduction of direct-to-consumer (DTC) advertising has led to charges that the public is lulled into ignoring the risks associated with prescription drugs and believing that pills are available for every ailment.

Disconnection between high industry profits and R&D spending. For years, the industry's explanation for its prices and profits related to having sufficient money to carry out new research, as well as sufficient profits to reward the inherent risks. Recent revelations that many companies spend more on promotion than on R&D, combined with the decline in the number of major new therapies, has made people skeptical of this claim. Even those who agree with it indicate to pollsters that they feel Americans are paying more than their fair share for the cost of drug development.

Fundamental distrust of the industry's ethics. The public realisation that research studies have been withheld from public view, or released in partial (and misleading) form, has created enormous pressures for industry to make information on all trials available via the internet. The delays in relabelling products, the precipitous withdrawal of widely marketed drugs and the failure to identify safety risks before approval (even when it was not scientifically possible to do so) gives support to the canard that companies put profits before people. And prosecutions of major companies for violations of a myriad of different laws seems to underscore the appearance of deficient basic ethics within the industry.

This catalog contains grossly overblown and unfair accusations. Unfortunately, there have been sufficient numbers of isolated examples to give the list credibility and to tarnish the entire industry. Public sentiment no longer appears willing to recognise the high costs of new drug development and to meet, on a national basis, the challenge of paying for medical advances that improve the quality of life and the savings of healthcare money.

22.2.6 Changing public perception of drug safety

There has been a tremendous increase over the years in the amount of knowledge available about a candidate drug at the time of NDA submission. The size of NDAs has grown enormously, and it is not uncommon for an NDA to contain data generated from scores of trials involving more than 10 000 patients, and sometimes several times that much. Much of this growth is in response to regulatory demands for a clearer delineation of the safety profile of a drug before approval.

Despite this record level of premarket risk information, new problems are invariably identified after approval. For many years, roughly 2–3% of the drugs approved by the FDA and by the United Kingdom regulators each year, ultimately are removed from the market for safety reasons. This situation is understandable and expected; in fact, recognition that the post-market experience inevitably reveals new adverse effects forms the basis for the requirement for post-marketing surveillance and other pharmacovigilance practices. It has always been a part of the tradeoff at the point of initial NDA approval, because the clinical trials cannot have realistically evaluated a drug in all the populations who may ultimately use it. Spontaneous reports from the entire population, plus Phase 4 studies, usually provide the first signals of new adverse events. No matter how large the number

of patients studied prior to marketing, discovery of new adverse events will always occur. Because of the very large size of the US market, relatively rare events may have a better opportunity to be discovered here earlier, and further examined in more formal studies.

Regrettably, the general public does not understand this fact. The layperson's view of drug risks might be summarised as follows:

1. Drugs should generally not have any serious or life-threatening risks (except for life-saving drugs; anticancer drugs have terrible toxicities, yet rarely provoke an outcry about side effects). Drugs for symptomatic relief or for life-style choices, especially for which there are alternatives, simply do not justify permanent injury or death.

2. The devil you knew is safer than the one you've just heard about. In the rofecoxib debate, for example, the media rarely attempted to quantify the number of life-threatening gastrointestinal bleeds caused by first generation NSAIDs but avoided by rofecoxib. Instead, the discussion focused entirely on the newly-identified cardiovascular risks.

3. Science should be able to reveal all side effects during drug development. The failure to do so suggests concealment by industry and/or incompetence by the FDA.

When drugs are withdrawn for toxicity, therefore, the public debates whether the standards for drug approval should be increased. Sponsors and the FDA are pressured to identify as many risks as possible prior to NDA approval. A point of dispute is whether these events make the Agency, or the Industry, or both, more risk-averse. Some industry members and observers believe so. They point to the natural caution of a regulatory agency that is subject to congressional criticism for appearing to have made a mistake. This problem is not new, of course, but new tools can aggravate it. For example, FDA reviewers now have access to electronic versions of the safety database in an NDA. Not surprisingly, this easier access has opened the door for *ad hoc* analyses and new safety concerns. The practice further raises the question whether there are any limits on the extent to which a sponsor must further explore potential risk signals derived from the clinical safety database.

In contrast, FDA officials have contended that the agency is more willing to admit (and leave) drugs on the market than other national authorities. They assert that the FDA can do so because it has been proactive in developing programmes to manage the known risks, when a drug with a narrow benefit/risk ratio comes up for approval.

As we have described, the genesis of FDA's approach to risk management occurred after a string of withdrawals of such widely used drugs as terfenadine, cisapride, bromfenac and troglitazone in the 1990s. Studies of the effects of new warnings and labelling changes demonstrated that they had done little to affect prescribing behaviour. The agency recognised that it needed new tools to identify safety issues, to minimise preventable risks and to inform physicians and patients about risks. The agency's position paper on a framework for risk management issued in 1999, and the proposed Guidances on Risk Management in 2003 and 2004, reveal some ongoing trends in FDA's philosophy on drug safety. In the proposed Premarketing Drug Safety document, the desire for extensive information and analysis of the safety of a product is expressed. Carried to its logical extreme, it appears to request very extensive testing and evaluation beyond the customary practice. The Risk Minimization Action Plan (proposed guidance) contains an implication for interventions beyond labelling more often than has previously been the case. Such an approach could lead to limitations on access to many novel products, at least in the early period after approval.

If risk management activities are used to permit the marketing of drugs that otherwise would be kept off because of serious safety concerns, and the activities are effective, the public will be better off. On the other hand, if risk minimisation tools are routinely applied to drugs that could be marketed without them, they could serve to deny access of physicians and patients to valuable and acceptably safe medicines. How the FDA will strike this balance remains to be seen.

22.3 Improvements Needed for the Future

From our discussion in the first part of this chapter, it is obvious that some of the industry's most serious problems could be solved if the development and approval processes were streamlined and facilitated so that unsuccessful drug candidates could be eliminated earlier, and successful candidates could, with appropriate safety, reach the market faster and at lower cost.

Despite numerous attempts in the past to streamline it, the drug development and approval process still takes far too long, is too expensive and is getting steadily more cumbersome. The process urgently needs to be speeded up. Incremental improvements (e.g. defining the optimal size of an IND) have worked for a while in the past, but the tendency for the system to accrete and bog down has become so persistent that bolder initiatives are needed to have any impact on speed and cost. For 30 years it has been recognised that such fundamental reforms are needed. The answer, we believe, is to work within the legal and regulatory framework of the current system, and to implement some of the best reforms that have already been proposed. It is the difficulty of implementation, rather than the lack of ideas, that has prevented progress and allowed the system itself to become an ever-larger impediment.

Our main proposals are

1. Simplify the initial IND filing, in order to facilitate, by partial deregulation, early-stage exploratory clinical development from Phase 1 through proof-of-concept in patients
2. At the NDA stage, make more use of the NDA's current conditional approval mechanisms, so that in a wider range of circumstances (including at the request of a sponsor) a drug may be approved for the market for limited indications, considerably earlier than it would be at present, on condition that the development programme continues and that the conditions of initial approval are enforced. In this way, the law's ultimate effectiveness and safety standards for a full approval are safeguarded, not compromised.

3. In addition, we have a number of smaller proposals that, taken together, would further facilitate the process.

22.3.1 Simplifying the IND process for early clinical studies through proof-of-concept

Contrary to what one would wish to see in an efficient clinical development process, the *de-facto* requirements for an IND continue to rise to the point where, in complexity and size, an IND today exceeds the size of some NDAs in the past. We recommend simplifying the IND requirements, so that key safety and early efficacy studies can be performed very early in humans with the same protections, but at less time and cost than they are today.

While the formal filing of a new IND is still relatively simple in principle, the amount of work that is actually required (or at least performed) to support it at present is much larger than an NDA used to be, well after the 1962 Amendments. The bureaucratic overhead that goes into managing the submissions and amendments, in both large pharmas and small startups, is excessive. The cost of impediments at this early stage is magnified because they contribute greatly to the front-loading of the clinical development costs that we have already described.

The filing of a full IND, with a formal coordinated writeup of all the supporting data, while necessary 40 years ago, is now an unnecessary requirement in the early-stage clinical programs of most large pharmas and CROs that do this work today. It is a barrier to the easy access to human studies that is needed for proof-of-concept studies (Phases 1 and 2a). There has been very little trouble in the past 20 years with early INDs filed by responsible individuals, corporations and institutions. The system can now be safety adjusted to recognise this fact, by scaling back the IND requirements for responsible entities, based on what has been learned in the past 40 years.

This is not a new idea. It was seriously considered 25 years ago in the hearings of the McMahon Commission in 1980.

It should be noted that our proposal goes considerably beyond the current proposal of FDA to create a looser 'Phase 0' stage for first-in-man pharmacokinetic and similar activities. Our proposal would cover all early human studies through clinical proof-of-concept, which usually occurs in Phase 2a. Only in the large pivotal studies (Phases 2b–3), when there is more assurance that the drug candidate has a solid chance of getting to an NDA submission, would the full formal IND filing be necessary. (These proposals are the opposite of what has been introduced by the EC Clinical trial Directive, see Chapter 17.)

The streamlined system would work like this:

• The IND filing step, and the oversight of proof-of-concept clinical research, would be safely implemented by cutting back the detail customarily required from pharma sponsors and others (i.e. CROs, Institutions, IRBs and perhaps other entities) that have been formally qualified as 'responsible' in this context. All such sponsors would have been previously screened by the agency, and accepted for the accelerated programme if qualified, based on the applicant's historical record with the agency.

• For sponsors that qualify for this new status, the IND and all studies under it would be allowed by simple notification to the FDA – rather than by FDA's scrutiny and formal allowance in each case. This system would be similar, in some respects, to the former German Hinterlegungsstelle ('Deposition'), whereby the sponsor made a simple deposition of the supporting data that the sponsor deemed sufficient, with no review or attention needed by the agency unless a problem arose. If a problem did arise, the data deposition package would be opened and reviewed by the agency, and the sponsor held liable (and, among other penalties, would lose its responsible status) if safety or other key deficiencies were found.

• The rationale for this proposal is that first-in-man and other early studies are of small size and are relatively safe when performed by experienced investigators; and that entities and individuals with a good track record and a repu-tation to lose have a powerful incentive to keep their record spotlessly clean and so retain their 'responsible' status privileges.

• For investigators and institutions that have not been qualified as 'responsible', the present IND system would apply unchanged.

22.3.2 Reforming the NDA by extending the option of provisional approval

While the standards of ultimate NDA approval based on effectiveness and safety should be care-fully maintained, existing regulations already provide for attaining full approval in stages. Our proposal is that these options should be made available in a wider range of circumstances, including at the option of the sponsor. That is, the sponsor would have the option of requesting earlier approval under, for example, a restricted range of uses or other post-market controls.

This proposal reflects the reality of many approvals today, plus the fact – not yet fully recognised – that in the past few decades there has arisen, outside the drug regulatory system, a set of additional utilisation controls of con-siderable power that can further direct drug use in many ways. That is, over the past 40 years, the marketplace has developed a power-ful, expanding set of utilisation controls (based on payment, marketing, managed care and information-feedback), that already function as a *de-facto* additional utilisation-control system, which can – and in some cases already does – act as an additional safeguard for the use of new drugs in the early post-marketing situation.

The conditional approval step could be integ-rated with the existing system of market-place utilisation controls, and thus be used as an option to expedite approvals for earlier access to prom-ising therapies. However, it would be important not to burden new drugs unnecessarily with con-ditional approval status if there is not a real reason to do so.

The agency's accession to a sponsor's request for an earlier approval, with conditions, would, in addition to helping patients, help those small sponsor companies and products for which approval in some form, even with extensive restrictions, is an increasingly necessary option. It would be particularly useful, for example, for patients who might benefit from orphan drugs and drugs developed by the numerous small biotechnology companies that have products in development for limited indications.

22.3.3 Improving success rates

As important as – or even more important than – speed of development, is the success rate of the overall process, which must be increased. It has been estimated (J DiMasi, personal communic-ation) that increasing the success rate by 10% across a portfolio of drugs at all stages of clin-ical development would have the same effect on development costs as reducing the development time by more than 20%.

22.3.4 Other opportunities for improvement in discovery and early development

Finally, we discuss here a further set of potential areas for improvement across a wide area of the drug development process.

Having better New Molecular Entity (NME) candidates and better ways of choosing which of them should enter into development would be an important step forward. Although the enormous increase in power of the biological and phar-maceutical sciences has increased the quality of development candidates over recent years, pre-diction of consistently successful ones still eludes us, and the overall success rate of drugs in clinical development has changed little over the last few decades. The overall success rate – from the Tufts CSDD data – remains at approximately 20%, des-pite other estimates that suggest an even lower range of 5–15%.

Much hope is currently held out for the poten-tial effects of biomarkers, including genomic and other molecular markers, in improving the quality of targets, drug candidates and their progression through early development.

At present, as we have discussed, these prom-ises are still somewhat hypothetical, but progress is being made. While we all have high hopes that the increasing sophistication of drug development sciences will solve the problems, particularly of success rate, it should also be borne in mind that the increasing cost being built into the system requires a continuous increase in success rates just to break even; and thus – if they fail to deliver – will further threaten the future of the pharma development enterprise. Given the enthusiasm and the clamor for front-loading the development process with more science, and despite the plausibility of this approach, this aspect needs to be carefully tracked and made to live up to its claims, to prevent the situation from collapsing.

22.3.4.1　FDA's skills

Using the increased skills and talents of the greater number of qualified staff now at FDA (made possible in particular by the budget expansions of PDUFA, and now in more concrete form in the agency's critical path initiative) is another avenue. DiMasi and Manocchia have shown that early and continuing discussions between the regulators and the regulated, in the form of FDA-sponsor conferences, facilitate drug approval. This is what one would expect if, by the time of filing an NDA, all the important questions had been asked and answered. FDA's critical path initiative is an obvious way in which the agency's skills and resources can be brought to bear, and the results of this effort will be followed with particular interest. Again, however, the amount and effect of front-end loading of the process needs to be carefully compared against the results.

22.3.4.2　Animal data

It may also be possible for time and money to be saved by eliminating requirements for animal toxicity data that are found to be no longer necessary. Excessive use of toxicity data has been criticised by some, reminiscent of the days when LD_{50} values in laboratory animals were routinely performed even when the precision sought in such studies was unnecessary for product development.

22.3.4.3　'Naturalistic' studies

The inclusion/exclusion criteria needed in formal clinical trials inevitably produce experimental populations that are not typical of patient populations in routine medical practice. More attention therefore needs to be paid to the 'naturalistic' study of drugs, after marketing, in general clinical practice. Such studies could lead to an increased understanding of both effectiveness and risk in the intended patient population. Benefits will almost certainly accrue by identifying empiric relations between genetic make-up and drug response, with the possibility of increasing benefit or decreasing harm. Progress in this area is unfortunately predicted too optimistically at present by scientists who should be aware of the length of time that will be required to achieve these goals, but nevertheless ultimate progress will be made if we apply ourselves to the task.

22.3.4.4　Direct-to-consumer advertising

At this time when DTC advertising is again coming under criticism, there needs to be continuing debate over its nature, effectiveness and overall effects. Whereas some patients do not wish to play an aggressive role in affecting their physicians' prescribing, others do. The latter, understandably, do not consider themselves naïve innocents who are too ill informed to play a useful role. And many physicians (perhaps most?) do not feel that they will be inevitably forced to prescribe badly because of patient pressures. On the other hand, there is scope for abuse here, and a balance needs to be identified and sought, particularly in the disclosure of side effects.

22.3.4.5　Secondary indications

The current restrictions by FDA on the advertising of secondary or tertiary indications (that is, unapproved by FDA) for drugs need to re-evaluated. Experience has taught us that often not all the uses of a drug are known at the time of first marketing, and indeed it is not unusual for later approved uses to be more important medically than the original indication.

On the other hand, the recent abuses and allegations of fraud that have occurred in manipulation of off-label drug use, resulting in the creation of the anti-kickback legislation and regulations, demonstrate that this is a complex matter that needs to be carefully controlled and adjusted to achieve the optimal balance between benefit and risk.

22.3.4.6   Incentives for obtaining new data

Because some additional uses may only be discovered late in a drug's patent life (or even after the patent has expired), a company may be reluctant to spend the time and money to obtain formal FDA approval of new uses primarily to benefit generic manufacturers. Optimal medical practice, however, calls for access to sound and persuasive data on new indications. Some method needs to be found to encourage sponsors to seek new indications during more of a product's patent life and – if possible – beyond.

The success of the various special-case areas of drug development regulation and performance, such as orphan drugs, cancer, and AIDS drugs, and the pediatric exclusivity extension could be a guide to how to approach – and what to avoid – in creating larger facilitatory approaches in the future.

22.4   Conclusions

After a difficult decade following the 1962 Amendments, the pharma industry and the FDA have in general worked well together, and the 35 years from 1970 to 2005 mark an era of unparalleled achievement in the modernisation of drug development and approval. The present system has achieved much in its near half-century of operation. Nevertheless, it is becoming in part a victim of its own successes, as the finely balanced processes are now paradoxically coming closer to bogging down under the weight of continually increasing requirements from many directions.

In the last 10 years, cracks have become obvious in the system, just when it should be flowering. The pharma industry's output of new drugs has slowed despite unprecedented investment in discovery and development; and at the same time the industry, and the drug development process itself, has acquired the most negative public image ever, mainly because of pricing, marketing and safety issues. The FDA, too, has come under criticism over drug safety questions, in part due to communication problems.

The causes of this unfortunate state of affairs are numerous, and require a variety of solutions as we have described in this chapter. Defining the roles of the industry and government in the pursuit of effective new therapies and their appropriate use is one of the areas where attention is needed in the future.

We may in part be a victim of our own successes. For example, pharma's well-honed coping skills, evolved to respond to the growing tendency for society to pile on regulatory requirements, and for the industry to accept and cope with almost any challenge thrust upon it, have hindered the necessary streamlining and reform efforts, while the system daily accretes more obligations for the industry and for the FDA.

International harmonisation has also turned out to be another effort that went far beyond its original aims, extending now into creating new regulations and becoming an end and career niche in itself. Some international safety consortia developed similar expansionist activities. The autonomy of these groups is creating problems as they expand, with Europe and the United States seeking to develop separate policies and rules, which not only defeats the original purpose of the harmonisation efforts, but could easily result in problems worse than the original harmonisation program was designed to cure. Overall, the regulatory bodies have made considerable efforts to support the spirit of harmonisation, but in practice, continue to devolve interpretations of some of the policies to the individual countries. For example, in FDA's recently proposed safety regulations, there are new definitions for periodic safety update reports (PSURs) that deviate from the generally expected formats already adopted in many countries.

More aggressive reforms are needed if pharma and regulatory agencies are to serve the public optimally. In this chapter we considered how some of these hindrances – in particular, regulation of early drug development and also the approval stage – could be addressed. As we have shown, there are steps of the early IND research that have become routine and could be deregulated, under appropriate controls, with beneficial effects. And at the NDA approval stage, a considerable benefit could be achieved by combining approval earlier in the development process with existing safeguards in drug utilisation controls necessary to guarantee safe use until enough experience is obtained to relax the initial marketing restrictions. There are many other areas that need to be addressed in addition to the ones we have considered here.

In summary, the main reforms we have suggested here – involving both the IND and NDA, are a start, but much more is needed to adjust the Pharma's productivity to the needs of society.

Drug development and regulation promises to be an interesting ride through the twenty-first century.

Acknowledgements

The authors wish to acknowledge the contributions of their friend and colleague Dr Louis Lasagna to the field of Clinical Pharmacology and to its wider applications in Regulation, Drug Development and Pharmaceutical Medicine. Dr Lasagna contributed to the previous edition of this chapter, and died in August 2003 as the present edition was being planned.

Further Reading

Center for the Study of Drug Development, Tufts University: *Outlook 2004* and other publications.

DiMasi JA. The value of improving the productivity of the drug development process: faster times and better decisions. *PharmacoEcon* 2002;**20**:1–10.

DiMasi JA. Risks in new drug development: approval success rates for investigational drugs. *Clin Pharmacol Ther* 2001;**69**:297–307.

DiMasi JA, Hansen RW, Grabowski HG. The price of innovation: new estimates of drug development costs. *J Health Econ* 2003;**22**:151–85.

DiMasi JA, Grabowski HG, Vernon J. R&D costs and returns by therapeutic category. *Drug Info J* 2004;**38**:211–23.

DiMasi JA, Manocchia M. Initiatives to speed new drug development and regulatory review: the impact of FDA-sponsor conferences. *Drug Info J* 1997;**31**:771–8.

DiMasi JA, Paquette C. The economics of follow-on drug development: trends in entry rates and the timing of development. *PharmacoEcon* 2004;**22**:1–14.

Food and Drug Administration Modernization Act of 1997 (FDAMA).

Food and Drug Administration. Innovation, Stagnation: Challenge and Opportunity on the Critical Path to New Medical Products, March 2004.

Jones JK. Broader Uses of Post-Marketing Surveillance. In *Drug Development, Regulatory Assessment and Post Marketing Surveillance*. Velo G, Wardell W, eds. New York–London: Plenum Press, 1981;203–16.

Jones JK National/International Systems for Postmarketing Surveillance. In Velo G, Wardell W, eds. *Drug Development, Regulatory Assessment and Post Marketing Surveillance*. New York–London: Plenum Press, 1981;233–40.

Jones JK. Joint Commission on Prescription Drug Use. In Velo G, Wardell W eds. *Drug Development, Regulatory Assessment and Post Marketing Surveillance*. New York–London: Plenum Press, 1981; 191–200.

Jones JK. Regulatory Use of Adverse Reactions. In *Detection and Prevention of Adverse Drug Reactions*. 1983 International Symposium, Stockholm, Skandia International Symposia, Almquist and Wiksall International, Stockholm, 1984;203–14.

Jones JK, Faich GA and Anello C. Post-Marketing Surveillance in the General Population – the U.S.A. In William H Inman, ed, *Monitoring for Drug Safety, 2nd edn*. Lancaster, U.K.: MTP Press Limited, 1985;153–63.

Jones JK, Idänpään-Heikkilä, JE. Adverse Reactions, Postmarketing Surveillance and Pharmacoepidemiology. In Burley DM, Clarke JM, Lasagna L, Edward Arnold, eds. *Pharmaceutical Medicine*. A Division of Hodder & Stoughton Publishers, 1993;145–80.

Kaitin K, Cairns C. The new drug approvals of 1999, 2000, and 2001: drug development trends a decade after passage of the prescription Drug User Fee Act of 1992. *Drug Information Journal* 2003;**4**:357–71.

Lasagna L. Who will adopt the orphan drug? *Regulation* 1979;**3**:27–32.

McMahon Commission Report. Commission on the Federal Drug Approval Process. Final Report 1982.

Reichart J. Biopharmaceutical approvals in the US increase. *Regul Aff J – Pharma* 2004;**15**(7):1–7.

Wardell W. The Drug Lag and American therapeutics: an international comparison. 22nd International Congress of Pharmacology, San Francisco, 1972.

Wardell W. Therapeutic implications of the drug lag. *Clin Pharmacol Ther* 1973;**14**:1022–34.

Wardell W, Lasagna L, Regulation and Drug Development, American Enterprise Institute for Public Policy Research, Washington, DC, 1975.

Wardell W, ed. *Controlling the Use of Therapeutic Drugs: An International Comparison*, Washington, DC: American Enterprise Institute for Public Policy Research, 1978.

www.FDA.gov (The history section of the FDA's website is particularly informative.)

CHAPTER 23

23 Regulatory and clinical trial systems in Japan

Yuichi Kubo

23.1 Introduction

Japan is the second largest country in terms of pharmaceutical market with the population exceeding 120 million. The importance of this market has been recognised for long, but many pharmaceutical companies have excluded this particular area from their global development strategy. One reason for such omission is the unique marketing/distributing rules that handicap new-comers. Another reason is the unique clinical trial system, represented by the now abolished general guideline that required the primary endpoint of a clinical study to be categorised to the final global improvement rate (FGIR), and by the old Japanese good clinical practice (GCP) that did not require study-site monitoring or auditing. The other obstacle is the notion of the Japanese that they are unique and are different in every aspect from the rest of world, and therefore, the clinical data obtained in foreign countries are not applicable to the Japanese population.

The marketing/distributing rules in Japan have become almost identical to those in the West, and GCP is updated in-line with the International Conference on Harmonisation (ICH) GCP. ICH discussion on ethnic factors established a concept that foreign clinical data are accepted for new drug application if there are no concerns about ethnic differences in the effect or adverse effect of the product.

Because of these changes, many multinational pharmaceutical companies include the Japanese market into their global development and marketing strategies. It is important to understand, however, that there are still many oddities for conducting clinical trial in Japan. Many of these are due to the difference in medical practice and/or attitude of the Japanese people towards effects and side effects of medicinal products, which may not harmonise with the West in a short period of time. Therefore, it is important to conduct a careful feasibility study before commencing clinical trials in Japan if global development is planned.

23.2 Regulatory Systems

23.2.1 Introduction

The procedures described below are essentially those that apply to the approval of ethical pharmaceutical products containing new chemical entities. Procedures for approval of drugs containing agents already listed in the Japanese pharmacopoeia, or which are modifications of already approved drugs, or are *in vitro* diagnostic agents are all subject to slightly different procedures. For a full description of these variations the reader is referred to 'Drug Approval and Licensing Procedures in Japan'.[1]

The basis of the regulatory review and the clinical trial system is established in 1977 after

The views expressed in this chapter are those of the authors and not necessarily those of Daiichi Pharmaceutical Co. Ltd.

significant amendment of the Pharmaceutical Affairs Law. Also the revised GCP based on ICH has become a legal requirement, effective from 1 April 1997. A clinical trial review procedure has been instigated with a 30-day review period before trial initiation. Although clinical trial applications were previously sent to the Ministry of Health and Welfare (MHW, now Ministry of Health, Labour and Welfare, MHLW), the hospital and in-house Institutional Review Boards also undertook active review.

Responsibility for regulatory review has been passed to an Incorporated Administrative Agency, the Pharmaceutical and Medical Devices Agency (PMDA). PMDA also intensively checks applications for GCP compliance and reliability compliance. Another important role of PMDA includes an advice to sponsors on clinical trials and on which result can be submitted at the time of a new drug application.

23.2.2 Type of approvals

Until March 2005, approvals fell into three categories, namely manufacturing approvals, import approvals and foreign manufacturing approvals. This will change from April 2005. Approval is no longer granted for manufacturing, import or foreign manufacturing, but for marketing, in-line with the approval system of Western countries. This change of the approval system has no direct effect on the clinical trial system, but may provide a chance to a foreign manufacturer seeking marketing opportunities in Japan.

23.2.3 Review process

The procedure by which applications are reviewed is described below and for all new drugs is shown schematically in Figure 23. 1.

Applications for marketing should be sent to MHLW. The application then passes to PMDA, where the application splits into two different routes, namely (1) good laboratory practice (GLP), GCP and reliability compliance check by Office of Conformity Audit and (2) application review by Offices of New Drug or Office of Biologics.

First, the Office of Conformity Audit will conduct a compliance review to ensure that the dossier meets the standards of GCP, GLP and reliability. The GCP compliance check is based on the inspection of both study sites and sponsor. For the submission of new active substance usually four study sites are inspected. If the pivotal studies are conducted overseas, the inspection may be conducted by MHLW instead of PMDA.

As well as GCP site inspections, an examination is undertaken of the raw or source data and records of Chemistry Manufacturing and Control (CMC), non-clinical and clinical reports that are the basis of the application. This is to ensure that the application dossier accurately reflects the source data. The procedure issued by PMDA details that list of raw data and records must be provided. The applicant is required to bring the data and records to PMDA on the specified days and when the examination finishes they should be retrieved. Therefore, the raw data and records stored at overseas sites are usually categorised as 'documents not to be submitted' and not subject to reliability review by PMDA. Instead, the MHLW may investigate the data from non-Japanese studies at the site of storage since submission of a photocopy of the data is not permitted.

Review of the submission dossier will begin simultaneously with the above-mentioned compliance check. Review is undertaken by one of the four evaluation office teams, which comprised experts from medicine, pharmaceutical sciences, veterinary sciences and statistics. The team also includes external experts. Evaluation meetings are held at which questions are raised by the reviewing team and the applicant has the opportunity to discuss issues with the reviewers. The reviewer in charge will prepare a report of the application for the next stage of the special review and interview.

Once the PDMA review is completed, the result is reported to the Evaluation and Licensing Division of MHLW. The report is then consulted to the Pharmaceutical Affairs Section of Pharmaceutical Affairs and Food Sanitation Council (PAFSC). Upon positive advise from PAFSC, the minister of MHLW grants the approval.

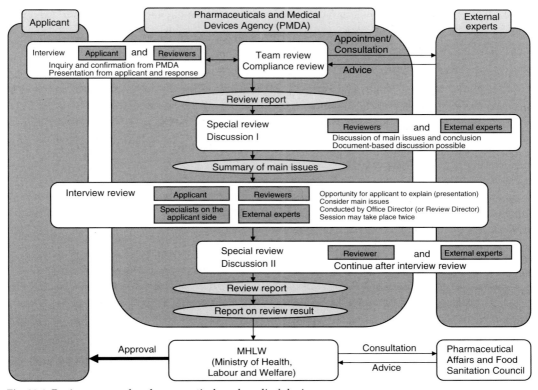

Fig. 23.1 Review process for pharmaceuticals and medical devices.

The period required from receipt to approval of the application is treated as that for handling of the standard clerical service, except for replying to PAFSC inquiries and that for correcting incomplete applications. The period for handling the standard clerical service is 12 months. The applicant also has another 12 months to respond to queries and requests from the agency.

23.2.4 Priority review

The priority review is applicable for orphan drugs, orphan medical devices and 'innovative drugs or medical devices that have been authorised to be highly necessary from a medical standpoint'. The standards to define orphan drugs are the following: (1) patient number of disease indicated for the drug concerned is less than 50 000; (2) excellent usefulness of the drug from the medical standpoint and (3) the development

and the future use of the drug is fairly feasible. The criteria for 'innovative drugs' other than the orphan drugs are that (1) the indicated diseases are serious and (2) the drug is clinically significantly superior to existing product.

The priority review system places the product in front of the review product queue and by this means expedites approval of the product. It is important to note that there is no intention in the system to reduce the scientific standard or quality of the application data.

23.2.5 Data requirements for marketing approval in Japan

The data requirements for the registration of new drugs were defined in the Pharmaceutical Affairs Law and its Enforcement Regulations. Practical guidelines were issued in PMSB Director General Notification No. 481 dated

8 April 1999, 'On Application for Drug Approval' and PMSB/ELD Notification No. 666 dated 8 April 1999, 'On Requirements for Application for Drug Approval', followed by ICH Common Technical Document guidelines, PMSB Director General Notification No. 481 dated 21 June 2001, 'On Application for Drug Approval' and PMSB Notification No. 899 dated 21 June 2001, 'On Requirements for Application for Drug Approval'.

The various data, which must be submitted with applications for approval to manufacture ethical drugs, were specified in these notifications (Tables 23.1 and 23.2).

The application should be in the format of common technical document (CTD), which became mandatory from July 2003. The regional specific requirements are in the Modules 1 and 5 of CTD, which are described below.

Module 1

• NDA Application Form (format based on Pharmaceutical Affairs Law Enforcement Regulations)
• Certificates (including statement by a responsible person supervising collection and preparation of application data, documents related to GLP and GCP, copy of a written contract of co-development)
• Patent Status Information
• Origin, background of the discovery and R&D history (formerly in the first part of Gaiyo. This can be described in Module 2 instead of in Module 1)
• Status of use in foreign countries
• List of other pharmaceuticals with similar pharmacological effect(s) and/or indications(s)
• Draft package insert (labelling)
• Documentation of non-proprietary name
• Format for designation of poisonous/deleterious pharmaceutical ingredients
• Draft protocol for post-marketing surveillance (if necessary)
• List of information/documents complied in the dossier.

In addition to Section 5.3.7 of Module 5 'Case Report Forms and Individual Patients

Listing', the following tabulations and charts are required:

• The list of subjects in the pivotal studies of dose setting/efficacy clinical studies
• The list of subjects with adverse reactions in all the submitted clinical studies
• The list of subjects with serious adverse reactions in all the submitted clinical studies
• The list of subjects with observed clinical data that are abnormal in all the submitted clinical studies
• The charts that illustrate progression of observed clinical test data that are abnormal.

If any consultation with PMDA (or formerly Drug Organisation) took place, the official records should be incorporated into Module 5.4.

Module 2 is termed GAIYO (which means summary in Japanese) as before and should be prepared in Japanese except for the figures and tables, if they are accompanied with translation of keywords. The original English reports are accepted in Modules 3, 4 and 5 and a Japanese summary is not required anymore.

After the approval of the product, the sponsor is requested to disclose GAIYO to the public except for the parts containing trade secrets and private information. The electronic version of GAIYO for disclosure can be obtained from: http://www.info.pmda.go.jp/info/syounin_index.html. (Please note that the homepage is written in Japanese.)

23.2.6 Clinical trial consultation

The PMDA consults with sponsors on the protocol and the issues relating to drug development. There are a number of categories of consultations for drug development stages, starting from pre-Phase 1 to pre-NDA and other consultations (see Table 23.3). These consultations should be based on the scientific knowledge of the product obtained within the consultation time and should clear the queries of sponsors either on the design of study protocol, concepts of development or rationale for submission. The consultations provide the merits of both of FDA

Table 23.1 Information required for new drug application in Japan

Type of drug	A			B			C			D							E			F						G
	1	2	3	1	2	3	1	2	3	1	2	3	4	5	6	7	1	2	3	1	2	3	4	5	6	1
Drug with new active ingredients	X	X	X	X	X	X	X	X	X	X	X	X	/	X	/	/	X	X	/	X	X	X	X	–	/	X
New combination prescription	X	X	X	–	–	X	X	X	X	X	X	–	–	–	/	–	X	/	/	X	X	X	X	–	/	X
Drug with new route of administration	X	X	X	–	–	X	X	X	X	X	X	–	/	X	/	/	X	/	/	X	X	X	X	–	/	X
Drugs with new ingredients	X	X	X	–	–	–	–	–	–	–	–	–	–	–	–	–	X	–	–	/	/	/	/	–	/	X
Drugs with new dosage forms	X	X	X	–	–	X	X	X	X	–	–	–	–	–	–	–	–	–	–	X	X	X	X	–	/	X
Drugs with new doses	X	X	X	–	–	X	–	–	–	–	–	–	–	–	–	–	X	–	–	X	X	X	X	–	/	X

Notes: Type of drug is defined in the Article 18–3, Paragraph 1, Item 1 of MHLW Ordinance.
For the Code in the right column, refer to Table 23.2.
X: required.
/ : required on a case-by-case basis, depending on individual new drug application.
–: note required in principle.

Table 23.2 Key Table for Table 23.1

A.	Data on the origin and background of the discovery, and conditions of use in foreign countries, etc.	Data on: 1. Origin and background of discovery 2. Conditions of use in foreign countries 3. Properties and comparative studies with other drugs
B.	Data on physical and chemical properties, specifications, testing methods, etc.	Data on: 1. Determination of structure 2. Physical and chemical properties, etc. 3. Specifications and testing methods
C.	Data on stability	Data on: 1. Long-term shelf-life tests 2. Stress tests 3. Accelerated tests
D.	Data on acute, subacute and chronic toxicity, teratogenicity and other types of toxicity	Data on: 1. Single-dose toxicity 2. Repeated-dose toxicity 3. Genotoxicity 4. Carcinogenicity 5. Developmental and reproductive toxicity 6. Local irritation 7. Other types of toxicity
E.	Data on pharmacological effects	Data on: 1. Tests supporting the efficacy 2. Genera pharmacology
F.	Data on absorption, distribution, metabolism and excretion	Data on: 1. Absorption 2. Distribution 3. Metabolism 4. Excretion 5. Biological equivalence
G.	Data on results of clinical studies	Clinical study results

meetings and EMEA scientific advice. The consultation is chargeable and the fee is shown in the table. PMDA prepares the official records of the consultation, which is attached to the new drug application and will be considered by the reviewers.

23.3 Clinical Trial Systems

23.3.1 Introduction

Based on Step 4 of the ICH GCP guideline of May 1996, the Japanese MHW prepared an amendment to the previous GCP guideline and this was issued as 'MHW Ordinance of the Standards for Good Clinical Practice' on 27 March 1997. This new GCP became effective as of 1 April 1997 with some moratoria [preparation of standard operating procedures (SOP) at medical institutes, source data verification, etc.], and full implementation was from 1 April 1998. Unlike the previous GCP guidelines, the new GCP is based on the revised Pharmaceutical Affairs Law of June 1996, which requires that the data for new drug applications are obtained at the standard set by the ministry, and therefore it is legally

Table 23.3 List of major consultation meetings offered by PMDA, as on April 2004

Category	Fee (in Japanese Yen)
Pre-Phase I meeting	2 349 900
Pre-early Phase II meeting	865 200
Pre-late Phase II meeting	1 678 700
End-of Phase II meeting	3 331 900
Pre-NDA meeting	3 333 000

obligatory to respect the new GCP in conducting clinical trials in Japan.

The new GCP follows the ICH GCP guideline but there are some unique aspects added in order to cope with Japanese medical and clinical practices. Although such modifications have been made, the concept of the ICH guidelines is maintained, and this caused significant change in clinical trial practice in Japan. The main points of the changes in clinical trial practice between the old and new GCP, as well as unique aspects of Japanese GCP and clinical trial practice are explained in the sections below.

23.3.2 Sponsor

The new GCP requires the sponsor to be fully responsible for all aspects of the clinical trial. This responsibility includes preparation of the study protocol, selection of investigators and study centres, monitoring and auditing, and writing the clinical reports. Under the old GCP system, most of the responsibility for conduct of the clinical trial fell upon the chief investigator and, in a sense, the sponsoring company was immune from such responsibility. This mechanism deprived Japanese pharmaceutical companies of incentives to build medical and other expertise within the company. As many Japanese pharmaceutical companies have little or no expertise in the clinical area, the new GCP guidelines require the sponsor to organise a study

team consisting of specialists for a variety of aspects.

23.3.3 Medical Advisor

There is serious shortage of medically qualified personnel in Japanese pharmaceutical companies, or worse is the fact that they do not recognise the importance of such expertise in-house. The new GCP requires sponsoring companies to either employ or contract medical professionals in order to obtain medical advice in preparing protocols and conducting clinical trials.

23.3.4 Other specialists

Other specialists include biostatisticians, regulatory affairs personnel, pharmacokineticists, medical writers and so on, but the new GCP does not specify those specialists. If the sponsoring company does not possess such expertise, the sponsor can give it on contract.

23.3.5 In-house study review board

The government had required that the sponsors should have their own in-house study review board to review the ethical aspects of clinical trial protocols. Such a requirement was based on the former Japanese GCP, which stipulates that the company should organise an internal formal body or mechanism that reviews and authorises its planned studies before submitting to either study centres or the MHW for clinical trial plan notification.

The new Japanese GCP no longer contains a clause to this effect, but it seems that the authorities favours the sponsor to maintain the procedures for an in-house study review board and to determine the appropriateness of the planned studies.

23.3.6 Contract research organisations

Contract research organisations (CROs) are formally recognised in the new GCP, as it explicitly stipulates that the sponsor may contract all or some parts of clinical trial activity to contract bodies, and in such a case the contract between the sponsor and the study site should be executed between the sponsor, the study site and the CRO. Since then, many CROs have been established and because of heavy demand of trial monitors and data management specialists by sponsoring companies, further growth of CROs in terms of number and size is expected.

23.3.7 Protocol development

The former requirement of categorised result of efficacy, called FGIR or utility and global utility rate (GUR) are not required anymore. For confirmation studies, a single objective, clinically meaningful endpoint should be identified. Where an objective endpoint is not available, subjective endpoints can be used instead. If the endpoint is not well established or subjective, it must be validated. Study investigators or others who are involved in evaluation should be well trained, and their variation of evaluation results should be within an acceptable range.

Surrogate endpoints should be carefully chosen, if they are required. Some surrogate endpoints, such as peak flow in asthma or haemoglobin A1c in diabetes mellitus, are well established and can be used in the confirmation studies. Conducting true endpoint study is difficult if it is not incorporated into global study because patient recruitment is still slow in Japan and hence relatively small number of study participants will be achieved in a reasonable time frame.

23.3.8 Study guidelines

It is always advised to check whether there is a specific guideline for evaluating a given medicinal product in the area of interest. Most of the study guidelines have not been updated for a long time, and caution should be exercised to confirm that the contents therein are already obsolete and therefore invalid.

The agency had requested sponsors to adhere to the guidelines strictly, but now it explicitly warns sponsors that the guidelines are

the guidelines at the time of their issue and the latest scientific standard will be applied when the agency reviews a new drug application.

23.3.9 Study design

A double-blind randomised study is recommended for the confirmation study unless there are substantial scientific reasons not to do so. In many cases, an active comparator is preferred to an inactive placebo, as evidence of similar efficacy to the premium priced product will be an advantage for obtaining favourable reimbursement price. Nevertheless, choice of the placebo increasing to demonstrates absolute efficacy of the drug and has been accepted by many study sites.

If conducting multinational studies in Japan, choice of an active comparator may be a difficult issue. There are many products that are not available, or their indication, dose and dosage or condition of use are different from other countries.

23.3.10 Selection of study centres and investigators

23.3.10.1 Study site

The new GCP requires clinical study sites to have enough facilities to conduct clinical trials and be able to cope in the case of emergency. Adequately trained staff should be available. The sites must prepare SOPs for accepting, reviewing and operating clinical trial. Additional SOPs are required for the operation of the Institutional Review Board (IRB). A clinical trial office and an office for IRB operation must be established in the study site. These requirements have been defined as the minimum requirements for any clinical trial to be conducted in hospitals equipped with ample resources, to manage many SOPs, and office staff for clinical trial and IRB.

The new GCP, however, also stipulates requirements when clinical sites give the above activities on contract to contractors. By this means the trial-related offices can be established among a collection of study sites if the sites are those of general practitioners or small clinics. The contractors are called site management organisations (SMOs), which establish a network of clinical trial sites and provide faster patient recruitment capability in therapeutic areas for general practitioners or small clinics.

23.3.10.2 Number of study sites and number of patients at each site

It was customary for confirmation studies that study centres were chosen on marketing grounds, as well as from a scientific aspect. Because many similar products were developed and launched, hospitals decided to list only those drugs that they had included in the development into their formulary. A vital issue for sponsoring companies is to get their product to be listed in the formulary of major hospitals, such as university hospitals or main regional hospitals. Therefore, the confirmation clinical study sites tend to spread all over Japan and favour at least one hospital in each prefecture (Japan consists of 43 prefectures). Although the number of participating hospitals is large, the number of patients involved in confirmation studies was rather limited, and therefore many studies were conducted with few patients per centre.

If the number of patients at each centre is small, doctors cannot gain experience in the study and they cannot compare the responses of patients to the study medications. Study monitors have to cover wide geographic area and large number of study-related personnel in order to monitor relatively small number of patients. This old practice might be expected to reduce the quality and credibility of the study.

Currently, the agency recommends sponsors to recruit more than 10 patients at each centre, and most of the study centres are able to accommodate this number. As the overall number of clinical trials has declined because of the new GCP guidelines and unfavourable pricing rules for the new products, with limited advantage over existing products, it has become relatively easy for the sponsors to meet such requirements than before.

23.3.10.3 Institutional Review Board

The new GCP guidelines has expanded the IRB constitution and its role in the clinical trial. The IRB must consist of more than five members and must include non-medical personnel and a person who does not relate to the study centre. There are no requirements regarding the balance of gender. The head of the institute can attend the IRB meetings but cannot be a member nor discuss or vote at the meeting.

The IRB is responsible for judging all studies to be conducted at the centre concerned by reviewing protocols, the informed consent sheet, the investigator's brochure and other materials relating to the conduct of clinical trials. The IRB is also responsible for monitoring whether the clinical trials are conducted in compliance with both GCP and IRB's requirements, if any. When the study period of a clinical trial exceeds 1 year the IRB should review the study every year. As the new GCP allows the study sponsor to pay a reasonable amount of money to the study subjects, the IRB is expected to review whether the amount and method of payment is reasonable and does not infringe upon the ethical aspects of the study. Also, the advertisement of a trial for patient recruitment is allowed, but the IRB's approval to implement this at the study centre is required.

The new GCP stipulates that many study centres may share an IRB or an IRB may be established by academic organisations to which medical centres can seek advice on the studies. As the maintenance and operation of full IRBs may be a burden to some medical institutes, it is likely that such 'public' IRBs will become a practical option.

23.3.10.4 Investigators

The new GCP clarifies the role of the investigators. They are expected to take an active part in the study from the planning stage. Previously, the number of patients and the study protocols were allotted to each centre by the chief investigator, but now it is the responsibility of investigators as to whether they accept the protocol and the number of patients to be recruited, and then take part in the study.

Preparation of the patient informed consent sheet is the responsibility of each investigator, although support of the sponsor is requested. The investigator can nominate sub-investigators and other supportive staff for the study and establish a study team. The member list of the study team should be submitted to, and confirmed by, the head of the institute. The investigator should endorse the study protocol and the study contract, and must comply with them. Any deviations from the protocol should be recorded and reported to both the head of the institute and the sponsor.

Selection of study investigators is difficult and involves many factors. Among the factors, possible patient recruitment would be the most important one. It is not easy to predict patient recruitment at the time of protocol discussion, because the attitude of patients towards clinical trial is not entirely in favour of participation. Whether the study site is acceptable in the light of GCP is another important issue for the choice of investigators. Although many centres are 'GCP compliant', close monitoring is required to confirm that such status is maintained during the conduct of clinical trial. GCP system in hospitals is maintained by a small number of competent staff, mostly by pharmacy staff, and therefore the retirement or movement of the main staff may change the situation.

23.3.11　Clinical trial plan notification

An outline of the data from non-clinical studies must be submitted to the PMDA with the protocol for the proposed clinical study before commencing the clinical trial. A notification is required for each protocol. The list of items required for 'Clinical Trial Plan Notification' is shown in Table 23.4. Furthermore, supplementary data must be added on entry to subsequent clinical phases, that is, general clinical trials and comparative trials. Such data are reviewed by the PMDA, and for this purpose the sponsor must wait for 30 days after submitting the initial notification before executing a contract with the medical institute. For a subsequent notification, the review period is reduced to 14 days. The notification also

Table 23.4 List of items required for 'Clinical Trial Plan Notification'

- Description of trial drug
- Manufacturing method
- Anticipated indications, dose and dosage
- Purpose of trial
- Trial details including study period
- Name and address of each study centre
- Names of all investigators
- Amount of clinical supply for each centre
- Reasons if the supply is free of charge
- (Name and address of local CT manager)

requires the names of all investigators, whether investigators or sub-investigators, and this list of investigators must be kept updated throughout the study period.

23.3.12　Contracts and funding

23.3.12.1　Head of study centre
Japanese GCP requires that the head of the medical institute and the sponsor must execute a study contract, and does not allow the investigator to directly contract with the sponsor. Historically, a clinical trial is considered as an activity of the hospital as a whole, not of an individual investigator. The reason behind this is that the investigator cannot conduct any study without the full support of hospital staff and access to hospital facilities. The head of the medical institute is responsible for organising an IRB in-house or to make it available outside the hospital, if the hospital is not large enough to maintain an IRB. Once the sponsoring company submits the clinical study plan to the hospital, the head of the medical institute should submit the study document to the IRB for their opinion. The head cannot be a member of the IRB, is not allowed to discuss or vote on the clinical trial, but nevertheless attendance to the IRB is not prohibited.

The head of the medical institute should sign the study contract after receiving a favourable opinion from the IRB. The head cannot accept the study if the IRB decision is not favourable.

Table 23.5 Essential clauses of the contract between study sponsor and medical institution

---

- Date of contract
- Name and address of person sponsoring clinical trial
- In the case where a part of the work is entrusted to a CRO, name and address of CRO, and range of the work entrusted
- Name and address of medical institution
- Name and title of persons responsible for contract
- Names and titles of investigators and others
- Period of clinical trial
- Target number of subjects
- Matters related to control of clinical trial drugs
- Matters related to preservation of records (including data)
- Maters related to report by sponsor and persons engaged at medical institution pursuant to the GCP
- Matters related to conservation of subjects' privacy
- Matters related to costs of clinical trials
- Statement that medical institution conduct the clinical trial in conformity with the protocol
- Statement that medical institution allow access to records (including documents) specified by GCP at request of the sponsor
- In the case where it is evident that medical institution adversely interfered with the proper clinical trial by violating GCP, protocol or the contract, the sponsor can cancel the contract
- Matters related to compensation to health damage to subjects
- Other matters necessary for ensuring that the clinical trial can be conducted properly and smoothly

---

GCP stipulates essential clauses of the contract (Table 23.5).

In addition to IRB members, the head of the institute must appoint a study drug manager, a document archiving manager and administration staff for both clinical trials and the IRB. In order to handle clinical trials in such a complex structure, SOPs for conducting clinical trials must be prepared at the hospital.

All serious adverse events, deviations from the protocol, extensions of study period or increase in patient numbers should be reported to the head of the institute by the investigator.

23.3.12.2   Clinical trial funding

The regulations on clinical trial funding differ among hospitals based on their background. For example, in national university hospitals there is a standard table that categorises clinical trial activities. (The national universities are incorporated as on April 2004.) To calculate the study budget, the activities are added up for each protocol and some hospital overheads, which cover general management costs, are also added. The entire study points are then multiplied by the index to change the points into actual currency. This index is set as 6000 yen (about 30 sterling pounds). Private university hospitals set a similar rule but with greater overheads.

23.3.13   Ethical issues

23.3.13.1   Informed consent

The patient's informed consent was required in the old GCP, with a wording of 'in writing as a rule'. A survey performed in the early 1990s showed that a limited number of informed consents were obtained in writing and the rest

Table 23.6 Items required in the IC form

- The fact that the clinical trial is conducted as a test
- Purpose of the clinical trial
- Name and title of the investigator, and contact site
- Methods of the clinical trial
- Anticipated efficacy of the clinical trial drugs and anticipated disadvantage to the subject
- Matters on other therapeutic methods
- Duration of participating in the clinical trial
- The fact that participation in the clinical trial can be withdrawn at any time
- The fact that the subject is never placed at any disadvantage by refusing to participate or withdrawal of participation
- The fact that monitor, auditor and the IRB can have access to source data on condition that the secret of the subjects is kept
- The fact that the secret related to the subject is kept
- Contact site of the medical institution in case of health damage
- Matters on compensation to health damage
- Necessary matters related to the clinical trial

were in the form of verbal agreements without witnesses. There was concern about whether patients understood the nature of clinical trials because the informed consent sheet was rarely provided to the patient and, even if it was provided, the explanations in the consent form might be too difficult for a layperson.

Based on the ICH guidelines, fully written informed consent is now required for all participating patients. If the patient cannot consent due to his/her health condition, a responsible caretaker is allowed to give consent in lieu of the patient.

The investigator should prepare an informed consent form for every study to be performed at the institute and should obtain an approval by the IRB that covers the institute. GCP listed a dozen points to be covered by the informed consent (IC) form (see Table 23.6). The new GCP allows a reasonable amount of payment to the patient, such as transport cost. Patients should allow clinical trial monitors, auditors, IRB members and inspectors from the regulatory authority to verify the source documents. This new requirement of obligatory written IC is regarded as a major challenge for the conduct of clinical trial in Japan. In Japan, patients are usually not informed of their medications and they are unaware of possible outcomes or side effects. As this is the normal practice in Japan, patients do not expect any detailed explanation of their conditions, or to participate in decision-making of treatment choices. Also, it must be borne in mind that in Japan verbal agreements or contracts are widely accepted, not only in the clinical setting, but also in society in general. It is easily imaginable in such an environment that patients may be frightened by a very detailed explanation of the disease, possible options of treatment including study drug, possible side effects (sometimes including fatalities) and compensation policy.

More recently, IC has become much popular not only for clinical studies, but also for daily medical practice, and patients are now much more accustomed to give their consent. Clinical studies become more visible to general public and the media reports studies with potential therapeutic benefit in a favourable manner. This is a significant change from the past when most media coverage of clinical studies were scandals or sensational without sound scientific reason.

23.3.13.2 Patient recruitment

Pharmaceutical Affairs Law prohibits advertisement of non-approved drugs, that is, clinical study drugs. But if the study drug is not identified, the sponsor can advertise the clinical trial itself in order to recruit patients.

Similarly, hospitals were not able to advertise their involvement into clinical studies. There are detailed regulations as to what hospitals can advertise, and they were amended in April 2001 so that the hospitals can recruit patients by means of mass media.

Patient recruitment advertisement often appears in major newspapers or leaflets, which are delivered with newspapers, as most households prescribe one or more major newspapers. Some CROs established call centres to handle patient/volunteer applications or queries regarding the clinical trial and introduction of participating hospitals.

23.3.13.3 Payment to the participating patients

Participation in a clinical study should be voluntary and there will be no payment unless the study provides no therapeutic benefit, such as tolerability/pharmacokinetic studies in healthy volunteers. When the new GCP was introduced, there was substantial discussion if patients were required to visit study sites more often than usual, for example, to attend additional examinations or treatments would it be fair to put all financial burden on the patients.

In Japan, when patients receive medical service they need to pay 30% of actual medical cost and the insurer pays the rest of the cost. There are ceilings of patient payment, if the patient's own payment exceeds predefined monthly limits or the patient falls into certain category, such as the elderly or those suffering from diseases designated as difficult to treat by the government. The body of insurers and sponsoring companies agreed that the sponsoring company of the trial must pay (1) all laboratory costs including

radiological imaging during the study period, (2) concomitant medication costs if such medication is used for the disease of concern in the study. For this purpose, the study period is defined as 'between the first day of dosing and the last day of dosing'.

In addition, many study sites set rules that patients should be paid for their attendance at clinical examination or treatment during the study. It is roughly considered as the reimbursement of travel cost. There are no statistics on the amount of these payments, but the majority of hospitals set a standard of about 40 Sterling pounds for each visit based on the protocol requirements.

23.3.14 Monitoring

The old GCP did not contain the word 'monitoring'. The lack of monitoring was based on the general view at the time of legislation (early 1980s) that 'the culprits are pharmaceutical companies'. The new GCP requires monitoring and on-site audit including source data verification (SDV) as in the ICH GCP guidelines. The difficulty in circumventing violation of privacy laws (medical law, criminal law and other related regulations) was resolved by obtaining an IC from the patient that allows sponsor's monitors, auditors, IRB members and inspectors from regulatory authorities to access the source record, provided that the subjects' privacy is respected.

The monitors put much emphasis on the SDV, as it is a new concept in the Japanese clinical trial scene. The way case record forms (CRFs) are prepared causes difficult problems in monitoring. Most of the CRFs used in Japan are in the format of booklets with 8–12 pages. Investigators fill them after completion of each case, or sometimes after completion of all cases. Therefore, there was a vague understanding that the SDV is a post-hoc confirmation of CRF against the source data. This view is changing and more emphasis is placed on the initiation and ongoing monitoring to confirm that investigators adhere to the study protocol. Visit-type CRFs and electronic CRFs are being introduced in this connection and this becomes possible as sponsors reinforce their data management capabilities and study sites/investigators introduce clinical study coordinators.

Once many sponsors started monitoring based on the new GCP, they found that they were heavily understaffed. In previous times, a monitor was able to take care of 15–20 centres all over Japan. Now, most sponsoring companies consider that the appropriate number of centres per monitor should be around five. This number reflects not only the workload of study-site monitoring but also complicated study initiation procedures required by new GCP and serious adverse reaction reporting procedures as some major hospitals require the personal presence of the monitor to report such events. The sponsors are also aware that there is mismatch in monitor's qualification, as most of monitors in major pharmaceutical companies are graduates, postgraduates or sometimes doctors in pharmaceutical/biosciences but they are not trained in the bedside settings. Their responsibilities are not limited to the monitoring but include the area of study planning, administration and medical writing, a few to mention. Sponsors recognise this is not idealistic situation, and they are introducing more medically trained monitors and separate other activities from them.

23.3.15   Clinical research coordinator

It is agreed in Japan that the key person for the successful conduct of clinical trials is the clinical research coordinator (CRC), equivalent to the study nurse or study coordinator. Despite lack of history of such a role and rather rigid labour environment in Japan, the concept of CRC is now well established and introduction of the CRC to hospitals is gradually progressing.

The role of the CRC is identical to that of European or American counterparts, or may be of more complex nature because of the complicated Japanese GCP and medical system. Many professional bodies, some backed up by regulatory body and academia, provide training courses for CRCs and recent statistics showed the number of trainee has exceeded 5000 and activities of

these graduates have enhanced the quality and productivity of clinical trial in Japan.

23.3.16   Audit

The new GCP requires that: 'sponsors shall compile plan and operating procedures on auditing and implement auditing in conformity with the plan and the procedures', thus auditors audit not only the sponsor's in-house process but also processes at study sites. Within the sponsoring company, usually all CRFs and study reports are subject to the audit. Study sites are selected for audit based on auditors SOP, usually based on sampling methodology. Audit certificate for each clinical trial is required to be incorporated into new drug submission dossier.

23.3.17   Safety issues

23.3.17.1   Serious adverse event reporting

All unexpected, serious and drug-related adverse events should be reported to MHLW, the investigators and study sites. The requirement to report to the MHLW is identical to ICH guidelines with an additional definition that adverse events include any suspicious infection related to a study drug. This addition reflects the bitter experience of spread of AIDS among haemophilia patients due to HIV-contaminated non-heat-treated human plasma products.

The agency reinforces the serious adverse event (SAE) reporting system rigorously during the clinical study and this is reiterated at the time of GCP inspection. Some hospitals require the chief investigator to acknowledge the report before submiting it to the hospital study office. As the number of study centres for each protocol is rather large in Japan, such a requirement is resource consuming for the sponsoring companies.

The occurrences of study suspension or obtaining additional written IC from participating patients based on new SAEs vary from one ethics committee to another. There is no clear rule for this, and the decision of sponsors whether they would suspend an entire study or not may be different among them. It is worthwhile to note that the SAE described here is not only life threatening or of potential harm for the entire study population but moderate or sometime mild adverse conditions, but, nevertheless, falls within the definition of serious.

23.3.17.2 Safety concerns

Concerns about safety of the study drug may characterise the Japanese clinical trial. In a Phase I study, the dose escalation stops at the level of expected therapeutic dose or double dose of it, and is never escalated to identify any toxicity (except for anticancer drugs). If toxicity is observed in a Phase I study, even if it is at the highest dose or under experimental conditions, further study will be difficult. Everybody in the clinical trial is used to handle study drugs with no safety problems and there is the general concept that the drug must be 'safe'.

This concept becomes an absolute requirement of drug development with Japanese companies developing many compounds that are an improvement over established products. Under such circumstances, the effect of the study drug is guaranteed and the major point of characterisation of the product is 'enhanced safety'. Sponsoring companies have tried to establish the therapeutic dose as low as possible so as to give a larger safety margin and a lower incidence of side effects. This attitude has led to lower dose levels of drugs in Japan than in the United States or Europe.

The situation is changing as a simultaneous development of a product between Europe, Japan and the United States becomes popular and the same level of side effects at the same dose and dosage conditions is expected.

23.4 Conclusion

Introduction of the new GCP and other study practices is aimed at bringing Japanese clinical studies to be accepted by the regulatory bodies worldwide. Hospitals, regulatory authorities and pharmaceutical industries have worked to change many aspects of clinical studies, and although it is hard work they are establishing the new clinical study system. There are dramatic improvement in the quality and reliability of clinical trials and the objectives of the new GCP are achieved in many ways. As the difference in medical practice or ethnic factors will, nevertheless, still remain, sponsors should consider incorporating such differences into their global development plan and conduct.

References

1. Drug Approval and Licensing Procedures in Japan 2001, Jiho Co., Ltd., Tokyo.
2. Pharmaceutical Administration and Regulation in Japan, March 2004, Japan Pharmaceutical Manufacturers Association. Available at http://www.jpma.or.jp/12english/parj/index.html.

Useful Websites

More information on regulatory affairs of Japan in English can be found at the following websites:

http://www.pmda.go.jp/index-e.html
http://www.mhlw.go.jp/english/index.html

CHAPTER 24

24 The regulation of therapeutic products in Australia

Janice Hirshorn and Deborah Monk

24.1 Introduction

The Commonwealth Therapeutic Goods Act 1989 (the Act) sets out the legal requirements for the import, export, manufacture and supply of therapeutic goods in Australia. It is supported by the Therapeutic Goods Regulations and various Orders and Determinations. The aim of this legislation is to provide a national framework for the regulation of therapeutic goods in Australia, so as to ensure their quality, safety, efficacy and timely availability.

The Therapeutic Goods Administration (TGA), as part of the Commonwealth Department of Health, has the responsibility for administering the Act. It applies a risk management approach to therapeutic goods regulation, which is intended to ensure public health and safety while minimising the regulatory burden and associated costs.

The TGA carries out a range of assessment and monitoring activities to ensure that all therapeutic goods available in Australia are of an acceptable standard:

- pre-market evaluation and approval of registered products intended for supply in Australia
- licensing of manufacturers in accordance with international standards under good manufacturing practice (GMP)
- post-marketing monitoring, through sampling, adverse event reporting, surveillance activities, and response to public inquiries
- development, maintenance and monitoring of the systems for listing of medicines
- the assessment of medicines for export.

The term 'therapeutic goods' includes prescription medicines, non-prescription medicines, complementary medicines and medical devices. The TGA also develops and implements national policies and controls for chemicals, gene technology, blood and blood products.

A product's 'risk' is determined by a number of factors, including whether:

- the medicine contains a substance scheduled in the Standard for the Uniform Scheduling of Drugs and Poisons (SUSDP)
- the medicine's use can result in significant side effects
- the medicine is used to treat life-threatening or very serious illnesses
- there may be any adverse effects from prolonged use or inappropriate self-medication.

The scheduling of drugs is performed under State and Territory (henceforth referred to as State) legislation controlling access to medicines, but is coordinated at a national level to ensure uniformity except in exceptional circumstances.

All therapeutic goods must be entered as either 'registered' goods or 'listed' goods on the Australian Register of Therapeutic Goods (ARTG) before they may be supplied in, or exported from, Australia unless they are exempt under the legislation.

Prescription medicines are medicines considered as having a higher level of risk. They must be registered on the ARTG, and the degree of assessment and regulation they undergo is rigorous and detailed, with sponsors being required to provide comprehensive safety, quality and efficacy data. They contain ingredients included in Schedule 4 (prescription) or Schedule 8 (controlled drugs) of the SUSDP, or are specified products such as sterile injectables. Biologics fall into the same overall approach – they are not handled separately.

Non-prescription medicines are medicines considered as having a lower level of risk than prescription medicines. They still must be registered on the ARTG, but undergo a lesser degree of evaluation. They contain ingredients included in Schedule 2 (pharmacy-only) or Schedule 3 (pharmacist-supervised supply) of the SUSDP. Non-prescription medicines have frequently been termed over-the-counter (OTC) medicines, and include analgesics, cough and cold products, and sunscreens.

Complementary medicines (also known as 'traditional' or 'alternative' medicines) include vitamin, mineral, herbal, aromatherapy and homoeopathic products. They may be registered or listed on the ARTG, depending on their ingredients and the claims made. Most complementary medicines are listed.

Medical devices also are required to be registered or listed if not exempt. The specified categories of implantable and other higher risk devices that require registration, rather than listing, must undergo a more comprehensive evaluation process.

All medicines and devices supplied solely for export are listed (not registered) on the ARTG.

For a new medicine to obtain public subsidy for patients in the community, the sponsor must successfully apply for the product to be included in the Pharmaceutical Benefits Scheme (PBS). Data are required on relative cost and effectiveness, and the scrutiny of this information according to prescribed criteria is described as the 'fourth hurdle', that is, in addition to quality, safety and efficacy requirements that medicines must overcome, to be readily available to the Australian public.

The Commonwealth Government has agreed to establish a joint therapeutic products regulatory agency with the New Zealand Government, scheduled to begin operation on 1 July 2006. Subsidy arrangements through the PBS and other mechanisms have been specifically excluded from these discussions.

24.2 The History of Prescription Medicine Regulation

24.2.1 Quality, safety and efficacy

The Commonwealth Department of Health was established in 1921, but most health-related activities at that time remained the responsibility of the States. The current name is the Department of Health and Ageing but its description frequently changes, so throughout this chapter the Department will be called the Department of Health and the relevant Commonwealth Government Minister will be called the Minister for Health.

The Therapeutic Substances Act 1937 gave the Minister for Health power to control the import and export of substances declared to be therapeutic substances in the Commonwealth Gazette.

The Therapeutic Substances Act 1953 repealed the 1937 Act and gave the Commonwealth control of the import into Australia and interstate trading of therapeutic substances and controlled therapeutic substances (drugs of addiction). It came into operation in 1956 and was administered by the Therapeutic Substances Branch of the Department of Health.

In 1959, the National Biological Standards Laboratory (NBSL) was established, to test therapeutic products imported into Australia or supplied under the PBS for compliance with quality and manufacturing standards, largely based on the British Pharmacopoeia.

In the wake of the thalidomide tragedy, the Australian Drug Evaluation Committee (ADEC) was established in 1963 as a statutory committee to advise the government on the regulation of drugs intended for marketing in Australia. The adverse drug reaction (ADR) reporting scheme and the Adverse Drug Reactions Advisory Committee (ADRAC) were also introduced.

Furthermore, Commonwealth legislation was reviewed to give the Commonwealth powers to require companies to submit specified data to establish the quality, safety and efficacy of imported therapeutic goods. The resultant Therapeutic Goods Act 1966 provided the basis for the regulation of pharmaceuticals in Australia for over 20 years.

The 'Guidelines for Preparing Applications for General Marketing or Clinical Investigational Use of a Therapeutic Substance' outlined information requirements for applications. Provision was also made for special Australian standards to apply where appropriate.

Some States had separate arrangements that covered the few locally manufactured products sourced from local active ingredients, as the Commonwealth's jurisdiction was limited to imports, exports and goods crossing State borders (although the last power was thought unlikely to sustain a prosecution if taken to court).

A Code of GMP was introduced in the late 1960s, covering principles and practices to be followed in the manufacture of therapeutic goods in Australia, but still relied upon State legislation and personnel for its enforcement.

The Customs (Prohibited Imports) Regulations were amended in 1970 to enable the Department of Health to further control importation through import permits for drug products.

The drug evaluation guidelines (known from 1976 as the NDF4 Guidelines) gradually became more detailed and were supplemented by appendices on specific issues such as bioavailability studies and bioequivalence. Rules were also introduced to address agency concerns that companies might manipulate the system, for example, by seeking review of data contained in a clinical trial application for a product that was already the subject of a general marketing application, thereby achieving speedier evaluation.

A revised clinical trial application evaluation scheme introduced in 1983 aimed for a response time of 45 working days for Phase I and early Phase II trials, and 80 working days for Phase II and Phase III trials, but in practice it took an average of 10 or 11 months from submission of data to receipt of written approval.

A Clinical Trial Exemption (CTX) Scheme was introduced in Australia in 1987, with the intention of encouraging clinical trial activity. However, in addition to the aforementioned TGA restrictions, which required all clinical trials of an active substance underway in Australia to be completed before the review of a general marketing application relating to that substance, the specified data package included requirements unique to Australia, and the 60 working day review period compared with a 35 calendar day review under the UK CTX Scheme.

Australia's drug evaluation system was increasingly criticised due to the 'drug lag' in availability of new and improved products in Australia, compared with other countries with well-regarded regulatory systems. Several government inquiries recommended streamlining and making better use of overseas experience. The pharmaceutical industry repeatedly expressed concern about the unique requirements that had led to significant delays in both the submission of applications and obtaining marketing approval, for example, requiring individual patient data (required in the United States but not in Europe) to be presented by parameter (uniquely to Australia) instead of by subject (as required in the United States).

By the late 1980s, it had also become clear that reliance on a combination of Commonwealth and State legislation was not the best way to ensure that desired standards were met. There were many complaints about loopholes and lack of uniformity. The way forward came from an unexpected source, namely, a court case that confirmed that the Commonwealth Government has powers over all corporations, and thus these powers could be used in relation to therapeutic goods matters even if they occurred within one State.

The Therapeutic Goods Act 1989 and Regulations came into effect on 15 February 1991, giving the Commonwealth more clearly defined regulatory authority. It changed the focus of control over therapeutic goods from the point of importation to the point of supply of the goods.

The Act applies to:

- all corporations who supply or manufacture medicines for supply (regardless of where) in Australia
- unincorporated parties who supply or manufacture medicines for supply in Australia outside their own state or territory
- all parties (whether incorporated or unincorporated) who supply medicines under the PBS
- all parties (whether incorporated or unincorporated) who import or export medicines.

Supportive State legislation is required only to cover activities of persons within one State, and specified areas (such as some aspects of labelling, packaging, distribution and fair trade) that are the responsibility of State governments.

Fees and charges were also introduced – through the Therapeutic Goods Act 1989 and Therapeutic Goods (Charges) Act 1989, respectively, and associated Regulations.

Pressure increased for the TGA to 'free up' the regulatory system for prescription medicines. In particular, the 1990 report by the Australian National Council on AIDS Working Party on the Availability of HIV/AIDS Treatments recommended that a notification scheme be introduced for clinical trials of unapproved products that had already been approved by respected agencies overseas.

In March 1991, the Commonwealth Government announced the introduction of an alternative clinical trial system. The Clinical Trial Notification (CTN) Scheme was introduced in May 1991, following recognition of the negative effects of discouraging trials of investigational drugs – on patients (who were unable to access possible treatments for potentially life-threatening illnesses) and on pharmaceutical industry investment in research and development (R&D) in Australia. The Government also announced a major review of drug evaluation processes in Australia.

Professor Peter Baume's report, 'A Question of Balance: Report on the Future of Drug Evaluation in Australia',[1] was released in July 1991, with a commitment from the Commonwealth Government to speedily implement all 164 recommendations in the stated time frames.

Key aspects were:

- the retention of Australian sovereignty in deciding which drugs might be marketed in Australia
- recognition that considerable streamlining of drug evaluation procedures could be achieved
- acceptance that international harmonisation was a concept whose 'time had come', and that considerable benefit could flow from improved cooperation with other comparable developed countries
- recognition that no drugs were totally risk free, and that the need for a system of controls relating to the quality, safety and efficacy of therapeutic goods must be balanced against the more recently highlighted need for timely availability
- recommendations for re-organisation of the TGA and its advisory committees, with a new management plan and increased emphasis on performance
- provision of a timeline for Australia to bring about the reform of its drug evaluation processes within the next 2 years.

Recommendations were also made to streamline the CTX Scheme for clinical trials and continue the CTN Scheme, with further assessment in the future.

Professor Baume noted that, in 1990, the TGA process of evaluation of new chemical entities (NCEs) was taking approximately twice as long as its target time of $16\frac{1}{2}$ months.

Following the Baume Report, changes were made to the Act and Regulations to introduce specific target evaluation times, together with a fee penalty of 25% if a decision on an application is not made within the specified period.

The statutory time frames led to a major reorganisation of TGA processes to focus on meeting them and complex measuring arrangements were introduced to ensure that only 'TGA working days' were included in the calculations. 'The clock' is stopped whenever questions are raised with the product sponsor, and only restarted when no queries are outstanding.

New data requirements came into force from 1993 that closely aligned Australian marketing applications with those in the European Community (EC). The 'Australian Guidelines for the Registration of Drugs – Volume 1: Prescription and Other Specified Drug Products' (AGRD1) specified that the document to support a prescription drug registration application should be compiled in accordance with the current version of 'The Rules Governing Medicinal Products in the European Community' Volumes II and III with Addenda and supplementary 'Notes for Guidance' published by the Committee for Proprietary and Medicinal Products (CPMP), and also described specific administrative requirements for registration applications in Australia.

Information about the overseas status of the product was also now sought as part of an application. The list of countries mentioned in this context in the AGRD1 included members of the Pharmaceutical Evaluation Report (PER) Scheme, other EC countries and the United States. Expert reports also began to be utilised in the evaluation of applications.

In June 2004 the 'Australian Regulatory Guidelines for Prescription Medicines' (ARGPM) were issued by the TGA to replace the AGRD1. Under the ARGPM the format for registration applications in Australia is the Common Technical Document (CTD) developed through the International Conference on Harmonisation (ICH).

On 30 September 2004, the ARTG included 10 514 registered medicines (6649 of which were Schedule 4 and Schedule 8 medicines), 16 868 listed medicines and 3148 export-listed medicines – a total of 30 530 medicines. It should be noted that this number reflects the separate inclusion of each strength, dosage form and brand as a distinct therapeutic item. There are also 30 455 medical devices on the Register, some of which are 'grouped', and some of which would be termed diagnostic products in other countries.

It is a requirement under the Act that a sponsor takes responsibility for each therapeutic item that is imported, exported, manufactured or supplied in or from Australia. The sponsor must be a corporation or person within Australia.

Sponsors must be able to substantiate all claims made by them about their therapeutic products. On 30 September 2004, there were 2411 sponsors of therapeutic goods on the ARTG.

24.2.2 Fees and charges

The Therapeutic Goods Act 1989 and Therapeutic Goods (Charges) Act 1989, respectively, and associated Regulations stipulate the fees and charges payable to TGA for processing applications, GMP inspections and annual licences. When fees and charges were first introduced in 1991 they were intended to cover 50% of the costs attributable to the TGA's responsibilities under the Therapeutic Goods Act, including those deemed to be 'for the public good'. It took some time to reach those levels – in 1992–3 only 28% of the TGA's relevant costs were covered.

By July 1996 the 50% target was reached, and the Commonwealth Government announced that fees and charges would increase over the following 3 years to raise industry's contribution to the Government's therapeutic goods programme from 50% to 75%. In 1997 the Government announced that the TGA would be required to recover 100% of its operating costs from 1998–9.

In 2005–6 the overall revenue raised by the TGA from fees and charges is forecast to be AUD\$67.6 million, of which the prescription medicines sector contributes approximately 60%.

Fees apply to almost all evaluation activities undertaken by TGA – not only to the review of general marketing applications but also to minor marketing-related matters, clinical trial applications and notifications, and GMP evaluations and inspections in Australia or overseas, but not to ADR assessments.

In 2002–3 there was a major revision of the fees and charges structure for prescription medicines to simplify the structure and to rebalance revenue obtained from pre-market and post-market activities to more closely reflect the actual costs. The new structure, effective from 1 July 2003, is no longer based on the number of pages of data submitted. A single evaluation fee is now charged for each type of application – NCE, extension of indications, new generic product, etc.

The new fee structure, which sees pre-market evaluation fees gradually reducing and post-market annual product registration charges increasing, is being phased in over 5 years. At the end of the transition period, revenue from pre-market evaluations will be 60% rather than 80% under the previous arrangements. The revised structure will make TGA's revenue less vulnerable to fluctuations in number of major applications.

The evaluation fee for an NCE will decrease from AUD$235 720 (pre 1 July 2003) to AUD$150 000 in 2007–8, dependent on further fees and charges negotiations as the new joint therapeutics agency with New Zealand is established. The evaluation fee for an NCE in 2004–5 is AUD$189 900. Sponsors are required to pay 75% of the evaluation fee at the time of submitting their application. The balance of 25% of the evaluation fee is payable when the TGA completes the evaluation within the legislated time frame.

There is no application fee but, if an application is withdrawn before it is accepted for evaluation, a screening fee of 20% of the evaluation fee up to a maximum of AUD$5850 currently applies.

Annual charges apply to maintaining each product on the ARTG. The annual charge for continuing registration of a prescription medicine will increase over the transition period to approximately AUD$4000 for a biological product and AUD$2500 for a non-biological in 2007–8, again dependent on the fees under the new joint agency arrangement. The annual charges in 2004–5 were AUD$3050 and AUD$1840, respectively.

24.2.3 Availability to the community

The authority for the Commonwealth Government to provide pharmaceutical benefits was introduced in the 1940s. Prior to that, except for the Federal scheme covering war veterans, health care was the province of the States.

The Commonwealth National Health Act 1953 (the National Health Act), together with the National Health (Pharmaceutical Benefits) Regulations, introduced the current framework for the operation of the PBS.

The Pharmaceutical Benefits Advisory Committee (PBAC) was established under Section 101 of the National Health Act, to give advice to the Minister for Health about products to be made available as pharmaceutical benefits. The minister is required to consider the PBAC's advice but is not required to follow its recommendations. The initial criteria for inclusion of new products on the PBS were comparative safety and efficacy.

Initially, 139 'lifesaving and disease preventing drugs' were provided under the scheme without charge to pension recipients and their dependants. By 1960, the scheme had expanded to include a wider range of drugs, and supply to the general public with some co-payment. PBS listing continued to be based primarily on medical considerations.

A non-statutory body called the Pharmaceutical Benefits Pricing Bureau (PBPB) was established in 1963 to make recommendations to government on the pricing of PBS-listed medicines.

Escalation of costs led to multiple measures to limit the increase in PBS expenditure, including the introduction of an authority system for new drugs from 1988. Co-payments were eventually also introduced for concessional patients – for disadvantaged patients in 1989 and for pensioners in 1990. Details of the early history of the PBS and the myriad of subsequent changes can be found in 'A History of the Pharmaceutical Benefits Scheme 1947–1992'.[2]

Amendments to the National Health Act in 1987 introduced the additional requirement for the PBAC to consider cost and effectiveness. Sponsors were encouraged to provide cost-effectiveness substantiation from 1991, and from 1 January 1993 it became mandatory to include pharmacoeconomic analyses in listing applications – the 'fourth hurdle'.

In 1988, the PBPB was replaced by the (also non-statutory) Pharmaceutical Benefits Pricing Authority (PBPA). The PBPA was required to review the prices of items on the PBS and consider items recommended by the PBAC for listing, taking eight factors in account. Factor (f) – the level of activity being undertaken by the company in Australia – was not to be considered in the price determination of each item, but through a separate allocation of funds to the companies that were successful in their proposals under the Pharmaceutical Industry Development Programe (the factor (f) programe).

When the factor (f) programe concluded in 1999, it was followed by the Pharmaceutical Industry Investment Programme (PIIP). Both schemes were intended to partially compensate participating companies for the price suppression imposed by the government in exercising its monopsony purchasing powers under the PBS. The PIIP funds of AUD$300 million over 5 years were awarded to nine companies who successfully applied for funding in return for increased R&D and/or production value-adding activity in Australia. The PIIP concluded in early 2004.

In 2002, the Parliamentary Secretary to the Treasurer requested the Productivity Commission, the government's review and advisory body on microeconomic policy and regulation, to investigate the rationale, effectiveness and efficiency of the programme. The commission's report recommended that there should be a programme to follow PIIP but that it should be modified to be oriented to reward only R&D investment, not production value-adding activity.

In September 2003, the Minister for Industry Tourism and Resources announced the new competitive grants programme, the Pharmaceuticals Partnerships Programme (P3), which provides AUD$150 million over 5 years from 1 July 2004 for successful applicants, who receive 30 cents for each additional dollar they spend on eligible R&D activities. The first of three rounds of P3 awards were announced in April 2004. Eleven pharmaceutical companies were offered funding of AUD$87 million. In April 2005, the Minister announced that seven pharmaceutical and biotechnology companies were successful in the second round of P3 funding for projects totalling AUD$ 46.8 million.

The overwhelming importance of gaining PBS-listing in order to achieve widespread availability and use of a prescription medicine in Australia is evident from information published by the Australian Institute of Health and Welfare (AIHW).[3] Expenditure on benefit-paid items under the PBS is the largest single component of total expenditure on pharmaceuticals. In 2001–2 the cost to government under the PBS, not including expenditure under the Repatriation Pharmaceutical Benefits Scheme (RPBS) was AUD$4181 million. This increased to an estimated AUD$4572 million in 2002–3 with the share of total cost of the PBS met by the Commonwealth being 84.2%.

Total expenditure on all pharmaceuticals in 2001–2 was estimated at AUD$10 304 million. This included AUD$1315 million on drugs used by hospitals in the provision of hospital services, which are not normally included in national estimates of expenditure on pharmaceuticals, but are included as part of estimates of expenditure on hospitals. The AUD$1315 million estimated expenditure comprised AUD$1105 million on drugs dispensed in public hospitals and AUD$210 million in private hospitals. Commonwealth expenditure on non-hospital pharmaceuticals was AUD$8989 million in 2001–2, comprising AUD$5586 million on benefit-paid pharmaceuticals and AUD$3320 million on other non-hospital pharmaceuticals.

In 2002–3 there were 158.5 million community PBS prescriptions – 132.7 million (83.7%) to concessional patients (pensioners, seniors, repatriation health beneficiaries) and 25.9 million to general patients. In addition, about 42.1 million prescriptions did not attract a subsidy – 26 million below the co-payment threshold and about 16.1 million 'private' prescriptions, that is, prescriptions for drugs not listed on the PBS or RPBS, for which the consumer pays the full cost of the medicine. Thus 79.0% of prescriptions were for items subsidised through the PBS.

Analysis of 2003–4 data shows that the Commonwealth Government contributed AUD$5001.1 million (84.2%) to the benefit-paid pharmaceuticals and individuals paid the remaining AUD$937.8 million. Concessional cardholders represented 79.5% of government expenditure and a total of 166 million PBS prescriptions were processed.

Eligibility for PBS is restricted to Australian residents and visitors from those countries with which Australia has a Reciprocal Health Care Agreement – currently, the United Kingdom (including Northern Ireland), Ireland, New Zealand, Malta, Italy, Sweden, the Netherlands and Finland. From May 2002, proof of eligibility by means of a Medicare card or passport has been an absolute requirement for the subsidy to be applied.

The Government has also decided to introduce a series of programmes aimed at 'preventing the unnecessary use of PBS-subsidised medicines' and 'reinforcing the commitment to evidence-based medicine'. These include 'a more detailed consideration process' for new PBS listings, ensuring greater compliance by doctors with PBS prescribing requirements, and the enhancement of PBS restrictions, to reduce prescriptions supplied to individuals in breach of PBS conditions. It also intends to strengthen measures to reduce pharmacy fraud and further encourage the use of generics.

On 1 February 2004, the Schedule of Pharmaceutical Benefits included more than 600 drug substances in 1500 forms and strengths (items) supplied as 2617 different drug products (brands). Restrictions apply to approximately 800 items and approximately 300 require authority prescriptions.

24.2.4 National Medicines Policy

The Australian National Medicines Policy aims to establish an appropriate balance between health, economic and industry objectives. It has four central elements:

- timely access to the medicines that Australians need, at a cost individuals and the community can afford
- medicines meeting appropriate standards of quality, safety and efficacy
- quality use of medicines
- maintaining a responsible and viable medicines industry.

Although these goals are not enshrined in legislation, they have become increasingly accepted by successive governments as a sound basis for informed policy decisions.

The Australian Pharmaceutical Advisory Council (APAC) provides the primary forum for the engagement of all stakeholders in discussion, debate and resolution of issues arising from the application of the National Medicines Policy, facilitating cooperation between stakeholders and addressing specific issues brought to it for deliberation.

Other groups focus on particular aspects, such as greater dissemination of information about the quality use of medicines.

24.3 Marketing Applications for Prescription Medicines

Prescription medicines and certain other high-risk medicines, such as injections, are evaluated for inclusion on the ARTG by the Drug Safety and Evaluation Branch (DSEB) of the TGA. The types of medicines that are evaluated by the DSEB are described in Schedule 10 of the Therapeutic Goods Regulations. Usually, medicines containing new active substances are evaluated by the DSEB for inclusion on the register as registrable goods. However, a sponsor can submit a justification for an alternative route of evaluation of a new active substance by another branch of the TGA as a non-prescription medicine, for example, where there is experience with the active ingredient in non-prescription medicines in other countries. Guidelines for providing such a justification are available at the TGA website at www.tga.gov.au (TGA website).

24.3.1 Applications for registration

The sponsor of a therapeutic product is responsible for submitting an application to the TGA for registration of the goods and, once the goods are registered, for compliance with conditions of registration such as reporting any adverse drug reactions.

As previously mentioned, Australia has closely aligned its data requirements for the registration of prescription medicines with those of the European Union. The ARGPM describes certain administrative requirements and provides technical guidance in addition to EU technical guidance, relevant to applications for registration in Australia. Under the ARGPM, if a sponsor prepares a dossier in the CTD format for submission in the European Union, this will be also accepted in Australia.

Where registration is being sought for a new drug to treat a life-threatening illness or to treat a condition for which no satisfactory alternative therapy exists, the TGA will accept the application in either US or EU format.

The TGA will accept dossiers in an electronic format, in addition to hard copy, following discussion with the sponsor. The TGA has been monitoring international developments in relation to applications in electronic formats and is expected to adopt any agreed international standard arising from the ICH process.

There is a formal process for consultation with the pharmaceutical industry on the adoption of each EU guideline in Australia. Australia has adopted the majority of guidelines published by the CPMP without amendment. Guidelines that have not been adopted usually concern labelling or the content of the Australian Product Information (PI) document. All of the EU guidelines that have been adopted or not adopted in Australia are listed on the TGA website. Any changes or additional comments on an EU guideline agreed between the industry and TGA are also published on the TGA website.

24.3.2 Categories of application

There are three categories of applications relating to prescription medicines.

Category 1 applications are defined as being those that do not meet the requirements of Category 2 or 3 applications. Essentially, Category 1 applications are those that include clinical, preclinical or bioequivalence data, such as applications to register goods containing a new active ingredient, a new generic product, a new strength, dosage form or route of administration.

Category 2 applications are defined as those that include clinical, preclinical or bioequivalence data for which there are two evaluation

reports from 'acceptable countries', where the submission is already approved. The evaluation reports must be independent (not based on each other) and the product must be identical in Australia and the 'acceptable countries', in respect to formulation, directions for use and indications. The countries identified as 'acceptable' for the purposes of providing evaluation reports are currently Canada, Sweden, the Netherlands, the United Kingdom and the United States. As the availability of evaluation reports would assist the TGA to evaluate an application, Category 2 applications are subject to shorter legislated evaluation times. However, as most sponsors submit applications for registration in Australia at the same time, or shortly after, they are submitted in the 'acceptable countries', it is rare for two evaluation reports to be available to qualify for a Category 2 application. Hence, almost no Category 2 applications are submitted.

Category 3 applications seek changes to the pharmaceutical data of goods already included on the ARTG, which do not need to be supported by clinical, preclinical or bioequivalence data.

Examples of Category 3 applications include changes to the specifications of the active ingredient, change of shelf life or storage conditions, and change of trade name.

It is a condition of registration that, with limited exceptions, no changes may be made to registered goods without prior approval from the TGA. An exception is that some narrowly specified changes to pharmaceutical and manufacturing aspects may be made without prior approval, as outlined in Appendices 12 and 13 (for biological products) of ARGPM. A number of general and specific conditions must be complied with under the 'self-assessable' changes provisions. These are primarily the proper validation of any change and the notification of the change to the TGA.

24.3.3 Evaluation time frames

The Therapeutic Goods Regulations specify time frames for completion of the evaluation of Category 1, 2 and 3 applications in 'working days', which excludes weekends and public holidays.

Category 1 applications are required to be:

- accepted for evaluation, or rejected, in 40 working days from receipt of the application and the application fee
- evaluated in 255 working days from the date of acceptance.

Category 2 applications are required to be:

- accepted for evaluation, or rejected, in 20 working days from receipt of the application and the application fee
- evaluated in 175 working days from the date of acceptance.

Category 3 applications are required to be approved or rejected or to have an objection raised within 45 working days of receipt of the application, or payment of the evaluation fee, whichever is the later day. There is no application acceptance period. If an objection to the application is raised, the applicant may respond and provide further information or data. A further 30 working days from receipt of this response is then allowed for consideration of the response before the application must be approved or rejected.

Under Section 31 of the Therapeutic Goods Act, the TGA may request a sponsor to provide additional information or seek clarification of information provided in a submission. Fee penalties apply only if the statutory evaluation period is not met. The evaluation times do not include the time frames for initial acceptance or rejection of an application or the time taken by the sponsor to respond to TGA Section 31 requests. They apply to each application as an absolute criterion, that is, not as an average performance target. The TGA has almost invariably met the legislated time frames.

In addition, in 2000 the TGA undertook to target the following *mean* evaluation times for different subtypes of Category 1 applications:

- new chemical entities–150 working days
- new generics, except 'own generics'–100 working days
- new indications–160 working days
- product information changes–90 working days
- other Category 1 applications–130 working days.

For applications finalised in the first quarter of calendar year 2004 the average elapsed time from submission of an application to registration, for an NCE, was approximately 64 weeks/15 months.

24.3.4   Confidentiality of submissions

Sponsors routinely require that data contained in their applications remain confidential. If another party requests access to such data under the provisions of the Commonwealth Freedom of Information Act 1982 (FOI Act), the Department of Health will consult with the sponsor to establish whether release of the information is possible, and enable the sponsor to request a review by the Administrative Appeals Tribunal (AAT) of any decision made by the TGA to release the information.

The TGA will not comply with demands for undertakings of confidentiality that seek to limit the lawful use or release of information by the TGA. The TGA will not accept confidentiality statements from sponsors that seek to prohibit the evaluator's access to departmental records of prior applications, and the accumulated knowledge and experience gained from the evaluation of previous applications. Examples of acceptable confidentiality statements are provided in ARGPM.

24.3.5   Data exclusivity

In 1998 an amendment to the Therapeutic Goods Act was enacted introducing data exclusivity provisions. Under Section 25A, the TGA must not use 'protected information' about other therapeutic goods when evaluating therapeutic goods for registration. Protected information is information lodged with an application to register goods containing a new active ingredient that is not currently, and has never been, included in the ARTG. Such information is protected for 5 years from the date of registration of the goods containing the new active ingredient. Thus products containing new actives are given 5 years data exclusivity.

At the time the data exclusivity amendments were being discussed, the pharmaceutical industry sought to extend the provisions to protect data relating to new indications, new dosage forms or routes of administration, but was unsuccessful.

The data exclusivity arrangements are primarily of interest to sponsors of products that are not otherwise protected by patent. A sponsor of a generic product may avoid the need for TGA to refer to protected information by submitting a full Category 1 application for registration, including preclinical and clinical data, although this would be unusual.

24.3.6 Orphan Drug Program

The Australian Orphan Drug Program was introduced in 1998. Through a cooperative arrangement with the US Food and Drug Administration (FDA), it intended to improve access to treatments for rare diseases in Australia by utilising US orphan drug evaluations as the basis for Australian approvals, where possible. It also waived evaluation fees for new medicines or indications designated as 'orphan'.

In order to be designated as an orphan drug in Australia, the prevalence of the disease to be treated is required to be equal to or less than 2000 affected individuals or, if the drug is a vaccine or *in vivo* diagnostic agent, the persons to whom the drug will be administered in Australia are equal to or less than 2000 per year. The prevalence limit in Australia is considerably lower than other countries' orphan drug programmes, both in absolute terms and as a proportion of the population.

Also, whereas the US Orphan Drug Program offers several incentives to sponsors to bring drugs to treat rare diseases to market, such as a period of market exclusivity, tax credits for clinical research costs, clinical research grants and waiver of FDA evaluation fees, the Australian programm offers a 100% reduction of the evaluation fee for a designated orphan drug but no research incentives. The TGA guideline does state that an orphan drug will be granted 5 years

market exclusivity, which can be shared by a clinically superior product, but this exclusivity is not supported by any legislation.

Since the Australian program commenced, 90 drugs have been designated as orphan drugs (as at 14 October 2004). In December 2001, a review of the Orphan Drug Program found that sponsors had lodged applications for marketing approval for 33 of the 42 drugs designated as orphan at the time, and 17 of 20 that had reached their conclusion were approved. Seven of these had been successful in obtaining government funding, as highly specialised drugs or under the life-saving drugs programme. Three drugs had been considered and rejected by the PBAC on the grounds of unacceptable cost-effectiveness.

The 2001 review found that there have been few opportunities for the TGA to utilise a review by the FDA. Of 215 orphan drugs granted marketing approval in the United States, only 63 had not already been approved for marketing in Australia or did not have an equivalent in Australia. Of these, the review stated that not more than a dozen would represent a significant gap in what has been approved for marketing in Australia, and most of these would fall into the category of 'like to have' rather than 'need to have because there is no alternative.' The review recommended a number of changes to the Australian Orphan Drug Program, primarily focusing on increasing the incentives for sponsors to bring orphan drugs to market by offering greater surety of obtaining public subsidy under the PBS. As at August 2005, the review recommendations had not been implemented. The full review report is available from the TGA website.

24.3.7 Priority evaluations

The Drug Safety Evaluation Board may allocate priority evaluation to applications for registration of important new medicines. The current criteria for priority evaluation are:

• the active ingredient is a new chemical entity
• the drug is indicated for the treatment or diagnosis of a serious, life-threatening or severely debilitating disease or condition

- there is clinical evidence that the drug may provide an important therapeutic gain.

Priority evaluation status does not give a definite, shorter evaluation period. Rather, the application is simply moved ahead in the queue of applications under evaluation. Discussions are currently underway to define a priority evaluation time frame and broaden the criteria for priority status.

24.3.8 Good manufacturing practice

It is a requirement of the Therapeutic Goods Act that all steps in the manufacture of a prescription medicine, including the manufacture of bulk active drugs and finished pharmaceutical products, are performed in manufacturing facilities of acceptable standards.

An updated list of manufacturing principles established under the Therapeutic Goods Act is available from the TGA website.

Manufacturing sites within Australia must comply with the Australian 'Code of GMP for Medicinal Products' – August 2002, which is based entirely on the international standard 'Guide to Good Manufacturing Practices for Medicinal Products', Version PH1/97 (Rev.3) 15 January 2002, published by the Pharmaceutical Inspection Cooperation Scheme (PIC/S). The ICH GMP Guide for Active Pharmaceutical Ingredients has also been adopted.

The TGA conducts regular inspections of Australian manufacturing operations to ensure compliance with the code of GMP. Scrutiny has increased, including unannounced inspections, since the major recall of a contract manufacturer's wide range of products in 2003 (see Section 24.3.20).

The standard of any steps of manufacture and quality control conducted outside Australia must also be shown to be acceptable for the inclusion of therapeutic goods on the ARTG. The TGA document 'Standard of Overseas Manufacturers' specifies what is regarded as acceptable evidence of GMP standards, and is available on the TGA website. The TGA will accept GMP certification only from countries where it is satisfied that the standard of GMP inspection is equivalent to GMP inspections in Australia.

Australia and the EC have entered into a Mutual Recognition Agreement (MRA) on conformity assessment of medicinal products. The TGA will accept a certificate of GMP compliance of a manufacturer issued under this MRA by the official inspection services of the EU countries. This follows on from Australia's work over many years with the Pharmaceutical Inspection Convention, now known as the PIC/S.

24.3.9 The evaluation process

Details of requirements for the registration of prescription medicines are contained in the ARGPM, which is available from the TGA website.

Submissions to register new prescription medicines in Australia undergo a two-stage process of evaluation by the DSEB – application acceptance and evaluation.

Prior to submitting an application for registration there is an opportunity for a sponsor to have a pre-submission meeting with TGA delegates to discuss the application. Pre-submission meetings are strongly recommended for complex applications, where there is some uncertainty as to whether the data package to be submitted will meet all Australian regulatory requirements, and for orphan drugs and literature-based submissions.

An application is screened for acceptance by the Application Entry Team of the DSEB. Although primarily intended to be an administrative check that the application is in the required format, the three main modules (quality data, non-clinical data and clinical data) are also briefly reviewed by the relevant evaluation sections to ensure that there are no major omissions of data.

Once an application has been accepted for evaluation, the Pharmaceutical Chemistry Evaluation Section, Toxicology Section and Clinical Evaluation Units evaluate the Module 3, 4 and 5 data, respectively. For applications relating to products of biological origin, a second copy of the Module 3 data is also evaluated by the TGA Laboratories (TGAL) Branch, which evaluates aspects such as laboratory methodology, method validation and shelf-life.

There are currently five clinical evaluation units within DSEB, each headed by a senior medical officer and supported by pharmacists. Applications are distributed among the five evaluation units based on the therapeutic area of the drug under evaluation. The DSEB contracts a number of external clinical evaluators who are specialist medical practitioners in the medical condition that the proposed new drug is intended to treat. External evaluators may also be contracted to evaluate the Module 4 data. The head of the clinical evaluation unit coordinates the evaluation and makes the final decision on marketing approval as a delegate under the Therapeutic Goods Act.

From receipt of an application until a final decision on an application, a DSEB evaluator may request additional information or clarification from the sponsor under Section 31 of the Act. During the period from issuing a Section 31 letter and receipt of responses to all questions, the clock is stopped and the elapsed time is not counted towards the TGA's statutory evaluation time frames. If several Section 31 requests overlap, the periods are not additive but the clock remains stopped until the final question is answered. A sponsor is given a time frame in which a Section 31 request should be answered. Justification for an extension of time may be discussed with the evaluator. If a sponsor considers that a Section 31 request is unreasonable they can discuss this with the delegate who issued the request. If the sponsor is unable to resolve the matter with the delegate, it may seek review under an additional, non-statutory appeal mechanism by a three-member Standing Arbitration Committee (SAC).

At the conclusion of evaluation of the Module 3, 4 and 5 data the evaluators prepare an evaluation report for each module. The evaluation reports are sent to the sponsor as they are received to allow comments to the delegate. Once the three evaluation reports are finalised, the delegate evaluates the reports and prepares an overview of the evaluation and a proposed decision for consideration by ADEC, which are also provided to the sponsor. The sponsor is given 10 working days from receipt of the overview and proposed decision to provide a response and submit any additional comment on the application to ADEC. This 'pre-ADEC response' is limited to six A4 pages.

24.3.10 Submission of new data

Two classes of new data may be submitted after an application has been accepted – additional data and supplementary data. Additional data are data identified at a pre-submission meeting that TGA agrees to accept during the course of an evaluation at a predetermined date, such as the results from an ongoing clinical study.

Supplementary data are clinical or preclinical data submitted at the initiation of the sponsor, after it has received either or both of the Module 4 and Module 5 evaluation reports. The sponsor must notify its intention to submit supplementary data within five working days of receipt of the last evaluation report. Only one submission of supplementary data is permitted for each of Modules 4 and 5, unless otherwise agreed by TGA in writing. Supplementary data will not be accepted after commencement of the pre-ADEC process, which is signified by the issuing of the delegates overview and recommendation. Acceptance of supplementary data is at the discretion of the TGA and is dependent upon mutual agreement to a 'clock stop'.

Up to 60 working days is allowed for all additional data and fees to be presented to the TGA following the sponsor's notification of intent; and up to 135 days may be taken for evaluation of the supplementary data after all data and fees have been received by TGA.

24.3.11 Australian Drug Evaluation Committee

The Australian Drug Evaluation Committee makes medical and scientific evaluations of drugs referred to it by the minister or the secretary, and gives advice to the minister or secretary in relation to the import, export, manufacture and distribution of therapeutic goods. It is important to note that ADEC has an advisory function and is not the final decision-maker. The TGA Delegate is guided by ADEC's advice but may make a decision contrary to ADEC's recommendations.

The ADEC comprises six or seven 'core' members – eminent practising physicians, pharmaceutical scientists and pharmacologists who attend each meeting. There are up to 20 'associate' members whose expertise is drawn on as appropriate to the applications under consideration at a particular meeting. ADEC members adhere to strict guidelines on competing interests, which effectively exclude a member from proceedings if they have any pecuniary interest in a pharmaceutical company whose product is under consideration or in any competitor company. Participation in company-sponsored clinical trials must also be declared, but does not necessarily exclude the member from proceedings. The ADEC 'Competing Interest Guidelines' are available from the TGA website. ADEC is supported by specialist sub-committees, which currently include the Pharmaceutical Subcommittee (PSC) and ADRAC.

The ADEC meets six times a year for 2-day meetings in February, April, June, August, October and December. For each application it receives the sponsor's covering letter, all evaluation reports, the delegate's overview and proposed decision, and the sponsor's pre-ADEC response. ADEC makes recommendations on applications referred to it for advice. This recommendation, termed an ADEC resolution, is sent to the sponsor five working days after the ADEC meeting. Ratified minutes of the meeting in which the resolution is made are available only after the next ADEC meeting, whereafter all positive recommendations relating to applications for registration are published in the Commonwealth Gazette and are posted on the TGA website. Occasionally, significant recommendations relating to a class of drugs or the content of the PI document are also published. The ADEC minutes are also provided to a number of overseas regulatory agencies.

Not all prescription medicine applications are referred to ADEC. Category 3 applications and some Category 1 applications may be dealt with entirely by the DSEB. An informal process has also been under trial, whereby some applications for which all the evaluators and the delegate recommend approval are not formally considered by ADEC prior to approval. ADEC is advised of the delegate's decision.

24.3.12 Post-ADEC and the delegate's decision

Following consideration by ADEC, if the delegate proposes to approve the application, he or she will communicate with the sponsor to address any outstanding issues, and the final PI will be negotiated. Once all outstanding matters are resolved, a marketing approval letter is issued by the delegate, which states the conditions of registration, together with the approved PI. A certificate of registration is also issued detailing the information included on the ARTG. The annual registration charge is payable following the registration.

If the delegate proposes to reject the application, a letter is sent to the sponsor advising of this intent, giving the reasons for the decision. A sponsor may appeal the initial decision of the delegate.

24.3.13 Appeals against marketing application decisions

Under Section 60 of the Therapeutic Goods Act, appeal mechanisms are available to sponsor companies to challenge decisions made by officers of the TGA. Prior to this legislation, an ADEC recommendation that a marketing application for a new product should not be approved could only be appealed to ADEC.

The decision of the secretary or delegate is called an initial decision. If the sponsor wishes to appeal an initial decision, it must do so within 90 calendar days of receiving advice of that decision. The appeal of the initial decision is directed to the minister, who generally appoints the TGA principal medical adviser to act as a delegate in considering that appeal, and the decision on the appeal must be issued within 60 days. The outcome of this stage is called a reviewable decision. Reviewable decisions are so-called because they may be appealed through the AAT. Eligible appeals to the AAT are defined in the Act and must be made within 28 calendar days of receiving advice on the minister's decision. This process has been used only a few times since 1991 and can be relatively complex and time consuming, and potentially expensive. Restrictions have been added over the years that strictly delineate the information that may be considered and the grounds for a successful appeal by this route.

24.3.14   Product information

The PI is the summary of the outcomes of the evaluation for registration, in the same way as the Summary of Product Characteristics (SPC) forms the basis for prescribing in the European Union. It is intended to provide appropriate information to health professionals for the safe and effective use of the product, and is negotiated between the delegate and sponsor following the ADEC meeting, taking into account ADEC's recommendations. Once approved by the delegate, the sponsor may not change any aspect of the PI without prior approval from the TGA, except in specific circumstances such as safety-related changes. Unlike the SPC, the PI is not subject to 5-yearly review, although this has been proposed.

Safety-related changes to the PI that may be made by the sponsor without prior approval are those that reduce the patient population or add a warning, precaution, contraindication or adverse event. They must be notified to the TGA within 5 days of implementation and the date of each safety-related change must be listed in the PI in addition to the TGA approval date.

Non-safety-related changes to the PI may only be made by the sponsor without approval if they are minor editorial matters such as changes to headings or relocation of text or a change consequent to self-assessable change made in accordance with ARGPM. These changes must also be notified to TGA within five working days.

For PI changes that require approval, DSEB accepts three main types of submission:

• conventional submissions, containing full study reports of clinical trials

• literature-based submissions
• hybrid submissions, comprising a mix of conventional and literature-based data.

The type of submission considered by DSEB to be appropriate for a PI update depends on the regulatory and clinical history of the drug in Australia and overseas, with special reference to the United Kingdom, United States, Sweden, Canada and the Netherlands. Submissions based on company sponsored clinical trials are usually required for drugs marketed for less than 5 years, whereas any of the three types of submission can be used for drugs marketed for more than 10 years. Drugs marketed between 5 and 10 years will be considered on a case by case basis, but it is generally expected that either a conventional or hybrid submission will be submitted.

Published non-clinical (Module 4) and clinical (Module 5) data may be used for either a literature-based submission or as the literature-based component of a hybrid submission. However, published reports rarely include sufficient validation information for pharmaceutical chemistry (Module 3) data to be accepted in the form of published literature. Conventional Module 3 data may accompany literature-based Module 4 and/or Module 5 data. Full guidelines on the preparation of literature-based submissions are available from the TGA website.

24.3.15   Paediatric indications

It is recognised internationally that there is a lack of information from proper investigations of the use of drugs in children, and a problem with the availability of paediatric-specific formulations, leading to drugs being used outside their approved indications and, at times, being reformulated by pharmacists to make them more suitable for use by children.

The TGA has endeavoured to encourage the submission of paediatric data packages by offering fee reductions for products that are not commercially viable or whose supply is in the public interest, waiving fees for orphan drugs and indications, and by accepting literature-based submissions. The TGA has also adopted internationally recognised ICH/EU guidelines dealing with paediatric data generation and facilitating the extrapolation of data from one patient population to another.

Sponsors are encouraged to consider whether their products are likely to be used in children and, if so, to discuss with the TGA how to make paediatric formulations available and to update PIs with information on paediatric use.

24.3.16 Consumer medicine information

Since 1993, all new prescription products (including changes to existing products that lead to a 'new' entry on the ARTG) have been required to also have a consumer medicine information (CMI) document, referred to in the Therapeutic Goods Regulations as a patient information document. From 1 January 2003, all prescription medicines have been required to have a CMI. The content of the CMI must be consistent with the PI and contain the information described in Schedule 12 to the regulations. CMI is also required for pharmacist-only (Schedule 3) medicines approved for registration since mid-1995, in accordance with Schedule 13 to the regulations.

Enormous effort has been invested in CMI development in Australia, with the aim of producing highly useful and usable information for consumers. Guidelines called 'Writing about medicines for people' (the usability guidelines) are in their second edition, providing guidance to sponsors on how to prepare CMIs with highly consistent usability. Unlike the European Union, Australian sponsors are not required to provide the CMI as a pack insert but may distribute the documents in a form that enables the CMI to be given to a person to whom a product is administered or dispensed. A system has been developed for electronic distribution of CMIs, so that they may be printed by doctors or pharmacists from their computer software.

24.3.17 Post-marketing responsibilities

The standard conditions of registration require the sponsor to inform the TGA of any adverse drug reactions and safety alerts related to their product of which they become aware.

The requirements for reporting adverse drug reactions to prescription medicines occurring in Australia or overseas are described in the Australian Pharmacovigilance Guideline, which is available at the TGA website.

For spontaneous reports of reactions occurring in Australia, serious reactions (whether expected or unexpected) should be reported immediately and in no case later than 15 calendar days of receipt of the report. Other reactions occurring in Australia should be reported on request or as line listings in a Periodic Safety Update Report (PSUR).

Reports of reactions occurring in other countries are not required to be routinely submitted to TGA. However, any significant safety issue or action that has arisen from an analysis of foreign reports, or has been taken by a foreign regulatory agency, must be reported to the TGA within 72 h.

Australia has harmonised its requirements for post-marketing reports with those of the CPMP/ICH 'Guideline on Periodic Safety Update Reports (CPMP/ICH/228/95)'. The timing and frequency of provision of PSURs has also been harmonised with the CPMP/ICH requirements. Thus an Australian sponsor may submit PSURs prepared to meet international regulatory requirements to the TGA. Post-marketing reports must be provided annually until the period covered by such reports is not less than 3 years from the date of the Australian marketing approval letter. No fewer than three annual reports are required. If a PSUR is not available, the Australian sponsor must prepare a post-marketing report.

Another condition of registration is that a product recall (or similar regulatory action) in any other country, that has relevance to the quality, safety and efficacy of the goods to be distributed in Australia, must be notified to the TGA immediately. Other conditions of registration include conditions related to the sampling and testing of products and manufacturing premises.

24.3.18 Products of gene technology

The Commonwealth Gene Technology Act 2000 came into force in 2001, introducing a national scheme for the regulation of genetically modi-fied (GM) organisms in Australia. The legislation regulates some GM products, but only where the products are not regulated by an existing agency. Thus, therapeutic goods that contain GM organisms or are products of GM organisms continue to be regulated by the TGA.

The Gene Technology Act requires the Gene Technology Regulator to be notified by other regulators such as the TGA about GM products approved for sale in Australia. For example, if the TGA approves a GM medicine for sale in Australia, this must be entered in the centralised, publicly available database of all GM organisms and GM products.

24.3.19 Products manufactured or tested using human embryos or human embryonic stem cells

In late 2003 an amendment to the Therapeutic Goods Regulations introduced new requirements for products registered on or after 1 July 2004 that are manufactured or tested using a human embryo or human embryonic stem cells (HESC). For products manufactured using a human embryo or HESC, or any material sourced from these materials, including any testing associated with the manufacture of the product, there must be a statement included in the PI and CMI disclosing this use.

In addition, where information is provided to the TGA as part of an application for registration of a prescription medicine that refers to use of human embryos, HESC or materials derived from human embryos or HESC in research undertaken in the development of the medicine, the PI and CMI must also include a statement to that effect.

The sponsor must provide a declaration on these matters in Module 1 of the application for registration.

24.3.20 Recalls

Recalls are handled by the Australian Recall Coordinator within the TGA according to the voluntary 'Uniform Recall Procedures for Therapeutic Goods', in conjunction with the States. The Australian Recall Coordinator also liaises with the Commonwealth Minister responsible for Consumer Affairs in relation to safety-related recalls of therapeutic goods, which must be notified within 48 h, in accordance with the Trade Practices Act 1974. A mandatory recall of faulty goods may be enforced where safety is involved.

In April/May 2003 the TGA forced the recall of approximately 1600 complementary medicines at retail level throughout Australia, due to concerns about the quality of their manufacture. The recalled products were manufactured in Australia by Pan Pharmaceuticals, principally as a contract manufacturer for other companies. The resultant publicity impacted around the world and highlighted the importance of effective implementation of GMP standards for all therapeutic products. In view of the issues raised by this massive recall, and to restore community confidence, an Expert Committee on Complementary Medicines in the Health System was established to consider a wide range of matters relating to complementary medicines. Their report was published in September 2003 and is available from the TGA website.

As a consequence of the regulatory action involving Pan Pharmaceuticals, amendments were made to the Therapeutic Goods Act to increase maximum penalties for a range of existing offences; create a range of new offences such as falsifying documents relating to therapeutic goods regulation; expand compulsory public notification and recall provisions; insert a 'fit and proper person' test in relation to manufacturing licences and conformity assessment certificates; require better identification of therapeutic goods in the event of a recall; and require inclusion of manufacturer details on the labels of medicines. The Therapeutic Goods Amendment Act (No. 1) 2003 took effect on 27 May 2003.

24.3.21 Counterfeit goods and tampering

Amendments were made to the Therapeutic Goods Act in mid-2000 to make it a specific offence to supply counterfeit therapeutic goods in Australia.

Also new offences were introduced under the Act for tampering with therapeutic goods or continuing to supply goods that may have been tampered with, and for failing to notify the TGA of any knowledge of actual tampering or threats associated with tampering.

24.3.22 Trans-Tasman Mutual Recognition arrangement

The Trans-Tasman Mutual Recognition Act 1997, developed under the policy of closer economic relations between Australia and New Zealand, came into force in 1998. The Act is intended to enhance Trans-Tasman trade by allowing goods available in one country to be acceptable in the other (and also recognise professional qualifications in both countries). A special exemption for therapeutic goods was immediately granted in recognition of the differences between the Australian and New Zealand regulatory systems. During the life of the special exemption, which must be renewed annually, the two countries' therapeutic goods agencies have been working towards resolving the special exemption in consultation with the industry, consumers, medical and pharmacy professions.

The Health Ministers in Australia and New Zealand agreed that harmonisation of regulatory requirements for therapeutic goods is the best option under the Trans-Tasman Mutual Recognition Arrangement. In December 2003, the two governments signed a treaty, which commits them to establishing a 'single world-class agency' and a 'regulatory regime consistent with international best practice for the regulation of quality, safety and efficacy or performance of therapeutic products.' The joint therapeutics regulatory agency, which will be responsible for implementing regulatory controls over the import, manufacture and supply of therapeutic products in both countries, is scheduled to begin operation on 1 July 2006.

It is anticipated that legislation establishing the new agency will be presented to both parliaments in early 2006, following release for public consultation of the Therapeutic Products Bill and associated rules in late 2005.

At the commencement of the new joint agency, all therapeutic products currently on the market in either Australia or New Zealand will be granted an interim product licence to continue to supply those products in that country. During the (proposed) 3-year transition period the sponsors of these products must apply for, and be granted, a full agency licence that will permit the products to be supplied in both Australia and New Zealand. For prescription medicines it is likely that there will be some differences between the registered details for products that are currently supplied in both countries. These differences will be analysed by sponsors to determine which of the details will apply to the full agency licensed product. The data that may be required to justify this selection is yet to be determined, but it is anticipated that, where a product or indication has been rejected by either TGA or Medsafe (New Zealand), more data or justification will be required to obtain the full agency licence.

There is considerable work ahead for the Australian and New Zealand industry in late 2005 and early 2006 to negotiate the final details for the new regulatory regime, including the fees and charges that will apply. It is currently both the Australian and New Zealand Governments' policy that the new agency will operate under 100% cost recovery, including paying for the establishment costs of the agency – approximately AUD$7 million to be repaid over 5 years through the fees and charges revenue.

24.4 Listing on the Pharmaceutical Benefits Section – the 'Fourth Hurdle'

Applications for listing a product on the PBS are generally submitted by the pharmaceutical company sponsor, which has the data required to support the application, to the Pharmaceutical Benefits section of the Department of Health. However, submissions from medical bodies, health professionals or members of the public may also be considered.

A product may not be listed on the PBS until marketing approval is granted. However, a sponsor may apply for PBS listing once the TGA delegate has recommended to ADEC that the product be granted marketing approval. Thus, consideration of a listing application can to some extent overlap with the final stages of evaluation of an application for marketing approval.

Products may not be subsidised under the PBS for unapproved indications, and some approved indications may not be subsidised.

24.4.1 The PBAC process

The PBAC assesses applications for listing on the PBS for reimbursement against criteria specified in the National Health Act. These criteria include safety and efficacy compared with other available treatments including non-drug therapies, and comparative cost-effectiveness.

The current 'Guidelines for the Pharmaceutical Industry on Preparation of Submissions to the PBAC including Major Submissions involving Economic Analyses' were published in 1995, and are available through www.health.gov.au/pbs (the PBS website), together with the 'Application to List' form (commonly referred to as PB11). The guidelines are currently being reviewed and updated with the intention of issuing revised guidelines following the November 2005 PBAC meeting.

Section 1 of the guidelines establishes the context of the submission. It asks for a description of the drug, its use on the PBS and the therapies that will be co-administered or substituted. Section 2 asks for the best available evidence on the clinical performance of the drug, including the scientific and statistical rigour of randomised trials, and a preliminary economic evaluation based on evidence from the randomised trials. Section 3 describes when extrapolation beyond the preliminary economic evaluation may be made and how adjustments can be made in a modelled economic evaluation. Section 4 requests a financial analysis from the perspective of the PBS and government health budgets.

The guidelines must be followed for major submissions to the PBAC to:

- list a new drug on the schedule of pharmaceutical benefits
- request a significant change to the listing of a currently restricted drug (including a new indication or a de-restriction)
- enable a review of the comparative cost-effectiveness of a currently listed drug in order to change a PBAC recommendation to the PBPA or its therapeutic relativity or price premium
- list a new formulation or strength of a currently listed drug for which a price premium is requested.

The guidelines are interpreted in a very prescriptive manner, and have been the subject of ongoing discussion. Improved health outcomes that are difficult to quantify, such as 'indirect' benefits, are accorded a low weighting. Also large head-to-head comparative studies with adequate power to yield significant differences may be required before superior outcomes are regarded as proven.

In April 2000 some sections of the guidelines were revised. An interim document to accompany the guidelines with two new appendices came into effect in June 2000 and introduced changes relating to the selection of randomised trial evidence from the literature and other searches, and the presentation of modelled economic evaluations. It is available from the PBS website.

On receipt of a major application for listing, the PBAC secretariat forwards the application to the Pharmaceutical Evaluation Section (PES). The PES evaluates these applications together with three external groups from academic institutions contracted for this work. The PES provides an evaluation report to the Economic Subcommittee (ESC) of the PBAC. The ESC reviews and interprets the economic analyses and advises the PBAC on these analyses. The PBAC also receives advice from the Drug Utilisation SubCommittee (DUSC).

The sponsor receives the PES evaluation and DUSC report approximately $2\frac{1}{2}$ weeks prior to the PBAC meeting at which the application will be considered. The sponsor's response to the overview and commentary must be sent to the PBAC secretariat within 1 week and are provided to the PBAC along with the ESC advice and the PES overview and commentary.

As with ADEC, conflict of interest guidelines are strictly applied to PBAC and its subcommittees. The membership of the PBAC was revised in 2001, allowing for a greater range of expertise to be included, and introducing restrictions on the length of term that members may serve. Amid some controversy, a member with pharmaceutical industry experience was included, in addition to medical practitioners and members with pharmacy and consumerist backgrounds. Following the untimely death of the pharmaceutical industry member, and the appointment of a new Minister for Health, the industry member was not replaced. In April 2004, the National Health Act was amended to increase the number of members of the PBAC to a maximum of 15, with five new members appointed in March 2005 to fill the new positions and replace retiring members.

The PBAC meets three times per annum, in March, July and November, as the culmination of the 17 week pre-meeting application cycle (see Section 4.8). Positive PBAC recommendations are published on the PBS website approximately 6 weeks after the PBAC meeting. If an application for listing is successful, the PBAC recommends the maximum quantity to be dispensed on each prescription and the number of repeat prescriptions. The PBAC may also recommend prescribing restrictions – an authority required item requires the prescriber to obtain prior approval from the Health Insurance Commission (HIC), by telephone or post, and restricted benefit items may only be prescribed for specified therapeutic uses.

24.4.2 Appeals against recommendations on PBS listing applications

The National Health Act does not include the option for PBAC recommendations to be appealed to the AAT. Generally, the only avenue is for the applicant to appeal to the PBAC.

Pharmaceutical Benefits Advisory Committee rejections, and the lack of available appeal mechanisms, have been increasingly challenged in recent years. One route available is to pursue a legal challenge to the Federal Court of Australia for a review of the decision. Most recently, in March 2000, the Federal Court rejected a pharmaceutical company's application to overturn the recommendation of the PBAC not to list a product on the scheme.

Following a review of the listing process in 2002, the opportunity for meetings between the PBAC and stakeholders was established. These meetings are not intended as an appeals mechanism but as a 'without prejudice', non-adversarial process to facilitate a resubmission by the sponsor. A stakeholder meeting may be sought where the drug is indicated for a serious disabling or life-threatening condition for which there is no other realistic management option. The 'Guidelines for Stakeholder Meetings' are available from the PBS website.

As an outcome of the Australia–United States Free Trade Agreement (AUSFTA), an Independent Review Mechanism has been introduced for negative PBAC recommendations.

24.4.3 Free Trade Agreement

On 18 May 2004 the Australian Trade Minister and the US Trade Representative signed a Free Trade Agreement between Australia and the United States. The AUSFTA came into force on 1 January 2005, following a formal exchange of letters between Australia and the United States on 17 November 2004 confirming that all domestic processes to implement the agreement had been completed. The full text of the agreement is available from the Department of Foreign Affairs and Trade website at www.dfat.gov.au/trade/negotiations/us_fta/final-text/index.html. The provisions relating to pharmaceuticals are contained in Annex 2C of the agreement and in a side letter to the agreement that confirms the outcomes of the negotiations relating to the PBS.

Annex 2C and the side letter outline that the following changes (in summary) will be made to enhance the processes for listing medicines on the PBS:

Annex 2C

- greater transparency of the listing process for applicants and the public
- a medicines working group to be established comprising officials from each government to promote discussion and understanding of the Annex
- enhanced dialogue between the TGA and the FDA with the view to expedite availability of innovative medicines
- companies to be permitted to provide truthful and not misleading information on their websites about medicines approved for sale

Side letter

- applicants will have the opportunity to consult with officials prior to submission, to respond fully to all reports or evaluations, and to have a hearing before the PBAC, and will receive information on the reasons for the PBAC's determination
- there will be an independent review process for PBAC determinations of listing applications where there is a negative recommendation
- the listing process will be streamlined and expedited, with more frequent revisions of the schedule of pharmaceutical benefits
- applicants will be allowed to apply for an adjustment to a reimbursement amount.

There has been considerable public debate concerning the impact of the AUSFTA on the PBS. Critics have claimed that the AUSFTA will increase the cost of medicines on the PBS. Both the government and industry have clearly stated that this will not be the case. Rather, it is intended that Australians will benefit from faster access to subsidies for innovative medicines through improvements to listing processes.

The prescription medicines industry has been working closely with government officials to implement the changes agreed under the AUSFTA through a working group established by the Minister for Health to advise on the implementation of Australia's commitments. In July 2004 the Minister released a public consultation document, which outlines the proposed independent review mechanism and describes principles to support the implementation of hearings before the PBAC and for enhancing transparency of PBAC recommendations. Further work is required to enable these changes to be implemented.

24.4.4 Pricing of products on the PBS

The PBPA makes recommendations to the Department of Health on the prices for new items that have been recommended for PBS listing by the PBAC. It also reviews the prices for all items listed on the Schedule of Pharmaceutical Benefits at least once per annum. The PBAC provides advice to the PBPA regarding comparison with other treatments and comparative cost-effectiveness.

The Commonwealth Government negotiates an agreed wholesale price with the pharmaceutical company sponsor, through a senior officer in the pharmaceutical benefits branch. This process applies to all products subsidised as PBS-listed items under Section 85 of the National Health Act, including products that are priced below the general patient co-payment.

A wholesaler margin is then set on the supplier's price, a pharmacist margin is applied to the wholesaler's price, and a pharmacist dispensing fee is also added, determined by the Pharmaceutical Benefits Remuneration Tribunal. Patients pay the co-payment (and any premiums) to the pharmacist when the PBS-listed medicine is dispensed, with the balance of the cost of the product being paid to the pharmacist by the government.

Consumers' contributions to the cost of their medicines are limited by safety net thresholds, which are adjusted annually in relation to the consumer price index (CPI). Under the PBS the maximum cost for a listed item on 1 January 2005 is AUD\$4.60 for concessional patients and AUD\$28.60 for general patients, except where a brand premium, therapeutic group premium (TGP) or special patient contribution applies.

There are two safety net thresholds. For general patients, once a patient has spent AUD\$874.90 on PBS medicines, the patient co-payment decreases to the concessional level of AUD\$4.60 for the rest of the calendar year. For concessional patients the safety net threshold is AUD\$239.20. Once concessional patients reach this level they receive PBS items free of charge for the rest of the calendar year. From 1 August 2003 information about the full cost of each item has been included on the label of the medicine, so that consumers will be better informed.

Determination of the agreed price for a product to be listed on the PBS is understandably one of the most contentious areas between the pharmaceutical industry and government. The pricing procedure and methods used by the PBPA in recommending prices for new items and in its annual review of prices of all items listed on the PBS, including Reference Pricing and Weighted Average Monthly Treatment Cost (WAMTC), are explained in a document that is available from the PBS website.

The PBPA sometimes recommends the use of price/volume arrangements, particularly where unit prices are reasonably high and there is the potential for significant volumes or where there is uncertainty about future volumes.

If the predicted annual cost to the government is greater than AUD\$5 million in 1 year, including consideration of the potential for prescribing outside of the agreed restrictions, the Department of Health must obtain the Department of Finance's agreement to the estimated costs. If the predicted annual cost to government is greater than AUD\$10 million, the listing must be approved by the Prime Minister and the Minister for Finance, in Addition to the Minister for Health.

The PBAC and PBPA also consider the prices of pharmaceuticals listed under Section 100 of the National Health Act, which allows for an alternative means of providing an adequate pharmaceutical service in circumstances where pharmaceutical benefits cannot be conveniently and efficiently supplied in the usual manner under the PBS. Drugs in this category, such as medicines for HIV/AIDS, are reviewed by the Highly Specialised Drugs Working Party and are generally supplied through different dispensing arrangements in public hospitals under agreements with the States, and exclude wholesaler involvement.

24.4.5 Brand premiums

Where there are two or more brands of the same form and strength of a drug listed on the PBS that are bioequivalent and hence interchangeable, the PBPA recommends the benchmark price for that drug, being the price of the lowest priced brand. Sponsors of the other brands may charge a premium above the benchmark price. Brands that are considered interchangeable are indicated in the schedule by alphabetic superscripts. The cost of the brand premium must be paid by the consumer in addition to any co-payment. A pharmacist may substitute brands to avoid a consumer paying a premium, provided the prescriber does not specifically prohibit this and the consumer agrees.

24.4.6 Special patient contribution arrangements

A sponsor may not seek to charge a product premium above the agreed listing price unless there is an alternative brand of the drug in the same form and strength listed on the PBS. If the sponsor and government cannot agree on a listing price for a new product, and there is no alternative listed on the PBS, the product cannot be listed with a brand premium. However, on rare occasions a special patient contribution can apply. This currently applies to only five PBS items.

24.4.7 Reference pricing and therapeutic group premiums

In 1998, the Commonwealth Government introduced TGPs, a form of reference pricing, to certain therapeutic drug classes listed on the Schedule of Pharmaceutical Benefits – H2 receptor antagonists, ACE inhibitors, HMG CoA reductase inhibitors (statins) and calcium channel blockers. Under this policy, the government agreed to subsidise all drug products in the therapeutic subgroup up to the price of the lowest priced product in the group, the benchmark. Different chemical entities in a therapeutic group were deemed to be equivalent for the purpose of pricing, including patented and out of patent products. If a sponsor chooses to charge a premium above the benchmark price, that premium must be paid by the consumer in addition to the co-payment. This premium does not count towards the PBS safety net threshold.

A prescriber may apply to the HIC for a TGP exemption for an individual patient for a particular product, if adverse effects or reactions are expected to occur with all of the benchmark priced products or the transfer to a benchmark priced product would cause patient confusion leading to problems with compliance. Pharmacists may not substitute between different chemical entities in a therapeutic group.

When the policy was introduced it was thought that some sponsors would maintain significant premiums for their products over the benchmark price. However, over time, many have reduced their price to the benchmark price or charged a reduced premium compared with the price prior to introduction of the TGP policy. The premiums currently range from AUD$7.01 to AUD$0.64 in three of the four groups, with no premium charged on any of the HMG CoA reductase inhibitors.

As part of the October 2004 Federal election campaign, the Prime Minister announced that from 1 April 2005 (later revises to 1 August 2005) new generic medicines listed on the PBS would be required to be listed at 12.5 percent below the current benchmark price. As a result of reference pricing arrangements this price reduction also applies to all products in the same reference pricing group. The price reduction will apply only to the first new brand of any PBS medicine listed, not to subsequent new brands of the same medicine, and will apply once only for each medicine including for medicines in a reference pricing group where the reduction has occurred as a flow-on from another medicine. Savings generated from this policy of over AUD $800 million over four years will be used to fund a Seniors policy announced in the election campaign.

If a company refuses to accept the 12.5 percent price reduction, a special patient Contribution (the difference between the existing price and the new benchmark price) will apply in addition to the usual patient copayment. If a prescriber considers that there is no clinically appropriate alternative for a particular patient, the government will pay the special contribution following the prescriber seeking authority from the HIC.

24.4.8 Time frames

It currently takes a minimum of 35 weeks from submission of an application for PBS listing to the time it may be prescribed as a PBS item if the application is successful the first time it is considered, although some of this process may overlap the final stages of registration approval.

Action	Weeks prior to PBAC meeting
Cut-off date for major submissions	17
PES evaluation and DUSC commentary sent to sponsor	7.5
Cut-off date for minor submissions	6–7
Pre-ESC and pre-DUSC responses provided by sponsors	6.5
DUSC meeting	5
ESC meeting	4.5
Restrictions Working Group (RWG) meeting	4
ESC, DUSC and RWG advice sent to sponsors	2
Pre-PBAC comments provided by sponsor	1
ESC report and sponsor comments sent to PBAC	1
PBAC meeting	0

Action	Weeks post-PBAC meeting
Verbal advice of recommendation given to sponsor	0.5
Written advice of recommendation sent to sponsor	3
Unratified minutes sent to sponsor	4–5
PBPA meeting	6
Approval by Minister for Health/parliamentary secretary	10–12
Closing date to amend Schedule of Pharmaceutical Benefits	14
Listing in the Schedule of Pharmaceutical Benefits	18

Products are frequently not launched in Australia until the outcome of the PBS listing application is known.

Before listing, the National Health Act also required that a product must have been cleared with respect to chemistry and quality control matters. This was undertaken by the TGAL. As a result of the post-PBAC review this requirement has recently been removed, recognising that the TGA marketing approval processes are sufficient.

24.4.9 Post-PBAC review

In August 2003, the Department of Health and Medicines Australia, representing the prescription medicines industry, commenced a joint review of the listing processes post-PBAC. The review's main objective was to 'advise on any necessary post-PBAC (pPBAC) changes … which would improve the efficiency and effectiveness of the entire process in order to achieve earliest possible subsidised access for consumers to cost-effective medicines, while minimising the regulatory burden on industry'.

The Post-PBAC Review Report was released in July 2004 by the Minister for Health. It is available at www.health.gov.au (the Department of Health website).

An implementation group was established to implement the recommendations, which were all accepted in principle. A key recommendation is to publish the Schedule of Pharmaceutical Benefits electronically to enable monthly listing updates. This will require significant upgrading of the department's information technology systems. It will take some time to fully implement all the recommendations.

24.5 Access to Medicines not Registered or Listed on the ARTG

Guidelines detailing the four avenues available for access to medicines not registered or listed on the ARTG are available through the following URLs:

- Clinical trials: www.tga.gov.au/docs/html/clintrials.htm
- Special access scheme: www.tga.gov.au/docs/html/sasinfo.htm
- Authorised prescriber: www.tga.gov.au/docs/html/authpres.htm
- Personal importation: www.tga.gov.au/docs/html/personalimp.htm.

24.5.1 Clinical trials

There are two schemes under which clinical trials involving therapeutic goods may be conducted in Australia – the Clinical Trial Notification (CTN) Scheme and the Clinical Trial Exemption (CTX) Scheme. These schemes are used for clinical trials involving any product not entered on the ARTG, or use of a registered or listed product in a clinical trial beyond the conditions of its marketing approval.

Clinical trials in which registered or listed medicines (or medical devices) are used within the conditions of their marketing approval are not subject to CTN or CTX requirements but still need to be approved by a Human Research Ethics Committee (HREC) before the trial may commence.

All CTN and CTX trials must have an Australian sponsor. The sponsor is that person, body, organisation or institution which takes overall responsibility for the conduct of the trial. It need not be a pharmaceutical company. The sponsor usually initiates, organises and supports a clinical study and carries the medicolegal responsibility associated with the conduct of the trial.

In 2003–4 there were 2378 CTN scheme notifications. It should be noted, however, that this does not indicate the number of different clinical trial protocols, which was approximately 560 in 2003–4. This contrasts with two CTX 50 working day applications in the same period and zero 30 working day applications.

24.5.1.1   The CTN scheme

Under the CTN scheme the sponsor of the clinical trial provides detailed information about the proposed trial to the principal investigator who submits an application to conduct the clinical trial to the HREC at the institution or other site at which the trial is proposed to be conducted. The clinical trial application generally includes the protocol, the investigator's brochure, related patient information, supporting data and the CTN form. HRECs usually have their own standard format for applications to conduct a CTN trial at their institution. The HREC evaluates the scientific and ethical validity of the proposed clinical trial and the safety and efficacy of the medicine in the context of its stage of development. The TGA does not evaluate any information about the clinical trial.

If the HREC approves the conduct of the clinical trial, the chairman of the HREC signs the CTN form. The institution or organisation at which the trial will be conducted, referred to as the approving authority, gives the final approval for the conduct of the trial at the site, having due regard to advice from the HREC and also must sign the CTN form. In some cases, the HREC can also be the approving authority for a particular trial site.

In signing the CTN form the signatories agree that they will comply with all legislative and regulatory requirements, that the trial will be conducted in accordance with the 'Note for Guidance on Good Clinical Practice' (GCP Guidelines) (CPMP/ICH/135/95), and the National Health and Medical Research Council (NHMRC) 'National Statement on the Ethical Conduct of Research Involving Humans' 1999 (National Statement), and that they will agree to release information to the TGA about the conduct of the trial in the event of an inquiry or audit of the trial.

The form is then submitted by the sponsor of the trial to the TGA, along with the appropriate notification fee. The current notification fee is AUD$240 for each notification, which can comprise a single site conducting a clinical trial, or multiple sites conducting the same trial notified together. Once the CTN form has been submitted to the TGA along with the relevant fee, the clinical trial may commence. The TGA acknowledges receipt of the CTN form and fee, which takes 2 or 3 days. Some sponsors choose to wait for receipt of this acknowledgement before commencing a trial, although this is not strictly necessary.

There is one CTN form for each site conducting the same clinical trial, such as multicentre trials. In some cases a composite site can be notified where a single HREC and approving authority have responsibility for all sites conducting the trial, such as a general practice network.

To assist the TGA to maintain a record of each CTN trial, the sponsor must subsequently notify the TGA of the date the trial was completed, the reason the trial ceased (e.g. concluded normally; insufficient recruits) and any changes to the trial with respect ot information previously submitted.

24.5.1.2   The CTX scheme

Under the CTX scheme, a sponsor submits an application to conduct clinical trials to both the TGA and the HREC at each institution or site at which it is proposed to conduct the clinical trial.

The TGA reviews the information about the product provided by the sponsor, including whether the medicine is under investigation or approved for marketing in other countries, proposed usage guidelines, a pharmaceutical data sheet and a summary of the preclinical data and clinical data.

There are two levels of evaluation of applications for clinical trials of medicines under the CTX scheme. A 30 working day period for evaluation of a CTX application applies when the supporting data relate only to chemical, pharmaceutical and biological issues. A 50 working day period applies for applications supported by chemical, pharmaceutical and biological, preclinical and clinical data. These evaluation times commence from the date of acceptance of the application or receipt of the appropriate fee. The fee for a 30 day CTX application is currently AUD$1240 and for a 50 day application AUD$15300.

If the TGA delegate raises an objection, trials may not proceed until the objection has been addressed to the delegate's satisfaction. Even if no objection is raised, the delegate usually provides comments on the accuracy or interpretation of the summary information supplied by the sponsor. The sponsor must forward these comments to the HREC(s) at sites at which the sponsor intends to conduct the trial.

As with the CTN scheme, the sponsor prepares information for submission by the principal investigator to the HREC at the institution or other site at which the trial is proposed to be conducted. The HREC in each host institution/ organisation is responsible for approving the proposed trial protocol after reviewing the summary information received from the sponsor and any additional comments from the TGA delegate. The approving authority gives the final approval for the conduct of the trial at the site, having due regard to advice from the HREC.

A sponsor may not commence a CTX trial until written advice has been received from the TGA regarding the application, and approval has been obtained from the HREC and the institution at which the trial will be conducted.

There are two forms relating to the CTX scheme that must be submitted to TGA by the sponsor. Part 1 is the formal CTX application and must be completed by the sponsor of the trial and submitted to TGA with data for evaluation. Part 2 is used to notify the commencement of each new trial conducted under the CTX as well as new sites in ongoing CTX trials. It requires the signature of the chairman of the HREC, the responsible person from the approving authority, the principal investigator and the sponsor, and must be submitted within 28 days of the commencement of supply of goods under the CTX. There is no fee for notification of additional trials.

Applications can be lodged simultaneously with the TGA and the institution(s) at which studies are proposed to be conducted. However, if the application is lodged simultaneously with the TGA and HREC(s), the sponsor is required to convey any TGA comments or revisions on the application and/or objections to the HREC(s).

The sponsor may conduct any number of clinical trials under the CTX application without further assessment by the TGA, provided use of the product in the trials falls within the original approved usage guidelines. However, HREC approval of each protocol and approval from the institution or organisation for the conduct of each trial are still required.

24.5.1.3 TGA investigation of clinical trials

In 2000, the Therapeutic Goods Regulations were amended to expand and strengthen the TGA's powers to require provision of information about the conduct of any clinical trial being conducted under the legislation, and to audit a clinical trial. These amendments were introduced following a review, which indicated that the TGA's powers were inadequate to enable it to thoroughly investigate complaints.

New provisions allow an authorised person to enter a site at which a clinical trial is being conducted and examine any thing at the site relating to the clinical trial, including any documents or records relating to the trial. The revised regulations also require the principal investigator to give assurances that the trial will be conducted in accordance with the Guidelines on Good Clinical Practice (GCP), and will comply with an audit of the trial by an authorised person.

24.5.1.4   Reporting adverse events and adverse drug reactions during clinical trials

Australia has largely harmonised its reporting requirements for adverse events and adverse drug reactions occurring during clinical trials with international requirements and has adopted, in principle, the 'Note for Guidance on Clinical Safety Data Management: Definitions and Standards for Expedited Reporting CPMP/ICH/377/95)' – in particular the definitions and reporting time frames.

Despite the TGA's adoption of these international requirements, the local interpretation of these guidelines in relation to reporting serious and unexpected adverse reactions must be adhered to. Sponsors of clinical trials are required to report to TGA single cases of serious and unexpected adverse reactions. Fatal or life-threatening ADRs should be reported within seven calendar days of the reaction first being notified to the sponsor. This should be followed by as complete a report as possible within eight additional calendar days. All other serious and unexpected ADRs should be reported to TGA within 15 calendar days of first knowledge of the sponsor.

Information should be provided in the form of a detailed summary in the ADRAC 'Blue Card' format. Even if initial information is scanty, these details should be forwarded to the TGA pending receipt and provision of further data. This procedure should be followed even when the medicine in question is the subject of an application for registration and under evaluation by the TGA.

Sponsors are not required, as a matter of routine, to submit individual patient reports to the TGA of suspected adverse drug reactions occurring with use of the same product in another country, even if a trial is ongoing at Australian sites. However, the TGA requires that sponsors advise the Experimental Drugs Section of DSEB within 72 h of any significant safety issue which has arisen from an analysis of overseas reports or action with respect to safety taken by another country's regulatory agency. This advice must include the basis for such action.

24.5.1.5   Good clinical practice and ethical conduct of clinical trials

The TGA's regulation of clinical trials involving new medicines requires adherence to international standards of ethical conduct and GCP.

In 2000, the TGA Guidelines on Good Clinical Research Practice 1991 were replaced by the CPMP/ICH GCP guidelines (see Section 24.5.1.1), with some amendments to reflect Australian regulatory requirements.

Furthermore, Australia has a strong framework in place to support the ethical conduct of clinical trials, provided by the NHMRC, its principal committees and HRECs. In June 2003, there were 226 registered HRECs in Australia – 125 hospital (public and private), 53 university, 23 government and 25 associated with professional and other bodies.

The strategic intent of the NHMRC is to provide leadership and work with other relevant organisations to improve the health of all Australians by:

• fostering and supporting a high quality and internationally recognised research base
• providing evidence based advice
• applying research evidence to health issues thus translating research into better health practice and outcomes
• promoting informed debate on health and medical research, health ethics and related issues.

A principal committee of the NHMRC, the Australian Health Ethics Committee (AHEC), provides guidance and support for HRECs in Australia, and is responsible for developing and publishing the 'National Statement on the Ethical Conduct of Research Involving Humans 1999', which replaced the previous 'NHMRC Statement on Human Experimentation and Supplementary Notes 1992'.

Compliance with the national statement is a requirement for all clinical trials conducted in Australia under the CTX and CTN schemes. The chairman of the HREC certifies that the HREC is constituted in accordance with guidelines issued by the NHMRC, has registered with the AHEC, and has approved the clinical trial in accordance with the guidance provided by the national statement.

The increased awareness of ethical issues relating to human research has led to the release in 2002 of the Human Research Ethics Handbook, including detailed commentary on the national statement and discussion of ethical and legal issues, to further assist HRECs to assess and facilitate the ethical conduct of research involving human participants, and resolve the challenges encountered during this process.

Both the national statement and the associated handbook are available at www.nhmrc.gov.au (the NHMRC website).

Currently, AHEC is working with HRECs around Australia to develop a nationally accepted clinical trial application format that will be acceptable to all HRECs. This will significantly benefit sponsors of clinical trials who currently have to prepare applications in different formats to meet individual HREC requirements, which delays submission of applications in Australia and adds to the workload.

24.5.1.6 Status of the Declaration of Helsinki

The clinical trial guidelines published by the TGA specify that all clinical trials must be conducted in accordance with the Declaration of Helsinki, October 1996. The World Medical Association updated the Declaration of Helsinki in October 2000 but these changes were not adopted in Australia due to concerns in relation to the interpretation of two new clauses.

Clause 29 has been interpreted to mean that it prohibits use of a placebo where there is a current therapy available. Clause 30 has been considered unrealistic as few sponsors would be willing to guarantee ongoing access to an experimental therapy at the conclusion of a clinical trial.

The AHEC has advised HRECs to continue to regard the national statement as the definitive guideline for the review and conduct of research in Australia. In October 2001 the WMA issued a note of clarification on the interpretation of its guideline on the ethical use of placebo-controlled trials. The note of clarification has reduced any differences between the national statement and the Declaration of Helsinki, but AHEC has advised HRECs that wherever there is doubt regarding the interpretation and application of various ethical guidelines, the National Statement should always take precedence.

24.5.1.7 Clinical trial compensation guidelines and indemnity

In order to promote a uniform approach to offering compensation to subjects and indemnity to investigators and institutions conducting clinical trials, Medicines Australia has published a 'Form of Indemnity for Clinical Trials' and 'Guidelines for Compensation for Injury Resulting from Participation in a Company-Sponsored Clinical Trial'. These documents are based on those published by the Association of the British Pharmaceutical Industry and are available from www.medicinesaustralia.com.au (the Medicines Australia website).

24.5.2 Special Access Scheme

The Special Access Scheme (SAS) allows for the import and supply of an unapproved therapeutic good to an individual patient on a case by case basis. The Scheme envisages two categories of patients – Category A patients, who are defined in the Regulations as 'persons who are seriously ill with a condition from which death is reasonably likely to occur within a matter of months, or from which premature death is reasonably likely to occur in the absence of early treatment', and Category B, all other patients. A medical practitioner can supply an unapproved product to a Category A patient without the approval of the TGA, but must inform the TGA within 4 weeks following supply. Thus, no prior approval is required from the TGA. For Category B patients, individual approval for each patient must be obtained from a TGA delegate or a delegate outside the TGA referred to as an external delegate.

Classification of a patient as Category A or B lies with the medical practitioner. However, the TGA may review, seek clarification and request information regarding the classification of patients under Category A.

A medical practitioner can supply any unapproved medicine to a Category A patient, except medicines listed in Schedule 9 of the SUSDP, which are primarily drugs of abuse such as heroin or cannabis.

Adverse event and ADR reporting requirements are similar to those for clinical trials, with greater emphasis on the prescriber being responsible for reporting any ADR to the TGA, the sponsor and HREC.

24.5.3   Authorised prescribers

Another avenue for limited access to an unapproved medicine is through the Authorised Prescriber provisions of the Act. A few specified medical practitioners are authorised by the TGA to prescribe a specific unapproved therapeutic good or class of unapproved therapeutic goods, to specified recipients or classes of recipients (identified by their medical condition) in their immediate care, without further approval from the TGA. The authorised prescriber must also have the endorsement of an appropriate HREC to supply the product.

A pharmaceutical company is not obliged to supply an unapproved product under the authorised prescriber provisions. If it does supply the specified product, the company must provide reports every six months of the amount of product supplied to authorised prescribers.

Adverse event and ADR reporting requirements are similar to those for clinical trials, with greater emphasis on the authorised prescriber being responsible for reporting any ADR to the TGA, the sponsor and HREC as the sponsor will not normally be actively monitoring the use of the product.

24.5.4   Personal importation

Individuals may personally import an unapproved therapeutic good by either bringing the goods with them as they enter Australia or arranging for someone outside Australia to send the goods to them. Personal importation may only be used for that person or their immediate family,

that is, the goods may not be given or sold to another person. Furthermore, the quantity that may be imported is restricted to 3 months' supply at one time and a total of 15 months' supply in a 12-month period at the manufacturer's recommended maximum dosage.

If a prescription medicine is to be imported in this way, the importer must have a prescription from a medical practitioner, unless the goods are being carried with the person.

Certain medicines may not be imported under the personal importation provisions, including drugs of abuse, such as narcotics, amphetamines and psychotropic substances, and anabolic substances, androgenic steroids and treatments for alcohol and drug addiction. There are also controls over certain other medicines including erythropoietin, growth hormones and gonadotrophins.

An individual cannot import injections that contain substances of human or animal origin (except insulin) without an SAS approval. The TGA considers that these injections represent a high risk from inadequately or improperly prepared materials (including a lack of sterility) and, therefore, approvals will only be granted to the supervising physician.

24.6   Presentation

Under the Therapeutic Goods Act, presentation means the way in which the goods are presented for supply, and includes matters relating to the name of the goods, the labelling and packaging of the goods, and any advertising or other informational material associated with the goods. The term label refers to the display of printed information on, or supplied with, the goods and their packaging, rather than the broader meaning applied in the United States, which includes approved uses of the product. Labels fall within the definition of advertising.

24.6.1   Standard for the Uniform Scheduling of Drugs and Poisons

The SUSDP lists drugs and poisons according to the recommended restrictions on their availability to the public. The categories of the SUSDP most relevant to medicines on the ARTG are:

- Schedule 8 – controlled drugs (e.g. strong analgesics, such as morphine)
- Schedule 4 – prescription only medicines
- Schedule 3 – non-prescription medicines for supply by pharmacists only
- Schedule 2 – non-prescription medicines the safe use of which may require advice from a pharmacist.

Schedules 5 and 6 of the SUSDP also include some therapeutic products, such as head lice preparations and some essential oils.

The National Drugs and Poisons Schedule Committee (NDPSC), established under the Therapeutic Goods Act, is responsible for the SUSDP, which includes requirements for signal headings, warning statements and safety directions to be included on the labels of medicines containing scheduled substances, and exemptions from scheduling gained by placement of specified warnings on labels.

Access to the substances listed in the SUSDP is usually restricted for a number of reasons, including toxicity, safety, and the risks and benefits associated with the use of the product.

The NDPSC decisions in relation to the SUSDP have no force in Commonwealth law. However, State legislation refers to or reflects the SUSDP (occasionally with some differences in some States) and may impose warning statements and other labelling and packaging requirements additional to those covered by Commonwealth legislation and associated Therapeutic Goods Orders (TGOs).

Medicines that are not scheduled in the SUSDP can be sold through any distribution outlet, such as a supermarket or health food store. Examples of medicines that are unscheduled include small packs of simple pain relievers, and most vitamins and minerals.

24.6.2 Labels and packaging

The labels of medicines are required to conform to TGO69: General Requirements for Labels for Medicines, except for goods solely for export or for use in clinical trials. The requirements include names and quantities of active ingredients, dosage form, batch number, expiry date, the registration or listing number (AUSTR or AUSTL number, respectively), identification of inactive ingredients, what labelling is adequate for special packs and small containers, and letter size and additional requirements in particular circumstances.

In addition, labels for medicines must conform to requirements for labelling described in the SUSDP. The 'Required Advisory Statements for Medicine Labels' (RASML) document has been established to enable the transfer of all mandatory label advisory statements from the SUSDP and the Therapeutic Goods Regulations to a new document, separate from, but linked to, TGO69.

Non-prescription medicines must, in addition, comply with TGO69A, which introduced performance-based labelling from 1 July 2004. Products with labels that have been designed in accordance with the industry code of practice, titled 'Labelling Code of Practice: Designing Usable Non-prescription Medicine Labels for Consumers', should achieve this aim. TGO69, TGO69A and RASML are available on the TGA website.

Certain medicines considered to have a high risk of poisoning children must be packaged in child-resistant packaging. The specified medicines and acceptable types of packaging are described in TGO33: Child-Resistant Containers. A replacement Therapeutic Goods Order, TGO65, is being phased in and will be in force from 1 July 2007.

Evaluation areas within the TGA responsible for the different categories of registered medicines make recommendations on the labelling of individual products as part of the registration process. Listed medicines are entered into the ARTG with a declaration from the sponsor that they meet the relevant standards and advertising requirements, and have acceptable presentations. Labels are not examined at the time of listing, but may be assessed following listing either as a result of a random review or if a problem arises.

24.6.3 Country of origin

Country of origin is generally not indicated on the labels of therapeutic goods marketed in Australia.

As prescription medicines are prescribed by a medical practitioner rather than purchased 'off the shelf' by the consumer, there is generally little incentive to convey origin information. Where manufacturers choose to do so, they must comply with State Fair Trading Acts, and the Commonwealth Trade Practices Act 1974.

Prior to December 1994, an 'essential character' test, was used to determine the validity of country of origin claims, in the context of Sections 52 and 53 (eb) of the Trade Practices Act 1974 in relation to false or misleading statements. However, in 1994 the Federal Court handed down a decision that effectively rejected the essential character test and created uncertainty about outcomes of future cases in this area.

In 1998, the Trade Practices Amendment (Country of Origin Representations) Act 1998 came into force. Manufacturers making unqualified statements about country of origin, such as 'Made in …' must be able to demonstrate substantial transformation and exceed a 50% production costs threshold. They, therefore, tend to use qualified claims, such as 'Made in Australia from local and imported ingredients', to ensure that labels are not misleading or deceptive.

24.6.4 Advertising

The Therapeutic Goods Act and Regulations, Trade Practices Act, and State legislation all contain sections relating to the promotion of therapeutic goods. In particular, the Therapeutic Goods Act specifies that advertising of a therapeutic good can only refer to the approved indications for that good.

Prescription medicines may only be advertised to healthcare professionals – they may not be advertised to consumers. Advertisements of prescription medicines directed at healthcare professionals are regulated under a self-regulatory Code of Conduct administered by Medicines Australia. First published in 1960, it includes standards for appropriate advertising, the behaviour of medical representatives, and relationships with healthcare professionals. The current edition (the 14th) of the Medicines Australia Code of Conduct is available from the Medicines Australia website. The Annual Report of the outcome of all complaints considered by the Code of Conduct Committee is also published on the website.

The Therapeutic Goods Advertising Code currently forms the basis for determining the acceptability of advertisements directed to consumers. All advertisements for therapeutic goods directed to consumers, published or broadcast in mainstream (designated) media, must be approved before publication or broadcast. The Minister for Health has delegated this responsibility to the Australian Self-Medication Industry and the Complementary Healthcare Council.

As part of the establishment of a single regulatory regime for therapeutic products in Australia and New Zealand, there will be a Trans-Tasman Advertising Scheme encompassing all therapeutic products. An Interim Advertising Council has developed, in consultation with all stakeholders, a Therapeutic Products Advertising Code (TPAC) which will become part of the legislative framework of the new joint agency. All advertising of therapeutic products, including advertising to health professionals and consumers in Australia and New Zealand will be legally required to comply with the TPAC. Industry Codes of Conduct, such as the Medicines Australia Code, which currently sets the standard for conduct of companies when engaged in marketing prescription medicines to health professionals in Australia, will be recognised as being part of the new advertising regime and enforceable by the joint regulatory agency. Advertising prescription medicines to consumers will continue to be prohibited in Australia but permitted in New Zealand under the new Trans-Tasman regulatory arrangements.

24.7 Patents

The Patents Act 1990 conveys a 20-year standard term of patent protection. From July 1999, holders of patents for a pharmaceutical substance have been permitted to apply for an extension beyond the standard term, as long as the application is made within 6 months of the first marketing approval of a pharmaceutical product containing the substance. The extension granted may be for no more than 5 years and will permit a maximum of 15 years protection after marketing approval. Sponsors of generic products containing that substance are permitted to undertake certain preparatory activities, known as 'springboarding', from the date the extension is granted.

The Commonwealth US Free Trade Agreement Implementation Act 2004 was passed on 13 August 2004 and received Royal Assent on 16 August 2004. It required amendment of the Therapeutic Goods Act to ensure that a generic manufacturer is not able to enter the market with a generic version of a medicine before a patent covering that product has expired. Applicants registering a generic medicine are required to provide a certificate to the Secretary of the Department of Health (effectively the TGA) stating either that they believe that the generic medicine would not infringe a valid patent or that they have given notice to the patent holder that they propose to market the generic medicine before the end of the patent term. These amendments commended when the AUSFTA came into force on 1 January 2005.

Prior to passing the Implementation Bill, the Federal Opposition successfully argued for certain further amendments to the Therapeutic Goods Act that imposes significant penalties on patent holders (up to $10 million) if they commence proceedings under the Patents Act 1990 against a generic manufacturer unless they are to be commenced in good faith, have reasonable prospects of success and will be commenced without reasonable delay.

24.8 Non-prescription Medicines and Complementary Medicines

Non-Prescription or OTC medicines are considered to be 'low risk' in comparison with prescription medicines. They are evaluated for quality, safety and efficacy by the TGA and the Medicines Evaluation Committee (MEC), in accordance with the 'Australian Regulatory Guidelines for OTC Medicines' 1 July 2003 (ARGOM) before they may be registered on the ARTG.

Complementary medicines are most frequently listed rather than registered, but this depends on the ingredients and claims made. The document 'Guidelines for Levels and Kinds of Evidence to Support Indications and Claims' was developed to assist sponsors in determining the appropriate evidence to support indications and claims made in relation to complementary medicines, sunscreens and other listable medicines, and is available from the TGA website. The Complementary Medicines Evaluation Committee (CMEC) provides scientific and policy advice relating to controls on the supply and use of complementary medicines, with particular reference to the quality and safety of products and, where appropriate, efficacy relating to the claims made.

A product's principal use and the claims made are also key determinants of whether it is deemed to be a medicine or a food, or a medicine or a cosmetic. Guidance on these distinctions are available from the TGA website.

24.9 Medical Devices

The Therapeutic Device Programe was established in 1984. In 1987, the Customs (Prohibited Imports) Regulations were amended to require the Department of Health's approval before devices in five 'designated' categories could be imported, and the Therapeutic Device Evaluation Committee (TDEC) was established.

The Commonwealth Government gradually introduced regulatory requirements for devices akin to those for medicines, especially where higher risks were associated to their use. These include formal guidelines for marketing and clinical trial applications, GMP requirements and an adverse event reporting scheme. However, TDEC is not as involved as ADEC in considering individual marketing applications.

When the Therapeutic Goods Act came into effect, most therapeutic devices were classified as listable goods. Registrable devices include implantable devices, biomaterials, intraocular lenses and fluids, intrauterine and other contraceptive devices, and drug infusion systems.

A MRA on standards and conformity assessment between Australia and the EC came into effect from 1999, covering eight industry sectors including GMP inspection and batch certification of medicinal products, and conformity assessment of medical devices.

The ECMRA applies to medical devices manufactured in the EC, Australia and New Zealand. It recognises the competence of designated conformity assessment bodies (CABs) in the EC to undertake conformity assessment of medical devices to Australian regulatory requirements, and the competence of the TGA to undertake assessment of medical devices for compliance with the requirements for certification (CE Marking) for entry onto the EC market.

Devices incorporating animal-derived tissues, radioactive materials, *in vitro* diagnostics and devices manufactured in other countries, such as the United States (even those devices that have CE marking) are excluded.

For registrable devices, the MRA included an 18-month transition period, to allow each party to gain confidence in the other's procedures and processes for pre-market assessment.

The Commonwealth Therapeutic Goods Amendment (Medical Devices) Act 2002 and the Therapeutic Goods (Medical Devices) Regulations 2002 came into effect from October 2002. Under the new harmonised requirements, most medical devices are classified into one of five classes – I, IIa, IIb, III and Active Implantable Medical Devices (AIMDs). All new medical devices are required to comply with the new requirements. All medical devices currently approved for use in Australia (i.e. those that were already on the ARTG as registered or listed devices) have until October 2007 to comply with the new requirements.

The TGA has also initiated development of two new regulatory frameworks for *in vitro* diagnostic devices (IVDs) and human tissues and cellular therapies, which will include *ex vivo* reagents, to be harmonised with international best practice. It is expected that implementation will occur from early 2006 for IVDs and mid-2006 for human tissues and cellular therapies.

Current details of the regulation of medical devices and diagnostics in Australia may be obtained through the TGA website.

References

1. Baume PE. A Question of Balance: Report on the Future of Drug Evaluation in Australia, Canberra AGPS 1991.
2. Sloan C. A History of the Pharmaceutical Benefits Scheme 1947–1992, Canberra AGPS 1995.
3. Australian Institute of Health and Welfare. Australia's Health 2004: The Ninth Biennial Health Report of the Australian Institute of Health and Welfare, Canberra AIHW 2004 (http://www.aihw.gov.au/publications/index.cfm/title/10014).

PART IV

Pharmacoeconomic and other issues

CHAPTER 25

25 | Economics of healthcare

CHAPTER 25

Carole Bradley and Jane R Griffin

25.1　Introduction

Economics is about the allocation of resources to production and the distribution of the outputs that result. Economics exists as a discipline because the resources available globally, nationally, regionally or to any industry, organisation or individual are finite. At the same time, it would appear that no amount of output could ever satisfy all human wants and desires. Taken together, this means that choices about the level of resources to allocate to various sectors of the economy or to the production of specific outputs within those sectors are unavoidable. Equally, choices about distribution cannot be escaped. Thus, economics is the science of making choices.

Health economics is the application of the discipline of economics to the topic of health. When viewed in this light, health economics becomes first and foremost a way of thinking based on the principles of scarcity and the need for choice. Although the techniques of economic appraisal (to be discussed later in this chapter) are the principal ways in which the discipline is applied, they are merely the 'toolkit'. The use of these tools without a proper understanding of the principles upon which they are based can be both ineffective and misleading.[1]

25.2　The Economics of the National Health Service

25.2.1　The key principles of health economics: output, cost and efficiency

25.2.1.1　The output of healthcare

Healthcare services are not normally provided for their own sake. Few people receive any direct satisfaction (utility) from consuming healthcare. Generally these services are demanded because of an expectation that they will have a positive impact on present or future health.

Consequently, the principal output of healthcare is 'health'. If health is viewed in the broadest sense of well-being then, if effective, interventions will make people better-off than they would have been in the absence of the interventions. In other words, effective interventions will normally increase the length or improve the quality life, or achieve some combination of the two.

The practical difficulties of viewing output in terms of health achieved is that health is notoriously difficult to define, measure and value. Broad definitions of health, such as a 'state of complete physical, mental and social well-being' given by the World Health Organisation, are unhelpful when trying to compare the effectiveness of alternative therapies or to compare the health gain from either of these with that of some wholly unrelated area of healthcare.

Consequently, in practice, intermediate measures of output are often used as surrogate markers for final (health) outputs. This is generally considered to be acceptable, provided there is an established link between the surrogate marker and health. Thus, the evidence that a reduction in the number of exacerbations requiring hospitalisation is a strong indication of improved health in asthma patients means that 'number of exacerbations requiring hospitalisation' is an acceptable output measure. The less well established the link between the surrogate marker and health, the less useful the marker.

25.2.1.2   The cost of producing health

By definition, resources are those things that contribute to the production of output. In terms of health services, the output 'health' is produced using resources, such as doctors, nurses, hospital beds, operating theatres, equipments and drugs. Money is needed in order to acquire these resources but, according to the above definition, money is not itself a resource as it only becomes productive if used to hire doctors, buy drugs, etc. Similarly, according to the above definition, resources can include the time of volunteers, informal care-takers or anything else that does not involve money payment but which, nevertheless, contributes to the production of health.[1]

A focus on resource use rather than money leads to a fundamental difference in how 'cost' is viewed in economics. Because resources are scarce, their commitment to any one use means sacrificing the benefits that could have been achieved if they had been used in an alternative way. In economics, cost is therefore equated to 'sacrifice', and the term 'opportunity cost' is used to emphasise the idea of an opportunity foregone. Money cost and opportunity cost may coincide – or they may not.

25.2.1.3   The basis on which resource allocation choices should be made – efficiency

Scarcity of resources means that it is not possible to do everything that we would like to do. Regardless of the level of resources currently being devoted to healthcare, it will always be possible to do more. This is due partly to the rapid development of new technologies, including pharmaceuticals, which allows more and more to be done each year, but also to the fact that resources devoted to healthcare incur opportunity costs elsewhere. The huge variety of human wants means that better health is not the only good thing that a society desires, and there are limits to how many other potential benefits society is willing to sacrifice in the pursuit of better health.

Scarcity means that resource allocation decisions cannot be avoided. If this is accepted, then it is clear that the basis on which these decisions are made should be explicit. Although economists do not claim to have the only – or even necessarily the best – answer for all choices that need to be made, at least economic criteria are explicit and hence open for criticism and debate.

The main criterion used in economic thinking is efficiency, which is about maximising the benefits from available resources. It concerns the relationship between inputs and outputs, that is, the most benefit for the least cost. Being efficient means getting as much health as possible from the available resources. Being inefficient means getting less. Viewed in this light, there is clearly an ethical justification for the pursuit of efficiency.

25.2.1.4   The acceptance of scarcity

A prerequisite to the use of health economics is an acceptance that no healthcare system can possibly do all things for all people. This means recognising explicitly that some form of prioritising is necessary and unavoidable. Such recognition has been slowly emerging over the past decade or so.

In the United Kingdom, annual expenditure on the National Health Service (NHS) is largely determined by government during public expenditure negotiations. Until recently, there has tended to be an implicit belief that this money (or the resources that this money could command) should be used to meet all health needs. Words such as rationing were avoided at all costs in official documents.

Whereas many in the United Kingdom would accept the need for rationing in the NHS, most would also wish to see additional resources made available. However, it is increasingly being recognised that although extra funding will ease the problem it cannot eliminate it. If need is believed to be the 'capacity to benefit from treatment', then clearly each new technological advance will increase need. Premature babies, born with low birthweights, that were previously incompatible with life only became 'in need' when the technology of neonatal intensive care allowed them to be saved. 'Need' is consequently a dynamic concept. As the pace of technological advance is unlikely to decrease, the gap between the need met (what is being achieved) and the total need (what could be achieved given infinite resources) will widen. Constantly increasing funding is, therefore, needed just to keep the gap from widening further, and as long as society has other needs (for education, defence, law and order, etc., as well as private consumption needs) closing the health needs gap completely will not be possible.

25.2.1.5 Prioritisation in operation

As a result of this growing acceptance of scarcity, explicit prioritisation is becoming an increasingly common feature of the British NHS. In the past decade, we have increasingly seen health authorities make clear choices about the kind of interventions that they will provide for their inhabitants. Many have gone so far as to remove certain procedures (e.g. tattoo removal, gender reorientation and fertility treatments) from the list of services that they will provide.

By the late 1990s, the issue of 'postcode prescribing' (patients being able to receive a particular treatment in one health authority but not if they resided in a neighbouring one) was a contributing factor in the election in Britain of the Labour government in 1997. The Labour party in their election manifesto promised to put an end to postcode prescribing, and since coming to power have endeavoured to establish measures to try and achieve this aim. One of these was the National Institute for Clinical Excellence (NICE; see Section 25.4.2). NICE was created to rationalise the system of care rationing in the NHS by using the evidence base on the clinical and cost-effectiveness of new products to determine whether the NHS would reimburse them. The government believed that this 'fourth hurdle' would control costs and eradicate postcode prescribing. In the event they were wrong about both these issues.

First, NICE's recommendations are as likely to increase expenditure as to reduce it. The purpose of their evaluations has been clearly stated as being to identify 'value for money', not whether the NHS could afford the intervention. Second, postcode rationing exists because the exercise of clinical discretion locally results in treatments being available in one place and not in another. As new products are accepted by NICE, local decision-makers have to decide, given their finite resources, which 'old' products and procedures to eradicate and which efficient products and services to provide. Local choices will inevitably vary, and as a consequence one form of postcode rationing will simply replace another.[2]

25.2.2 Health service costs

The earliest developments in health economics concentrated on measuring the cost of healthcare. The work of Abel-Smith and Titmus for the Guillebaud Committee in 1955[3] showed that rather than the NHS becoming too expensive, in reality the share that the NHS was taking up had fallen at a time when the population had grown. Since then the share of national income spent on the NHS has risen, but international comparisons, set out in Table 25.1, show that the United Kingdom remains a relatively low spender on healthcare services. As Figure 25.1 shows, this is partly explained by the strong positive correlation between total national income and the

Table 25.1 Total health expenditure as a percentage of GDP

	1975	1985	1995	1998	2002
Australia	7.0	7.5	8.2	8.6	9.1
Canada	7.1	8.3	9.3	9.3	9.6
France	6.8	8.3	9.6	9.4	9.7
Germany	8.8	9.3	10.2	10.3	10.9
Italy	6.2	7.0	7.9	8.2	8.5
Japan	5.6	6.7	7.2	7.4	7.8
Spain	4.7	5.4	7.0	7.0	7.6
United Kingdom	5.5	5.9	6.9	6.8	7.8
United States	7.8	10.0	13.2	12.9	14.6

Source: OECD Health Database

amount spent on healthcare. Clearly, richer countries can afford to spend more on healthcare services. However, as the diagram demonstrates, even on this basis the United Kingdom falls below countries with comparable incomes. The NHS in the United Kingdom, if nothing else, is relatively low cost.

25.3 Measuring the Value

The increasing use of pharmacoeconomic analyses as tools in health policy decision-making has highlighted the fact that the 'value' of a drug (or service) cannot be assessed solely on the basis of its acquisition cost. Rather, a drug's value should be considered relative to other therapies (or services) that are used for the same condition, and should include both the costs and clinical consequences associated with each. An important thing to remember when reading the following section is that all references to 'cost' refer to the total costs associated with a treatment pathway, and not solely the acquisition cost of the drug.

25.3.1 Types of analysis

The underlying premise of pharmacoeconomic analyses is that fiscal resources are scarce and that there is a need to make decisions based on

the relative value of different interventions in creating better health and/or longer life. There are five main analytical techniques used to evaluate the incremental value of products.[4] These are: cost–consequence analysis (CCA), cost-effectiveness analysis (CEA), cost–benefit analysis (CBA), cost-minimisation analysis (CMA), and cost–utility analysis (CUA). Although the identification and valuation of the cost component (numerator) of these analyses are similar, it is the identification and valuation of the consequences (denominator) that truly differentiate these analytic techniques. A brief description of each of these techniques follows.

25.3.1.1 Cost–consequence analysis

The CCA is the most disaggregated of all the economic analyses and places the greatest interpretive burden on decision-makers. The incremental costs and clinical consequences of the drugs being compared are simply listed, with no indication of the relative importance of any of their components (e.g. a CCA involving drugs used in stroke prevention would include drug costs, hospital costs, other costs, such as those associated with any special monitoring necessary, number of strokes observed, the number of deaths observed, the rate of clinically meaningful side effects, etc.). CCAs are often presented alongside other analytical techniques, such as CEAs.

25.3.1.2 Cost-effectiveness analysis

In CEA, the total cost and the total benefits, measured in terms of an efficacy parameter, associated with two or more treatment pathways are added, and the increment is calculated. The incremental costs are then compared (in a ratio) with incremental outcomes (as measured in physical or natural units). Physical and natural units can include both intermediate (surrogate) clinical endpoints (e.g. millimetres of mercury blood pressure reduction, changes in FEV_1) or final endpoints (e.g. deaths averted or life-years gained). In a study that assessed the cost per deaths due to pulmonary embolism averted, Hull and associates[5] reported that subcutaneous administration of

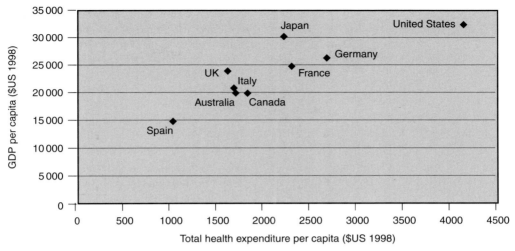

Fig. 25.1 Relationship between total health spending per capita and GDP per capita, 1998. *Source*: OECD Health Data 2001.

low-dose heparin starting 2 hours before surgery was a cost-effective approach to prophylaxis compared with the four alternative regimens. It should be noted that although this study is somewhat dated, it was included because a critical assessment of this chapter can be found in Drummond.[6]

25.3.1.3 Cost–benefit analysis

In CBA, monetary values are assigned to the health consequences so that the overall ratio is expressed completely in financial terms (e.g. pounds, dollars, euros). In principle, CBA allows policy- and decision-makers to make allocative comparisons and decisions across divergent sectors (e.g. healthcare and transportation). Notwithstanding this advantage, the valuation of health outcomes can be problematic (e.g. what monetary value do you assign to a life-year gained?) and therefore CBAs tend to be performed less frequently than other analytic types. Trollfors[7] examined the cost–benefit of infant vaccination with a conjugated *Haemophilus influenzae* type b (HIB) vaccine versus no vaccination (i.e. the 'do nothing' option). After taking into account the value of lives lost, the study author concluded that the widespread vaccination of infants for HIB was cost-effective and that it saved lives and reduced human suffering.

25.3.1.4 Cost-minimisation analysis

Cost-minimisation analysis are performed when the clinical outcomes (e.g. efficacy and safety) of the comparator groups are virtually identical and for all practical purposes can be considered to be equal. Because no decision can be made based on differences in the clinical endpoints, decisions are based on the incremental costs of the treatment pathways. Such was the case in a study that assessed the cost-effectiveness of treating proximal deep vein thromboses (DVT) at home with low molecular weight heparin versus standard heparin in hospital therapy. A cost-minimisation approach was chosen for this analysis because the results from a comparative clinical trial confirmed that there were no statistically significant differences in safety or efficacy between the two treatment groups. The study authors concluded that for patients with acute proximal DVTs, treatment at home with low molecular weight heparin was less costly than hospital treatment with standard heparin.[8]

25.3.1.5 Cost-utility analysis (CUA)

The CUA is a form of cost-effectiveness analysis in which the health outcomes are measured in terms of quality-adjusted life-years (QALYs) gained. The QALY is a measure that associates *quantity* of life (e.g. survival data and life expectancy) with *quality* of life, by amalgamating them into a single index. One QALY is equal to a year of full life quality. Because of its universal denominator that allows comparisons across divergent areas, CUA is a tool that can (in theory) be used by policy-makers to determine the best way to spend their limited resources. In an attempt to assess the value of introducing a rehabilitation programme to the standard care of patients with chronic respiratory disease, Griffiths and colleagues[9] assessed the incremental cost utility of the rehabilitation programme versus standard care. The results of the analysis indicated that the incremental cost of adding rehabilitation to standard care was £152 and the incremental utility was 0.030 QALYs per patient. The study authors concluded that the pulmonary rehabilitation programme produced cost per QALY ratios within the bounds considered to be cost-effective and would probably result in financial benefits to the health service.

In summary, there are five types of analysis that can be used to assess the incremental cost-effectiveness of a drug or service. The type performed is generally predicated by the therapeutic area being evaluated, the research question being addressed and the clinical data available. For example, whereas a CBA (which converts clinical effect into monetary terms) may not be considered (for ethical reasons) to be the best choice for oncology or HIV-related evaluations, a CUA (which takes into account both quality of life and survival duration) may be considered appropriate.

25.3.2 Measuring the benefits

When used in an economic milieu, the term 'benefit' can mean different things to different groups, even when referring to the same drug or service. For a person who suffers from migraines the benefit of a new effective, rapid onset anti-migraine therapy is that he or she may be able to alleviate the headaches more rapidly than with their current medication. Employers may benefit because their staff remain productive, and

accident and emergency departments may benefit because migraineurs do not end up in their waiting rooms seeking treatment.

The assessment of the clinical benefit of medicines is generally understood by clinicians, regulatory authorities and reimbursement authorities alike. Everyone instinctively understands the clinical benefit of decreasing a hypertensive patient's blood pressure to 130/90 or the benefit in reducing the number of strokes. However, in an era of increasing healthcare costs and funding decisions, there is a need not only to illustrate the clinical benefit of a drug, but to translate that clinical outcome into an economic benefit.

As previously mentioned, the actual acquisition cost of a drug or service should not be used in isolation to determine the value of a drug. Value should be assessed in an analysis that takes into account all consequences (both positive and negative) that result from use of the therapy. For example, if a therapy eliminates the need for surgery, the cost of the surgery would be eliminated from the overall treatment pathway. However, if the same therapy results in an adverse event that requires specific laboratory monitoring, the cost of the laboratory tests would be added into the treatment pathway. The accurate identification and valuation of resource items that result from the use of that therapy are extremely important components of economic analysis.

Cost identification often involves the development of a probability or decision tree of the therapeutic pathway that describes all relevant downstream events related to use of that therapy and its comparator(s). Once the relevant resources are identified and measured (e.g. number of physician visits, treatment of side effects, number and duration of hospital visits, etc.), local costs/prices can be applied to those resources to determine the overall cost of that intervention. The scope of the resources (and costs) included in an analysis is determined by the perspective (or intended audience) of the study.

Perspectives can be very broad (i.e. societal) or extremely narrow (e.g. the casualty department in a particular hospital), depending on the analytical question posed (e.g. is drug W a cost-effective option to drug X, in the treatment of disease Y, in hospital Z?). It should be noted that an economic analysis may be performed using several different perspectives, and that a drug may be considered cost-effective from one perspective and not when assessed from a different perspective. For example, drugs or services that affect or influence a patient's ability to work may be cost-effective from a societal perspective owing to a reduction in productivity losses; however, these drugs may or may not be considered cost-effective from the perspective of a healthcare system.

When assessing a drug from the societal perspective, the following resource items should be included. This list is provided as an example only, and should not be considered exhaustive.

- Health system items (e.g. drugs, physicians and other healthcare workers, hospitalisations, laboratory tests, surgeries, etc.)
- Social services items (e.g. home help)
- Spillover costs on other sectors (e.g. additional educational costs related to the proportion of children who survive neonatal intensive care units with learning disabilities)
- Costs that fall on the patient and family (e.g. loss of wages, transportation).

Analyses from the healthcare system perspective (e.g. Ministry or Department of Health) would include only those costs that are paid by that system.

Resource items can be identified and measured using several different techniques, each having both positive and negative attributes. These techniques include (but are not limited to) direct measurement in clinical trials,[10,11] direct measurement in activity-based costing exercises,[12] retrospective database assessment, direct measurement in disease registries and physician/healthcare professional estimation. The amount of economic data collected as part of clinical trials has increased substantially over the last few years, with a recent survey reporting the inclusion of pharmcoeconomics in up to 71% of both Phase III and IV studies.[13] It should be recognised that prior to regulatory authority approval, in most cases the only product-specific

utilisation data available for inclusion in economic analyses is collected during the Phase II and III clinical trials. Because of forced treatment compliance and protocol-driven physician visits and tests, such data may not necessarily reflect real-world resource utilisation patterns and real-world clinical benefit.

In summary, there is more to demonstrating the benefit of a drug than proving its clinical efficacy or looking at its acquisition cost. Such a demonstration involves translating both positive and negative clinical consequences into resource/fiscal consequences and then comparing these to other drugs or therapies commonly used for that indication. The identification, measurement and valuation of resource items associated with drug therapy are extremely important components of economic analysis, and attention should be paid to these areas when evaluating such studies. Economic analyses should be reported in such a manner that the reader can determine whether the treatment patterns and costs described are relevant to those in his or her country or area.

25.3.3 Evaluating economic analyses

In recent years there has been a dramatic increase in the number of studies published in the scientific literature that purport to be economic analyses. As with all areas of research, the quality of studies varies and care should be taken when reviewing published (and unpublished) economic analyses. Studies have shown that although improving over time, the general quality of many published economic analyses is still poor.[14,15]

As when evaluating the published medical literature, results from economic analyses should not be taken at face value. Claims of cost-effectiveness must be supported by assessments against appropriate comparators. Analyses comparing against placebo should be viewed with caution unless the drug or therapy in question is the very first treatment available for that disease. Reports should be detailed, clear and transparent. It is crucial that readers are able

Box 25.1   Ten questions to ask of any published study

1. Was a well-defined question posed in answerable form?

2. Was a comprehensive description of the competing alternatives given? (i.e. can you tell who? did what? to whom? where? and how often?)

3. Was the effectiveness of the programme of services established?

4. Were all the important and relevant costs and consequences for each alternative identified?

5. Were costs and consequences measured accurately in appropriate physical units (e.g. hours of nursing time, number of physician visits, lost workdays, gained life-years)?

6. Were costs and consequences valued credibly?

7. Were costs and consequences adjusted for differential timing?

8. Was an incremental analysis of costs and consequences of alternatives performed?

9. Was allowance made for the uncertainty in the estimates of costs and consequences?

10. Did the presentation and discussion of study results include all issues of concern to users?

Adapted from Drummond et al.[6]

to follow exactly what was done (with justification) throughout the analysis. Care should also be taken to determine that the type of analysis performed (e.g. CEA, CBA) corresponds with the analytical technique purported to be used in the study. Zarnke and colleagues[16] sampled the published literature to assess whether evaluations labelled as CBAs met the contemporary definition using CBA methodology. They reported that 53% of the 95 studies assessed were reclassified as cost comparisons because health outcomes were not appraised. Several authors have developed checklists that are useful when evaluating the overall quality of an economic analysis.[6,17] One of the best-known checklists is given in Box 25.1.

These checklists are useful tools that prompt the reader systematically to pose simple questions which aid in the critical assessment of the study. The first question prompts the reader to consider the overall validity of the research question. Did the investigators explain the problem

and why it has not been adequately addressed? Are both the costs and the consequences of the drug under investigation included? Is the analysis incremental? Is the viewpoint (or perspective) of the analysis stated, and is it valid? The research question is well defined if it states the perspective and alternatives and makes it clear that both costs and consequences were to be compared.

The second question addresses the issue of relevant treatment comparators and the justification for those comparators. When discussing the issue of comparators, pharmacoeconomic guidelines worldwide state that (at a minimum) the drug in question must be compared with the standard treatment or usual regimen. It should be noted that, unlike regulatory authorities, most decision-makers do not consider placebo to be a relevant comparator. When assessing the comprehensiveness of the description, the reader must decide whether the relevant alternatives have been compared. In order to do this, the reader must first identify the primary objective of the drug or service targeted for the evaluation.

An economic analysis does not measure the clinical-effectiveness of a drug or its comparator: rather, it reports the fiscal consequences associated with their use. Question three serves as a reminder to the reader that the clinical data included in the economic analysis should be based on appropriately conducted clinical studies (considering both methodological rigour and generalisability), and that the study report should establish the clinical effectiveness of the treatments under investigation.

Question four addresses one of the most important issues in the critical assessment of economic analyses, that is, the issue of identification and inclusion/exclusion of resources. As discussed in the previous section, the actual scope of the resources included should match the (stated) perspective of the analysis. It is important to note that it is not always possible to measure and value all the costs and consequences of the alternatives; however, a comprehensive list of the most important and relevant ones should be provided, along with justification for any major omissions. For example, a new drug has several side effects with similar rates of occurrence. One side effect results in a transient cough, another results in a gastrointestinal (GI) bleed. Given the scope of the total costs/resources involved, an economic analysis of this drug could probably justify non-inclusion of the treatment costs associated with the cough because such a cost would represent a very small percentage of overall costs and its exclusion would not change the overall conclusion of the analysis. However, because of the significant impact of even one hospitalisation, the costs associated with the GI bleed must be included.

Questions five and six address the actual identification, quantification and valuation of resources and costs. Resources previously identified as being relevant to the analysis have to be collected, measured and reported in appropriate units. For example, if blood tests are determined to be a resource that is important to the analysis, the actual number of each specific test performed must be recorded (e.g. five CBCs). Because of differing treatment regimens across regions or countries, it is extremely important that there is full disclosure of each resource identified, along with the frequency of use. Such 'resource dictionaries' allow the person critically evaluating the analysis to determine whether the treatment patterns in the analysis accurately reflect treatment patterns in their area. In addition, the unit cost/price for each resource should be provided, along with the source of each value. The provision of unit prices/costs allows the reader to determine whether the relative costs shown in the analysis are similar to those found in his or her area.

Economic analyses may evaluate the effect of drugs or therapies over several years, and because economic analyses operate in the present, the costs and consequences that occur in the future have to be adjusted to reflect their present-day values. This process is called discounting – discounting basically assumes that one unit of monetary (or health outcome) value is worth more today than it will be worth in the future, therefore, future units have to be reduced to reflect this expected decrease in value. Question seven addresses the issue of differential timing and whether discounting of future costs and consequences has occurred. As a rule of thumb, economic analyses that are less than or equal to 1 year in duration are not discounted, as it is assumed that the relative value of items would not change within a year. It should also be noted that discount rates used in analyses vary from country to country. Justification should be provided for the rate used in the analysis.

Question eight addresses another extremely important area in economic analysis – that is, whether the analysis is incremental. For an analysis to be a truly meaningful comparison it is necessary to examine the additional costs that one drug or therapy imposes over another, compared with the additional effects or benefits it delivers. As with the issue of choice of the comparator drug, most economic guidelines worldwide stipulate that an economic analysis must be incremental.

Economic analyses (models) are only as good as their ability to represent reality at the level needed to draw useful conclusions. Because all economic evaluations contain some degree of imprecision, there is value in varying the parameters or estimates that have the greatest degree of uncertainty (i.e. perform a sensitivity analysis). Sensitivity analyses should be performed on the estimates that have the greatest degree of imprecision in order to see if the overall results are dependent on that parameter.

The final question asks about the 'validity' of the conclusions drawn by the study authors. Were the conclusions based on some overall index or ratio of costs to consequences, and was the index interpreted intelligently? Did the study authors provide benchmarks to aid in the interpretation of the study, and was the robustness of the conclusions discussed in light of results of the sensitivity and/or statistical analyses? Was subgroup analysis undertaken where relevant? Were the results compared with those of others who have investigated the same question? Were the limitations of the study and the generalisability of the results discussed? Were other relevant factors in the decision to adopt the intervention discussed (e.g. distribution, ethics)? And

Incremental effectiveness of drug A compared to drug B

	More	Same	Less
More	??	XX	XX
Same	vv	??	XX
Less	vv	vv	??

(row label axis: Incremental cost* of drug A compared to drug B)

*   Cost refers to total expected expenditures that result from use of the drug.
vv   Generally speaking, products fitting this profile would be considered
        cost-effective.
??   Products fitting this profile may be considered cost-effective, depending
        on the magnitude of the ratio.
XX   Products fitting this profile are not considered to be cost-effective.

Fig. 25.2 Assessment of the incremental cost-effectiveness of treatment options. (Adapted from Reference 6.)

finally, did the authors discuss implementation issues?

In summary, in a critical assessment of an economic analysis, careful attention should be paid to the choice of analytical technique, the relevance of the comparator and the identification, measurement and valuation of resources, ensuring that the latter components are relevant to the stated viewpoint of the analysis. Published checklists are useful tools that aid in the assessment of these analyses.

25.3.4 Interpreting cost-effectiveness ratios

Once the 'validity' of an analysis has been determined, it is up to the reader to decide whether or not the drug or service is a cost-effective treatment option in their setting. The fact that the majority of economic analyses (especially those found in the published literature) are performed in a setting that is different from that of the reader emphasises the need for transparency in reporting. Readers need to be able to assess whether the treatment patterns, the

resources identified and the unit costs associated with those resources are applicable to their setting.

Figure 25.2 provides a simple 'rule of thumb' reference as to whether a drug could potentially be considered to be a cost-effective option in therapy.

Drugs that are more (or equally) effective than the comparator drug (or service) *and* which have total costs that are either equal to or less than those of the comparator drug are generally considered to be a cost-effective option. It should be noted that if a drug is both more effective and has lower overall costs than the comparator, it is said to *dominate* the alternative. Readers should be aware that in cases of dominance some study authors will not provide the cost-effectiveness ratio: rather, they will simply state that the comparator drug was dominated.

This somewhat simplistic explanation becomes more complex when we consider drugs that are both more effective and more expensive, as is the case with many (most?) new therapies. Above or below what fiscal threshold are drugs considered cost-effective? There is no simple answer to this question because funding decisions are often made in response to fiscal (budgetary) realities at that point in time, even when considering drugs that are deemed to be cost-effective.

Notwithstanding these issues, attempts have been made to identify and quantify acceptability thresholds.[18,19] Laupacis and associates[18] proposed that new therapies be classified into one of five grades of recommendation based on the magnitude of their incremental benefits (see Box 25.2).

In summary, the assessment of whether or not a drug or therapy is cost-effective is often somewhat subjective, depending on the financial burden that the decision-maker is willing to assume. These decisions cannot and should not be made in isolation: rather, the costs and consequences of the therapy under investigation must be considered relative to existing usual or gold standard practices.

25.4 Compulsory Economic Evaluation: The Ultimate Measure

The most extreme way of ensuring that economic evaluations are undertaken and that the results affect service delivery is to make economic appraisal a compulsory part of the process of

---

Box 25.2   Proposed Acceptability Threshold

Grade	Description of incremental cost-effectiveness ratio	Recommendations
A	The new therapy is either equally or more effective and less costly than existing therapies (i.e. is dominant)	There is compelling evidence for adoption and appropriate utilisation of the new therapy
Ba	The new therapy is more effective than the existing one and costs less than $20 000 per QALY gained	There is strong evidence for adoption and appropriate utilisation of the new therapy
Bb	The new therapy is less effective than the existing one but its introduction would save more than $100 000 per QALY gained	
Ca	The new therapy is more effective than the existing one and costs $20 000–100 000 per QALY gained	There is moderate evidence for adoption and appropriate utilisation of the new therapy
Cb	The new therapy is less effective than existing one, but its introduction would save $20 000–100 000 per QALY gained	
Da	The new therapy is more effective than the existing one and and costs more than $100 000 per QALY gained	There is weak evidence for adoption and appropriate utilisation of the new therapy
Db	The new therapy is less effective than existing one, but its introduction would save less than $20 000 per QALY gained	
E	The new therapy is less effective than or is as effective as the existing therapy and is more costly	Compelling evidence for rejection

Adapted from Laupacis *et al.*[18]

getting the intervention approved for practice. Several countries have made attempts to achieve this objective, with varying degrees of success. These countries include Australia, Canada, the Netherlands and the United Kingdom. For the purposes of this chapter we have chosen to focus on the approaches of the home countries of the two authors, namely Canada and the United Kingdom.

25.4.1 Canada

The year 1994 can be considered a landmark year with regard to health economics in Canada, with both the Ontario and the Canadian Coordinating Office of Health Technology Assessment (CCOHTA) guidelines being published during that year.[4,20] Since their introduction, the role of these guidelines has evolved. Initially used as guidance for research, their role has expanded to a point where all provinces mandate that pharmaceutical manufacturers include economic evaluations based on the principles set out in these guidelines in their drug formulary submissions.[21]

Although economic analyses are not required to obtain regulatory approval for pharmaceutical products in Canada, as previously mentioned, they are required by many of the provincial drug formularies and private drug plan insurers as part of their formulary decision-making process. The importance of inclusion in a formulary (especially the provincial formularies) to the success of new and existing drugs cannot be overstated. There is one basic 'truism' that exists in countries such as Canada, which is that unless your drug is a so-called 'lifestyle' drug (i.e. one for which patients are willing to pay out of pocket), provincial formulary inclusion is essential for its overall (commercial) success. This is because most physicians (especially general and family practitioners) will not prescribe a drug until it is included in their local province's formulary.

Although the requirement for economic analyses may be seen by many to be 'another hurdle' used to reduce access to new medicines, it should also be viewed as a means to demonstrate the value of the new medicine. Prior to the requirement for economic analyses, the value of a drug was often solely determined by its potential impact on the decision-maker's drug budget. The net result of this method of decision-making was the non-reimbursement of many highly effective (albeit) expensive drugs. Since the introduction of economic requirements, it has become harder for formulary decision-makers to reject a drug solely because of its acquisition cost and potential budgetary impact.

25.4.1.1 Common Drug Review

The publicly funded provincial drug formularies in Canada subsidise the cost of prescription drugs to people who are eligible for coverage under these programmes. With new drugs constantly emerging on the market, health policy-makers and drug plan managers need clear answers to the following questions: *Does a new drug provide a clinical advantage over existing products? Is it cost-effective? Will it benefit certain patient groups?*

Until recently, each province sought to answer these questions individually, using local expert formulary review committees that reviewed the clinical and cost-effectiveness evidence and made province specific listing recommendations. In an attempt to reduce this duplication of efforts, all Federal, Provincial and Territorial Ministers of Health (with the exception of Quebec) formed an alliance that was tasked with solving this issue. In September 2003, operating under the auspices of CCOHTA, the Common Drug Review (CDR) programme was launched. The CDR programme provides a forum that reduces the duplication associated with drug formulary reviews. Under this new programme, when a pharmaceutical company wants to apply for provincial drug formulary coverage, a single submission is sent to the CDR (as opposed to the previous process that involved sending out submissions to each province). This submission is then evaluated during a 6-month process by pharmacists, physicians and health economists. Results of these evaluations are then reviewed by the Canadian Expert Drug Advisory Committee (CEDAC). Based on this review, CEDAC provides a public recommendation regarding their listing recommendation for the drug under review. In addition to the 'list or do not list recommendation', the committee will make recommendations regarding reimbursement criteria/restrictions. These recommendations are then forwarded to each participating drug plan. It should be noted that a positive recommendation for listing from CDR does not guarantee formulary listing as each province will then make a listing decision based on their plan's mandate, priorities and resources – the incremental cost impact on the drug formulary is an important component of this decision. The health ministers associated with each participating drug plan have publicly committed that they will not reimburse a drug that receives a negative review from CDR – in other words, 'no means no, yes means maybe'. More information about the CDR can be found at the following website: http://www.ccohta.ca/.

25.4.2 The United Kingdom

25.4.2.1 The National Institute of Clinical Excellence

The NICE was established as a Special Health Authority in April 1999. In establishing NICE, the Labour government hoped to improve standards of patient care and reduce inequalities in access to innovative treatments (i.e. postcode prescribing).

The NICE was to achieve these aims by providing guidance to the NHS on the effectiveness and cost of clinical interventions. This would be done by appraising new and existing technologies, developing disease-specific clinical guidelines and by supporting clinical audit. Perhaps unsurprisingly, it is the work of NICE in the technology appraisals arena that has dominated its work programme since 1999 and generated the most controversy both within and outside the United Kingdom.

For the purposes of this chapter the focus will be on the technology appraisals. However, for details of other aspects of the institute's work and their procedures, the NICE website is a useful source of material (http://www.nice.org.uk/).

The scope for the technology appraisals was set out in the Department of Health discussion paper *'Faster Access to Modern Treatment: How NICE Appraisal will Work'*. This document clearly states that it would be 'desirable to cover all kinds of clinical intervention on an equal basis', and in particular all medicines and medical devices; all therapeutic interventions and programmes of care; products and processes to diagnose and prevent disease and population screening programmes. In the discussion paper it is openly acknowledged that the principles of technology appraisal will be easier to implement in some areas than others and the example of the medical devices industry, where the evidence base in terms of randomised clinical trials may be more limited, is cited. However, this does not fully explain why the vast majority of technology appraisals carried out to date have been on pharmaceuticals. Ease of undertaking an appraisal should not be a requirement for an assessment to take place.

The selection of a technology for appraisal is undertaken by the Department of Health and the National Assembly of Wales. This selection is based upon one or more of the following criteria.

1. Is the technology likely to result in a significant health benefit, taken across the NHS as a whole, if given to all patients for whom it is indicated?
2. Is the technology likely to result in a significant impact on other health-related government policies (e.g. reduction in health inequalities)?
3. Is the technology likely to have a significant impact on NHS resources (financial or other) if given to all patients for whom it is indicated?
4. Is the institute likely to be able to add value by issuing national guidance? For instance, in the absence of such guidance is there likely to be significant controversy over the interpretation or significance of the available evidence on clinical and cost effectiveness?

Details of the technology appraisal process itself can be found on the website but briefly, when a technology appraisal is referred from the Department of Health and the National Assembly of Wales all possible stakeholders are identified (stakeholders can be manufacturers, professional bodies and patient groups). They are then consulted on the scope of the appraisal. An independent review of the published literature is commissioned and submissions (both written and oral) are received from the stakeholders. The appraisal committee considers all this information and consults on its provisional views (appraisal consultation document) via the institute's website. The appraisal committee reconsiders it in the light of the comments and produces a final appraisal determination, which is again placed on the website. Stakeholders can appeal against it if they consider that the institute and the guidance have not fulfilled a number of criteria (details of the appeal process can be found on the website). Guidance is finally issued direct to the NHS.

The institute has set out quite clearly the data it wishes to see presented in a submission from a stakeholder. For each of the three main groups of stakeholders, patient/carer groups, healthcare professional groups, and manufacturers and sponsors, there is a separate set of guidelines. These may be accessed via the NICE website and should be essential reading for all those involved in the preparation of a submission.

The advent of NICE heralds a new era in which evidence about cost-effectiveness is formally required to help determine whether new interventions should be made available at public expense. However, definitive 'yes/no' decisions about market access have major implications for pharmaceutical companies. Economic information available at launch can only provide initial guidance about value for money. Further evidence on cost-effectiveness in real-world use will also be required.

25.4.2.2 The Scottish Medicines Consortium

The Scottish Medicines Consortium (SMC) was established in 2001 with the remit to provide advice to NHS Boards and their Area Drug and Therapeutics Committees across Scotland about the status of all newly licensed medicines, all new formulations of existing medicines and any major new indications for established products. The SMC process (full details of which are available on their website http://www.scottishmedicines.org.uk/) requires pharmaceutical companies to complete a new product submission form. The aim is to make a recommendation soon after the launch

of the product involved. The timescales involved usually require a submission to be made ahead of product launch. The entire process is extremely quick and it is possible for a decision to be made in 3 months from the manufacturer's submission. However, even a positive recommendation from SMC does not mean that the product will necessarily go onto formularies if other equivalent treatments already exist.

In 2004, the SMC made a total of 74 assessments of which 31 (42%) were considered 'acceptable for use', 24 (32%) were 'acceptable for restricted use' and 19 (26%) were 'not recommended'.[22]

25.4.2.3 The All Wales Medicines Strategy Group

The remit of the All Wales Medicines Strategy Group (AWMSG) is similar to the SMC in that its function is to provide advice to the Minister for Health and Social Services (Wales) in 'an effective, efficient and transparent manner on strategic medicines management and prescribing' (AWMSG website). It currently differs from the SMC in that while it only reviews newly licensed medicines these products should cost over £2000 per patient per year. However, it is anticipated that in the near future the AWMSG will be moving to a process and review strategy which will be essentially the same as that of the SMC. Further information about the AWMSG process can be found on their website (www.wales.nhs.uk/awmsg/).

25.5 Conclusion

We live in an era in which the value of medicines can no longer be assumed and the phrase 'evidence based' is no longer restricted to the realm of academics. The increasing financial burden on our healthcare systems has prompted decision-makers around the world to demand that the pharmaceutical industry provide proof of the value of new drugs being introduced into the market. Decision-makers in certain countries (e.g. Australia and Canada) have taken this requirement a step further by linking reimbursement approval to the provision of such evidence. Therefore, the provision of well-performed, credible analyses is vital for the future of present and future pharmaceutical products.

Most (if not all) companies within the pharmaceutical industry have recognised that such requirements are now a permanent part of doing business, and are developing internal health economics expertise, both on a global (corporate) and on a country-specific level. It should be noted that because of the multidisciplinary nature of this area of research, pharmaceutical company-based health economists cannot operate in isolation from the other disciplines within the company. It is therefore vital that pharmaceutical physicians understand the basic principles of health economic evaluations in order to work with the health economists in the development of high-quality analyses.

References

1. Cohen D. The impact of health economics on health policy, health services and decision-making. In: Salek S, ed. *Pharmacoeconomics and Outcome Assessment – A Global Issue*. Haslemere: Euromed Communications Ltd, 1999.
2. Maynard A. NICE mess? *Pharm Times* 2001;**22**.
3. Abel-Smith B, Titmus R. *The Cost of the National Health Service in England and Wales*. Oxford: Oxford University Press, 1956.
4. Canadian Coordinating Office for Health Technology Assessment (CCOHTA). *Guidelines for Economic Evaluation of Pharmaceuticals: Canada*. Ottawa: CCOHTA 1997 http://www.ccohta.ca/
5. Hull RD, Hirsh J, Sackett DL, *et al*. Cost-effectiveness of primary and secondary prevention of fatal pulmonary embolism in high-risk surgical patients. *CMAJ* 1982;**127**:990–5.
6. Drummond M, O'Brien B, Stoddart G, *et al*. *Methods for the Economic Evaluation of Health Care Programmes, 2nd edn*. Oxford: Oxford Medical Press, 1997.
7. Trollfors B. Cost-benefit analysis of general vaccination against haemophilus influenzae type b in Sweden. *Scand J Infect Dis* 1994;**26**:611–14.
8. O'Brien B, Levine M, Willan A, *et al*. Economic evaluation of outpatient treatment with low-molecular-weight heparin for proximal vein thrombosis. *Arch Intern Med* 1999;**159**:2298–304.

9. Griffiths TL, Phillips CJ, Burr SD, *et al*. Cost effectiveness of an outpatient multidisciplinary pulmonary rehabilitation programme. *Thorax* 2001;**56**:779–84.
10. Mauskopf J, Schulman K, Bell L, *et al*. A strategy for collecting pharmacoeconomic data during Phase **9**:II/III clinical trials. *PharmacoEconomics* 1996; 264–77.
11. Coyle D, Drummond MF. Analyzing differences in the costs of treatment across centers within economic evaluations. *Int J Tech Assess Health Care* 2001;**17**:155–63.
12. Doyle JJ, Casciano JP, Arikian SR, *et al*. Full-cost determination of different levels of care in the intensive care unit. *PharmacoEconomics* 1996;**10**:395–408.
13. DiMasi JA, Caglarcan E, Wood-Armany M. Emerging role of pharmcoeconomics in the research and development decision making process. *PharmacoEconomics* 2001;**19**:753–66.
14. Bradley CA, Iskedjian M, Lanctôt KL, *et al*. Quality assessment of economic evaluations in selected pharmacy, medical, and health economics journals. *Ann Pharmacother* 1995;**29**:681–6.
15. Iskedjian M, Trakas K, Bradley CA, *et al*. Quality assessment of economic evaluations published in *PharmacoEconomics*: the first four years (1992 to 1995). *PharmacoEconomics* 1997;**12**: 685–94.
16. Zarnke KB, Levine MA, O'Brien BJ. Cost-benefit analyses in the health care literature: don't judge a study by its label. *J Clin Epidemiol* 1997;**50**: 813–22.
17. Sacristán JA, Soto J, Galende I. Evaluation of pharmacoeconomic studies: utilization of a checklist. *Ann Pharmacother* 1993;**27**:1126–33.
18. Laupacis A, Feeny D, Detsky A, *et al*. How attractive does a technology have to be to warrant adoption and utilization? Tentative guidelines for using clinical and economic evaluations. *CMAJ* 1992;**146**: 473–81.
19. Holloway RG, Benesch CG, Rahilly CR, *et al*. A systematic review of cost-effectiveness research of stroke valuation and treatment. *Stroke* 1999;**30**: 1340–9.
20. Ontario Ministry of Health. Ontario guidelines for economic analysis of pharmaceutical products. 1994; http://www.gov.on.ca/health/english/pub/drugs/drugpro/economic.html
21. Glennie JL, Torrance GW, Baladi JF, *et al*. The revised Canadian guidelines for the economic evaluation of pharmaceuticals. *PharmacoEconomics* 1999;**15**: 459–68.
22. NHS Scotland. Scottish Medicines consortium Annual Report 2003–2004.

26 Controls on NHS medicines prescribing and expenditure in the UK (a historical perspective) with some international comparisons

John P Griffin and Jane R Griffin

26.1   Introduction

There is a well-defined system of pharmaceutical distribution in the United Kingdom that is controlled by a licensing system covering manufacture, wholesale and retail supply. For every medicinal product there has to be a product licence (PL) or marketing authorisation (MA), and the product may only be manufactured (or imported) and distributed for sale in accordance with that licence. In addition, manufacturers are required to hold a manufacturer's licence and those who deal in medicines wholesale must hold a wholesale dealer's licence. An important factor in the control of the manufacture of human medicines in the United Kingdom is the activities of the Medicines Inspectorate of the Department of Health (DoH). Premises are inspected before a manufacturer's licence is granted, and at regular intervals thereafter. Withdrawal of licences and, rarely, prosecutions can result, if standards are not maintained. In this respect the DoH gives detailed guidance regarding good manufacturing practice (GMP).

The distribution of medicines from manufacturer to retailer is mainly a private function, the wholesaler covering their costs and earning their profit through the margin allowed in the retail price. The wholesale dealer's licence, among other things, seeks to ensure adequate record keeping, in case a batch of medicines has to be recalled.

In the United Kingdom, prescriptions are required for all medicines supplied under the National Health Service (NHS) and for all prescription-only medicines. Prescriptions may only be written by a doctor or dentist registered in the United Kingdom.

The UK NHS is financed primarily out of taxation and is available to all permanent residents. Most people are registered with a general medical practitioner (under contract with the NHS and paid mainly on a capitation basis), who provides primary care and is the normal route of referral to hospital and specialist services, whether in the NHS or the private sector. A small minority of the population obtain some or all of their medical treatment privately, mainly through insurance schemes.

As part of primary care, general practitioners (GPs) are free to prescribe virtually any medicine they consider desirable for the patient, with the exception of medicines in certain therapeutic categories covered by the 1985 and 1992 Selected List restrictions (see below).

In some mainly rural areas the doctor may also dispense the medicines prescribed, but more usually the patient takes the prescription to a community pharmacist, also under contract with the NHS, who dispenses the medicines and claims reimbursement at predetermined rates. Unless they are exempt, patients pay a prescription charge at the time of dispensing.

From April 1985, within certain therapeutic categories, general medical practitioners have been restricted in the medicines they may prescribe under the NHS to those included in a limited list. The excluded medicines are generally those that can be purchased directly by the patient without a prescription, that is, minor analgesics, but also include some prescription items, such as benzodiazepine sedatives and tranquillisers. The principle underlying this economy measure is that, in theory, for the therapeutic categories concerned, the only medicines prescribable at NHS expense should be those that meet a real clinical need at the lowest cost. The list will remain under review by an expert advisory committee, the Advisory Committee on National Health Services Drugs. For medicines no longer available under the NHS but for which a prescription is necessary, it is open to the doctor to prescribe these and to the patient to pay for them privately. These measures have, for all practical purposes, introduced a 'need clause' into the British drug regulations.

The prescribing practices of general practitioners are monitored. After dispensing, the prescriptions are sent to one central point for authorisation of reimbursement, and thus it is possible to analyse each practitioner's prescribing habits and costs (PACT). A summary is sent to each practitioner, together with a note of the area and national averages. If a practitioner's costs are significantly different from the average this may be discussed with him or her by a doctor from the Regional Medical Service of the DoH.

26.2 The NHS and Community Care Act 1990

Until 1 April 1991, the key features for the procurement of medicines in the Family Practitioner (GP) Service (FPS) were as follows: GPs were independent contractors to the Family Practitioner Committees (FPCs) with freedom to prescribe without cash constraints. The FPCs reported directly to the DoH and were responsible for paying GPs for the provision of primary health services. A small group of Regional Medical Services Officers (RMSOs) reported directly to the DoH and were responsible for ensuring economical prescribing of medicines by GPs. The non-dispensing GP was not involved in the procurement of medicines. The pharmacist bought and dispensed the product and was reimbursed by the Prescription Pricing Authority (PPA) on behalf of FPCs. The Regional Health Authority (RHA) had responsibility for the FPS.

Under the system introduced by the NHS and Community Care Act 1990, the Government set an overall budget for GP prescribing, putting a cash restraint on the FPS medicines bill for the first time. The RHAs took over responsibility for the FPCs. Each RHA received a share of the overall drug budget and was responsible for allocating the budget to the newly named Family Health Service Authority (FHSA, formerly FPC). The FHSA set indicative amounts for medicines for each GP and was responsible for monitoring GPs' prescribing against that set amount.

In these circumstances, the main concern of FHSAs was to stay within their budget. They had little incentive to tackle the problem of under-prescribing, whereby GPs could give better patient care by spending more on medicines. Medical audit and FHSA visits were likely to be directed at high-spending practices rather than low-spending ones. After all, it must be borne in mind that one of the declared objectives of the original White Paper 'Working for Patients' was to exert 'downward pressure' on the NHS Medicines Bill. This Act operated in tandem with the other measures that have been taken since the inception of the NHS in 1948 to control NHS medicines expenditure.

26.3 The Problem of the Rising NHS Medicines Bill

The costs of health care are rising in all developed countries, and despite the fact that in the United Kingdom since the inception of the NHS in 1948, the cost of pharmaceuticals has been hovering at about 10% of the total, it has been the target of successive governments for savings. This is because health spending is made up of 70% fixed costs, which are difficult to change, and 30% variable costs. Pharmaceutical expenditure has historically been around one-third of the variable cost element and as such has been judged to be an obvious target for reduction and control. However, in the last few years there has been some increase in the proportion of the NHS budget spent on medicines, from 10.5% in 1990 to some 12% in 1998. Although there has been a significant increase in the average net ingredient cost of each prescription, the major cause of the rise has been an increase in the annual number of prescriptions, from some 500 million to 750 million for the United Kingdom over the last 10 years (OHE Compendium of Health Statistics 2004–2005 16th edition). Much of this increase has been due to the demands of an ageing population.

The methods used to control NHS medicines expenditure have been on both the supply side by attempting to reduce costs and the demand side by attempting to restrict volume. The 10 distinct measures taken by successive UK governments since 1948 to attempt to do this will be reviewed in chronological order.

26.4 Prescription Charges for NHS Medicines

Prescription charges were first introduced in the United Kingdom in 1952, and are collected by the pharmacist when a doctor's prescription is dispensed. The money collected is *not* offset against the cost of the medicines prescribed but is allocated to the cost of running the pharmaceutical services. (The prescription charges levied in 1994 funded only 6% of the cost of pharmaceutical services). Prescription charges should therefore be regarded as a revenue-raising exercise rather than a genuine co-payment for medicines dispensed.

In 1948, when the NHS was established by the then Minister of Health, Aneurin Bevan, during the Labour Government of Clement Attlee, all prescriptions were supplied free of charge. A charge of 1s 0d (£0.05) per prescription, irrespective of the number of items, was eventually introduced in 1952. Shortly after this the charge was changed to 1s 0d (£0.05) per item on the prescription.[1,2]

For a short period between 1965 and 1968, under the Labour government of Harold Wilson, prescription charges were abolished. In 1968, however, charges were reintroduced and the concept of exemptions was introduced.

In 1971, when the prescription charge was £0.20, the proportion of prescriptions that were exempted was 52% of the total; of these, 32% were for the elderly (men over 65 and women over 60) and 20% were for non-age related reasons. In 1995, 89% of prescriptions were exempt from charge, 45% on grounds of age, which means that 44% of prescriptions were exempt from charge for non-age related reasons.

The list of grounds for exemption from a prescription charge in the United Kingdom is extensive. The social grounds are low income, children below the age of 16 years, people in full-time education up to 19 years of age, pregnant women and women in the puerperium following either a live or still birth, old age (women over 60, men over 65, but since October 1995 men over 60) and war pensioners.

In addition, for social policy reasons, since July 1975 prescriptions for oral contraceptives have also been exempt from charges. The medical grounds for exemption from prescription charge are diabetes mellitus, diabetes insipidus, hypopituitarism, hypothyroidism, hypoparathyroidism, hypoadrenalism, myasthenia gravis, epilepsy and permanent fistula, for example colostomy, ileostomy. In addition, police personnel can claim back from their employing authority any prescription charge they incur.

There are illogicalities in the system, as a patient who is exempt from paying a prescription charge gets all medicines free, even if the prescription is for the treatment of an illness unrelated to the medical condition for which the exemption has been allowed, for example, a millionaire with diabetes mellitus would be exempt from a prescription charge for a bottle of aspirins, whereas a parent with a chronic medical condition not on the exemption list would have to pay a charge for medicines prescribed for his or her chronic condition, for example, rheumatoid arthritis, parkinsonism or hypertension. (This can to some extent be mitigated by purchase of an annual prescription season ticket, which for a flat sum covers the cost of all prescription charges for medicines and devices for the ensuing 12 months).

In the 25 years from 1979 to 2004, there were annual increases in the prescription charge, from £0.20 per item to £6.40 per item. The government has attempted to use this tax to raise revenue and as an unsuccessful deterrent to patients demanding a prescription at each visit to their doctor. Since about 85% of prescriptions are exempt from charge, this latter objective has been deemed to be ineffective. This has been largely due at times to high levels of unemployment – at times in excess of 3 million – during this period, which has also meant that the unemployed and their families have been exempt from prescription charges. In addition, unemployment also contributes to or is associated with ill health and demands for health care.[3]

In October 1995, the European Court of Justice in Luxembourg ruled on equal treatment for men and women regarding the age at which they should be exempted from paying an NHS prescription charge. Until then the exemption from the prescription charge had been linked to the state pensionable age of 60 years for women and 65 for men. Men are now exempt from the age of 60, at an estimated cost of £30 million per year in 1995 for lowering the age and £10 million for refunds for those men between 60 and 65 years who had paid for a prescription in the preceding 3 months.[4]

Another criticism of the current level of prescription charges is that in 1994, nearly 60% of prescribed medicines could either be purchased from a pharmacist for less than the prescription charge, or had a net ingredient cost (NIC) less than the prescription charge.

Both physicians and economists, have called for reform of the prescription charge exemptions for both social and medical conditions.[5–7] It has been pointed out that if the exemptions were reduced from 89% to 55% – the level that applied when they were first introduced – and the charge actually reduced to £2.50 per item, then £250 million per annum extra could be collected at the 1995 prescribing level of 500 million items per year.[5] Changes in the current system would not only have to be logical but politically acceptable, and there is no indication that the political will to introduce changes is growing.

Rationalisation of the exemptions from prescription charges and a variation of the current season ticket scheme linked to annual registration with a general practice have been proposed.[6,7]

In conclusion, charges for NHS prescriptions should be regarded as a tax rather than co-payment for the medicines prescribed. They have been inefficient as a deterrent on the demand side owing to the high level of exemptions. The application of the principle of exemption has led to legal action before the European courts on grounds of sex discrimination. Furthermore, a potential legal challenge exists on the grounds of social inequities and unfairness in selecting certain illnesses as worthy of exemption but not others, and is under consideration by patient pressure groups.

26.5 The Pharmaceutical Price Regulation Scheme

The prices of medicines sold to the NHS are controlled in the United Kingdom by the PPRS,[8,9] negotiated periodically every 5 to 6 years by the DoH with the Association of the British Pharmaceutical Industry (ABPI), for example in 1979, 1986, 1993 and 1999. The PPRS controls the maximum – *but not guaranteed* – profits that pharmaceutical companies make on the capital they have invested in plant for research, development and manufacturing for sales made to the NHS. (Capital employed by the individual companies is allocated between that devoted to NHS sales and that for non-NHS sales and exports).

The scheme was proposed in 1957, in an attempt by the pharmaceutical industry to stave off more draconian measures by the government of the day. It was known as the voluntary price regulation scheme (VPRS) that was neither voluntary nor a price regulation scheme. It was a profit regulation scheme. By the mid-1970s its name had been changed to the Pharmaceutical Price Regulation Scheme (PPRS), but it still retained a level of inaccuracy even until the 1993 agreement. However, the most recent negotiation between the DoH and ABPI in 1999 was in effect no longer a voluntary agreement because of the statutory powers and penalties behind it. This leaves a lot less room for negotiation and flexibility. The 1999–2004 PPRS, which is in accordance with the provisions of the Health Act 1999 Section 33, leaves no room for uncertainty. It changes the status of the PPRS and makes it more formulaic.[10]

The scheme applies to all companies supplying NHS medicines prescribed by medical or dental practitioners or nurses qualified to prescribe. Generic medicines, whose price is determined by the Drug Tariff, are excluded, as are the over-the-counter (OTC) medicines, and sales of medicines derived from private (non-NHS) prescriptions.

26.5.1 Annual financial returns

Each company with sales to the NHS of more than £1 million per annum has to supply financial information and those with sales of between £1 million and £25 million will have to supply full audited accounts. Companies with NHS sales greater than £25 million will have to submit a full annual financial return (AFR). Products with NHS sales of greater than £100 000 and £500 000 will have to be specifically identified. These annual returns cover the overall sales to the NHS and the costs incurred, such as research and development expenditure, manufacturing costs, general administrative costs, promotional expenditure and capital employed. (Details of *specific* produce costs or sales are not required.)

26.5.2 Profitability

The reasonableness of the maximum return on capital (ROC) earned by individual companies on home sales of NHS medicines is a matter for negotiation within a published range of 17% for level 1 and 21% for level 2, having regard to the nature and scale of the company's relevant investment and activities, and associated long-term risks.

26.5.3 Margin of tolerance

The allowable returns on capital will be associated with a margin of tolerance (MOT). Companies will be able to retain profits of up to 140% of the level 2 (21%) ROC target calculated by reference to level 2 allowances. Companies will not be granted price increases unless they are forecasting profits less than 50% of their level 1 (17%) ROC target calculated by reference to the level 1 allowances.

The MOT will not be available to a scheme member for any year in which it has had a price increase agreed by the Department. Where a scheme member exceeds its level 1 target profit for a year in which it has received a price increase, all profits above the level 1 target will be repayable. Where a price increase is agreed by the Department in the second half of a year, the Department may decide that the MOT will not be available to a scheme member for the year following the increase.

If the Department's assessment of an AFR shows profits in excess of the MOT, it will negotiate one or more of the following:

• price reductions, during the accounting year following that covered by the return, to bring prospective profits down to an acceptable level, on the basis of available forecasts;
• repayments of that amount of past profits that is agreed to exceed the MOT;
• a delay or restriction of price increases agreed for the company, or both.

26.5.4 Profitability of companies with small capital base in UK

Prior to 1999, PPRS companies with a negligible capital base in the United Kingdom had their profits assessed on a return on sales basis, which ranged from 3.75 to 4.25%.

Scheme members will now be able to include capital employed in their AFR on the basis of its inclusion in UK statutory accounts, by injection or by imputation in the transfer price. This will enable some companies that have been assessed as return on sales (ROS) companies under the 1993 scheme to be assessed as ROC companies under this agreement.

Alternatively, for scheme members whose AFR home sales exceed their average assessed home capital employed (excluding any capital imputation from the transfer price) by a factor of 3.5 or more, a target rate of profit will be set by dividing the ROC target rate by a factor of 3.5. The assessment of the returns of scheme members who elect for the ROS option will take account of the MOT on transfer price profit.

These changes in the 1999 PPRS have been introduced to enable the DoH to control transfer pricing arrangements, which ABPI has long resisted.

26.5.5   The export disincentive

Profits allowed on sales of prescription medicines in the United Kingdom are limited to a target return on assets related to UK sales.

Manufacturing assets used for NHS products are normally allocated between home sales to the NHS and exports pro rata to cost of sales. Costs must be computed on a fully allocated basis, that is, overheads are spread on a consistent basis between home and export products.

The effect of an increased proportion of exports is to allocate an increased proportion of the manufacturing assets to exports and, by definition, a reduced share to the United Kingdom. Thus the asset base on which target UK profit is computed is reduced.

At the same time an increased proportion of exports will allocate an increased proportion of annual fixed manufacturing overheads to export sales and hence a reduced proportion to UK NHS sales. The effect of this will be to reduce the cost of sales charged to the United Kingdom, with a consequent increase in profit.

The effect of these two factors constitutes a double disadvantage for any company wishing to increase its proportion of exports, as its UK NHS asset base is reduced and at the same time its national UK profits are increased.

For a company below its target rate of return this will reduce the price increase it can apply for, and if it is over its target return it will increase the amount it pays back to the DoH or the amount by which it will have to reduce prices.

This disincentive is particularly relevant for large tender business where multinationals typically have several manufacturing sources they can consider. Increasingly they are placing the business in countries where the impact of the domestic market is either cost neutral or has a cost-positive impact.

The export disincentive is becoming increasingly relevant in the context of the single European market, where the number of manufacturing facilities is being reduced by many multinationals and those that remain acquire substantial export business within the Community.

Under the most recent revision of the PPRS, the DoH will allocate 7.5% of the net value of each company's non-research and development fixed assets and its manufacturing infrastructure costs to its NHS sales before the balance is apportioned between home and export sales.[11]

26.5.6   Pricing of major new products

New products introduced following a major application for a product licence from the United Kingdom Licensing Authority may be priced at the discretion of the company on entering the market. This will have to take account of costs of research and development and the competition in the marketplace.

26.5.7   Promotional expenditure

Allocated expenditure by companies on product promotion is limited. The aggregate sales promotional allowance will be set as a percentage of *total* industry NHS sales. The distribution of the aggregate between individual companies is made on the basis of a formula agreed between the DoH and ABPI, for example, in the 1999 agreement promotional expenditure was allocated between three component parts.

1. Basic allowance of £464 000 per company.
2. A percentage of NHS sales allowance of 3% for level 1 and 6% for level 2.
3. An individual product servicing allowance of £58 000 for three products, £46 000 for a further three products, £35 000 for a further three products, and a £23 000 allowance for the 10th and subsequent products. These allowances only apply to products with NHS sales greater than £100 000 per annum. These figures, agreed in October 1999, are subject to adjustment based on level of inflation.

26.5.8   Research and development expenditure

Under the 1999 revision of the PPRS, each company's research and development expenditure allowance will be 20% (level 2) of the company's sales to the NHS for assessing profitability under the scheme [however, a maximum of 17% (level 1) will be allowed for assessing applications from companies seeking a price increase].

For a maximum of 12 in-patent active substances, each with an individual sales level to the NHS of £500 00 or more, a company will be able to add 0.25% of total NHS turnover to their PPRS research and development allowance for each such active substance. Thus a company could achieve a maximum allowance of 23% of NHS sales as its research and development allowance.[10]

26.5.9   The 2004 revision of the PPRS

In the summer of 2004, it was variously but widely rumoured that the pharmaceutical industry was facing a 6% price cut, or a 10% price cut phased over 10 years, or a 6% price cut over 2 years. In November 2004, when the details of the revised PPRS were announced for companies with sales to the NHS of over £10 million

per annum there was to be a 7.0% price cut. The price cuts were graded so that smaller companies with annual turnover of less than £1 million were exempt from price cuts, those with an annual turnover of under £3.5 million had a 3.5% price cut enforced. Companies with annual turnover of under £9 million had to cut prices by 6.3%.

The threshold at which companies had to submit AFRs was increased from £1 million to £5 million annual sale of goods to the NHS.

The allowable Research and Development allowance was increased by 5%.

The 2004 revision of the PPRS continued to allow companies launching a product that has been the subject of a major application for a MA to be priced at the discretion of the company (see Section 26.5.6). This freedom is cherished by the industry (see Section 26.5.10).

26.5.10   Assessment of the PPRS

The weaknesses of the PPRS are clear from the above outline. These are first, the export disincentive, which discourages pharmaceutical companies from sourcing export orders from UK manufacturing sites, so that multinationals with several alternative sourcing arrangements will avoid using the United Kingdom. This is clearly disadvantageous for both jobs and UK balance of payments.

The promotional formula and the capping of allowable promotional expenses operate in favour of the pharmaceutical companies with large existing sales to the NHS, and to the disadvantage of small companies or companies wishing to start up business in the United Kingdom.

The cap on allowable research and development costs to 20% of NHS sales is a disincentive to conducting research in the United Kingdom at levels above this. Small and middle-sized companies are penalised more than the pharmaceutical giants by this provision. It also favours companies who have products in patent being sold to the NHS 'but whose current pipe-line may be weak, no financial provision is made to encourage companies with a strong pipe-line to bring them forward more effectively other than an offer of "jam tomorrow". The position of companies marketing 'in-patent' products that have been licensed from other companies rather than their own research is unclear.

A number of non-UK European-based companies have criticised the rate of return on capital (ROC) on the basis that it favours companies with a large capital base in the United Kingdom and could therefore be regarded as an incentive to invest in the United Kingdom, which is contrary to European Union legislation.

The same group of companies have regarded the PPRS as discriminatory, as companies with a significant capital investment in the United Kingdom have their profits determined as return on capital base, whereas others that have a large investment in the European Union as a whole may operate in the United Kingdom as sales companies only. In this situation, these companies are treated on a percentage profit on sales, which are less favourable terms.

Some US-owned companies with large UK operations have been particularly vociferous in their criticism of the PPRS.

In terms of curtailing NHS expenditure on medicines the effectiveness of the PPRS is more difficult to assess: it has the power to restrict price increases and 'claw back' excess profits, and the opportunities for the DoH to enforce these powers has been increased in the 1999 revision of the PPRS. The amount of money 'clawed back' from companies each year has been insignificant in the past compared to the overall medicines expenditure, but this will change.

In general, the pharmaceutical industry would regard the freedom to price new products without awaiting the outcome of protracted negotiations – that can delay marketing for months or even years in some European Union countries – as a major advantage that counterbalances the system's many faults. This freedom was maintained in the 1999 revision of the PPRS.

In a recent assessment of various pricing and profit cost containment schemes Scherer(2004)[2] makes the point that most such schemes are a dis- incentives for innovation; his view of the PPRS is less unfavourable "less impairment of such incentives would be expected with a system such as that used in Great Britain under which

drug companies are allowed a generous profit rate of return on their assets, including capitalised research and development investments, even that system, however, baises the results against smaller but innovative drug companies,. . . .

Achieving the best trade-off between technological progress and the affordability of drugs remains a challenging goal."

26.6 The Drug Tariff and Reference Pricing

The Drug Tariff operated by the DoH was the first reference price system. Introduced in the early 1950s, the tariff price represents the price that the Prescription Pricing Authority operates on when reimbursing pharmacists and dispensing doctors for the cost of materials dispensed, whether drugs, dressings or devices. The average price for each generic formulation is determined as an average of the prices of the largest four or five manufacturers for each generic formulation (generics in the United Kingdom being generally unbranded). The community pharmacist who dispenses the prescribed generic is reimbursed at the tariff price. The pharmacist therefore does not purchase generic preparations from manufacturers whose price is above the tariff price. This effectively forces a downward price spiral for generics, as their tariff price was originally determined on a yearly basis but is now done as frequently as each month.

The prices of generic medicines must inevitably rise in the near future as manufacturers move to produce patient packs, which will be required to contain patient information leaflets. Under EC legislation, bulk containers will almost inevitably be phased out of production (except perhaps for hospital use).

The concept of the UK's Drug Tariff has been adapted into the various European Reference Price models, namely the grouping together of similar products usually containing the same active substance – or members of the same therapeutic group, for example, beta-adrenergic blocking agents – and then setting a maximum cost that the payer will reimburse for any product in that group. In Germany there are 435 therapeutic groups of products covered by their reference price scheme. Reference pricing has already been introduced into France, Netherlands, New Zealand and some provinces of Canada. Reference pricing fits well with the prevailing US belief that the key to capping health care expenditure is to offer financial incentives to patients. Reference pricing does just that, and in fact it has already been used in the States of Massachusetts and Delaware in their Medicaid Programmes.

Wherever reference pricing in any form has been implemented, the reference price becomes the effective market price.

26.7   Contract Purchase of Medicines from Cheap Sources

In the early 1960s, when Enoch Powell was Minister of Health in Macmillan's Conservative government, the DoH bought large quantities of tetracycline from Poland for NHS hospital use. This was found to be clinically ineffective and of substandard quality; a public outcry in the medical press followed. The cheap drugs exercise was not repeated, but bulk hospital purchase at competitive contract prices continues, and this leads to wide discrepancies between the hospital price and the price charged to prescriptions written in the primary healthcare sector.

26.8   The MacGregor Committee

In the late 1960s, the DoH set up 'The Standing Committee on the Classification of Proprietary Preparations' under the Chairmanship of Prof Alastair Gould MacGregor. The committee became known as the MacGregor Committee.

The committee classified products subject to monographs in the British Pharmacopoeia (BP), British Pharmaceutical Codex (BPC) and the British National Formulary (BNF) as 'Category M-Products'. Acceptable products other than monograph preparations were 'Category A-Products'. All other products were 'Category B-Products', these were considered less effective or more toxic than those in 'Categories M or A' or their efficacy was regarded as unproven.

In practice most combination products were regarded as undesirable and were relegated to 'Category B' status. The deliberations of the MacGregor Committee were published as 'Proplist' that went through regular editions. The pages referring to 'Category B-Products' had a black corner to the top of the page and they appeared in 'Proplist' after 'Category M and A Products'. Pressure was exerted by local health authorities on doctors not to prescribe 'Category B' preparations, and to use 'Category M Products' as a preference to both 'Category A and B preparations'. Category A products were usually branded medicines and were more costly than the generic monographed preparations. Proplist was an early attempt to encourage doctors to prescribe generically and cheaply, thus exerting downward pressure on prescribing costs.

26.9   Generic Substitution

In the United Kingdom, generic substitution was raised as a means of reducing the NHS medicines bill in the Greenfield Report of 1983, but was not implemented.

Generic substitution has however been implemented by a number of reimbursement authorities, both insurance based schemes as in the United States and nationally run health care schemes, for example, Sweden (introduced October 2002) and Finland (introduced 1st April 2003) both countries health care schemes claim very considerable savings of the order of 5% of national expenditure on medicines. Sweden is considering extending the scheme to lead to compulsory generic prescribing.

26.10   Enforced Price Reductions

In December 1983, the then Health Minister announced measures to cut industry profits and reduce the NHS medicines bill, then running at £1.3 billion per year, by £100 million. In November 1984, further measures were taken by reducing the ROC allowed under the PPRS from 25% to a range of 15–17%. ROC was raised to

17–21% in two stages under the 1986 renegotiation of the PPRS. In 1993, due to renegotiation of the PPRS the ROC was left unchanged, but a price reduction of 2.5% on pharmaceuticals was enforced. This was negotiated by ABPI to be achieved by a 2.5% reduction overall on each company's products, but could be modulated by taking a larger reduction on some products than on others. The alternative to price reductions was for companies to present the DoH with a cheque equivalent to 2.5% of its sales to the NHS, a solution accepted but not favoured by the DoH, as the money disappeared into Treasury Funds and so did not offer any real advantage to the Department.

In the 1999 PPRS negotiations, as a part of the agreement, the DoH imposed a 4.5% price reduction on sales to the NHS. This was equivalent to a loss of sales by the industry of £200 million. Because the 1999 revision of the PPRS permits companies to modulate these enforced price reductions across their product range, it could be expected that companies would do so in such a way that competition from parallel-traded products would be reduced, maximum price reductions being applied to those products that were currently being most affected by parallel trade. The 2004 PPRS enforced a 7% price cut on the pharmaceutical industry.

26.11   Limited or Selected Lists

The first limited list proposals were announced in November 1984 and proposed that a list of 31 products was adequate to meet 'all clinical needs in the seven therapeutic areas of indigestion remedies, laxatives, analgesics, cold and cough remedies, vitamin preparations, tonics and benzodiazepines'. In the event, when the proposals became operational in April 1985, the initial list had been expanded to 129 products, and later to 160 products. The remaining products reimbursable on the NHS could only be dispensed if prescribed by their generic as opposed to their brand names.

The saving from the original limited list exercise in its first year of operation was claimed to

be £75 million, and Ministers of Health over the next 10 years have been unable to quantify what, if any, the savings that took place in subsequent years, despite a series of parliamentary questions seeking this information.

If 10% of patients previously receiving prescriptions for an antacid were prescribed a H_2 antagonist such as cimetidine or ranitidine, this claimed savings would not have been achieved. The growth in the H_2 antagonist market was rapid at this time, and some of this growth must have been due to such escalation of prescribing.

In November 1992, the Secretary of State for Health announced the extension of the limited list procedure to further 10 therapeutic categories, namely antidiarrhoeals, appetite suppressants, treatments for allergic disorders, hypnotics and anxiolytics, treatments for vaginal and vulval conditions, contraceptives, treatment for anaemia, topical antirheumatics, treatments for ear and nose conditions and treatments for all skin conditions. These measures were announced despite repeated undertakings by a series of Conservative Secretaries of State for Health that the government had no intention of extending the limited list, and despite the fact that the DoH remains unable to quantify the savings achieved from the limited list exercise in the original seven categories.

The second limited list operation affecting 10 therapeutic categories announced in November 1992, became an exercise to reduce the prices of products to preconceived 'reasonable levels', these being delegated by Health Ministers to the Advisory Committee on NHS Drugs chaired by a Department of Health official and having outside members from the medical and pharmaceutical professions. The achievement of this exercise has been to inveigle a number of companies into agreeing price reductions in exchange for their product's continuing to be presentable in the NHS. This exercise has therefore amounted to a reference price system with a non-transparent method of fixing the price. It is therefore probable that the second phase of the limited list operation was in breach of the Transparency Directive (89/105/EEC). (The price reductions achieved under this exercise were not permitted to be counted towards the 2.5% overall price reduction imposed as part of the 1993 PPRS agreement).

The Advisory Committee on NHS Drugs, when examining oral contraceptives as one of the classes involved in the second phase of the limited list exercise, formed a preliminary position that the more expensive third-generation oral contraceptives should be precluded from availability on NHS prescription on grounds of cost. The outcry from women's groups, family planning practitioners and the medical profession was such that these proposals were never implemented.

26.12 The Indicative Prescribing Scheme and GP Fundholding

The indicative prescribing scheme (IPS) and GP fundholding were both introduced in 1991. These schemes were described by Whalley and co-workers in *PharmacoEconomics* in 1992 and 1995, including the various incentives offered to both fundholders and non-fundholders to reduce their prescribing costs by allowing a proportion of the 'saving' to be used on other projects in the practice.[3,4] Their effects were summarised by Whalley as follows:

The IPS has generally failed to control the rise in drug costs because of unrealistic targets, organisational difficulties (inducing the lack of adequate data to set budgets properly) and because there was neither incentive nor penalty to encourage compliance on the part of the general practitioner (GP). The IPS stresses cost containment, and makes little allowance for the consideration of quality or appropriateness of prescribing.

GP fund holding, in contrast, has reduced the rate of rise of drug cost in participating GP practices, although it has not actually reduced drug costs ... Although there is a commitment on the part of the government to encourage and make use of data about economic evaluations of drug therapy and other medical interventions, so far the emphasis has been exclusively on cost containment.

26.13 The Development of Primary Care Groups (PCGs)

The labour government elected in May 1997, committed itself to abolishing the concept of fundholding practices. This was not because of any fundamental disagreement with the concept of primary care commissioning *per se*, but rather because of the inevitable 'two-tierism' in service provision between fundholders and non-fundholders that resulted. In December 1997, the government produced its own White Paper entitled *The New NHS – Modern. Dependable*. When this document was first published it seemed to be signalling a new direction, but however much of the content could be described largely as a repackaging of existing (Conservative) policy, psychologically it felt different. The evolution of PCGs can clearly be traced back to the fundholding initiative begun in 1991. Halpen expressed the opinion of many NHS commentators when be wrote:

The Government use of PCGs as a mechanism for managing primary care is no more than a continuation of the policies of the previous government. Although GP fundholders revelled in their initial freedoms, it is clear that the move towards total purchasing (in whatever guise) was a clear precursor of PCGs.

However, the Labour government has clearly stamped its mark on PCGs and essentially the changed philosophy behind them. The following quote from the White Paper summarises some of their thinking as follows:

[PCGs] will have control over resources but will have to account for how they have used them in improving efficiency and quality. The new role envisaged for GPs and community nurses will build on some of the most successful recent developments, in primary care. These professionals have seized opportunities to extend their role in recent years ... Despite its limitations, many innovative GPs and their fund managers have used the fundholding scheme to sharpen the responsiveness of some hospital services and to extend the range of services available in their own surgeries. But the fundholding scheme had also proved bureaucratic and costly. It has allowed development to take place in a fragmented way, outside a coherent strategic plan.

It has artificially separated responsibility for emergency and planned care, and given advantage to some patients at the expense of others. So the government wants to keep what has worked about fundholding but discard what has not.

There are a couple of key differences between fundholding and PCGs. First, the unified budget. The White Paper did not set out much detail about the implications and consequences of a unified budget, but its importance should not be underestimated. Its implications for general practice and the NHS as a whole are probably only equalled by the clinical governance initiative (Royce). The government perceive the unified budget and clinical governance as the principal vehicle by which the long-standing problems of successive governments – cost constraint and medical practice variation – can be tackled. As Majeed and Malcolm (1999) writing in the *BMJ*, concluded:

The main factor behind the introduction of unified budgets is the belief that making general practitioners accountable for cost as well as the quality of health care will prove an effective method of tackling many of the problems facing the NHS.

Another key difference is that fundholding was always vulnerable to the charge that it was creating a two-tier NHS, but there is no opt out clause for general practices with the development of PCGs. Together with the unified budget, this means that resource decisions taken by one practice in a PCG have a direct impact on others. They are no longer islands, and practices have to be concerned with how well the PCG is doing as a whole and with any poorly performing practices within it, as the bottom line is that a PCG can be dragged down by them.

This helps to explain why GP involvement makes or breaks the Labour Government's reforms. It boils down to simple economics: GPs, principally through their referral and prescribing decisions, commit the vast majority of PCGs' (and consequently NHS) resources. Ultimately, under the new NHS reforms, it is the GP who will have to take responsibility for limiting (and in many cases reversing) the growth

in prescribing costs and hospital expenditure. In the ever changing world of NHS organisation there is the opportunity for PCGs to apply to become Primary Care Trusts (PCTs) that provides greater autonomy.

26.14 Changing the Legal Status of Medicines from Prescription only to Over-the-Counter Availability

Speaking at the Annual Pharmaceutical Conference on this matter in November 1993, Dr Brian Mawhinney, the UK Minister for Health, stated that self-medication 'encourages people to be more interested in and committed to their own health; [and] it empowers individuals with greater freedom to determine for themselves what medicines they will use'.

The theoretical advantages to the government are clear. First, by switching more medicines from being prescription only (POM) to over-the-counter (OTC) or pharmacy sale (P) and encouraging patients to self-medicate, it might be anticipated that the country's medicines bill would be reduced. Second, by encouraging patients to purchase their own medicine it obviates the need for a GP consultation, the main object of which was to obtain a prescription. However, although many items are available considerably cheaper than the prescription change, approximately 89% of prescription items were dispensed free. Thus, there is little incentive for most patients to purchase their medicines as OTC.

In June 1997, DGIII of the European Commission circulated a consultation document entitled 'A Guideline on Changing the Classification for the Supply of a Medicinal Product for Human Use'. The objective of this was to ensure that the route of sale will be the same in all member states of the European Union. The grounds for making decisions on route of supply are based on safety considerations, and for medicines for purchase directly by the patient stringent requirements for information are proposed. (The Commission document does not consider economic grounds for change of status).[15]

26.15   Encouragement to Prescribe Generically

A number of the above government initiatives have resulted in changing doctors' prescribing habits towards a greater use of generic formulations. Doctors are currently happier to prescribe generics as they have become more convinced of their quality. 'This was probably not unrelated to the fact that in the year ending August 1993, 80% of generic medicine sales in the United Kingdom originated from subsidiaries of the four multinational manufacturers Rhône Poulenc Rorer, Hoechst, Fisons and Ivax'.[16]

In 1993, the overall shape of the NHS market by value of products dispensed was as follows: generics accounted for 11% by value and over 41% by volume; prescriptions for medicines still within patent accounted for 26% by value but only 7% by volume. The bulk of the NHS prescription market, 63% by value and 52% by volume was made up of active substances that were out of patent but still being prescribed by brand name.

In 1993, 7% of the 530 million prescriptions dispensed were for products in patent. On the basis of these products coming off patent, the DoH believed that by the year 2000, 60% of prescriptions would be dispensed generically. In a reply to a question in the House of Commons, the Minister of Health stated that for 1994–1995 more than 50% of GP prescriptions dispensed in England and Wales were written generically, with GP fundholders writing 55.3% by generic name and non-fundholders 50.5%. However, the highest figure recorded by the Office of Health Economics was 46% for the year 1998.

Overall, the government policies have been directed towards cheap drugs and a drive towards generic prescribing, and this has been successful to a very large extent. It is, however, unfortunate that this policy has deterred doctors from prescribing newer in-patent products. In a study of the uptake of new chemical entities in 20 countries in 1993 a more rapid uptake expressed as percentage of all prescriptions filled with products marketed in the previous five years was seen in 17 countries compared to the United Kingdom.[17,18]

26.16   The National Institute for Clinical Excellence

It was repeatedly claimed throughout the 1990s that the uptake of therapeutic advances in the United Kingdom was sub-optimal.[19–21] In the year 1990, only 38% of the UK medicines bill was for products launched onto the market in the previous 20 years, thus 62% of medicines by value prescribed on the NHS were active substances introduced into the UK market earlier than 1970.[18] It was claimed that 'cost reducing philosophies and constraints have resulted in the under use of therapeutic advances in the United Kingdom'.[19]

In 1993, The Advisory Council on Science and Technology said 'that innovations, which are recognised as offering significant economic and/or quality of life advantages should be fully funded by the NHS'.[21] It was also pointed out that pressures by the DoH to prescribe cheaply was not the same as cost effective prescribing.[22]

In 1997, the British Government proposed in the White Paper 'The New NHS:Modern and Dependable' that the 'National Institute for Clinical Excellence' (NICE) should be established;[23] a proposal endorsed by Griffin.[24]

The NICE was established as a Special Health Authority in April 1999. In establishing NICE, the Labour Government hoped to improve standards of patient care and reduce inequalities in access to innovative treatments ('Postcode Prescribing'). NICE was to achieve these aims by providing guidance to the NHS on the effectiveness and cost of clinical interventions. This would be done by the appraisal of new and existing technologies, and developing disease specific clinical guidelines and supporting clinical audit. Perhaps unsurprisingly it is the work of NICE in the technology appraisal arena that has dominated its work programme since 1999 and generated most debate within and outside the United Kingdom.

Pharmaceuticals and other products and procedures are selected for appraisal by NICE, by the DoH and The National Assembly for Wales on the basis of the extent to which such technologies are likely to result in:

1. a significant health benefit, taken across the NHS as a whole, for example, might reduce hospital admissions or bed occupancy;
2. a significant impact on other health related Government policies, for example, a new approach to smoking cessation;
3. a significant impact on NHS resources, for example, in vitro fertilization (IVF).

NICE meets a medical need. If millions of patients are under-medicated something has to be done to rectify the situation. However, NICE guidance aimed at under medication and 'Post-code Prescribing' has added some £700 million to the NHS bill for pharmaceuticals.[25] By the end of 2004, NICE had issued more than 250 Appraisals and had announced the appointment of an Executive Director with the responsibility for implementing NICE appraisals.

It is inevitable that the increased cost of the NHS medicines bill will result in the introduction of measures elsewhere to curtail these rises. These measures have undoubtedly influenced the changes to the PPRS agreement of 2004, that is, enforced price reductions, and possibly changes to the operation of the Drug Tariff.

The Labour Prime Minister, Mr Blair, gave an under taking that the NHS would follow NICE guidance. Under the current rules the DoH and the Welsh Assembly must make funding available for implementation of NICE appraisals within 3 months of their publication, unless instructed to the contrary.

NICE recommendations will have a major impact on the direction of industry research and development. It will also have major impact on politicians and civil servants who run the NHS, since NICE recommendations have already had considerable cost implications.

The influence of the recommendations made by NICE are international and its decisions are closely monitored by other similar bodies (e.g. Canadian Coordinating Office for Health Technical Assessments (CCOHTA) and Pharmaceutical Benefits Advisory Committee (PBAC)) across the world and as a consequence the NICE website is achieving around 35 000 hits per day.[26] The

impact of their decisions can be seen most clearly in the uptake (or otherwise) in sales of appraised products and classes of drugs across the world.

26.17 The European Transparency Directive

Under Directive 89/105/EEC 'relating to transparency of measures regulating the scope of national health insurance systems'[27] all measures introduced by national governments to control expenditure on medicines will have to be compatible with EU rules.

The Directive applies to *any* national measures to control price or restrict the range of products covered by national health insurance systems. The specific articles of the Directive cover the various schemes operational within the Community and demands that objective and verifiable criteria are met in their implementation (see also page 532 Chapter 17.15.4).

The Transparency Directive does not lay down a requirement for harmonisation of procedures, nor does it imply a need to harmonise prices within the Community, and even if harmonisation of prices were achieved the Directive does not mean that there would be harmonisation of Health Service reimbursement.

As long as price differences exist between Member States of the European Community, parallel importing or parallel trading of medicinal products from Member States with lower prices to those with higher prices will take place. In fact, parallel trading in medicinal products could be called importation of another Member State's price constraints. The European Commission and Member States' Health Authorities not only condone but covertly encourage parallel trading. This creates considerable problems for pharmaceutical companies. The United Kingdom's DoH claws back a percentage of the reimbursement due from the PPA to reduce the windfall profits made by pharmacists buying cheaply from parallel traders.

At present, healthcare systems remain a national prerogative and are subject to national rather than European controls, but operated within the broad scope of the Transparency

Directive. However, future changes in the direction of greater pan-European harmonisation can be envisaged.

26.18   Supply of Controlled Drugs

Special arrangements apply to the prescribing of drugs of dependence in the United Kingdom under the provisions of the Misuse of Drugs Act 1971. Drugs controlled include cocaine, dipipanone, diamorphine (heroin), methadone, morphine, opium, pethidine, phencyclidine, lysergide (LSD), amphetamines, barbiturates, cannabis, codeine, pholcodine and certain drugs related to the amphetamines, such as chlorphentermine and diethylpropion.

For all controlled drugs, prescriptions must be signed and dated by the prescriber and the following particulars included in the prescriber's own handwriting: name and address of patient, form and strength of preparation as appropriate, total quantity in both words and figures and dose.

Only medical practitioners who hold a special licence issued by the Home Secretary may prescribe diamorphine, dipipanone or cocaine for addicts; other practitioners must refer the addict to a treatment centre. This stipulation only applies to addicts and does not preclude the prescription of diamorphine or cocaine for the relief of pain due to organic disease or injury (see also page 531 Chapter 17.15.3).

26.19   The British National Formulary

The greatest influence on doctors to prescribe well is the provision of high quality information. This has been achieved over the last decades by the British National Formulary BNF.

During the Second World War 1939–1945, it was imperative to exercise stict economy in prescribing, and in 1941, the then Minister of Health, Dr Charles Hill, introduced the National War Formulary as 'a select range of medicaments sufficient in range to meet the ordinary requirements of therapeutics for doctors in the community and in hospital'. After the creation of the NHS in 1948, the BNF was published jointly by the British Medical Association and the Pharmaceutical society of Great Britain, appearing first in 1949 and then every 3 years until 1979.

In 1975, a paper was produced by the Professional Head of Medicines Division of the Department of Health and Social Security (DHSS)(now DoH) for consideration by the Medicines Commission. It was proposed that a new style BNF should be produced because the DHSS was concerned that doctors were being unduly influenced by promotional material produced by the pharmaceutical industry that was leading to an escalating medicines bill for the NHS. It was suggested that the 'New Style BNF' should fulfill the following criteria:

1. No longer be selective but give information on all medicines available for prescribing by doctors.
2. Give information on the price of medicines.
3. Draw attention to certain unsuitable products.
4. Be compact enough to fit into the pocket.
5. Be kept up to date.

Initially it was proposed that the Medicines Commission should publish this, but neither the BMA or the Pharmaceutical Society were willing to surrender copyright.

Negotiations between the DHSS, the BMA and the Pharmaceutical Society started in 1975, during which the DHSS gave an undertaking to produce a new edition of the BNF every 6 months that would be distributed free to all doctors and pharmacists. A Joint Formulary Committee (JFC) was set up under Prof Owen Wade as Chairman with three members of the JFC appointed by the BMA, three by the Pharmaceutical Society and three by the DHSS. The role of the JFC was to commission therapeutic reviews of each body system disease areas from several experts and to produce an authoritative synthesis. The first new style BNF appeared on the 26th February 1981. It was comprehensive and drew attention to over 600 products in small print considered undesirable by the JFC. Pricing information was initially given in a price banding by letter, for example, A being 20p upto G for the most expensive course of treatment in excess of 450p. In later editions actual prices were given in a format that allowed strict comparisons between treatments.

Table 26.1 Healthcare expenditure and medicines expenditure as % GDP and comparative cost of medicines (OECD Health Data 2000 and 2001)

Country	Medicine prices according to a model in which 100 sets the average price for the year 2000	Pharmaceutical expenditure per head in US$ for the year 2000	Spending on healthcare as % GDP, in ( ) spending on medicines as % GDP	
Austria	98	277	8.2	(1.2)
Belgium	93	318	8.8	(1.4)
Denmark	101	174	8.4	(0.8)
Finland	95	221	6.8	(1.0)
France	94	446	9.3	(1.7)
Germany	114	283	10.3	(1.3)
Greece	71	—	8.4	(1.4)
Italy	93	307	7.9	(1.7)
Japan	—	361	7.5	(1.3)
Netherlands	108	224	8.7	(1.0)
Norway	94	183	8.5	(0.9)
Portugal	92	—	—	—
Spain	84	238	7.0	(1.5)
Sweden	103	220	7.6	(1.2)
Switzerland	133	214	10.4	(0.8)
United Kingdom	126	229	6.9	(1.1)
USA	—	451	12.9	(1.4)

In the 24 years since it was first published in the current format, editions have appeared every 6 months and it has become generally regarded as the most influential guide to good prescribing practice.

The BNF Joint Formulary Committee as of May 2005 will publish a Paediatric version annually. It will comprise monographs on safe and effective medicines for use in children, even if usage in children is not included in the summary of product characteristics (SPC).

26.20 International Comparisons

The effectiveness of various measures to contain expenditure on medicines in the United Kingdom can only be assessed in the context of the situation in other European Union countries. Table 26.1 gives data for the total expenditure on health care as a percentage of gross domestic product (GDP),

expenditure on medicines as a percentage of total healthcare spend, the national pharmaceutical industry's research and development expenditure in euro-millions, the general price index and the medicines price index nationally compared to a European price of 100, and the national pharmaceutical consumption per capita expressed as defined daily doses (DDD). These comparisons are based on Organisation for Economic Cooperation and Development (OECD) Health Data 2000.

The United Kingdom is seen from these figures to be a country with a comparatively low per-capita consumption of medicines, to have a high medicines price index and a strong pharmaceutical research base, therefore the various measures to contain medicines expenditure would appear to have had their greatest impact on the demand side.

Three of the four countries with the highest industry research and development spend have the highest medicines price index. France is the exception in this respect but has the highest per capita level of medicine consumption. Expressed in another way, the three largest spenders on health care as a percentage of GDP are France, Switzerland and Germany, which are three of the four countries where the pharmaceutical industry invests most in research and development.

Conversely, in countries where the population is relatively small and where individual consumption of medicines is low and pharmaceutical industry investment is also low, the government is able to enforce low prices for medicines. These countries are typified by the Netherlands, Norway, Finland and Denmark. Sweden, where there is significant pharmaceutical research, is atypical of the rest of Scandinavia and the medicines price index and medicine consumption are approximately the European average.

It would appear that the national governments' desires to impose draconian measures to control pharmaceutical prices and/or consumption is modulated by financial/fiscal necessity not to damage its national researched-based industry. Balancing such conflicting demands has been the key to the strength of the PPRS scheme as it was in its inception. It remains to be seen whether this has been retained or lost following the 2004 revision, which now has a legal basis.

The US Government believes that the various European pharmaceutical pricing systems constitute barriers to free trade. The ambition of the US Trade Representative is to liberalise pharmaceutical pricing systems anywhere in the world. A provision in the newly enacted Medicare reform legislation requires the US Trade Representative to use trade negotiations – specifically those recently involving Australia – 'as a way to achieve the elimination of Government measures such as price controls and reference pricing'. It is therefore paradoxical to see various US states Medicaid systems adopting both generic substitution and Massachusets and Delaware introducing reference price schemes. On 26th November 2003, Australia's Minister for Trade, Mark Vaile, pointed out that Australia's Pharmaceutical Benefits Scheme negotiated prices with pharmaceutical companies, just as health plans do in the United States. Mr Vaile stated that such negotiations were 'fundamental policy of our government and consecutive governments in Australia'.

References

1. Office of Health Economics. *Compendium of Health Statistics, 9th edn.* London: Office of Health Economics, 1998.
2. Prescription Pricing Authority Annual Reports, 1994/5.
3. Griffin JR. *The Impact of Unemployment on Health.* Briefing No 29. London: Office of Health Economics, 1993.
4. Warden J. Men can have free prescriptions at 60. *BMJ* 1995;**311**:1118.
5. Griffin TD. Patient contribution to the cost of prescribed medicines in Europe. In: Griffin JP, O'Grady J, Wells FO, eds. *The Textbook of Pharmaceutical Medicine, 2nd edn.* Belfast: Queens University, 1995;581–94.
6. Griffin JP. Increasing cost of medicines. *Lancet* 1993;**341**:1156–7.
7. Green DG, Lucas DA. *Medicard: A Better Way to Pay for Medicines.* London: Institute of Economic Affairs Health and Welfare Unit, Choice in Welfare No 16, 1993.
8. Department of Health. *The Pharmaceutical Price Regulation Scheme.* London: HMSO, 1993. Reference number Det DH 004643, 9/93.
9. ABPI. *A Guide to the Pharmaceutical Price Regulation Scheme (PPRS).* London: Association of the British Pharmaceutical Industry, 1993.
10. *The Pharmaceutical Price Regulation Scheme.* ABPI and Department of Health. www.doh.gov.uk/pprs.htm
11. Butler S. Will PPRS R&D benefits compensate for price cut in UK? *Scrip* 1999;**2457**:4.
12. Scherer F.M. The pharmaceutical Industry-Prices and Profits. *N Engl J Med* 2004;**351**:927–32.
13. Bligh J, Whalley T. The UK indicative prescribing scheme. *PharmacoEconomics* 1992;**2**:137–52.
14. Whalley T, Wilson R, Bligh J. Current prescribing in primary care in the UK. *PharmacoEconomics* 1995;**7**:320–31.
15. European Commission Director General III. *A Guideline on Changing the Classification for the Supply of a Medicinal Product for Human Use.* 12 July 1997.

16. Walker R. Generic medicines: reducing cost at the expense of quality? *PharmacoEconomics* 1995;**7**:375–7.

17. Griffin JP. *Is therapeutic conservatism cost effective prescribing?* European Federation of Pharmaceutical Industries Associations, General Assembly 1993 3rd session: Health Objectives and Cost Control.

18. Griffin JP. New drugs and their Impact on Health Care. Report on the Workshop New Provider Structures for Health insurance and Tax – Based Health care Systems, WHO Collaborating Centre for Public Health Research. Kiel 27–30th Nov 1995. Publ WHO, Keil, 1996;71–83.

19. Griffin JP, Griffin TD, The economic implications of Therapeutic conservatism. In: George Teeling Smith ed., *'Innovative Competition in Medicine: A Shumpetarian analysis of the Pharmaceutical industry and the NHS'*, London: Office of Health Economics Whitehall, 1991;85–96.

20. Griffin JP, Griffin TD. The Economic implications of Therapeutic conservatism. *J Royal College of Physicians of London* 1993;**27**:121–6.

21. Griffin JP. Therapeutic conservatism: more costly in the long-term. *PharmacoEconomics* 1995;**7**:378–87.

22. Advisory Council on Science and Technology. A Report on Medical Research and Health. London: Her Majesty's Stationary Office, 1993;28.

23. Department of Health. The New NHS: Modern and Dependable. London: CM3807 Publ Stationary Office Ltd., 1997.

24. Griffin JP. The Need for Pharmaco Economic Evaluations in the NHS. *PharmacoEconomics* 1998;**14**: 241–50.

25. Brown PJ. NICE is here to stay. *Scrip* 2004;**2917**.

26. Rawlins M. Treading a fine Line. *Scrip Magazine* October 2003;65–7.

27. European Commission Directive 89/105 EEC. Relating to transparency of measures regulating the scope of national health insurance systems. *Official Journal of the European Communities* 1989.

Recommended Further Reading

Halpen S. Doctoring the truth? Milburn lets the cats out of the bag. *Br J Health Care Mgt* 1998;**4**:426.

Majeed A, Malcolm L. Unified budgets for primary care groups. *BMJ* 1999;**319**:772.

Royce R. *Primary Care and the NHS Reforms: A Manager's View*. London: Office of Health Economics, 2000.

Moskowitz DB. Another rocky road for Pharma R&D. *Scrip Magazine* July/August 2004;37–39

Brown PJ. Fiddling with prices. *Scrip Magazine* June 2004;3–4.

Appendix 1
Declaration of Helsinki

The Declaration of Helsinki, one of the most significant documents on medical ethics, was adopted by the World Medical Association (WMA) at its 18th General Assembly in Helsinki in June 1964. The first revision of the document was endorsed by the WMA at its 29th General Assembly in Tokyo in 1975. The most significant addition in terms of the conduct of medical research was the requirement that independent committees (ethics committees) review research protocols. At the second revision adopted at the 35th WMA General Assembly in Venice in 1983 the changes were fairly minor. The third revision was adopted at the 48th WMA General Assembly in Somerset West, South Africa in 1996, which was amended at the 52nd WMA General Assembly held in 2000 at Edinburgh. This version introduced a number of changes including reference to the vexed principle of the use of placebos in therapeutic trials.

A very useful review of the history and development of the Declaration of Helsinki in the last four decades from its evolution from the principles enunciated in the Nuremberg Code of 1947 to the current version has been published in the *British Journal of Clinical Pharmacology*[1] and is recommended reading, it includes the texts of the various versions of the Declaration.

The current version of the Declaration is reproduced in the following page.

1. Carlson RV, Boyd KM, Webb D. The Revision of the Declaration of Helsinki: past, present and future. *Brit J Clin Pharmacol* 2004;**57**:695–713.

WORLD MEDICAL ASSOCIATION DECLARATION OF HELSINKI

Ethical Principles for Medical Research Involving Human Subjects

---

Adopted by the 18th WMA General Assembly
Helsinki, Finland, June 1964
and amended by the
29th WMA General Assembly, Tokyo, Japan, October 1975
35th WMA General Assembly, Venice, Italy, October 1983
41st WMA General Assembly, Hong Kong, September 1989
48th WMA General Assembly, Somerset West, Republic of
South Africa, October 1996 and the
52nd WMA General Assembly, Edinburgh, Scotland, October 2000

A. Introduction

1. The World Medical Association has developed the Declaration of Helsinki as a statement of ethical principles to provide guidance to physicians and other participants in medical research involving human subjects. Medical research involving human subjects includes research on identifiable human material or identifiable data.

2. It is the duty of the physician to promote and safeguard the health of the people. The physician's knowledge and conscience are dedicated to the fulfillment of this duty.

3. The Declaration of Geneva of the World Medical Association binds the physician with the words, 'The health of my patient will be my first consideration,' and the International Code of Medical Ethics declares that, 'A physician shall act only in the patient's interest when providing medical care which might have the effect of weakening the physical and mental condition of the patient.'

4. Medical progress is based on research which ultimately must rest in part on experimentation involving human subjects.

5. In medical research on human subjects, considerations related to the well-being of the human subject should take precedence over the interests of science and society.

6. The primary purpose of medical research involving human subjects is to improve prophylactic, diagnostic and therapeutic procedures and the understanding of the aetiology and pathogenesis of disease. Even the best proven prophylactic, diagnostic, and therapeutic methods must continuously be

challenged through research for their effectiveness, efficiency, accessibility and quality.

7. In current medical practice and in medical research, most prophylactic, diagnostic and therapeutic procedures involve risks and burdens.

8. Medical research is subject to ethical standards that promote respect for all human beings and protect their health and rights. Some research populations are vulnerable and need special protection. The particular needs of the economically and medically disadvantaged must be recognized. Special attention is also required for those who cannot give or refuse consent for themselves, for those who may be subject to giving consent under duress, for those who will not benefit personally from the research and for those for whom the research is combined with care.

9. Research investigators should be aware of the ethical, legal and regulatory requirements for research on human subjects in their own countries as well as applicable international requirements. No national ethical, legal or regulatory requirement should be allowed to reduce or eliminate any of the protections for human subjects set forth in this Declaration.

B. Basic principles for all medical research

10. It is the duty of the physician in medical research to protect the life, health, privacy, and dignity of the human subject.

11. Medical research involving human subjects must conform to generally accepted scientific principles, be based on a thorough knowledge of the scientific literature, other relevant sources of information, and on adequate laboratory and, where appropriate, animal experimentation.

12. Appropriate caution must be exercised in the conduct of research which may affect the environment, and the welfare of animals used for research must be respected.

13. The design and performance of each experimental procedure involving human subjects should be clearly formulated in an experimental protocol. This protocol should be submitted for consideration, comment, guidance, and where appropriate, approval to a specially appointed ethical review committee, which must be independent of the investigator, the sponsor or any other kind of undue influence. This independent committee should be in conformity with the laws and regulations of the country in which the research experiment is performed. The committee has the right to monitor ongoing trials. The researcher has the obligation to provide monitoring information to the committee, especially any serious adverse events. The researcher should also submit to the committee, for review, information regarding funding, sponsors, institutional affiliations, other potential conflicts of interest and incentives for subjects.

14. The research protocol should always contain a statement of the ethical considerations involved and should indicate that there is compliance with the principles enunciated in this Declaration.

15. Medical research involving human subjects should be conducted only by scientifically qualified persons and under the supervision of a clinically competent medical person. The responsibility for the human subject must always rest with a medically qualified person and never rest on the subject of the research, even though the subject has given consent.

16. Every medical research project involving human subjects should be preceded by careful assessment of predictable risks and burdens in comparison with foreseeable benefits to the subject or to others. This does not preclude the participation of healthy volunteers in medical research. The design of all studies should be publicly available.

17. Physicians should abstain from engaging in research projects involving human subjects unless they are confident that the risks involved have been adequately assessed and

can be satisfactorily managed. Physicians should cease any investigation if the risks are found to outweigh the potential benefits or if there is conclusive proof of positive and beneficial results.

18. Medical research involving human subjects should only be conducted if the importance of the objective outweighs the inherent risks and burdens to the subject. This is especially important when the human subjects are healthy volunteers.

19. Medical research is only justified if there is a reasonable likelihood that the populations in which the research is carried out stand to benefit from the results of the research.

20. The subjects must be volunteers and informed participants in the research project.

21. The right of research subjects to safeguard their integrity must always be respected. Every precaution should be taken to respect the privacy of the subject, the confidentiality of the patient's information and to minimize the impact of the study on the subject's physical and mental integrity and on the personality of the subject.

22. In any research on human beings, each potential subject must be adequately informed of the aims, methods, sources of funding, any possible conflicts of interest, institutional affiliations of the researcher, the anticipated benefits and potential risks of the study and the discomfort it may entail. The subject should be informed of the right to abstain from participation in the study or to withdraw consent to participate at any time without reprisal. After ensuring that the subject has understood the information, the physician should then obtain the subject's freely-given informed consent, preferably in writing. If the consent cannot be obtained in writing, the non-written consent must be formally documented and witnessed.

23. When obtaining informed consent for the research project the physician should be particularly cautious if the subject is in a dependent relationship with the physician or

may consent under duress. In that case the informed consent should be obtained by a well-informed physician who is not engaged in the investigation and who is completely independent of this relationship.

24. For a research subject who is legally incompetent, physically or mentally incapable of giving consent or is a legally incompetent minor, the investigator must obtain informed consent from the legally authorized representative in accordance with applicable law. These groups should not be included in research unless the research is necessary to promote the health of the population represented and this research cannot instead be performed on legally competent persons.

25. When a subject deemed legally incompetent, such as a minor child, is able to give assent to decisions about participation in research, the investigator must obtain that assent in addition to the consent of the legally authorized representative.

26. Research on individuals from whom it is not possible to obtain consent, including proxy or advance consent, should be done only if the physical/mental condition that prevents obtaining informed consent is a necessary characteristic of the research population. The specific reasons for involving research subjects with a condition that renders them unable to give informed consent should be stated in the experimental protocol for consideration and approval of the review committee. The protocol should state that consent to remain in the research should be obtained as soon as possible from the individual or a legally authorized surrogate.

27. Both authors and publishers have ethical obligations. In publication of the results of research, the investigators are obliged to preserve the accuracy of the results. Negative as well as positive results should be published or otherwise publicly available. Sources of funding, institutional affiliations and any possible conflicts of interest should be declared in the publication. Reports of experimentation not in accordance with the

principles laid down in this Declaration should not be accepted for publication.

C. Additional principles for medical research combined with medical care

28. The physician may combine medical research with medical care, only to the extent that the research is justified by its potential prophylactic, diagnostic or therapeutic value. When medical research is combined with medical care, additional standards apply to protect the patients who are research subjects.

29. The benefits, risks, burdens and effectiveness of a new method should be tested against those of the best current prophylactic, diagnostic, and therapeutic methods. This does not exclude the use of placebo, or no treatment, in studies where no proven prophylactic, diagnostic or therapeutic method exists.

30. At the conclusion of the study, every patient entered into the study should be assured of access to the best proven prophylactic, diagnostic and therapeutic methods identified by the study.

31. The physician should fully inform the patient which aspects of the care are related to the research. The refusal of a patient to participate in a study must never interfere with the patient physician relationship.

32. In the treatment of a patient, where proven prophylactic, diagnostic and therapeutic methods do not exist or have been ineffective, the physician, with informed consent from the patient, must be free to use unproven or new prophylactic, diagnostic and therapeutic measures, if in the physician's judgement it offers hope of saving life, re-establishing health or alleviating suffering. Where possible, these measures should be made the object of research, designed to evaluate their safety and efficacy. In all cases, new information should be recorded and, where appropriate, published. The other relevant guidelines of this Declaration should be followed.

Appendix 2
Code of Practice for the Pharmaceutical Industry

CODE OF PRACTICE
for the
PHARMACEUTICAL INDUSTRY
2003 Edition

Contents

In the Code of Practice, guidance on the interpretation of the Code appears as supplementary information to the text against a pale grey background.

Material in Appendix 2 was reproduced with permission from The Association of the British Pharmaceutical Industry.

CODE OF PRACTICE
for the
PHARMACEUTICAL INDUSTRY

Introduction

Promoting Health

The commitment of Britain's pharmaceutical industry to providing high quality effective medicines brings major benefits to both the health of the nation and the country's economy.

The National Health Service spends more than £8.6 billion a year on medicines, yet this represents less than 13 per cent of its total expenditure. Medicine exports are worth over £10 billion a year – the United Kingdom's third largest foreign exchange earner in manufactured goods. Nearly a quarter of the world's top 100 medicines were discovered in Britain.

Investment into researching and developing new products in the UK is now running at around £3.2 billion a year and each new medicine takes an average of ten to twelve years to develop before it is authorized for use by doctors, with no guarantee of commercial success. It is vital therefore that the pharmaceutical industry keeps the medical profession informed about its products and promotes their rational use.

The Association of the British Pharmaceutical Industry and its Code of Practice

The Association of the British Pharmaceutical Industry (ABPI) is the trade association representing manufacturers of prescription medicines. It was formed in 1930 and now represents about eighty companies which supply nearly 80 per cent of the medicines used by the National Health Service.

The ABPI Code of Practice for the Pharmaceutical Industry has been regularly revised since its inception in 1958 and is drawn up in consultation with the British Medical Association, the Royal Pharmaceutical Society of Great Britain and the Medicines and Healthcare products Regulatory Agency of the Department of Health.

It is a condition of membership of the ABPI to abide by the Code in both the spirit and the letter. Companies which are not members of the Association may give their formal agreement to abide by the Code and accept the jurisdiction of the Prescription Medicines Code of Practice Authority and about seventy have done so. Thus the Code is accepted by virtually all pharmaceutical companies operating in the UK.

The ABPI encourages pharmaceutical companies to try to settle inter-company disputes between themselves before submitting complaints to the Authority.

Ensuring High Standards

The aim of the Code of Practice for the Pharmaceutical Industry is to ensure that the promotion of medicines to members of the health professions and to administrative staff is carried out in a responsible, ethical and professional manner. The Code recognises and seeks to achieve a balance between the needs of patients, industry, health professionals and the general public, bearing in mind the political and social environment within which the industry operates and the statutory controls governing medicines.

Strong support is given to the Code by the industry with all companies devoting considerable resources to ensure that their promotional activities comply with it. Any complaint made against a company under the Code is regarded as a serious matter by both that company and the industry as a whole. A number of sanctions may be applied against a company ruled in breach of the Code.

Companies must ensure that all relevant personnel are appropriately trained in the requirements of the Code and have strict internal procedures under which all promotional material and activities are reviewed to ensure compliance with the Code and the appropriate legal requirements. The Code reflects and extends well beyond the legal requirements controlling the advertising of medicines.

The Code incorporates the principles set out in:

- the International Federation of Pharmaceutical Manufacturers Associations' (IFPMA) Code of Pharmaceutical Marketing Practices
- the European Federation of Pharmaceutical Industries and Associations' (EFPIA) European Code of Practice for the Promotion of Medicines
- the European Directive on the advertising of medicinal products for human use (92/28/EEC) (now consolidated as Articles 86 to 100 of Directive 2001/83/EC)

- the World Health Organisation's Ethical criteria for medicinal drug promotion.

Guidance on the interpretation of the Code appears as supplementary information to the text against a pale blue background.

Monitoring the Code of Practice

The Code is administered by the Prescription Medicines Code of Practice Authority which is responsible for the provision of advice, guidance and training on the Code as well as for the complaints procedure. Complaints which are made under the Code about promotional material or the promotional activities of companies are considered by the Code of Practice Panel and, where required, by the Code of Practice Appeal Board. Reports on completed cases are published quarterly by the Authority in its Code of Practice Review which is available on request.

Complaints about the promotion of medicines should be submitted to the Director of the Prescription Medicines Code of Practice Authority, 12 Whitehall, London SW1A 2DY, telephone 020-7930 9677, facsimile 020-7930 4554.

PROVISIONS OF THE CODE OF PRACTICE

CODE OF PRACTICE

Clause 1   Scope of the Code and Definition of Certain Terms

1.1 This Code applies to the promotion of medicines to members of the United Kingdom health professions and to appropriate administrative staff and to information made available to the general public about medicines so promoted.

The Code also applies to a number of areas which are non-promotional.

It does not apply to the promotion of over-the-counter medicines to members of the health professions when the object of that promotion is to encourage their purchase by members of the general public.

1.2 The term 'promotion' means any activity undertaken by a pharmaceutical company or with its authority which promotes the prescription, supply, sale or administration of its medicines.

It includes:

- journal and direct mail advertising
- the activities of representatives including detail aids and other printed material used by representatives
- the supply of samples
- the provision of inducements to prescribe, supply, administer, recommend or buy medicines by the gift, offer or promise of any benefit or bonus, whether in money or in kind
- the provision of hospitality for promotional purposes
- the sponsorship of promotional meetings
- the sponsorship of scientific meetings including payment of traveling and accommodation expenses in connection therewith

SUPPLEMENTARY INFORMATION

Clause 1.1   Scope of the Code

For the purposes of the application of the Code, the United Kingdom includes the Channel Islands and the Isle of Man.

The Code applies to the promotion of medicines to members of the health professions and to appropriate administrative staff as specified in Clause 1.1. This includes promotion at meetings for UK residents held outside the UK. It also applies to promotion to UK health professionals and administrative staff at international meetings held outside the UK, except that the promotional material distributed at such meetings will need to comply with local requirements.

Some of the requirements of the Code are not necessarily related to promotion. Examples include declaration of sponsorship in Clause 9.10, certain aspects of the provision of medicines and samples in Clause 17 and the provision of information to the public in clause 20.

The Code does not apply to the promotion of over-the-counter medicines to members of the health professions when the object of that promotion is to encourage their purchase by members of the general public as specified in Clause 1.1. Thus, for example, an advertisement to doctors for an over-the-counter medicine does not come within the scope of the Code if its purpose is to encourage doctors to recommend the purchase of the medicine by patients. Where the advertisement is designed to encourage doctors to prescribe the medicine, then it comes within the scope of the Code.

Advertisements for over-the-counter medicines to pharmacists are outside the scope of the Code. Advertisements to pharmacists for other medicines come within the scope of the Code.

CODE OF PRACTICE

- the provision of information to the general public either directly or indirectly
- all other sales promotion in whatever form, such as participation in exhibitions, the use of audio-cassettes, films, records, tapes, video recordings, radio, television, the Internet, electronic media, interactive data systems and the like.

It does not include:

- replies made in response to individual enquiries from members of the health professions or appropriate administrative staff or in response to specific communications from them whether of enquiry or comment, including letters published in professional journals, but only if they relate solely to the subject matter of the letter or enquiry, are accurate and do not mislead and are not promotional in nature
- factual, accurate, informative announcements and reference material concerning licensed medicines and relating, for example, to pack changes, adverse-reaction warnings, trade catalogues and price lists, provided they include no product claims
- measures or trade practices relating to prices, margins or discounts which were in regular use by a significant proportion of the pharmaceutical industry on 1 January 1993
- summaries of product characteristics
- European public assessment reports
- the labelling on medicines and accompanying package leaflets insofar as they are not promotional for the medicines concerned; the contents of labels and package leaflets are covered by regulations
- statements relating to human health or diseases provided there is no reference, either direct or indirect, to specific medicines.

1.3 The term 'medicine' means any branded or unbranded medicine intended for use in humans which requires a marketing authorization.

SUPPLEMENTARY INFORMATION

Clause 1.1   Journals with an International Distribution

The Code applies to the advertising of medicines in professional journals which are produced in the UK and/or intended for a UK audience.

International journals which are produced in English in the UK are subject to the Code even if only a small proportion of their circulation is to a UK audience. It is helpful in these circumstances to indicate that the information in the advertisement is consistent with the UK marketing authorization.

It should be noted that the Medicines and Healthcare products Regulatory Agency's guidance notes on advertising and promotion differ from the above in that they state that advertising material in professional publications intended for circulation, whether wholly or partly, in the UK (whether or not in the English language) must comply with UK legislation and with the UK marketing authorization for the product.

Where a journal is produced in the UK but intended for distribution solely to overseas countries local requirements and/or the requirements of the International Federation of Pharmaceutical Manufacturers Associations' (IFPMA) Code of Pharmaceutical Marketing Practices should be borne in mind.

Clause 1.1   Advertising to the Public and Advertising Over-the-Counter Medicines to Health Professionals and the Retail Trade

The promotion of medicines to the general public for self medication is covered by the Code of Standards of Advertising Practice for Over-the-Counter Medicines of the Proprietary Association of Great Britain (PAGB). The PAGB also has a Code of Practice for Advertising Over-the-Counter Medicines to Health Professionals and the Retail Trade.

CODE OF PRACTICE

1.4 The term 'health professional' includes members of the medical, dental, pharmacy and nursing professions and any other persons who in the course of their professional activities may prescribe, supply or administer a medicine.

1.5 The term 'over-the-counter medicine' means those medicines or particular packs of medicines which are primarily advertised to the general public for use in self medication.

1.6 The term 'representative' means a representative calling on members of the health professions and administrative staff in relation to the promotion of medicines.

SUPPLEMENTARY INFORMATION

Clause 1.1 Promotion to Administrative Staff

The provisions of the Code apply in their entirely to the promotion of medicines to appropriate administrative staff except where the text indicates otherwise. For example, the prescribing information required under Clause 4 must be included in promotional material provided to administrative staff but it is not permissible to provide samples of medicines to them as this is proscribed by Clause 17.1.

Particular attention is drawn to the provisions of Clause 12.1 and the supplementary information to that clause, which concern the appropriateness of promotional material to those to whom it is addressed.

Clause 1.2 Replies Intended for Use in Response to Individual Enquiries

Replies intended for use in response to enquiries which are received on a regular basis may be drafted in advance provided that they are used only when they directly and solely relate to the particular enquiry. Documents must not have the appearance of promotional material.

Clause 1.6 Representatives

'Medical representatives' and 'generic sales representatives' are distinguished in Clause 16.3 relating to examinations for representatives.

Clause 2 Discredit to, and Reduction of Confidence in, the Industry

Activities or materials associated with promotion must never be such as to bring discredit upon, or reduce confidence in, the pharmaceutical industry.

Clause 2 Discredit to, and Reduction of Confidence in, the Industry

A ruling of a breach of this clause is a sign of particular censure and is reserved for such circumstances.

CODE OF PRACTICE

SUPPLEMENTARY INFORMATION

Clause 3   Marketing Authorization

3.1 A medicine must not be promoted prior to the grant of the marketing authorization which permits its sale or supply.

3.2 The promotion of a medicine must be in accordance with the terms of its marketing authorization and must not be inconsistent with the particulars listed in its summary of product characteristics.

Clause 3   Marketing Authorization

The legitimate exchange of medical and scientific information during the development of a medicine is not prohibited provided that any such inform-ation or activity does not constitute promotion which is prohibited under this or any other clause.

Clause 3   Promotion at International Meetings

The promotion of medicines at international meetings held in the UK may on occasion pose certain problems with regard to medicines or indications for medicines which do not have a marketing authorization in the UK although they are so authorized in another major industrialised country.

The display and provision of promotional material for such medicines is permitted at international meetings in the UK provided that the following conditions are met:

- *the meeting must be a truly international meet-ing of high scientific standing with a significant proportion or attendees from outside the UK*
- *the medicine or indication must be relevant and proportional to the purpose of the meeting*
- *promotional material for a medicine or indica-tion that does not have a UK marketing author-ization must be clearly and prominently labelled to that effect*
- *in relation to an unlicensed indication, UK approved prescribing information must be read-ily available for a medicine authorized in the UK even though it will not refer to the unlicensed indication*
- *the name must be given of at least one major industrialised country (such as EU member states, EFTA countries, Australia, Canada, Israel, Japan, New Zealand, South Africa and the United States of America) in which the medicine or indication is authorized and it must be stated that registration conditions differ from country to country*

- *the material is certified in accordance with Clause 14, except that the signatories need certify only that in their belief the material is a fair and truthful presentation of the facts about the medicine.*

Clause 3.1 Advance Notification of New Products or Product Changes

Health authorities and health boards and their equivalents, trust hospitals and primary care trusts and groups need to estimate their likely budgets two to three years in advance in order to meet Treasury requirements and there is a need for them to receive advance information about the introduction of new medicines, or changes to existing medicines, which may significantly affect their level of expenditure during future years.

At the time this information is required, the medicines concerned (or the changes to them) will not be the subject of marketing authorizations (though applications will often have been made) and it would thus be contrary to the code for them to be promoted. Information may, however, be provided on the following basis:

(i) *the information must relate to:*

   (a) *a product which contains a new active substance, or*

   (b) *a product which contains an active substance prepared in a new way, such as by the use of biotechnology, or*

   (c) *a product which is to have a significant addition to the existing range of authorized indications, or*

   (d) *a product which has a novel and innovative means of administration*

(ii) *information should be directed to those responsible for making policy decisions on budgets rather than those expected to prescribe*

(iii) *whether or not a new medicine or a change to an existing medicine is the subject of a marketing authorization in the UK must be made clear in advance information*

(iv) *the likely cost and budgetary implications must be indicated and must be such that they will make significant differences to the likely expenditure of health authorities and trust hospitals and the like*

(v) *only factual information must be provided which should be limited to that sufficient to provide an adequate but succinct account of the product's properties; other products should be only be mentioned to put the new product into context in the therapeutic area concerned*

(vi) *the information may be attractively presented and printed but should not be in the style of promotional material-product specific logos should be avoided but company logos may be used; the brand name of the product may be included in moderation but it should not be stylized or used to excess*

(vii) *the information provided should not include mock up drafts of either summaries of product characteristics or patient information leaflets*

(viii) *if requested, further information may be supplied or a presentation made.*

Clause 3.2 Unauthorized Indications

The promotion of indications not covered by the marketing authorization for a medicine is prohibited by this clause.

CODE OF PRACTICE

Clause 4 Prescribing Information and Other Obligatory Information

4.1 The prescribing information listed in Clause 4.2 must be provided in a clear and legible manner in all promotional material for a medicine except for abbreviated advertisements (see Clause 5) and for promotional aids which meet the requirements of Clause 18.3.

The prescribing information must be positioned for ease of reference and must not be presented in a manner such that the reader has to turn the material round in order to read it, for example by providing it diagonally or around the page borders.

The prescribing information must form part of the promotional material and must not be separate from it.

4.2 The prescribing information consists of the following:

- the name of the medicine (which may be either a brand name or a generic name)
- a quantitative list of the active ingredients, using approved names where such exist, or other non-proprietary names; alternatively, the non-proprietary name of the product if it is the subject of an accepted monograph
- at least one authorized indication for use consistent with the summary of product characteristics
- a succinct statement of the information in the summary of product characteristics relating to the dosage and method of use relevant to the indications quoted in the advertisement and, where not otherwise obvious, the route of administration
- a succinct statement of the side-effects, precautions and contra-indications relevant to the indications in the advertisement, giving, in an abbreviated form, the substance of the relevant information in the summary of product characteristics

Clause 4.1 Prescribing Information and Summaries of Product Characteristics

Each promotional item for a medicine must be able to stand alone. For example, when a 'Dear Doctor' letter on a medicine is sent in the same envelope as a brochure about the same medicine, each item has to include the prescribing information. It does not suffice to have the prescribing information on only one of the items. The inclusion of a summary of product characteristics moreover does not suffice to conform with the provisions of this clause.

The prescribing information must be consistent with the summary of product characteristics for the medicine.

Clause 4.1 legibility of prescribing information

The prescribing information is the essential information which must be provided in promotional material. It follows therefore that the information must be given in a clear and legible manner which assists readability.

Legibility is not simply a question of type size. The following recommendations will help to achieve clarity:

- *type size should be such that a lower case letter 'x' is no less than 1 mm in height*
- *lines should be no more than 100 characters in length, including spaces*
- *sufficient spaces should be allowed between lines to facilitate easy reading*
- *a clear style of type should be used*
- *there should be adequate contrast between the colour of the text and the background*
- *dark print on a light background is preferable*
- *emboldening headings and starting each section on a new line aids legibility.*

CODE OF PRACTICE

- any warning issued by the Medicines Commission, the Committee on Safety of Medicines or the licensing authority, which is required to be included in advertisements
- the cost (excluding VAT) of either a specified package of the medicine to which the advertisement relates, or a specified quantity or recommended daily dose, calculated by reference to any specified package of the product, except in the case of advertisements in journals printed in the UK which have more than 15 per cent of their circulation outside the UK and audio-visual advertisements and prescribing information provided in association with them
- the legal classification of the product
- the number of the relevant marketing authorization and the name and address of the holder of the authorization or the name and address of the part of the business responsible for its sale or supply.

The information specified above in relation to dosage, method of use, side effects, precautions and contra-indications and any warning which is required to be included in advertisements, must be placed in such a position in the advertisement, that its relationship to the claims and indications for the product can be appreciated by the reader.

4.3 In addition, the non-proprietary name of the medicine or a list of the active ingredients using approved names where such exist must appear immediately adjacent to the most prominent display of the brand name in bold type of a size such that a lower case 'x' is no less than 2 mm in height or in type of such a size that the non-proprietary name or list of active ingredients occupies a total area no less than that taken up by the brand name.

4.4 In the case of audio-visual material such as films, video recordings and such like and in the case of inter-active data systems, the prescribing

SUPPLEMENTARY INFORMATION

Clause 4.1   Electronic Journals

The first part of an advertisement in an electronic journal, such as the banner, is often the only part of the advertisement that is seen by readers. It must therefore include a clear, prominent statement as to where the prescribing information can be found. This should be in the form of a direct link. The first part is often linked to other parts and in such circumstances the linked parts will be considered as one advertisement.

If the first part mentions the product name then this is the most prominent display of the brand name and the non-proprietary name of the medicine or a list of the active ingredients using approved names where such exist must appear immediately adjacent to the most prominent display of the brand name. The size must be such that the information is easily readable. If the product is one that is required to show an inverted black triangle on its promotional material then the black triangle symbol should also appear adjacent to the product name. That is not, however, a requirement of the code (see supplementary information to Clause 4.3). The requirement of Clause 10 that promotional material and activities should not be disguised should also be borne in mind.

Clause 4.1   Advertisements for Devices

Where an advertisement relates to the merits of a device used for administering medicines, such as an inhaler, which is supplied containing a variety of medicines, the prescribing information for one only need be given if the advertisement makes no reference to any particular medicine.

Full prescribing information must, however, be included in relation to each particular medicine which is referred to.

CODE OF PRACTICE

information may be provided either:

- by way of a document which is made available to all persons to whom the material is shown or sent, or
- by inclusion on the audio-visual recording or in the interactive data system itself.

When the prescribing information is included in an interactive data system instructions for accessing it must be clearly displayed.

4.5 In the case of audio material, ie. material which consists of sound only, the prescribing information must be provided by way of a document which is made available to all persons to whom the material is played or sent.

4.6 In the case of promotional material included on the Internet, there must be a clear, prominent statement as to where the prescribing information can be found.

In the case of an advertisement included in an independently produced electronic journal on the Internet, there must be a clear and prominent statement in the form of a direct link between the first page of the advertisement and the prescribing information.

The non-proprietary name of the medicine or the list of active ingredients, as required by Clause 4.3, must appear immediately adjacent to the brand name at its first appearance in a size such that the information is readily readable.

4.7 In the case of a journal advertisement where the prescribing information appears overleaf, at either the beginning or the end of the advertisement, a reference to where it can be found must appear on the outer edge of the other page or double page spread of the advertisement in a type size such that a lower case 'x' is no less than 2 mm in height.

SUPPLEMENTARY INFORMATION

Clause 4.1 Prescribing Information at Exhibitions

The prescribing information for medicines promoted on posters and exhibition panels at meetings must either be provided on the posters or panels themselves or must be available at the company stand. If the prescribing information is made available at the company stand, this should be referred to on the posters or panels.

Clause 4.3 Non-Proprietary Name

'Immediately adjacent to . . .' means immediately before, immediately after, immediately above or immediately below.

It should be noted that in a promotional letter the most prominent display of the brand name will usually be that in the letter itself, rather than that in prescribing information provided on the reverse of the letter.

Clause 4.3 Black Triangle Symbol

Certain medicines are required to show an inverted black triangle on their promotional material, other than promotional aids, to denote that special reporting is required in relation to adverse reactions. This is not a Code of Practice or a statutory requirement.

The agreement between the Committee on Safety of Medicines and the ABPI on the use of the black triangle is that:

The symbol should always be black and its size should normally be not less than 5 mm per side but with a smaller size of 3 mm per side for A5 size advertisements and a larger size of 7.5 mm per side for A3 size advertisements:

- *the symbol should appear once and be located adjacent to the most prominent display of the name of the product*
- *no written explanation of the symbol is necessary.*

CODE OF PRACTICE

4.8 In the case of printed promotional material consisting of more than four pages, a clear reference must be given to where the prescribing information can be found.

4.9 Promotional material other than advertisements appearing in professional publications must include the date on which the promotional material was drawn up or last revised.

Clause 5 Abbreviated Advertisements

5.1 Abbreviated advertisements are advertisements which are exempt from the requirement to include prescribing information for the advertised medicine, provided that they meet with the requirements of this clause.

5.2 Abbreviated advertisements may only appear in professional publications i.e. publications sent or delivered wholly or mainly to members of the health professions and/or appropriate administrative staff. A loose insert in such a publication cannot be an abbreviated advertisement.

Abbreviated advertisements are not permitted in audio-visual material or in interactive data systems or on the Internet, including journals on the Internet.

5.3 Abbreviated advertisements must be no larger than 420 square centimetres in size.

5.4 Abbreviated advertisements must provide the following information in a clear and legible manner:

- the name of the medicine (which may be either a brand name or a generic name)

SUPPLEMENTARY INFORMATION

Clause 4.4 Prescribing Information on Audio-Visual Material

Where prescribing information is shown in the audio-visual material as part of the recording, it must be of sufficient clarity and duration so that it is easily readable. The prescribing information must be an integral part of the advertisement and must appear with it. It is not acceptable for the advertisement and the prescribing information to be separated by any other material.

Clause 4.9 Dates on Loose Inserts

A loose insert is not regarded for this purpose as appearing in the professional publication with which it is sent and must therefore bear the date on which it was drawn up or last revised.

Clause 5.2 Abbreviated Advertisements – Professional Publications

Abbreviated advertisements are largely restricted to journals and other such professional publications sent or delivered wholly or mainly to members of the health professions etc. A promotional mailing or representative leavepiece cannot be an abbreviated advertisement and an abbreviated advertisement cannot appear as part of another promotional item, such as in a brochure consisting of a full advertisement for another of the company's medicines.

Diaries and desk pads bearing a number of advertisements are considered to be professional publications and may include abbreviated advertisements for medicines. Similarly, video programmes and such like sent to doctors etc may be considered professional publications and an abbreviated advertisement may be affixed to the side of the video cassette or included on the box containing the video. The prescribing information must, however, be made available for any advertisement for a medicine appearing on audio-visual material or in an interactive data system or on the Internet, including journals on the Internet. Such advertisements cannot be deemed abbreviated advertisements.

CODE OF PRACTICE

- the non-proprietary name of the medicine or a list of the active ingredients using approved names? where such exist
- at least one indication for use consistent with the summary of product characteristics
- the legal classification of the product
- any warning issued by the Medicines Commission, the Committee on Safety of Medicines or the licensing authority which is required to be included in advertisements
- the name and address of the holder of the marketing authorization or the name and address of the part of the business responsible for its sale or supply
- a statement that further information is available on request to the holder of the marketing authorization or that it may be found in the summary of product characteristics.

5.5 In addition, the non-proprietary name of the medicine or a list of the active ingredients using approved names where such exist must appear immediately adjacent to the most prominent display of the brand name in bold type of a size such that a lower case 'x' is no less than 2 mm in height or in type of such a size that the non-proprietary name or list of active ingredients occupies a total area no less than that taken up by the brand name.

5.6 Abbreviated advertisements may in addition contain a concise statement consistent with the summary of product characteristics, giving the reason why the medicine is recommended for the indication or indications given.

SUPPLEMENTARY INFORMATION

Clause 5.5   Non-Proprietary Name

'Immediately adjacent to . . .' means immediately before, immediately after, immediately above or immediately below.

Clause 5.5   Black Triangle Symbol

Certain medicines are required to show an inverted black triangle on their promotional material, other than promotional aids, to denote that special reporting is required in relation to adverse reactions. This is not a Code of Practice or a statutory requirement.

The agreement between the Committee on Safety of Medicines and the ABPI on the use of the black triangle is that:

They symbol should always be black and its size should normally be not less than 5 mm per side but with a smaller size of 3 mm per side for A5 size advertisements and a larger size of 7.5 mm per side for A3 size advertisements:

- *the symbol should appear once and be located adjacent to the most prominent display of the name of the product*
- *no written explanation of the symbol is necessary.*

Clauses 5.4, 5.5 and 5.6   Abbreviated Advertisements – Permitted Information

The contents of abbreviated advertisements are restricted as set out in Clauses 5.4, 5.5 and 5.6 and the following information should not therefore be included in abbreviated advertisements:

- *marketing authorization numbers*
- *references*
- *dosage particulars*
- *details of pack sizes*
- *cost.*

CODE OF PRACTICE

There may be exceptions to the above if the information provided, for example the cost, of the medicine or the frequency of its dosage or its availability as a patient pack, is given as the reason why the medicine is recommended for the indication or indications referred to in the advertisement.

Artwork used in abbreviated advertisements must not convey any information about a medicine which is additional to that permitted under Clauses 5.4, 5.5 and 5.6.

Telephone numbers may be included in abbreviated advertisements.

Clause 6 Journal Advertising

6.1 Where the pages of a two page advertisement are not facing, neither must be false or misleading when read in isolation.

In a three page advertisement, neither the double page spread nor the preceding or succeeding single page must be false or misleading when read in isolation.

6.2 No advertisement taking the form of a loose insert in a journal may consist of more than a single sheet of a size no larger than the page size of the journal itself, printed on one or both sides.

6.3 No issue of a journal may bear advertising for a particular product on more than three pages.

Clause 6 Journal Advertisements

See Clause 4 and in particular Clause 4.7 regarding the requirements for prescribing information in journal advertisements.

A two or three page journal advertisement is one where the pages follow on continuously without interruption by intervening editorial text or other copy. Thus, for example, promotional material on two successive right and pages cannot be a single advertisement. Each such page would need to be treated as a separate advertisement for the purposes of prescribing information.

Similarly, if promotional material appears on the outer edges of the left and right hand pages of a double page spread, and the promotional material is separated by intervening editorial matter, then again each page would need to be treated as a separate advertisement.

Clause 6.2 Advertising on the Outside of Journals

Advertising such as cards stapled to a journal and 'wrap-arounds' must not have a greater surface area than that outlined for loose inserts under Clause 6.2.

CODE OF PRACTICE

Clause 6.3   Limitation on Number of Pages of Advertising

Advertisements taking the form of inserts, whether loose or bound in, count towards the three pages allowed by Clause 6.3. A loose insert printed on both sides counts as two pages.

A summary of product characteristics is permitted as an insert in addition to the three pages of advertising which is allowed.

Inserts and supplements which are not advertisements as such, though they may be regarded as promotional material, for example reports of conference proceedings, are not subject to the restriction of Clauses 6.2 and 6.3.

Clause 7 Information, Claims and Comparisons

7.1 Upon reasonable request, a company must promptly provide members of the health professions and appropriate administrative staff with accurate and relevant information about the medicines which the company markets.

7.2 Information, claims and comparisons must be accurate, balanced, fair, objective and unambiguous and must be based on an up-to-date evaluation of all the evidence and reflect that evidence clearly. They must not mislead either directly or by implication.

7.3 A comparison is only permitted in promotional material if:

- it is not misleading
- medicines or services for the same needs or intended for the same purpose are compared
- one or more material, relevant, substantiable and representative features are compared
- no confusion is created between the medicine advertised and that of a competitor or between the advertiser's trade marks, trade names, other distinguishing marks and those of a competitor

Clause 7   General

The application of this clause is not limited to information or claims of a medical or scientific nature. It includes inter alia, information or claims relating to pricing and market share. Thus, for example, any claim relating to the market share of a product must be substantiated without delay upon request as required under Clause 7.5.

It should be borne in mind that claims in promotional material must be capable of standing alone as regards accuracy etc. In general claims should not be qualified by the use of footnotes and the like.

Clause 7.2   Misleading Information, Claims and Comparisons

The following are areas where particular care should be taken by companies:

- *claims for superior potency in relation to weight are generally meaningless and best avoided unless they can be linked with some practical advantage, for example, reduction in side-effects or cost of effective dosage.*

CODE OF PRACTICE

- the trade marks, trade names, other distinguishing marks, medicines, services, activities or circumstances of a competitor are not discredited or denigrated
- no unfair advantage is taken of the reputation of a trade mark, trade name or other distinguishing marks of a competitor
- medicines or services are not presented as imitations or replicas of goods or services bearing a competitor's trade mark or trade name.

7.4 Any information, claim or comparison must be capable of substantiation.

7.5 Substantiation for any information, claim or comparison must be provided without delay at the request of members of the health professions or appropriate administrative staff. It need not be provided, however, in relation to the validity of indications approved in the marketing authorization.

7.6 When promotional material refers to published studies, clear references must be given.

7.7 When promotional material refers to data on file, the relevant part of this data must be provided without delay at the request of members of the health professions or appropriate administrative staff.

7.8 All artwork including illustrations, graphs and tables must conform to the letter and spirit of the Code. Graphs and tables must be presented in such a way as to give a clear, fair, balanced view of the matters with which they deal, and must not be included unless they are relevant to the claims or comparisons being made.

7.9 Information and claims about side-effects must reflect available evidence or be capable of substantiation by clinical experience. It must not be stated that a product has no side-effects, toxic hazards or risks of addiction. The word 'safe' must not be used without qualification.

SUPPLEMENTARY INFORMATION

- *the use of data derived from in-vitro studies, studies in healthy volunteers and in animals.* *Care must be taken with the use of such data so as not to mislead as to its significance. The extrapolation of such data to the clinical situation should only be made where there is data to show that it is of direct relevance and significance*
- *economic evaluation of medicines.* *The economic evaluation of medicines is a relatively new science. Care must be taken that any claim involving the economic evaluation of a medicine is borne out by the data available and does not exaggerate its significance*

To be acceptable as the basis of promotional claims, the assumptions made in an economic evaluation must be clinically appropriate and consistent with the marketing authorization

Attention is drawn to guidance on good practice in the conduct of economic evaluations of medicines which has been given by the Department of Health and the ABPI and which is available upon request from the Prescription Medicines Code of Practice Authority

- *emerging clinical or scientific opinion.* *Where a clinical or scientific issue exists which has not been resolved in favour of one generally accepted viewpoint, particular care must be taken to ensure that the issue is treated in a balanced manner in promotional material*
- *hanging comparisons* *whereby a medicine is described as being or stronger or suchlike without stating that with which the medicine is compared must not be made*
- *price comparisons.* *Price comparisons, as with any comparison, must be accurate, fair and must not mislead. Valid comparisons can only be made where like is compared with like. It follows therefore that a price comparison should be made on the basis of the equivalent dosage requirement for the same indications. For example, to compare the cost per ml for topical preparations is likely to mislead unless it can be shown that their usage*

CODE OF PRACTICE

7.10 Exaggerated or all-embracing claims must not be made and superlatives must not be used except for those limited circumstances where they relate to a clear fact about a medicine. Claims should not imply that a medicine or an active ingredient has some special merit, quality or property unless this can be substantiated.

7.11 The word 'new' must not be used to describe any product or presentation which has been generally available, or any therapeutic indication which has been generally promoted, for more than twelve months in the UK.

SUPPLEMENTARY INFORMATION

rates are similar or, where this is not possible, for the comparison to be qualified in such a way as to indicate that usage rates may vary.

- **stastical information.** *Care must be taken to ensure that there is a sound statistical basis for all information, claims and comparisons in promotional material. Differences which do not reach statistical significance must not be presented in such a way as to mislead.*

Instances have occcured where claims have been based on published papers in which the arithmetic and/or statistical methodology was incorrect. Accordingly, before statistical information is included in promotional material it must have been subjected to statistical appraisal.

Clause 7.3   Comparisons

The Code does not preclude the use of other companies' brand names when making caomparisons.

Clause 7.6   References

Clause 7.6 applies to references to published material, including the use of quotations, tables, graphs and other illustrative matters.

Clause 7.8   Artwork, Illustrations, Graphs and Tables

Care must be taken to ensure that artwork does not mislead as to the nature of a medicine or any claim or comparison and that it does not detract from any warnings or contraindications. For example, anatomical drawings used to show results from a study must not exaggerate those results and depictions of children should not be used in relation to products not authorized for use in children in any way which might encourage such use.

Particular care should be taken with graphs and tables to ensure that they do not mislead, for example by their incompletness or by the use of suppressed zeros or unusual scales. Differences which do not reach statistical significance must not be presented in such a way as to mislead.

SUPPLEMENTARY INFORMATION

Graphs and tables must be adequately labelled so that the information presented can be readily understood. If a graph, table or suchlilke is taken form a published paper but has not been reproduced in its entirety, the graph must clearly be labelled as having been adapted from the paper in question (See also Clause 7.6). Any Such adaptation must not distort or mislead as to the significance of that graph, table etc. It should also be noted that if a table, graph etc in a paper is unacceptable in terms of the requirements of the Code, because, for example, it gives a visually misleading impression as to the data shown, then it must not be used or reproduced in promotional material.

Clause 7.9 Use of the Word 'Safe'

The restrictions on the word 'safe' apply equally to grammatical derivatives of the word such as 'safety'. For example, 'demonstrated safety' or 'proven safety' are prohibited under this clause.

Clause 7.10 Superlatives

Superlatives are those grammatical expressions which denote the highest quality or degree, such as best, strongest, widest etc. A claim that a product was 'the best' treatment for a particular condition, for example, could not be substantiated as there are too many variables to enable such a sweeping claim to be proven. The use of a superlative is acceptable only if it can be substantiated as a simple statement of fact which can be very clearly demonstrated, such as that a particular medicine is the most widely prescribed in the UK for a certain condition, if this is not presented in a way which misleads as to its significance.

SUPPLEMENTARY INFORMATION

Clause 7.10 Use of the Words 'The' and 'Unique'

In certain circumstances the use of the word 'the' can imply a special merit, quality or property for a medicine which is unacceptable under this clause if it cannot be substantiated. For exanple, a claim that a product is 'The analgesic' implies that it is in effect the best, and might not be acceptable under this clause.

Similarly, great care needs to be taken with the use of the word 'unique'. Although in some circumstances the word unique may be used to describe some clearly defined special feature of a medicine, in many instances it is not possible to substantiate the claim as the claim itself is so ill defined.

CODE OF PRACTICE

SUPPLEMENTARY INFORMATION

Clause 8   Disparaging References

8.1 The medicines, products and activities of other pharmaceutical companies must not be disparaged.

8.2 The health professions and the clinical and scientific opinions of health professionals must not be disparaged.

Clause 8.1   Disparaging References

Much pharmaceutical advertising contains comparisons with other products and, by the nature of advertising, such comparisons are usually made to show an advantage of the advertised product over its comparator. Provided that such critical references to another company's products are accurate, balanced, fair etc, and can be substantiated, they are acceptable under the code.

Unjustified knocking copy in which the products or activities of a competitor are unfairly denigrated is prohibited under this clause.

Attention is drawn to the requirements for comparisons set out in clauses 7.2 to 7.5.

Clause 9   High Standards, Format, Suitability and Causing Offence, Sponsorship

9.1 High standards must be maintained at all times.

9.2 All material and activities must recognise the special nature of medicines and the professional nature of the audience to which they are directed and must not be likely to cause offence.

9.3 The name or photograph of a member of a health profession must not be used in any way that is contrary to the conventions of that profession.

9.4 Promotional material must not imitate the devices, copy, slogans or general layout adopted by other companies in a way that is likely to mislead or confuse.

9.5 Promotional material must not include any reference to the Medicines Commission, the Committee on Safety of Medicines, the Medicines and Healthcare products Regulatory Agency, the Medicines Control Agency or the licensing authority, unless this is specifically required by the licensing authority.

Clauses 9.1 and 9.2   Suitability and Taste

The special nature of medicines and the professional audience to which the material is directed require that the standards set for the promotion of medicines are higher than those which might be acceptable for general commodity advertising.

It follows therefore that certain types, styles and methods of promotion, even where they might be acceptable for the promotion of products other than medicines, are unacceptable.

These include:

- *the display of naked or partially naked people for the purpose of attracting attention to the material or the use of sexual imagery of that purpose*
- *'teaser' advertising whereby promotional material is intended to 'tease' the recipient by eliciting an interest in something which will be following or will be available at a later date without providing any actual information about it*
- *the provision of rubber stamps to doctors for use as aids to prescription writing*
- *the provision of private prescription forms preprinted with the name of a medicine.*

CODE OF PRACTICE

9.6 Reproductions of official documents must not be used for promotional purposes unless permission has been given in writing by the appropriate body.

9.7 Extremes of format, size or cost of promotional material must be avoided.

9.8 Postcards, other exposed mailings, envelopes or wrappers must not carry matter which might be regarded as advertising to the general public, contrary to Clause 20.1.

9.9 The telephone, text messages, email, telemessages and facsimile must not be used for promotional purposes, except with the prior permission of the recipient.

9.10 Material relating to medicines and their uses, whether promotional in nature or not, which is sponsored by a pharmaceutical company must clearly indicate that it has been sponsored by that company.

The only exception to this is market research material which need not reveal the name of the company involved but must state that it is sponsored by a pharmaceutical company.

SUPPLEMENTARY INFORMATION

Clause 9.8   Reply Paid Cards

Reply paid cards which are intended to be returned to companies through the post and which relate to a medicine which may not legally be advertised to the general public should not bear both the name of the medicine and information as to its usage but may bear one or the other.

Clause 9.10   Declaration of Sponsorship

The declaration of sponsorship must be sufficiently prominent to ensure that readers of sponsored material are aware of it at the outset.

Clause 9.10   Market Research

Where market research is carried out by an agency on behalf of a pharmaceutical company, the agency must reveal the name of its client to the Prescription Medicines Code of Practice Authority when the Authority requests it to do so. When commissioning market research, a company must take steps to ensure that its identity would be so made know to the Authority should a request for that information be made.

CODE OF PRACTICE

Clause 10   Disguised Promotion

10.1 Promotional material and activities must not be disguised.

10.2 Market research activities, post-marketing surveillance studies, clinical assessments and the like must not be disguised promotion.

Clause 10.1 Disguised Promotional Material

Promotional material sent in the guise of personal communications, for example by using envelopes or postcards addressed in real or facsimile handwriting is inappropriate. Envelopes must not be used for the dispatch of promotional material if they bear words implying that the contents are non-promotional, for example that the contents provide information relating to safety.

Advertisements in journals must not resemble editorial matter. Care must also be taken with company sponsored reports on meeting and the like to ensure that they are not disguised promotion. Sponsorship must be declared in accordance with Clause 9.10.

Clause 10.2 Guidelines for Company Sponsored Safety Assessment of Marketed Medicines

Attention is drawn to the Guidelines for Company Sponsored Safety Assessment of Marketed Medicines (SAMM) which have been produced jointly by the ABPI, the British Medical Association, the Committee on Safety of Medicines, the Medicines and Healthcare products Regulatory Agency and the Royal College of General Practitioners. These state that SAMM studies should not be undertaken for the purposes of promotion.

Clause 10.2   Market Research

Market research is the collection and analysis of information and must be unbiased and non-promotional. The use to which the statistics or information is put may be promotional. The two phases must be kept distinct.

Attention is drawn to guidelines – The Legal and Ethical Framework for Healthcare Market Research – produced by the British Healthcare Business Intelligence Association in consultation with the ABPI.

CODE OF PRACTICE

Market research material should be examined to ensure that it does not contravene the Code.

Where market research is carried out by an agency on behalf of a pharmaceutical company, the agency must reveal the name of its client to the Prescription Medicines Code of Practice Authority when the Authority requests it to do so. When commissioning market research, a company must take steps to ensure that its identity would be so made known to the Authority should a request for that information be made.

Clause 11 Provision of Reprints and the Use of Quotations

11.1 Reprints of articles in journals must not be provided unsolicited unless the articles have been refereed.

11.2 Quotations from medical and scientific literature, or from personal communications must accurately reflect the meaning of the author.

11.3 Quotations relating to medicines taken from public broadcasts, for example on radio and television, and from private occasions, such as medical conferences or symposia, must not be used without the formal permission of the speaker.

11.4 The utmost care must be taken to avoid ascribing claims or views to authors when these no longer represent the current views of the authors concerned.

Clause 11.1 Provision of Reprints

The provision of an unsolicited reprint of an article about a medicine constitutes promotion of that medicine and all relevant requirements of the Code must therefore be observed. Particular attention must be paid to the requirements of Clause 3.

When providing an unsolicited reprint of an article about a medicine, it should be accompanied by prescribing information.

Clause 11.2 Quotations

Any quotation chosen by a company for use in promotional material must comply with the requirements of the Code itself. For example, to quote from a paper which stated that a certain medicine was 'safe and effective' would not be acceptable even if it was an accurate reflection of the meaning of the author of the paper, as it is prohibited under Clause 7.9 of the Code to state without qualification in promotional material that a medicine is safe.

Care should be taken in quoting from any study or the like to ensure that it does not mislead as to overall significance. (See Clause 7.2 which prohibits misleading information, claims etc in promotional material.) Attention is drawn to the provisions of Clause 7.6 which requires that when promotional material refers to published studies clear references must be given to where they can be found.

CODE OF PRACTICE

Clause 11.4   Current Views of Authors

If there is any doubts as to the current view of an author, companies should check with the author prior to its use in promotional material.

Clause 12 Distribution of Promotional Material

12.1 Promotional material should only be sent or distributed to those categories of persons whose need for, or interest in, the particular information can reasonably be assumed.

12.2 Restraint must be exercised on the frequency of distribution and on the volume of promotional material distributed.

12.3 Mailing lists must be kept up-to-date. Requests to be removed from promotional mailing lists must be complied with promptly and no name may be restored except at the addressee's request or with their permission.

Clause 12.1   Distribution of Promotional Material

Promotional material should be tailored to the audience to whom it is directed. For example, promotional material devised for general practitioners might not be appropriate for hospital doctors and, similarly, material devised for clinicians might not be appropriate for use with National Health Service administrative staff.

Clause 12.2   Frequency of Mailings

The style of mailings is relevant to their acceptability to doctors and criticism of their frequency is most likely to arise where their informational content is limited or where they appear to be elaborate and expensive. A higher frequency rate will be accepted for mailings on new products than for others.

Clause 13 Scientific Service Responsible for Information

Companies must have a scientific service to compile and collate all information, whether received from medical representatives or from any other source, about the medicines which they market.

CODE OF PRACTICE

SUPPLEMENTARY INFORMATION

Clause 14   Certification

14.1 Promotional material must not be issued unless its final form, to which no subsequent amendments will be made, has been certified by two persons on behalf of the company in the manner provided by this clause. One of the two persons must be a registered medical practitioner or, in the case of a product for dental use only, a registered medical practitioner or a dentist. The other must be a pharmacist or some other appropriately qualified person or a senior official of the company or an appropriately qualified person whose services are retained for that purpose.

14.2 All meetings which involve travel outside the UK must be certified in advance in a manner similar to that provided for by Clause 14.1.

14.3 The names of those nominated, together with their qualifications, shall be notified in advance to the Product Information and Advertising Unit of the Post Licensing Division of the Medicines and Healthcare products Regulatory Agency and to the Prescription Medicines Code of Practice Authority. The names and qualifications of designated alternative signatories must also be given. Changes in the names of nominees must be promptly notified.

14.4 The certificate for promotional material must certify that the signatories have examined the final form of the material and that in their belief it is in accordance with the requirements of the relevant advertising regulations and this Code, is not inconsistent with the marketing authorization and the summary of product characteristics and is a fair and truthful presentation of the facts about the medicine.

Material which is still in use must be recertified at intervals of no more than two years to ensure that it continues to conform with the relevant advertising regulations and the Code.

Clause 14.1   Certification

An acceptable way to comply with Clause 14.1 is for the final proof to be certified but this is not obligatory provided that which is certified is in its final form to which no subsequent amendments will be made.

All promotional material must be certified in this way including audio and audio-visual material, promotional material on databases, interactive data systems and the Internet, promotional aids and representatives' technical briefing materials.

Other material issued by companies which relates to medicines but which is not intended as promotional material for those medicines per se, for example, corporate advertising, press releases, market research material, financial information to inform shareholders, the stock exchange and the like, and educational material for patients etc, should be examined to ensure that it does not contravene the Code or the relevant statutory requirements.

Account should be taken of the fact that a non-promotional item can be used for a promotional purpose and therefore come within the scope of the Code.

In certifying audio and audio-visual material and promotional material on databases, interactive systems and the Internet, companies must ensure that a written transcript of the material is certified including reproductions of any graphs, tables and the like that appear in it. In the event of a complaint, a copy of the written material will be requested.

The guidelines on company procedures relating to the Code which are on page 40 give further information on certification.

See also the supplementary information to Clause 3 on promotion at international conferences regarding the certification of such material.

CODE OF PRACTICE

The certificate for meetings involving travel outside the UK must certify that the signatories have examined all the proposed arrangements for the meeting and that in their belief the arrangements are in accordance with the relevant advertising regulations and the Code.

14.5 Companies shall preserve all certificates. In relation to certificates for promotional material, the material in the form certified and information indicating the persons to whom it was addressed, the method of dissemination and the date of first dissemination must also be preserved. In relation to certificates for meetings involving travel outside the UK, details of the programme, the venue, the reasons for using the venue, the audience, the anticipated and actual costs and the nature of the hospitality and the like must also be preserved.

Companies shall preserve certificates and the relevant accompanying information for not less than three years after the final use of the promotional material or the date of the meeting and produce them on request from the Medicines and Healthcare products Regulatory Agency or the Prescription Medicines Code of Practice Authority.

SUPPLEMENTARY INFORMATION

Clause 14.1 Joint Ventures and Co-Promotion

In a joint venture in which a third party provides a service on behalf of a number of pharmaceutical companies, the pharmaceutical companies involved are responsible for any activity carried out by that third party on their behalf.

It follows therefore that the pharmaceutical companies involved should be aware of all aspects of the service carried out on their behalf and take this into account when certifying the material or activity involved. Similarly if two or more pharmaceutical companies organise a joint meeting each company should ensure that the arrangements for the meeting are acceptable.

Under co-promotion arrangements whereby companies jointly promote the same medicine and the promotional material bears both company names, each company should certify the promotional material involved as they will be held jointly responsible for it under the Code.

Clause 14.2 Meetings involving Travel outside the UK

When certifying meetings which involve travel outside the UK, the signatories should ensure that all the arrangements are examined, including the programme, the venue, the reasons for using that venue, the intended audience, the anticipated cost and the nature of the hospitality and the like.

Clause 14.5 Retention of Documentation

Companies should note that the Medicines and Healthcare products Regulatory Agency is entitled to request particulars of an advertisement, including particulars as to the content and form of the advertisement, the method of dissemination and the date of first dissemination, and such a request is not subject to any time limit. This does not apply to the certificates themselves in respect of which the three year limit in Clause 14.5 is applicable.

CODE OF PRACTICE

Clause 15 Representatives

15.1 Representatives must be given adequate training and have sufficient scientific knowledge to enable them to provide full and accurate information about the medicines which they promote.

15.2 Representatives must at all times maintain a high standard of ethical conduct in the discharge of their duties and must comply with all relevant requirements of the Code.

15.3 Representatives must not employ any inducement or subterfuge to gain an interview. No fee should be paid or offered for the grant of an interview.

15.4 Representatives must ensure that the frequency, timing and duration of calls on health professionals, administrative staff in hospitals and health authorities and the like, together with the manner in which they are made, do not cause inconvenience. The wishes of individuals on whom representatives wish to call and the arrangements in force at any particular establishment, must be observed.

15.5 In an interview, or when seeking an appointment for one, representatives must at the outset take reasonable steps to ensure that they do not mislead as to their identity or that of the company they represent.

15.6 Representatives must transmit forthwith to the scientific service referred to in Clause 13 any information which they receive in relation to the use of the medicines which they promote, particularly reports of side-effects.

15.7 Representatives must be paid a fixed basic salary and any addition proportional to sales of medicine must not constitute an undue proportion of their remuneration.

SUPPLEMENTARY INFORMATION

Clause 15 Representatives

All provisions in the Code relating to the need for accuracy, balance, fairness, good taste etc apply equally to oral representations as well as to printed material. Representatives must not make claims or comparisons which are in any way inaccurate, misleading, disparaging, in poor taste etc, or which are outside the terms of the marketing authorization for the medicine or are inconsistent with the summary of product characteristics. Indications for which the medicine does not have a marketing authorization must not be promoted.

Attention is drawn to the provisions of Clause 9.9 which prohibit the use of the telephone, text message, email, telemessages and facsimile for promotional purposes, except with the prior permission of the recipient.

Clause 15 Contract Representatives

Companies employing or using contract representatives are responsible for their conduct and must ensure that they comply with the provisions of this and all other relevant clauses in the Code, and in particular the training requirements under Clauses 15.1, 16.1, 16.2 and 16.3.

Clause 15.3 Hospitality and Payments for Meetings

Attention is drawn to the requirements of Clauses 18 and 19 which prohibit the provision of any financial inducement for the purposes of sales promotion and require that any hospitality provided is secondary to the purpose of a meeting, is not out of proportion to the occasion and does not extend beyond members of the health professions or appropriate administrative staff.

Meetings organised for groups of doctors, other health professionals and/or appropriate administrative staff which are wholly or mainly of a social or sporting nature are unacceptable.

CODE OF PRACTICE

15.8 Representatives must provide, or have available to provide if requested, a copy of the summary of product characteristics for each medicine which they are to promote.

15.9 Companies must prepare detailed briefing material for medical representatives on the technical aspects of each medicine which they will promote. A copy of such material must be made available to the Medicines and Healthcare products Regulatory Agency and the Prescription Medicines Code of Practice Authority on request. Briefing material must comply with the relevant requirements of the Code and, in particular, is subject to the certification requirements of Clause 14.

Briefing material must not advocate, either directly or indirectly, any course of action which would be likely to lead to a breach of the Code.

15.10 Companies are responsible for the activities of their representatives if these are within the scope of their employment even if they are acting contrary to the instructions which they have been given.

SUPPLEMENTARY INFORMATION

Representatives organising meetings are permitted to provide appropriate hospitality and/or to meet any reasonable, actual costs which may have been incurred. For example, if the refreshments have been organised and paid for by a medical practice the cost may be reimbursed as long as it is reasonable in relation to what was provided and the refreshments themselves were appropriate for the occasion.

Donations in lieu of hospitality are unacceptable as they are inducements for the purpose of holding a meeting. If hospitality is not required at a meeting there is no obligation or right to provide some benefit of an equivalent value.

Clause 15.3   Donations to Charities

Donations to charities in return for representatives gaining interviews are prohibited under Clause 15.3.

Clause   15.3   Items   Delivered   by Representatives

Reply paid cards which refer to representatives delivering items which have been offered to health professionals or appropriate administrative staff should explain that there is no obligation to grant the representative an interview when the item is delivered. This is to avoid the impression that there is such an obligation, which would be contrary to Clause 15.3 which prohibits the use of any inducement to gain an interview.

Clause 15.3   General Medical Council

The General Medical Council is the regulatory body for the medical profession and is responsible for giving guidance on standards of professional conduct and on medical ethics. In its guidance, the Council advises doctors that 'You must act in your patients' best interests when making referrals and providing or arranging treatment or care. So you must not ask for or accept any inducement, gift or hospitality which may affect or be seen to affect your judgement'.

SUPPLEMENTARY INFORMATION

Clause 15.4 Frequency and Manner of Calls on Doctors

The numbers of calls made on a doctor and the intervals between successive visits are relevant to the determination of frequency.

Companies should arrange that intervals between visits do not cause inconvenience. The number of calls made on a doctor by a representative each year should not normally exceed three on average. This does not include the following which may be additional to those three visits:

- attendance at group meetings, including audio-visual presentation and the like
- a visit which is requested by a doctor or a call which is made in order to respond to a specific enquiry
- a visit to follow up a report of an adverse reaction.

Representatives must always endeavour to treat doctors' time with respect and give them no cause to believe that their time might have been wasted. If for any unavoidable reasons, an appointment cannot be kept, the longest possible notice must be given.

SUPPLEMENTARY INFORMATION

Clause 15.8 Provision of Summary of Product Characteristics

If discussion on a medicine is initiated by the person or persons on whom a representative calls, the representative is not obliged to have available the information on that medicine referred to in this clause.

Clause 15.9 Briefing Material

The detailed briefing material referred to in this clause consists of both the training material used to instruct medical representatives about a medicine and the instructions given to them as to how the product should be promoted.

CODE OF PRACTICE

Clause 16   Training

16.1 All relevant personnel including members of staff concerned in any way with the preparation or approval of promotional material or of information to be provided to members of the UK health professions and to appropriate administrative staff or of information to be provided to the public, must be fully conversant with the requirements of the Code.

16.2 Representatives must pass the appropriate ABPI representatives examination, as specified in Clause 16.3. Prior to passing the appropriate examination, they may be engaged in such employment for no more than two years, whether continuous or otherwise.

16.3 The Medical Representatives Examination is appropriate for, and must be taken by, representatives whose duties comprise or include one or both of:

- calling upon doctors and/or dentists
- the promotion of medicines on the basis, *inter alia*, of their particular therapeutic properties.

The Generic Sales Representatives Examination is appropriate for, and must be taken by, representatives who promote medicines primarily on the basis of price, quality and availability.

16.4 The following exemptions apply in relation to Clause 16.2:

- persons who were employed as medical representatives on 1 October 1979 are exempt from the need to take the Medical Representatives Examination
- persons with an acceptable professional qualification, for example in pharmacy, medicine or nursing, who were employed as medical representatives at an time before 1 October 1984, are exempt from the need to take the Medical Representatives Examination

SUPPLEMENTARY INFORMATION

Clause 16.1   Training

Extensive in house training on the Code is carried out by companies and by the Prescription Medicines Code of Practice Authority.

In addition, the Authority runs seminars on the Code which are open to all companies and personnel from advertising agencies, public relations agencies and the like which act for the pharmaceutical industry. Details of these seminars can be obtained from the Authority.

Clause 16.2   Time Allowed to Pass Examination

Prior to passing the appropriate ABPI examination, representatives may be engaged in such employment for no more than two years, whether continuous or otherwise and irrespective of whether with one company or with more than one company. A representative cannot, for example, do eighteen months with one company and eighteen months with another and so on, thus avoiding the examination.

In the event of extenuating circumstances, such as prolonged illness or no or inadequate opportunity to take the examination, the Director of the Prescription Medicines Code of Practice Authority may agree to the continued employment of a person as a representative past the end of the two year period, subject to the representative passing the examination within a reasonable time.

Service as a representative prior to 1 January 1996 does not count towards the two year limit on employment as a representative prior to passing the appropriate examination.

CODE OF PRACTICE

- persons who were employed as Generic Sales Representatives on 1 January 1993 are exempt from the need to take the Generic Sales Representatives Examination
- persons who were employed as representatives on 1 January 1996 who had not previously been required to take an examination because they neither promoted generic medicines nor called on doctors and/or dentists are exempt from the need to take either examination.

16.5 Persons who have passed the Medical Representatives Examination whose duties change so as to become those specified in Clause 16.3 as being appropriate to the Generic Sales Representatives Examination are exempt from the need to take that examination.

Persons who have passed the Generic Sales Representatives Examination whose duties change so as to become those specified in Clause 16.3 as being appropriate to the Medical Representatives Examination must pass that examination within two years of their change of duties.

16.6 Details of the numbers of medical and generic sales representatives who have passed the respective examinations above, together with the examination status of others, must be provided to the Prescription Medicines Code of Practice Authority on request.

Clause 17 Provision of Medicines and Samples

17.1 Samples of a product may be provided only to a health professional qualified to prescribe that product. They must not be provided to administrative staff.

17.2 No more than ten samples of a particular medicine may be provided to an individual health professional during the course of a year.

17.3 Samples may only be supplied in response to written requests which have been signed and dated.

SUPPLEMENTARY INFORMATION

Clause 16.3 Medical Representatives and Generic Sales Representatives

The ABPI examinations for medical representatives and generic sales representatives are based on a syllabus published by the ABPI which covers, as appropriate, subjects such as body systems, disease processes and pharmacology, the classification of medicines and pharmaceutical technology. Information on the National Health Service and pharmaceutical industry forms an additional core part of the syllabus. The syllabus is complementary to, and may be incorporated within, the company's induction training which is provided to representatives as a pre-requisite to carrying out their function.

Every effort should be made to ensure that representatives are entered for the appropriate ABPI examination as soon as possible and certainly within their first year of employment. Delaying entry into the second year can lead to representatives failing to pass within the two year period allowed.

Clause 17 Definition of Sample

A sample is a small supply of a medicine provided to health professionals so that they may familiarise themselves with it and acquire experience in dealing with it. A sample of a medicine may be provided only to a health professional qualified to prescribe that particular medicine.

A small sample which is provided only for identification or similar purposes and which is not intended to be used in treatment may be provided to any health professional but is otherwise subject to the requirements of Clause 17.

CODE OF PRACTICE

SUPPLEMENTARY INFORMATION

17.4 A sample of a medicine must be no larger than the smallest presentation of the medicine on the market in the UK.

17.5 Each sample must be marked 'free medical sample – not for resale' or words to that effect and must be accompanied by a copy of the summary of product characteristics.

17.6 The provision of samples is not permitted for any medicine which contains a substance listed in any of Schedules I, II or IV to the Narcotic Drugs Convention (where the medicine is not a preparation listed in Schedule III to that Convention) or a substance listed in any of Schedules I to IV of the Psychotropic Substances Convention (where the medicine is not a preparation which may be exempted from measures of control in accordance with Paragraphs 2 and 3 of Article 3 of that Convention).

17.7 Samples distributed by representatives must be handed direct to the health professionals requesting them or persons authorized to receive them on their behalf.

17.8 The provision of medicines and samples in hospitals must comply with individual hospital requirements.

17.9 Companies must have adequate systems of control and accountability for samples which they distribute and for all medicines handled by representatives.

17.10 Medicines which are sent by post must be packed so as to be reasonably secure against being opened by young children. No unsolicited medicine must be sent through the post.

17.11 Medicines may not be sold or supplied to members of the general public for promotional purposes.

Titration packs, free goods and bonus stock provided to pharmacists and others are not samples. Neither are starter packs classified as samples. This is because they are not for the purposes described above.

Starter packs are small packs designed to provide sufficient medicine for a primary care prescriber to initiate treatment in such circumstances as a call out in the night or in other instances where there might be some undesirable or unavoidable delay in having a prescription dispensed. It follows from this that the types of medicines for which starter packs are appropriate are limited to those where immediate commencement of treatment is necessary or desirable, such as analgesics and antibiotics. Starter packs are not samples and should not be labelled as such. The quantity of medicine in a starter pack should be modest, only being sufficient to tide a patient over until their prescription can be dispensed.

Titration packs are packs containing various strengths of a medicine for the purpose of establishing a patient on an effective dose.

Clause 17.3   Sample Requests

This clause does not preclude the provision of a pre-printed sample request form bearing the name of the product for signing and dating by the applicant.

All signed and dated written requests for samples should be retained for not less than one year.

Clause 17.9   Control and Accountability

Companies should ensure that their systems of control and accountability relating to medicines held by representatives cover such matters as the security of delivery to them, the security of medicines held by them, the audit of stocks held by them, including expiry dates, and the return to the companies of medicines no longer to be held by representatives.

CODE OF PRACTICE

Clause 18   Gifts and Inducements

18.1 No gift, benefit in kind or pecuniary advantage shall be offered or given to members of the health professions or to administrative staff as an inducement to prescribe, supply, administer, recommend or buy any medicine, subject to the provisions of Clause 18.2.

18.2 Gifts in the form of promotional aids and prizes, whether related to a particular product or of general utility, may be distributed to members of the health professions and to appropriate administrative staff, provided that the gift or prize is inexpensive and relevant to the practice of their profession or employment.

18.3 The prescribing information for a medicine as required under Clause 4 does not have to be included on a promotional aid if the promotional aid includes no more than the following about the medicine:

- the name of the medicine
- an indication that the name of the medicine is a trade mark
- the name of the company responsible for marketing the product.

SUPPLEMENTARY INFORMATION

Clause 18.1 Provision of Medical and Educational Goods and Services

Clause 18.1 does not prevent the provision of medical and educational goods and services which will enhance patient care or benefit the National Health Service. The provision of such goods or services must not be done in such a way as to be an inducement to prescribe, supply, administer, recommend or buy any medicine. They must not bear the name of any medicine but may bear a corporate name.

The following guidance is intended to assist companies in relation to medical and educational goods and services.

1(i) The role of medical/generic representatives in relation to the provision of goods and services supplied in accordance with the supplementary information to Clause 18.1 needs to be in accordance with the principles set out below. In this context companies should consider using staff other than medical/generic representatives.

(ii) If medical/generic representatives provide, deliver or demonstrate medical and educational goods and services then this must not be linked in any way to the promotion of products.

(iii) The acceptability of the role of medical/generic representatives will depend on the nature of the goods and services provided and the method of provision.

(iv) The nature of the service provider, the person associated with the provision of medical and educational goods and services, is important ie is the service provider a medical/generic representative or is the service provider some other appropriately qualified person, such as a sponsored registered nurse? If the goods and services require patient contact, for example either directly or by identification of patients from patient records and the like, then medical/generic representatives must not

SUPPLEMENTARY INFORMATION

be involved. Only an appropriately qualified person, for example a sponsored registered nurse, not employed as a medical/generic representative, may undertake activities relating to patient contact and/or patient identification. Medical/generic representatives could provide administrative support in relation to the provision of a screening service, but must not be present during the actual screening and must not discuss or help interpret individual clinical findings.

(v) Neither the company nor its medical/generic representatives may be given access to data/records that could identify, or could be linked to, particular patients.

(vi) Sponsored health professionals should not be involved in the promotion of specific products. Registered nurses, midwives and health visitors are required to comply with the Nursing & Midwifery Council Code of professional conduct. This code requires, inter alia, that registration status is not used in the promotion of commercial products or services.

2 The remuneration of those not employed as medical/generic representatives but who are sponsored or employed as service providers in relation to the provision of medical and educational goods and services must not be linked to sales in any particular territory or place or to sales of a specific product or products and, in particular. may not include a bonus scheme linked to such sales. Bonus schemes linked to a company's overall national performance, or to the level of service provided, may be acceptable.

3 Companies must ensure that patient confidentiality is maintained at all times and that data protection legislation is complied with.

4 Service providers must operate to detailed written instructions provided by the company. It is recommended that these should be similar to the briefing material for representatives as

SUPPLEMENTARY INFORMATION

referred to in Clause 15.9 of the Code. The written instructions should set out the role of the service provider and should cover patient confidentiality issues. Instructions on how the recipients are to be informed etc should be included. The written instructions must not advocate, either directly or indirectly, any course of action which would be likely to lead to a breach of the Code.

5 Service providers must abide by the principle set out in Clause 15.5 of the Code that in an interview, or when seeking an appointment, reasonable steps must be taken to ensure that they do not mislead as to their identity or that of the company they represent.

6 A recipient of a service must be provided with a written protocol to avoid misunderstandings as to what the recipient has agreed. The identity of the sponsoring pharmaceutical company must be given. For example, a general practitioner allowing a sponsored registered nurse access to patient records should be informed in writing of any data to be extracted and the use to which those data will be put.

7 Any printed material designed for use in relation to the provision of medical and educational goods and services must be non-promotional. It is not acceptable for such materials to promote the prescription, supply, sale or administration of the sponsoring company's medicines: Nor is it acceptable for materials to criticise competitor products as this might be seen as promotional. All printed materials must identify the sponsoring pharmaceutical company.

8 Materials relating to the provision of medical and educational goods and services, such as internal instructions, external instructions, the written protocol for recipients and printed material etc, must be examined by the Code of Practice signatories within companies to ensure that the requirements of the Code are met as recommended in the supplementary information to Clause 14.1 of the Code.

SUPPLEMENTARY INFORMATION

A copy of the materials must be made available to the Prescription Medicines Code of Practice Authority on request.

9 Companies are recommended to inform relevant parties such as NHS trusts, health authorities, health boards and primary care organisations of their activities where appropriate. This is particularly recommended where companies are proposing to provide medical and educational goods and services which would have budgetary implications for the parties involved. For example the provision of a screening service for a limited period might mean that funds would have to be found in the future when company sponsorship stopped. Another example might be the provision of diagnostic or laboratory services and the like, which the NHS trust, health authority, health board or primary care organization would normally be expected to provide.

Clause 18.1   General Medical Council

The General Medical Council is the regulatory body for the medical profession and is responsible for giving guidance on standards of professional conduct and on medical ethics. In its guidance, the Council advises doctors that 'You must act in your patients' best interests when making referrals and providing or arranging treatment or care. So you must not ask for or accept any inducement, gift or hospitality which may affect or be seen to affect your judgement'.

Clause 18.1   Terms of Trade

Measures or trade practices relating to prices, margins and discounts which were in regular use by a significant proportion of the pharmaceutical industry on 1 January 1993 are outside the scope of the Code (see Clause 1.2) and are excluded from the provisions of this clause. Other trade practices are subject to the Code. The terms 'prices', 'margins' and 'discounts' are primarily financial terms.

SUPPLEMENTARY INFORMATION

Schemes which enable health professionals to obtain personal benefits, for example gift vouchers for high street stores, in relation to the purchase of medicines are unacceptable even if they are presented as alternatives to financial discounts.

The Royal Pharmaceutical Society of Great Britain has issued guidance in relation to the acceptance of gifts and inducements to prescribe or supply. The Society states that pharmacists accepting items such as gift vouchers, bonus points, discount holidays, sports equipment etc would be in breach of the Society's Code of Ethics and advises pharmacists not to participate in such offers.

Clause 18.1   Package Deals

Clause 18.1 does not prevent the offer of package deals whereby the purchaser of particular medicines receives with them other associated benefits, such as apparatus for administration, provided that the transaction as a whole is fair and reasonable and the associated benefits are relevant to the medicines involved.

Clause 18.1   Donations to Charities

Donations to charities made by companies in return for health professionals' attendance at company stands at meetings or offered as rewards for completing and returning quiz cards in mailings and such like are not unacceptable under this clause provided that the level of donation for each individual is modest, the money is for a reputable charity and any action required of the health professional is not inappropriate. Any donation to a charity must not constitute a payment that would otherwise be unacceptable under the Code. For example, it would not be acceptable for a representative to pay into a practice equipment fund set up as a charity as this would be a financial inducement prohibited under Clause 18.1. Donations to charities in return for representatives gaining interviews are also prohibited under Clause 15.3 of the Code.

SUPPLEMENTARY INFORMATION

Any offer by a company of a donation to a charity which is conditional upon some action by a health professional must not place undue pressure on the health professional to fulfil that condition. At all times the provisions of Clauses 2 and 9.1 must be kept in mind.

Clause 18.2   Gifts

Items provided on long term or permanent loan to a doctor or a practice are regarded as gifts and are subject to the requirements of this clause.

Gifts must be inexpensive and relevant to the recipients' work. An 'inexpensive' gift means one which has cost the donor company no more that £6, excluding VAT.

Items of general utility which have been held to be acceptable gifts to doctors as being inexpensive and of relevance to their work include pens, pads, diaries, nail brushes, surgical gloves, desk trays, calendars, a peak flow whistle, walking sticks and desk clocks.

Items which are for use in the home, and have no use in the ordinary course of the practice of medicine or any other health profession, such as table mats, are unacceptable. Other examples of items which have been found unacceptable are neck cushions, plant seeds, road atlases and compact discs of music which were not considered relevant items and an x-ray light box and an age-sex register on grounds of costs.

Names of medicines should not be used on promotional aids when it would be inappropriate to do so, for example, when it might mislead as to the nature of the item.

Certain independently produced medical/educational publications such as textbooks have been held to be acceptable gifts under Clause 18.2 of the Code. The content of publications used in this way has to be considered carefully and must comply with the Code as regards any references to the donor's or competitors' products. It might be possible to give certain medical/educational publications in accordance with the supplementary

SUPPLEMENTARY INFORMATION

information to Clause 18.1 – Provision of Medical and Educational Goods and Services.

Clause 18.2   Competitions and Quizzes

The use of competitions, quizzes and suchlike for the purposes of sales promotion are not necessarily an unacceptable form of promotion. Any competition must, however, be in good taste and must not involve any subject matter which is inappropriate for the promotion of a medicine as required under Clause 9.2. A competition is more likely to be considered acceptable if its subject matter is clearly related to the practice of medicine and pharmacy.

Any competition used for promotional purposes must be a bona fide test of skill and must recognise the professional standing of the recipients.

The provisions of Clause 18.2 · apply to the provision of competition prizes. Prizes of a higher value than would ordinarily be acceptable for a promotional aid are acceptable where the competition is a serious one and the prizes are few in number, relevant to the potential recipient's work and not out of proportion to the skill required in the competition. The maximum acceptable cost to the donor of a prize in a promotional competition is £100, excluding VAT.

Gladstone bags, a desk clock and a business card holder are examples of prizes which have been found acceptable in particular competitions or quizzes.

Computer equipment and a substantial travel award offered as a prize in a promotional competition are examples of prizes which have been found unacceptable on grounds of cost.

Attention is drawn to the fact that the items listed above as acceptable competition prizes or gifts are instances where the particular examples in question were found acceptable. It does not mean that any such item is automatically acceptable under the Code.

SUPPLEMENTARY INFORMATION

Clause 18.2 Gifts to or for use by Patients

Some items distributed as promotional aids are intended for use by patients and these are not generally unacceptable provided that they meet the requirements of Clause 18.2; for example, puzzles and toys for a young child to play with during a visit to the doctor.

Other items which may be made available to patients, for example by completing a request card enclosed with a medicine, should meet the relevant principles set out in Clause 18.2, that is they should be inexpensive and related to either the condition under treatment or general health. Care must be taken that any such activity meets all the requirements of the Code and in particular Clause 20.

No gift or promotional aid for use by patients must be given for the purpose of encouraging patients to request a particular medicine.

SUPPLEMENTARY INFORMATION

Clause 18.3 Promotional Aids – Name of the Medicine

The name of the medicine means the brand name or the non-proprietary name. Both names may be included but it is not obligatory to include both. A promotional aid may bear the names of more than one medicine.

Clause 18.3 Prescribing Information on Note Pads and Calendars

If a promotional aid consists of a note pad or calendar in which the individual pages bear advertising material, there is no need for the individual pages to comply with Clause 4 provided that the information required by that clause is given elsewhere; for example, on the cover.

CODE OF PRACTICE

Clause 19   Meetings and Hospitality

19.1 Companies must not provide hospitality to members of the health professions and appropriate administrative staff except in association with scientific meetings, promotional meetings, scientific congresses and other such meetings. Hospitality must be secondary to the purpose of the meeting. The level of hospitality offered must be appropriate and not out of proportion to the occasion. The costs involved must not exceed that level which the recipients would normally adopt when paying for themselves. It must not extend beyond members of the health professions or appropriate administrative staff.

19.2 Payments may not be made to doctors or groups of doctors, either directly or indirectly, for rental for rooms to be used for meetings.

19.3 When meetings are sponsored by pharmaceutical companies, that fact must be disclosed in all of the papers relating to the meetings and in any published proceedings. The declaration of sponsorship must be sufficiently prominent to ensure that readers are aware of it at the outset.

SUPPLEMENTARY INFORMATION

Clause 19.1   Meetings and Hospitality

The provision of hospitality includes the payment of reasonable, actual travel costs which a company may provide to sponsor a delegate to attend a meeting. The payment of travel expenses and the like for persons accompanying the delegate is not permitted.

The payment of reasonable honoraria and reimbursement of out of pocket expenses, including travel, for speakers, is permissible.

Pharmaceutical companies may appropriately sponsor a wide range of meetings. These range from small lunchtime audio-visual presentations in a group practice, hospital meetings and meetings at postgraduate education centers, launch meetings for new products, management training courses, meetings of clinical trialists, patient support group meetings, satellite symposia through to large international meetings organised by independent bodies with sponsorship from pharmaceutical companies.

With any meeting, certain basic principles apply:

- *the meeting must have a clear educational content*
- *the hospitality associated with the meeting must be secondary to the nature of the meeting, must be appropriate and not out of proportion to the occasion and*
- *any hospitality provided must not extend to a spouse or other such person unless that person is a member of the health professions or appropriate administrative staff and qualifies as a proper delegate or participant at the meeting in their own right*
- *spouses and other accompanying persons, unless qualified as above, may not attend the actual meeting and may not receive any associated hospitality at the company's expense; the entire costs which their presence involves are the responsibility of those they accompany.*

SUPPLEMENTARY INFORMATION

Administrative staff may be invited to meetings where appropriate. For example, receptionists might be invited to a meeting in a general practice when the subject matter related to practice administration.

A useful criterion in determining whether the arrangements for any meeting are acceptable is to apply the question 'would you and your company be willing to have these arrangements generally known?' The impression that is created by the arrangements for any meeting must always be kept in mind.

Meetings organized for groups of doctors, other health professionals and/or for administrative staff which are wholly or mainly of a social or sporting nature are unacceptable.

Meetings organised by pharmaceutical companies which involve UK health professionals at venues outside the UK are not necessarily unacceptable. There have, however, to be valid and cogent reasons for holding meetings at such venues. As with meetings held in the UK, in determining whether such a meeting is acceptable or not, consideration must also be given to the educational programme, overall cost, facilities offered by the venue, nature of the audience, hospitality provided and the like. As with any meeting it should be the programme that attracts delegates and not the associated hospitality or venue.

The requirements of the Code do not apply to the provision of hospitality other than to those referred to in Clause 19.1. For example, a company could provide hospitality at a meeting of organic chemists. They are neither health professionals nor appropriate administrative staff.

Clause 19.1 Certification of Meetings

Pharmaceutical companies must ensure that all meetings which are planned are checked to see that they comply with the Code. Companies must have a written document that sets out their policies on meetings and hospitality and the associated allowable expenditure. In addition, meetings which involve travel outside the UK must be formally certified as set out in Clause 14.2 of the Code.

SUPPLEMENTARY INFORMATION

Clause 19.1 General Medical Council

The General Medical Council is the regulatory body for the medical profession and is responsible for giving guidance on standards of professional conduct and on medical ethics. In its guidance, the Council advises doctors that 'You must act in your patients' best interests when making referrals and providing or arranging treatment or care. So you must not ask for or accept any inducement, gift or hospitality which may affect or be seen to affect your judgement'.

Clause 19.1 Continuing Professional Development (CPD) Meetings and Courses

The provisions of this and all other relevant clauses in the Code apply equally to meetings and courses organized or sponsored by pharmaceutical companies which are continuing professional develpment (CPD) approved, such as postgraduate education allowance (PGEA) approved meetings and courses. The fact that a meeting or course has CPD approval does not mean that the arrangements are automatically acceptable under the code. The relevant provisions of the Code and, in particular, those relating to hospitality, must be observed.

Clause 19.2 Payment of Room Rental

This provision does not preclude the payment of room rental to postgraduate medical centres and the like.

Payment of room rental to doctors or groups of doctors is not permissible even if such payment is made to equipment funds or patients' comforts funds and the like or to charities or companies.

Clause 19.3 Sponsorship and Reports of Meetings

Attention is drawn to Clause 9.10 which requires that all material relating to medicines and their uses, whether promotional or not, which is sponsored by a pharmaceutical company must clearly indicate that it has been sponsored by that company.

It should be noted that where companies are involved in the sponsorship and/or distribution of reports on meetings or symposia etc, these reports may constitute promotional material and thus be fully subject to the requirements of Code.

CODE OF PRACTICE

Clause 20   Relations with the General Public and the Media

20.1 Medicines must not be advertised to the general public if they are prescription only medicines or are medicines which, though not prescription only, may not legally be advertised to the general public. This prohibition does not apply to vaccination campaigns carried out by companies and approved by the health ministers.

20.2 Information about medicines which is made available to the general public either directly or indirectly must be factual and presented in a balanced way. It must not raise unfounded hopes of successful treatment or be misleading with respect to the safety of the product.

Statements must not be made for the purpose of encouraging members of the public to ask their doctors to prescribe a specific medicine.

20.3 Requests from individual members of the public for information or advice on personal medical matters must be refused and the enquirer recommended to consult his or her own doctor.

20.4 The introduction of a new medicine must not be made known to the general public until reasonable steps have been taken to inform the medical and pharmaceutical professions of its availability.

20.5 Companies are responsible for information about their products which is issued by their public relations agencies.

SUPPLEMENTARY INFORMATION

Clause 20.1   Advertising of Medicines to the General Public

The advertising of prescription only medicines to the general public is also prohibited by the Advertising Regulations.

The promotion of medicines to the general public for self medication purposes is covered by the Code of Standards of Advertising Practice for Over-the-Counter Medicines of the Proprietary Association of Great Britain (PAGB).

Methods of sale of medicines through pharmacies are also covered by the Code of Ethics of the Royal Pharmaceutical Society of Great Britain.

Clause 20.2   Information to the General Public

This clause allows for the provision of non-promotional information about prescription medicines to the general public either in response to a direct inquiry from an individual, including inquiries from journalists, or by dissemination of such information via press conferences, press announcements, television and radio reports, public relations activities and the like. It also includes information provided by means of posters distributed for display in surgery waiting rooms etc.

Any information so provided must observe the principles set out in this clause, that is, it should be factual, balanced and must not be made for the purpose of encouraging members of the public to ask their doctors to prescribe a specific medicine. It must not constitute the advertising of medicines to the general public prohibited under Clause 20.1. The provisions of Clause 20.3 must be observed if an inquiry is from an individual member of the public.

It is good practice to include the summary of product characteristics with a press release or press pack relating to a medicine.

Particular care must be taken in responding to approaches from the media to ensure that the provisions of this clause are upheld.

SUPPLEMENTARY INFORMATION

In the event of a complaint which relates to the provisions of this clause, companies will be asked to provide copies of any information supplied, including copies of any relevant press releases and the like. This information will be assessed to determine whether it fulfils the requirements of this clause.

European public assessment reports, summaries of product characteristics and package leaflets may be provided to members of the public on request.

Companies may provide members of the health professions with leaflets concerning a medicine with a view to their provision to patients to whom the medicine has already been prescribed, provided that such a leaflet is factual and non-promotional in nature.

A company may conduct a disease awareness or public health campaign provided that the purpose is to encourage members of the public to seek treatment for their symptoms while in no way promoting the use of a specific medicine. Particular care must be taken where the company's product, even though not named, is the only medicine relevant to the disease or symptoms in question.

Attention is drawn to the Disease Awareness Campaigns Guidelines produced by the Medicines and Healthcare products Regulatory Agency.

Clause 20.2   Financial Information

Information made available in order to inform shareholders, the Stock Exchange and the like by way of annual reports and announcements etc. may relate to both existing medicines and those not yet marketed. Such information must be factual and presented in a balanced way.

Clause 20.2   Approval of Information

Information on medicines made available under this clause should be examined to ensure that it does not contravene the Code or the relevant statutory requirements.

SUPPLEMENTARY INFORMATION

Clause 20.3   Requests for Information or Advice on Personal Medical Matters

This clause prohibits the provision of information or advice on personal medical matters to individual members of the general public requesting it. The intention behind this prohibition is to ensure that companies do not intervene in the patient/doctor relationship by offering advice or information which properly should be in the domain of the doctor. However, information may be given, including information on medicines prescribed for the enquirer, provided that it complies with the requirements of Clauses 20.1 and 20.2 and does not impinge on the principle behind this clause. For example, answering requests by members of the public as to whether a particular medicine contains sucrose or some other inactive ingredient, or whether there would be problems associated with drinking alcohol whilst taking the medicine or whether the medicine should be taken before or after a meal, is acceptable. The situation with enquiries relating to side-effects, the indications for a medicine and such like is not as clear cut and particular caution is required in dealing with them.

All requests from members of the general public need to be handled with great care and a decision taken as to whether the company can responsibly answer the enquiry.

Requests from patients for information may in some instances best be handled by passing the information to the patients' doctors for discussion with them rather than providing the information direct to the patients concerned.

CODE OF PRACTICE

SUPPLEMENTARY INFORMATION

Clause 21   The Internet

21.1 Access to promotional material directed to a UK audience provided on the Internet in relation to prescription only medicines, or medicines which, though not prescription only, may not legally be advertised to the general public, must be limited to health professionals and appropriate administrative staff.

21.2 Information or promotional material about medicines covered by Clause 21.1 above which is placed on the Internet outside the UK will be regarded as coming within the scope of the Code if it was placed there by a UK company or an affiliate of a UK company or at the instigation or with the authority of such a company and it makes specific reference to the availability or use of the medicine in the UK.

21.3 Information about medicines covered by Clauses 21.1 and 21.2 above which is provided on the Internet and which can be accessed by members of the public must comply with Clause 20.2 of the Code.

21.4 Notwithstanding the provisions of Clauses 21.1 and 21.3 above, a medicine covered by Clause 21.1 may be advertised in a relevant independently produced electronic journal intended for health professionals or appropriate administrative staff which can be accessed by members of the public.

21.5 European public assessment reports, summaries of product characteristics and package leaflets for medicines covered by Clause 21.1 above may be included on the Internet and be accessible by members of the public provided that they are not presented in such a way as to be promotional in nature.

Clause 21.4   Advertisements in Electronic Journals

It should be noted that the Medicines and Healthcare products Regulatory Agency's guidance notes on advertising and promotion state that each page of an advertisement for a prescription only medicine should be clearly labelled as intended for health professionals.

CODE OF PRACTICE

21.6 It should be made clear when a user is leaving any of the company's sites, or sites sponsored by the company, or is being directed to a site which is not that of the company.

Clause 21.6   Sites liked via Company Sites
Sites linked via company sites are not necessarily covered by the Code.

Clause 22   Compliance with Undertakings

When an undertaking has been given in relation to a ruling under the Code, the company concerned must ensure that it complies with that undertaking.

PRESCRIPTION MEDICINES CODE OF PRACTICE AUTHORITY
CONSTITUTION AND PROCEDURE
Operative in respect of complaints received on and after 1 July 2003

INTRODUCTION

The Code of Practice for the Pharmaceutical Industry is administered by the Prescription Medicines Code of Practice Authority. The Authority is responsible for the provision of advice, guidance and training on the Code of Practice as well as for the complaints procedure. It is also responsible for arranging for conciliation between companies when requested to do so and for scrutinising journal advertising on a regular basis. Complaints made under the Code about promotional material or the promotional activities of companies are considered by the Code of Practice Panel and, where required, by the Code of Practice Appeal Board. Reports on cases are published quarterly by the Authority and are available on request.

The names of individuals complaining from the pharmaceutical industry are kept confidential. In exceptional cases it may be necessary for a company know the identity of the complainant so that the matter can be properly investigated. Even in these instances, the name of the complainant is only disclosed with the complainant's permission.

Complaints about the promotion of medicines should be submitted to the Director of the Prescription Medicines Code of Practice Authority, 12 Whitehall, London SW1A 2DY, telephone 020-7930 9677, facsimile 020-7930 4554.

STRUCTURE AND RESPONSIBILITIES

1 Prescription Medicines Code of Practice Authority

1.1 The Prescription Medicines Code of Practice Authority is responsible for the administration of the Code of Practice for the Pharmaceutical Industry including the provision of advice, guidance and training on the Code. It is also responsible for arranging for conciliation between companies when requested to do so and for scrutinising journal advertising on a regular basis.

1.2 The Authority also administers the complaints procedure by which complaints made under the Code are considered by the Code of Practice Panel and, where required, by the Code of Practice Appeal Board.

1.3 The Authority is appointed by and reports to the Board of Management of The Association of the British Pharmaceutical Industry (ABPI) and consists of the Director, Secretary and Deputy Secretary.

1.4 The Director has the authority to request copies of any relevant material from a pharmaceutical company, including copies of the certificates authorizing any such material and copies of relevant briefing material for representatives.

1.5 The Authority may consult the Appeal Board upon any matter concerning the Code or its administration.

2 Code of Practice Panel – Constitution and Procedure

2.1 The Code of Practice Panel consists of members of the Prescription Medicines Code of Practice Authority and meets as business requires to consider complaints made under the Code.

2.2 Two members of the Authority form a quorum for a meeting of the Panel. Decisions are made by majority voting. The Director or, in his absence, the Secretary, acts as Chairman of the Panel and has both an original and a casting vote.

2.3 The Director may obtain expert assistance in any field. Expert advisers who are consulted may be invited to attend a meeting of the Panel but have no voting rights.

3 Code of Practice Appeal Board – Constitution

3.1 The Code of Practice Appeal Board and its Chairman are appointed by the Board of Management of the ABPI. The appointment of independent members to the Appeal Board is made following consultation with the Medicines and Healthcare products Regulatory Agency.

3.2 The Appeal Board comprises:
- an independent, legally qualified Chairman
- three independent medical members appointed in consultation with the British Medical Association, one with recent experience as a general practitioner and one with recent experience as a hospital consultant
- one independent pharmacist appointed following consultation with the Royal Pharmaceutical Society of Great Britain

- one member representative of the interests of patients
- one member from an independent body involved in providing information on medicines
- four medical directors or medically qualified senior executives from pharmaceutical companies
- eight directors or senior executives from pharmaceutical companies.

3.3 The Chairman of the Appeal Board is appointed for a term of five years which may be renewed. Members of the Appeal Board are each appointed for a term of three years which may be renewed.

3.4 The Director is responsible for providing appropriate administrative support to the Appeal Board.

The Director, Secretary and Deputy Secretary of the Authority may be present at a meeting of the Appeal Board during the consideration of an appeal or a report from the Code of Practice Panel made under Paragraph 8 below only at the invitation of the Chairman and with the agreement of the party or parties involved in the appeal or report in question.

4 Code of Practice Appeal Board – Procedure

4.1 The Code of Practice Appeal Board meets as business requires to consider appeals under the Code and any other matter which relates to the Code. The Appeal Board receives reports on all complaints which have been submitted under the Code and details of the action taken on them.

4.2 The Chairman and seven members of the Appeal Board constitute a quorum. Two of those present must be independent members, at least one of whom must be medically qualified, and there must also be present

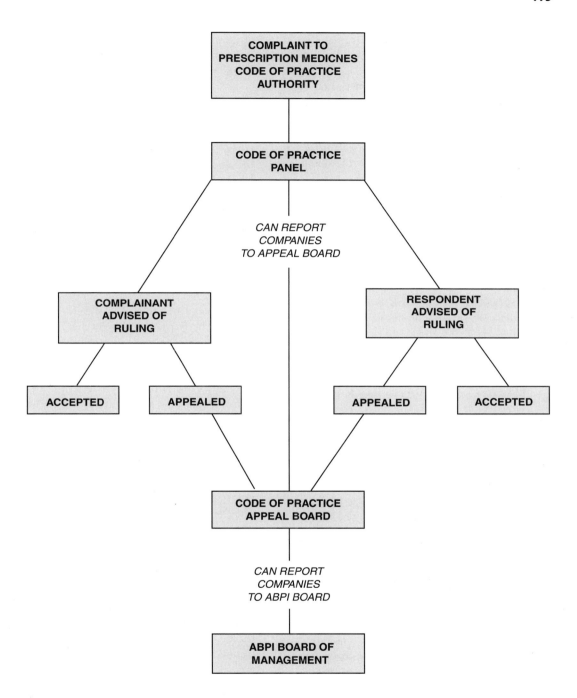

at least one medically qualified member from a pharmaceutical company.

In the event that a quorum cannot be attained for the consideration of a case because of the number of members barred under Paragraph 4.4 below, or for any other reason, the Chairman may co-opt appropriate persons to the Appeal Board so as to enable a quorum to be achieved.

4.3 Decisions are made by majority voting. The Chairman has both an original and a casting vote.

4.4 If a member of the Appeal Board is concerned in a case either as complainant or respondent, that member does not receive copies of the papers circulated in connection with the case and is required to withdraw from the Appeal Board during its consideration.

Members of the Appeal Board are also required to declare any other interest in a case prior to its consideration. The Chairman determines whether it is appropriate for that member to remain for the consideration of the case.

4.5 The Chairman may obtain expert assistance in any field. Expert advisers may be invited to attend a meeting of the Appeal Board but have no voting rights.

4.6 When an appeal is considered by the Appeal Board, both the complainant and the respondent company are entitled to appear or be represented.

The first presentation in relation to a ruling which is appealed is made by the appellant.

A company may not be represented before the Appeal Board by a representative who is also a member of the Appeal Board except with the consent of the Chairman. Such consent may be given only if the member of the Appeal Board can satisfy the Chairman that no other person within his company can properly represent it in the case in question.

4.7 Where an appeal is brought which is concerned with an issue of fact between a complainant and the company concerned which cannot be properly resolved without the oral evidence of the persons directly involved, the Chairman may invite such persons to attend and give evidence.

COMPLAINTS PROCEDURE

5 Action on Complaints

5.1 When the Director receives information from which it appears that a company may have contravened the Code, the chief executive of the company concerned is requested to comment on the matters of complaint.

If a complaint concerns a matter closely similar to one which has been the subject of a previous adjudication, it may be allowed to proceed at the discretion of the Director if new evidence is adduced by the complainant or if the passage of time or a change in circumstances raises doubts as to whether the same decision would be made in respect of the current complaint. The Director should normally allow a complaint to proceed if it covers matters similar to those in a decision of the Code of Practice Panel which was not the subject of appeal to the Code of Practice Appeal Board.

If a complainant does not accept a decision of the Director that a complaint should not be proceeded with because a similar complaint has been adjudicated upon previously and nothing has changed in the meantime, then the matter is referred to the Chairman of the Appeal Board for his decision which is final.

If, in the view of the Director, a complaint does not show that there may have been a breach of the Code, the complainant shall be so advised. If the complainant does not accept that view, the matter is referred to the Chairman of the Appeal Board for his decision which is final.

5.2 When the complaint is from a pharmaceutical company, the complaint must be signed or authorized in writing by the company's chief executive and must state those clauses of the Code which are alleged to have been breached.

5.3 Upon receipt of a complaint, the company concerned has ten working days in which to submit its comments in writing.

6 Establishment of *Prima Facie* Case and Consideration by the Code of Practice Panel

6.1 Upon receipt of the comments from the respondent company, the Director must determine whether there is a *prima facie* case to answer under the Code. If, in the view of the Director, no *prima facie* case has been established the complainant and the respondent company are so advised. If the complainant does not accept that view, the matter is referred to the Chairman of the Code of Practice Appeal Board for his decision which is final.

If the complainant submits further evidence which, in the view of the Director, shows that there may have been a breach of the Code, then the respondent company shall be invited to comment on that further evidence. Upon receipt of the further comments from the respondent company, the Director must determine whether a *prima facie* case has been established. If, in the view of the Director, no *prima facie* case has been established the complainant and the respondent company are so advised. If the complainant does not accept that view, the matter is referred to the Chairman of the Code

of Practice Appeal Board for his decision which is final.

6.2 Once it has been determined that a *prima facie* case exists, the case is referred to the Code of Practice Panel to determine whether or not there has been a breach of the Code.

7 Code of Practice Panel: Rulings

7.1 Where the Code of Practice Panel rules that there is a breach of the Code, the complainant and the respondent company are so advised in writing and are given the reasons for the decision.

The respondent company has ten working days to provide a written undertaking that the promotional activity or use of the material in question (if not already discontinued or no longer in use) will cease forthwith and that all possible steps will be taken to avoid a similar breach of the Code in the future. This undertaking must be signed by the chief executive of the company or with his or her authority and must be accompanied by details of the actions taken by the company to implement the undertaking, including the date on which the promotional material was finally used or appeared and/or the last date on which the promotional activity took place.

The company must also pay within twenty working days an administrative charge based on the number of matters ruled in breach of the Code.

If an appeal is subsequently lodged by the respondent company, the complainant will be sent a copy of the initial comments and enclosures submitted by the respondent company in relation to the complaint. If the respondent company objects to this because it regards part of the material as being confidential, and the matter cannot be settled by the Director, then it will be referred to the Chairman of the Code of Practice Appeal Board for his decision which is final.

7.2 Where the Panel rules that there is no breach of the Code, the complainant and the respondent company are so advised in writing and are given the reasons for the decision. Where the complaint is from a pharmaceutical company, the complainant must pay within twenty working days an administrative charge based on the number of matters alleged and ruled not to be in breach of the Code.

When advised of the outcome, the complainant will be sent a copy of the comments and enclosures submitted by the respondent company in relation to the complaint. If the respondent company objects to this because it regards part of the material as being confidential, and the matter cannot be settled by the Director, then it will be referred to the Chairman of the Code of Practice Appeal Board for his decision which is final.

7.3 The complainant or the respondent company may appeal against rulings of the Panel to the Code of Practice Appeal Board. Appeals must be lodged within ten working days of the notification of the ruling of the Panel and must be accompanied by reasons as to why the Panel's ruling is not accepted. These reasons will be circulated to the Appeal Board.

If the respondent company accepts one or more of the Panel's rulings of breaches of the Code, but appeals one or more other such rulings, then within ten working days of notification of the Panel's rulings it must provide the undertaking required by Paragraph 7.1 above in respect of the ruling or rulings which it is not appealing.

7.4 Where an appeal is lodged by the complainant, the respondent company has ten working days to comment on the reasons given by the complainant for the appeal and

these comments will be circulated to the Appeal Board.

The complainant has five working days to comment on the respondent company's comments upon the reasons given by the complainant for the appeal and these comments will be circulated to the respondent company and the Appeal Board.

In the event that the respondent company objects to certain of its comments being made available to the complainant on the grounds of confidentiality, and the matter cannot be settled by the Director, then the matter will be referred to the Chairman of the Appeal Board who will decide whether those particular comments can be included in the evidence which goes before the Appeal Board. The Chairman's decision is final.

7.5 Where an appeal is lodged by the respondent company, the complainant has ten working days to comment on the reasons given by the respondent company for the appeal and these comments will be circulated to the respondent company and the Appeal Board.

In the event that the respondent company objects to certain details of its appeal being made available to the complainant on the grounds of confidentiality, and the matter cannot be settled by the Director, then the matter will be referred to the Chairman of the Appeal Board who will decide whether those particular details can be included in the evidence which goes Before the Appeal Board. The Chairman's decision is final.

8 Code of Practice Panel: Reports to the Code of Practice Appeal Board

8.1 Failure to comply with the procedures set out in Paragraphs 5, 6 and 7 above shall be reported to the Code of Practice Appeal Board for consideration in relation to the provisions of Paragraph 12.1 below.

8.2 The Code of Practice Panel may also report to the Appeal Board any company whose conduct in relation to the Code, or in relation to a particular case before it, warrants consideration by the Appeal Board in relation to the provisions of Paragraphs 10.3, 10.4 and 12.1 below. Such a report to the Appeal Board may be made notwithstanding the fact that a company has provided an undertaking requested by the Panel.

8.3 Where the Panel reports a company to the Appeal Board under the provisions of Paragraphs 8.1 and 8.2 above, the company concerned is provided with a copy of the report prior to its consideration and is entitled to have a representative or representatives appear before the Appeal Board to state the company's case.

A company may not be represented before the Appeal Board by a representative who is also a member of the Appeal Board except with the consent of the Chairman. Such consent may be given only if the member of the Appeal Board can satisfy the Chairman that no other person within his company can properly represent it in the matter in question.

9 Action on Complaints about Safety from the Medicines and Healthcare products Regulatory Agency

9.1 In the event of the Medicines and Healthcare products Regulatory Agency making a complaint which relates to the safety or proper use of a medicine, and requesting that an advertisement be withdrawn, the respondent company has five working days to respond with its comments.

9.2 If the Code of Practice Panel upholds the complaint, the company is required to suspend the advertisement or practice forthwith pending the final outcome of the case.

10 Code of Practice Appeal Board: Rulings

10.1 Where the Code of Practice Appeal Board rules that there is no breach of the Code, the complainant and the respondent company are so advised in writing and are given the reasons for the decision.

Where a complainant pharmaceutical company appeals and the Appeal Board upholds the ruling that there was no breach of the Code, the complainant pharmaceutical company must pay within twenty working days an administrative charge based on the number of matters taken to appeal on which no breach is ruled.

Where a respondent company appeals and the Appeal Board rules that there was no breach of the Code, the complainant pharmaceutical company must pay within twenty working days an administrative charge based on the number of matters taken to appeal on which no breach is ruled.

10.2 Where the Appeal Board rules that there is a breach of the Code, the respondent company is so advised in writing and is given the reasons for the decision. The respondent company then has five working days to provide a written undertaking providing the information specified in Paragraph 7.1 above.

The company must also pay within twenty working days an administrative charge based on the number of matters ruled in breach of the Code.

10.3 A company ruled in breach of the Code may also be required by the Appeal Board to take steps to recover items given in connection with the promotion of a medicine. Details of the action taken must be provided in writing to the Appeal Board.

10.4 Where a company is ruled in breach of the Code the Appeal Board may require an audit of the company's procedures in relation to the Code to be carried out by the Prescription Medicines Code of Practice Authority and following that audit, decide whether to impose requirements on the company concerned to improve its procedures in relation to the Code.

10.5 Where a company not in membership of the ABPI fails to comply with the procedures set out in Paragraphs 5, 6, 7 or 10 and indicates that it no longer wishes to accept the jurisdiction of the Authority, the Appeal Board may decide that the company should be removed from the list of non member companies which have agreed to abide by the Code and the Medicines and Healthcare products Regulatory Agency advised that responsibility for that company under the Code can no longer continue to be accepted.

The Board of Management of the ABPI must be advised that such action has been taken.

11 Reports by the Prescription Medicines Code of Practice Authority

Failure to comply with the procedures set out in Paragraph 10 above shall be reported to the Code of Practice Appeal Board for consideration in relation to the provisions of Paragraph 12.1 below.

Where such a report is made, the company concerned is provided with a copy of the report prior to its consideration and is entitled to have a representative or representatives appear before the Appeal Board to state the company's case.

A company may not be represented before the Appeal Board by a representative who is also a member of the Appeal Board except with the consent of the Chairman. Such consent may be given only if the member of the Appeal Board can satisfy the Chairman

that no other person within his company can properly represent it in the matter in question.

12 Code of Practice Appeal Board: Reports to the ABPI Board of Management

12.1 Where the Code of Practice Appeal Board considers that the conduct of a company in relation to the Code or a particular case before it warrants such action, it may report the company to the Board of Management of the ABPI for it to consider whether further sanctions should be applied against that company. Such a report may be made notwithstanding the fact that the company has provided an undertaking requested by either the Code of Practice Panel or the Appeal Board.

12.2 Where such a report is made to the Board of Management, the Board of Management may decide:

- to reprimand the company and publish details of that reprimand
- to require an audit of the company's procedures in relation to the Code to be carried out by the Prescription Medicines Code of Practice Authority and following that audit, decide whether to impose requirements on the company concerned to improve its procedures in relation to the Code
- to require the company to publish a corrective statement
- to suspend or expel the company from the ABPI or
- in the case of companies not in membership of the ABPI, to remove the company from the list of non member companies which have agreed to abide by the Code and to advise the Medicines and Healthcare products Regulatory Agency that responsibility for that company under the Code can no longer continue to be accepted.

12.3 If a member of the Board of Management is concerned in a case which has led to the report, as either complainant or respondent, that member does not receive a copy of the report and is required to withdraw from the Board of Management during its consideration.

Members of the Board of Management are also required to declare any other interest in a report prior to its consideration. The President (or Chairman in the absence of the President) determines whether it is appropriate for that member to remain for the consideration of the report.

12.4 Where a report is made to the Board of Management under Paragraph 12.1 above, the company concerned is provided with a copy of the report prior to its consideration and is entitled to have a representative or representatives appear before the Board of Management to state the company's case.

13 Case Reports

13.1 At the conclusion of any case under the Code, the complainant is advised of the outcome and a report is published summarising the details of the case.

13.2 The respondent company and the medicine concerned are named in the report.

In a case where the complaint was initiated by a company or by an organisation or official body, that company or organisation or official body is named in the report. The information given must not, however, be such as to identify any individual person.

13.3 A copy of the report on a case is made available to both the complainant and the respondent company prior to publication. Any amendments to the report suggested by these parties are considered by the

Director, consulting with the other party where appropriate. If either party does not accept the Director's decision as to whether or not a report should be amended, the matter is referred to the Chairman of the Code of Practice Appeal Board for his decision which is final.

13.4 Copies of all case reports are submitted to the Appeal Board and the Board of Management of the ABPI for information prior to publication.

Copies of the published reports are sent to the Medicines and Healthcare products Regulatory Agency, the Office of Fair Trading, the British Medical Association, the Royal Pharmaceutical Society of Great Britain and the Editors of the BMJ and The Pharmaceutical Journal. Copies of the published reports are also available to anyone on request.

GENERAL PROVISIONS

14 Time Periods for Responding to Matters under the Code

The number of working days within which companies or complainants must respond to enquiries etc, from the Prescription Medicines Code of Practice Authority, as referred to in the above procedures, are counted from the date of receipt of the notification in question.

An extension in time to respond to such notifications may be granted at the discretion of the Director.

15 Withdrawal of Complaints and Notices of Appeal

15.1 A complaint may be withdrawn by a complainant with the consent of the respondent company up until such time as the respondent company's comments on the complaint have been received by the

Prescription Medicines Code of Practice Authority, but not thereafter.

15.2 Notice of appeal may be withdrawn by a complainant with the consent of the respondent company up until such time as the respondent company's comments on the reasons for the appeal have been received by the Authority, but not thereafter.

15.3 Notice of appeal may be withdrawn by a respondent company at any time but if notice is given after the papers relating to its appeal have been circulated to the Code of Practice Appeal Board, then the higher administrative charge will be payable.

16 Code of Practice Levy and Charges

16.1 An annual Code of Practice levy is paid by members of the ABPI. The levy together with the administrative charges referred to in Paragraphs 7 and 10 above and the charges for audits carried out in accordance with Paragraphs 10.4 and 12.2 above are determined by the Board of Management of the ABPI subject to approval at a General Meeting of the ABPI by a simple majority of those present and voting.

16.2 Administrative charges are payable only by pharmaceutical companies and companies are liable for such charges whether they are members of the ABPI or not.

There are two levels of administrative charge.

The lower level is payable by a company which accepts either a ruling of the Code of Practice Panel that it was in breach of the Code or a rejection by the Panel of its allegation against another company. The lower level is also payable by a complainant company if a ruling of the Panel that there

was a breach of the Code is subsequently overturned by the Code of Practice Appeal Board and by a respondent company if a ruling of the Panel that there was no breach of the Code is subsequently overturned by the Appeal Board.

The higher level is paid by a company which unsuccessfully appeals a decision of the Panel.

16.3 Where two or more companies are ruled in breach of the Code in relation to a matter involving co-promotion, each company shall be separately liable to pay three-quarters only of the aidministrative charge which would otherwise be payable.

16.4 The number of administrative charges which apply in a case is determined by the Director. If a campany does not agree with the Director's decision, the matter is referred to the Chairman of the Appeal Board for his decision which is final.

16.5 Failure to pay any of the charges provided for by this paragraph must be reported by the Director to the Appeal Board or the Board of Management of the ABPI as appropriate.

17 Possible Breaches identified by the Code of Practice Panel or Code of Practice Appeal Board

17.1 Where the Code of Practice Panel or the Code of Practice Appeal Board identifies a possible breach of the Code which has not been addressed by the complainant in a case, the respondent company is invited to comment. The company has ten working days to respond in writing.

17.2 If the company accepts that there is a breach of the Code, the company is requested to provide an undertaking providing the information specified in Paragraph 7.1

above. No administrative charge shall be payable in these circumstances and there shall be no case report on the matter in question.

17.3 If the company does not accept that there is a breach of the Code and, having considered the company's comments, the Director decides that there is no *prima facie* case to answer under the Code, then the procedure is brought to a close. There shall be no case report on the matter in question.

17.4 If the company does not accept that there is a breach of the Code but, having considered the company's comments, the Director considers that a *prima facie* case has been established, the procedures under Paragraph 6.2 above onwards shall be followed.

18 Scrutiny of Advertisements

18.1 A sample of advertisements issued by pharmaceutical companies is scrutinised by the Prescription Medicines Code of Practice Authority in relation to the requirements of the Code on a continuing basis.

18.2 Where a *prima facie* breach of the Code is identified under this procedure, the company concerned is requested to comment in writing within ten working days of receipt of the notification.

18.3 If the company accepts that there is a breach of the Code, the company is requested to provide an undertaking providing the information specified in Paragraph 7.1 above. No administrative charge shall be payable in these circumstances and there shall be no case report on the matter in question.

18.4 If the company does not accept that there is a breach of the Code and, having

considered the company's comments, the Director decides that there is no *prima facie* case to answer under the Code, then the procedure is brought to a close. There shall be no case report on the matter in question.

18.5 If the company does not accept that there is a breach of the Code but, having considered the company's comments, the Director considers that a *prima facie* case has been established, the procedures under Paragraph 6.2 above onwards shall be followed.

19 Provision of Advice and Conciliation

19.1 The Prescription Medicines Code of Practice Authority is available to provide informal guidance and advice in relation to the requirements of the Code and, where appropriate, may seek the views of the Code of Practice Appeal Board.

19.2 Companies wishing to seek the assistance of a conciliator with the view to reaching agreement on inter-company differences about promotion may contact the Director for advice and assistance.

20 Amendments to the Code of Practice and Constitution and Procedure

20.1 The Code of Practice for the Pharmaceutical Industry and this Constitution and Procedure may be amended by a simple majority of those present and voting at a General Meeting of the ABPI.

20.2 The views of the Prescription Medicines Code of Practice Authority and the Code of Practice Appeal Board must be sought on any proposal to amend the Code or this Constitution and Procedure. The views of the Medicines and Healthcare products Regulatory Agency, the British Medical Association and the Royal Pharmaceutical

Society of Great Britain must also be invited.

20.3 The Prescription Medicines Code of Practice Authority and the Code of Practice Appeal Board may, in the light of their experience, make recommendations for amendment of the Code and this Constitution and Procedure.

21 Annual Report

An annual report of the Prescription Medicines Code of Practice Authority is published each year with the approval of the Code of Practice Appeal Board. This report includes details of the work of the Authority, the Code of Practice Panel and the Appeal Board during that year.

GUIDELINES ON COMPANY PROCEDURES RELATING TO THE CODE OF PRACTICE

Paragraphs 10.4 and 12.2 of the Constitution and Procedure for the Prescription Medicines Code of Practice Authority authorize respectively the Code of Practice Appeal Board and the Board of Management of The Association of the British Pharmaceutical Industry to require an audit of a company's procedures in relation to the Code of Practice for the Pharmaceutical Industry to be carried out by the Prescription Medicines Code of Practice Authority.

Set out below are guidelines on company procedures which are regarded as representing good practice in this regard. They are minimum requirements and will need to be adapted to fit in with the arrangements at any particular company.

1) Certification of Promotional Material

Procedures must ensure that:

- promotional material is not issued until its final form has been certified in accordance with Clause 14 of the Code
- the names of signatories are notified in advance to the Product Information and Advertising Unit of the Post Licensing Division of the Medicines and Healthcare products Regulatory Agency and to the Prescription Medicines Code of Practice Authority (Clause 14.3)
- the form of certificate encompasses at least the requirements of Clause 14.4
- material still in use is recertified at intervals of no more than two years (Clause 14.4)
- the certificates, together with the material in the form certified and information as to whom it was addressed, the method of dissemination and the date of first dissemination are preserved for at least three years after final use (Clause 14.5).

Each certificate should bear a reference number with the same reference number appearing on the promotional material in question so that there can be no doubt as to what has been certified. A particular reference number should relate to only one item of promotional material.

Different sizes and different layouts of a piece of promotional material should be separately certified and each should have its own unique reference number.

2) Representatives' Briefing and Training Materials

The certification requirements of Clause 14 of the Code which are covered above apply also to briefing material prepared for representatives in accordance with Clause 15.9. Briefing material includes the training material used to instruct medical representatives about a medicine and the instructions given to them as to how the product should be promoted.

Procedures must ensure that no such material is used or issued prior to certification.

3) Representatives' Expenses

There should be a clearly laid down procedure for approval and payment of representatives' expenses and expenditure on meetings and hospitality and the like. A system should be in place for an audit on a systematic or random basis which will check the nature of the expenditure which has been incurred and assess whether that expenditure was in accordance with the requirements of the Code.

4) Representatives' Training

Procedures must ensure that:

- representatives are adequately trained in relation to every product which they are to promote (Clause 15.1)
- representatives are not employed as medical representatives or generic sales representatives unless they have passed the relevant examination as provided for in Clauses 16.2 and 16.3 of the Code, or have the benefit of an exemption, or have been in such employment for less than two years (whether continuous or otherwise and irrespective of whether with one company or with more than one company)
- contract representatives are only employed or used if they comply with the requirements of Clauses 16.2 and 16.3 as regards examination status.

Representatives should be provided with written instructions on the application of the Code to their work even if they are also provided with an actual copy of it. Their instructions should cover such matters as the company's policies on meetings and hospitality, and the associated allowable expenditure, and the specific requirements for representatives in Clause 15 of the Code. It should be made clear how reporting to the 'scientific service' of the company is to be carried out in relation to information about the medicines which they promote which comes to their notice, particularly reports of side-effects (Clause 15.6).

It should be made clear to representatives as to whether, and in what circumstances, they can themselves write letters (or prepare other written materials) which mention particular products and are thus almost certain to be considered promotional material.

Such items must be certified, either in advance by way of proforma letters or by certifying each individual letter or other item, and must bear prescrbing information in accordance with Clause 4.1

5) Training Generally

It should be ensured that all relevant personnel, including members of staff concerned in any way with the preparation or approval of promotional material or of information to be provided to members of the UK health professions or to appropriate administrative staff or of information to be provided to the public, are fully conversant with the requirements of the Code (Clause 16.1).

Appropriate arrangements should be in place for training on the requirements of the Code. These may be internal arrangements for appropriate staff members but key personnel should attend one of the seminars organised by the Prescription Medicines Code of Practice Authority.

Adequate arrangements should be in place to ensure that any information as to changes to the Code etc, including reports of decided cases, provided by the Authority are circulated to relevant personnel.

6) Provision of Medicines and Samples

Procedures should ensure that the requirements of Clause 17 are complied with.

Clause 17.9 requires companies to have adequate systems of control and accountability for samples and for all medicines handled by representatives. Similarly, there should be an adequate system to control the number of samples of a particular product given to a particular health professional in the course of a year (Clause 17.2).

7) Gifts and Inducements

Procedures should ensure that Clause 18 rlelating to gifts and inducements is complied with and that promotional gifts or prizes comply with Clauses 18.2 and 18.3.

Promotional gifts and prizes must be certified in accordance with Clause 14.

8) Meetings and Hospitality

A company must have a written document that sets out its policies on meetings and hospitality and the associated allowable expenditure and must ensure that all meetings that it plans are checked to see that they comply with Clause 19.

Meetings which involve travel outside the UK must be formerly certified in advance in accordance with Clause 14.2.

A company's procedures should cover its own meetings, those which it sponsors and the sponsorship of attendance at meetings.

9) Breaches of the Code

In the event of a company being found in breach of the Code, procedures should ensure that adequate steps are taken to ensure that relevant information about it is communicated internally to appropriate members of staff.

Procedures must be in place to ensure that promotional material found to be in breach of the Code is quickly and entirely withdrawn from use. They should include checks that claims etc found to be in breach do not also appear in other formats, such as exhibition stands, which might otherwise be overlooked.

Companies are advised to keep written records of he action taken to withdraw material.

10) Co-Promotion

Adequate provision should be made in co-promotion agreements and the like to ensure that the Code is complied with. Where companies jointly promote the same product and the promotional material bears both company names, each company must certify the promotional material involved as the companies concerned will be held jointly responsible for it under the Code (supplementary information to Clause 14.1).

11) Non-Promotional Items

Procedures should ensure that any item or activity regarded as non-promotional in nature is vetted by an appropriate member of staff familiar with the Code with a view to determining whether it is indeed non-promotional (supplementary information to Clause 14.1).

Account should be taken of the fact that a non-promotional item can be used for a promotional purpose and therefore come within the scope of the Code.

LEGISLATION, OTHER CODES *and* GUIDELINES

LEGISLATION

The Medicines Act 1968
   Part VI Promotion of Sales of Medicinal Products

The Medicines (Advertising) Regulations 1994
   1994 No. 1932

The Medicines (Advertising) Amendment
Regulations 1996
   1996 No. 1552

The Medicines (Monitoring of Advertising)
Regulations 1994
   1994 No. 1933

The Medicines (Advertising and Monitoring of
Advertising) Amendment Regulations 1999
   1999 No. 267

The Medicines (Monitoring of Advertising)
Amendment Regulations 1999
   1999 No. 784

The Control of Misleading Advertisements
Regulations 1988
   1988 No. 915

The Control of Misleading Advertisements
(Amendment) Regulations 2000
   2000 No. 914

European Directive 92/28/EEC of 31 March 1992 on
the advertising of medicinal products for human use
(now consolidated as Articles 86 to 100 of
Directive 2001/83/EC)

OTHER CODES

International

IFPMA Code of Pharmaceutical Marketing Practices
   (International Federation of Pharmaceutical
   Manufacturers Associations)

EFPIA European Code of Practice for the Promotion
of Medicines
   (European Federation of Pharmaceutical Industries
   and Associations)

WHO Ethical Criteria for Medicinal Drug Promotion,
Geneva 1988
   (ISBN 92 4 154239 X)
   (World Health Organisation)

IPCAA Code of Conduct
   (International Pharmaceutical Congress Advisory
   Association)

United Kingdom

The British Code of Advertising, Sales Promotion and
Direct Marketing
   (Committee of Advertising Practice/
   Advertising Standards Authority)

Code of Practice for Advertising Over-the-Counter
Medicines to Health Professionals and the Retail Trade
   (Proprietary Association of Great Britain – PAGB)

Code of Standards of Advertising Practice for Over-
the-Counter Medicines
   (Proprietary Association of Great Britain – PAGB)

BMA Handbook of Medical Ethics
   (British Medical Association)

General Medical Council 'Good medical practice'

Department of Health 'Code of Conduct for NHS
Managers'

Department of Health 'Commercial sponsorship –
Ethical standards for the NHS'

Nursing & Midwifery Council 'Code of professional
conduct'

Royal Pharmaceutical Society of Great Britain 'Code of
Ethics'

GUIDELINES

Advertising and Promotion of Medicines in the UK
(Medicines and Healthcare products Regulatory
Agency Guidance Note No. 23)

Disease Awareness Campaigns Guidelines
(Medicines and Healthcare products Regulatory
Agency)

Guidance on Good Practice in the Conduct of
Economic Evaluations of Medicines
(Department of Health/ABPI)

Guidelines for Company-Sponsored Safety Assessment
of Marketed Medicines
(Medicines and Healthcare products Regulatory
Agency/Committee on Safety of Medicines/
Royal College of General Practitioners/British
Medical Association/ABPI)

Guidelines for Phase IV Clinical Trials (ABPI)

Guidelines on Standards for Medical Information
Departments
(Association of Information Officers in the
Pharmaceutical Industry)

Medicines which are Promoted for Use during
Pregnancy – Guidance for the Pharmaceutical
Industry
(Medicines and Healthcare products Regulatory
Agency)

Relationships between the Medical Profession and the
Pharmaceutical Industry (ABPI)

The Legal and Ethical Framework for Healthcare
Market Research
(British Healthcare Business Intelligence
Association/ABPI)

Appendix 3

Guidelines and Documentation for Implementation of Clinical Trials

CLINICAL TRIAL AGREEMENT FOR PHARMACEUTICAL INDUSTRY SPONSORED RESEARCH IN NHS TRUSTS

This agreement dated **day of** **20..**

is between

[. . . insert name . . .] NHS TRUST, of [. . . insert address . . .]
(Hereinafter known as the 'NHS Trust')

AND

[. . . insert name . . .], of [. . . insert address . . .]

(Hereinafter known as the 'Sponsor')

NOW

WHEREAS the Sponsor is a pharmaceutical company involved in the research, development, manufacture and sale of medicines for use in humans

WHEREAS the Sponsor is developing new treatments for patients with [. . . insert disease . . .]

WHEREAS the NHS Trust is concerned with the diagnosis, treatment and prevention of disease and clinical research for the improvement of healthcare

WHEREAS the NHS Trust has a particular interest and expertise in [. . . insert disease . . .]

WHEREAS the Sponsor wishes to contract with the NHS Trust to undertake a sponsored clinical trial entitled:

. . . insert title . . .

It is agreed that the NHS Trust and Sponsor shall participate in the aforementioned clinical trial in accordance with this Agreement.

1 DEFINITIONS

1.1   The following words and phrases have the following meanings:

'Clinical Trial' means the investigation to be conducted at the Trial Site in accordance with the Protocol numbered [. . . insert identification number . . .].

'Clinical Trial Subject' means a person recruited to participate in the Clinical Trial.

'Confidential Information' means in the case of obligations imposed upon the NHS Trust under clauses 6.2 and 12.8 any and all information relating to the Clinical Trial including the Investigational Medicinal Product and in the case of obligations imposed upon the Parties under clause 6.2 all information concerning the arrangements contemplated by this Agreement or the business affairs of one Party that it discloses to the other Party pursuant to or in connection with this Agreement.

'ICH GCP' means the ICH Harmonised Tripartite Guideline for Good clinical Practice (CPMP/ICH/135/95) together with such other good clinical practice requirements as are specified in Directive 2001/20/EC of the European Parliament and the Council of 4 April 2001 relating to medicinal products for human use and in guidance published by the European Commission pursuant to such Directive.

'Intellectual Property Rights' means patents, trademarks, copyrights, rights to extract information from a database, design rights and all rights or forms of protection of a similar nature or having equivalent or the similar effect to any of them which may subsist anywhere in the world, whether or not any of them are registered and including applications for registration of any of them.

'Investigational Medicinal Product' means [. . . insert details of study drug/control material . . .] as defined in the Protocol.

'Know How' means all technical and other information which is not in the public domain, including but not limited to information comprising or relating to concepts, discoveries, data, designs, formulae, ideas, inventions, methods, models, procedures, designs for experiments and tests and results of experimentation and testing, processes, specifications and techniques, laboratory records, clinical data, manufacturing data and information contained in submissions to regulatory authorities.

'Monitor' means one or more persons appointed by the Sponsor to monitor compliance of the Clinical Trial with ICH GCP and to conduct source data verification.

'NHS Trust' means the [. . . insert name . . .] NHS Trust that is a signatory to this Agreement.

'Party' means the Sponsor, or the NHS Trust and 'Parties' shall mean both of them.

'Protocol' means the description of the Clinical Trial and all amendments thereto as the Parties may from time to time agree. Such amendments will be signed by the Parties and form a part of this Agreement.

'R & D Office' means the NHS Trust department responsible for the administration of this Clinical Trial on behalf of the NHS Trust.

'Site File' means the file maintained by the Site Principal Investigator containing the documentation specified in section 8 of ICH GCP (edition CPMP/ICH/135/95).

'Site Principal Investigator' means the person who will lead and co-ordinate the work of the Clinical Trial at the Trial Site on behalf of the NHS Trust or any other person as may be agreed from time to time between the Parties as a replacement.

'Sponsor' means the corporate entity that is a signatory to this Agreement.

'Timelines' means the dates set out in Appendix 2 hereto as may be amended by agreement between the Parties and Timeline shall mean any one of such dates.

'Trial Site(s)' means any premises occupied by the NHS Trust.

1.2   Any reference to a statutory provision shall be deemed to include reference to any statutory modification or re-enactment of it.

2   SITE PRINCIPAL INVESTIGATOR

2.1   The NHS Trust represents that it is entitled to procure and the NHS Trust will procure the Services of [. . . insert name of investigator . . .] to act as Site Principal Investigator and shall ensure the performance of the obligations of the Site Principal Investigator set out in this Agreement.

2.2   The NHS Trust represents that the Site Principal Investigator has the necessary expertise to perform the Clinical Trial and that the Site Principal Investigator meets and will continue to meet the conditions set out at Appendix 6 to this Agreement.

2.3   The NHS Trust shall notify the Sponsor if [. . . insert name of investigator . . .] ceases to be employed by or associated with the NHS Trust, and shall use its best endeavours to find a replacement acceptable to both the Sponsor and the NHS Trust. If no mutually acceptable replacement can be found the Sponsor may terminate this Agreement pursuant to clause 12.3 below.

3   CLINICAL TRIAL GOVERNANCE

3.1   The Sponsor shall inform the NHS Trust and the Site Principal Investigator of the name and telephone number of the Monitor and the name of the person who will be available as a point of contact. The Sponsor shall also provide the Site Principal Investigator with an emergency number to enable adverse event reporting at any time.

3.2   The Parties shall comply with all laws and statutes applicable to the performance of the Clinical Trial including, but not limited to, the Human Rights Act 1998, the Data Protection Act 1998, the Medicines Act 1968, and with all relevant guidance relating to medicines and clinical trials from time to time in force including, but not limited to the ICH GCP, the World Medical Association Declaration of Helsinki entitled 'Ethical Principles for Medical Research Involving Human Subjects' (1996 version) and the NHS Research Governance Framework for Health and Social Care of March 2001, as amended from time to time.

3.3   The Sponsor shall comply with all guidelines from time to time in force and published by the Association of the British Pharmaceutical Industry in relation to clinical trials and in particular those entitled 'Clinical Trial Compensation Guidelines' (1991) a copy of which is set out in Appendix 3.

3.4   The Sponsor shall not commit (and warrants that in entering into the Agreement it has not committed) any of the following facts:

     3.4.1   provide or offer to provide to any person in the employment of the NHS Trust any gift or consideration not contemplated by the financial arrangements set out at clause 10 below in relation to the negotiation or performance of this Agreement or any other contract with the NHS Trust.

     3.4.2   make payment or agree to make payment of any commission to any person in the employment of the NHS Trust whether in relation to this Agreement or any other contract with the NHS Trust.

3.5   If the Sponsor or any of his employees, agents or sub-contractors, or any person acting on their behalf, commits any of the acts referred to in clause 3.4 above or commits any offence under the Prevention of Corruption Acts 1889 to 1916, in relation to this or any other agreement with the NHS Trust or an authority that is a health service body within the meaning given by Section 4(2) of the National Health Service and Community Care Act 1990, the NHS Trust shall be entitled, in addition to any other remedy available, to terminate this Agreement with immediate effect.

3.6   Should there be any inconsistency between the Protocol and the other terms of this Agreement the terms of the Protocol shall prevail to the extent of such inconsistency.

4   OBLIGATIONS OF THE PARTIES

4.1   The Site Principal Investigator shall be responsible for obtaining and maintaining all approvals from the relevant local research ethics committee for the conduct of the Clinical Trial and the Site Principal Investigator shall keep the Sponsor fully apprised of the progress of ethics committee submissions and shall upon request provide the Sponsor with all correspondence relating to such submissions. The Site Principal Investigator shall not consent to any change in the Protocol requested by a relevant ethics committee without the prior written consent of the Sponsor.

4.2   The Parties shall conduct the Clinical Trial in accordance with:

     (i)   the Protocol a copy of which for the purposes of identification appears at Appendix 1 to this Agreement;

     (ii)   the current marketing authorisation for the Investigational Medicinal Product or, as the case may be, Clinical Trial Certificate or Clinical Trial Exemption Certificate applicable to the Clinical Trial; and

     (iii)   the terms and conditions of the approval of the relevant [. . . insert name . . .] Ethics Committee(s).

and the NHS Trust shall ensure that neither administration of the Investigational Medicinal Product to any Clinical Trial Subject nor any other clinical intervention mandated by the Protocol takes place in relation to any such Clinical Trial Subject until it is satisfied that all relevant regulatory and ethics committee approvals have been obtained.

4.3   The Sponsor shall make available to the Site Principal Investigator copies of the documentation referred to in sub-paragraphs (i) and (ii) of clause 4.2 above and the Site Principal Investigator shall include such documents together with the Ethics Committee approvals in the Site File.

4.4 The Site Principal Investigator shall inform the Sponsor immediately upon learning of the existence of any of financial arrangement or interest between the Site Principal Investigator and the Sponsor of the type described at paragraph (f) of Appendix 6 hereto and for the purposes of the obligation contained in such paragraph the Sponsor shall advise the Site Principal Investigator in writing of the completion date of the Clinical Trial.

4.5 Neither the NHS Trust nor the Site Principal Investigator shall permit the Investigational Medicinal Product to be used for any purpose other than the conduct of the Clinical Trial and upon termination or expiration of this Agreement all unused Investigational Medicinal Product shall, at the Sponsor's option, either be returned to the Sponsor or disposed of in accordance with the Protocol.

4.6 The NHS Trust shall recruit [... insert number ...] Clinical Trial Subjects to participate in the Clinical Trial and the Parties shall conduct the Clinical Trial in accordance with the Timelines.

4.7 In the event that the Clinical Trial is part of a multi-centre clinical trial (which for the purposes of this Agreement shall mean that at least one other institution is taking part) the Sponsor may amend the number of Clinical Trial Subjects to be recruited pursuant to clause 4.6 above as follows:

4.7.1 if in the reasonable opinion of the Sponsor recruitment of Clinical Trial Subjects is proceeding at a rate below that required to enable the relevant Timeline to be met the Sponsor may by notice to the NHS Trust require recruitment at the Trial Site to cease and the terms of the Agreement shall relate thereafter to the number of Clinical Trial Subjects who have been accepted for treatment in the Clinical Trial at the date of such notice; or

4.7.2 if recruitment of Clinical Trial Subjects is proceeding at a rate above that required to meet the relevant Timeline the Sponsor may with the agreement of the NHS Trust increase the number of Clinical Trial Subjects to be recruited.

4.8 The NHS Trust shall permit the Monitor access to the records of Clinical Trial Subjects for monitoring and source data verification, such access to be arranged at mutually convenient times and on reasonable notice. The Sponsor will report on the Clinical Trial activity to the NHS Trust R & D Office, the frequency of reports to be [... insert period as appropriate to the Protocol ...]. The Sponsor will alert the R & D Director of the NHS Trust promptly to significant issues (in the opinion of the Monitor) relating to the conduct of the Clinical Trial. In the event that the Sponsor reasonably believes there has been any research misconduct in relation to the Clinical Trial the NHS Trust and the Site Principal Investigator shall provide all reasonable assistance to any investigation into any alleged research misconduct undertaken by or on behalf of the Sponsor. At its conclusion, the Sponsor and the R&D Director of the NHS Trust shall review the conduct of the Clinical Trial at the Trial Site, such review to take place within 3 months of Trial Site close-out.

4.9 The NHS Trust shall ensure that any clinical samples required to be tested during the course of the Clinical Trial are tested in accordance with the Protocol and at a laboratory approved by the Sponsor.

4.10   Upon completion of the Clinical Trial (whether prematurely or otherwise) the Site Principal Investigator shall [provide the Sponsor with/co-operate with the Sponsor in producing] a report of the Clinical Trial detailing the methodology, results and containing an analysis of the results and drawing appropriate conclusions.

4.11   Neither the NHS Trust nor the Site Principal Investigator shall during the term of this Agreement conduct any other trial which might adversely affect the NHS Trust's ability to perform its obligations under this Agreement.

5   LIABILITIES AND INDEMNITY

5.1   In the event of any claim or proceeding in respect of personal injury made or brought against the NHS Trust by a Clinical Trial Subject, the Sponsor shall indemnify the NHS Trust, its servants, agents and employees in accordance with the terms of the indemnity set out at Appendix 4 hereto.

5.2   The Sponsor shall indemnify the NHS Trust, its servants, agents and employees against all claims, proceedings, costs and expenses (including reasonable legal costs) in respect of loss of or damage to property which is the result of negligence on the part of the Sponsor or of a breach by the Sponsor of any of its obligations under this Agreement, save to the extent that any such loss or damage is the result of negligence on the part of the NHS Trust, its servants, agents or employees or of a breach of the obligations of the NHS Trust under this Agreement.

5.3   The NHS Trust shall indemnify the Sponsor, its servants, agents and employees against all claims, proceedings, costs and expenses (including reasonable legal costs) in respect of loss of or damage to property which is the result of negligence on the part of the NHS Trust or of a breach by the NHS Trust of its obligations under this Agreement, save to the extent that any such loss or damage is the result of negligence on the part of the Sponsor, its servants, agents or employees or of a breach of the obligations of the Sponsor under this Agreement.

5.4   Where a Party is required to provide an indemnity under clause 5.2 or (as the case may be) clause 5.3 above, that Party shall have the right to take over full care and control of the defence to any claim or proceeding by a third party, said defence to be at the sole expense of the indemnifying Party. The indemnifying Party shall be entitled to use legal counsel of his choice. The indemnifying Party shall keep the other Party fully informed of the progress of any such claim or proceeding, will consult fully with the other Party on the nature of any defence to be advanced, and will not compromise or settle any such claim or proceeding (whether by admission, statement or payment) nor will it conduct itself in such a way as could prejudice the defence of any such claim or proceeding without the written approval of the other Party, such approval not to be unreasonably withheld. Each Party will give the other written notice of any claim or proceeding brought against it with respect to any matter to which it may be entitled to indemnification under clause 5.2 or (as the case may be) clause 5.3 above and each Party will also use its best endeavours to inform the other Party promptly of any circumstances thought likely to give rise to any such claim or proceeding. Each Party will give to the other Party such help as may reasonably be required for the conduct and prompt handling of any such claim or proceeding.

5.5   In no circumstances shall either Party be liable to the other in contract, tort (including negligence or breach of statutory duty) or otherwise howsoever arising or whatever the cause thereof, for any loss of profit, business, reputation, contracts, revenues or anticipated savings for any special, indirect or consequential damage of any nature, which arises directly or indirectly from any default on the part of either Party. Nothing in this clause shall affect the responsibility of either Party in relation to death or personal injury caused by the negligence of that Party or its servants, agents or employees.

5.6   For the purpose of the indemnity provided in clause 5.2 above, the expression 'agents' shall include, but shall not be limited to, any person providing services to the NHS Trust under a contract for services or otherwise.

5.7   The Sponsor will take out appropriate insurance cover or will provide evidence to the satisfaction of the NHS Trust of self-insurance in respect of its potential liability under clauses 5.1 and 5.2 above and such cover shall be for a minimum of £[... insert amount ...] in respect of any one occurrence or series of occurrences arising from one event. The Sponsor shall produce to the NHS Trust, on request, copies of insurance policies or other evidence thereof together with evidence that such policies remain in full force and effect. The terms of any insurance or the amount of cover shall not relieve the Sponsor of any liabilities under this Agreement.

6   CONFIDENTIALITY

6.1   Medical confidentiality
        The Parties agree to adhere to the principles of medical confidentiality in relation to Clinical Trial Subjects involved in the Clinical Trial. Personal data shall not be disclosed to the Sponsor by the NHS Trust save where this is required directly or indirectly to satisfy the requirements of the Protocol or for the purpose of monitoring or adverse event reporting. The Sponsor shall not disclose the identity of Clinical Trial Subjects to third parties without prior written consent of the Clinical Trial Subject, in accordance with the requirements of the Data Protection Act 1998 and the principles set out in the Report of the Caldicott Committee on the review of patient identifiable information dated December 1997, a copy of which the NHS Trust shall supply to the Sponsor on request.

6.2   Confidential information

        6.2.1   The NHS Trust and the Sponsor shall ensure that only those of its officers and employees directly concerned with the carrying out of this Agreement have access to the Confidential Information and each Party undertakes to treat as strictly confidential and not to disclose to any third party any Confidential Information save where disclosure is required by a regulatory authority or by law and not to make use of any Confidential Information other than in accordance with this Agreement without the prior written consent of the other Party.

        6.2.2   In the event of a Party visiting the establishment of the other Party, the visiting Party undertakes that any further information relating to other clinical trials which may come to the visiting Party's knowledge as a result of any such visit, shall be kept strictly confidential and that any such information will not be disclosed to any third party or made use of in any way by the visiting Party without prior written permission of the other Party.

6.2.3   The obligations of confidentiality set out in this clause 6.2 shall not apply to Confidential Information which is (i) published or generally available to the public through no fault of the receiving Party, (ii) in the possession of the receiving Party prior to the date of this Agreement and is not subject to a duty of confidentiality, (iii) independently developed by the receiving Party and is not subject to a duty of confidentiality, (iv) obtained by the receiving Party from a third party not subject to a duty of confidentiality.

6.3   This clause 6 shall continue to apply after the expiry or termination of this Agreement.

7   PUBLICITY

The Sponsor will not use the name of the NHS Trust, nor of any member of the NHS Trust's staff, in any publicity, advertising or news release without the prior written approval of an authorised representative of the NHS Trust, such approval not to be unreasonably withheld. The NHS Trust will not use the name of the Sponsor nor of any of its employees, in any publicity without the prior written approval of the Sponsor.

8   PUBLICATION

8.1   The Sponsor recognises that the NHS Trust and Site Principal Investigator have a responsibility under the Research Governance Framework for Health and Social Care to ensure that results of scientific interest arising from the Clinical Trial are appropriately published and disseminated. The Sponsor agrees that employees of the NHS Trust shall be permitted to present at symposia, national or regional professional meetings, and to publish in journals, theses or dissertations, or otherwise of their own choosing, methods and results of the Clinical Trial subject to the publication policy described in the Protocol. If the Clinical Trial is multi-centred (as defined in clause 4.7 above), any publication based on the results obtained at the Trial Site (or a group of sites) shall not be made before the first multi-centre publication. If a publication concerns the analyses of sub-sets of data from a multi-centred Clinical Trial the publication shall make reference to the relevant multi-centre publication(s).

8.2   Upon completion of the Clinical Trial, and any prior publication of multi-centre data, or when the Clinical Trial data are adequate (in Sponsor's reasonable judgement), the NHS Trust may prepare the data deriving from the Clinical Trial for publication. Such data will be submitted to the Sponsor for review and comment prior to publication. In order to ensure that the Sponsor will be able to make comments and suggestions where pertinent, material for public dissemination will be submitted to the Sponsor for review at least sixty (60) days (or the time limit specified in the Protocol if longer) prior to submission for publication, public dissemination, or review by a publication committee.

8.3   The NHS Trust agrees that all reasonable comments made by the Sponsor in relation to a proposed publication by the NHS Trust will be incorporated by the NHS Trust into the publication.

8.4   During the period for review of a proposed publication referred to in clause 8.2 above, the Sponsor shall be entitled to make a reasoned request to the NHS Trust that publication be delayed for a period of up to six (6) months from the date of first submission to the Sponsor in order to enable the Sponsor to take steps to protect its proprietary information and the NHS Trust shall not unreasonably withhold its consent to such a request.

9 INTELLECTUAL PROPERTY

9.1   All Intellectual Property Rights and Know How owned by or licensed to NHS Trust prior to and after the date of this Agreement other than any Intellectual Property Rights and Know How arising from the Clinical Trial is and shall remain the property of the NHS Trust.

9.2   All Intellectual Property Rights and Know How owned by or licensed to the Sponsor prior to and after the date of this Agreement other than any Intellectual Property Rights and Know How arising out of the Clinical Trial is and shall remain the property of the Sponsor.

9.3   All Intellectual Property Rights and Know How arising from the Clinical Trial shall vest in or be exclusively licensed to the Sponsor in accordance with clauses 9.4 and 9.5 below.

9.4   The NHS Trust hereby assigns its rights in all Intellectual Property Rights and, to the extent possible in all Know How, arising out of the Clinical Trial to the Sponsor and at the request and expense of the Sponsor, the NHS Trust and the Site Principal Investigator shall execute all such documents and do all such other acts and things as the Sponsor may reasonably require in order to vest fully and effectively all such Intellectual Property Rights and Know How in the Sponsor or its nominee.

9.5   NHS Trust and Site Principal Investigator shall promptly disclose to the Sponsor any and all Know How generated pursuant to this Agreement and undertake not to use such Know How other than for the purposes of this Agreement without the prior written consent of the Sponsor, such consent not to be unreasonably withheld. NHS Trust hereby grants to the Sponsor an exclusive, worldwide, irrevocable, fully paid up royalty free licence under such Know How (to the extent such Know How is not assigned pursuant to clause 9.4 above) to exploit the same for any purpose whatsoever.

10 FINANCIAL ARRANGEMENTS

10.1   Arrangements relating to the financing of this Clinical Trial by the Sponsor are set out in Appendix 5 hereto.

10.2   All payments will be made according to the schedule contained in Appendix 5 on presentation of a VAT invoice to the Sponsor by the NHS Trust.

10.3   The Sponsor shall make payment within thirty (30) days of the date of receipt of the invoice mentioned in Clause 10.2 above.

10.4   Any delay in the payment of the payee invoices by the Sponsor will incur an interest charge on any amounts overdue of 2 per cent per month above the National Westminster Bank plc base rate prevailing on the date the payment is due.

11 TERM

This Agreement will remain in effect until completion of the Clinical Trial, close-out of the Trial Site and completion of the obligations of the Parties under this Agreement or earlier termination in accordance with this Agreement.

12   EARLY TERMINATION

12.1   Either the Sponsor or the NHS Trust (the Terminating Party) may terminate this Agreement with immediate effect at any time if the other Party (the Defaulting Party) is:

    12.1.1   in breach of any of the Defaulting Party's obligations hereunder (including a failure without just cause to meet a Timeline) and fails to remedy such breach where it is capable of remedy within 28 days of a written notice from the Terminating Party specifying the breach and requiring its remedy;

    12.1.2   declared insolvent or has an administrator or receiver appointed over all or any part of its assets or ceases or threatens to cease to carry on its business.

12.2   A Party may terminate this Agreement on notice to the other Party with immediate effect if it is reasonably of the opinion that the Clinical Trial should cease in the interests of the health of Clinical Trial Subjects involved in the Clinical Trial.

12.3   The Sponsor may terminate this Agreement on notice to the NHS Trust if [. . . insert name of investigator . . .] is no longer able (for whatever reason) to act as Site Principal Investigator and no replacement mutually acceptable to the NHS Trust and the Sponsor can be found.

12.4   The Sponsor may terminate this Agreement immediately upon notice in writing to the NHS Trust for reasons not falling within clauses 12.1, 12.2 or 12.3 above, save that in such circumstances the provisions of clause 12.6 below shall also apply. In all such circumstances the Sponsor shall confer with the Site Principal Investigator and use its best endeavours to minimise any inconvenience or harm to Clinical Trial Subjects caused by the premature termination of the Clinical Trial.

12.5   In the event of early termination of this Agreement by the Sponsor, pursuant to clauses 12.2, 12.3 and 12.4 and subject to an obligation on the NHS Trust and the Site Principal Investigator to mitigate any loss, the Sponsor shall pay all costs incurred and falling due for payment up to the date of termination, and also all expenditure falling due for payment after the date of termination which arises from commitments reasonably and necessarily incurred by the NHS Trust for the performance of the Clinical Trial prior to the date of termination, and agreed with the Sponsor.

12.6   In the event of early termination pursuant to clause 12.4 above the Sponsor shall make a compensatory payment in accordance with Appendix 5.

12.7   In the event of early termination if payment (whether for salaries or otherwise) has been made by the Sponsor to the NHS Trust in advance for work not completed such monies shall be applied to termination related costs and in the case of termination pursuant to clause 12.4 above towards the compensatory payment payable pursuant to clause 12.6 and the remainder of the monies shall be returned forthwith to the Sponsor.

12.8   At close-out of the Trial Site following termination or expiration of this Agreement the NHS Trust shall immediately deliver to the Sponsor all Confidential Information and any other unused materials provided to the NHS Trust pursuant to this Agreement.

12.9   Termination of this Agreement will be without prejudice to the accrued rights and liabilities of the Parties under this Agreement.

13   RELATIONSHIP BETWEEN THE PARTIES

13.1   Neither Party may assign its rights under this Agreement or any part thereof without the prior written consent of the other Party and neither Party may sub-contract the performance of all or any of its obligations under this Agreement without the prior written consent of the other Party. Any party who so sub-contracts shall be responsible for the acts and omissions of its sub-contractors as though they were its own.

13.2   Nothing shall be construed as creating a partnership, contract of employment or relationship of principal and agent between the Parties.

14   AGREEMENT AND MODIFICATION

14.1   Any change in the terms of this Agreement shall be valid only if the change is made in writing, agreed and signed by the Parties.

14.2   This Agreement including its Appendices contains the entire understanding between the Parties and supersedes all other negotiations representations and undertakings whether written or oral of prior date between the Parties relating to the Clinical Trial which is the subject of this Agreement.

15   FORCE MAJEURE

Neither Party shall be liable to the other Party or shall be in default of its obligations hereunder if such default is the result of war, hostilities, revolution, civil commotion, strike, epidemic, accident, fire, wind, flood or because of any act of God or other cause beyond the reasonable control of the Party affected. The Party affected by such circumstances shall promptly notify the other Party in writing when such circumstances cause a delay or failure in performance ('a Delay') and where they cease to do so. In the event of a Delay lasting for [. . . insert number . . .] weeks or more the non-affected Party shall have the right to terminate this Agreement immediately by notice in writing to the other Party.

16   NOTICES

Any notices under this Agreement shall be in writing, signed by the relevant Party to this Agreement and delivered personally, by courier or by recorded delivery post.

Notices to the Sponsor shall be addressed to:

[. . . insert address . . .]

Notices to the NHS Trust shall be addressed to:

[. . . insert address . . .]

17   RIGHTS OF THIRD PARTIES

Nothing in this Agreement is intended to confer on any person any right to enforce any term of this Agreement which that person would not have had but for the Contracts (Rights of Third Parties) Act 1999.

18   WAIVER

No failure, delay, relaxation or indulgence by any Party in exercising any right conferred on such Party by this Agreement shall operate as a waiver of such right, nor shall any single or partial exercise of any such right nor any single failure to do so, preclude any other or future exercise of it, or the exercise of any other right under this Agreement.

19   DISPUTE RESOLUTION

19.1   In the event of a dispute the Parties agree to attempt to settle it by mediation in accordance with the Centre for Effective Dispute Resolution Model Mediation Procedure. To initiate a mediation a Party must give notice in writing (ADR Notice) to the other Party requesting mediation in accordance with this clause. The Parties shall seek to agree the nomination of the mediator, but in the absence of agreement he shall be nominated by the President for the time being of the British Medical Association. The mediation will start no later than [20] days after date of the ADR Notice. If the dispute is not resolved within [30] days of the ADR Notice a Party may by written notice to the other refer the dispute to arbitration in accordance with clause 19.2 below.

19.2   If the Parties are unable to settle a dispute arising out of or in connection with this Agreement by mediation the dispute shall be finally settled by arbitration in accordance with the UNCITRAL Arbitration Rules as at present in force (the 'UNCITRAL Rules'). The Notice of Arbitration shall be served in accordance with Article 3 of the UNCITRAL Rules and a single arbitrator shall be appointed by agreement of the Parties or in the absence of agreement, by the President for the time being of the British Medical Association. The seat of arbitration shall be London and the language of the arbitral proceedings shall be English. All and any awards of the arbitrators shall be made in accordance with the UNCITRAL Rules in writing and shall be binding on the Parties who expressly exclude all and any rights of appeal from all and any awards to the extent that such exclusion may be validly made.

20   GOVERNING LAW

This Agreement shall be interpreted and governed by English Law.

Signed on behalf of the:

SPONSOR: ....

　　　　　　　...   Date: ....
　　　　　　　(Print name and position)

Signed on behalf of the:

NHS TRUST   ....

　　　　　　　...   Date: ....
　　　　　　　(Print name and position)

Authorised signatory (Chief Executive, Director of R&D, or Finance Director)

APPENDIX 1

Append The Protocol

APPENDIX 2

TIMELINES FOR PARTIES

Milestone	Sponsor responsibility	Site responsibility	Target date
Provision of materials for Ethics Committee submission	X		
Ethics Committee submission	[X]	X	
Trial Site initiation visit	X	X	
First Clinical Trial Subject recruited		X	
Last Clinical Trial Subject recruited		X	
All CRF queries submitted	X		
All CRF queries completed		X	

APPENDIX 3

[COPY OF 'CLINICAL TRIAL COMPENSATION GUIDELINES']

APPENDIX 4

FORM OF INDEMNITY

1. The Sponsor indemnifies and holds harmless the NHS Trust and its employees and agents against all claims and proceedings (to include any settlements or ex gratia payments made with the consent of the Parties hereto and reasonable legal and expert costs and expenses) made or brought (whether successfully or otherwise):

    1.1 by or on behalf of Clinical Trial Subjects and (or their dependants) against the NHS Trust or any of its employees or agents for personal injury (including death) to Clinical Trial Subjects arising out of or relating to the administration of the product(s) under investigation or any clinical intervention or procedure provided for or required by the Protocol to which the Clinical Trial Subjects would not have been exposed but for their participation in the Clinical Trial;

    1.2 by the NHS Trust its employees or agents or by or on behalf of a Clinical Trial Subject for a declaration concerning the treatment of a Clinical Trial Subject who has suffered such personal injury.

2. The above indemnity by the Sponsor shall not apply to any such claim or proceeding:

    2.1 to the extent that such personal injury (including death) is caused by the negligent or wrongful acts or omissions or breach of statutory duty of the NHS Trust, its employees or agents;

    2.2 to the extent that such personal injury (including death) is caused by the failure of the NHS Trust, its employees, or agents to conduct the Clinical Trial in accordance with the Protocol;

    2.3 unless as soon as reasonably practicable following receipt of notice of such claim or proceeding, the NHS Trust shall have notified the Sponsor in writing of it and shall, upon the Sponsor's request, and that the Sponsor's cost, have permitted the Sponsor to have full care and control of the claim or proceeding using legal representation of its own choosing;

    2.4 If the NHS Trust, its employees, or agents shall have made any admission in respect of such claim or proceeding or taken any action relating to such claim or proceeding prejudicial to the defence of it without the written consent of the Sponsor such consent not to be unreasonably withheld provided that this condition shall not be treated as breached by any statement properly made by the NHS Trust, its employees or agents in connection with the operation of the NHS Trust's internal complaint procedures, accident reporting procedures or disciplinary procedures or where such a statement is required by law.

3. The Sponsor shall keep the NHS Trust and its legal advisors fully informed of the progress of any such claim or proceeding, will consult fully with the NHS Trust on the nature of any defence to be advanced and will not settle any such claim or proceeding without the written approval of the NHS Trust (such approval not to be unreasonably withheld).

4. Without prejudice to the provisions of paragraph 2.3 above, the NHS Trust will use its reasonable endeavours to inform the Sponsor promptly of any circumstances reasonably sought likely to give rise to any such claim or proceeding of which it is directly aware and shall keep the Sponsor reasonably informed of developments in relation to any such claim or proceeding even where the NHS Trust decides not to make a claim under this indemnity. Likewise, the Sponsor shall use its reasonable endeavours to inform the NHS Trust or any circumstances and shall keep the NHS Trust reasonably informed of developments in relation to any such claim or proceeding made or brought against the Sponsor alone.

5. The NHS Trust and the Sponsor will each give to the other such help as may reasonably be required for the official conduct and prompt handling of any claim or proceeding by or on behalf of Clinical Trial Subjects (or their dependants) or concerning such a declaration as is referred to in paragraph 1.2 above.

6. Without prejudice to the foregoing if injury is suffered by a Clinical Trial Subject while participating in the Clinical Trial, the Sponsor agrees to operate in good faith the guidelines published in 1991 by the Association of the British Pharmaceutical Industry and entitled 'Clinical Trial Compensation Guidelines' and shall request the Site Principal Investigator to make clear to the Clinical Trial Subjects that the Clinical Trial is being conducted subject to the Association guidelines.

7. For the purpose of this indemnity, the expression 'agents' shall be deemed to include without limitation any nurse or other health professional providing services to the NHS Trust under a contract for services or otherwise and any person carrying out work for the NHS Trust under such a contract connected with such of the NHS Trust's facilities and equipment as are made available for the Clinical Trial.

APPENDIX 5

FINANCIAL ARRANGEMENTS

APPENDIX 6

CONDITIONS APPLICABLE TO THE SITE PRINCIPAL INVESTIGATOR

(a)   he is free to participate in the Clinical Trial and there are no rights which may be exercised by or obligations owed to any third party which might prevent or restrict his performance of the obligations detailed in this Agreement.

(b)   he is not involved in any regulatory or misconduct litigation or investigation by the Food and Drug Administration, the Medicines Control Agency, the European Medicines Evaluation Agency, the General Medical Council or other regulatory authorities. No data produced by him in any previous clinical study has been rejected because of concerns as to its accuracy or because it was generated by fraud.

(c)   he has considered, and is satisfied that, facilities appropriate to the Clinical Trial are available to him at the Trial Site and that he is supported, and will continue to be supported, by medical and other staff of sufficient number and experience to enable the NHS Trust to perform the Clinical Trial efficiently and in accordance with its obligations under the Agreement.

(d)   he carries medical liability insurance (or the NHS Trust carries medical liability insurance covering him) and details and evidence of the coverage will be provided to Sponsor upon request.

(e)   during the Clinical Trial, he will not serve as an investigator or other significant participant in any clinical trial for another sponsor if such activity might adversely affect his ability to perform his obligations under this Agreement.

(f)   neither he, nor his spouse nor any dependent children, have entered into and will not enter into any financial arrangements with the Sponsor to hold financial interests in the Sponsor that are required to be disclosed pursuant to the US Code of Federal Regulations Title 21, Part 54, namely (i) any financial arrangement whereby the value of the compensation paid in respect of the performance of the Clinical Trial could be influenced by the outcome of the Clinical Trial (as defined in 21 CFR 54.2(a)), (ii) any proprietary interest in the product being tested (as defined in 21 CFR 54.2(c)), (iii) any significant equity interest in the Sponsor (as defined in 21 CFR 54.2(b)) and (iv) any significant payments from the Sponsor such as grants to fund ongoing research, compensation in the form of equipment, retainers for ongoing consultation or honoraria (as defined in 21 CFR 54.2(f)). In the case of subparagraphs (iii) and (iv) the Site Principal Investigator understands that such prohibitions relate to the period that the Site Principal Investigator is carrying out the Clinical Trial and for 1 year following completion of the Clinical Trial.

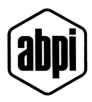

FORM OF INDEMNITY FOR CLINICAL STUDIES

To: **[Name and address of sponsoring company] ('the Sponsor')**

From: **[Name and address of health authority/health board/NHS Trust] ('the Authority')**

Re: **Clinical study No ( ) with [name of product]**

1.   It is proposed that the Authority should agree to participate in the above sponsored study ('the Study') involving [patients of the Authority] [non-patient volunteers] ('the Subjects') to be conducted by [name of investigator(s)] ('the Investigator') in accordance with the protocol annexed, as amended from time to time with the agreement of the Sponsor and the Investigator ('the Protocol'). The Sponsor confirms that it is a term of its agreement with the Investigator that the Investigator shall obtain all necessary approvals of the applicable Local Research Ethics Committee and shall resolve with the Authority any issues of a revenue nature.

2.   The Authority agrees to participate by allowing the Study to be undertaken on its premises utilising such facilities, personnel and equipment as the Investigator may reasonably need for the purpose of the Study.

3.   In consideration of such participation by the Authority, and subject to paragraph 4 below, the Sponsor indemnifies and holds harmless the Authority and its employees and agents against all claims and proceedings (to include any settlements or ex gratia payments made with the consent of the parties hereto and reasonable legal and expert costs and expenses) made or brought (whether successfully or otherwise).

    (a)   by or on behalf of Subjects taking part in the Study (or their dependants) against the Authority or any of its employees or agents for personal injury (including death) to Subjects arising out of or relating to the administration of the product(s) under investigation or any clinical intervention or procedure provided for or required by the Protocol to which the Subjects would not have been exposed but for their participation in the Study.

    (b)   by the Authority, its employees or agents or by or on behalf of a Subject for a declaration concerning the treatment of a Subject who has suffered such personal injury.

4.   The above indemnity by the Sponsor shall not apply to any such claim or proceeding:

    4.1   to the extent that such personal injury (including death) is caused by the negligent or wrongful acts or omissions or breach of statutory duty of the Authority, its employees or agents.

    4.2   to the extent that such personal injury (including death) is caused by the failure of the Authority, its employees, or agents to conduct the Study in accordance with the Protocol.

    4.3   unless as soon as reasonably practicable following receipt of notice of such claim or proceeding, the Authority shall have notified the Sponsor in writing of it and shall, upon the Sponsor's request, and at the Sponsor's cost, have permitted the Sponsor to have full care and control of the claim or proceeding using legal representation of its own choosing.

    4.4   if the Authority, its employees, or agents shall have made any admission in respect of such claim or proceeding or taken any action relating to such claim or proceeding prejudicial to the defence of it without the written consent of the Sponsor such consent not to be unreasonably withheld provided that this condition shall not be treated as breached by any statement properly made by the Authority, its employees or agents in connection with the operation of the Authority's internal complaint procedures, accident reporting procedures or disciplinary procedures or where such statement is required by law.

5.   The Sponsor shall keep the Authority and its legal advisers fully informed of the progress of any such claim or proceeding, will consult fully with the Authority on the nature of any defence to be advanced and will not settle any such claim or proceeding without the written approval of the Authority (such approval not to be unreasonably withheld).

6.   Without prejudice to the provisions of paragraph 4.3 above, the Authority will use its reasonable endeavours to inform the Sponsor promptly of any circumstances reasonably thought likely to give rise to any such claim or proceeding of which it is directly aware and shall keep the Sponsor reasonably informed of developments in relation to any such claim or proceeding even where the Authority decides not to make a claim under this indemnity. Likewise, the Sponsor shall use its reasonable endeavours to inform the Authority of any such circumstances and shall keep the Authority reasonably informed of developments in relation to any such claim or proceeding made or brought against the Sponsor alone.

7.   The Authority and the Sponsor will each give to the other such help as may reasonably be required for the efficient conduct and prompt handling of any claim or proceeding by or on behalf of Subjects (or their dependants) or concerning such a declaration as is referred to in paragraph 3(b) above.

8.   Without prejudice to the foregoing if injury is suffered by a Subject while participating in the Study, the Sponsor agrees to operate in good faith the Guidelines published in 1991 by The Association of the British Pharmaceutical Industry and entitled 'Clinical Trial Compensation Guidelines' (where the Subject is a patient) and the Guidelines published in 1988 by the same Association and entitled 'Guidelines for Medical Experiments in non-patient Human Volunteers' (where the subject is not a patient) and shall request the Investigator to make clear to the Subjects that the Study is being conducted subject to the applicable Association Guidelines.

9. For the purpose of this indemnity, the expression 'agents' shall be deemed to include without limitation any nurse or other health professional providing services to the Authority under a contract for services or otherwise and any person carrying out work for the Authority under such a contract connected with such of the Authority's facilities and equipment as are made available for the Study under paragraph 2 above.

10. This indemnity shall be governed by and construed in accordance with English/Scots* law.

SIGNED on behalf of the Health Authority/Health Board/NHS Trust

....

Chief Executive/District General Manager

SIGNED on behalf of the Company

....

Dated ....

* Delete as appropriate

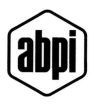

FORM OF INDEMNITY FOR CLINICAL STUDIES

From: **('the Sponsor')**

To: **('the Trust')**

Re:

1. It is proposed that the Trust should agree to participate in the above sponsored study ('the Study') involving patients of the Trust ('the Subjects') to be conducted by .... ('the Investigator') in accordance with the protocol annexed, as amended from time to time with the agreement of the Sponsor and the Investigator ('the Protocol'). The Sponsor confirms that it is a term of its agreement with the Investigator that the Investigator shall obtain all necessary approvals of the applicable Local Research Ethics Committee and shall resolve with the Trust any issues of a revenue nature.

2. The Trust agrees to participate by allowing the Study to be undertaken on its premises utilising such facilities, personnel and equipment as the Investigator may reasonably need for the purpose of the Study.

3. In consideration of such participation by the Trust and subject to paragraph 4 below, the Sponsor indemnifies and holds harmless the Trust and its employees and agents against all claims and proceedings (to include any settlements or *ex gratia* payments made with the consent of the parties hereto and reasonable legal and expert costs and expenses) made or brought (whether successfully or otherwise):-

    (a) by or on behalf of Subjects taking part in the Study (or their dependants) against the Trust or any of its employees and agents for personal injury (including death) to Subjects arising out of or relating to the administration of the product(s) under investigation or any clinical intervention or procedure provided for or required by the Protocol to which the Subjects would not have been exposed but for their participation in the Study.

    (b) by the Trust, its employees or agents or by or on behalf of a Subject for a declaration concerning the treatment of a Subject who has suffered such personal injury.

4. The above indemnity by the Sponsor shall not apply to any such claim or proceeding:

(a) to the extent that such personal injury (including death) is caused by the negligent or wrongful acts or omissions or breach of statutory duty of the Trust, its employees, or any agents;

(b) to the extent that such personal injury (including death) is caused by the failure of the Trust, its employees, or any agents to conduct the Study within the NHS in accordance with the Protocol;

(c) unless as soon as reasonably practicable following receipt of notice of such claim or proceeding, the Trust shall have notified the Sponsor in writing of it and shall, upon the Sponsor's request, and at the Sponsor's cost, have permitted the Sponsor to have full care and control of the claim or proceeding using legal representation of its own choosing;

(d) if the Trust, its employees, or agents shall have made any admission in respect of such claim or proceeding or taken any action relating to such claim or proceeding prejudicial to the defence of it without the written consent of the Sponsor such consent not to be unreasonably withheld provided that this condition shall not be treated as breached by any statement properly made by the Trust, its employees or agents in connection with the operation of the Trust's internal complaint procedures, accident reporting procedures or disciplinary procedures or where such statement is required by law.

5. The Sponsor shall keep the Trust and its legal advisers fully informed of the progress of any such claim or proceeding, will consult fully with the Trust on the nature of any defence to be advanced and will not settle any such claim or proceeding without the written approval of the Trust (such approval not to be unreasonably withheld).

6. Without prejudice to the provisions of paragraph 4(c) above, the Trust will use its reasonable endeavours to inform the Sponsor promptly of any circumstances reasonably thought likely to give rise to any such claim or proceeding of which it is directly aware and shall keep the Sponsor reasonably informed of developments in relation to any such claim or proceeding even where the Trust decides not to make a claim under this indemnity. Likewise, the Sponsor shall use its reasonable endeavours to inform the Trust of any such circumstances and shall keep the Trust reasonably informed of developments in relation to any such claim or proceeding made or brought against the Sponsor alone.

7. The Trust and the Sponsor will each give to the other such help as may reasonably be required for the efficient conduct and prompt handling of any claim or proceeding by or on behalf of Subjects (or their dependants) or concerning such a declaration as is referred to in paragraph 3(b) above.

8. Without prejudice to the foregoing if injury is suffered by a Subject while participating in the study, the Sponsor agrees to operate in good faith the Guidelines published in 1991 by The Association of the British Pharmaceutical Industry and entitled 'Clinical Trial Compensation Guidelines' (where the subject is a patient) and the 'Guidelines for Medical Experiments on Non-Patient Human Volunteers' (where the Subject is not a patient) and shall request the Investigator to make clear to the Subjects that the Study is being conducted subject to the applicable Association Guidelines.

9. For the purpose of this indemnity, the expression 'agents' shall be deemed to include without limitation any nurse or other health professional providing services to the Trust under a contract for services or otherwise and any person carrying out work for the Trust under such a contract connected with such of the Trust's facilities and equipment as are made available for the study under paragraph 2 above.

10. This indemnity shall be governed by and construed in accordance with Scots law.

SIGNED for and on behalf of the NHS Trust

SIGNED ....

PRINTED ....

Chief Executive

DATED ....

SIGNED for and on behalf of the Sponsor

SIGNED ....

PRINTED ....

DATED ....

ABPI GUIDELINE ON ADVERTISING FOR SUBJECTS FOR CLINICAL TRIALS

As a result of a number of enquiries to the Medical Affairs Department of the Association of the British Pharmaceutical Industry (ABPI) and the recognition that the media was being increasingly used to advertise for subjects for clinical trials, the ABPI Medical Committee set up a Task Group to develop these guidelines.

Recently the European Commission (EC) have included an appendix on advertising for trial subjects in the detailed guidance on the application to be submitted for an ethics committee opinion on a clinical trial on a medicinal product for human use. The ABPI guideline set out below takes into account the views of the Medical Committee and additional guidance from the EC guideline.

Research Ethics Committees (RECs) should be invited to review all materials used to recruit subjects for all phases of clinical trials, including, but not limited to:

1. Television and radio advertisements.

2. Letters, posters, newsletters, etc.

3. Newspaper advertisements.

4. Internet web sites.

1 Essential Information for an Advertisement

1. A statement indicating that the study involves research.

2. A contact name and phone number for the subject to contact.

3. Some of the eligibility criteria.

4. The likely duration of the subject's participation for a specific study.

5. That the advertisement has been approved by an ethics committee.

6. That your general practitioner will be informed that you are taking part in the clinical trial.

7. That any response to the advertisement will be recorded but will not indicate any obligation.

2 Additional Permitted Content

1. The purpose of the research may be described.

2. The location of the research.

3. The company or institution involved may be named if appropriate.

3   Statements That Should Not Be Used

1.   Implied or expressed claims of safety or efficacy.

2.   Undue emphasis on reimbursement but mention of reimbursement is permitted.

3.   Any express or implied claim that the research is FDA or MCA approved.

4.   Use of the term 'new' unless qualified, i.e. 'new research medicine', 'new investigational medicine'.

5.   The compound's name.

6.   Care should be taken to ensure that advertisements are in no way promotional for the medicine concerned.

The ethics committee approval of any advertising material should be kept with the master study file.

GUIDELINES FOR COMPANY-SPONSORED SAFETY ASSESSMENT OF MARKETED MEDICINES (SAMM)

Introduction

It is well-recognised that there is a continuous need to monitor the safety of medicines as they are used in clinical practice. Spontaneous reporting schemes (e.g. the UK yellow card system) provide important early warning signals of potential drug hazards and also provide a means of continuous surveillance. Formal studies to evaluate safety may also be necessary, particularly in the confirmation and characterisation of possible hazards identified at an earlier stage of drug development. Such studies may also be useful in identifying previously unsuspected reactions.

Scope of guidelines

These guidelines apply to the conduct of all company-sponsored studies which evaluate the safety of marketed products. They take the place of previous guidelines on post-marketing surveillance which were published in 1988 (*BMJ*, 296: 399–400). Studies performed under those guidelines were found to have some notable limitations (*BMJ*, 1992, 304: 1470–1472) and these new guidelines have been prepared in response to the problems identified. The major changes may be summarised as follows:

(1) The scope of the guidelines has been expanded to include all company-sponsored studies which are carried out to evaluate safety of marketed medicines. It should be emphasised that this includes both studies conducted in general practice and in the hospital setting. The name of the guidelines has been changed to reflect the emphasis on safety assessment rather than merely surveillance.

(2) The guidelines have been developed to provide a framework on which a variety of data collection methods can be used to improve the evaluation of the safety of marketed medicines. Whilst it is recognised that the design used needs to be tailored to particular drugs and hazards, the guidelines define the essential principles which may be applied in a variety of situations. The study methods in this field continue to develop and therefore there will be a need to review regularly these guidelines to ensure that they reflect advances made in the assessment of drug safety.

The guidelines have been formulated and agreed by a Working Party which includes representation from the Medicines Control Agency (MCA), Committee on Safety of Medicines (CSM), Association of the British Pharmaceutical Industry (ABPI), British Medical Association (BMA) and the Royal College of General Practitioners (RCGP). Other guidelines exist for the conduct of 'Phase IV clinical trials' where the medication is provided by the sponsoring company (see section 2(b) below). Some of these studies will also meet the definition of a SAMM study (see below) and should therefore also comply with the present guidelines.

1   Definition of Safety Assessment of Marketed Medicines

(a)   Safety assessment of marketed medicines (SAMM) is defined as 'a formal investigation conduc-
        ted for the purpose of assessing the clinical safety of marketed medicine(s) in clinical practice'.

(b)   Any study of a marketed drug which has the evaluation of clinical safety as a specific objective
        should be included. Safety evaluation will be a specific objective in postmarketing studies either
        when there is a known safety issue under investigation and/or when the numbers of patients to
        be included will add significantly to the existing safety data for the product(s). Smaller studies
        conducted primarily for other purposes should not be considered as SAMM studies. However,
        if a study which is not conducted for the purpose of evaluating safety unexpectedly identifies a
        hazard, the manufacturer would be expected to inform the MCA immediately and the section
        of these guidelines covering liaison with regulatory authorities would thereafter apply.

        In cases of doubt as to whether or not a study comes under the scope of the guidelines the
        sponsor should discuss the intended study plan with the MCA.

2   Scope and Objectives of SAMM

(a)   SAMM may be conducted for the purpose of identifying previously unrecognised safety issues
        (hypothesis-generation) or to investigate possible hazards (hypothesis-testing).

(b)   A variety of designs may be appropriate including observational cohort studies, case-
        surveillance or case-control studies. Clinical trials may also be used to evaluate the safety
        of marketed products, involving systematic allocation of treatment (for example randomisa-
        tion). Such studies must also adhere to the current guidelines for Phase IV clinical trials.

(c)   The design to be used will depend on the objectives of the study, which must be clearly defined
        in the study plan. Any specific safety concerns to be investigated should be identified in the
        study plan and explicitly addressed by the proposed methods.

3   Design of studies

Observational cohort studies

(a)   The population studied should be as representative as possible of the general population of
        users, and be unselected unless specifically targeted by the objectives of the study (for example
        a study of the elderly). Exclusion criteria should be limited to the contraindications stated in
        the data sheet or summary of product characteristics (SPC). The prescriber should be provided
        with a data sheet or SPC for all products to be used. Where the product is prescribed outside
        the indications on the data sheet, such patients should be included in the analysis of the study
        findings.

(b)   Observational cohort studies should normally include appropriate comparator group(s). The
        comparator group(s) will usually include patients with the disease/indication(s) relevant to
        the primary study drug and such patients will usually be treated with alternative therapies.

(c)   The product(s) should be prescribed in the usual manner, for example on an FP10 form written
        by the general practitioner or through the usual hospital procedures.

(d) Patients must not be prescribed particular medicines in order to include them in observational cohort studies since this is unethical (see section 15 of the 'Guidelines on the Practices of Ethics Committees in Medical Research involving Human Subjects', Royal College of Physicians, 1990).

(e) The prescribing of a drug and the inclusion of the patient in a study are two issues which must be clearly separated. Drugs must be prescribed solely as a result of a normal clinical evaluation, and since such indications may vary from doctor to doctor a justification for the prescription should be recorded in the study documents. In contrast, the inclusion of the patient in the study must be solely dependent upon the criteria for recruitment which have been specifically identified in the study procedures. Any deviation from the study criteria for recruitment could lead to selection bias.

(f) The study plan should stipulate the maximum number of patients to be entered by a single doctor. No patient should be prospectively entered into more than one study simultaneously.

Case-control studies

(g) Case-control studies are usually conducted retrospectively. In case-control studies comparison is made between the history of drug exposure of cases with the disease of interest and appropriate controls without the disease. The study design should attempt to account for known sources of bias and confounding.

Case-surveillance

(h) The purpose of case-surveillance is to study patients with diseases which are likely to be drug-related and to ascertain drug exposure. Companies who sponsor such studies should liaise particularly closely with the MCA in order to determine the most appropriate arrangements for the reporting of cases.

Clinical trials

(i) Large clinical trials are sometimes useful in the investigation of post-marketing safety issues and these may involve random allocation to treatment. In other respects, an attempt should be made to study patients under as normal conditions as possible. Exclusion criteria should be limited to the contraindications in the data sheet or SPC unless they are closely related to the particular objectives of the study. Clinical trials must also adhere to the current guidelines for Phase IV clinical trials (see 2(b) above). Studies which fulfil the definition of SAMM but are performed under a clinical trial exemption (CTX) or under the clinical trial on a marketed product (CTMP) scheme are within the scope of these guidelines.

4 Conduct of studies

(a) Responsibility for the conduct and quality of company-sponsored studies shall be vested in the company's medical department under the supervision of a named medical practitioner registered in the United Kingdom, and whose name shall be recorded in the study documents.

(b)   Where a study is performed for a company by an agent, a named medical practitioner registered in the United Kingdom shall be identified by the agent to supervise the study and liaise with the company's medical department.

(c)   Consideration should be given to the appointment of an independent advisory group(s) to monitor the safety information and oversee the study.

5   Liaison with regulatory authorities

(a)   Companies proposing to perform a SAMM study are encouraged to discuss the draft study plan with the Medicines Control Agency (MCA) at an early state. Particular consideration should be given to specific safety issues which may require investigation.

(b)   Before the study commences a study plan should be finalised which explains the aims and objectives of the study, the methods to be used (including statistical analysis) and the record keeping which is to be maintained. The company shall submit the study plan plus any proposed initial communications to doctors to the MCA at least one month before the planned start of the study. The MCA will review the proposed study and may comment. The responsibility for the conduct of the study will, however, rest with the sponsoring pharmaceutical company.

(c)   The company should inform the MCA when the study has commenced and will normally provide a brief report on its progress at least every six months, or more frequently if required by MCA.

(d)   The regulatory requirements for reporting of suspected adverse reactions must be fulfilled. Companies should endeavour to ensure that they are notified of serious suspected adverse reactions and should report these to the MCA within 15 days of receipt. Events which are not suspected by the investigator to be adverse reactions should not be reported individually as they occur. These and minor adverse reactions should be included in the final report.

(e)   A final report on the study should be sent to the MCA within 3 months of follow-up being completed. Ideally this should be a full report but a brief report within 3 months followed by a full report within 6 months of completion of the study would normally be acceptable. The findings of the study should be submitted for publication.

(f)   Companies are encouraged to follow MCA guidelines on the content of progress reports and final reports.

6   Promotion of medicines

(a)   SAMM studies should not be conducted for the purposes of promotion.

(b)   Company representatives should not be involved in SAMM studies in such a way that it could be seen as a promotional exercise.

7   Doctor participation

(a)   Subject to the doctor's terms of service, payment may be offered to the doctor in recompense for his time and any expenses incurred according to the suggested scale of fees published by the BMA.

(b)   No inducement for a doctor to participate in a SAMM study should be offered, requested or given.

8   Ethical issues

(a)   The highest possible standards of professional conduct and confidentiality must always be maintained. The patient's right to confidentiality is paramount. The patient's identity in the study documents should be codified and only his or her doctor should be capable of decoding it.

(b)   Responsibility for the retrieval of information from personal medical records lies with the consultant or general practitioner responsible for the patient's care. Such information should be directed to the medical practitioner nominated by the company or agent, who is thereafter responsible for the handling of such information.

(c)   Reference to a Research Ethics Committee is required if patients are to be approached for information, additional investigations are to be performed or if it is proposed to allocate patients systematically to treatments.

9   Procedure for complaints

A study which gives cause for concern on scientific, ethical or promotional grounds should be referred to the MCA, ABPI and the company concerned. Concerns regarding possible scientific fraud should be referred to the ABPI. They will be investigated and, if appropriate, referred to the General Medical Council.

10   Review of Guidelines

The Working Party will review these guidelines as necessary.

Association of the British Pharmaceutical Industry (ABPI)
British Medical Association (BMA)
Committee on Safety of Medicines (CSM)
Medicines Control Agency (MCA)
Royal College of General Practitioners (RCGP)

REPORTING OF SUSPECTED ADVERSE DRUG REACTIONS: THE ROLE OF THE MEDICAL REPRESENTATIVE

What are a company's responsibilities in respect of safety information it receives back on its medicines?

The ABPI Code of Practice, in line with European Directive 75/319/EEC, calls for an efficient transfer of information on adverse drug reactions. In the case of defective medicines, an ABPI 'Batch Recall of Pharmaceutical Products' system is in operation. In the ABPI Expanded Syllabus, batch recall is referred to in the 'Pharmaceutical Technology' section and adverse drug reactions in the 'Pharmacology and Classification of Medicines' and the 'Pharmaceutical Industry and the NHS' sections.

Relevant sections of the ABPI Code of Practice are:

Clause 13 *Scientific Service Responsible for Information*
Companies must have a scientific service to compile and collate all information, whether received from medical representatives or from any other source, about the medicines which they market.

Clause 15.6 *Representatives*
Representatives must transmit forthwith to the scientific service referred to in Clause 13 any information which they receive in relation to the use of the medicines which they promote, particularly reports of side-effects.

What is an adverse drug reaction?

A reaction which is harmful and unintended and which occurs at doses normally used in man for the prophylaxis, diagnosis, or treatment of disease or the modification of physiological function.

What is your own responsibility?

As the company's representative you have an important role to play in the process of collecting information on possible adverse reactions and quality defects to the products we market. You will often be the only contact that a healthcare professional has with the company, and it is known that some healthcare staff report suspected adverse reactions only to the representative.

Your involvement in this reporting process will help to emphasise the importance of your role in providing a service to medicine and patient care.

Why collect information on suspected ADRs?

There are two main reasons why a company needs to collect this information:

- The company requires information in order to establish and monitor the safety profile of a product. At the time a new product is first marketed its efficacy has been well defined. As a relatively small number of patients will have taken part in clinical trials during the development of a new medicine, it is likely that only the more common side-effects will have been identified. It is only after larger scale use of the product in normal clinical practice that less common reactions may be detected and an indication of the more common side-effects determined.

- The company has a legal obligation to report all suspected serious ADRs occurring in the European Union to the Licensing Authority within 15 days of the receipt from any health professional. Serious and unexpected suspected ADRs are required to be reported from outside the EU within 15 days of receipt from health professionals. All other ADRs should be reported in the periodic safety updates.

Reporting of ADRs

The detection and recording of ADRs is of vital importance and doctors are urged to report adverse reactions direct to the Committee on Safety of Medicines (CSM) as follows:

- For medicines introduced recently – as indicated by an inverted black triangle (▼) in the product entry in the British National Formulary, MIMS and the ABPI Data Sheet Compendium – doctors and hospital pharmacists are asked to report **all** suspected reactions. This includes any adverse or any unexpected event, however minor, which could conceivably be attributed to the medicine. Reports should be made despite uncertainty about a cause or relationship, irrespective of whether or not the reaction is well recognised and even when other medicines have been taken concurrently. (The legal position for the pharmaceutical industry requires the reporting of all serious ADRs from the UK or other EU countries, and of all serious and unexpected ADRs from countries outside the EU).

  The CSM decides when the black triangle can be removed (usually after two years), the decision being based on experience in use. Note that references to new formulations or presentations of an established medicine will not usually require a black triangle.

- For established medicines, doctors and hospital pharmacists are asked to report serious suspected reactions including those that are fatal, life-threatening, disabling, incapacitating or which result in hospital admission or prolong hospitalisation for in-patients. They should be reported even if the effect is well recognised.

What is a 'yellow card'?

Yellow prepaid letter cards for reporting adverse reactions are available from the CSM at a Freepost address.

'Yellow cards' are also found in the back of the British National Formulary, with the ABPI Data Sheet Compendium, and interleaved with National Health Service General Practitioner FP10 prescription forms.

What company action is taken on reports of suspected ADRs?

All reports on suspected ADRs are co-ordinated and assessed in the company's Medical Department and/or Pharmacovigilance Unit. As much relevant information as possible is obtained from the doctor concerned to enable physicians and scientists to assess the case and determine whether the reaction was caused by the product. A special company ADR card which is often similar to the CSM 'yellow card' may be sent to the doctor to be completed with the required details.

Pharmaceutical companies are now required to report all serious suspected ADRs to the CSM within 15 calendar days of receipt of the original information by the representative or other appropriate employee. Companies are also now obliged to submit reports received from 'all health professionals (doctors, dentists, coroners, pharmacists and nurses)' (ref: The Medicines for Human Use (Marketing Authorisations etc) Regulations 1994). All reports are retained by the company and the information used to build up a well-defined safety profile of a medicine so the company can advise prescribing doctors as necessary.

What is the doctor's responsibility?

Some reports of suspected ADRs come directly to the Medical Department from doctors, and other health professionals, e.g. pharmacists, dentists and nurses. Doctors are requested to report suspected ADRs to the CSM on 'yellow cards', as described above.

However, it is known that many suspected ADRs are not reported by doctors – some estimates put the proportion notified to the CSM as only 1–25 per cent of total 'reportable' reactions.

The CSM issues a briefing sheet on Adverse Drug Reaction reporting to all prescribing doctors and a section on Adverse Reactions to Drugs is contained in the Section of the British National Formulary relating to 'Guidance on Prescribing'.

What if a doctor mentions a suspected ADR?

When a doctor or hospital pharmacist tells you of a suspected ADR to a company product there is a recommended course of action to follow:

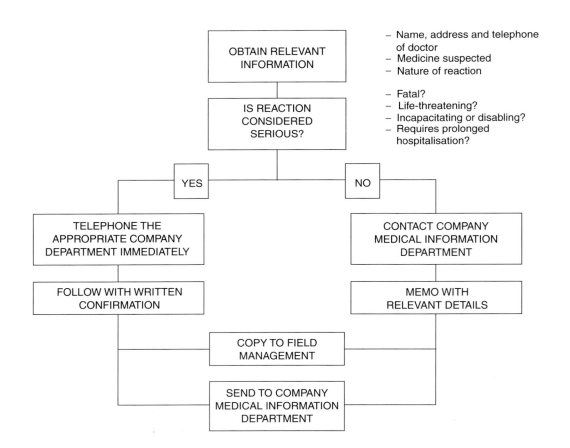

Note: It is as well to inform doctors who report ADRs to medical representatives that the company is legally obliged to report the ADR to the CSM in 15 calendar days, and that a rapid reply would be appreciated if further information is required.

Committee on Safety of Medicines

The Committee on Safety of Medicines (CSM) was established in 1970 under section 4 of the Medicines Act 1968. Its Terms of Reference are:

- To give advice with respect to safety, quality and efficacy in relation to human use of any substance or article (not being an instrument, apparatus or appliance) to which any provision of the Medicines Act 1968 is applicable.

- To promote the collection and investigation of information relating to adverse reactions for the purpose of enabling such advice to be given.

The work of the CSM involves:

(i) advising the Licensing Authority (UK Health Ministers) of whether on the grounds of safety, quality, and efficacy, medicinal products should be allowed to enter or remain upon the market – the authority is statutorily required to consult the Committee where for example it is minded to refuse the grant of a marketing authorisation on these grounds.

(ii) a statutory responsibility for collecting and investigating information on adverse drug reactions.

The CSM has 30 members and meets fortnightly, but by using a pairing system members are only asked to attend once a month. The term of office of the current Committee will expire on 31 December 1998.

There are three sub-committees of the CSM: Biologicals; Chemistry, Planning and Standards; and Pharmacovigilance.

There is a 24 hour Freephone service available to all parts of the UK for advice and information on suspected adverse drug reactions: contact the National Yellow Card Information Service at the MCA on 0800 731 6789.

The following addresses and phone numbers may be useful:

Medicines Control Agency, CSM Freepost, London SW8 5BR (0800 731 6789).

Regional Centres:

CSM Mersey, Freepost, Liverpool, L3 3AB (0151 794 8113)
CSM Northern, Freepost 1085, Newcastle upon Tyne, NE1 1BR (0191 232 1525)
CSM Wales, Freepost, Cardiff, CF4 1ZZ (01222 744181)
CSM West Midlands, Freepost SW2991, Birmingham, B18 7BR (no phone number)

FURTHER READING

- British National Formulary published every six months by the British Medical Association and the Royal Pharmaceutical Society of Great Britain

- Reporting Adverse Drug Reactions – A BMA Policy Document published by the British Medical Association in 1996. Price £5.95

- British Recall of Pharmaceutical Products – 2nd edition 1994 published by the ABPI

- Code of Practice for the Pharmaceutical Industry 1998 published by the ABPI for the Prescription Medicines Code of Practice Authority

Appendix 4

Directive 2001/20/EC of the European Parliament and of the Council of 4 April 2001

DIRECTIVE 2001/20/EC OF THE EUROPEAN PARLIAMENT AND OF THE COUNCIL

of 4 April 2001

on the approximation of the laws, regulations and administrative provisions of the Member States relating to the implementation of good clinical practice in the conduct of clinical trials on medicinal products for human use

Only European Community legislation printed in the paper edition of the *Official Journal of the European Union* is deemed authentic.

THE EUROPEAN PARLIAMENT AND THE COUNCIL OF THE EUROPEAN UNION,

Having regard to the Treaty establishing the European Community, and in particular Article 95 thereof,

Having regard to the proposal from the Commission ([1]),

Having regard to the opinion of the Economic and Social Committee ([2]),

Acting in accordance with the procedure laid down in Article 251 of the Treaty ([3]),

Whereas:

(1) Council Directive 65/65/EEC of 26 January 1965 on the approximation of provisions laid down by law, regulation or administrative action relating to medicinal products ([4]) requires that applications for authorisation to place a medicinal product on the market should be accompanied by a dossier containing particulars and documents relating to the results of tests and clinical trials carried out on the product. Council Directive 75/318/EEC of 20 May 1975 on the approximation of the laws of Member States relating to analytical, pharmacotoxicological and clinical standards and protocols in respect of the testing of medicinal products ([5]) lays down uniform rules on the compilation of dossiers including their presentation.

(2) The accepted basis for the conduct of clinical trials in humans is founded in the protection of human rights and the dignity of the human being with regard to the application of biology and medicine, as for instance reflected in the 1996 version of the Helsinki Declaration. The clinical trial subject's protection is safeguarded through risk assessment based on the results of toxicological experiments prior to any clinical trial, screening by ethics committees and Member States' competent authorities, and rules on the protection of personal data.

(3) Persons who are incapable of giving legal consent to clinical trials should be given

([1]) OJ C 306, 8.10.1997, p. 9 and
OJ C 161, 8.6.1999, p. 5.

([2]) OJ C 95, 30.3.1998, p. 1.

([3]) Opinion of the European Parliament of 17 November 1998 (OJ C 379, 7.12.1998, p. 27). Council Common Position of 20 July 2000 (OJ C 300, 20.10.2000, p. 32) and Decision of the European Parliament of 12 December 2000. Council Decision of 26 February 2001.

([4]) OJ 22, 9.2.1965, p. 1/65. Directive as last amended by Council Directive 93/39/EEC (OJ L 214, 24.8.1993, p. 22).

([5]) OJ L 147, 9.6.1975, p. 1. Directive as last amended by Commission Directive 1999/83/EC (OJ L 243, 15.9.1999, p. 9).

special protection. It is incumbent on the Member States to lay down rules to this effect. Such persons may not be included in clinical trials if the same results can be obtained using persons capable of giving consent. Normally these persons should be included in clinical trials only when there are grounds for expecting that the administering of the medicinal product would be of direct benefit to the patient, thereby outweighing the risks. However, there is a need for clinical trials involving children to improve the treatment available to them. Children represent a vulnerable population with developmental, physiological and psychological differences from adults, which make age- and development-related research important for their benefit. Medicinal products, including vaccines, for children need to be tested scientifically before widespread use. This can only be achieved by ensuring that medicinal products which are likely to be of significant clinical value for children are fully studied. The clinical trials required for this purpose should be carried out under conditions affording the best possible protection for the subjects. Criteria for the protection of children in clinical trials therefore need to be laid down.

(4) In the case of other persons incapable of giving their consent, such as persons with dementia, psychiatric patients, etc., inclusion in clinical trials in such cases should be on an even more restrictive basis. Medicinal products for trial may be administered to all such individuals only when there are grounds for assuming that the direct benefit to the patient outweighs the risks. Moreover, in such cases the written consent of the patient's legal representative, given in cooperation with the treating doctor, is necessary before participation in any such clinical trial.

(5) The notion of legal representative refers back to existing national law and consequently may include natural or legal persons, an authority and/or a body provided for by national law.

(6) In order to achieve optimum protection of health, obsolete or repetitive tests will not be carried out, whether within the Community or in third countries. The harmonisation of technical requirements for the development of medicinal products should therefore be pursued through the appropriate fora, in particular the International Conference on Harmonisation.

(7) For medicinal products falling within the scope of Part A of the Annex to Council Regulation (EEC) No 2309/93 of 22 July 1993 laying down Community procedures for the authorisation and supervision of medicinal products for human and veterinary use and establishing a European Agency for the Evaluation of Medicinal Products ([1]), which include products intended for gene therapy or cell therapy, prior scientific evaluation by the European Agency for the Evaluation of Medicinal Products (hereinafter referred to as the 'Agency'), assisted by the Committee for Proprietary Medicinal Products, is mandatory before the Commission grants marketing authorisation. In the course of this evaluation, the said Committee may request full details of the results of the clinical trials on which the application for marketing authorisation is based and, consequently, on the manner in which these trials were conducted and the same Committee may go so far as to require the applicant for such authorisation to conduct further clinical trials. Provision must therefore be made to allow the Agency to have full information on

([1]) OJ L 214, 24.8.1993, p. 1. Regulation as amended by Commission Regulation (EC) No 649/98 (OJ L 88, 24.3.1998, p. 7).

the conduct of any clinical trial for such medicinal products.

(8)   A single opinion for each Member State concerned reduces delay in the commencement of a trial without jeopardising the well-being of the people participating in the trial or excluding the possibility of rejecting it in specific sites.

(9)   Information on the content, commencement and termination of a clinical trial should be available to the Member States where the trial takes place and all the other Member States should have access to the same information. A European database bringing together this information should therefore be set up, with due regard for the rules of confidentiality.

(10) Clinical trials are a complex operation, generally lasting one or more years, usually involving numerous participants and several trial sites, often in different Member States. Member States' current practices diverge considerably on the rules on commencement and conduct of the clinical trials and the requirements for carrying them out vary widely. This therefore results in delays and complications detrimental to effective conduct of such trials in the Community. It is therefore necessary to simplify and harmonise the administrative provisions governing such trials by establishing a clear, transparent procedure and creating conditions conducive to effective coordination of such clinical trials in the Community by the authorities concerned.

(11) As a rule, authorisation should be implicit, i.e. if there has been a vote in favour by the Ethics Committee and the competent authority has not objected within a given period, it should be possible to begin the clinical trials. In exceptional cases raising especially complex problems, explicit written authorisation should, however, be required.

(12) The principles of good manufacturing practice should be applied to investigational medicinal products.

(13) Special provisions should be laid down for the labelling of these products.

(14) Non-commercial clinical trials conducted by researchers without the participation of the pharmaceuticals industry may be of great benefit to the patients concerned. The Directive should therefore take account of the special position of trials whose planning does not require particular manufacturing or packaging processes, if these trials are carried out with medicinal products with a marketing authorisation within the meaning of Directive 65/65/EEC, manufactured or imported in accordance with the provisions of Directives 75/319/EEC and 91/356/EEC, and on patients with the same characteristics as those covered by the indication specified in this marketing authorisation. Labelling of the investigational medicinal products intended for trials of this nature should be subject to simplified provisions laid down in the good manufacturing practice guidelines on investigational products and in Directive 91/356/EEC.

(15) The verification of compliance with the standards of good clinical practice and the need to subject data, information and documents to inspection in order to confirm that they have been properly generated, recorded and reported are essential in order to justify the involvement of human subjects in clinical trials.

(16) The person participating in a trial must consent to the scrutiny of personal information during inspection by competent authorities and properly authorised persons, provided that such personal information is treated as strictly

confidential and is not made publicly available.

(17)   This Directive is to apply without pre-judice to Directive 95/46/EEC of the European Parliament and of the Council of 24 October 1995 on the protection of individuals with regard to the processing of personal data and on the free move-ment of such data (^{1}).

(18)   It is also necessary to make provision for the monitoring of adverse reactions occur-ring in clinical trials using Community surveillance (pharmacovigilance) proced-ures in order to ensure the immediate cessation of any clinical trial in which there is an unacceptable level of risk.

(19)   The measures necessary for the imple-mentation of this Directive should be adopted in accordance with Council Decision 1999/468/EC of 28 June 1999 laying down the procedures for the exer-cise of implementing powers conferred on the Commission (^{2}),

HAVE ADOPTED THIS DIRECTIVE:

Article 1

Scope

1.   This Directive establishes specific provi-sions regarding the conduct of clinical trials, including multi-centre trials, on human sub-jects involving medicinal products as defined in Article 1 of Directive 65/65/EEC, in particular relating to the implementation of good clinical practice. This Directive does not apply to non-interventional trials.

2.   Good clinical practice is a set of interna-tionally recognised ethical and scientific quality

(^{1})   OJ L 281, 23.11.1995, p. 31.
(^{2})   OJ L 184, 17.7.1999, p. 23.

requirements which must be observed for design-ing, conducting, recording and reporting clinical trials that involve the participation of human subjects. Compliance with this good practice provides assurance that the rights, safety and well-being of trial subjects are protected, and that the results of the clinical trials are credible.

3.   The principles of good clinical practice and detailed guidelines in line with those principles shall be adopted and, if necessary, revised to take account of technical and scientific progress in accordance with the procedure referred to in Article 21(2).

These detailed guidelines shall be published by the Commission.

4.   All clinical trials, including bioavailability and bioequivalence studies, shall be designed, conducted and reported in accordance with the principles of good clinical practice.

Article 2

Definitions

For the purposes of this Directive the following definitions shall apply:

(a)   'clinical trial': any investigation in human subjects intended to discover or verify the clinical, pharmacological and/or other pharmacodynamic effects of one or more investigational medicinal product(s), and/or to identify any adverse reactions to one or more investigational medicinal product(s) and/or to study absorption, distribution, metabolism and excretion of one or more investigational medicinal product(s) with the object of ascertaining its (their) safety and/or efficacy;

This includes clinical trials carried out in either one site or multiple sites, whether in one or more than one Member State;

(b)   'multi-centre clinical trial': a clinical trial conducted according to a single protocol but at more than one site, and therefore by more than one investigator, in which the trial sites may be located in a single Member State, in a number of Member States and/or in Member States and third countries;

(c) 'non-interventional trial': a study where the medicinal product(s) is (are) prescribed in the usual manner in accordance with the terms of the marketing authorisation. The assignment of the patient to a particular therapeutic strategy is not decided in advance by a trial protocol but falls within current practice and the prescription of the medicine is clearly separated from the decision to include the patient in the study. No additional diagnostic or monitoring procedures shall be applied to the patients and epidemiological methods shall be used for the analysis of collected data;

(d) 'investigational medicinal product': a pharmaceutical form of an active substance or placebo being tested or used as a reference in a clinical trial, including products already with a marketing authorisation but used or assembled (formulated or packaged) in a way different from the authorised form, or when used for an unauthorised indication, or when used to gain further information about the authorised form;

(e) 'sponsor': an individual, company, institution or organisation which takes responsibility for the initiation, management and/or financing of a clinical trial;

(f) 'investigator': a doctor or a person following a profession agreed in the Member State for investigations because of the scientific background and the experience in patient care it requires. The investigator is responsible for the conduct of a clinical trial at a trial site. If a trial is conducted by a team of individuals at a trial site, the investigator is the leader responsible for the team and may be called the principal investigator;

(g) 'investigator's brochure': a compilation of the clinical and non-clinical data on the investigational medicinal product or products which are relevant to the study of the product or products in human subjects;

(h) 'protocol': a document that describes the objective(s), design, methodology, statistical considerations and organisation of a trial. The term protocol refers to the protocol, successive versions of the protocol and protocol amendments;

(i) 'subject': an individual who participates in a clinical trial as either a recipient of the investigational medicinal product or a control;

(j) 'informed consent': decision, which must be written, dated and signed, to take part in a clinical trial, taken freely after being duly informed of its nature, significance, implications and risks and appropriately documented, by any person capable of giving consent or, where the person is not capable of giving consent, by his or her legal representative; if the person concerned is unable to write, oral consent in the presence of at least one witness may be given in exceptional cases, as provided for in national legislation.

(k) 'ethics committee': an independent body in a Member State, consisting of healthcare professionals and non-medical members, whose responsibility it is to protect the rights, safety and wellbeing of human subjects involved in a trial and to provide public assurance of that protection, by, among other things, expressing an opinion on the trial protocol, the suitability of the investigators and the adequacy of facilities, and on the methods and documents to be used to inform trial subjects and obtain their informed consent;

(l) 'inspection': the act by a competent authority of conducting an official review of documents, facilities, records, quality assurance arrangements, and any other resources that are deemed by the competent authority to be related to the clinical trial and that may be located at the site of the trial, at the sponsor's and/or contract research organisation's facilities, or at other establishments which the competent authority sees fit to inspect;

(m) 'adverse event': any untoward medical occurrence in a patient or clinical trial subject administered a medicinal product and which does not necessarily have a causal relationship with this treatment;

(n) 'adverse reaction': all untoward and unintended responses to an investigational medicinal product related to any dose administered;

(o) 'serious adverse event or serious adverse reaction': any untoward medical occurrence or effect that at any dose results in death, is life-threatening, requires hospitalisation or prolongation of existing hospitalisation, results in persistent or significant disability or incapacity, or is a congenital anomaly or birth defect;

(p) 'unexpected adverse reaction': an adverse reaction, the nature or severity of which is not consistent with the applicable product information (e.g. investigator's brochure for an unauthorised investigational product or summary of product characteristics for an authorised product).

Article 3

Protection of clinical trial subjects

1. This Directive shall apply without prejudice to the national provisions on the protection of clinical trial subjects if they are more comprehensive than the provisions of this Directive and consistent with the procedures and timescales specified therein. Member States shall, insofar as they have not already done so, adopt detailed rules to protect from abuse individuals who are incapable of giving their informed consent.

2. A clinical trial may be undertaken only if, in particular:

(a) the foreseeable risks and inconveniences have been weighed against the anticipated benefit for the individual trial subject and other present and future patients. A clinical trial may be initiated only if the Ethics Committee and/or the competent authority comes to the conclusion that the anticipated therapeutic and public health benefits justify the risks and may be continued only if compliance with this requirement is permanently monitored;

(b) the trial subject or, when the person is not able to give informed consent, his legal representative has had the opportunity, in a prior interview with the investigator or a member of the investigating team, to understand the objectives, risks and inconveniences of the trial, and the conditions under which it is to be conducted and has also been informed of his right to withdraw from the trial at any time;

(c) the rights of the subject to physical and mental integrity, to privacy and to the protection of the data concerning him in accordance with Directive 95/46/EC are safeguarded;

(d) the trial subject or, when the person is not able to give informed consent, his legal representative has given his written consent after being informed of the nature, significance, implications and risks of the clinical trial; if the individual is unable to write, oral consent in the presence of at least one witness may be given in exceptional cases, as provided for in national legislation;

(e)   the subject may without any resulting detriment withdraw from the clinical trial at any time by revoking his informed consent;

(f)   provision has been made for insurance or indemnity to cover the liability of the investigator and sponsor.

3.   The medical care given to, and medical decisions made on behalf of, subjects shall be the responsibility of an appropriately qualified doctor or, where appropriate, of a qualified dentist.

4.   The subject shall be provided with a contact point where he may obtain further information.

Article 4

Clinical trials on minors

In addition to any other relevant restriction, a clinical trial on minors may be undertaken only if:

(a)   the informed consent of the parents or legal representative has been obtained; consent must represent the minor's presumed will and may be revoked at any time, without detriment to the minor;

(b)   the minor has received information according to its capacity of understanding, from staff with experience with minors, regarding the trial, the risks and the benefits;

(c)   the explicit wish of a minor who is capable of forming an opinion and assessing this information to refuse participation or to be withdrawn from the clinical trial at any time is considered by the investigator or where appropriate the principal investigator;

(d)   no incentives or financial inducements are given except compensation;

(e)   some direct benefit for the group of patients is obtained from the clinical trial and only where such research is essential to validate data obtained in clinical trials on persons able to give informed consent or by other research methods; additionally, such research should either relate directly to a clinical condition from which the minor concerned suffers or be of such a nature that it can only be carried out on minors;

(f)   the corresponding scientific guidelines of the Agency have been followed;

(g)   clinical trials have been designed to minimise pain, discomfort, fear and any other foreseeable risk in relation to the disease and developmental stage; both the risk threshold and the degree of distress have to be specially defined and constantly monitored;

(h)   the Ethics Committee, with paediatric expertise or after taking advice in clinical, ethical and psychosocial problems in the field of paediatrics, has endorsed the protocol; and

(i)   the interests of the patient always prevail over those of science and society.

Article 5

Clinical trials on incapacitated adults not able to give informed legal consent

In the case of other persons incapable of giving informed legal consent, all relevant requirements listed for persons capable of giving such consent shall apply. In addition to these requirements, inclusion in clinical trials of incapacitated adults who have not given or not refused informed consent before the onset of their incapacity shall be allowed only if:

(a)   the informed consent of the legal represent-ative has been obtained; consent must rep-resent the subject's presumed will and may be revoked at any time, without detriment to the subject;

(b)   the person not able to give informed legal consent has received information accord-ing to his/her capacity of understand-ing regarding the trial, the risks and the benefits;

(c)   the explicit wish of a subject who is capable of forming an opinion and assessing this information to refuse participation in, or to be withdrawn from, the clinical trial at any time is considered by the invest-igator or where appropriate the principal investigator;

(d)   no incentives or financial inducements are given except compensation;

(e)   such research is essential to validate data obtained in clinical trials on persons able to give informed consent or by other research methods and relates directly to a life-threatening or debilitating clinical condi-tion from which the incapacitated adult concerned suffers;

(f)   clinical trials have been designed to min-imise pain, discomfort, fear and any other foreseeable risk in relation to the dis-ease and developmental stage; both the risk threshold and the degree of distress shall be specially defined and constantly monitored;

(g)   the Ethics Committee, with expertise in the relevant disease and the patient population concerned or after taking advice in clin-ical, ethical and psychosocial questions in the field of the relevant disease and patient population concerned, has endorsed the protocol;

(h)   the interests of the patient always prevail over those of science and society; and

(i)   there are grounds for expecting that administering the medicinal product to be tested will produce a benefit to the patient outweighing the risks or produce no risk at all.

Article 6

Ethics Committee

1.   For the purposes of implementation of the clinical trials, Member States shall take the measures necessary for establishment and operation of Ethics Committees.

2.   The Ethics Committee shall give its opinion, before a clinical trial commences, on any issue requested.

3.   In preparing its opinion, the Ethics Committee shall consider, in particular:

(a)   the relevance of the clinical trial and the trial design;

(b)   whether the evaluation of the anticip-ated benefits and risks as required under Article 3(2)(a) is satisfactory and whether the conclusions are justified;

(c)   the protocol;

(d)   the suitability of the investigator and supporting staff;

(e)   the investigator's brochure;

(f)   the quality of the facilities;

(g)   the adequacy and completeness of the written information to be given and the procedure to be followed for the pur-pose of obtaining informed consent and the justification for the research on persons incapable of giving informed consent as regards the specific restrictions laid down in Article 3;

(h) provision for indemnity or compensation in the event of injury or death attributable to a clinical trial;

(i) any insurance or indemnity to cover the liability of the investigator and sponsor;

(j) the amounts and, where appropriate, the arrangements for rewarding or compensating investigators and trial subjects and the relevant aspects of any agreement between the sponsor and the site;

(k) the arrangements for the recruitment of subjects.

4. Notwithstanding the provisions of this Article, a Member State may decide that the competent authority it has designated for the purpose of Article 9 shall be responsible for the consideration of, and the giving of an opinion on, the matters referred to in paragraph 3(h), (i) and (j) of this Article.

When a Member State avails itself of this provision, it shall notify the Commission, the other Member States and the Agency.

5. The Ethics Committee shall have a maximum of 60 days from the date of receipt of a valid application to give its reasoned opinion to the applicant and the competent authority in the Member State concerned.

6. Within the period of examination of the application for an opinion, the Ethics Committee may send a single request for information supplementary to that already supplied by the applicant. The period laid down in paragraph 5 shall be suspended until receipt of the supplementary information.

7. No extension to the 60-day period referred to in paragraph 5 shall be permissible except in the case of trials involving medicinal products for

gene therapy or somatic cell therapy or medicinal products containing genetically modified organisms. In this case, an extension of a maximum of 30 days shall be permitted. For these products, this 90-day period may be extended by a further 90 days in the event of consultation of a group or a committee in accordance with the regulations and procedures of the Member States concerned. In the case of xenogenic cell therapy, there shall be no time limit to the authorisation period.

Article 7

Single opinion

For multi-centre clinical trials limited to the territory of a single Member State, Member States shall establish a procedure providing, notwithstanding the number of Ethics Committees, for the adoption of a single opinion for that Member State.

In the case of multi-centre clinical trials carried out in more than one Member State simultaneously, a single opinion shall be given for each Member State concerned by the clinical trial.

Article 8

Detailed guidance

The Commission, in consultation with Member States and interested parties, shall draw up and publish detailed guidance on the application format and documentation to be submitted in an application for an ethics committee opinion, in particular regarding the information that is given to subjects, and on the appropriate safeguards for the protection of personal data.

Article 9

Commencement of a clinical trial

1. Member States shall take the measures necessary to ensure that the procedure described in this Article is followed for commencement of a clinical trial.

The sponsor may not start a clinical trial until the Ethics Committee has issued a favourable opinion and inasmuch as the competent authority of the Member State concerned has not informed the sponsor of any grounds for non-acceptance. The procedures to reach these decisions can be run in parallel or not, depending on the sponsor.

2.   Before commencing any clinical trial, the sponsor shall be required to submit a valid request for authorisation to the competent authority of the Member State in which the sponsor plans to conduct the clinical trial.

3.   If the competent authority of the Member State notifies the sponsor of grounds for non-acceptance, the sponsor may, on one occasion only, amend the content of the request referred to in paragraph 2 in order to take due account of the grounds given. If the sponsor fails to amend the request accordingly, the request shall be considered rejected and the clinical trial may not commence.

4.   Consideration of a valid request for authorisation by the competent authority as stated in paragraph 2 shall be carried out as rapidly as possible and may not exceed 60 days. The Member States may lay down a shorter period than 60 days within their area of responsibility if that is in compliance with current practice. The competent authority can nevertheless notify the sponsor before the end of this period that it has no grounds for non-acceptance.

No further extensions to the period referred to in the first subparagraph shall be permissible except in the case of trials involving the medicinal products listed in paragraph 6, for which an extension of a maximum of 30 days shall be permitted. For these products, this 90-day period may be extended by a further 90 days in the event of consultation of a group or a committee in accordance with the regulations and procedures of the Member States concerned. In the case of xenogenic cell therapy there shall be no time limit to the authorisation period.

5.   Without prejudice to paragraph 6, written authorisation may be required before the commencement of clinical trials for such trials on medicinal products which do not have a marketing authorisation within the meaning of Directive 65/65/EEC and are referred to in Part A of the Annex to Regulation (EEC) No 2309/93, and other medicinal products with special characteristics, such as medicinal products the active ingredient or active ingredients of which is or are a biological product or biological products of human or animal origin, or contains biological components of human or animal origin, or the manufacturing of which requires such components.

6.   Written authorisation shall be required before commencing clinical trials involving medicinal products for gene therapy, somatic cell therapy including xenogenic cell therapy and all medicinal products containing genetically modified organisms. No gene therapy trials may be carried out which result in modifications to the subject's germ line genetic identity.

7.   This authorisation shall be issued without prejudice to the application of Council Directives 90/219/EEC of 23 April 1990 on the contained use of genetically modified micro-organisms [1] and 90/220/EEC of 23 April 1990 on the deliberate release into the environment of genetically modified organisms [2].

8.   In consultation with Member States, the Commission shall draw up and publish detailed guidance on:

(a)   the format and contents of the request referred to in paragraph 2 as well as the documentation to be submitted to support that request, on the quality and manufacture of the investigational medicinal

---

[1]   OJ L 117, 8.5.1990, p. 1. Directive as last amended by Directive 98/81/EC (OJ L 330, 5.12.1998, p. 13).
[2]   OJ L 117, 8.5.1990, p. 15. Directive as last amended by Commission Directive 97/35/EC (OJ L 169, 27.6.1997, p. 72).

product, any toxicological and pharma-cological tests, the protocol and clinical information on the investigational medicinal product including the investigator's brochure;

(b)   the presentation and content of the proposed amendment referred to in point (a) of Article 10 on substantial amendments made to the protocol;

(c)   the declaration of the end of the clinical trial.

Article 10

Conduct of a clinical trial

Amendments may be made to the conduct of a clinical trial following the procedure described hereinafter:

(a)   after the commencement of the clinical trial, the sponsor may make amendments to the protocol. If those amendments are substantial and are likely to have an impact on the safety of the trial subjects or to change the interpretation of the scientific documents in support of the conduct of the trial, or if they are otherwise significant, the sponsor shall notify the competent authorities of the Member State or Member States concerned of the reasons for, and content of, these amendments and shall inform the ethics committee or committees concerned in accordance with Articles 6 and 9.

On the basis of the details referred to in Article 6(3) and in accordance with Article 7, the Ethics Committee shall give an opinion within a maximum of 35 days of the date of receipt of the proposed amendment in good and due form. If this opinion is unfavourable, the sponsor may not implement the amendment to the protocol. If the opinion of the Ethics Committee is favourable and the competent authorities of the Member States have raised no

grounds for non-acceptance of the above-mentioned substantial amendments, the sponsor shall proceed to conduct the clinical trial following the amended protocol. Should this not be the case, the sponsor shall either take account of the grounds for non-acceptance and adapt the proposed amendment to the protocol accordingly or withdraw the proposed amendment;

(b)   without prejudice to point (a), in the light of the circumstances, notably the occurrence of any new event relating to the conduct of the trial or the development of the investigational medicinal product where that new event is likely to affect the safety of the subjects, the sponsor and the investigator shall take appropriate urgent safety measures to protect the subjects against any immediate hazard. The sponsor shall forthwith inform the competent authorities of those new events and the measures taken and shall ensure that the Ethics Committee is notified at the same time;

(c)   within 90 days of the end of a clinical trial the sponsor shall notify the competent authorities of the Member State or Member States concerned and the Ethics Committee that the clinical trial has ended. If the trial has to be terminated early, this period shall be reduced to 15 days and the reasons clearly explained.

Article 11

Exchange of information

1.   Member States in whose territory the clinical trial takes place shall enter in a European database, accessible only to the competent authorities of the Member States, the Agency and the Commission:

(a)   extracts from the request for authorisation referred to in Article 9(2);

(b) any amendments made to the request, as provided for in Article 9(3);

(c) any amendments made to the protocol, as provided for in point a of Article 10;

(d) the favourable opinion of the Ethics Committee;

(e) the declaration of the end of the clinical trial; and

(f) a reference to the inspections carried out on conformity with good clinical practice.

2.   At the substantiated request of any Member State, the Agency or the Commission, the competent authority to which the request for authorisation was submitted shall supply all further information concerning the clinical trial in question other than the data already in the European database.

3.   In consultation with the Member States, the Commission shall draw up and publish detailed guidance on the relevant data to be included in this European database, which it operates with the assistance of the Agency, as well as the methods for electronic communication of the data. The detailed guidance thus drawn up shall ensure that the confidentiality of the data is strictly observed.

Article 12

Suspension of the trial or infringements

1.   Where a Member State has objective grounds for considering that the conditions in the request for authorisation referred to in Article 9(2) are no longer met or has information raising doubts about the safety or scientific validity of the clinical) trial, it may suspend or prohibit the clinical trial and shall notify the sponsor thereof.

Before the Member State reaches its decision it shall, except where there is imminent risk, ask the sponsor and/or the investigator for their opinion, to be delivered within one week.

In this case, the competent authority concerned shall forthwith inform the other competent authorities, the Ethics Committee concerned, the Agency and the Commission of its decision to suspend or prohibit the trial and of the reasons for the decision.

2.   Where a competent authority has objective grounds for considering that the sponsor or the investigator or any other person involved in the conduct of the trial no longer meets the obligations laid down, it shall forthwith inform him thereof, indicating the course of action which he must take to remedy this state of affairs. The competent authority concerned shall forthwith inform the Ethics Committee, the other competent authorities and the Commission of this course of action.

Article 13

Manufacture and import of investigational medicinal products

1.   Member States shall take all appropriate measures to ensure that the manufacture or importation of investigational medicinal products is subject to the holding of authorisation.

In order to obtain the authorisation, the applicant and, subsequently, the holder of the authorisation, shall meet at least the requirements defined in accordance with the procedure referred to in Article 21(2).

2.   Member States shall take all appropriate measures to ensure that the holder of the authorisation referred to in paragraph 1 has permanently and continuously at his disposal the services of at least one qualified person who, in accordance with the conditions laid down in Article 23 of the second Council Directive

75/319/EEC of 20 May 1975 on the approximation of provisions laid down by law, regulation
or administrative action relating to proprietary
medicinal products (^{1}), is responsible in particular for carrying out the duties specified in
paragraph 3 of this Article.

3.   Member States shall take all appropriate
measures to ensure that the qualified person
referred to in Article 21 of Directive 75/319/EEC,
without prejudice to his relationship with the
manufacturer or importer, is responsible, in the
context of the procedures referred to in Article 25
of the said Directive, for ensuring:

(a)   in the case of investigational medicinal
       products manufactured in the Member
       State concerned, that each batch of medi-
       cinal products has been manufactured
       and checked in compliance with the
       requirements of Commission Directive
       91/356/EEC of 13 June 1991 laying down
       the principles and guidelines of good man-
       ufacturing practice for medicinal products
       for human use (^{2}), the product specification
       file and the information notified pursuant
       to Article 9(2) of this Directive;

(b)   in the case of investigational medicinal
       products manufactured in a third coun-
       try, that each production batch has been
       manufactured and checked in accord-
       ance with standards of good manufac-
       turing practice at least equivalent to
       those laid down in Commission Direct-
       ive 91/356/EEC, in accordance with the
       product specification file, and that each
       production batch has been checked in
       accordance with the information notified
       pursuant to Article 9(2) of this Directive;

(c)   in the case of an investigational medicinal
       product which is a comparator product
       from a third country, and which has a

marketing authorisation, where the documentation certifying that each production
batch has been manufactured in conditions
at least equivalent to the standards of good
manufacturing practice referred to above
cannot be obtained, that each production
batch has undergone all relevant analyses,
tests or checks necessary to confirm its
quality in accordance with the information notified pursuant to Article 9(2) of this
Directive.

Detailed guidance on the elements to be taken
into account when evaluating products with the
object of releasing batches within the Community
shall be drawn up pursuant to the good manufacturing practice guidelines, and in particular
Annex 13 to the said guidelines. Such guidelines
will be adopted in accordance with the procedure referred to in Article 21(2) of this Directive
and published in accordance with Article 19a of
Directive 75/319/EEC.

Insofar as the provisions laid down in (a), (b)
or (c) are complied with, investigational medicinal products shall not have to undergo any
further checks if they are imported into another
Member State together with batch release certification signed by the qualified person.

4.   In all cases, the qualified person must certify in a register or equivalent document that
each production batch satisfies the provisions of
this Article. The said register or equivalent document shall be kept up to date as operations are
carried out and shall remain at the disposal of the
agents of the competent authority for the period
specified in the provisions of the Member States
concerned. This period shall in any event be not
less than five years.

5.   Any person engaging in activities as the
qualified person referral to in Article 21 of
Directive 75/319/EEC as regards investigational
medicinal products at the time when this Directive is applied in the Member State where that
person is, but without complying with the conditions laid down in Articles 23 and 24 of that

---

(^{1}) OJ L 147, 9.6.1975, p. 13. Directive as last amended
       by Council Directive 93/39/EC (OJ L 214, 24.8.1993,
       p. 22).
(^{2}) OJ L 193, 17.7.1991, p. 30.

Directive, shall be authorised to continue those activities in the Member State concerned.

Article 14

Labelling

The particulars to appear in at least the official language(s) of the Member State on the outer packaging of investigational medicinal products or, where there is no outer packaging, on the immediate packaging, shall be published by the Commission in the good manufacturing practice guidelines on investigational medicinal products adopted in accordance with Article 19a of Directive 75/319/EEC.

In addition, these guidelines shall lay down adapted provisions relating to labelling for investigational medicinal products intended for clinical trials with the following characteristics:

— the planning of the trial does not require particular manufacturing or packaging processes;

— the trial is conducted with medicinal products with, in the Member States concerned by the study, a marketing authorisation within the meaning of Directive 65/65/EEC, manufactured or imported in accordance with the provisions of Directive 75/319/EEC;

— the patients participating in the trial have the same characteristics as those covered by the indication specified in the abovementioned authorisation.

Article 15

Verification of compliance of investigational medicinal products with good clinical and manufacturing practice

1. To verify compliance with the provisions on good clinical and manufacturing practice. Member States shall appoint inspectors to inspect the sites concerned by any clinical trial conducted, particularly the trial site or sites, the manufacturing site of the investigational medicinal product, any laboratory used for analyses in the clinical trial and/or the sponsor's premises.

The inspections shall be conducted by the competent authority of the Member State concerned, which shall inform the Agency; they shall be carried out on behalf of the Community and the results shall be recognised by all the other Member States. These inspections shall be coordinated by the Agency, within the framework of its powers as provided for in Regulation (EEC) No 2309/93. A Member State may request assistance from another Member State in this matter.

2. Following inspection, an inspection report shall be prepared. It must be made available to the sponsor while safeguarding confidential aspects. It may be made available to the other Member States, to the Ethics Committee and to the Agency, at their reasoned request.

3. At the request of the Agency, within the framework of its powers as provided for in Regulation (EEC) No 2309/93, or of one of the Member States concerned, and following consultation with the Member States concerned, the Commission may request a new inspection should verification of compliance with this Directive reveal differences between Member States.

4. Subject to any arrangements which may have been concluded between the Community and third countries, the Commission, upon receipt of a reasoned request from a Member State or on its own initiative, or a Member State may propose that the trial site and/or the sponsor's premises and/or the manufacturer established in a third country undergo an inspection. The inspection shall be carried out by duly qualified Community inspectors.

5. The detailed guidelines on the documentation relating to the clinical trial, which shall

constitute the master file on the trial, archiving, qualifications of inspectors and inspection procedures to verify compliance of the clinical trial in question with this Directive shall be adopted and revised in accordance with the procedure referred to in Article 21(2).

Article 16

Notification of adverse events

1.   The investigator shall report all serious adverse events immediately to the sponsor except for those that the protocol or investigator's brochure identifies as not requiring immediate reporting. The immediate report shall be followed by detailed, written reports. The immediate and follow-up reports shall identify subjects by unique code numbers assigned to the latter.

2.   Adverse events and/or laboratory abnormalities identified in the protocol as critical to safety evaluations shall be reported to the sponsor according to the reporting requirements and within the time periods specified in the protocol.

3.   For reported deaths of a subject, the investigator shall supply the sponsor and the Ethics Committee with any additional information requested.

4.   The sponsor shall keep detailed records of all adverse events which are reported to him by the investigator or investigators. These records shall be submitted to the Member States in whose territory the clinical trial is being conducted, if they so request.

Article 17

Notification of serious adverse reactions

1.   (a)   The sponsor shall ensure that all relevant information about suspected serious unexpected adverse reactions that are fatal or life-threatening is recorded and reported as soon as possible to the competent authorities in all the Member States concerned, and to the Ethics Committee, and in any

case no later than seven days after knowledge by the sponsor of such a case, and that relevant follow-up information is subsequently communicated within an additional eight days.

(b)   All other suspected serious unexpected adverse reactions shall be reported to the competent authorities concerned and to the Ethics Committee concerned as soon as possible but within a maximum of fifteen days of first knowledge by the sponsor.

(c)   Each Member State shall ensure that all suspected unexpected serious adverse reactions to an investigational medicinal product which are brought to its attention are recorded.

(d)   The sponsor shall also inform all investigators.

2.   Once a year throughout the clinical trial, the sponsor shall provide the Member States in whose territory the clinical trial is being conducted and the Ethics Committee with a listing of all suspected serious adverse reactions which have occurred over this period and a report of the subjects' safety.

3.   (a)   Each Member State shall see to it that all suspected unexpected serious adverse reactions to an investigational medicinal product which are brought to its attention are immediately entered in a European database to which, in accordance with Article 11(1), only the competent authorities of the Member States, the Agency and the Commission shall have access.

(b)   The Agency shall make the information notified by the sponsor available to the competent authorities of the Member States.

Article 18

Guidance concerning reports

The Commission, in consultation with the Agency, Member States and interested parties, shall draw up and publish detailed guidance on the collection, verification and presentation of adverse event/reaction reports, together with decoding procedures for unexpected serious adverse reactions.

Article 19

General provisions

This Directive is without prejudice to the civil and criminal liability of the sponsor or the investigator. To this end, the sponsor or a legal representative of the sponsor must be established in the Community.

Unless Member States have established precise conditions for exceptional circumstances, investigational medicinal products and, as the case may be, the devices used for their administration shall be made available free of charge by the sponsor.

The Member States shall inform the Commission of such conditions.

Article 20

Adaptation to scientific and technical progress

This Directive shall be adapted to take account of scientific and technical progress in accordance with the procedure referred to in Article 21(2).

Article 21

Committee procedure

1.   The Commission shall be assisted by the Standing Committee on Medicinal Products for Human Use, set up by Article 2b of Directive 75/318/EEC (hereinafter referred to as the Committee).

2.   Where reference is made to this paragraph, Articles 5 and 7 of Decision 1999/468/EC shall apply, having regard to the provisions of Article 8 thereof.

The period referred to in Article 5(6) of Decision 1999/468/EC shall be set at three months.

3.   The Committee shall adopt its rules of procedure.

Article 22

Application

1.   Member States shall adopt and publish before 1 May 2003 the laws, regulations and administrative provisions necessary to comply with this Directive. They shall forthwith inform the Commission thereof.

They shall apply these provisions at the latest with effect from 1 May 2004.

When Member States adopt these provisions, they shall contain a reference to this Directive or shall be accompanied by such reference on the occasion of their official publication. The methods of making such reference shall be laid down by Member States.

2.   Member States shall communicate to the Commission the text of the provisions of national law which they adopt in the field governed by this Directive.

Article 23

Entry into force

The Directive shall enter into force on the day of its publication in the Official Journal of the European Communities.

Article 24

Addressees

This Directive is addressed to the Member States.

Done at Luxembourg, 4 April 2001.

For the European Parliament	*For the Council*
The President	*The President*
N. FONTAINE	B. ROSENGREN

Index

Note: page numbers in *italics* refer to figures, those in bold refer to tables.